**Anesthesia for
Congenital Heart Disease**

Dedication

This book is dedicated to Arthur S. Keats, M.D., the first anesthesiologist for cardiovascular surgery at Texas Children's Hospital and the Baylor College of Medicine. In 1955 Dr. Keats, with Dr. Denton A. Cooley and Dr. Dan McNamara, began a remarkable era, pioneering many techniques in diagnosis and treatment of congenital heart disease, particularly in infants. Dr. Keats is an inspiring figure who faced the daunting task of caring for these critically ill patients without the technology available today; his skill and compassion in producing remarkable results attests to the fact that he is a true giant in our field. We are proud to call him the founder of our service at Texas Children's Hospital. We lost a pioneer and a giant in our field when Dr. Keats passed away in 2007; he is sorely missed.

This book is also dedicated to Susheela Sangwan, M.D., who dedicated her life to the care of patients with congenital heart disease. Her excellence in clinical care and teaching skills resulted in significant contributions to the development of pediatric cardiac anesthesia.

Anesthesia for Congenital Heart Disease

Editor-in-Chief

Dean B. Andropoulos, M.D., M.H.C.M.
Chief of Anesthesiology
Texas Children's Hospital
Professor, Anesthesiology and Pediatrics
Baylor College of Medicine
Houston, TX
USA

Editors

Stephen A. Stayer, M.D.
Medical Director of Perioperative Services
Texas Children's Hospital
Professor, Anesthesiology and Pediatrics
Baylor College of Medicine
Houston, TX
USA

Isobel Russell, M.D., Ph.D.
Chief of Cardiac Anesthesia
Moffitt-Long Hospitals
Professor of Anesthesia
University of California, San Francisco
San Francisco, CA
USA

Emad B. Mossad, M.D.
Director of Pediatric Cardiovascular Anesthesiology
Texas Children's Hospital
Professor of Anesthesiology and Pediatrics
Baylor College of Medicine
Houston, TX
USA

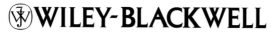

WILEY-BLACKWELL
A John Wiley & Sons, Ltd., Publication

This edition first published 2004, © 2010 by Blackwell Publishing Ltd

Blackwell Publishing was acquired by John Wiley & Sons in February 2007. Blackwell's publishing program has been merged with Wiley's global Scientific, Technical and Medical business to form Wiley-Blackwell.

Registered office
John Wiley & Sons Ltd, The Atrium, Southern Gate, Chichester, West Sussex, PO19 8SQ, UK

Editorial offices:
9600 Garsington Road, Oxford, OX4 2DQ, UK
The Atrium, Southern Gate, Chichester, West Sussex, PO19 8SQ, UK
111 River Street, Hoboken, NJ 07030-5774, USA

For details of our global editorial offices, for customer services and for information about how to apply for permission to reuse the copyright material in this book please see our website at www.wiley.com/wiley-blackwell

Library of Congress Cataloging-in-Publication Data

Anesthesia for congenital heart disease / edited by Dean B. Andropoulos . . . [et al.]. – 2nd ed.
    p. ; cm.
    Includes bibliographical references and index.
    ISBN 978-1-4051-8634-6
    1. Congenital heart disease–Surgery.   2. Congenital heart disease in children–Surgery.   3. Anesthesia in cardiology.   4. Pediatric anesthesia.   I. Andropoulos, Dean B.
    [DNLM: 1. Heart Defects, Congenital–surgery.   2. Anesthesia–methods.   3. Child.
4. Infant.
WS 290 A579 2010]
    RD598.A576 2010
    617.9′67412–dc22
                                                                          2009013377

A catalogue record for this book is available from the British Library.

Set in 9.5/12pt Palatino by Aptara® Inc., New Delhi, India
Printed and bound in Singapore by Fabulous Printers Pte Ltd

1   2010

Contents

Contents

Contributors

Dean B. Andropoulos, M.D., M.H.C.M.
Chief of Anesthesiology
Texas Children's Hospital
Professor, Anesthesiology and Pediatrics
Baylor College of Medicine
Houston, TX
USA

Elumalai Appachi, M.D.
Medical Director, Pediatric Intensive Care Unit
Cleveland Clinic
Cleveland, OH
USA

Philip D. Arnold, B.M., F.R.C.A.
Consultant in Pediatric Cardiac Anaesthesia
Jackson Rees Department of Anaesthesia
Royal Liverpool Children's NHS Trust
Alder Hey Hospital
Liverpool, UK

Victor C. Baum, M.D.
Professor of Anesthesiology & Pediatrics
Executive Vice-Chair
Director, Cardiac Anesthesia
University of Virginia
Charlottesville, VA
USA

M. Gail Boltz, M.D.
Clinical Professor, Department of Anesthesia
Lucile Packard Children's Hospital
Stanford University School of Medicine
Stanford, CA
USA

Kathryn K. Collins, M.D.
Associate Professor of Pediatrics
Department of Pediatrics, Section of Cardiology
University of Colorado at Denver and Health Sciences Center
The Children's Hospital
Aurora, CO
USA

Laura K. Diaz, M.D.
Attending Cardiac Anesthesiologist
The Children's Hospital of Philadelphia
Assistant Professor of Anesthesia
University of Pennsylvania School of Medicine
Philadelphia, PA
USA

Duncan G. de Souza, M.D.
Staff Cardiac Anesthesiologist
Assistant Professor of Anesthesiology
University of Virginia
Charlottesville, VA
USA

James A. DiNardo, M.D., F.A.A.P.
Director, Anesthesia Fellowship Program
Senior Associate in Cardiac Anesthesia
Children's Hospital, Boston
Associate Professor of Anaesthesia
Harvard Medical School
Boston, MA
USA

Brain W. Duncan, M.D.
Staff Physician, Departments of Pediatric and Congenital Heart
Surgery, Biomedical Engineering, Molecular Cardiology, and the
    Transplantation Center
Cleveland Clinic
Cleveland, OH
USA

Ralph Gertler, M.D.
Staff Anesthesiologist
Institute of Anesthesiology and Intensive Care
German Heart Centre of the State of Bavaria and the Technical
University Munich
Munich, Germany

Gregory B. Hammer, M.D.
Professor of Anesethesia and Pediatrics
Lucile Packard Children's Hospital

Contributors

Stanford University School of Medicine
Stanford, CA
USA

Dolly D. Hansen, M.D.
Emeritus Senior Associate in Cardiac Anesthesia
Children's Hospital, Boston
Emeritus Associate Professor of Anaesthesia
Harvard Medical School
Boston, MA
USA

Paul R. Hickey, M.D.
Anesthesiologist-in-Chief
Children's Hospital Boston
Professor of Anaesthesia
Harvard Medical School
Boston, MA
USA

Helen M. Holtby, M.B. B.S., F.R.C.P.C.
Director of Cardiovascular Anaesthesia
The Hospital for Sick Children
Assistant Professor
Department of Anaesthesia
Toronto, Canada

Javier Joglar, M.D.
Staff Pediatric Cardiovascular Anesthesiologist, Texas Children's
   Hospital
Assistant Professor, Anesthesiology and Pediatrics
Baylor College of Medicine
Houston, TX
USA

Jeffrey J. Kim, M.D.
Assistant Professor of Pediatrics
Department of Pediatrics, Division of Pediatric Cardiology
Baylor College of Medicine
Texas Children's Hospital
Houston, TX
USA

Peter C. Laussen, M.B.B.S.
Senior Associate in Anesthesia
Children's Hospital Boston
Professor of Anaesthesia
Harvard Medical School
Boston MA
USA

Andreas W. Loepke, M.D., Ph.D.
Staff Anesthesiologist
Cincinnati Children's Hospital Medical Center
Assistant Professor of Clinical Anesthesia and Pediatrics
University of Cincinnati School of Medicine
Cincinnati, OH
USA

Bruce E. Miller, M.D.
Director, Pediatric Cardiac Anesthesiology
Children's Healthcare of Atlanta at Egleston
Associate Professor of Anesthesiology
Emory University School of Medicine
Atlanta, GA
USA

Wanda C. Miller-Hance, M.D.
Professor of Pediatrics and Anesthesiology
Department of Pediatrics, Divisions of Anesthesiology and
   Pediatric Cardiology
Department of Anesthesiology
Baylor College of Medicine
Associate Director for Pediatric Cardiovascular Anesthesia
Director of Intraoperative Echocardiography
Texas Children's Hospital
Houston, TX
USA

Emad B. Mossad, M.D.
Director of Pediatric Cardiovascular Anesthesiology
Texas Children's Hospital
Professor of Anesthesiology and Pediatrics
Baylor College of Medicine
Houston, TX
USA

Pablo Motta, M.D.
Staff Pediatric Cardiovascular Anesthesiologist
Texas Children's Hospital
Assistant Professor, Anesthesiology and Pediatrics
Baylor College of Medicine
Houston, TX
USA

Susan C. Nicolson, M.D.
Chief, Division of Cardiothoracic Anesthesia
The Children's Hospital of Philadelphia
Professor of Anesthesia, University of Pennsylvania School of
   Medicine
Philadelphia, PA
USA

Kirsten C. Odegard, M.D.
Senior Associate in Anesthesia
Children's Hospital Boston
Associate Professor in Anaesthesia
Harvard Medical School
Boston, MA
USA

Chandra Ramamoorthy, M.B., B.S.; F.F.A. (UK)
Professor, Department of Anesthesia
Lucile Packard Children's Hospital
Stanford University School of Medicine
Stanford, CA
USA

Stephen J. Roth, M.D., M.P.H.
Medical Director, Cardiovascular Intensive Care Unit
Lucile Packard Children's Hospital,
Associate Professor of Pediatrics
Stanford University School of Medicine
Stanford, CA
USA

Kathryn Rouine-Rapp, M.D.
Professor of Clinical Anesthesia
Department of Anesthesia and Perioperative Care
University of California
San Francisco, CA
USA

Isobel A. Russel, M.D., Ph.D.
Chief of Cardiac Anesthesia
Moffitt-Long Hospitals
Professor of Anesthesia
University of California, San Francisco
San Francisco, CA
USA

Michael L. Schmitz, M.D.
Director, Pediatric Cardiac Anesthesia
Arkansas Children's Hospital
Professor, Anesthesiology and Pediatrics
University of Arkansas for Medical Sciences
Little Rock, AR
USA

Anshuman Sharma, M.D., F.F.A.R.C.S.I., M.B.A.
Associate Professor, Department of Anesthesiology
Washington University School of Medicine
St Louis Children's Hospital
St Louis, MO
USA

James P. Spaeth, M.D.
Director of Cardiac Anethesia
Cincinnati Children's Hospital Medical Center
Associate Professor of Clinical Anesthesia and Pediatrics
University of Cincinnati School of Medicine
Cincinnati, OH
USA

Stephen A. Stayer, M.D.
Medical Director of Perioperative Services
Texas Children's Hospital
Professor, Anesthesiology and Pediatrics
Baylor College of Medicine
Houston, TX
USA

James M. Steven, M.D., S.M.
Senior Vice President for Medical Affairs
Chief Medical Officer
The Children's Hospital of Philadelphia
Attending Cardiac Anesthesiologist
Associate Professor of Anesthesia

University of Pennsylvania School of Medicine
Philadelphia, PA
USA

Sugantha Sundar, M.D.
Staff Cardiac Anesthesiologist
Director, Adult Cardiothoracic Anesthesia Fellowship
Beth Israel Deaconess Medical Center
Assistant Professor of Anaesthesia
Harvard Medical School
Boston, MA
USA

Sana Ullah, M.D.
Staff Pediatric Cardiac Anesthesiologist
Arkansas Children's Hospital
Associate Professor of Anesthesiology
University of Arkansas for Medical Sciences
Little Rock, AR
USA

David F. Vener, M.D.
Staff Pediatric Cardiovascular Anesthesiologist
Texas Children's Hospital
Associate Professor, Anesthesiology and Pediatrics
Baylor College of Medicine
Houston, TX
USA

Glyn D. Williams, M.B.Ch.B., F.F.A.
Associate Professor, Department of Anesthesiology
Lucile Packard Children's Hospital
Stanford University School of Medicine
Stanford, CA
USA

Scott G. Walker, M.D.
Director Pediatric Cardiac Anesthesia
Riley Hospital for Children
Associate Professor of Clinical Anesthesia
Indiana University School of Medicine
Indianapolis, IN
USA

Ivan Wilmot, M.D.
Postdoctoral Fellow in Pediatric Cardiology
Department of Pediatrics, Division of Pediatric Cardiology
Baylor College of Medicine
Texas Children's Hospital
Houston, TX
USA

Maria Markakis Zestos, M.D.
Chief of Anesthesiology
Children's Hospital of Michigan
Assistant Professor of Anesthesiology
Wayne State University School of Medicine
Detroit, MI
USA

Preface

In the 5 years since the publication of *Anesthesia for Congenital Heart Disease*, there has been continual progress in the advancement of the science and art of caring for these complicated patients. The collaboration of anesthesiologists, surgeons, cardiologists, intensivists, neonatologists, neurologists, nurses, perfusionists, and specialists in adult congenital heart disease is a shining example of true multidisciplinary patient care, education, and research to discover the basic knowledge and the breakthroughs that will improve not only survival, but also quality of life for these patients. This second edition is thoroughly updated with extensive new material and references. Also, we have recognized the need for anesthesiologists who care for these patients to have a broad based knowledge of the embryology and development of congenital cardiac defects, and so have added a chapter addressing this critical topic. Patient outcome data have assumed critical importance in all of medicine, and to recognize the need for education in this area we have added a chapter on "Quality, Outcomes, and Databases in Congenital Cardiac Anesthesia." The burgeoning field of mechanical support of the pediatric circulation necessitated a separate chapter on this topic that thoroughly reviews the indications, complications, and devices available for this complex and expensive therapy. The expanding scope of invasive cardiac catheterization procedures necessitated a major expansion of this chapter, including new information on "hybrid" procedures involving both surgery and catheterization. The book cover, depicting a pediatric ventricular assist device, and the hybrid Stage I operation for hypoplastic left heart syndrome, acknowledges the importance of the latter two developments. Finally, to facilitate access to this new edition, Wiley-Blackwell has made the full text of the book available in electronic book form on the Wiley Interscience Web Site: HYPERLINK "http://www.wileyinterscience.com" www.wileyinterscience.com.

Since the publication of the first edition, the Congenital Cardiac Anesthesia Society (CCAS) has been founded, within the Society for Pediatric Anesthesia in the USA. The CCAS mission is to advance the anesthetic care of all patients with congenital heart disease through education, research, training, and advocacy. The CCAS is a society of energetic physicians with deep commitment to provide the highest quality care for these complicated patients, and to educate anesthesiologists in their care and contribute to the breakthroughs that will improve their lives. It is to these hardworking professionals that we dedicate the second edition of this book.

Dean B. Andropoulos, M.D.
Stephen A. Stayer, M.D.
Isobel A. Russell, M.D.
Emad B. Mossad, M.D.
November 2009

Acknowledgements

The editors would like to acknowledge the outstanding editorial assistance of Rose Palomares, Texas Children's Hospital and Baylor College of Medicine, for her extensive efforts with formatting and finalizing chapter manuscripts, preparation of references, and obtaining many permissions for reproduction of figures.

We would like to thank the extraordinary group of anesthesiologists and their associates, for their labors in writing the chapters of this book. They have all taken the time from their incredibly stressful, busy and typically overextended schedules to share their immense expertise in these pages. Their efforts will serve well all who provide anesthesia care to patients with congenital heart disease.

We would also each like to acknowledge the encouragement of our families, and in particular our spouses: Julie Andropoulos, Marce Stayer, John Russell, and Mona Mossad. Each of them has supported us and our respective families through the many hours of weekend and evening work so that we could complete this text.

1 History, education, outcomes, and science

1

History of anesthesia for congenital heart disease

Dolly D. Hansen, M.D. and Paul R. Hickey, M.D.

Children's Hospital, Boston and Harvard Medical School, Boston, Massachusetts, USA

Introduction

Over the last 65 years, pediatric cardiac anesthesia has developed as a subspecialty of pediatric anesthesia, or a subspecialty of cardiac anesthesia, depending on one's perspective. It is impossible to describe the evolution of pediatric cardiac anesthesia without constantly referring to developments in the surgical treatment of congenital heart disease (CHD) because of the great interdependency of the two fields. As pediatric anesthesia developed over the years, surgical treatments of children with CHD were invented, starting with simple surgical ligation of a patent ductus arteriosus (PDA) to sophisticated, staged repair of complex intracardiac lesions in low-birth-weight neonates requiring cardiopulmonary bypass (CPB) and circulatory arrest. Practically, every advance in surgical treatment of CHD had to be accompanied by changes in anesthetic management to overcome challenges that impeded successful surgical treatment or mitigated morbidity associated with surgical treatment.

This history will mostly be organized around the theme of how anesthesiologists met these new challenges using the then-available anesthetic armamentarium. The second theme running through this story is the slow change of interest and focus from just events in the operating room

(OR) to perioperative care in its broadest sense, including perioperative morbidity. The last theme is the progressive reduction in the age of patients routinely presenting for anesthesia and surgery from the 9-year-old undergoing the first PDA ligation in 1938 [1] to the fetus recently reported in the *New York Times* in 2002 who had aortic atresia repaired in utero [2]. Interestingly, both patients had had their cardiac procedures at the same institution.

This story will be told working through the different time frames—the first years: 1938–1954; CPB and early repair: 1954–1970; deep hypothermic circulatory arrest (DHCA) and introduction of prostaglandin E$_1$ (PGE$_1$): 1970–1980; hypoplastic left heart syndrome (HLHS): 1980–1990; refinement and improvement in mortality/morbidity: 1990–2000.

The first years: 1938–1954

These years began with the ligation of the PDA and continued with palliative operations. The first successful operation for a CHD occurred in August 1938 when Robert E. Gross ligated the PDA of a 9-year-old girl. The operation and the postoperative course were smooth, but because of the interest in the case, the child was kept in the hospital until the 13th day. In the report of the case, Gross mentions that the operation was done under cyclopropane anesthesia, and continues: "The chest was closed, the lung being re-expanded with positive pressure anesthesia

Anesthesia for Congenital Heart Disease 2nd edition. Edited by
Dean Andropoulos, Stephen Stayer, Isobel Russell and Emad Mossad.
© 2010 Blackwell Publishing.

just prior to placing the last stitch in the intercostal muscles."

A nurse using a "tight-fitting" mask gave the anesthetic. There was no intubation and of course no postoperative ventilation. The paper does not mention any particular pulmonary complications, so it cannot have been much different from ordinary postoperative course of the day [1].

In 1952 Dr Gross published a review of 525 PDA ligations where many, if not all, of the anesthetics were administered by the same nurse anesthetist, under surgical direction [3]. Here he states: "[F]ormerly we employed cyclopropane anesthesia for these cases, but since about half of the fatalities seemed to have been attributable to cardiac arrest or irregularities under this anesthetic, we have now completely abandoned cyclopropane and employ ether and oxygen as a routine." It is probably correct that cyclopropane under these circumstances with insufficient airway control were more likely to cause cardiac arrhythmias than ether. An intralaryngeal airway was used which also served "to facilitate suction removal of any secretions from the lower airway" (and we may add, the stomach). Dr Gross claims that the use of this airway reduced the incidence of postoperative pulmonary complications. Without having a modern, rigorous review of this series, it is hard to know what particular anesthetic challenges other than these confronted the anesthetist, but we may assume that intraoperative desaturation from the collapsed left lung, postoperative pulmonary complications, and occasional major blood loss from an uncontrolled, ruptured ductus arteriosus were high on the list.

The next operation to be introduced was billed as "corrective" for the child with cyanotic CHD and was the systemic to pulmonary artery shunt. The procedure was proposed by Helen Taussig as an "artificial ductus arteriosus" and first performed by Albert Blalock at Johns Hopkins Hospital in 1944. In a very detailed paper, Drs Blalock and Taussig described the first three patients to undergo the Blalock–Taussig shunt operation. Dr Harmel anesthetized the first and third patients, using ether and oxygen in an open drop method for the first patient and cyclopropane through an endotracheal tube for the third patient. The second patient was given cyclopropane through an endotracheal tube by Dr Lamont. Whether patient #1 and #3 were intubated is unclear, but it is noted that in all three cases positive pressure ventilation was used to reinflate the lung [4]. Interestingly, in this early kinder and gentler time, the surgical and pediatric authors reporting the Blalock–Taussig operation acknowledged by name the pediatricians and house officers who took such good care of the children postoperatively but still did not acknowledge in their paper the contribution of the anesthesiologists Lamont and Harmel.

Although intubation of infants was described by Gillespie as early as 1939, it is difficult to say exactly at what time intubations became routine [5].

Drs Harmel and Lamont, who were anesthesiologists, reported in 1946 on their anesthetic experience with 100 operations for congenital malformations of the heart "in which there is pulmonary artery stenosis or atresia." They reported 10 anesthetic-related deaths in the series, so it is certain that they encountered formidable anesthetic problems in these surgical procedures [6]. This is the first paper we know of published in the field of pediatric cardiac anesthesia.

In 1952 Damman and Muller reported a successful operation in which the main pulmonary artery was reduced in size and a band placed around the artery in a 6-month-old infant with single ventricle (SV). It is mentioned that morphine and atropine were given preoperatively, but no further anesthetic agents are mentioned. At that time infants were assumed to be oblivious to pain so we can wonder what was used beyond oxygen and restraint [7].

Over the next 20 years many palliative operations for CHD were added and a number of papers appeared describing the procedures and the anesthetic management. In 1948 McQuiston described the anesthetic technique used at Children's Memorial Hospital in Chicago [8]. This is an excellent paper for its time, but a number of the author's conclusions are erroneous, although they were the results of astute clinical observations and the current knowledge at the time. The anesthetic technique for shunt operations (mostly Potts' anastomosis) is discussed in some detail, but is mostly of historical interest today. McQuiston explained that he had no experience with anesthetic management used in other centers, such as the pentothal–N_2O–curare used at Minnesota or the ether technique used at the Mayo clinic. McQuiston used heavy premedication with morphine, pentobarbital and atropine, and/or scopolamine; this is emphasized because it was important "to render the child sleepy and not anxious." The effect of sedation with regard to a decrease in cyanosis (resulting in making the child look pinker) is noted by the authors. They also noted that children with severe pulmonic stenosis or atresia do not decrease their cyanosis "because of very little blood flow," and these children have the highest mortality.

McQuiston pointed out that body temperature control was an important factor in predicting mortality and advocated the use of moderate hypothermia, i.e., "refrigeration" with ice bags, because of a frequently seen syndrome of hyperthermia. McQuiston worked from the assumption that hyperthermia is a disease in itself, but did not explore the idea that the rise in central temperature might be a symptom of low cardiac output with peripheral vasoconstriction. Given what we now know of shunt physiology, it is interesting to speculate that this "disease" was caused by pulmonary hyperperfusion after the opening of what would now be considered as an excessively large shunt, stealing a large portion of systemic blood flow.

In 1950 Harris described the anesthetic technique used at Mount Zion Hospital in San Francisco. He emphasized the use of quite heavy premedication with morphine, atropine, and scopolamine. The "basal anesthetic agent" was Avertin (tribromoethanol). It was given rectally and supplemented with N_2O/O_2 and very low doses of curare. Intubation was facilitated by cyclopropane. The FiO_2 was changed according to cyanosis, and bucking or attempts at respiration were thought to be due to stimulation of the hilus of the lung. This was treated with "cocainization" of the hilus [9].

In 1952 Dr Robert M. Smith discussed the circulatory factors involved in the anesthetic management of patients with CHD. He pointed out the necessity to understand the pathophysiology of the lesion and also "the expected effect of the operation upon this unnatural physiology." That is, he recognized that the operations are not curative. The anesthetic agents recommended were mostly ether following premedication.

While most of these previous papers had been about Tetralogy of Fallot (TOF), Dr Smith also described the anesthetic challenges of surgery for coarctation of the aorta. He emphasized the hypertension following clamping of the aorta and warned against excessive bleeding in children operated on at older ages using ganglionic blocking agents. This bleeding was far beyond what anesthesiologists now see in patients operated on at younger ages, before development of substantial collateral arterial vessels [10].

The heart–lung machine: 1954–1970

From 1954 to 1970 the development of what was then called the "heart–lung machine" opened the heart to surgical repair of complex intracardiac congenital heart defects. At the time, the initial high morbidity of early CPB technology seen in adults was even worse in children, particularly smaller children weighing less than 10 kg. Anesthetic challenges multiplied rapidly in association with CPB coupled with early attempts at complete intracardiac repair. The lung as well as the heart received a large share of the bypass-related injuries leading to increased postoperative pulmonary complications. Brain injury began to be seen and was occasionally reported, in conjunction with CPB operations, particularly when extreme levels of hypothermia were used in an attempt to mitigate the morbidity seen in various organ systems after CPB.

In Kirklin's initial groundbreaking report of intracardiac surgery with the aid of a mechanical pump–oxygenator system at the Mayo Clinic, the only reference to anesthetic management is a brief remark that ether and oxygen were given [11]. In Lillehei's description of direct vision intracardiac surgery in man using a simple, disposable artificial oxygenator, there is no mention of anesthetic management [12]. What strikes a "modern" cardiac anesthesiologist in these two reports is the high mortality: 50% in Kirklin's series and 14% in Lillehei's series. All of these patients were children with CHD ranging in age from 1 month to 11 years. Clearly, such mortality and the associated patient care expense would not be tolerated today.

At that time, pediatric anesthesia was performed with open drop ether administration and later with ether using different nonrebreathing systems. Most anesthetics were given by nurses under the supervision of the surgeon. The first physician anesthetist to be employed by a Children's Hospital was Robert M. Smith in Boston in 1946.

The anesthetic agent to come into widespread use after ether was cyclopropane; in most of the early textbooks, it was the recommended drug for pediatric anesthesia. Quite apart from being explosive, cyclopropane was difficult to use. It was obvious that CO_2 absorption was necessary with cyclopropane to avoid hypercarbia and acidosis, which might precipitate ventricular arrhythmias. However, administration with a Waters' absorber could be technically difficult especially as tracheal intubation was considered dangerous to the child's "small, delicate airway."

In all the early reports it is noted or implied that the patients were awake (more or less) and extubated at the end of the operation. In the description of the postoperative course, respiratory complications were frequent, in the form of either pulmonary respiratory insufficiency or airway obstruction. This latter problem was probably because "the largest tube, which would fit through the larynx" was used. Another reason may have been that the red rubber tube was not tissue tested. The former problem was probably often related to the morbidity of early bypass technology on the lung.

Arthur S. Keats, working at the Texas Heart Institute and Texas Children's Hospital with Denton A. Cooley, had much experience with congenital heart surgery and anesthesia from 1955 to 1960, and provided the most extensive description of the anesthetic techniques used in this era [13, 14]. He described anesthesia for congenital heart surgery without bypass in 150 patients, the most common operations being PDA ligation, Potts operation, atrial septectomy (Blalock–Hanlon operation), or pulmonary valvotomy. Premedication was with oral or rectal pentobarbital, chloral hydrate per rectum, intramuscular meperidine, and intramuscular scopolamine or atropine. Endotracheal intubation was utilized, and ventilation was assisted using an Ayres T-piece, to-and-fro absorption system, or circle system. Cyclopropane was used for induction, and a venous cutdown provided vascular access. Succinylcholine bolus and infusion were used to maintain muscle relaxation. Light ether anesthesia was used for maintenance until the start of chest closure, and then 50% N_2O used as needed during chest closure. Of note is that the electrocardiogram, ear oximeter, and intra-arterial blood pressure recordings were used for monitoring during this period, as well as arterial blood gases and measurements of electrolytes and hemoglobin. The next year he published his experiences with 200 patients undergoing surgery for CHD with CPB, almost all of whom were children. Ventricular septal defect (VSD), atrial septal defect (ASD), tetralogy of Fallot (TOF), and aortic stenosis were the most common indications for surgery. The anesthetic techniques were the same as above, except that d-tubocurare was given to maintain apnea during bypass.

Perfusion rates of 40–50 mL/kg/min were used in infants and children, and lactic acidemia after bypass (average 4 mmol/L) was described. No anesthetic agent was added during bypass, and "patients tended to awaken during the period of bypass," but apparently without recall or awareness. Arrhythmias noted ranged from frequent bradycardia with cyclopropane and succinylcholine to junctional or ventricular tachycardia, ventricular fibrillation (VF), heart block, and rapid atrial arrhythmias. Treatments included defibrillation, procainamide, digitalis, phenylephrine, ephedrine, isoproterenol, and atopine. Eleven of 102 patients with VSD experienced atrioventricular block. Epicardial pacing was attempted in some of these patients but was never successful. Fresh citrated whole blood was used for small children throughout the case, and transfusion of large amounts of blood was frequently necessary in small infants. Mortality rate was 13% in the first series (36% in the 42 patients less than 1-yr-old) and 22.5% in the second series (47.5% in the 40 patients less than 1-yr-old). Causes of death included low cardiac output after ventriculotomy, irreversible VF, coronary air emboli, postoperative atrioventricular block, hemorrhage, pulmonary hypertension, diffuse atelectasis, and aspiration of vomitus. No death was attributed to the anesthetic alone. Reading these reports provides an appreciation of the daunting task of providing anesthesia during these pioneering times.

Tracheostomy after cardiac operations was not unusual and in some centers it was done "prophylactically" a week before the scheduled operation. These practices were certainly related to primitive (in present terms) techniques and equipment used for both endotracheal intubation and CPB. Postoperative ventilatory support did not become a routine until later when neonatologists and other intensive care specialists had proven it could be done successfully. Successful management of prolonged respiratory support was first demonstrated in the great epidemics of poliomyelitis in Europe and the USA in 1952–1954 [15].

Halothane was introduced in clinical practice in the mid-1950s and it became rapidly the most popular agent in pediatric anesthesia, mostly because of the smooth induction compared to the older agents. Halothane was also widely used for pediatric cardiac anesthesia in spite of its depressive effect on the myocardium and the significant risk of arrhythmias. Halothane is no longer available, and the newer inhalational agents isoflurane and sevoflurane are now the mainstays of pediatric cardiac cases in US academic centers.

During this period, adult cardiac anesthesiologists following the practice reported by Edward Lowenstein in 1970 [16] began to use intravenous anesthesia based on opiates. Initially, morphine in doses up to as much as 1 mg/kg was given with 100% oxygen and this technique became the anesthetic of choice for adult cardiac patients, but vasodilation and hypotension associated with its use slowed the incorporation of this technique into pediatric cardiac anesthesia until the synthetic opiates became available.

Before CPB was yet developed, or when it still carried high morbidity and mortality, a number of modalities were used to improve the outcome for infants. One was inflow occlusion (IO) and another was the hyperbaric chamber. IO was useful and, if well managed, an elegant technique. The secret was the organization of the efforts of the entire operative team, and the technique required the closest cooperation between surgeon and anesthesiologists. The technique was as follows.

The chest was opened in the midline. After pericardiotomy, a side clamp was placed on the right atrial (RA) free wall and an incision made in the RA or proximal on the pulmonary artery prior to placing the vascular clamps used to occlude caval return. Prior to application of the clamps, patients were hyperventilated with 100% O_2. During IO, the superior vena cava (SVC) and inferior vena cava (IVC) inflow were occluded, ventilation held, the RA or the pulmonary artery clamp released; the heart was allowed to empty and the septum primum excised or the pulmonic valve dilated. After excision of the septum or valvotomy, one caval clamp was released initially to de-air the atrium. The RA side clamp or the pulmonary artery clamp was then reapplied and the other caval clamp released. The heart was resuscitated with bolus calcium gluconate (range 30–150 mg/kg) and bicarbonate (range 0.3–3 mEq/kg). Occasionally, inotropes were administered, most often dopamine. It was important to titrate the inotropes so as not to aggravate rebound hypertension caused by endogenous catecholamines. The duration of the IO was between 1 and 3 minutes—terrifying minutes for the anesthesiologist, but quickly over.

Another modality used to improve the survival after shunt operations, pulmonary artery banding, and atrial septectomy, was to operate in the hyperbaric chamber, thereby benefiting from the increased amount of physically dissolved oxygen. It was a cumbersome affair operating in crowded and closed quarters. There was room for only two surgeons, two nurses, one anesthesiologist, and one baby, as the number of emergency oxygen units limited access. Retired navy divers ran the chamber and kept track of how many minutes the personnel had been in the hyperbaric chamber in the previous week. Help was not readily available because the chamber was buried in a subbasement and people had to be sluiced in through a side arm that could be pressurized. The chamber was pressurized to 2–3 atm so it was unpleasantly hot while increasing the O_2 pressure and cold while decreasing the pressure; people with glasses were at a disadvantage. It did not seem to add to survival and was abandoned circa 1974.

Anesthesia was a challenge in the hyperbaric chamber. The infants were anesthetized with ketamine and nitrous oxide. As the pressure in the chamber increased, the concentrations of N_2O had to be decreased to avoid the hypotension and bradycardia that occurred rapidly.

Also in this era, the first infant cardiac transplant was performed by Kantrowitz in 1967 [17]. The recipient was an 18-day-old, 2.6-kg patient with severe Ebstein's anomaly, who had undergone a Potts shunt on day 3 of life. The donor was an anencephalic newborn. The anesthetic technique is not described, and the infant died 7 hours postoperatively of pulmonary dysfunction.

The era of deep hypothermic circulatory arrest and the introduction of PGE₁: 1970–1980

About 1970 physiological repair of CHD or "correction" had begun to come of age. In the adult world, coronary bypass operations and valve replacement spurred interest in cardiac anesthesia, which centered increasingly on use of high-dose narcotics and other pharmacological interventions. As synthetic opiates with fewer hypotensive side effects became available, their use spread into pediatric cardiac anesthesia late in the 1970s and 1980s.

Children were still treated as "small adults" because major physiological differences were not yet well appreciated, particularly as they related to CPB morbidity. CPB was rarely employed during surgery on children weighing less than 20 lb because of the very high mortality and morbidity that had been experienced in the early years. The notion of repairing complex CHD in infancy was getting attention but was hindered by technical limitations of surgical techniques, CPB techniques, and anesthetic challenges in infants. Theoretically, physiological repair early in life provides a more normal development of the cardiovascular and pulmonary systems and might avoid palliation all

together. The advantage of this was that the sequelae after palliation, for instance distorted pulmonary arteries after shunts and pulmonary artery banding, might be avoided. Pulmonary artery hypertension following Waterston and Potts shunts occurred as a result of increased pulmonary blood flow and resulted in pulmonary obstructive disease. This would not develop if the defect were physiologically repaired at an early age. Furthermore, parents could be spared the anxiety of repeated operations and the difficulties of trying to raise a child with heart that continued to be impaired.

The perceived need for early repair, together with the high mortality of bypass procedures, in infants and small children led to the introduction of DHCA. It was first practiced in Kyoto, Japan, but spread rapidly to Russia, the West Coast of the USA at Seattle, and from there to Midwestern and other US pediatric centers. As an example of the difficulties this presented to anesthesiologists, the introduction of DHCA in practice at Children's Hospital in Boston is useful. The newly appointed chief of cardiovascular surgery at the Children's Hospital in Boston was Aldo R. Castaneda, M.D., Ph.D., one of the first supporters of early total correction of CHD, who quickly embraced DHCA as a tool to accomplish his goals for repair in infants. He immediately, in 1972, introduced DHCA into practice at Children's Hospital in Boston and the rather shocked anesthesia department had to devise an anesthetic technique to meet this challenge, aided only by a couple of surgical papers in Japanese that Dr Castaneda kindly supplied to the anesthesia department. These papers had, of course, little reference to anesthesia.

The first description of the techniques of DHCA from Japan in the English literature was Horiuchi's from 1968 [18]. They used a simple technique with surface cooling and rewarming during resuscitation, using ether as the anesthetic agent, without intubation. In 1972 Mori reported details of their technique for cardiac surgery in neonates and infants using deep hypothermia, again in a surgical publication. Their anesthetic technique was halothane/N_2O combined with muscle relaxant; CO_2 was added to the anesthetic gas during cooling and rewarming (pH-stat) to improve brain blood flow. The infants were surface cooled with ice bags and rewarmed on CPB [19].

Surprisingly, given the enormity of the physiological disturbances and challenges presented by DHCA, very few articles describing an anesthetic technique for DHCA were published, perhaps because DHCA and early correction was not widely accepted. A paper from Toronto described an anesthetic regime with atropine premedication occasionally combined with morphine [20]. Halothane and 50% N_2O were used, combined with d-tubocurare or pancuronium. CO_2 was added to "improve tissue oxygenation by maintaining peripheral and cerebral perfusion." The infants were cooled with surface cooling

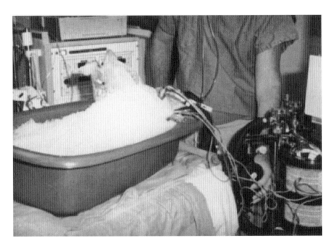

Figure 1.1 Infant submerged in ice water

(plastic bags with melting ice) and rewarmed on CPB. It was noted that 6 of the 25 infants had VF when cooled to below 30°C.

Given the lack of any scientific data or studies to guide anesthetic management of such cases, a very simple technique with ketamine–O_2–N_2O and curare supplemented by small amounts of morphine (0.1–0.3 mg/kg) was used at Children's Hospital in Boston. This was the way infants were anesthetized for palliative cardiac surgical procedures in the hyperbaric chamber at Boston Children's. The infants were surface cooled in a bathtub filled with ice water to a core temperature of approximately 30°C. The bathtub was a green plastic bucket (for dishwashing) bought at a Sears-Roebuck surplus store, keeping things as simple as possible (Figure 1.1). This method was used in hundreds of infants over the next couple of years and only one infant developed VF in the ice water bathtub. This was an infant with TOF who suffered a coronary air embolus either from a peripheral IV or during an attempted placement of a central venous line. In retrospect, it is amazing that so few papers were published about the anesthetic management of this procedure that rapidly was seen to be lifesaving. The little material that was published about these techniques was restricted to surgical journals and did not describe or make any attempt to study the anesthetic techniques used for DHCA. The published surgical articles were largely unknown to cardiac and pediatric anesthesiologists.

It was during these 10 years that the "team concept" developed with cardiologists, cardiac surgeons, and anesthesiologists working together in the OR and the ICU in the larger centers. These teams were facilitated by the anesthesiologists' "invasion" of weekly cardiology–cardiac surgeons conferences where the scheduled operations for the week were discussed. Dr Aldo Castaneda, the chief surgeon at Boston's Children's Hospital, was a leader in the

creation of a cardiac team concept for pediatric cardiac surgery.

During the first year of using DHCA in Boston, it was noticed that a number of the infants had "funny, jerky" movements of the face and tongue. A few also had transient seizures during the postoperative period, but as they had normal EEGs at 1-year follow-up, it was felt that significant cerebral complications were not a problem. In view of knowledge developed subsequently, these clues to neurological damage occurring during and after pediatric cardiac surgery involving DHCA were overlooked. In hindsight maybe it will be more correct to say these clues were ignored, thus a great opportunity to study this problem was delayed for almost two decades. The issue of neurological damage with DHCA was raised repeatedly by surgeons such as John Kirklin, but was not really studied until the group at Boston Children's Hospital led by Jane Newburger and Richard Jonas systematically followed a cohort of infants who had the arterial switch operation in the late 1980s using DHCA techniques [21]. In the late 1980s and early 1990s, Greeley and coworkers at Duke performed a series of human studies delineating the neurophysiological response to deep hypothermia and circulatory arrest [22]. These studies provided the crucial data in patients from which strategies for cooling and rewarming, length of safe DHCA, blood gas management, and perfusion were devised to maximize cerebral protection.

Those ongoing studies were followed by a number of studies comparing DHCA with hypothermic low-flow perfusion, with different hematocrit in the perfusate and with different pH strategies during hypothermic CPB, pH-stat versus alpha-stat.

During those years, the ketamine–morphine anesthetic technique had been supplanted by fentanyl-based high-dose narcotic techniques. For the neurologic outcome studies, the anesthetic technique was very tightly controlled, using fentanyl doses of 25 mcg/kg at induction, incision, onset of bypass and on rewarming, in addition to pancuronium. From the beginning of this period, surgical results as measured by mortality alone were excellent with steady increases in raw survival statistics. Because anesthetic techniques were evolving over this period of time, it was difficult to definitely ascribe any outcome differences to different anesthetic agents. A 1984 study of 500 consecutive cases of cardiac surgery in infants and children looked at anesthetic mortality and morbidity. Both were very low, so low in fact that they were probably not universally believed [23].

As the new synthetic opioids such as fentanyl and sufentanil were developed, they replaced morphine to provide more hemodynamic stability in opiate-based anesthetic techniques for cardiac patients. In 1981 Gregory and his associates first described the use of "high-dose" fentanyl,

30–50 mcg/kg, combined with pancuronium in 10 infants undergoing PDA ligation. It is noteworthy that transcutaneous oxygen tension was measured as part of this study. This paper was in fact the introduction of high-dose narcotics in pediatric cardiac anesthesia [24].

The technique was a great success; one potential reason for that success was demonstrated 10 years later in Anand's paper showing attenuation of stress responses in infants undergoing PDA ligation who were given lesser doses of fentanyl in a randomized, controlled study [25].

During this same period, synthetic opioids were replacing morphine in adult cardiac surgery. This technique slowly and somewhat reluctantly made its way into pediatric anesthesia [26], replacing halothane and morphine, which had previously been the predominant choice of pediatric anesthesiologists dealing with patients with CHD. In the years from 1983 to 1995, a number of papers were published showing the effect of different anesthetic agents on the cardiovascular system in children with CHD. Ketamine, nitrous oxide, fentanyl, and sufentanil were systematically studied. Some misconceptions stemming from studies of adult patients were corrected, such as the notion that N_2O combined with ketamine raises pulmonary artery pressure and pulmonary vascular resistance (PVR) [27]. On the other hand, the role of increased P_{CO_2} or lower pH in causing higher PVR was also demonstrated and that subsequently became important in another connection [28]. A number of studies done at this time demonstrated in a controlled fashion the earlier clinical observation (Harmel and McQuiston in the late 1940s) [6,29] that in cyanotic patients the O_2 saturation would rise during induction of anesthesia, almost irrespective of the agent used [30]. These events only reinforce the value of acute clinical observation and provide an example of how the interpretation of such observations may well change as new knowledge is discovered.

PDA and the introduction of PGE₁

In the mid-1970s several discoveries were made and introduced into clinical practice that turned out to be of great importance to the pediatric cardiac anesthesiologist and the rest of the cardiac team, the most important being the discovery that PGE_1 infused intravenously prevented the normal ductal closure [31]. These developments revolved around the role of the PDA in the pathophysiology of both cyanotic and acyanotic CHD. The critical role of PDA closing and opening in allowing early neonatal survival of infants with critical CHD began to be appreciated and clinicians sought methods of either keeping the PDA open or closing it, depending on what type of critical CHD the neonate was born with and the role of patency of the ductus arteriosis in the CHD pathophysiology. In some cases, particularly in very small neonates, the im-

portance of closing the PDA was increasingly appreciated and in other cases, the critical importance of maintaining the patency of a PDA was appreciated.

As the survival of very small premature infants began to improve, mostly because of technical improvements with the use of a warmed isolette and improved mechanical ventilation for preemies, it became apparent that in many of these infants the PDA would not undergo the normal closure over time. As the understanding of these infants' physiological problems improved and more infants survived, the role of continued patency of the PDA in neonates needing mechanical ventilation was appreciated. This led to medical therapy directed at promoting ductal closure using aspirin and indomethacin.

When such attempts failed, it was increasingly understood that necrotizing enterocolitis in the preemie was associated with decreased mesenteric blood flow secondary to the "steal" of systemic blood flow into the pulmonary circulation through a PDA. Thus in cases when the PDA failed to close in premature infants, the need for operative treatment of the PDA in preemies arose as prophylaxis for necrotizing enterocolitis.

Pediatric and cardiac anesthesiologists were now faced with the task of anesthetizing these tiny preemies safely. This involved maintaining body temperature in infants of 1 kg or less with very large surface area/volume ratios. Intraoperative fluid restriction was important and low levels of FIO_2 were used to decrease the risk of retinopathy of prematurity. As the decade progressed these issues emerged and were addressed. In 1980 Neuman [32] described the anesthetic management of 70 such infants using an O_2/N_2O muscle relaxant anesthesia technique with no mortality. Low FIO_2 was used to reduce the risk of retrolental fibroplasia and precautions were taken to prevent heat loss. In those days before AIDS became a wide concern, 40% of the infants received blood transfusion. Interestingly, the question of whether to operate in the NICU or the OR for closure of the PDA in the preemie was discussed at that time and remains unsettled today.

The PDA lesion presents an interesting story. In 1938 it was the first of the CHD lesions to be successfully treated surgically [1]. In the mid-1970s it was closed with medical therapy, first with aspirin and later with indomethacin. It was the first CHD lesion to be treated in the catheterization laboratory using different umbrella devices or coils [33]. Presently, if surgical closure is necessary, it is often done using a minimally invasive, thoracoscopic video-assisted technique [34]. Thoracoscopy has the benefit of using four tiny incisions to insert the instruments, avoiding an open thoracotomy and limiting dissection and trauma to the left lung. At the same time, this latest development of surgical technique required the anesthesiologist to again change the anesthetic approach to these patients. Unlike adult anesthesiologists who can use double-lumen endotracheal tubes for thoracoscopic procedures, pediatric anesthesiologists caring for 1–3-kg infants undergoing PDA ligation do not have the luxury of managing the left lung [34]. Another problem posed by thoracoscopic PDA ligation in the infant is the emerging need for neurophysiological monitoring of recurrent laryngeal nerve's innervation of the muscles of the larynx to avoid injury, a known complication of PDA surgery [35]. The last issue is tailoring the anesthetic so that the children are awake at the end of the operation, can be extubated, and spend an hour or so in the postanesthesia care unit, bypassing the cardiac intensive care unit. In fact, in 2001 a group led by Hammer at Stanford published the first description of true outpatient PDA ligation in two infants aged 17 days and 8 months [36]. These patients were managed with epidural analgesia, extubated in the OR, and discharged home 10 hours postoperatively. This report brings PDA closure full circle from a 13-day hospital stay following an ether mask anesthetic for an open thoracotomy to a day surgery procedure in an infant undergoing an endotracheal anesthetic for a thoracoscopic PDA ligation.

Maintaining patency of the PDA using PGE_1 is probably now of considerably greater importance than its closure both numerically and in terms of being life-sustaining in neonates with critical CHD. The introduction of PGE_1 suddenly improved the survival rate of a large number of neonates with CHD having lesions that require ductal patency to improve pulmonary blood flow, or to improve systemic blood flow distal to a critical coarctation of the aorta. The introduction of PGE_1 into clinical practice for therapy of neonatal CHD substantially changed the life of the pediatric cardiac surgeon and the pediatric cardiac anesthesiologist, as frequent middle-of-the-night shunt operations with extremely cyanotic infants almost immediately became a thing of the past. These operations were particularly daunting when one realizes that these procedures were most common before the availability of pulse oximetry; the only warning signs of impending cardiovascular collapse were the very dark color of the blood and preterminal bradycardia. To get an arterial blood gas with a PaO_2 in the low teens was not uncommon and PaO_2 measurements in single digits in arterial blood samples from live neonates during such surgical procedures were recorded. Even more dramatic was the disappearance of the child with critical post-ductal coarctation. These infants were extremely acidotic with pH of 7.0 or less at the start of the procedure (if it was possible to obtain an arterial puncture); they looked mottled and almost dead below the nipples. With the advent of PGE_1 therapy, they were resuscitated medically in the ICU and could be operated on the following day in substantially better condition than previously.

But the introduction of PGE_1 had an effect that was not clearly foreseen except maybe by some astute cardiologists. Survival of a number of these neonates presented pediatric cardiologists and cardiac surgeons (and then anesthesiologists) with rare and severe forms of CHD that had hitherto been considered a "rare" pathological diagnosis. Foremost among these were the infants with HLHS and some forms of interrupted aortic arch. As further experience was gained, it became obvious that these forms of disease were not so rare, but infants who had survived with those forms of CHD were very rare.

The story of HLHS: 1980–1990

As mentioned above, the introduction of PGE_1 brought major changes to pediatric cardiac anesthesia, solving some problems and at the same time bringing new challenges for the cardiac team. New diagnoses of CHD presented for treatment and were recognized; some had been known previously but had until then presented insurmountable obstacles to any effective therapy.

One of these was HLHS. It had been accurately described in 1958 by Noonan and Nadas but only as a pathological diagnosis [37]. The syndrome is a ductus-dependent lesion and had 100% mortality within a few days to weeks when the ductus underwent physiological closure. HLHS was therefore of no practical interest from a therapeutic standpoint until ductal patency could be maintained. When it became possible to keep the ductus arteriosus patent with PGE_1, these neonates rapidly became a problem that could not easily be ignored. In the beginning, most of the infants were misdiagnosed as having sepsis and being in septic shock, few babies reached the tertiary center without a telltale Band-Aid, indicating a lumbar puncture to rule out sepsis.

But even with the ability to diagnose the defect in a live neonate temporarily kept alive with a PGE_1 infusion, the outlook was not much better. There was no operation devised, and in some centers such neonates were kept viable on a PGE_1 infusion for weeks and even months in the (usually) vain attempt to get them to grow large enough for some surgical procedure to be attempted.

In the next years, several centers tried different approaches with ingenious conduits, trying to create an outlet from the right ventricle to the aorta and the systemic circulation.

Those were also the years where President Ronald Reagan's Baby Doe regulations were in effect. Anyone who thought an infant was being mistreated, i.e., not operated upon, could call a "Hot Line Number" which was posted in all neonatal ICUs to report the physicians "mistreatment" of the infant. Fortunately, this rule died a quiet death after a few chaotic years [38].

In the meantime, the search for a palliative operation went on, also spurred by the increasing success of the

Fontan operation, which had been introduced in 1970 [39]. This meant that there now was a theoretical endpoint for HLHS as well as for other forms of SV physiology. It was William Norwood at Boston Children's Hospital who was the first not only to devise a viable palliation but also to complete the repair with a Fontan operation the following year [40]. The publication of this landmark paper spurred considerable discussion. Many cardiologists and surgeons took the position that this operative procedure represented experimental and unethical surgery and that these infants "were better off dead."

The current approach to these infants varies from multistage physiological repair with palliation followed by Fontan operation. Another alternative is neonatal transplantation as proposed by the group at Loma Linda in California [41]. Some cardiologists are still advocates of conservative "comfort care" for neonates with HLHS.

With eventual survival of about 70% being achieved in many centers, these infants can no longer be written off as untreatable. Now the question is more about quality of survival, especially intellectual development. It is also recognized that many have both chromosomal and nonchromosomal anomalies in both the cerebral and gastrointestinal systems [42].

As was the case from the beginnings of pediatric cardiac surgery, this new patient population presented a management dilemma for the anesthesiologists; they posed a new set of problems that required solution before acceptable operative results could be achieved. It was obvious that patients with HLHS were hemodynamically unstable before CPB because of the large volume load on the heart coupled with coronary artery supply insufficiency. The coronary arteries in HLHS are supplied from the PDA retrograde through a hypoplastic ascending and transverse aorta that terminates as a single "main" coronary artery. A common event at sternotomy and exposure of the heart was VF secondary to mechanical stimulation. This fibrillation was sometimes intractable, necessitating emergent CPB during internal cardiac massage. This was not an auspicious beginning to a major experimental open-heart procedure.

It was during these years that the transition from morphine–halothane–N_2O to high-dose narcotic technique with fentanyl or sufentanil combined with 100% oxygen took place. This technique seemed to provide some protection against the sudden VF events. Despite this modest progress in getting patients successfully onto CPB, it soon became painfully clear to us that we had not made much progress in treating this lesion when we tried to wean the patients from bypass. The infants were still unstable coming off bypass and severely hypoxemic, and it took some time before we discovered a way to deal with the problem.

A chance observation led us to a solution. We noticed that infants who came off bypass with low PaO_2 (around 30 mmHg) after the HLHS repair often did well, while the ones with immediate "excellent gases" (PaO_2 of 40–50 mmHg or better) became progressively unstable in the ICU a couple of hours later, developing severe metabolic acidosis and dying during the first 24 hours.

This observation combined with discussions with the cardiologists about PVR and systemic vascular resistance made us attempt to influence these resistances to assure adequate systemic flow. In retrospect, infants with low PO_2 after bypass had smaller pulmonary artery shunts and adequate systemic blood flow, while those with larger pulmonary shunts and higher initial PO_2 levels after weaning from bypass tended to "steal" systemic blood flow through the pulmonary artery shunt. This would occur in the postoperative period, as the PVR remained elevated as a result of CPB before returning to more normal levels. These observations led to the technique of lowering the FIO_2 sometimes as low as 0.21 and to allow hypoventilation to increase PVR in patients that had larger size shunts placed to supply adequate systemic blood flow as part of what became known as the Norwood operation [43]. A different technique used at other institutions to deal with this problem was to add CO_2 to the anesthetic gas flow, increasing PVR and continuing to use "normal ventilation" in children that had larger shunts placed and excessive pulmonary blood flow [44]. Both techniques represented different approaches to the same problem: finding ways of dealing with the need to carefully balance PVR and systemic vascular resistance after bypass in a fragile parallel circulation in the post-bypass period where dynamic changes were taking place in ventricular function.

These observations, and the subsequent modifications in anesthetic and postoperative management, improved the survival for the stage I palliation (Norwood procedure). It should be noted that the pediatric cardiac anesthesiologist was a full, contributing partner in the progressive improvement in outcome of this very complex and challenging lesion. More important, the techniques developed and the knowledge gained in this process also simplified the management of other patients with parallel circulation and SV physiology. The obvious example is truncus arteriosus where the "usual" ST depression and frequent VF that occurred intraoperatively almost always can be avoided. Any decrease in PVR during anesthesia in a child with unrepaired truncus arteriosus can lead to pulmonary "steal" of systemic blood flow and decreased diastolic pressure through the common trunk to the aorta and pulmonary artery, resulting in hypotension and insufficient systemic blood flow expressed initially as coronary insufficiency and ST depression (or elevation).

During the same decade the surgical treatment of transposition of the great arteries (TGA) underwent several changes. The Mustard operations (as one type of atrial switch procedure) were feared because of the risk of SVC obstruction as a complication of this surgical procedure. At the end of a Mustard procedure, it was not uncommon to see a child with a grotesquely swollen head who had to be taken back to the OR for immediate reoperation. Many of those children suffered brain damage, especially when reoperation was delayed. This resulted from low-perfusion pressure during bypass because of venous hypertension in the internal jugular veins and SVC. The extent and prevalence of such damage was never systematically studied. The arterial pressure during bypass and in the immediate post-bypass period in the OR tended to be low and the pressure in SVC high. An article from Great Ormond Street in London demonstrated arrested hydrocephalus in Mustard patients [45]. The Senning operation (another variant of the atrial switch approach to TGA) was better, but those children could develop pulmonary venous obstruction acutely in the OR, after the procedure or progressively after hospital discharge. When the diagnosis was not promptly made and acted upon, these infants were often quite sick by the time they came to reoperation.

The successful application of the arterial switch procedure described by Jatene then began to revolutionize operations for TGA [46]. It eliminated the risk of obstruction of the pulmonary and systemic venous return seen after the Mustard and Senning procedures. It also diminished the incidence of the subsequent sick sinus syndrome, a complication that might develop in the first 10 years postoperatively resulting from the extensive atrial suture lines and reconstructions required by these "atrial" switch procedures. The introduction of the arterial switch operation again involved anesthesiologists. The initial attempts at arterial switch operations in many institutions resulted in substantial numbers of infants who had severe myocardial ischemia and even frank infarcts. This resulted from a variety of problems with the coronary artery transfer and reimplantation into the "switched" aorta that had been moved to the left ventricle outflow tract. Pediatric cardiac anesthesiologists gained extensive experience with intraoperative pressor and inotropic support and nitroglycerine infusions. They were expected by surgeons to provide support to get infants through what later turned out to be iatrogenically caused myocardial ischemia. As surgeons learned to handle coronary artery transfers and reanastomoses well, these problems largely disappeared, along with the need for major pressor and inotropic support and for nitroglycerine infusion inappropriately directed at major mechanical obstructions in the coronary arterial supply. The arterial switch operation has now been refined at most centers to the point where it is largely "routine" and presents for the most part, no unique anesthetic challenges.

It was during the same time period that a randomized strictly controlled study of stress response in infants undergoing cardiac surgery while anesthetized with high-dose sufentanil was performed. It showed that a high-dose narcotic technique would suppress but not abolish stress responses. It also seemed to show a reduction in morbidity and possibly mortality [47]. However, when the study was repeated 10 years later, these results did not quite hold up. It must be pointed out that the patient population was older and refinement of bypass technique had occurred [48].

Fontan and the catheterization laboratory: 1990–2000

After the anesthetic technique and preoperative management of the stage I palliation had been refined and we had been encouraged by the initial successes of stage II, problems arose. The Fontan operation became problematic as it was applied to younger patients with a great variety of SV types of CHD. Many of the patients had seemingly perfect Fontan operations but in the cardiac intensive care unit they developed low cardiac output and massive pleural and pericardial effusions postoperatively. Many died in the postoperative period despite a variety of different support therapies; their course over the first 24–48 hours was relentlessly downward and could only be reversed by taking them back to the OR, reversing the Fontan operation and reconstructing a systemic to pulmonary artery shunt. It was hard for the caretakers of those infants to accept such losses of children they had known from birth. They were our little friends and we knew the families too. All kinds of maneuvers were tried to avoid the above sequence of events, from early extubation to the use of a G-suit to improve venous return to the heart. In some centers, a large balloon was placed tightly around the child's lower body and intermittently inflated by a Bird respirator asynchronous with ventilation.

After a couple of years, two innovations changed the outlook. Both were linked to the understanding that a major limitation of the Fontan operation was the need for a normal or near normal PVR to allow survival through the postoperative period when CPB had caused, through release of a variety of inflammatory mediators and cytokines, a marked elevation of PVR in the early postoperative period. When this bypass-related increase in PVR was associated with younger age (less than 2 yr of age) at the time a Fontan was attempted, the higher baseline PVR of the infant made the bypass-related PVR worse and resulted in inadequate pulmonary blood flow and (single) ventricular filling in the early postoperative period, leading to a cycle of low cardiac output, pulmonary and systemic edema, further increases in PVR, acidosis, and death.

One solution was to interpose a bidirectional cavopulmonary anastomosis (BDG) 6–12 months before completion of the Fontan operation. This procedure, increasingly known as a "hemi-Fontan," directed only half of the systemic venous return through the lungs at a time when the infant's PVR had not fallen to normal levels and by preserving an alternative pathway for (single) ventricular filling through systemic venous return not routed through the lungs. This enabled the patients to maintain reasonable cardiac output although a bit "blue" during the early postoperative period, when the PVR had been elevated by CPB. However, this made a third operation, the completion of the Fontan, necessary.

The other innovation was the "fenestrated" Fontan where a small fenestration in the atrial baffle allowed systemic venous return to bypass the lungs as a right-to-left shunt, thereby maintaining ventricular filling and systemic cardiac output during the early postoperative period of high PVR. Over time the fenestration closed as PVR fell and shunting decreased. Alternatively, a device delivered during an interventional cardiac catheterization could close the fenestrations.

This whole process of testing the applicability of the Fontan principle and various modifications of the Fontan operation to a wide variety of types of severe cyanotic CHD involved another set of challenges for the pediatric cardiac anesthesiologist and collaboration between anesthesiology, cardiology, and surgery. The net result of a great deal of work and collaboration among these groups was that the outlook for the HLHS patients and indeed for all children with SV defects improved locally and as these improvements spread and were amplified by work done in other centers, the improvement became national and international. In some institutions the preferred treatment was and is neonatal transplantation. Its limits are the long waiting time for a transplant, the unavoidable mortality during the waiting period and the ongoing morbidity of neonatal heart transplants, a lifetime of immunosuppression therapy, and the accelerated risk of coronary artery disease seen in heart transplants, even in young children.

The collaboration with pediatric cardiologists around postoperative care of HLHS, Fontan patients, and others spread naturally to the cardiac catheterization laboratory. As pediatric cardiologists began to develop interventional procedures, the need for more control and support of vital functions became apparent. Previously, nurses operating under the supervision of the cardiologist performing the catheterizations had sedated the children for the procedures. In many institutions this involved high volumes of cases sedated by specially trained nurses, while in others with smaller pediatric case loads the practice of using general anesthesia for children undergoing cardiac catheterizations had been routine.

The interventional cardiologists turned to pediatric cardiac anesthesiologists for help in managing these patients while the cardiologists themselves were dealing with the complex demands of doing interventional procedures in infants and children with CHD. As was the case with newly devised pediatric cardiac surgical procedures, the development of interventional procedures for CHD in the cardiac catheterization lab posed a whole new and different set of problems and challenges for pediatric cardiac anesthesia. Not the least of these was providing anesthesia and vital function support in the dark and difficult environment of the cardiac catheterization laboratory. The introduction of dilation techniques for pulmonary arteries and veins, mitral and aortic valves, and most recently, the dilation of fetal atretic aortic valves in utero along with device closure of the PDA, ASD, and VSD all placed progressively more demands on the anesthesiologists, who became more and more involved in these procedures.

The development of another set of interventional procedures, the use of radio frequency ablation to deal with arrhythmias in the pediatric patient, illustrates the progressive complexity and difficulty of anesthesia care in these patients. Used initially only on healthy teenagers with structurally normal hearts but having paroxysmal atrial tachycardia (PAT), anesthesia care was quite straightforward. Now, in contrast, many of these radio frequency ablation procedures are done in children with complex CHD, repaired or unrepaired, and frequently the children (or adults) may be quite cyanotic or have low cardiac output [49]. At present in Children's Hospital, Boston, the cardiac cath laboratory and the cardiac MRI unit present close to 1000 anesthesia cases per year over and above cardiac surgical cases.

But with all those development the defects remain the same. If we look at the relative distribution of cases in 1982 and 2008, we see the same diagnosis and pretty much the same numerical relationship between the major groups. As Helen Taussig remarked in her paper about the global distribution of cardiac diagnosis only surgical interventions change the numbers [50]. This we can see in the rise in numbers of Norwood and Fontan operations (Table 1.1).

2000–2010 and the future

Tempora mutantur et nos in illis: "Time changes and we develop with time." It has been 71 years since Robert Gross first ligated a PDA and we have seen amazing developments in the treatment of CHD. Concomitantly, anesthesiology has evolved and slowly defined pediatric anesthesia, then cardiac anesthesia and now in the past two decades, pediatric cardiac anesthesia has developed as a

Table 1.1 Cardiovascular surgery at Children's Hospital, Boston

	Total cases	
	1982 (*N* = 538)	2008 (*N* = 942)
Septal defects	27%	20.1%
VSD repair	12%	7.5%
ASD repair	9.6%	8.6%
CAVC repair	5.9%	4%
Cavopulmonary connection	3%	8.5%
Fontan procedure	3%	5.4%
Bidirectional glenn		3.1%
Systemic outflow obstruction	29%	27.1%
Coarctation	7.7%	5.1%
Transposition of great arteries		5.6%
Senning	7%	0%
Arterial switch operation		5.6%
LVOT repair	11.7%	13.8%
Norwood procedure	3%	2.5%
Pulmonary outflow obstruction	13%	18.2%
Tetralogy of Fallot repair	7.6%	6.8%
Conduit placement/revision	2.8%	2.3%
Other RVOT reconstruction	1.6%	9%
Pacemaker, AICD placement	5%	3.8%
Patent ductus arteriosus	8%	6.2%
Miscellaneous	15%	16.1%

distinct and separate area of subspecialization. There is no doubt that the current, "older" generation of pediatric cardiac anesthesiologists has played a major role in moving forward the whole field of treatment of CHD. This generation added to the knowledge of the physiology of CHD, and the effects of anesthetic agents. This knowledge helped enable surgeons and cardiologists to develop new treatments in ways that are not always obvious or dramatic, but nonetheless are important and essential to the progress made in this period.

The last decade has seen many changes driven by the availability of new technology; these too provide new challenges for the pediatric cardiac anesthesiologist to solve. Two-dimensional echocardiography has improved diagnosis both within and outside the OR and provided more challenges and opportunities for the pediatric cardiac anesthesiologist. Transesophageal echocardiography (TEE) is of special concern for the pediatric cardiac anesthesiologist. Its utility in congenital heart surgery was demonstrated in the late 1980s by the studies of several groups in Japan and the USA, including Russell and Cahalan at the University of California, San Francisco. The TEE interpretation of complex CHD and judgment of the adequacy of intraoperative repairs is considerably more challenging in CHD than in adult acquired heart disease. Many centers have called upon pediatric echocardiographers to make such judgments rather than have the pe-

diatric cardiac anesthesiologist be responsible for that as well as for managing the patient in the post-bypass period. Also in contrast to adults, the TEE transducer may cause airway obstruction, alter left atrial pressure, or even extubate the child in the middle of an operation "under the drapes."

Similarly, the emerging availability of cardiac magnetic resonance imaging for diagnosis and follow-up of CHD patients has compounded the difficulties of providing anesthesia and monitoring in an intense magnetic field with limited patient access, but requiring anesthesia to be delivered to patients with severe, complex CHD under difficult conditions. Such technological advances come at a high price and it is hard to see how innovations like the long and expensive search for a method of treatment of HLHS would be justified today.

Another technical innovation of great importance driving pediatric cardiac anesthesia is extracorporeal membrane oxygenation (ECMO) (Figure 1.2). Use of rapid response ECMO for children with CHD who suffer cardiopulmonary collapse postoperatively, cannot be weaned from CPB, or need to be supported as a bridge to heart transplantation has proven very effective in reducing mortality rates to astonishingly low levels.

In the history of development of pediatric cardiac anesthesia, there is a long way between the baby in the ice bath being prepared for DHCA and the complex technology necessary for ECMO resuscitation.

A significant challenge for the current generation of pediatric cardiac anesthesiologists is to help reduce the cost of care. One of the primary ways to reduce perioperative cost is limit ICU and ventilator time. This translates into increased demands and expectations for early extubation, preferably in the operation room.

Such changes in care have risks associated with them that will require careful assessment considering the

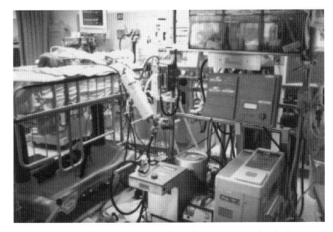

Figure 1.2 Infant on extracorporeal membrane oxygenation in the cardiac intensive care unit

advantages achieved with postoperative ventilation and sedation. For example, arrhythmias and cardiac arrest following endotracheal suctioning in the ICU postoperatively almost disappeared when heavy sedation with fentanyl prevented major swings in pulmonary artery pressure with suctioning [51,52]. Careful selection of patients for early extubation and judicious use of shorter acting anesthetic agents may allow lengths of stay to be shortened without increasing risks. In some studies, early extubation after relatively simple operations has in fact proven to be safe when using new short-acting anesthetic agents like sevoflurane and remifentanil, particularly when better pain control is also employed.

Other advances such as limiting the total dose of anesthetic agents by developing ways to monitor depth of anesthesia so as to give sufficient doses to prevent awareness and attenuate stress responses while avoiding awareness during CPB are being explored, but remain elusive [53].

The past decade has seen the continuing organization of the field of pediatric cardiac anesthesiology into a discrete subspecialty. The formation of the Congenital Cardiac Anesthesia Society (CCAS) (www.pedsanesthesia.org/ccas/) in the USA in 2005, which now has more than 350 members, provides a forum for subspecialized educational meetings, a national database of congenital cardiac anesthesia cases (see Chapter 3), and has initiated an effort to define adequate postgraduate training in pediatric cardiac anesthesia [54] (see Chapter 2). CCAS is a society organized within the larger Society for Pediatric Anesthesia, indicating that this specialty has chosen to align itself more closely with pediatric anesthesiology, than with adult cardiac anesthesiology, although important common interests and principles exist in all three of these specialties who care for patients with CHD.

The past decade has also seen a pushing of the envelope to devise new surgical and interventional catheterization approaches that cross the boundaries of the traditional care of patients with CHD. Two such approaches are in transuterine fetal cardiac catheter intervention (see Chapter 14), and hybrid stage I Norwood palliation (see Chapter 28). Pediatric cardiac anesthesiologists have an integral role in designing and carrying out these procedures; fetal cardiac intervention for aortic valve stenosis or HLHS with intact atrial septum requires the anesthesia team to induce general anesthesia for the pregnant mother, and also analgesia and muscle relaxation for the fetus, with fetal monitoring by ultrasound [55]. The hybrid stage I palliation in the catheterization laboratory requires the anesthesiologist to anticipate and treat significant hemodynamic perturbations, blood loss, and arrhythmias during the procedure while managing neonatal SV physiology without CPB and providing an anesthetic technique that provides for the possibility of early tracheal extubation [56,57].

In the past, the outcome criterion most emphasized for treatment of CHD has been survival. Now that survival rates are very good and getting better for almost all forms of CHD, attention has turned to the quality of that survival. Recent concern about the effect of anesthetic agents on the developing brain has prompted extensive efforts to study the magnitude of the effect of these agents, the mechanism of the effect, and whether alternative agents or protective strategies are warranted [58]. Neonatal cardiac surgery patients, who must have surgery at a vulnerable age and also potentially suffer from brain injury from cyanosis, bypass techniques, inflammation, or low cardiac output, are a particularly important focus of study. Pediatric cardiac anesthesiologists are involved in research to ameliorate these effects, including brain imaging, and long-term neurodevelopmental outcome studies [59,60].

As part of the trend of increasing long-term survival, the patient care group growing most rapidly at most centers is the adult with CHD. This is the somewhat unexpected result as care in childhood improves and more and more of these patients survive to adulthood and even into old age. At many institutions, special programs have been created to treat these patients and the problems they face. These problems include complications, reoperations, and socioeconomic barriers to normal education, employment, and creation of families. The question of pregnancy and anesthetic management of delivery for these patients is also evolving. It is unclear who is most qualified to provide anesthesia for such patients during labor and delivery. But suddenly the pediatric cardiac anesthesiologist may have to care for adults [61] (see Chapter 15).

Although much progress has been in the development of pediatric cardiac anesthesia to provide safe anesthetic care and improve outcome of treatment of CHD in the OR and catheterization laboratory for patients of all ages, much remains to be done. One can say with certainty that the intimate connection between advances in therapy, surgical or medical, and the anesthesia support services required to make those therapeutic advances possible will continue to present new challenges to the pediatric cardiac anesthesiologist. The pediatric cardiac anesthesiologists will in turn meet those challenges and in the process find ways to make still more improvements. Thus we progress in our art and science.

References

1. Gross RE, Hubbard JP (1939) First surgical ligation of a patent ductus arteriosus. JAMA 1112:729–731.
2. Grady D (2002) Operation on a fetus's heart valve called a "science fiction" success. *New York Times*, February 25, Section A:1.

3. Gross RE (1952) The patent ductus arteriosus. Observations on diagnosis and therapy in 525 surgically treated cases. JAMA 12:472–482.

4. Blalock A, Taussig HB (1954) The surgical treatment of malformation of the heart in which there is pulmonary stenosis or pulmonary atresia. JAMA 251:2124–2138.

5. Gillespie NA (1939) Endotrachial anaesthesia in infants. Brit J Anaest 17:2–12.

6. Harmel MH, Lamont A (1946) Anesthesia in the surgical treatment of congenital pulmonic stenosis. Anesthesiology 7:477–498.

7. Muller WH, Jr., Damman JF (1946) The treatment of certain congenital malformations of the heart by the creation of pulmonic stenosis to reduce pulmonary hypertension and excessive pulmonary blood flow. Surg Gyn Obstet 95:213–219.

8. McQuiston WO (1948) Anesthetic problems in cardiac surgery in children. Anesthesiology 10:590–600.

9. Harris AJ (1950) Management of anesthesia for congenital heart operations in children. Anesthesiology 11:328–332.

10. Smith RM (1952) Circulatory factors affecting anesthesia in surgery for congenital heart disease. Anesthesiology 13:38–61.

11. Kirklin JW, DuShane JW, Patrick RT, et al. (1955) Intracardiac surgery with the aid of a mechanical pump-oxygenator system (gibbon type): report of eight cases. Mayo Clin Proc 30:201–206.

12. Lillehei CW, DeWall RA, Read RC, et al. (1956) Direct vision intracardiac surgery in man using a simple, disposable artificial oxygenator. Chest 29:1–7.

13. Telford J, Keats AS (1957) Succinylcholine in cardiovascular surgery of infants and children. Anesthesiology 18:841–848.

14. Keats AS, Kurosu Y, Telford J, Cooley DA (1958) Anesthetic problems in cardiopulmonary bypass for open heart surgery. Experiences with 200 patients. Anesthesiology 19:501–514.

15. Lassen H (1953) A preliminary report on the 1952 epidemic of poliomyelitis in Copenhagen with special reference to the treatment of acute respiratory insufficiency. Lancet 1(6749):37–41.

16. Lowenstein E, Hallowell P, Levine FH, et al. (1969). Cardiovascular response to large doses of intravenous morphine in man. N Engl J Med 281:1389–1393.

17. Kantrowitz A, Haller JD, Joos H, et al. (1968) Transplantation of the heart in an infant and an adult. Am J Cardiol 22:782–790.

18. Horiuchi T (1963) Radical operation for ventricular septal defect in infancy. J Thorac Cardiovasc Surg 46:180–190.

19. Mori A, Muraoka R, Yokota Y, et al. (1972) Deep hypothermia combined with cardiopulmonary bypass for cardiac surgery in neonates and infants. J Thorac Cardiovasc Surg 64:422–429.

20. Steward DJ, Sloan IA, Johnston AE (1974) Anaesthetic management of infants undergoing profound hypothermia for surgical correction of congenital heart defects. Can Anaesth Soc J 21:15–22.

21. Newburger JW, Jonas RA, Wernovsky G, et al. (1993) A comparison of the perioperative neurologic effects of hypothermic circulatory arrest versus low-flow cardiopulmonary bypass in infant heart surgery. N Engl J Med 329:1057–1064.

22. Greeley WJ, Kern FH, Ungerleider RM, et al. (1991) The effect of hypothermic cardiopulmonary bypass and total circulatory arrest on cerebral metabolism in neonates, infants, and children. J Thorac Cardiovasc Surg 101:783–794.

23. Hickey PR, Hansen DD, Norwood WI, Castaneda AR (1984) Anesthetic complications in surgery for congenital heart disease. Anesth Analg 63:657–664.

24. Robinson S, Gregory GA (1981) Fentanyl-air-oxygen anesthesia for ligation of patent ductus arteriosus in preterm infants. Anesth Analg 60:331–334.

25. Anand KJ, Sippell WG, Aynsley-Green A (1987) Randomised trial of fentanyl anaesthesia in preterm babies undergoing surgery. Effects on the stress response. Lancet 1:62–66.

26. Hickey PR, Hansen DD (1984) Fentanyl- and sufentanil-oxygen-pancuronium anesthesia for cardiac surgery in infants. Anesth Analg 63:117–124.

27. Hickey PR, Hansen DD, Cramolini GM, et al. (1985) Pulmonary and systemic hemodynamic responses to ketamine in infants with normal and elevated pulmonary vascular resistance. Anesthesiology 62:287–293.

28. Chang AC, Zucker HA, Hickey PR, Wessel DL (1995) Pulmonary vascular resistance in infants after cardiac surgery. Role of carbon dioxide and hydrogen ion. Crit Care Med 23:568–574.

29. McQuiston WO (1949) Anesthetic problems in cardiac surgery in children. Anesthesiology 10:590–600.

30. Greeley WJ, Bushman GA, Davis DP, Reves JG (1986) Comparative effects of halothane and ketamine on systemic arterial oxygen saturation in children with cyanotic heart disease. Anesthesiology 65:666–668.

31. Heymann MA (1981) Pharmacologic use of prostaglandin E1 in infant with congenital heart disease. Am Heart J 101:837–843.

32. Neuman GG, Hansen DD (1980) The anaesthetic management of preterm infants undergoing ligation of patent ductus arteriosus. Can Anaesth Soc J 27:248–253.

33. Wessel DL, Keane JF, Parness I, Lock JE. (1988) Outpatient closure of the patent ductus arteriosus. Circulation 77:1068–1071.

34. Lavoie J, Burrows FA, Hansen DD (1996) Video-assisted thoracoscopic surgery for the treatment of congenital cardiac defects in the pediatric population. Anesth Analg 82:563–567.

35. Odegard KC, Kirse DJ, del Nido PJ, et al. (2000) Intraoperative recurrent laryngeal nerve monitoring during video-assisted throracoscopic surgery for patent ductus arteriosus. J Cardiothorac Vasc Anesth 14:562–564.

36. Uezono S, Hammer GB, Wellis V, et al. (2001) Anesthesia for outpatient repair of patent ductus arteriosus. J Cardiothorac Vasc Anesth 15:750–752.

37. Noonan JA, Nadas AS (1958) The hypoplastic left heart syndrome. An analysis of 101 cases. Pediatric Clin North Am 5:1029–1056.

38. Angell M (1983) Handicapped children. Baby Doe and Uncle Sam. N Engl J Med 309:659–661.

39. Fontan F, Baudet E (1971) Surgical repair of tricuspid atresia. Thorax 26:240–248.

40. Norwood WI, Lang P, Hansen DD (1983) Physiologic repair of aortic atresia-hypoplastic left heart syndrome. N Engl J Med 308:23–26.

41. Bailey LL, Nehlsen-Cannarella SL, Doroshow RW, et al. (1986) Cardiac allotransplantation in newborns as therapy for hypoplastic left heart syndrome. N Engl J Med 315: 949–951.

42. Natowicz M, Chatten J, Clancy R, et al. (1988) Genetic disorders and major extracardiac anomalies associated with the hypoplastic left heart syndrome. Pediatrics 82: 698–706.

43. Hansen DD, Hickey PR (1986) Anesthesia for hypoplastic left heart syndrome. Use of high-dose fentanyl in 30 neonates. Anesth Analg 65:127–132.

44. Tabbutt S, Ramamoorthy C, Montenegro LM, et al. (2001) Impact of inspired gas mixtures on preoperative infants with hypoplastic left heart syndrome during controlled ventilation. Circulation 104:I159-I164.

45. Dillon T, Berman W, Jr., Yabek SM, et al. (1986) Communicating hydrocephalus. A reversible complication of the Mustard operation with serial hemodynamics and long-term follow-up. Ann Thorac Surg 41:146–149.

46. Jatene AD, Fontes VF, Paulista PP, et al. (1975) Successful anatomic correction of transposition of the great vessels. A preliminary report. Arq Bras Cardiol 28:461–464.

47. Anand KJ, Hansen DD, Hickey PR (1990) Hormonal-metabolic stress responses in neonates undergoing cardiac surgery. Anesthesiology 73:661–670.

48. Gruber EM, Laussen PC, Casta A, et al. (2001) Stress response in infants undergoing cardiac surgery. A randomized study of fentanyl bolus, fentanyl infusion, and fentanyl-midazolam infusion. Anesth Analg 92:882–890.

49. Javorski JJ, Hansen DD, Laussen PC, et al. (1995) Paediatric cardiac catheterization. innovations. Can J Anaesth 42:310–329.

50. Taussig HB (1982) World survey of the common cardiac malformations. Developmental error or genetic variant? Am J Cardiol 50:544–559.

51. Shim C, Fine N, Fernandez R, Williams MH (1969) Cardiac arrhythmias resulting from tracheal suctioning. Ann Intern Med 71:1149–1153.

52. Hickey PR, Hansen DD, Wessel DL, et al. (1985) Blunting of stress responses in the pulmonary circulation of infants by fentanyl. Anesth Analg 64: 1137–1142.

53. Kussman BD, Gruber EM, Zurakowski D, et al. (2001) Bispectral index monitoring during infant cardiac surgery. relationship of BIS to the stress response and plasma fentanyl levels. Paediatr Anaesth 11: 663–669.

54. DiNardo JA, Baum VC, Andropoulos DB (2009) A proposal for training in pediatric cardiac anesthesia. Anesth Analg in press.

55. Tworetzky W, Marshall AC (2004) Fetal interventions for cardiac defects. Pediatr Clin North Am 51:1503–1513.

56. Galantowicz M, Cheatham JP (2005) Lessons learned from the development of a new hybrid strategy for the management of hypoplastic left heart syndrome. Pediatr Cardiol 26:190–199.

57. Caldarone CA, Benson L, Holtby H, et al. (2007) Initial experience with hybrid palliation for neonates with single-ventricle physiology. Ann Thorac Surg 84:1294–1300.

58. Loepke AW, Soriano SG (2008) An assessment of the effects of general anesthetics on developing brain structure and neurocognitive function. Anesth Analg 106; 1681–1707.

59. Nelson DP, Andropoulos DB, Fraser CD (2008) Perioperative neuroprotective strategies. Semin Thorac Cardiovasc Surg Pediatr Card Surg Annu 49–56.

60. Andropoulos DB, Stayer SA, Hunter JV, et al. (2007) Isoflurane, midazolam, and fentanyl do not injure the developing brain in neonatal cardiac surgery. Anesthesiology 107:A219.

61. Perloff JK, Warnes CA (2001) Challenges posed by adults with repaired congenital heart disease. Circulation 103:2637–2643.

2

Education for anesthesia in patients with congenital cardiac disease

Sugantha Sundar, M.D. and James, A. DiNardo, M.D., F.A.A.P.
Beth Israel Deaconness Medical Center, Children's Hospital Boston, Harvard Medical School, Boston, Massachusetts, USA

Introduction

Because of worldwide advances in pediatric cardiology, cardiac surgery, cardiac anesthesia, and cardiac intensive care over the last 30 years, survival of children with congenital heart disease (CHD) into adulthood has increased to approximately 95% [1]. The need for greater coordination and integration between pediatric and adult services and a long-term health care delivery system is obvious for this patient population [2,3]. In addition, there is a need for the establishment of a multi-institutional database to assist in assessment of health care outcomes and transitioning guidelines for patients with CHD as they reach adulthood [4]. Anesthesiologists, as an integral part of any system caring for patients with CHD, are often called upon to care for patients ranging in age from neonates to adults. Unfortunately, pediatric cardiothoracic anesthesia or more precisely anesthesia for patients with CHD as a specialty would be "homeless" due to lack of representation in the currently existent major anesthesia professional societies were it not for the recent establishment of the Congenital Cardiac Anesthesia Society (CCAS) [5,6].

Anesthesia for Congenital Heart Disease 2nd edition. Edited by
Dean Andropoulos, Stephen Stayer, Isobel Russell and Emad Mossad.
© 2010 Blackwell Publishing.

Why teach and learn congenital cardiac anesthesia?

There is currently no established curriculum for education in the care of patients with CHD. Establishment of a curriculum is complicated by the fact that very few anesthesiologists engage in a practice limited solely to the care of pediatric patients undergoing cardiac surgery. By necessity, most pediatric cardiothoracic anesthesiologists devote some portion of their time to the care of general pediatric patients or to the care of adult cardiothoracic surgical patients. In addition, while it is acknowledged that intraoperative transesophageal echocardiography (TEE) has become an essential component of the comprehensive care of CHD patients [7], at present no formal examination or certification process exists for pediatric TEE and there has been debate as to who (cardiologist or anesthesiologist) is best qualified to perform perioperative pediatric TEE [8,9]. Further complicating this issue is that while the American Society of Echocardiography acknowledges that many pediatric cardiovascular anesthesiologists have received appropriate training and have sufficient experience to interpret pediatric perioperative TEE, they recommend that a second trained individual in pediatric cardiovascular anesthesia or pediatric TEE be available in order that undivided attention can be paid to both the TEE findings and the anesthetic care of the patient [10].

Standardized clinical education helps to standardize patient care, simplifies evaluation of quality of care issues, encourages financial accountability and use of evidence-based strategies [11], and may improve surgical outcome by consolidating clinical experience in established centers [12].

Current model of teaching and learning in congenital cardiac anesthesia

Currently, teaching and learning in congenital cardiothoracic anesthesia more closely resembles an apprenticeship model than an established training program [13]. Training in congenital cardiothoracic anesthesia generally commences after completion of fellowship training in either pediatric anesthesia or adult cardiothoracic anesthesia, but this is by no means standardized. Training (curriculum, case number and composition, duration, faculty expertise and experience) is variable among institutions. No requisites to demonstrate competence exist and there is no board certification process. In short, training is most commonly determined by where and with whom one trains.

Curriculum for teaching and learning congenital cardiac anesthesia

Curriculum development should employ a logical, systematic approach linked to specific health care needs. The Kern model of curriculum development for medical education could be used to develop a curriculum to teach and learn congenital cardiothoracic anesthesia [14]. This is a six-step approach and consists of the following steps:
1 Problem identification and general needs assessment
2 Needs assessment of targeted learners
3 Goals and objectives
4 Educational strategies
5 Implementation
6 Evaluation and feedback

Problem identification and general needs assessment

Identification and characterization of the health care problem

- Whom does it affect?
- What does it affect?
- What is the qualitative and quantitative importance of the effects?

Teaching and learning in congenital cardiothoracic anesthesia education must encompass the management of the entire spectrum of interventions (palliation to complete repair), outcomes (all sequela and residua), and age range (neonate to adult) inherent to the CHD population. Most traditionally trained pediatric anesthesiologists and adult cardiothoracic anesthesiologists do not have the expertise to manage the unique set of problems presented by this diverse patient population. Although a relationship of clinical outcomes to the training and education level of the health care provider has yet to be demonstrated, yet there is potential for a structured curriculum to positively impact quality of care and allocation of health care resources.

General needs assessment

- What is currently being done?
- What personal and environmental factors affect the problem?
- Ideally what should be done?
- What are the key differences between the current and ideal approaches?

The current state of anesthesiology training in CHD has recently been characterized. In a telephone and electronic mail survey of anesthesia residency program directors ($n = 131$), Accreditation Council for Graduate Medical Education (ACGME) accredited pediatric anesthesia fellowship directors ($n = 45$), adult cardiothoracic anesthesia fellowship directors ($n = 71$: 44 ACGME accredited, 27 non-ACGME accredited), and 12-month pediatric cardiac anesthesia fellowship training program directors ($n = 3$), the following responses summarize training in the USA [15]. Hands-on experience with pediatric cardiac anesthesia during basic anesthesia training is described as "nonexistent" or "rare" in 50% of ACGME-accredited residency programs. In the remaining programs typical exposure is during the CA-2 and CA-3 years with residents caring for 5–10 patients requiring procedures with cardiopulmonary bypass (CPB). In a few programs, residents care for as many as 20–30 such patients. Pediatric anesthesia fellows in all 45 ACGME-accredited programs have at least a 2-month cardiac experience during the 12-month fellowship. The typical fellowship experience involves 30–50 CPB cases. In two-thirds of the programs this exposure occurs in 1-month blocks, in the remainder the experience is distributed throughout the year. Approximately one quarter of the pediatric fellows use elective time to obtain an additional month or two of experience. Presently, only 13 of the 44 ACGME-accredited and 1 of the 27 nonaccredited fellowships in adult cardiothoracic anesthesia have a mandatory exposure to pediatric cardiac anesthesia with the remaining programs offering an elective experience of varying duration. Typical mandatory exposure is 1–2 months with 20–30 CPB cases. The words "rarely" or "occasionally" were most commonly used by the individuals surveyed to describe the frequency with which adult cardiothoracic anesthesia fellows use available elective time to pursue training in pediatric cardiac anesthesia. Besides the three known 12-month pediatric cardiac anesthesia fellowships (two in the USA, one in the UK), there are several programs in the USA offer additional training in pediatric cardiac anesthesia for intervals of 3–12 months on an ad hoc basis [15].

A survey of pediatric cardiothoracic anesthesiologists in the UK reported that majority of the practitioners had at least two additional years of training in the fields of general pediatric, adult cardiothoracic and pediatric cardiothoracic anesthesia, as well as pediatric intensive care and had spent time gaining experience overseas [16]. A similar experience for future trainees was recommended with recognition that implementation of such a competency-based training would be difficult with the New Deal and the European Working Time Directive [16]. In 2004 the National Heart Lung and Blood Institute recommended outreach and educational programs for adults with CHD, development of adult CHD regional centers, technology development to support advances in imaging and modeling of abnormal structure and function, and a consensus on appropriate training for physicians to provide care for adults with CHD [17]. Table 2.1 compares this ideal approach to what is the best available summary of the current approach.

Needs assessment of targeted learners

The following points should be addressed to obtain adequate needs assessment:
- What proficiencies (cognitive, affective, and psychomotor skills) currently exist among learners?
- Previous training and experiences of fellows and residents in congenital cardiothoracic anesthesia

- Current training and experiences already planned for trainees
- Resources available to learners (patients and clinical experiences, information resources, computers, audiovisual equipment, role models, teachers, mentors)
- Perceived deficiencies and learning needs
- Characteristics of the learners and barriers to learn and teach

At the present time there are no reports of needs assessment for a curriculum development in congenital cardiothoracic anesthesia in the medical literature. An initial such needs assessment could be accomplished in the form of a Delphi system, in which global expert opinion as to curriculum needs is sought. It is an economical way of accessing experts in the field and imposes few geographical limitations [18]. The nominal group technique (also known as the expert panel), and the consensus development conference could also be utilized; however, these methodologies are more difficult to organize and are time consuming.

Goals and objectives

Goals and objectives by necessity must be specific and measurable. They should measure the knowledge (cognitive), attitude (affective), and competence (psychomotor) of the learners. The goals and objectives can be developed on the basis of the ACGME core competencies suggested for residency programs. The goals and objectives should reflect the relationship of the educational process to the degree of participation of the learners as well as the faculty response to the developed curriculum.

Table 2.1 Current and ideal state of education and training in anesthesia for pediatric and congenital heart disease

	Patients	Health care professionals	Medical educators	Society
Current	Educational material available at medical center where patient receives care	No standardized training of physicians Formation of the Congenital Cardiac Anesthesia Society Apprenticeship type model No training for noncardiac anesthesiologists	Continuing medical education seminars as part of national meetings	Support groups exist for various congenital lesions
Ideal	A national system by which care is transitioned from pediatric to adult care setting Education of patients for self-advocating	Standardized training of physicians Certification and recertification examinations Incorporation of basic knowledge in congenital cardiac disease in anesthesia residency programs	Faculty development programs	Development of health care quality measures in measuring outcome

A summary of proposed goals and objectives for training in congenital cardiothoracic anesthesiology is as follows:

What is the minimum level of anesthesia training required?

- Subspecialty training in congenital cardiothoracic anesthesiology should begin after satisfactory completion of a residency program in anesthesiology accredited by the ACGME or other training judged suitable by the Program Director. This track would be consistent with other subspecialty training areas in anesthesiology.
- Trainees could enter the training following completion of an ACGME-accredited adult cardiothoracic anesthesia fellowship of 12 months duration after anesthesia residency.
- Trainees could enter the training following completion of an ACGME-accredited pediatric anesthesia fellowship of 12 months duration after anesthesia residency.
- Subspecialty training in congenital cardiothoracic anesthesiology could be part of an 18-month continuum in conjunction with an ACGME-accredited pediatric anesthesia fellowship or adult cardiothoracic anesthesiology fellowship after successful completion of an anesthesia residency [15] (Figure 2.1).

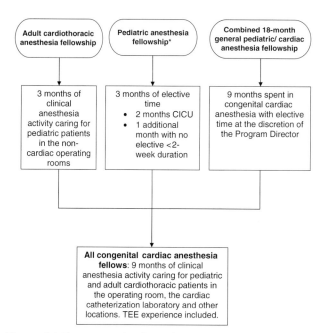

Figure 2.1 Three proposed pathways for entering fellowship training in pediatric cardiac anesthesia. * Time spent in pediatric cardiac anesthesia during a pediatric anesthesia fellowship may be counted toward the 9-month requirement at the discretion of the Pediatric Cardiac Anesthesia Program Director (Reproduced with permission from Reference [15])

What are the goals the learners will achieve?

To achieve goals the program must be structured to ensure optimal patient care while providing trainees the opportunity to develop skills in clinical care, judgment, teaching, and research [15].

The following goals and objectives are valuable:
- The subspecialist in congenital cardiothoracic anesthesiology should be proficient in providing anesthesia care for patients both pediatric and adults undergoing congenital cardiothoracic and vascular surgery as well as anesthesia for noncardiac surgery.
- Conduct of preoperative patient evaluation; interpret imaging, cardiovascular, and pulmonary diagnostic test data.
- Experience of anesthesia for patients undergoing non-operative diagnostic and interventional cardiac, thoracic, and electrophysiological procedures. Examples include angiography, arrhythmia mapping and ablation, stent placements, and device closures.
- The clinical curriculum should include competency in the management of CPB, pharmacological and mechanical hemodynamic support as well as extracorporeal circulation.
- An advanced skill level in perioperative TEE should be developed.
- Postoperative critical care, including ventilatory support, extracorporeal circulatory support, pharmacologic hemodynamic support as well as pain management.

To meet these goals, the program should expose fellows to a wide variety of clinical problems in children and adults with CHD, which are necessary for the development of these clinical skills.

What is the ideal duration, case quantity and scope of training?

The following represents suggested guidelines for the minimum clinical scope and duration of training [15]:
- Nine months of clinical anesthesia activity caring for patients with congenital cardiothoracic problems in the operating room, the cardiac catheterization laboratory, and other locations.
  - This experience should include a minimum of 100 anesthetic procedures, the majority of which must require CPB. At least 50 of these patients should be infants from birth to 1 year of age, and should include at least 25 neonates (≤1 month of age). The trainee should also care for at least 25 adults (≥18 years of age).
  - This experience should also include a minimum of 50 patients undergoing diagnostic procedures (cardiac catheterization, echocardiography, MRI, etc.), as well as therapeutic procedures in the catheterization

laboratory (arrhythmia ablation, pacemaker insertion, septal defect closure and valve dilatation, etc.).
- ○ This experience should include a structured intraoperative TEE experience consistent with the practice of intraoperative TEE in the participating program.
- Fellows entering the congenital cardiothoracic anesthesia fellowship following completion of an adult cardiothoracic anesthesia fellowship must complete a 3-month rotation caring for children in the general, noncardiac operating rooms to enhance their pediatric anesthesia skills.
- Fellows entering the congenital cardiothoracic anesthesia fellowship following completion of a pediatric anesthesia fellowship or as part of the 18-month congenital cardiothoracic anesthesiology program will complete:
  - ○ A 2-month experience managing pediatric cardiothoracic surgical patients in a critical care (ICU) setting. This experience may include the management of nonsurgical cardiothoracic patients. The fellow should actively participate in the management of patients on extracorporeal membrane oxygenation.
  - ○ One month of elective rotations (none less than 2 weeks in duration) from the following categories:
    - – Echocardiography (TEE and/or transthoracic echocardiography)
    - – Extracorporeal perfusion technology
    - – Research
- Experience should be obtained in the preoperative evaluation of pediatric and adult cardiothoracic patients. The fellow should understand how to use information from diagnostic studies and how to recognize when additional studies and/or consultations are indicated.

Relationship to other anesthesiology programs

The congenital cardiothoracic anesthesiology program should function in direct association with an ACGME-accredited core anesthesiology program, adult cardiothoracic anesthesiology, or with a pediatric anesthesiology program [15]. A congenital cardiothoracic anesthesiology program may be conducted in either a general hospital or a children's hospital. There must be within the same institution a fully accredited core anesthesiology program or an adult cardiothoracic anesthesiology program or pediatric anesthesiology program with which the congenital cardiothoracic anesthesiology program is associated.

The division of responsibilities between trainees in the core anesthesiology program and an associated fellowship program(s) in adult cardiothoracic anesthesiology and/or pediatric anesthesiology must be clearly delineated. The presence of congenital cardiothoracic anesthesiology fellows must not compromise the clinical experience and number of cases available to pediatric anesthesiology fellows and/or core anesthesiology residents. There must be close cooperation between the core anesthesiology program, the adult cardiothoracic anesthesiology program and/or the pediatric anesthesiology program, and the congenital cardiothoracic anesthesiology program.

Didactic components

The didactic curriculum provided through lectures, conferences, and workshops should supplement clinical experience as necessary for the fellow to acquire the knowledge to care for cardiothoracic patients with CHD and conditions outlined in the guidelines for the minimum clinical experience for each fellow. The didactic components should include the following areas, with emphasis on how cardiothoracic diseases affect the administration of anesthesia and life support to cardiothoracic patients with CHD.

These represent guidelines for the minimum didactic experience for each fellow [15]:
- Embryological and morphological development of the cardiothoracic structures; nomenclature of CHD
- Pathophysiology, pharmacology, and clinical management of patients with all adult and pediatric CHD, including single ventricle lesions, septal defects, defects of semilunar and atrioventricular valves, left- and right-sided obstructive lesions, transposition of the great vessels, defects of systemic and pulmonary venous return, cardiomyopathies, vascular rings and tracheal lesions
- Pathophysiology, pharmacology, and clinical management of patients requiring heart, lung, and heart–lung transplantation, including immunosuppressant regimes and selection criteria
- Noninvasive cardiovascular evaluation: electrocardiography, echocardiography, cardiovascular CT, and MRI imaging
- Cardiac catheterization procedures and diagnostic interpretation; invasive cardiac catheterization procedures, including balloon dilatations and stent placement; device closure of septal defects, patent ductus arteriosus and baffle leaks, and arrhythmia ablation
- Preanesthetic evaluation and preparation of pediatric and adult cardiothoracic patients
- Pharmacokinetics and pharmacodynamics of medications prescribed for medical management of pediatric and adult cardiothoracic patients
- Perianesthetic monitoring methods both noninvasive and invasive, including use of ultrasound guidance: intra-arterial, central venous, mixed venous saturation, cardiac output determination, transesophageal and epicardial echocardiography, neurological monitoring, including near infrared cerebral oximetry, transcranial Doppler, and processed electroencephalograms

- Pharmacokinetics and pharmacodynamics of anesthetic medications prescribed for cardiothoracic patients. Pharmacokinetics and pharmacodynamics of medications prescribed for management of hemodynamic instability: inotropes, chronotropes, vasoconstrictors, vasodilators
- Extracorporeal circulation (including CPB, low-flow CPB, deep hypothermic circulatory arrest, antegrade cerebral perfusion, extracorporeal membrane oxygenation), myocardial preservation, effects of extracorporeal circulation on pharmacokinetics and pharmacodynamics, cardiothoracic, respiratory, neurological, metabolic, endocrine, hematological, renal, and thermoregulatory effects of extracorporeal circulation and coagulation/anticoagulation before, during, and after extracorporeal circulation
- Circulatory assist devices: left and right ventricular assist devices and biventricular assist devices
- Pacemaker and automated internal cardiac defibrillator (AICD) insertion and modes of action
- Perioperative ventilator management: intraoperative anesthetic and critical care unit ventilators and techniques
- Pain management of pediatric and adult cardiothoracic surgical patients. Postanesthetic critical care of pediatric and adult cardiothoracic surgical patients
- Research methodology and statistical analysis
- Quality assurance and improvement
- Ethical and legal issues
- Practice management

Educational strategies

The next step is the development of educational strategies to implement the developed curriculum in congenital cardiothoracic anesthesia. The following is a suggestion list of educational strategies that could be employed on the basis of different domains in the curriculum.

Methods for achieving cognitive objectives
- Readings
- Lectures
- Audiovisual materials
- Discussion
- Programmed learning

Methods for achieving affective objectives
- Exposure to challenging clinical and ethical situations and learning to manage leadership skills, communication, task delegation, backup behavior and cross-training
- Facilitation of openness, introspection, and reflection
- Role models

Methods for achieving psychomotor objectives
- Supervised clinical experiences

- Simulations: artificial models, role plays, standardized patients
- Audio or visual reviews of skills

There should be provision to facilitate self-directed learning in the form of self-assessment, information searching, critical appraisal, clinical decision making, independent learning projects, personal learning plans or contracts, formulating and answering ones own questions, and role modeling. Conferences, including lectures, interactive conferences, hands-on workshops, morbidity and mortality conferences, cardiac catheterization conferences, echocardiography conferences, cardiothoracic surgery case review conferences, journal reviews, and research seminars should be regularly attended by the trainee. While the faculty should be the leaders of the majority of the sessions, active participation by the fellow in the planning and production of these conferences is essential. Attendance at multidisciplinary conferences, especially in cardiovascular medicine, pulmonary medicine, cardiothoracic surgery, vascular surgery, and pediatrics relevant to cardiothoracic anesthesiology should be encouraged. Provision of an opportunity for fellows to participate in research or other scholarly activities is vital to success of the educational strategies employed. The fellows must be encouraged to complete a minimum of one academic assignment. Projects may include grand rounds presentations, preparation and publication of review articles, book chapters, and manuals for teaching or clinical practice, clinical research investigation, or similar scholarly activities. A faculty supervisor must be in charge of each project.

Advances in the World Wide Web have created multiple opportunities for educational material to be easily shared [19]. Most of the content material developed could be posted on the Internet with password-protected access. Since the number of physicians training to be providers of anesthesia for CHD is small, this option is attractive. Interesting case discussions, sharing of echocardiographic images, and recent articles pertaining to this area could be posted on the Internet as well [20]. The MedEdPORTAL, Health Education Assets Library (HEAL), CCAS Web site, and Multimedia Educational Resource for Learning and Online Teaching are some currently available resources that could house the curricular material related to congenital cardiothoracic anesthesia. However, given this wealth of potential educational resources, it is important to keep in mind that the learner should be physically and mentally involved in the learning process [21].

The use of simulation in medical education is also gaining popularity. Simulation allows complex clinical tasks to be broken down into their component parts [22–24]. Simulation-based medical education (SBME) can contribute considerably to improving medical care by boosting medical professionals' performance and enhancing patient safety [25]. Many surgical specialties are seeking simulation as a method for teaching and learning as well as evaluation [26]. There is a role for simulation in learning procedural skills especially in the climate of decreasing clinical exposure [27,28]. There is also evidence in the surgical literature that virtual reality training can improve operating room performance [29]. Consideration should be given to the use of a clinical skills laboratory to preteach some of the skills necessary in the management of a complex patient population [30].

Anesthesia for CHD is a high risk, low error tolerance field [31]. The fundamental knowledge and skills that congenital cardiothoracic anesthesiologists will need to master if they are to increase their capacity to attain higher levels of performance is enormous. A clinical microsystems model to facilitate the development of the fundamental knowledge and skills using the action-learning theory and sound education principles to provide the opportunity to learn, test, and gain some degree of mastery may prove useful [32].

Implementation

Once a curriculum has been developed, implementation is the next challenge. It is the role of the Program Director to ensure successful implementation. The Program Director in conjunction with the faculty is responsible for the general administration of the program, and for the establishment and maintenance of a stable educational environment. Continuity of leadership is an important component of program stability and the length of appointments for both the Program Director and program faculty should reflect this reality. The Program Director must possess the requisite specialty expertise, as well as documented educational and administrative abilities. The Program Director must have training and/or clinical experience in providing anesthesia care for congenital cardiothoracic surgical patients that meets or exceeds that associated with the completion of the 1-year congenital cardiothoracic anesthesiology program.

The Program Director must:
• Identify resources
• Obtain support
• Develop administrative mechanisms to support the curriculum
• Anticipate and address barriers
• Plan to introduce the curriculum first in a pilot phase, then as a transition phase, and finally as full implementation

At each participating institution, there must be a sufficient number of faculty with documented qualifications to instruct and supervise adequately all fellows in the program. Although the number of faculty members involved in teaching will vary, at least three faculty members should be involved, and these should be equal to or greater than two full-time equivalents, including the Program Director. A ratio of no fewer than one full-time equivalent faculty member to one subspecialty fellow shall be maintained. The physician faculty must possess the requisite specialty expertise, competence in clinical care, teaching abilities, as well as documented educational and administrative abilities and experience in their field. There must be evidence of active participation by qualified physicians with training and/or expertise in congenital cardiothoracic anesthesiology beyond the requirement for completion of a core anesthesiology residency. The faculty should have training and experience that would generally meet or exceed that associated with the completion of a 1-year congenital cardiothoracic anesthesiology program. Faculty in cardiology, cardiothoracic surgery, pediatrics, intensive care, and pulmonary medicine could provide teaching in multidisciplinary conferences. The responsibility for establishing and maintaining an environment of inquiry and scholarship of discovery, dissemination, and application rests with the faculty, and an active research component must be included in each program. There must be faculty development programs to facilitate their growth and development as educators and teachers [33].

Additional necessary professional, technical, and clerical personnel must be provided to support the program. The program must ensure that adequate resources (e.g., sufficient laboratory space and equipment, computer and statistical consultation services) are available.

Evaluation and feedback

Evaluation and feedback are essential to the health and growth of a curriculum. The goal of evaluation in medical education remains the development of reliable measurements of student performance which, as well as having predictive value for subsequent clinical competence, also have a formative, educational role [34].

Currently, there are evaluation processes in place in various medical specialties that incorporate ACGME core competencies [35–47]. With adoption of the ACGME core competencies as the sole evaluation tool, there is the risk that the ability to evaluate higher-level clinical competence by assessing trainee sensitivity to clinical context will be lost [38]. Most of current assessment modalities for physicians and trainees reliably test core knowledge and basic skills. Adequate evaluation of professionalism, interpersonal skills, lifelong learning and incorporating core knowledge to clinical practice is more challenging [39,40].

The three most commonly used assessment methods are (1) subjective assessment by supervising clinicians, (2) multiple choice examinations to evaluate factual knowledge and abstract problem solving, and (3) standardized patient assessments of physical examination and technical and communication skills. Consideration should be given to incorporating the following newer modalities of assessment [39]:

- Clinical reasoning
- Exercises to assess use of medical literature
- Long station standardized patient exercises
- Simulated continuity [41]
- Assessment by patients and families [42]
- Mentored self-assessment
- Remediation based on a learning plan
- Numerous patient care quality measures in assessing the educational effectiveness and performance [43]

Trainee evaluation involves evaluation of knowledge, psychomotor skills, and affective competencies. The most commonly used knowledge evaluation methods are:

- Rating forms
- Essays on respondent's experience
- Written or computer-based tests
- Written test knowledge can be assessed with:
  ○ Posttest
    - Pretest and posttest
    - Controlled pretest and posttest
    - Randomized controlled posttest (experimental tool)
    - Randomized control pretest and posttest (experimental tool)
- Oral examinations
- Questionnaires
- Individual interview
- Performance audits

While all these methodologies can be used to assess the cognitive components of the educational exercise, they do not effectively evaluate the psychomotor and affective components in the curriculum [44]. Psychomotor skills may be evaluated by the following methods:

- Self-assessment forms
- Portfolios of videotapes
- Direct observation

Affective abilities relevant to the program may be assessed by:

- Teamwork exercises
- Peer assessment of professionalism
- Clinical situations that involve clinical uncertainty
- Group interview/discussion

The evaluative process for congenital cardiothoracic anesthesia trainees should promote an emphasis on learning, inspire confidence in the trainee, enhance the trainee's ability to self-monitor, and drive the institution toward self-assessment and curricular change when necessary [45]. The primary endpoint should be the ability to demonstrate trainee competence to the patients. There may be a role for incorporating the Cambridge Model for assessing practice performance into evaluating trainees in congen-

ital cardiothoracic anesthesia [46]. This is a modification of the Miller's pyramid that evaluates a trainee on the basis of the following paradigm: knows, knows how, shows how, does [47].

While the evaluative process generally focuses on the competency of the trainees, it is important to point out that evaluation of the curriculum, of the faculty and teaching staff, and of the sponsoring institution and its resources is important as well.

Keeping some of the previously discussed principles in mind, the following evaluative process for congenital cardiothoracic anesthesia training programs is suggested.

Fellow

Formative evaluation

The faculty must evaluate in a timely manner the fellows whom they supervise. In addition, the fellowship program must demonstrate that it has an effective mechanism for assessing fellow performance throughout the program and for utilizing the results to improve fellow performance. At a minimum, faculty responsible for teaching must provide critical evaluations of each fellow's progress and competence at the end of 6 and 12 months of training.

- Assessment should include the use of methods that produce an accurate assessment of fellows' competence in patient care, medical knowledge, practice-based learning and improvement, interpersonal and communication skills, professionalism, and systems-based practice.
- Assessment should include the regular and timely performance feedback to fellows that includes at least semi-annual written evaluations. Such evaluations are to be communicated to each fellow in a timely manner and maintained in a record that is accessible to each fellow. The Program Director or designee must inform each fellow of the results of the evaluations at least every 6 months during training, advise the fellow of areas needing improvement, and document the communication.
- Assessment should include the use of assessment results, including evaluation by faculty, patients, peers, self, and other professional staff, to achieve progressive improvements in fellows' competence and performance.
- Assessments should include essential character attributes, acquired character attributes, and fund of knowledge, clinical judgment and clinical psychomotor skills, as well as specific tasks and skills for patient management and critical analysis of clinical situations.
- Periodic evaluation of patient care (quality assurance) is mandatory. Subspecialty fellows in congenital cardiothoracic anesthesiology should be involved in continuing quality improvement and risk management.

Final evaluation

The Program Director must provide a final evaluation for each fellow who completes the program. This evaluation must include a review of the fellow's performance during the final period of education, and should verify that the fellow has demonstrated sufficient professional ability to practice competently and independently. The final evaluation must be part of the fellow's permanent record maintained by the institution. Subspecialty fellows in congenital cardiothoracic anesthesiology must obtain overall satisfactory evaluations at the completion of 12-month training to receive credit for training.

Faculty

Faculty should be evaluated for clinical teaching. These evaluations should be valid, reliable, efficient, and feasible. The faculty has to be evaluated on knowledge, clinical competence, teaching effectiveness, and professional attributes by the learner [48]. The performance of the faculty must be evaluated by the program no less frequently than at the midpoint of the accreditation cycle, and again prior to the next site visit. The evaluations should include a review of their teaching abilities, commitment to the educational program, clinical knowledge, and scholarly activities. This evaluation must include annual written confidential evaluations by fellows. The 12 learning outcomes model based on "what teachers do, how they do it, and what affects what they do" can serve as a framework for faculty evaluation [49]. The Clinical Teaching Effectiveness Instrument is another modality useful for evaluating faculty [50].

Program

The educational effectiveness of a program must be evaluated at least annually in a systematic manner.

1 Representative program personnel (at a minimum the Program Director, representative faculty, and one fellow) must be organized to review program goals and objectives, and the effectiveness with which they are achieved. This group must conduct a formal documented meeting at least annually for this purpose. In the evaluation process, the group must take into consideration written comments from the faculty, the most recent report of the graduate medical education committee of the sponsoring institution, and the fellows' confidential written evaluations. If deficiencies are found, the group should prepare an explicit plan of action, which should be approved by the faculty and documented in the minutes of the meeting.
2 The program should use fellow performance and outcome assessment in its evaluation of the educational

effectiveness of the fellowship program. Performance of program graduates on the certification examination should be used as one measure of evaluating program effectiveness. The program should maintain a process for using assessment results together with other program evaluation results to improve the fellowship program.

Curriculum maintenance and enhancement

Once a curriculum in congenital cardiothoracic anesthesia has been developed, the next challenge is curriculum maintenance. The following data can be collected and utilized to assess how well a curriculum is functioning:
• Program evaluation
• Learner/faculty/patient questionnaires
• Objective measures of skills and performance
• Focus group of learners, faculty, staff, and patients
• Systematically collected data
• Regular/periodic meetings with learners, faculty
• Special retreats and strategic planning sessions
• Site visits
• Informal observation of curricular components, learners, faculty, and staff
• Informal discussions with learners, faculty, and staff
Congenital cardiothoracic anesthesia is a subspecialty in which there are significant interactions between anesthesiologists and cardiac surgeons, cardiologists, radiologists, and other pediatric subspecialists. Close collaboration between these domains is vital to the growth and development of the subspecialty. Furthermore, curriculum enrichment and growth is dependant on both intra- and intersubspecialty collaboration [51,52].

Dissemination

There is a need for a comprehensive curriculum in congenital cardiothoracic anesthesia in all areas of the industrialized world [6]. Local adaptation of a core curriculum will be necessary to deal with technological and cultural care delivery constraints. The following should be considered as regards dissemination of core curriculum material:
• What core material should be disseminated?
• How should the material be disseminated (presentations, multi-institutional interest groups, educational clearinghouses, computerized communication systems, instructional videotapes or audiotapes, instructional computer software, publication and diffusion of innovation)?
• What resources are required (time and effort, personnel, equipment/facilities, funds)?

Role of professional societies

At present CCAS, in conjunction with the Society of Pediatric Anesthesia (SPA) has taken the lead in development of a core curriculum for fellowship training in congenital cardiothoracic anesthesia [15]. Close future collaboration with the Society of Cardiovascular Anesthesiologists (SCA) will be necessary. Collaboration with the ACGME, RRC, and the American Board of Anesthesiology will be necessary as the subspecialty matures to the point where it becomes a board certifiable specialty in its own right. Since many of the children with CHD survive to adulthood and develop adult cardiothoracic disease, the American Heart Association as well as the American College of Cardiology may be able to provide significant input into developing a holistic approach to the care of this complex patient population. A significant proportion of this patient population will go on to become pregnant and hence the American College of Obstetricians as well as the Society for Obstetric Anesthesia and Perinatology will need to contribute to the development of a curriculum.

Conclusions

Developing durable, new curricula will be challenging in the highly specialized area of congenital cardiothoracic anesthesia. Use of a systematic approach to its development will facilitate efficient teaching and learning in this complex discipline. It is important to develop programs that give faculty the necessary skills to develop curricula and that provide mentoring [53,54]. Finally, the challenge of transitioning trainees from fellow (learner) to faculty (provider and teacher) in congenital cardiothoracic anesthesia will be ongoing [55].

References

1. Warnes CA (2005) The adult with congenital heart disease: born to be bad? J Am Coll Cardiol 46:1–8.
2. Webb G (2005) Improving the care of Canadian adults with congenital heart disease. Can J Cardiol 21:833–838.
3. Dearani JA, Connolly HM, Martinez R, et al. (2007) Caring for adults with congenital cardiac disease: successes and challenges for 2007 and beyond. Cardiol Young 17 (Suppl 2):87–96.
4. Fernandes SM, Landzberg MJ (2004) Transitioning the young adult with congenital heart disease for life-long medical care. Pediatr Clin North Am 51:1739–1748.
5. de Souza DG, Baum VC (2007) An orphan subspecialty, or whither pediatric cardiac anesthesia? J Cardiothorac Vasc Anesth 21:171–173.
6. Baum VC, de Souza DG (2007) Beginning a career in pediatric cardiac anesthesia: up the creek, but where's the paddle? Paediatr Anaesth 17:407–409.
7. Sundar S, Dinardo JA (2008) Transesophageal echocardiography in pediatric surgery. Int Anesthesiol Clin 46:137–155.
8. Sangwan S, Au C, Mahajan A (2001) Pro: pediatric anesthesiologists should be the primary echocardiographers for pediatric patients undergoing cardiac surgical procedures. J Cardiothorac Vasc Anesth 15:388–390.
9. Moran AM, Geva T (2001) Con: pediatric anesthesiologists should not be the primary echocardiographers for pediatric patients undergoing cardiac surgical procedures. J Cardiothorac Vasc Anesth 15:391–393.
10. Ayres NA, Miller-Hance W, Fyfe DA, et al. (2005) Indications and guidelines for performance of transesophageal echocardiography in the patient with pediatric acquired or congenital heart disease: report from the task force of the Pediatric Council of the American Society of Echocardiography. J Am Soc Echocardiogr 18:91–8.
11. Murray E, Gruppen L, Catton P, et al. (2000) The accountability of clinical education: its definition and assessment. Med Educ 34:871–879.
12. Gauvreau K (2007) Reevaluation of the volume–outcome relationship for pediatric cardiac surgery. Circulation 115:2599–2601.
13. Hargreaves DH (1996) Transforming the apprenticeship model of training. Br J Hosp Med 55:342–343.
14. Windish DM, Gozu A, Bass EB, et al. (2007) A ten-month program in curriculum development for medical educators: 16 years of experience. J Gen Intern Med 22:655–661.
15. DiNardo JA, Baum VC, Andropoulos DB (2009) A proposal for training in pediatric cardiac anesthesia. Anesth Analg Aug 27. [Epub ahead of print]
16. White MC, Murphy TW (2007) Postal survey of training in pediatric cardiac anesthesia in the United Kingdom. Paediatr Anaesth 17:421–425.
17. Williams RG, Pearson GD, Barst RJ, et al. (2006) Report of the National Heart, Lung, and Blood Institute Working Group on research in adult congenital heart disease. J Am Coll Cardiol 47:701–707.
18. Elwyn G, O'Connor A, Stacey D, et al. (2006) Developing a quality criteria framework for patient decision aids: online international Delphi consensus process. Br Med J 333 (7565):417.
19. Gorman PJ, Meier AH, Rawn C, Krummel TM (2000) The future of medical education is no longer blood and guts, it is bits and bytes. Am J Surg 180:353–356.
20. Russell IA, Rouine-Rapp K, Stratmann G, Miller-Hance WC (2006) Congenital heart disease in the adult: a review with internet-accessible transesophageal echocardiographic images. Anesth Analg 102:694–723.
21. Grunwald T, Clark D, Fisher SS, et al. (2004) Using cognitive task analysis to facilitate collaboration in development of simulator to accelerate surgical training. Stud Health Technol Inform 98:114–120.
22. Issenberg SB, Scalese RJ (2008) Simulation in health care education. Perspect Biol Med 51:31–46.
23. Issenberg SB, McGaghie WC, Petrusa ER, et al. (2005) Features and uses of high-fidelity medical simulations that lead to effective learning: a BEME systematic review. Med Teach 27:10–28.

24. Issenberg SB, McGaghie WC, Hart IR, et al. (1999) Simulation technology for health care professional skills training and assessment. JAMA 282:861–866.

25. Ziv A, Ben-David S, Ziv M (2005) Simulation based medical education: an opportunity to learn from errors. Med Teach 27:193–199.

26. Satava RM (2008) Historical review of surgical simulation—a personal perspective. World J Surg 32:141–148.

27. Kneebone R (2005) Evaluating clinical simulations for learning procedural skills: a theory-based approach. Acad Med 80:549–553.

28. Grantcharov TP, Kristiansen VB, Bendix J, et al. (2004) Randomized clinical trial of virtual reality simulation for laparoscopic skills training. Br J Surg 91:146–150.

29. Seymour NE, Gallagher AG, Roman SA, et al. (2002) Virtual reality training improves operating room performance: results of a randomized, double-blinded study. Ann Surg 236:458–463.

30. Bradley P, Postlethwaite K (2003) Setting up a clinical skills learning facility. Med Educ 37 (Suppl 1): 6–13.

31. Bacha EA (2007) Patient safety and human factors in pediatric cardiac surgery. Pediatr Cardiol 28:116–121.

32. Batalden PB, Nelson EC, Edwards WH, et al. (2003) Microsystems in health care: part 9. Developing small clinical units to attain peak performance. Jt Comm J Qual Saf 29:575–585.

33. Houston TK, Ferenchick GS, Clark JM, et al. (2004) Faculty development needs. J Gen Intern Med 19:375–379.

34. Wass V, Van Der Vleuten C, Shatzer J, Jones R (2001) Assessment of clinical competence. Lancet 357 (9260):945–949.

35. Hamdy H, Prasad K, Williams R, Salih FA (2003) Reliability and validity of the direct observation clinical encounter examination (DOCEE). Med Educ 37:205–212.

36. Howley LD (2004) Performance assessment in medical education: where we've been and where we're going. Eval Health Prof 27:285–303.

37. Swing SR (2002) Assessing the ACGME general competencies: general considerations and assessment methods. Acad Emerg Med 9:1278–1288.

38. Huddle TS, Heudebert GR (2007) Taking apart the art: the risk of anatomizing clinical competence. Acad Med 82:536–541.

39. Epstein RM, Hundert EM (2002) Defining and assessing professional competence. JAMA 287:226–235.

40. Govaerts MJ, Van Der Vleuten CP, Schuwirth LW, Muijtjens AM (2007) Broadening perspectives on clinical performance assessment: rethinking the nature of in-training assessment. Adv Health Sci Educ Theory Pract 12:239–260.

41. Schuwirth LW, Van Der Vleuten CP (2003) The use of clinical simulations in assessment. Med Educ 37 (Suppl 1):65–71.

42. Spencer J, Blackmore D, Heard S, et al. (2000) Patient-oriented learning: a review of the role of the patient in the education of medical students. Med Educ 34:851–857.

43. Swing SR, Schneider S, Bizovi K, et al. (2007) Using patient care quality measures to assess educational outcomes. Acad Emerg Med 14:463–473.

44. van Dalen J, Kerkhofs E, Verwijnen GM, et al. (2002) Predicting communication skills with a paper-and-pencil test. Med Educ 36:148–153.

45. Sargeant J (2008) Toward a common understanding of self-assessment. J Contin Educ Health Prof 28:1–4.

46. Rethans JJ, Norcini JJ, Baron-Maldonado M, et al. (2002) The relationship between competence and performance: implications for assessing practice performance. Med Educ 36:901–909.

47. Miller MD (1997) Office procedures. Education, training, and proficiency of procedural skills. Prim Care 24:231–240.

48. Snell L, Tallett S, Haist S, et al. (2000) A review of the evaluation of clinical teaching: new perspectives and challenges. Med Educ 34:862–270.

49. Hesketh EA, Bagnall G, Buckley EG, et al. (2001) A framework for developing excellence as a clinical educator. Med Educ 35:555–564.

50. Copeland HL, Hewson MG (2000) Developing and testing an instrument to measure the effectiveness of clinical teaching in an academic medical center. Acad Med 75:161–166.

51. Parsell G, Bligh J (1998) Interprofessional learning. Postgrad Med J 74:89–95.

52. Wickey GS, Andrade O, Diaz MR (1992) An inter-American congenital heart disease program. J Cardiothorac Vasc Anesth 6:181–184.

53. Gozu A, Windish DM, Knight AM, et al. (2008) Long-term follow-up of a 10-month programme in curriculum development for medical educators: a cohort study. Med Educ 42:684–692.

54. Kalet A, Krackov S, Rey M (2002) Mentoring for a new era. Acad Med 77:1171–1172.

55. McKinstry B, Macnicol M, Elliot K, Macpherson S (2005) The transition from learner to provider/teacher: the learning needs of new orthopaedic consultants. BMC Med Educ 5:17.

3

Quality, outcomes, and databases in congenital cardiac anesthesia

David F. Vener, M.D.
Texas Children's Hospital, Baylor College of Medicine, Houston, Texas, USA

Introduction

Anesthesia practitioners have long been at the forefront of patient safety initiatives in the operating room and beyond. Technological innovations such as pulse oximetry and end-tidal capnography have combined with better trainee and practitioner education to dramatically increase the safety of our patients and the quality of our anesthesia. As a result of these systematic changes, anesthesia-related patient morbidity and mortality has steadily declined across all patient populations. Efforts to delineate the frequency of complications related to anesthesia in patients undergoing congenital cardiac surgery have been difficult because of the low occurrence of this surgery compared to other surgeries on children and the relatively rare incidence of anesthesia-related complications in this population. Even the busiest of cardiac anesthesia services at major North American pediatric institutions will each only have contact with 1000–2000 congenital cardiac patients per year and many of these cases are nonsurgical such as diagnostic and interventional catheterizations and radiology imaging procedures.

In order to better quantify both the incidence of complications and the outcomes of surgical procedures, the Society of Thoracic Surgeons (STS) database committee

Anesthesia for Congenital Heart Disease 2nd edition. Edited by
Dean Andropoulos, Stephen Stayer, Isobel Russell and Emad Mossad.
© 2010 Blackwell Publishing.

established a nationwide (and now international) voluntary and anonymous registry of congenital cardiac cases and outcomes in the 1990s [1]. Of the 122 locations in the USA and 8 locations in Canada that provide surgical care for congenital cardiac lesions in 2008, the database now has over 70 centers submitting their information during the annual data harvest, including almost every major cardiac center, with more centers joining annually. As of the 2007 report, the registry held information on over 60,000 patient procedures. This data serves as an important resource for determining nationwide outcomes on a given congenital cardiac lesion and can help establish benchmarks by which individual hospitals and surgeons can compare their results against aggregate data from around North America on a lesion-by-lesion, complexity and age-adjusted basis. These benchmarking efforts will strengthen programs that are doing a good job of serving this highly complex patient population and allow hospitals that are not as successful to see where they can improve their results. The State of Florida, for example, has now mandated participation in this type of database as a requirement for participation in state-run insurance programs such as Medicaid. Some private insurers such as United Healthcare have established "Centers of Excellence" to facilitate referrals within their systems and to maximize their patient outcomes and satisfaction while minimizing the added expense of complications (https://www.geoaccess.com/uhc/po/Default.asp; accessed July 24, 2009) [2, 3]. Demonstration of superior outcomes through benchmarking is one element of the requirements for consideration as a preferred referral center.

Other important efforts that have come out of the STS congenital cardiac surgical database include working groups that have established the consensus guidelines for defining lesion nomenclature, morbidity, and mortality [4]. All of these efforts have been coordinated internationally with other groups such as the European Association of Cardiothoracic Surgeons to eventually allow the free flow of comparative data across national boundaries. Additionally, work is ongoing to span specialties to involve pediatric cardiology, cardiac anesthesia, intensive care, and governmental agencies. Because many of the patients undergoing congenital cardiac surgery may have their procedures at multiple institutions, the various groups have worked to develop a Health Insurance Portability and Accountability Act (HIPAA)-compliant confidential patient identifier system that will allow the same patient to be tracked both geographically and longitudinally, which heretofore has not been possible. Other ongoing efforts include attempting to incorporate state and national death indices to track patient mortality beyond the initial postoperative period and capture mortality information on patients lost to follow-up. Much work remains to be done to ensure patient confidentiality while at the same time enabling comprehensive data capture.

The Congenital Cardiac Anesthesia Society (CCAS) was incorporated in 2005 and one of its first initiatives was to approach the STS in 2005 about developing anesthesia information to be included in the STS data set. It was felt by the board members of the CCAS that working in a cooperative effort with the STS would be more efficient financially and logistically for both groups rather than establishing parallel databases with large amounts of data overlap. The STS has been very forthcoming and supportive of this collaboration and sees it as a model for future incorporation of additional specialties that share the same patients such as pediatric interventional cardiology and pediatric cardiac critical care medicine.

One of the key benefits of utilizing an annual data submission process across multiple institutions is that it will allow for far more contemporaneous examination of patient outcomes. Recent publications from two centers with a long history of anesthesia data collection, Children's Hospital, Boston, and the Mayo Clinic (Rochester, MN) illustrate the difficulties with single-center record keeping [5, 6]. Their data, critically important as it is, represents time periods ranging from 6 years (Boston) to 17 years (Mayo). During these time spans multiple factors may change that significantly alter patient outcomes and potential complications. For example, personnel changes and experience (physician, nursing, and ancillary staff), surgical technique modifications, pharmacologic changes, technical advances with better monitoring and equipment, and more sophisticated complication

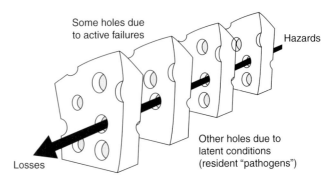

Figure 3.1 The "Swiss cheese" model of accident causation (Reproduced with permission from Reference [7])

detection and tracking all impact patient outcome statistics. In examining low-frequency events, the only way in which to properly determine their occurrence is to investigate large numbers of patients. Since no single center can provide sufficient patients as a denominator in a short period of time, it is necessary to either lengthen the time period studied (with the weaknesses mentioned above) or increase the denominator by expanding the patient base by making the data multi-institutional. One goal of the STS–CCAS collaboration is specifically to do the latter.

Errors and outcomes in surgery and anesthesia

The perioperative management of patients with congenital heart disease is fraught with times where even small decision-making errors may have catastrophic outcomes. James Reason has described the "Swiss Cheese Model" for evaluating patient complications due to human errors [7]. For a complication to occur, all the "holes" in the cheese have to line up – i.e., a sequential failure of various defense mechanisms in place to prevent, recognize, and/or treat unwanted physiological changes (Figure 3.1). Many "anesthesia" complications are multifactorial in origin and it can be difficult to assign the relative contributions of different clinical services. For example, failure to successfully separate from cardiopulmonary bypass may be due to issues such as technical difficulty or bleeding (surgery), inotrope management (anesthesia and surgery), ventilator management (anesthesia), or underlying patient physiology such as intractable pulmonary hypertension. These system factors are further exacerbated if there are communication difficulties between the various parties, including surgeons, anesthesiologists, perfusionists, cardiologists, and the pre- and postoperative medical and nursing teams [8].

de Leval and colleagues investigated the impact of human factors and teams on surgical outcomes in congenital cardiac patients focusing on the neonatal arterial switch operation (ASO) as a marker for complex, high-risk surgery [9]. Patient and procedural data were collected on 243 operations performed by 21 UK cardiac surgeons in 16 centers over 18 months. Of these 243 patients, case study data were collected on 173 ASOs by two human factors researchers who followed each case from time of induction of anesthesia until care was transferred to the intensive care team. The observed adverse events were subsequently divided into major and minor events depending on their impact on the safety of the patient. Multivariate logistic regression analyses determined that, after adjustment for patient factors, the total number of minor and major events per case were both strong predictors of the probability of death and near miss ($P < 0.001$). The authors concluded that minor events go largely unnoticed by the operating room team and are therefore left uncompensated. A subsequent analysis of the same data suggests that minor events impede the operating room team's ability to compensate for future major events [10].

In addition to the organizational factors, pediatric cardiac surgery procedures have a low error tolerance. The Bristol Royal Infirmary Inquiry and the Manitoba Inquiry reports both recognized the importance of human factors and systems research in improving pediatric cardiac surgical outcomes [11–13]. The report of the Manitoba Pediatric Cardiac Surgery Inquest found that "serious organizational and personnel problems experienced by the Health Sciences Center's Pediatric Cardiac Surgery Program during 1993 and throughout 1994 contributed to the deaths of these children." Galvan et al. recently published an initial observational study on complications in this complex patient population and recorded on average 1.8 major compensated and 9 minor compensated complications per case [14]. These complications were observed during the surgeries but were all recognized and treated by the medical team before injury resulted—all the "holes" in the Swiss Cheese did not line up because one or more of the various systems in place to prevent patient injury worked appropriately. Barach et al. reported on a comprehensive process map that they outlined the multiple steps involved in congenital cardiac anesthetic care and identified the potential sites for safety interventions [15]. They observed 108 open chest cardiac surgeries and found that communication failures were the most common underlying cause of major events. Examples of the organizational and human factors challenges that Barach et al. observed include:

- Unplanned transfusion of blood products correlated with a breakdown of communication between the anesthesia team, the nurses, and the perfusionist.

- Failure to identify a nonfunctioning infusion pump was directly related to poor communication between the anesthesia attending physician and resident who was performing several tasks simultaneously.
- Detection of increased chest tube bleeding was delayed and may have been related to suboptimal communication between residents and the attending physician.

"Near misses" are important as they are 10–100 times more common than documented adverse events and yet share the same organizational and cognitive sources of error as major adverse events [16]. Determining the frequency and nature of "Near miss" events is potentially far more important than just looking at system failures resulting in patient injury. However, "Near Miss" analysis is difficult as it requires a trained, independent observer to accompany the patient through the entire care continuum.

Closed claim analysis in anesthesia

The American Society of Anesthesiology has sponsored multiple investigations using a "closed claims" analysis method to identify areas of concern for anesthesia providers, including claims for death and brain injury, central venous line injuries, nerve injury, and airway injury [17–22]. These reports have not generally examined the effects of age or type of surgery and do not have a denominator that is needed to determine the incidence of injury. Jimenez et al. used the closed claims data to investigate pediatric anesthesia liability and segregated the data by type of surgery [22]. This report found that thoracic and cardiac surgeries accounted for slightly less than 10% of all claims that were settled. This figure probably represents a disproportionately high number because of the relative paucity of thoracic and cardiac surgeries compared to all surgeries performed on pediatric patients. Malpractice data are a very insensitive tool for determining the incidence or causality of complications, as so many different factors apart from medical error determine whether or not a claim is initiated or settled. The denominator of pediatric patients undergoing surgical and diagnostic procedures with anesthesia in the USA is not measurable with any accuracy due to the lack of a central reporting mechanism. Examining the caseload at children's hospitals is insufficient because many procedures are performed in mixed adult–pediatric general hospitals, ambulatory surgical centers, or physician offices. Furthermore, there are well-known weaknesses to using the closed claim data. These analyses rely upon the presence of a settled malpractice claim to be included and the period examined may span decades during which significant changes in anesthesia, medical, and surgical practice have occurred.

Pediatric and congenital cardiac anesthesia

In 2007 three major manuscripts concerning cardiac arrest in children were published: one of which focused on children with congenital heart disease and the other two on children undergoing all types of surgical and nonsurgical procedures [5, 6,23]. The Pediatric Perioperative Cardiac Arrest (POCA) registry was a multi-institutional effort in which participants anonymously reported all episodes of cardiac arrest in children 18 years of age and younger resulting in chest compressions or death at the time of surgery or within 24 hours. This project was begun in 1994 and data collection and analysis continued through 2004, at that time further data collection was put on hiatus. Subsequent examination of the detailed data forms allowed the investigators to assess the relative contribution of anesthesia to the cardiac arrest or death. The most recent publication from the POCA group was a follow-up to their original publication in 2000 [24].

The investigators at Children's Hospital, Boston, have been collecting anesthetic data on their own patients since January 2000. The publication of this data through December 31, 2005, as part of an internal quality assurance program, represents a significant effort to determine contemporary complications specific to pediatric cardiac anesthesia, both in the operating rooms and in outlying locations such as the cardiac catheterization or radiology suites [5]. One of the difficulties associated with determining causality in this patient population is the interdependent nature of anesthesia, surgery, and patient physiology. The authors examined each incident with a panel of three pediatric cardiac anesthesiologists, and a subsequent review by a pediatric cardiac surgeon, before assigning causality. Children's Hospital, Boston, reported that in their series of 5213 cardiac patients from 2000 to 2005, there were 41 arrests in 40 patients for an overall frequency of 0.79%, with anesthesia playing a significant role in 11 of the 41 cases, or in other words, 21.1 cardiac arrests per 10,000 anesthetics. This compares to their previously reported anesthesia-related incidence of 2.7 cardiac arrests or death per 10,000 anesthetics in all patients during roughly the same time period [25].

Another institution with a long history of anesthesia data collection, the Mayo Clinic in Rochester, Minnesota, has also recently reviewed their experience with cardiac arrests in children [23]. A consistent factor in all of these studies is that children with underlying congenital cardiac defects are at a much higher risk of arrest than children without these defects. The incidence of arrest at the Mayo Clinic for children during noncardiac procedures was 2.9 per 10,000 versus 127 per 10,000 for children undergoing cardiac procedures, a 30-fold increase in risk. This data,

however, does not attempt to assign anesthesia causality and therefore represents all risks. Subanalysis related to causality, age, and type of surgery further stratified their data. Of their 92,881 patients, 4242 were for cardiac procedures. Among the 54 children who suffered a cardiac arrest or death undergoing a cardiac procedure, age played a significant role, with neonates having the highest risk. Anesthesia was not identified as a causative factor in any of the cardiac surgical arrests or deaths.

As is evident from the newest data, even the busiest of programs have a low frequency of anesthesia-related cardiac arrests or death because of the low incidence of these events. As a consequence, it is necessary to harvest data over many years to collect any meaningful numbers, during which time major changes in patient management may occur. For example, the initial POCA study attributed many arrests to the use of the anesthetic agent halothane, a known cardiac depressant. By the time of the follow-up publication 7 years later, halothane had been replaced almost entirely in North America by sevoflurane, an anesthetic agent with significantly less cardiotoxicity at the typically administered doses. Likewise, there has been a trend in recent years toward intraoperative or early extubation of cardiac patients. This trend is probably safe, but there have been no large-scale studies to validate the concept or determine what, if any, complications may be occurring in these patients.

One of the only mechanisms for accurately determining the incidence and outcomes of low frequency events is to aggregate large amounts of data from multiple sources. To that end, the CCAS has joined with the Society of Thoracic Surgeons Congenital Database Task Force to incorporate anesthesia-specific data points into their surgical registry, which is now the largest single reporting site for children and adults undergoing surgical repair of congenital cardiac malformations and their sequelae in North America.

The Congenital Cardiac Anesthesia Society

The CCAS was formed in 2005 by representatives from many of the busiest congenital cardiac surgical programs in North America, including Children's Hospital in Boston, Children's Hospital of Philadelphia, the Hospital for Sick Children in Toronto, Texas Children's Hospital in Houston, Lucille Packard Children's Hospital at Stanford University in Palo Alto, California, the Cleveland Clinic Children's Hospital, Children's Healthcare of Atlanta Sibley Heart Center, Arkansas Children's Hospital, Children's Hospital Los Angeles, CS Mott Children's Hospital in Ann Arbor, Michigan, and others. The CCAS is a subsidiary organization of the Society for Pediatric Anesthesia and is also affiliated with the Society for Cardiac Anesthesia. Membership is open to all individuals providing anesthesia-related care for children with heart defects or an interest in the field. In addition to education, a major function of the organization is the development of this database.

The Joint Congenital Cardiac Anesthesia Society—Society of Thoracic Surgeons Database Initiative

After discussions with all interested parties, in order to minimize the redundancy of information and take advantage of a shared data structure, the data fields for the database were selected in coordination with the existing data fields in the databases of the Society of Thoracic Surgeons Congenital Heart Surgery Database and the European Association for Cardio-Thoracic Surgery. For an additional fee, Society of Thoracic Surgeons Congenital Surgery Database participants may elect to submit their anesthetic data to be pooled anonymously with the other participating centers during their annual harvest of data. The Joint Congenital Cardiac Anesthesia Society—Society of Thoracic Surgeons Database will therefore become an optional module of the Society of Thoracic Surgeons Congenital Heart Surgery Database.

The symbiotic relationship between congenital cardiac surgery and congenital cardiac anesthesia supports the creation of a common database for these subspecialties. Multiple potential benefits can be realized through the development of this joint database:
- Minimization of data entry burden
- Minimization of costs associated with data entry
- Minimization of the cost associated with database maintenance
- Utilization of common nomenclature based on the International Pediatric and Congenital Cardiac Code (www.ipccc.net)
- Utilization of common database fields
- Utilization of common database definitions
- Utilization of common database standards
- Development of common strategies to report outcomes
- Development of common quality improvement initiatives

The proposed fields of data are shown in Table 3.1. These fields will be reviewed periodically and modified as necessary. At the time of the writing of this manuscript, the CCAS is awaiting final approval of the documents coordinating their efforts with the Society of Thoracic Surgeons before data collection begins. Interested parties may contact the author directly or receive more information about the CCAS at the following website: www.pedsanesthesia.org/ccas.

International efforts

Efforts are ongoing to make this initiative a global project. Initial collaborative discussions have taken place with Dr Ehrenfried Schindler of Germany about the possibility of linking this initiative with the European Association of Cardiothoracic Anaesthesiologists (www.eacta.org). The final selection of database fields will be made through a collaborative effort involving surgeons and cardiologists from Europe and North America. Input from other continents is certainly welcome as well. It is certainly possible and desirable that the planned anesthesia module of the Society of Thoracic Surgeons Congenital Heart Database has an identical module in the congenital heart database of the European Association for Cardio-Thoracic Surgery and the European Congenital Heart Surgeons Association. These European and North American congenital heart surgery databases have functioned as sister databases with identical nomenclature and database fields and definitions [26, 27]. The incorporation of anesthetic data into the effort should follow a similar strategy. This project should also ideally spread beyond North America and Europe. Efforts to involve Africa, Asia, Australia, and South America are necessary and already underway under the leadership of the World Society for Pediatric and Congenital Heart Surgery [28]. The possible eventual creation of a World Society for Pediatric and Congenital Disease might further support the globalization of these efforts. In the interim, globalization of the collaborative surgery and anesthesia initiative is certainly supported by multiple entities:
- The Multi-Societal Database Committee for Pediatric and Congenital Heart Disease
- The International Nomenclature Committee for Pediatric and Congenital Heart Disease
- The World Society for Pediatric and Congenital Heart Surgery
- The Society of Thoracic Surgeons
- The European Association for Cardio-Thoracic Surgery
- The European Congenital Heart Surgeons Association
- The Congenital Heart Surgeons' Society
- Congenital Cardiac Anesthesia Society
- The European Association of Cardiothoracic Anesthesiologists

The creation of a joint cardiac surgery and anesthesia database is another step toward the ultimate goal of creating a database for congenital heart disease that spans both geographical and subspecialty boundaries.

Table 3.1 The proposed fields of data for the Joint Congenital Cardiac Anesthesia Society—Society of Thoracic Surgeons Database Initiative

Patient information
  Location of procedure
  Primary anesthesiology attending | Name
  Secondary anesthesiology attending | Name
  Fellow or resident present | Yes/no
  CRNA/SRNA present | Yes/no
  Patient body surface area | Calculated

Preoperative medications
  Drop down list of common medications | Patient is on For 24 hours prior to operating room (OR)
  Preoperative sedation | Yes/no; medication used
  Time of transport from ICU/floor | Hours:minutes (HH:MM)
  Time of induction | Hours:minutes (HH:MM)

Monitoring
  Preoperative baseline oxygen saturation | %
  Arterial line | Percutaneous/cutdown/none
  Central pressure monitoring | Percutaneous/cutdown/transthoracic/none
  Neurologic monitoring | None/BIS/NIRS/TCD/SSEP/EEG
  Lowest recorded core intraoperative temperature | Degrees Celsius
  Transesophageal echocardiography | Yes/no

Anesthetic technique
  Induction | Inhalation/intravenous/intramuscular
  Primary induction agent | List of medications
  Primary maintenance agent | List of medications
  Regional anesthetic | Yes/no: type (caudal/epidural/spinal); single/continuous

Airway
  Airway type | None/nasal cannula/endotracheal tube (ETT)/double lumen endobronchial tube (EBT)/laryngeal mask airway (LMA)/other
  Airway size | mm
  Cuffed | Yes/no
  Airway site | None/oral/nasal/tracheostomy

Transfusion | No/yes (if yes then continue below)
  Packed red blood cells (PRBC) | Volume or units
  Platelets | Volume or units
  Fresh frozen plasma (FFP) | Volume or units
  Cryoprecipitate | Volume or units
  Whole blood | Volume or units
  Activated factor VII | Yes/no

Intraoperative pharmacology
  Drop down list of medications | All common intraoperative/intraprocedural medications

Pharmacology at transfer to ICU/PACU
  Drop down list of medications | All common intraoperative/intraprocedural medications

ICU/PACU care
  Time of ICU/PACU arrival | Hours:minutes (HH:MM)
  Initial FIO_2 | %
  ECMO | Yes/no
  Initial pH | units
  Initial SpO_2 | %
  Temperature on Arrival | Degrees Celsius
  Need for Pacemaker | Yes/no

Morbidity/Mortality
  None | No/yes (if yes then continue below)
Anesthesia-related morbidity | Only events occurring during time of anesthetic care or related directly to anesthetic care

Table 3.1 *Continued*

Airway: Pulmonary	Dental injury
	Respiratory arrest either preoperatively, intra- or postoperatively requiring unanticipated airway support
	Unanticipated difficult intubation/reintubation
	Postextubation stridor or subglottic stenosis requiring therapy
	Unintended extubation in OR or during patient transfer
	Endotracheal tube migration requiring repositioning
	Airway/pulmonary injury related to ventilation
Vascular	Arrhythmia during central venous line placement requiring therapy
	Difficult vascular access (>1 hour of attempted access)
	Hematoma requiring cancellation or additional surgical exploration
	Inadvertent arterial puncture with hematoma or hemodynamic consequence
	Myocardial perforation or injury with central venous line placement
	Vascular compromise secondary to line placement (such as blue leg or venous obstruction)
	Pneumothorax during central venous line placement
Regional anesthetic	Bleeding at site or with aspiration
	Inadvertent intrathecal puncture
	Local anesthetic toxicity
	Neurologic injury
Pharmacology	Anaphylaxis/anaphylactoid reaction
	Nonallergic drug reaction
	Inadvertent drug administration (wrong drug)
	Inadvertent drug dosing (right drug, wrong dose)
	Intraoperative recall
	Malignant hyperthermia
	Protamine reaction requiring pharmacologic intervention
Cardiac*	Cardiac arrest after admit to OR and prior to incision
	Unexpected cardiac arrest not related to surgical manipulation
Transesophageal echocardiography (TEE)	Esophageal bleeding or rupture during TEE placement or manipulation
	Esophageal chemical burn
	Airway or vascular compromise during TEE placement/manipulation requiring removal of TEE
	Accidental extubation during TEE manipulation
Positioning	Patient falling out of either transport bed or OR table to floor
	Neurologic Injury resulting from patient positioning during anesthetic care

*Cardiac arrest defined as loss of perfusion/oxygenation requiring CPR.

References

1. Jacobs J, Wernovsky G, Elliot M (2007) Analysis of outcomes for congenital cardiac disease: can we do better? Cardiol Young 17 (Suppl 2):145–158.
2. Florida Department of Health, Childrens Medical Services Cardiac Facilities Standards, December 2005. Available at: http://www.cms-kids.com/providers/cardiac.html. Accessed July 24, 2009.
3. Quintessenza J, Jacobs J, Morrell V (2003) Issues in regionalization of pediatric cardiovascular care. Prog Pediatr Cardiol 18 (1):49–53.
4. Jacobs J, Jacobs M, Mavroudis C, et al. (2009) What is operative morbidity? Defining complications in a surgical registry database: a report of the STS Congenital Database Taskforce and the Joint EACTS-STS Congenital Database Committee. Ann Thorac Surg in press.
5. Odegard KC, DiNardo JA, Kussman BD, et al. (2007) The frequency of anesthesia-related cardiac arrests in patients with congenital heart disease undergoing cardiac surgery. Anesth Analg 105:335–343.
6. Bhananker S, Ramamoorthy C, Geiduschek J, et al. (2007) Anesthesia-related cardiac arrest in children: update from the Pediatric Perioperative Cardiac Arrest Registry. Anesth Analg 105:344–350.

7. Reason JT, Carthey J, de Leval MR (2001) Diagnosing "vulnerable system syndrome": an essential prerequisite to effective risk management. Qual Health Care 10 (Suppl 2): ii21–ii25.

8. Bognar A, Barach P, Johnson J, et al. (2008) Errors and the burden of errors: attitudes, perceptions, and the culture of safety in pediatric cardiac surgical teams. Ann Thorac Surg 85:1374–1381.

9. de Leval MR, Carthey J, Wright DJ, et al. (2000) Human factors and cardiac surgery: a multicenter study. J Thorac Cardiovasc Surg 119:661–672.

10. Carthey J, de Leval MR, Reason JT (2001) The human factor in cardiac surgery: errors and near misses in a high technology domain. Ann Thorac Surg 72:300–305.

11. Manitoba Pediatric Cardiac Surgery Inquest (2001). Available at: http://www.pediatriccardiacinquest.mb.ca/pdf/pcir_intro.pdf. Accessed July 24, 2009.

12. Walsh K, Offen N (2001) A very public failure: lessons for quality improvement in healthcare organizations from the Bristol Royal Infirmary. Qual Health Care 10:250–256.

13. Kennedy I (2001). Learning from Bristol: the report of the public inquiry into children's heart surgery at the Bristol Royal Infirmary 1984–1995. Command Paper: CM 5207. Available at: http://www.bristol-inquiry.org.uk/. Accessed July 24, 2009.

14. Galvan C, Bacha E, Mohr J, Barach P (2005) A human factors approach to understanding patient safety during pediatric cardiac surgery. Prog Pediatr Cardiol 20:13–20.

15. Barach P (2008) What is new in patient safety and how it will affect your practice? [Private Communication from Author].

16. Barach P, Small DS (2000) Reporting and preventing medical mishaps: lessons from non-medical near miss reporting systems. BMJ 320:753–763.

17. Domino K, Posner K, Caplan R, Cheney R (1999) Awareness during anesthesia: a closed claims analysis. Anesthesiology 90:1053–1061.

18. Cheney F, Domino K, Caplan R, Posner K (1999) Nerve injury associated with anesthesia: a closed claims analysis. Anesthesiology 90:1062–1069.

19. Domino K, Posner K, Caplan R, Cheney F (1999) Airway injury during anesthesia: a closed claims analysis. Anesthesiology 91:1703–1711.

20. Domino K, Bowdle T, Posner K, et al. (2004) Injuries and liability related to central vascular catheters: a closed claims analysis. Anesthesiology 100:1411–1418.

21. Cheney F, Posner K, Lee L, et al. (2006) Trends in anesthesia-related death and brain damage: a closed claims analysis. Anesthesiology 105:1081–1086.

22. Jimenez N, Posner K, Cheney F, et al. (2007) An update on pediatric anesthesia liability: a closed claims analysis. Anesth Analg 104:147–153.

23. Flick RP, Sprung J, Harrison TE (2007) Perioperative cardiac arrests in children between 1988 and 2005 at a tertiary referral center: a study of 92,881 patients. Anesthesiology 106:226–237.

24. Morray JP, Geiduscheck J, Ramamoorthy C, et al. (2000) Anesthesia-related cardiac arrest in children: initial findings of the Pediatric Perioperative Cardiac Arrest (POCA) Registry. Anesthesiology 93:6–14.

25. Zglesweski SE, Graham D, Hickey PR, et al. (2006) Anesthesia-related cardiac arrest: five year analysis at an academic pediatric medical center. Anesthesiology 105:A134, (Abstract).

26. Jacobs JP, Maruszewski B, Tchervenkov CI, et al. (2005) The current status and future directions of efforts to create a global database for the outcomes of therapy for congenital heart disease. Cardiol Young 15 (Suppl 1):190–198.

27. Jacobs JP, Jacobs ML, Maruszewski B, et al. (2005) Current status of the European Association for Cardio-Thoracic Surgery and the Society of Thoracic Surgeons Congenital Heart Surgery Database. Ann Thorac Surg 80:2278–2283.

28. Jacobs JP, Anderson RH (2007) From the editors – news and comments: World Society for Pediatric and Congenital Heart Surgery Inaugural Meeting. Cardiol Young 17:1–2.

4

Embryology, development, and nomenclature of congenital heart disease

Ivan Wilmot, M.D.
Texas Children's Hospital, Baylor College of Medicine, Houston, Texas, USA

Wanda C. Miller-Hance, M.D.
Texas Children's Hospital, Baylor College of Medicine, Houston, Texas, USA

Introduction

The pathogenesis of congenital heart disease is poorly understood. Developmental mechanisms involving cell migration, hemodynamic function, cell death, and extracellular matrix proliferation have all been proposed in the etiology of cardiovascular malformations. Multiple genetic pathways have been identified that contribute to cardiac development and whose disruption may result

Anesthesia for Congenital Heart Disease 2nd edition. Edited by
Dean Andropoulos, Stephen Stayer, Isobel Russell and Emad Mossad.
© 2010 Blackwell Publishing.

in structural defects [1–6]. These genetic controls influence cardiac-specific mechanisms such as cardiogenesis, looping of the heart tube, chamber specification, septation, conotruncal and aortic arch development, valvular formation, and ventricular function [4,7].

It is well recognized that a foundation in human embryology, in particular in the areas of cardiac morphogenesis and normal development, provides a window into the complex series of events that may result in abnormalities of the cardiovascular system. As such, a basic understanding of embryology and critical events during the different stages of cardiac development should be of relevance to those who care for patients with congenital heart disease.

This chapter provides an overview of the normal developmental program of the cardiovascular system, highlighting important events during cardiac morphogenesis and consequences of abnormal development, as relevant to the practice of cardiovascular anesthesiology. The data presented derives from a combination of descriptive or classic embryology, experimental work on other species, and current knowledge regarding human cardiac development. Lastly, basic concepts on the related, challenging subject of congenital heart disease nomenclature are reviewed.

Cardiac embryology and normal development

The heart represents the first functional organ in the embryo. It has been reported that cardiac development in most vertebrates follows a similar pattern from the formation of the cardiogenic plate to the complex fully developed pump, with minor variations across species.

The critical stages of cardiovascular development in the human encompass events between the second and eighth weeks of gestation (Color Plate 4.1). The sections that follow emphasize main aspects of embryologic development of the heart and great vessels during this period. To facilitate this discussion, a perspective that focuses on the origin and evolving changes of the major cardiovascular structures throughout embryonic development has been selected over a strict chronological approach. For a more exhaustive review of the subject, the reader is referred to several outstanding resources (http://pie.med.utoronto.ca/HTBG; accessed July 25, 2009) [8,9–13].

Early cardiogenesis

The earliest developmental stage of the heart and vascular system is seen following the second week of gestation. On the 15th day of gestation, mesoderm is derived from ectoderm. The mesoderm or "middle skin" will in turn give rise to the various cardiovascular structures (Color Plate 4.2). On the 18th day of gestation, mesodermal-derived cardiogenic crescent forms the precursor to the heart (Figure 4.1a). Cavitation of the mesoderm results in formation of the intraembryonic celom, from which all body cavities including pericardial, pleural, and peritoneal will be eventually derived.

Straight heart tube

On the 15th day of gestation, the cardiogenic crescent has developed into the primitive heart tube [15]. Blood in this midline tube enters caudally via the inflow and exits cranially via the outflow tract. It is the linear heart tube that gives rise to the atria, ventricles, bulbus cordis, and truncus arteriosus (Figure 4.1b). The bulbus cordis and truncus arteriosus contribute to formation of the ventricles and great vessels, respectively.

Cardiac looping

On the 21st day of gestation, cardiac loop formation takes place. The straight heart tube is fixed at both the sinus venosus and truncus arteriosus ends by pericardium. Differential growth of the straight heart tube results in the sinus venosus segment positioned posteriorly, the common ventricle positioned anteriorly, and the bulbus cordis positioned anterior and superiorly. This accounts for cardiac looping and the ventricular relationship (Figure 4.2).

Looping of the tube to the right gives rise to the normal ventricular relationship (d-loop), where the right ventricle is ultimately positioned rightward (Figure 4.1c). In contrast, looping to the left results in an abnormal ventricular relationship (l-loop), where the right ventricle is positioned leftward (l-looped ventricles) (Figure 4.1d). Molecular cues determining cardiac looping remain poorly understood.

Atrial septation

Atrial septation begins in the fourth week of gestation, and continues into the fifth week (Color Plate 4.3). The septum primum arises initially, being formed from tissue in growth along the superior aspect of the atria. In a curtain-like fashion, the primum septum extends inferiorly toward the endocardial cushions. Two foramena are associated with the septum primum: the superior foramen or ostium secundum and the inferior foramen primum. The foramen secundum arises from perforations in the septum primum and remains open until birth. The foramen primum is transient, as continued growth of the septum primum and endocardial cushions obliterates this communication.

The septum secundum forms during the fifth and sixth weeks of gestation, arising to the right of the septum primum. Similarly to the septum primum, the septum secundum extends inferiorly. The foramen secundum is closed by the inferiorly extending septum secundum. The superior septum secundum and inferior septum primum create the foramen of ovale.

In fetal life, the foramen ovale acts as a one-way valve, allowing oxygenated blood from inferior vena cava to course from the right atrium to the left atrium. In the postnatal circulation, functional closure of the foramen ovale results when left atrial pressure exceeds that of the right atrium. This takes place as the septum primum moves against the septum secundum. Fusion of the septum primum and septum secundum following birth results in

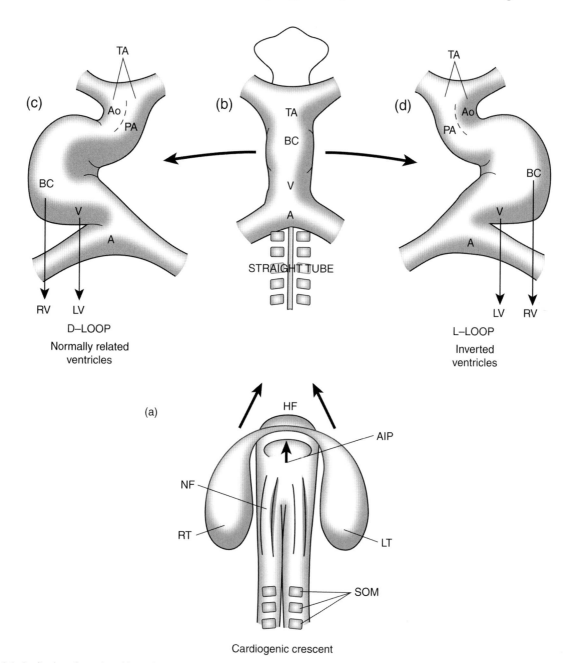

Figure 4.1 Cardiac loop formation. (a) Cardiogenic crescent of precardiac mesoderm. (b) Straight heart tube or preloop stage. (c) *d*-Loop, with normally related ventricles. (d) *l*-Loop, with inverted (mirror image) ventricles. A, atrium; AIP, anterior intestinal portal; Ao, aorta; BC, bulbus cordis; HF, head fold; LT, left; LV, morphologic left ventricle; NF, neural fold; PA, main pulmonary artery; RT, right; RV, morphologic right ventricle; SOM, somites; TA, truncus arteriosus (Reprinted with permission from Reference [14])

anatomic closure of the foramen ovale and complete atrial septation.

Development and incorporation of the sinus venosus

Initially, the segment corresponding to the sinus venosus is positioned in the midline of the posteriorly positioned primordial atrium. On the 26th day of gestation, two horns of the sinus venosus develop: the right and left horns (Color Plate 4.4a). The right horn is connected to the right umbilical, vitelline, anterior and common cardinal veins, and inferior vena cava. The left horn is connected to the left umbilical, vitelline, and anterior and common cardinal veins. There is a progressive shift of venous blood drainage from left- to right-sided structures. This results

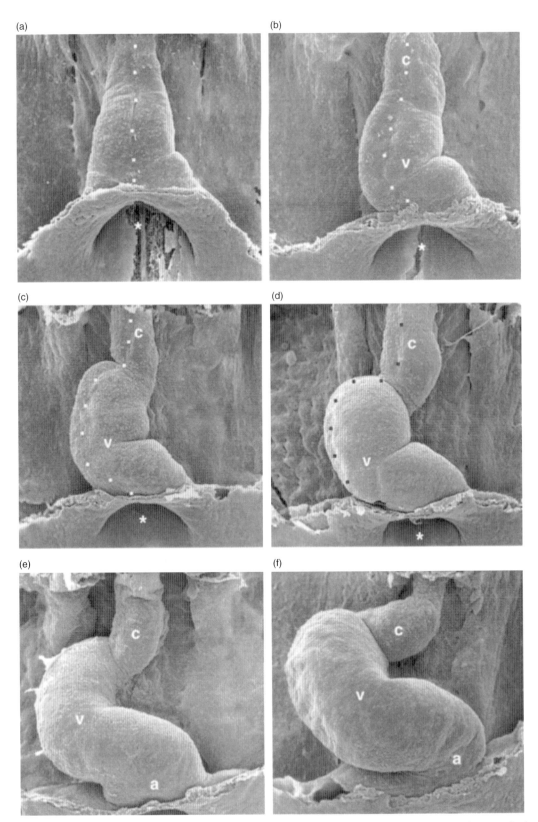

Figure 4.2 Looping of the heart tube in the chick embryo. (a, b) Ventral view demonstrating the primitive heart tube just prior to cardiac looping. The ventral midline of the primitive heart tube is marked by the dotted line. (c–f) Looping is the result of lengthening of the heart tube. Looping to the right is accompanied by twisting, allowing for the original ventral surface of the primitive heart to become the outer curvature of the looped heart. These forces contribute to the formation of atrioventricular and bulboventricular sulci. Various cardiac regions can be identified during this transition, including the atrium (a), conus arteriosus (c), and the primitive ventricle (v). The anterior intestinal portal is indicated by the asterisk (Reprinted with permission from Reference [8])

in an enlarging right horn and the sinoatrial orifice moving rightward, toward the primordial atrium. This process culminates in the incorporation of the right horn of the sinus venosus into the future right atrium (Color Plate 4.4b).

The smooth portion of the mature right atrium, the sinus venarum, is derived from sinus venosus (Color Plate 4.4c). The rough atrial appendage and conical muscular pouch of the right atrium are derived from the primordial atrium. Internally, the demarcation between the smooth, sinus venarum and the rough, primordial atrium is evidenced by a ridge of tissue, the crista terminalis. This is also present externally by a groove, the sulcus terminalis. Both the right anterior cardinal and common cardinal veins will form the superior vena cava during the eighth week of gestation. The right horn receives all the blood from the head and neck via the superior vena cava, and from the caudal regions and placenta through the inferior vena cava. The smaller left horn becomes the coronary sinus.

The sinus venosus contributes to the conduction system of the heart. The sinoatrial node develops from the sinus venosus during the fifth week of gestation. It is located along the high right atrium at the junction of the right atrium and superior vena cava. The atrioventricular node develops from the inferior portion of the sinus venosus in combination with cells from the atrioventricular region. The atrioventricular node arises slightly superior to the endocardial cushions (refer to other sections below) with the atrioventricular bundle coursing into the ventricles.

Development of the systemic veins

The development of the veins associated with the heart occurs during the fourth week of gestation. Three paired veins drain blood into the tubular heart: the vitelline, umbilical, and common cardinal veins (Color Plates 4.5, 4.6a, and 4.7).

The vitelline veins return poorly oxygenated blood from the yolk sac. The umbilical veins carry oxygenated blood from the placenta to the sinus venosus portion of the developing heart. As the liver develops, the umbilical veins lose their connection with the heart (Color Plate 4.6b). The left umbilical vein courses through the liver with the right umbilical vein degenerating at the end of the embryonic period. The caudal portion of the left umbilical vein between the liver and sinus venosus degenerates. The inferior portion of the left umbilical vein becomes the ductus venosus, bypassing the liver parenchyma, and enters the inferior vena cava.

The cardinal veins return deoxygenated blood from the body of the embryo to the sinus venosus. The superior and inferior cardinal veins join to form the common cardinal vein. The superior vena cava eventually develops from the right anterior cardinal vein and common cardinal vein as previously described (Color Plate 4.6c). The subcardinal and supracardinal veins subsequently largely replace the posterior cardinal veins. The subcardinal veins give rise to a segment of the inferior vena cava among other structures. During the seventh week of gestation, the supracardinal veins appear. The cranial portions of the supracardinal veins in turn give rise to the azygous and hemiazygous veins. The caudal portion of the left supracardinal veins degenerates with the right portion becoming the inferior portion of the inferior vena cava.

The inferior vena cava arises as a result of a shift of primordial venous drainage from the left to right side of the body (Color Plate 4.7). The inferior vena cava is composed of four main segments each originating from primordial vascular structures. This consists of the hepatic segment (derived from the right vitelline vein), prerenal segment (derived from the right subcardinal vein), renal segment (derived from the subcardinal and supracardinal anastomosis), and postrenal segment (derived from the right supracardinal vein).

Development of the pulmonary veins

Pulmonary development begins as a ventral outgrowth from the foregut, termed the respiratory diverticulum. The respiratory diverticulum develops with its most caudal segments represented by lung buds. A capillary plexus called the splanchnic plexus surrounds the lung buds (Figure 4.3).

The primitive pulmonary veins arise from the splanchnic plexus. The pulmonary venous plexus shares venous drainage with the splanchnic plexus, which is connected to the cardinal and umbilical venous systems in early development. Thus, the initial pulmonary venous drainage is via the cardinal and umbilical venous systems [17,18]. A primordial endocardial outgrowth from the superior margin of the left atrium forms the primordial pulmonary vein. It is the connection of this primordial pulmonary vein with the pulmonary venous plexus that allows pulmonary venous blood to flow into the left atrium. Once this connection to the left atrium is established, the pulmonary venous plexus loses its connection with the cardinal and umbilical veins. Persistence of this connection is considered to result in anomalous pulmonary venous drainage [19].

The left atrium is largely derived from the incorporation of the pulmonary veins. As the primordial pulmonary vein and its branches are incorporated into the primordial atrium, the four pulmonary veins incorporate into the left atrial wall. Areas of the left atrium derived from the pulmonary veins are smooth, whereas those derived from primordial atrium (left atrial appendage) are rough.

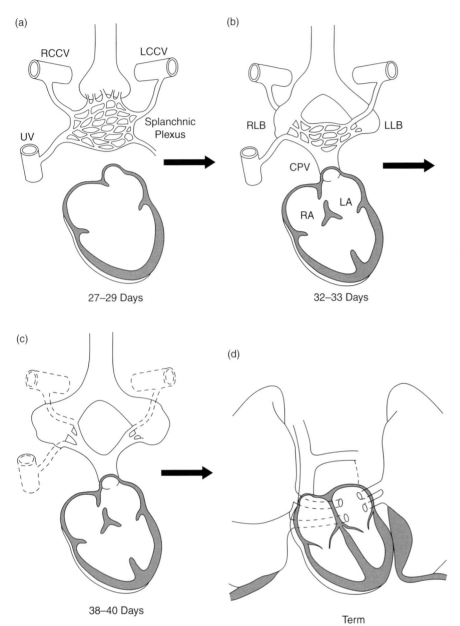

Figure 4.3 Development of the Pulmonary Veins. (a) At 27–29 days of gestation, the primordial lung buds are enmeshed by the vascular plexus of the foregut (splanchnic plexus). No direct connection to the heart is present at this stage. Instead, the multiple connections are present to the umbilicovitelline and cardinal venous systems. A small evagination can be seen in the posterior wall of the left atrium to the left of the developing septum secundum. (b) By the end of the first month of gestation, the common pulmonary vein establishes a connection between the pulmonary venous plexus and the sinoatrial portion of the heart. At this time, the connections between the pulmonary venous plexus and the splanchnic venous plexus are still patent. (c) Subsequently, the connections between the pulmonary venous plexus and the splanchnic venous plexus involute. (d) The common pulmonary vein (CPV) incorporates into the left atrium so that the individual pulmonary veins connect separately and directly to the left atrium. LA, left atrium; LCCV, left common cardinal vein; LLB, left lung bud; RA, right atrium; RCCV, right common cardinal vein; RLB, right lung bud; UV, umbilical vein (Reprinted with permission from Reference [16])

Development of the atrioventricular valves

Development of mesenchymal tissue swellings or endocardial cushions along the atrioventricular canal begins in the fourth week of gestation (Color Plate 4.8). The superior and inferior endocardial cushions are found in continuity with the interatrial and interventricular septa [20]. Simultaneous in growth of the lateral endocardial cushions results in the formation of separate right and left atrioventricular valves. In addition to the endocardial cushions, additional embryonic structures that contribute to the formation of the atrioventricular valves include the dextrodorsal conal crest and the ventricular walls.

The cushions perform a valve like function occluding blood flow from the ventricle into the atria during systole (Color Plate 4.9) [21]. Initially, these regions are muscular in nature, and through a process of cellular differentiation they become thin and membranous (Color Plate 4.7) [22].

Ventricular development and septation

Ventricular septation begins in the fifth week of gestation and continues into the seventh week (Color Plate 4.10). The primordial interventricular septum arises from a median muscular ridge between the right and left ventricles. Increased growth and dilation of the ventricles, combined with fusion of the medial ventricular wall, result in enlargement of the muscular ventricular septum. A crescentic interventricular foramen between the free edge of the septum and endocardial cushion exists up until the seventh week of gestation. Closure of the primary interventricular foramen (bulboventricular foramen) results from tissue in growth from the right bulbar ridge, left bulbar ridge, and the endocardial cushion.

The membranous portion of the interventricular septum is derived from tissue in growth from the right side of the endocardial cushion to the muscular region of the interventricular septum. The atrioventricular septum, or region of the septum that separates the right atrium from the left ventricle, originates from the inferior cushion of the atrioventricular canal.

Cavitation of the ventricular walls begins during the fifth week of gestation. This results in an increase in the ventricular sizes. Several of the remaining muscle bundles will form the trabeculae carneae (muscle bundles on the ventricular free wall), whereas others will contribute to the future papillary muscles and their chordal attachments to the atrioventricular valves. With respect to the embryologic origin of the ventricles, it has been suggested that the inlet region originates from the endocardial cushions, the trabecular area from the primordia of the trabecular portion of the ventricles, and the outlet region from conal tissue [23]. Other studies propose that the inlet and trabecular components are derived from the same primary ventricular septum [24].

Partitioning of the bulbus cordis and truncus arteriosus

Extensive experimental studies in the chick embryo have provided insight into the development of the conus and truncus arteriosus [25–27]. These observations strongly suggest that these sequences are similar in chick and man.

Neural crest cells originating in the posterior rhombencephalon are known to migrate into the pharyngeal arches. Continued migration of these cells contributes to the formation of the conus and great arteries (aorta, aortopulmonary septum), carotids, subclavian arteries, ductus arteriosus, and cardiac ganglia as follows [28–31]. It is thus not surprising that the neural crest has been implicated in the pathogenesis of several cardiovascular anomalies [32].

Partitioning of the bulbus cordis and truncus arteriosus begins in the fifth week of gestation (Color Plate 4.10). Neural crest cells migrate into both the bulbus cordis and truncus arteriosus forming bulbar and truncal ridges, respectively. These ridges undergo 180° of spiraling causing the formation of a spiral aortopulmonary septum. Development of these ridges into the aortopulmonary septum separate the future aorta from the pulmonary artery. The pulmonary artery courses around the aorta. The bulbus

cordis contributes to the development of both ventricles. In the right ventricle, it forms the conus arteriosus (infundibulum that gives rise to the pulmonary trunk). In the left ventricle, it forms the aortic vestibule (aortic cavity inferior to the aortic valve). Partitioning of the bulbus cordis and truncus arteriosus nears completion in the sixth week of gestation.

At the end of fifth week of gestation, the interventricular foramen is still patent (ventricular septal defect). The heart is largely septated into a double or parallel circulation at this stage. The third, fourth, and sixth aortic arches are present. The dorsal aorta and ductus arteriosus are formed. Continued neural crest cell migration aids in the formation of the infundibulum and great vessels. The right and left ventricles continue to develop at this stage. The aorta, left ventricle, and mitral valve align with the interventricular foramen. On the 32nd day of gestation, the main pulmonary artery and ascending aorta septate, and shortly thereafter the atrioventricular valves septate. The right ventricle enlarges at this time with concurrent movement of the interventricular septum leftward. The interventricular septum aligns underneath the atrioventricular canal as it moves leftward. Failure of this interventricular alignment has been implicated in the etiology of double outlet right ventricle.

Semilunar valve development and great artery relationships

The semilunar valves derived from subendocardial tissue swellings in the aortic and pulmonary trunk. These swellings subsequently become hollow and form the valve cusps.

On the 30th day of gestation, the pulmonary valve begins its movement to it final position, anterior and leftward of the aorta. This migration continues through the 36th day of gestation. During the course of this complex of process, various observations have been made regarding the position of the great arteries with respect to each other that resemble known abnormal great artery relationships. On the 30th to 32nd day of gestation, the semilunar valve relationship is similar to that of *d*-transposition of the great arteries. On the 33rd day of gestation, the semilunar valve relationship is side-by-side similar to that seen in Taussig–Bing malformation. On the 34th day of gestation, the semilunar valve relationship resembles that seen in tetralogy of Fallot.

Fates of the vitelline and umbilical arteries

Development of the dorsal aortae, vitelline, and umbilical arteries is complete by the fourth week of gestation. The vitelline artery, supplying the yolk sac, will in turn supply the primordial gut. In the mature fetus, the vitelline artery will form the celiac artery, superior mesenteric artery, and inferior mesenteric artery. The umbilical arteries transport poorly oxygenated blood from the body of the fetus to the placenta. These paired umbilical arteries will in turn form the internal iliac arteries (proximally), superior vesical arteries (proximally), and degenerate distally to form the medial umbilical ligament.

Development of the aortic arches

The aortic sac, aortic arches, and dorsal aortae contribute to the development of the mature aortic arch (Color Plate 4.11). Six pairs of aortic arches have been identified in the human embryo. Aortic arch development begins with the first pair of arches forming in the beginning of the fourth week of gestation. By the 26th day of gestation, the *first aortic arches* have involuted. A portion of these contributes to the development of the maxillary and external carotid arteries. At this time the second and third arches are formed, and the fourth and six arches are beginning formation. The *second aortic arches* eventually disappear, only a dorsal portion persists giving rise to the stapedial artery. The *third aortic arch*es contribute to the development of the carotid arteries.

It is during the sixth and seventh weeks of development in which the aortic arch orchestra of events lead to the development of the arch and its branching pattern. This series of events if altered can lead to vascular anomalies. The *fourth aortic arch* forms a portion of the aortic arch, innominate and proximal right subclavian artery. The *fifth aortic arch* regresses during normal development. The first, third, fourth, and six aortic arches contribute to the formation of the mature arch. The *sixth aortic arch* forms the proximal left and right pulmonary arteries, and ductus arteriosus. The *seventh intersegmental artery* gives rise to the left subclavian artery. A summary of the aortic arches and their future vascular structures can be found in Table 4.1. A graphic animation of the development of the aor-

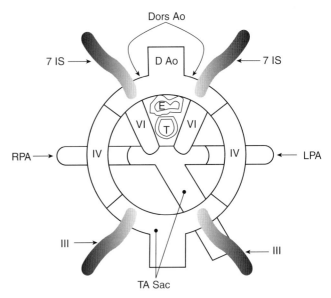

Figure 4.4 Totipotential aortic arch and pulmonary components. Edwards diagram depicting hypothetical representation of double aortic arch to illustrate the potential contribution of nearly all embryonic arches to components of the definitive arch system. D Ao, descending aorta; Dors Ao, dorsal aortae; E, esophagus; LPA, left pulmonary artery; RPA, right pulmonary artery; T, trachea; TA Sac, truncoaortic sac aortic and pulmonary artery components; III, IV, VI refer to third, fourth, sixth embryonic arches, respectively; 7 IS, seventh intersegmental artery (Reprinted with permission from Reference [34])

tic arches can be found at www.indiana.edu/~anat550/cvanim/aarch/aarch.html.

Various normal interruptions of the aortic arch system occur. These include involution of the right ductus arteriosus or sixth arch, involution of the ductus caroticus (dorsal aorta segment between the third and fourth arches), and involution of the right dorsal aorta distal to the seventh intersegmental artery (part of the embryonic right subclavian artery) [33]. This series of interruptions results in a left aortic arch. The totipotential aortic arch, or Edwards diagram, is often used to describe both normal and abnormal aortic arch development (Figure 4.4). This graphic representation can also be used to facilitate the understanding of vascular ring malformations.

Aortic arch sidedness is defined by the course of the arch over the mainstem bronchus. A left aortic arch courses over the left mainstem bronchus. Arch sidedness is also dependent on which of the dorsal aortic arches regresses. Namely, if the left dorsal aortic arch persists, the result is a left aortic arch; if the right dorsal arch persists, the result is a right aortic arch. If both arches persist, the result is a double aortic arch.

Intersegmental arteries

The aortic arch arises from the aortic sac as a paired structure. The paired dorsal aortae soon fuse, caudal to the

Table 4.1 Future vascular structures of the aortic arches

First aortic arch	Maxillary artery, external carotid arteries
Third aortic arch	Common carotid arteries
	Internal carotid arteries
Fourth aortic arch	Proximal right subclavian artery
	Transverse aortic arch (between left common carotid and left subclavian artery)
Sixth aortic arch	Proximal left and right pulmonary artery
	Ductus arteriosus
Seventh intersegmental artery	Distal right subclavian artery
	Left subclavian artery

pharyngeal arches, to form a single dorsal aorta. Arising from the dorsal aorta are at least 30 intersegmental arteries. These vessels provide blood supply to anterior body structures. The anterior intersegmental arteries in the neck join to form the vertebral arteries. The majority of the connections between the intersegmental arteries and dorsal aorta eventually regress. In the thorax, however, the dorsal intersegmental arteries persist as intercostal arteries. In the abdomen, several of these persist as lumbar arteries, where the fifth pair of lumbar intersegmental arteries forms the common iliac arteries.

Development of the coronary arteries

The coronary arteries appear relatively late during cardiac development. During early cardiac morphogenesis, nutrients to the cardiac mass are derived directly from surrounding circulating blood, and subsequently from intramyocardial communications, also termed sinusoids. The appearance of subepicardial vascular networks during the fifth week of development is thought to give rise to the distal coronary vasculature

Theories regarding the origin of the proximal coronary arteries are more controversial [35]. Several different mechanisms have been implicated [36–39]. These include penetration of the subepicardial vascular networks across the aortic wall to reach the aortic sinuses and the existence of coronary buds around the arterial trunks that eventually communicate with the subepicardial vascular network (Figure 4.5). The former concept appears most likely to be the case.

Types of circulation

Fetal circulation

Early circulation

On the 26th to 28th day of gestation, the heartbeat in the human is thought to begin. This is the initiation of the true circulation. Blood flows from the morphologic right atrium to the left atrium, to the left ventricle, to the right ventricle, and across the truncus arteriosus. Blood then courses through the aortic sac from which the aortic arches arise. Flow through the aortic arches and dorsal aorta supplies the developing embryo with nutrients. Paired umbilical arteries course toward the placenta where oxygen and nutrients are absorbed. Oxygenated blood from the placenta courses via the umbilical vein to the heart. The vitelline, umbilical, and cardinal veins return blood to the sinus venosus portion of the developing heart to begin the course again.

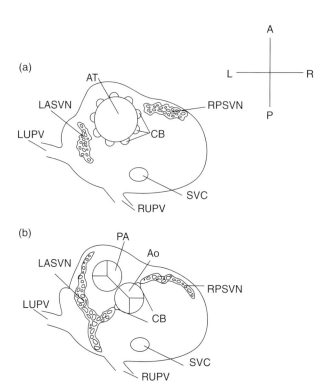

Figure 4.5 Schematic drawing of the heart demonstrating the embryologic development of the coronary arteries. (a) Illustration showing the development of the coronary buds along the walls of the arterial trunk and the development of the subepicardial vascular network. (b) Graphic demonstrating the disappearance of most of the coronary buds, with persistence of only those related to the aortic sinuses, presumed to establish connections with the subepicardial vascular network. CB, coronary buds; AT, arterial trunk; RPSVN, right posterior subepicardial vascular network; LASVN, left anterior subepicardial vascular network; SVC, superior vena cava; RUPV, right upper pulmonary vein; LUPV, left upper pulmonary vein; Ao, aorta; PA, pulmonary artery; A, anterior; P, posterior; L, left; R, right (Reprinted with permission from Reference [10])

Late circulation

Critical structures in the fetal circulation include the ductus venosus, foramen ovale, and ductus arteriosus. Oxygenated blood from the inferior vena cava blood bypasses the liver largely through the ductus venosus. This blood, directed by the Eustachian valve across the foramen ovale into the left atrium, is ejected by the left ventricle into the aorta. Deoxygenated blood from the upper body returns to the right atrium flowing preferentially into the right ventricle. In the setting of high pulmonary vascular resistance, the blood ejected by the right ventricle bypasses the lungs via the ductus arteriosus. Thus, in the fetal circulation the pulmonary vascular resistance is high, the systemic vascular resistance is low (placenta), and blood flow is shunted in the right to left direction at the foramen ovale and ductus arteriosus [40].

Transitional circulation

Several rapid changes occur in the circulation following birth. The previous neonatal parallel circulation transitions into separate pulmonary and systemic circulations arranged in series [41].

A simple initial breath and clamping of the cord initiates this transition. The pulmonary vasculature vasodilates in response to oxygen and the pulmonary vascular resistance decreases dramatically. The combination of lung expansion and pulmonary vasodilation results in increased pulmonary blood flow. This in turn increases left atrial filling. The decreased pulmonary vascular resistance in combination with the increased systemic vascular resistance (following removing the placenta from the systemic circulation) results in increased left atrial pressures, and decreased right atrial pressures. This combination causes closure of the foramen ovale. The oxygen tension increases as the source of oxygen supply transitions from the placenta to the lungs. The increased oxygen tension initiates constriction of the ductus arteriosus. The ductus arteriosus usually closes within 10–15 hours after birth in term infants, and functional closure occurs by 72 hours. Closure of the ductus venosus occurs within a few days following birth. In the transitional circulation, the pulmonary vascular resistance is low, the systemic vascular resistance is high, and blood flow is no longer shunting at the level of the foramen ovale.

Postnatal circulation

Following birth the pulmonary vascular resistance continues to decrease [42]. Closure of the ductus arteriosus allows the pulmonary artery systolic pressure to decrease below that of the aorta. Remodeling of the pulmonary vascular smooth muscle causes this decrease. The pulmonary vascular pressures decrease to near adult levels by 4 weeks of age. The pulmonary vascular resistance also declines, nearing adult levels by 3–6 months of age.

The pulmonary vascular resistance decreases and the systemic vascular resistance remain elevated during the neonatal period. The relative balance between the pulmonary and systemic resistances can be altered in children with congenital heart disease and may be influenced by drugs, inspired oxygen concentration, ventilation, and acid–base status. Structural defects causing excessive left to right shunting may increase pulmonary blood flow and pulmonary artery pressures. This left to right shunting may become clinically apparent as the pulmonary vascular resistance declines at 4 weeks of age.

Although in normal infants obliteration of the communications present during fetal life at the atrial level (foramen ovale) and great arteries (ductus arteriosus) is expected and of no consequence, it is important to consider that this may not be the case in those with structural pathology. A number of congenital cardiac malformations require patency of the ductus arteriosus and/or an intracardiac communication to sustain life following birth. Persistence of these fetal structures may allow blood to bypass a congenital cardiac defect. Clinically, children with such lesions may become symptomatic or critically ill during the period when the circulation evolves from the transitional to the neonatal pattern.

Defects resulting from abnormal cardiac development

Defects of cardiac positioning

Cardiac malpositions may result from extrinsic or intrinsic factors [43]. Dextrocardia represents a positional abnormality. This is considered to result from the rightward rotation of the cardiac mass. This condition may or may not be associated with other defects. Dextrocardia with situs solitus (also known as isolated dextrocardia) is frequently associated with severe cardiac anomalies that include atrioventricular discordance (*l*-looped ventricles), single ventricle, transposition of the great arteries, and heterotaxy syndrome. Dextrocardia with situs inversus is less likely to be accompanied by cardiac defects.

Defects of atrial septation

Defects resulting from the abnormal formation of the atrial septum are relatively common [44]. Atrial septal defects can occur in isolation, or may be seen within the context of associated cardiac anomalies. Five types of interatrial communications are recognized including patent foramen ovale, ostium secundum defect, ostium primum defect, sinus venosus defect, and common atrium. A patent foramen ovale may be found in up to 25% of the population. It results from failure of fusion of the primum and secundum septae. Ostium secundum defects are the most common type of atrial septal defects. These result from a combination of excessive resorption of the septum primum and large foramen ovale defects. Ostium primum defects are seen in up to 20% of patients with Trisomy 21. These are associated with cleft mitral valves and endocardial cushion defects. Primum defects result from lack of fusion of the primum septum with the absent endocardial cushion. Sinus venosus defects are rare resulting from defects in the sinus venosus portion of the atrial septum. They are associated with partial anomalous pulmonary venous connections. Complete absence of the atrial septum results in a common atrium. This may be seen in heterotaxy syndrome.

Defects of the atrioventricular canal and atrioventricular valves

Atrioventricular canal defects, also referred to as atrioventricular septal defects or endocardial cushion defects, result from failure of fusion of the superior and inferior endocardial cushions [22,45]. These defects can vary in severity and complexity [46]. Generally, the pathology involves a combination of the following: an atrial communication, a ventricular communication, and abnormal development of the atrioventricular valves. The complete form of defect involves all three of these above-mentioned components and a common atrioventricular valve. The less severe forms involve only one or two of the above defects. Children with canal type defects may have displacement of the conduction system. Knowledge of the abnormal conduction system course can help avoid injury during surgical interventions. Atrioventricular septal defects are often associated with Trisomy 21. Nearly 80% of all infants with atrioventricular septal defects have a chromosomal anomaly, syndrome, nonsyndromic organ anomaly, or deformation [47].

Tricuspid and mitral valve defects result from failure of normal formation of the two separate valves, chordae tendinae, and ventricular cavitation. Ebstein anomaly results in an apically displaced tricuspid valve with an atrialized portion of the right ventricle. The tricuspid valve is often dysplastic and regurgitant [48]. Valve stenosis may be seen. Isolated mitral valve anomalies in children are relatively rare.

Defects of ventricular septation

Ventricular septal defects are one of the most common types of congenital heart lesions [49]. These defects encompass four major regions or portions of the septum: membranous, muscular, inlet, and outlet. Defects in the membranous septum (referred to as membranous or perimembranous) predominate. These result from failure of fusion of endocardial tissue in growth, aorticopulmonary septum, and muscular septum. Muscular defects are the second most common type of defects in the ventricular septum. These can be single or multiple and can be located anywhere along the muscular portion of the septum. Multiple muscular defects in close proximity or that may coalesce together may be referred to as "Swiss cheese" defects. Defects in the inlet ventricular septum are associated with endocardial cushion defects. These result from failure of fusion of the medial endocardial cushions and formation of the inlet ventricular septum. Outlet defects may also be referred to as conal, supracristal, subarterial or doubly committed defects. These are located in the right ventricular outflow tract immediately below the pulmonary valve. When examined from the left ventricular aspect, these defects lie just below the right coronary cusp. This anatomic relationship can lead to aortic valve prolapse or herniation into the defect and associated aortic insufficiency.

Defects of conotruncal development and semilunar valve formation

Defects of conotruncal development and semilunar valve formation account for a large number of congenital heart defects [50, 51]. These include truncus arteriosus, *d*-transposition of the great arteries, tetralogy of Fallot, and aortopulmonary window. Several of these conotruncal malformations have been linked to abnormal aortopulmonary septation under the influence of the neural crest [29,52,53].

Truncus arteriosus results from failed formation of the truncal ridges and aorticopulmonary septum. A single aorticopulmonary trunk with underlying ventricular septal defect gives rise to the pulmonary, coronary, and systemic circulations [54]. Several subtypes of this anomaly exist with variations based on the anatomic origin of the pulmonary arteries and aortic arch abnormalities.

Failure of spiral septation of the aorticopulmonary septum can result in several congenital cardiac defects. Both transposition of the great arteries and tetralogy of Fallot can be explained by this mechanism. Transposition of the great vessels is thought to be the result of failed spiral septation. This results in the pulmonary artery arising from the posterior left ventricle and the aorta originating from the anterior right ventricle [55]. Tetralogy of Fallot results from unequal partitioning of the aorta and pulmonary artery. Anterior deviation of the conal septum results in a diminutive right ventricular outflow tract, overriding aorta, and secondary right ventricular hypertrophy [56]. Failure of fusion of the conal septum with the bulbus cordis results in the ventricular level communication seen in this defect. Pulmonary atresia may be considered the most severe form of tetralogy. Extreme anterior deviation of the aorticopulmonary septum and conal septum in this case results in lack of a pulmonary outflow tract.

An aortopulmonary window results from failed aorticopulmonary septation. In this defect there is a communication between the aorta and pulmonary arteries, but an intact interventricular septum [57].

Defects in aortic arch development

Normal aortic arch development relies on orchestrated development and regression of the aortic arches. Failure of normal development or regression can lead to a number of aortic arch anomalies.

Two developmental events that can result in aortic arch obstruction include hypoplasia of the arch and the presence of ductal tissue in the aorta at its site of insertion.

The aortic arch is derived proximally from the aortic sac, distally from the fourth aortic arch, and at the isthmus from the fourth and sixth aortic arches. Failure of development of each of these segments can lead to aortic arch hypoplasia or interruption. Although the specific level of arch obstruction is variable among these lesions, perfusion to the lower body in often ductal dependent. Therefore, ductal constriction prior to the recognition of the severe pathology can be life threatening.

Aortic arch anomalies can result in a vascular ring, double aortic arch, or pulmonary artery sling [58]. These variations in the arrangement of the great arteries can be further explained by considering the embryologic development of the aortic arch and pulmonary arteries, facilitated by the hypothetical Edwards diagram discussed previously of this chapter (Figure 4.6).

The embryonic aortic arches encircle the embryonic foregut (trachea and esophagus). Normal development results in regression of the right sixth aortic arch, and involution of the right dorsal aorta, thus avoiding formation of a vascular ring. Failure of this normal development or regression can lead to variations in pathologic anatomy that result in vascular encirclement or compression of the trachea and/or esophagus, in some cases associated to obstructive symptoms.

Selected defects in aortic arch development are listed in Table 4.2. We initiate this discussion reviewing variants associated with a left aortic arch. The formation of a left aortic arch with an aberrant or retroesophageal subclavian artery (branching pattern: right carotid, left carotid, left subclavian, and anomalous right subclavian artery) is the result of abnormal regression of the right fourth aortic arch. This is the most common arch variant occurring in 0.5% of the general population. The right sixth aortic arch regresses normally in this defect, and no vascular ring is formed. In contrast, a left aortic arch with retroesophageal diverticulum of Kommerell also has abnormal regression of the right fourth aortic arch, but persistence of the right sixth aortic arch as the right ligamentum arteriosum. This defect results in a vascular ring encircling the trachea and esophagus.

The formation of a right aortic arch with mirror image branching is the result of regression of the left dorsal aorta. The branching pattern in this case is as follows: first arch vessel, left innominate artery that branches into left subclavian and left carotid arteries; second vessel, right carotid artery; and third vessel, right subclavian artery. This variant is almost invariably associated with intracardiac disease.

A right aortic arch with retroesophageal diverticulum of Kommerell results from regression of the fourth aortic arch, persistence of the left sixth arch as the ligamentum arteriosus and of the left dorsal aorta. This results in a vascular ring. A right aortic arch with aberrant subclavian

Table 4.2 Aortic arch Anomalies

Anomaly	Cause
Left aortic arch with retroesophageal right subclavian artery (aberrant right subclavian artery)	Absence of right fourth aortic arch
Left aortic arch with retroesophageal diverticulum of Kommerell	Absence of right fourth aortic arch, persistence of right sixth arch (right ligamentum arteriosum)
Right aortic arch with mirror image branching	Absence of left dorsal aorta
Right aortic arch with diverticulum of Kommerell	Absence of left fourth aortic arch, persistence of left sixth arch (left ligamentum arteriosum)
Right aortic arch with retroesophageal left subclavian artery (aberrant left subclavian artery)	Absence of the left fourth and sixth aortic arches
Double aortic arch	Persistence of right and left fourth aortic arches

artery (branching sequence: left carotid, right carotid, right subclavian, and anomalous left subclavian artery) can be accounted for by the regression of the left fourth and sixth aortic arches. The absence of the left sixth arch, or ductal arch, prevents formation of a vascular ring. Many of these patients have conotruncal malformations. The formation of a double aortic arch is the result of persistence of both the right and fourth aortic arches. The presence of both arches results in a vascular ring. Frequently the left arch is atretic. This anomaly is associated with symptomatology in infancy related to tracheal and esophageal compression.

A cervical aortic arch occurs when the arch extends into the soft tissues of the neck, above the level of the clavicle. This rare anomaly has been also referred to as "high aortic arch." Various arrangements including normal and anomalous arch branching patterns, in addition to pathology such as aortic arch obstruction, have been reported in affected patients. A number of embryologic explanations (atresia of the fourth primitive aortic arch associated with persistence of the third arch, failure of normal caudal aortic arch migration) have been proposed to account for the various subtypes.

Defects in coronary artery development

Normal coronary arteries arise from epicardial blood islands in the sulci of the developing heart. These in turn connect to the sinuses of valsalva and form capillary networks with veins connected to the coronary sinus. Buds from the pulmonary arteries also connect to the coronary arteries, but regress during normal development.

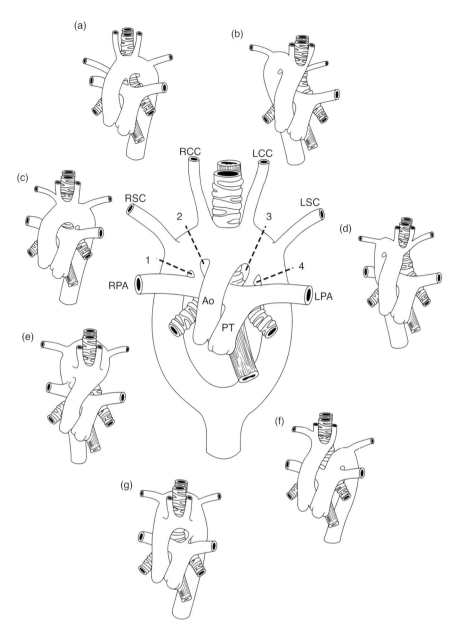

Figure 4.6 Hypothetical double aortic arch. During development, interruptions may occur at various sites (1–4), which give rise to different anatomic patterns of arch anatomy. If interruption occurs at site 1, a normal left aortic arch forms (a). If interruption occurs at site 4, a right aortic arch with mirror image branching is formed (d). Interruption at site 2 and 3 result in a left aortic arch with aberrant right subclavian artery (a) or right aortic arch with aberrant left subclavian artery (b), respectively. If neither arch is interrupted, double aortic arch with either a right descending aorta (e) or left descending aorta (g) results. Two interruptions may occur in the hypothetical double aortic arch, giving rise to interruption of the aortic arch. One example is shown (f) in which the double arches were interrupted at sites 1 and 3, resulting in aortic interruption distal to the left carotid artery. Ao, aorta; LCC, left common carotid artery; LPA, left pulmonary artery; LSC, left subclavian artery; PT, pulmonary trunk; RCC, right common carotid artery; RPA, right pulmonary artery; RSC, right subclavian artery (Reprinted with permission from Reference [59])

Persistence of this pulmonary connection can lead to anomalous origin of the left coronary artery from the pulmonary artery [60]. Affected children become symptomatic as the pulmonary vascular resistance declines following birth. The diminished perfusion pressure of the left coronary artery accounts for myocardial ischemia and systolic functional impairment.

Defects of the venous system

Defects of the superior and inferior vena cava rarely occur [61]. Among these defects, persistence of the left superior vena cava draining into the coronary sinus is most common. This occurs secondary to persistence of the left anterior and common cardinal veins. Interruption of the inferior vena cava with azygous and hemiazygous continuation of flow into the right atrium may be seen, most frequently in the setting of complex congenital heart disease. This is thought to be secondary to failure of formation of the hepatic portion of the inferior vena cava.

Defects in pulmonary venous drainage

During the early stages of human development, the vascular plexus of the foregut, also known as the splanchnic plexus, which forms the pulmonary vasculature, has no direct connection to the heart. Defective development or regression of the pulmonary venous plexus and its connection to the primordial or common pulmonary vein can lead to anomalous pulmonary venous connections and drainage.

Anomalous pulmonary venous drainage can occur in a total or partial manner [16]. In total anomalous pulmonary venous connection, the pulmonary veins drain into the right atrium or other venous structures. In partial pulmonary venous drainage, at least one vein empties normally into the left atrium with one or more pulmonary veins draining elsewhere. In some instances, mixed anomalous drainage may be present, with pulmonary venous connection to various sites.

Nomenclature and segmental analysis of congenital cardiac defects

Nomenclature in congenital and pediatric cardiology varies widely. Several names may be used to refer to the same anatomic structure, pathologic finding or lesion. This variability may be quite confusing.

Recent efforts at standardization of nomenclature in pediatric and congenital heart disease by the Nomenclature Working Group have resulted in the development of the International Pediatric and Congenital Cardiac Code (IPCCC) [62]. The objective of this endeavor has been to provide an all-inclusive, international cohesive and comprehensive system of pediatric cardiovascular and congenital heart disease nomenclature (www.ipccc.net). This should allow for a number of benefits including enhanced communication among health care providers, facilitation of patient care, teaching, case reporting, data collection and analysis, multicenter assessment of clinical outcomes, risk stratification, and others.

For the purpose of the discussion that follows, a segmental approach to nomenclature of congenital heart disease is used. This approach, developed by Van Praagh and colleagues, documents the structure of the cardiac components and their relations. While the majority of congenital heart defects can be explained by this segmental classification scheme, others such as heterotaxy syndromes (a condition characterized by abnormal arrangement of organs or viscera) are often more difficult to precisely define. A discussion of common terminology and a brief introduction to the segmental approach to congenital heart disease follows.

Cardiac position

Cardiac positioning in the thoracic cavity refers to location of the cardiac mass and direction of the apex. The alignment from the base to the apex of the heart is used to determine the cardiac position within the thorax. Levocardia describes a heart with its cardiac apex pointing to the left side of the chest. A mesocardic heart has its cardiac apex pointing straight inferiorly, whereas a dextrocardia refers to a heart with its apex pointing to the right. The term mirror image dextrocardia describes a dextrocardic heart in the setting of situs inversus (see below).

Displacement of the heart into the right or left thoracic cavity is described as dextropositioning or levopositioning, respectively. This type of positioning is determined regardless of the hearts base to apical axis orientation. In this way a levocardic heart may be dextropositioned. Mesopositioning refers to a heart positioned in the midline of the chest.

Sequential segmental analysis

A sequential segmental approach to classifying congenital heart defects was initially proposed by Van Praagh and subsequently endorsed by others. The segmental approach to congenital heart disease documents the anatomy of the heart in terms of three mayor components (the atria chambers, the ventricles, and arterial trunks) and evaluates their relationship to each other [63–66]. A three-letter code, depicted in brackets, is utilized to describe the atrial, ventricular, and arterial segments.

The term situs refers to the normal placement of an organ in the plane of bilateral symmetry. The situs of an organ may be defined as solitus (S), inversus (I), or ambiguous (A). As the atrial situs rarely differs from the visceral situs, one may refer to this as visceroatrial situs.

Atrial segment

The atrial segment of the heart is divided into the right and left atria. The atrial relationship may be identified by the unique right and left atrial morphology. However, the visceral relationship may assist in identifying the atrial relationship as well.

Atrial morphology is used to identify the atrial situs. The right atrium receives connections with the superior and inferior vena cava, coronary sinus, and contains a smooth sinusal portion between the crista terminalis and atrial septum. The trabecular portion of the right atrium extends from the crista terminalis to the base of the atrial appendage. This appendage is broad based with a blunt tip. In contrast, the left atrium is smooth and receives pulmonary venous drainage. The left atrial appendage is narrow, and fingerlike. The systemic and pulmonary venous drainage may be anomalous, and cannot be relied upon to definitively determine atrial morphology. Thus, the atrial appendages are primarily used to define atrial morphology [67].

Visceral anatomy may be used to aid in defining the atrial morphology. The atrial situs usually follows that of the viscera. In visceral situs solitus, the trilobed right lung with its eparterial bronchial pattern and liver are right sided [68]. The bilobed left lung with its hyparterial bronchial pattern and spleen are left sided. The normal right mainstem bronchus has a shorter more vertical orientation (eparterial), whereas the normal left mainstem bronchus is longer and more horizontal in orientation (hyparterial). In situs inversus, the trilobed right lung and the major lobe of the liver are left sided, whereas the spleen and stomach are right sided. This is the mirror image of the normal relationship. In situs ambiguus, there is a tendency toward duplication of either right-sided or left-sided structures. In bilateral right sidedness, or right visceroatrial isomerism, both atria lungs and bronchi are morphologically right sided. Conversely in bilateral left sidedness, or left visceroatrial isomerism, both atria lungs and bronchi are morphologically left sided. It must be emphasized that organ location or situs can differ, and discordance of the situs of the different organs can exist. Visceroatrial situs ambiguous may be seen in children with heterotaxy syndrome.

Ventricular segment

Analysis of the ventricular segment includes the location of the ventricles, and the relative spatial relationship to the atria. Ventricular looping, as previously discussed, can result in either d-looped or l-looped ventricles. In the normal d-loop, the morphologic right ventricle is right sided, whereas in l-loop the morphologic right ventricle is left sided. l-Looped ventricles may also be referred to as ventricular inversion.

Ventricular morphology is used to identify the location of the ventricles. The right ventricle is characterized by a trileaflet atrioventricular valve (tricuspid valve), consisting of a septal, anterosuperior, and posterior leaflet. The tricuspid valve is displaced inferiorly relative to the mitral valve, and is termed septophillic secondary to its septal leaflet attachments that connect to the interventricular septum. The densely trabeculated right ventricle consists of several papillary muscles. The pulmonary valve rests on this muscular infundibulum above the tricuspid valve. The left ventricle is characterized by a bileaflet atrioventricular valve (mitral valve), consisting of anterior and posterior leaflets. The left ventricle is characterized by its smooth and contains two prominent papillary muscles. The anterolateral and posteromedial papillary muscles have chordal attachments to both the anterior and posterior mitral valve leaflets. The aortic valve and mitral valve share fibrous continuity in the normal heart.

In a biventricular heart, the position of the atria relative to the ventricles may be described as concordant, or discordant. A concordant relationship exists when the right atrium connects to the right ventricle. This is obviously the case of the normal heart. An example of this also exists in mirror image dextrocardia. In this case, the cardiac apex is rightward and the atrioventricular relationship is concordant. In contrast, a discordant relationship is present when the right atrium connects to the left ventricle. In isolated l-looped ventricles (isolated ventricular inversion), the atrioventricular relationship is discordant. In children with single ventricle, the atrioventricular relationship may differ.

Arterial segment

Analysis of the arterial segment includes the relationship of the great arteries to each other, and relative to the ventricles. In normally related great arteries, the pulmonary artery is anterior and courses leftward prior to bifurcating into the left and right branches. The aorta is rightward and posterior with respect to the pulmonary artery, giving rise to the coronary arteries, head and neck vessels.

The ventriculoarterial connection may be described as concordant, discordant, double outlet, or single outlet. In ventriculoarterial concordance, the pulmonary artery arises from the right ventricle and the aorta from the left ventricle. In ventriculoarterial discordance, the pulmonary artery arises from the left ventricle and the aorta from the right ventricle. The term double outlet is used when both great arteries arise from one ventricle, or one vessel arises from the ventricle and the second overrides the septum by over 50%. Other criteria include the lack of fibrous continuity between the mitral valve and adjacent semilunar valve. In a single outlet relationship, a single great artery arises from the ventricle, and the other is atretic. Examples of this include pulmonary atresia and aortic atresia.

Analysis of the spatial relationship of the aorta relative to the pulmonary artery is important. In the normal relationship, the pulmonary valve sits anterior and leftward relative to the aortic valve. In d-transposition of the great arteries, the aortic valve is anterior and rightward of the pulmonary valve. In a similar fashion, in l-transposition the aortic valve is seated anterior and leftward of the pulmonary valve. Other abnormal spatial relationships may be referred to as side-by-side arrangements and malpositions.

In summary, the segmental approach to congenital heart disease nomenclature can be used to describe the majority of defects. The heart can be divided into atrial, ventricular, and great vessel segments. These three cardiac segments can be represented in a simplified three-letter system. Atrial segments are represented by S (solitus), I (inversus), and A (ambiguous). Ventricular segments are represented by D (d-looping) and L (l-looping). Arterial segments are represented by S (solitus), D (d-transposition), and L (l-transposition). Thus, the normal heart with atrial situs solitus, d-looped ventricles, and arterial situs solitus would be represented as {S, D, S}. Similarly, *d*-transposition of the great arteries would be referred to as {S, D, D}.

Summary

Caring for patients with structural malformations is an important aspect of cardiovascular anesthesia practice, representing the main focus for those who specialize in the case of children with heart disease. The spectrum of pathology in congenital heart disease ranges widely between relatively simple to complex defects. The ability to provide optimal care to these patients relies to a significant extent upon an understanding of the anatomic abnormalities, altered pathophysiology, and hemodynamic consequences of the disease.

This chapter has presented basic concepts in normal cardiac embryology and development, as a basis for the understanding of the complexity of events that take place during normal cardiac morphogenesis and the likely alterations that may result in the various congenital cardiac malformations. It is hoped that this overview of normal and altered cardiovascular development, in addition to the discussion regarding congenital heart disease nomenclature, will enhance the overall knowledge of the practicing anesthesiologist on the subject.

References

1. Anderson PA (1995) The molecular genetics of cardiovascular disease. Curr Opin Cardiol 10:33–43.
2. Benson DW, Basson CT, MacRae CA (1996) New understandings in the genetics of congenital heart disease. Curr Opin Pediatr 8:505–511.
3. Burn J, Goodship J (1996) Developmental genetics of the heart. Curr Opin Genet Dev 6:322–325.
4. Olson EN, Srivastava D (1996) Molecular pathways controlling heart development. Science 272:671–676.
5. Srivastava D (2001) Genetic assembly of the heart: implications for congenital heart disease. Annu Rev Physiol 63:451–469.
6. Sander TL, Klinkner DB, Tomita-Mitchell A, et al. (2006) Molecular and cellular basis of congenital heart disease. Pediatr Clin North Am 53:989–1009.
7. Poelmann RE, Gittenberger-de Groot AC (2008) Cardiac development. Sci World J 8:855–858.
8. Larsen WJ, Sherman LS, Potter SS, et al. (2008) Human Embryology. Churchill Livingstone, Philadelphia.
9. Gittenberger-de Groot AC, Bartelings MM, DeRuiter MC (1995) Overview: cardiac morphogenesis. In: Clark EB, Markwarld RR, Takao A (eds) Developmental Mechanisms of Heart Disease. Futura, Mount Kisco, New York, pp. 157–169.
10. Valdes-Cruz LM, Cayre RO (1999) Embryologic development of the heart and great vessels. In: Valdes-Cruz LM, Cayre RO (eds) Echocardiographic Diagnosis of Congenital Heart Disease: An Embryologic and Anatomic Approach. Lippincott-Raven Publishers, Philadelphia, p. 15.
11. Abdulla R, Blew GA, Holterman MJ (2004) Cardiovascular embryology. Pediatr Cardiol 25:191–200.
12. Kirby ML (2007) Cardiac Development. Oxford University Press, New York.
13. Moore KL, Persaud TVN (2007) The Developing Human: Clinically Oriented Embryology, 8th edn. Saunders Publishing, Philadelphia.
14. Van Praagh R, Weinberg PM, Matsuoka R, et al. (1983) Malpositions of the heart. In: Adams FH, Emmanouilides GC (eds) Heart Disease in Infants, Children, and Adolescents, 3rd edn. Williams and Wilkins, Baltimore.
15. Markwald RR (1995) Overview: formation and early morphogenesis of the primitive heart tube. In: Clark EB, Markwald RR, Takao A (eds) Developmental Mechanisms of Heart Disease. Futura Publishing, Armonk, New York, pp. 149–155.
16. Geva T, Van Praagh S (2008) Anomalies of the pulmonary veins. In: Allen HD, Driscoll DJ, Shaddy RE, Feltes TF (eds) Moss and Adams' Heart Disease in Infants, Children and Adolescents: Including the Fetus and Young Adult, 7th edn. Lippincott Williams & Wilkins, Philadelphia, pp. 761–792.
17. Edwards JE (1953) Pathologic and developmental considerations in anomalous pulmonary venous connection. Proc Staff Meet Mayo Clin 28:441–452.
18. Neill CA (1956) Development of the pulmonary veins; with reference to the embryology of anomalies of pulmonary venous return. Pediatrics 18:880–887.
19. Lucas RVJ, Anderson RC, Amplatz K, et al. (1963) Congenital causes of pulmonary venous obstruction. Pediatr Clin North Am 10:781–836.
20. De la Cruz MV, Gimenez-Ribotta M, Saravalli O, et al. (1983) The contribution of the inferior endocardial cushion of the atrioventricular canal to cardiac septation and to the development of the atrioventricular valves: study in the chick embryo. Am J Anat 166:63–72.
21. Thompson RP, Losada Cabrera MA, Fitzharris TP (1989) Embryology of the cardiac cushion tissue. In: Aranega A, Pexieder T (eds) Correlations between Experimental Cardiac Embryology and Teratology and Congenital Cardiac Defects. Universidad de Granada, Granada, Spain, pp. 147–169.
22. Van Mierop, LH, Alley RD, Kausel HW, et al. (1962) The anatomy and embryology of endocardial cushion defects. J Thorac Cardiovasc Surg 43:71–83.
23. Bartelings MM, Wenink AC, Gittenberger-De Groot AC, et al. (1986) Contribution of the aortopulmonary septum to the muscular outlet septum in the human heart. Acta Morphol Neerl Scand 24:181–192.
24. Lamers WH, Wessels A, Verbeek FJ, et al. (1992) New findings concerning ventricular septation in the human heart. Implications for maldevelopment. Circulation 86:1194–1205.
25. De la Cruz MV, Sanchez Gomez C, Arteaga MM, et al. (1977) Experimental study of the development of the truncus and the conus in the chick embryo. J Anat 123:661–686.
26. Bockman DE, Redmond ME, Waldo K, et al. (1987) Effect of neural crest ablation on development of the heart and arch arteries in the chick. Am J Anat 180:332–341.

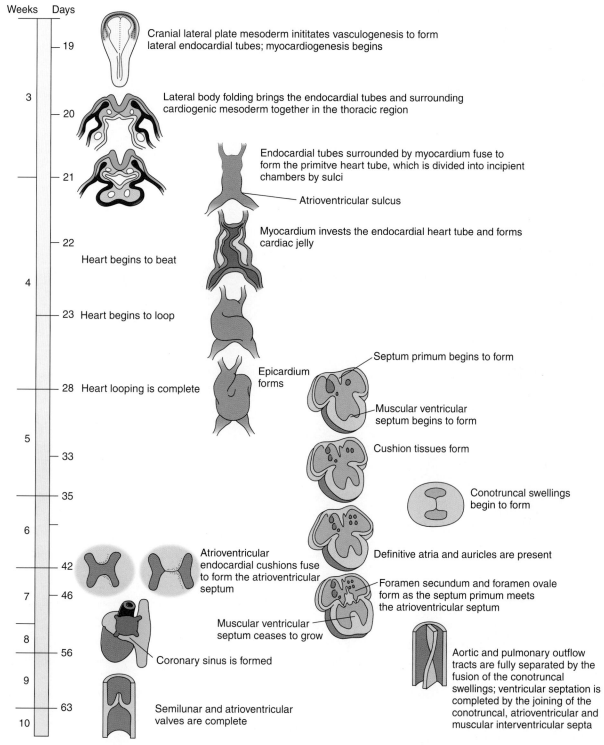

Weeks	Days	
3	19	Cranial lateral plate mesoderm inititates vasculogenesis to form lateral endocardial tubes; myocardiogenesis begins
	20	Lateral body folding brings the endocardial tubes and surrounding cardiogenic mesoderm together in the thoracic region
4	21	Endocardial tubes surrounded by myocardium fuse to form the primitve heart tube, which is divided into incipient chambers by sulci
		Atrioventricular sulcus
	22	Myocardium invests the endocardial heart tube and forms cardiac jelly
		Heart begins to beat
	23	Heart begins to loop
	28	Heart looping is complete
5	33	
	35	
6		
7	42	
	46	
8	56	
9		
10	63	

Epicardium forms

Septum primum begins to form

Muscular ventricular septum begins to form

Cushion tissues form

Conotruncal swellings begin to form

Atrioventricular endocardial cushions fuse to form the atrioventricular septum

Definitive atria and auricles are present

Foramen secundum and foramen ovale form as the septum primum meets the atrioventricular septum

Muscular ventricular septum ceases to grow

Coronary sinus is formed

Aortic and pulmonary outflow tracts are fully separated by the fusion of the conotruncal swellings; ventricular septation is completed by the joining of the conotruncal, atrioventricular and muscular interventricular septa

Semilunar and atrioventricular valves are complete

Plate 4.1 Timeline of the formation of the heart (Reprinted with modifications from Reference [8], modified with permission)

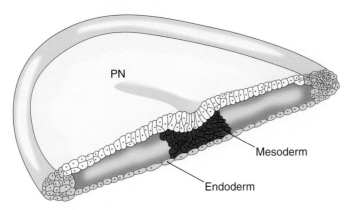

Plate 4.2 Cardiogenic mesoderm. The mesodemal layer is depicted as it emerges from the primitive streak during gastrulation. This layer gives rise to the cardiac progenitor cells. PN, primitive node (Reprinted with modifications from Reference [8], modified with permission)

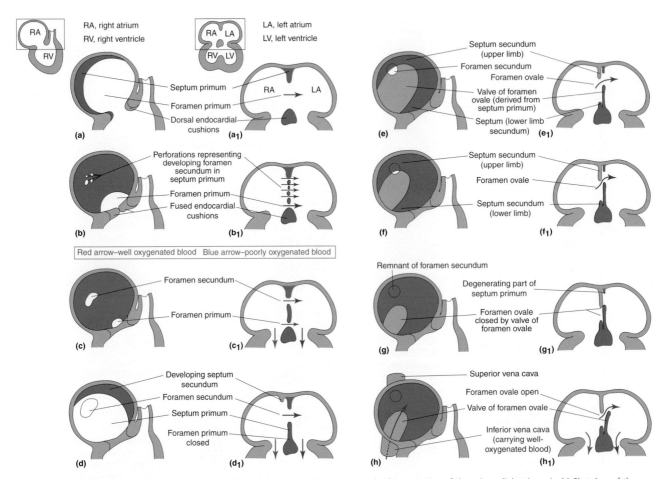

Plate 4.3 Atrial Septation. Diagrammatic representation of the progressive stages involved in septation of the primordial atrium. (a–h) Sketches of the developing interatrial septum as viewed from the right side. (a₁–h₁) coronal sections of the interatrial septum. As the septum secundum extends inferiorly, it overlaps the opening in the septum primum (foramen secundum). (g₁ and h₁) depicts the valve of the oval foramen. When right atrial pressure exceeds that in the left atrium, blood moves from the right to the left side of the heart. When pressures are equal or higher in the left atrium, the flap closes (h₁) (Reprinted with permission from Reference [13])

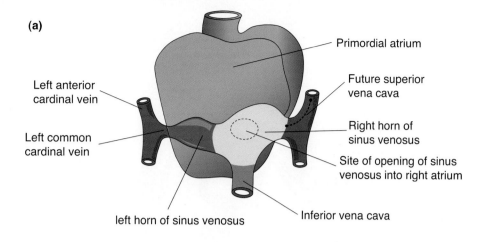

(a)

Primordial atrium

Future superior vena cava

Right horn of sinus venosus

Site of opening of sinus venosus into right atrium

Left anterior cardinal vein

Left common cardinal vein

left horn of sinus venosus

Inferior vena cava

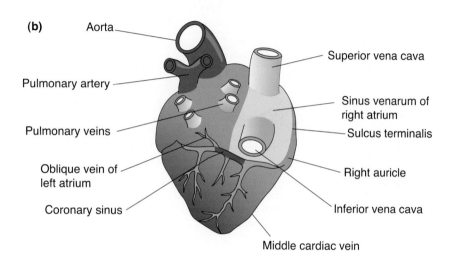

(b)

Aorta

Pulmonary artery

Pulmonary veins

Oblique vein of left atrium

Coronary sinus

Superior vena cava

Sinus venarum of right atrium

Sulcus terminalis

Right auricle

Inferior vena cava

Middle cardiac vein

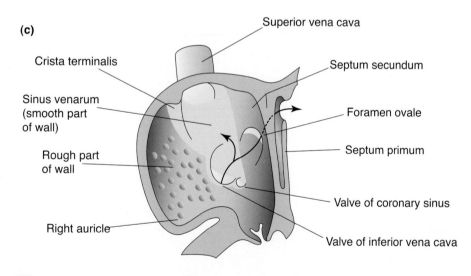

(c)

Superior vena cava

Crista terminalis

Sinus venarum (smooth part of wall)

Rough part of wall

Right auricle

Septum secundum

Foramen ovale

Septum primum

Valve of coronary sinus

Valve of inferior vena cava

■ Left horn of sinus venosus   □ Right horn of sinus venosus

Plate 4.4 Fate of the sinus venosus. (a) Diagrammatic illustration of dorsal view of the heart (approximately 26 days) demonstrating the primordial atrium and sinus venosus. (b) Dorsal view at 8 weeks after incorporation of the right sinus horn into right atrium. The left sinus horn has become the coronary sinus. (c) Internal view of the fetal right atrium showing (i) the smooth part of the wall of the right atrium (sinus venarum) derived from the right sinus horn and (ii) the crista terminalis and the valves of the inferior vena cava and coronary sinus derived from the right sinuatrial valve. The primordial right atrium becomes the right auricle, a conical muscular pouch (Reprinted with permission from Reference [13])

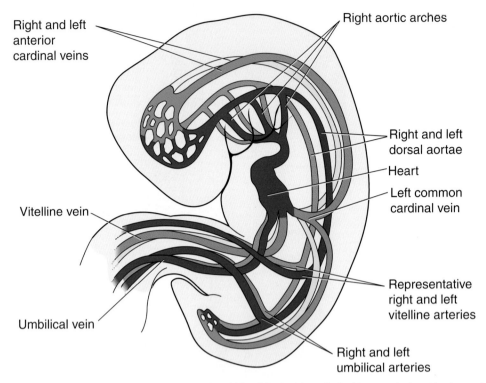

Right and left
anterior
cardinal veins

Right aortic arches

Right and left
dorsal aortae

Heart

Left common
cardinal vein

Vitelline vein

Representative
right and left
vitelline arteries

Umbilical vein

Right and left
umbilical arteries

Plate 4.5 Schematic depiction of the embryonic vascular system in the middle of the fourth week. At this stage, the heart has begun to beat and circulate blood. The outflow tract is now connected to four pairs of aortic arches and the paired dorsal aortae that circulate blood to the head and trunk. Three pairs of veins, umbilical, vitelline, and cardinal veins, deliver blood to the inflow region of the heart (Reprinted with permission from Reference [8])

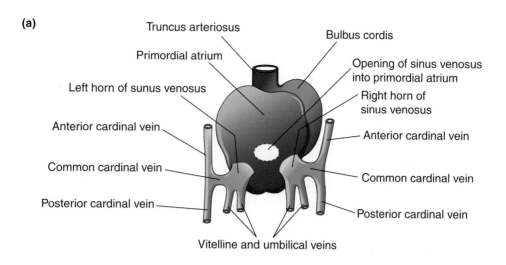

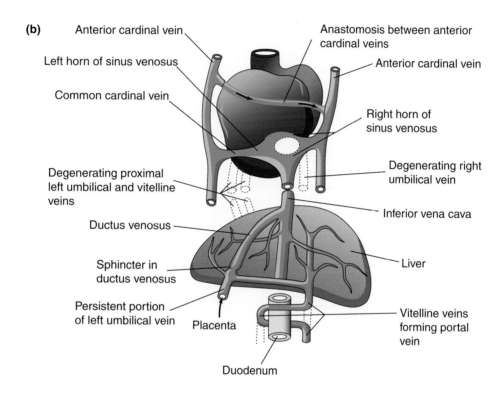

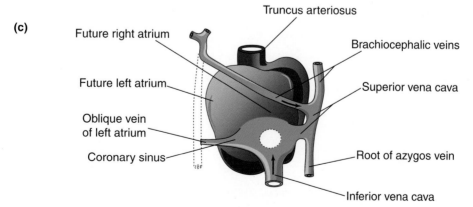

Plate 4.6 Dorsal views of the developing heart. (a) During the fourth week (approximately 24 days), showing the primordial atrium, sinus venousus, and venous drainage. (b) At 7 weeks, illustrating the enlarged right sinus horn and venous circulation through the liver (organs are not drawn to scale). (c) At 8 weeks, indicating the adult derivatives of the cardinal veins (Reprinted with permission from Reference [13])

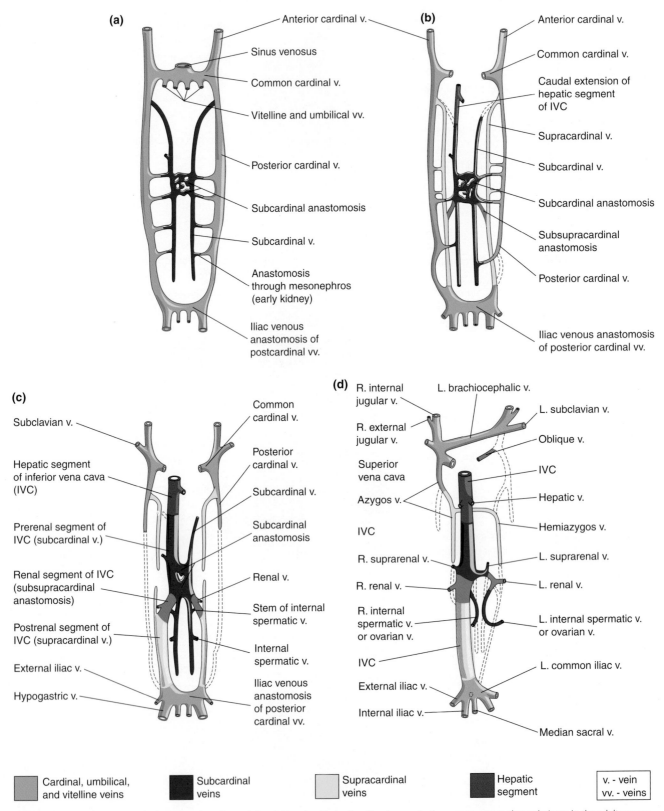

Plate 4.7 Primordial veins in the human embryo (ventral views). Drawing illustrating the changes in the venous system that culminate in the adult venous pattern. Initially, three systems of veins are present: the umbilical veins from the chorion, the vitelline veins from the umbilical vesicle (yolk sac), and the cardinal veins from the body of the embryo. Subsequently, the subcardinal veins appear, and finally the supracardinal veins develop. (a) At 6 weeks. (b) At 7 weeks. (c) At 8 weeks. (d) Adult (Reprinted with permission from Reference [13])

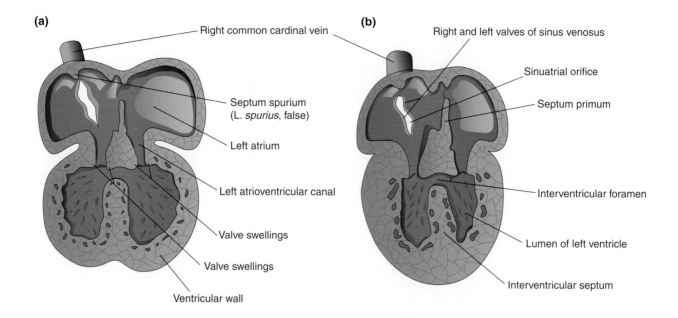

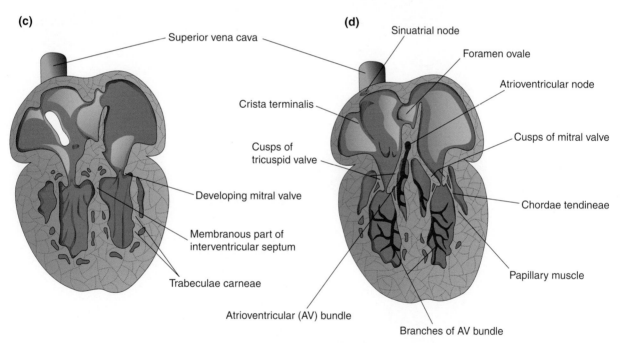

(a)

Right common cardinal vein

Septum spurium
(L. *spurius*, false)

Left atrium

Left atrioventricular canal

Valve swellings

Valve swellings

Ventricular wall

(b)

Right and left valves of sinus venosus

Sinuatrial orifice

Septum primum

Interventricular foramen

Lumen of left ventricle

Interventricular septum

(c)

Superior vena cava

Crista terminalis

Cusps of
tricuspid valve

Developing mitral valve

Membranous part of
interventricular septum

Trabeculae carneae

Atrioventricular (AV) bundle

(d)

Sinuatrial node

Foramen ovale

Atrioventricular node

Cusps of mitral valve

Chordae tendineae

Papillary muscle

Branches of AV bundle

Plate 4.8 Schematic sections of the heart illustrating successive stages in the development of the atrioventricular valves, tendinous cords, and papillary muscles. (a) At 5 weeks. (b) At 6 weeks. (c) At 7 weeks. (d) At 20 weeks (Reprinted with permission from Reference [13])

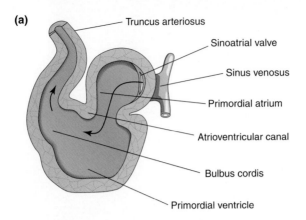

(a)
- Truncus arteriosus
- Sinoatrial valve
- Sinus venosus
- Primordial atrium
- Atrioventricular canal
- Bulbus cordis
- Primordial ventricle

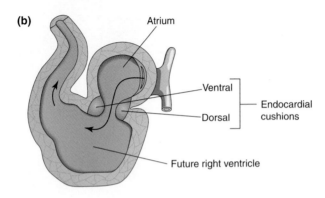

(b)
- Atrium
- Ventral
- Dorsal
- Endocardial cushions
- Future right ventricle

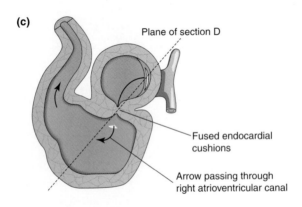

(c)
- Plane of section D
- Fused endocardial cushions
- Arrow passing through right atrioventricular canal

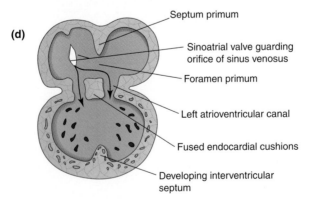

(d)
- Septum primum
- Sinoatrial valve guarding orifice of sinus venosus
- Foramen primum
- Left atrioventricular canal
- Fused endocardial cushions
- Developing interventricular septum

Plate 4.9 Sagittal sections of the primordial heart during the fourth and fifth weeks illustrating blood flow through the heart and division of the atrioventricular canal. (a–c) The *arrows* are passing through the sinuatrial orifice. (d) Coronal section of the heart at the plane shown in (c). Note that the interatrial and interventricular septa have started to develop (Reprinted with permission from Reference [13])

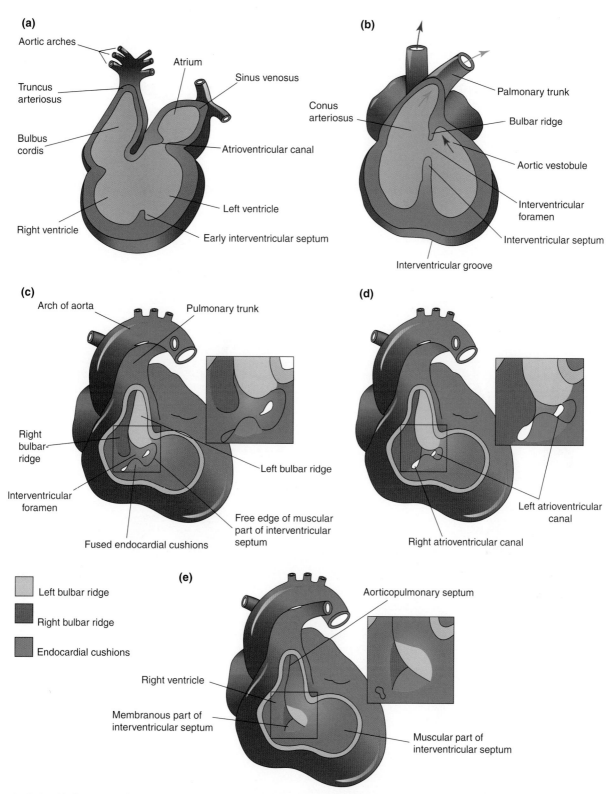

(a)
Aortic arches
Truncus arteriosus
Bulbus cordis
Right ventricle
Atrium
Sinus venosus
Atrioventricular canal
Left ventricle
Early interventricular septum

(b)
Conus arteriosus
Palmonary trunk
Bulbar ridge
Aortic vestobule
Interventricular foramen
Interventricular septum
Interventricular groove

(c)
Arch of aorta
Pulmonary trunk
Right bulbar ridge
Left bulbar ridge
Interventricular foramen
Free edge of muscular part of interventricular septum
Fused endocardial cushions

(d)
Left atrioventricular canal
Right atrioventricular canal

Left bulbar ridge
Right bulbar ridge
Endocardial cushions

(e)
Aorticopulmonary septum
Right ventricle
Membranous part of interventricular septum
Muscular part of interventricular septum

Plate 4.10 Graphic illustrations of the incorporation of the bulbus cordis into the ventricles and partitioning of the bubus cordis and truncus arteriosus. (a) Sagittal section at 5 weeks showing the bulbus cordis as one of the segments of the primordial heart. The primordial interventricular septum is noted. (b) Schematic coronal section at 6 weeks, after the bulbus cordis has been incorporated into the ventricles to become the conus arteriosus (infundibulum) of the right ventricle and the aortic vestibule of the left ventricle. The arrow indicates the direction of blood flow. The interventricular septum and interventricular foramen are depicted. (c–e) Schematic representation of closure of the interventricular foramen and formation of the membranous portion of the interventricular septum. The walls of the truncus arteriosus, bulbus cordis, and right ventricle have been removed. (c) At 5 weeks, showing the bulbar ridges and fused endocardial cushions. (d) At 6 weeks, showing how proliferation of subendocardial tissue diminishes the interventricular foramen. (e) At 7 weeks, showing the fused bulbar ridges, the membranous region of the interventricular septum formed by extensions of tissue from the right side of the endocardial cushions, and closure of the interventricular foramen (Reprinted with permission from Reference [13])

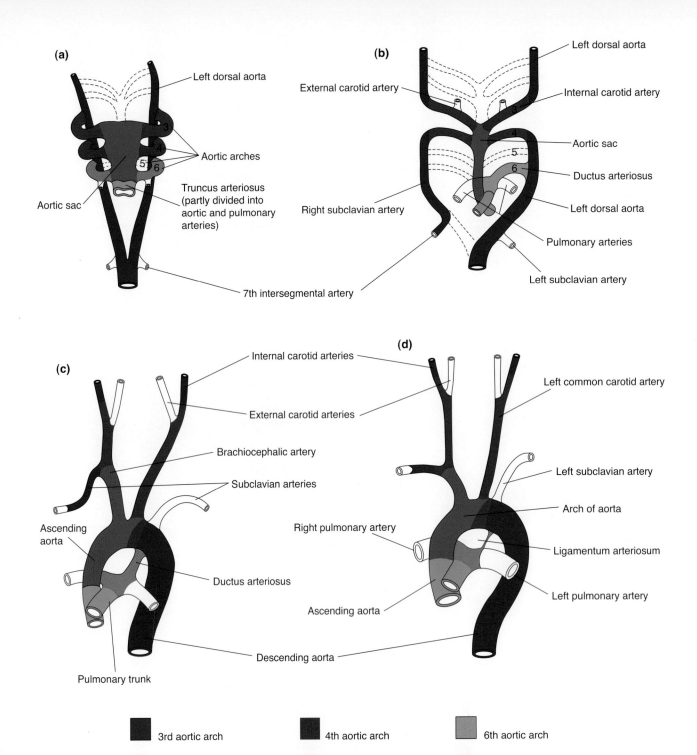

Plate 4.11 Graphical representation of the arterial changes that result during transformation of the truncus arteriosus, aortic sac, pharyngeal arch arteries, and dorsal aortas into the adult arterial pattern. (Vessels not colored are not derived from these structures.) (a) Pharyngeal arch arteries at 6 weeks; by this stage, the first two pairs of the arteries have largely disappeared. (b) Pharyngeal arch arteries at 7 weeks; the parts of the dorsal aortas and pharyngeal arch arteries that normally disappear are indicated with broken lines. (c) Arterial arrangement at 8 weeks. (d) Sketch of the arterial vessels of a 6-month-old infant. Note that the ascending aorta and pulmonary arteries are considerably smaller in (c) than in (d). This represents the relative flow through these vessels at the different stages of development. The ductus arteriosus normally becomes functionally closed with in the first few days after birth, eventually becoming the ligamentum arteriosum, as shown in (d) (Reprinted with permission from Reference [13])

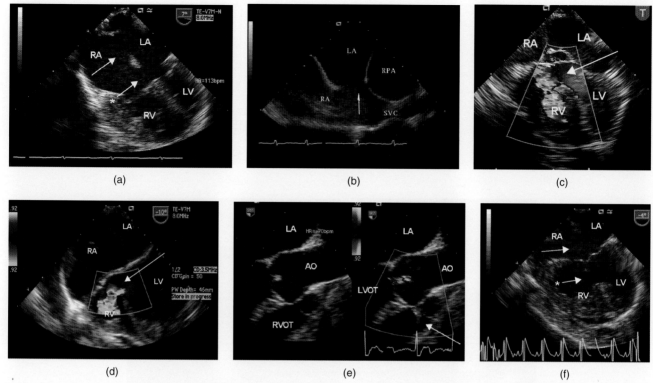

Plate 11.1 Representative echocardiographic images of septal defects. (a) Secundum and primum atrial septal defects: four-chamber view demonstrating secundum (*arrow*) and primum atrial septal defects (*arrow with asterisk*). (b) Sinus venosus atrial septal defect: bicaval view displaying sinus venosus defect at entrance of superior vena cava into the right atrium. A dilated tight pulmonary artery is seen as it courses behind the superior vena cava.
(c) Perimembranous ventricular septal defect: color flow Doppler depicts left-to-right shunting through a defect in the membranous septum (*arrow*). (d) Inlet ventricular septal defect: color flow Doppler displays large amount of ventricular level shunting across a posteriorly located, large inlet defect. (e) Supracristal ventricular septal defect: *left* panel depicts the aortic long-axis view displaying mild dilation of the anterior aortic sinus and early valve prolapse in a patient with a small supracristal VSD (also referred to as conal or doubly committed subarterial defect). *Right* panel displays a small color Doppler jet (blue signal marked by *arrow*) that represents left-to-right shunting across the defect. (f) Complete atrioventricular septal (canal) defect: four-chamber view of complete atrioventricular septal defect demonstrates defect ostium primum ASD (*arrow*) and inlet VSD (*arrow with asterisk*). AO, aorta; ASD, atrial septal defect; LA, left atrium; LV, left ventricle; SVC, superior vena cava; RA, right atrium; RV, right ventricle; RPA, right pulmonary artery; RVOT, right ventricular outflow tract; LVOT, left ventricular outflow tract

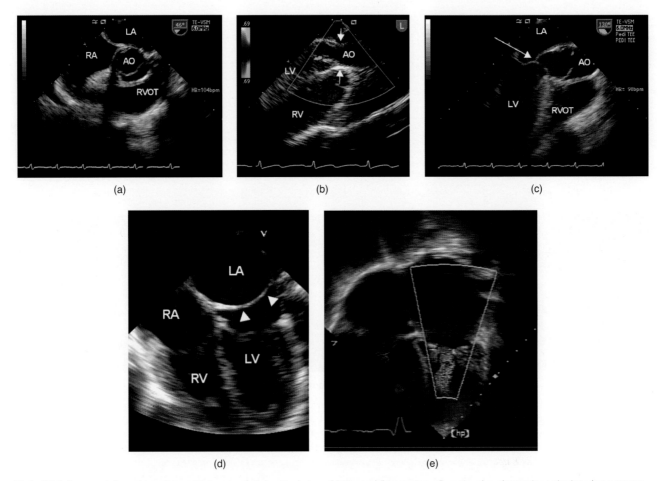

Plate 11.2 Representative echocardiographic images of obstructive lesions. (a) Bicuspid (bicommissural) aortic valve: short-axis aortic view demonstrates "fish mouth" appearance of bicuspid aortic valve in systolic frame. (b) Supravalvar aortic stenosis: aortic long-axis view demonstrating the typical hourglass deformity at the sinotubular region (*arrows*) in a patient with supravalvar aortic stenosis. A tiny jet of aortic regurgitation is shown by color Doppler. (c) Sub and valvar aortic stenosis: aortic long-axis view displaying multiple levels of left ventricular outflow tract obstruction. A fibromuscular ridge (*arrow*) is noted in addition to systolic doming of the aortic valve cusps. (d) Cor triatriatum: four-chamber view displays the obstructive membrane in the left atrium (*arrows*) that divides the cavity into proximal and distal portions (*arrows*). (e) Mitral stenosis: four-chamber view in patient with severe mitral stenosis demonstrating narrow color jet across mitral inflow. Note mosaic pattern of color Doppler signal consistent with aliased (turbulent), high velocity flow across the valve. AO, aorta; LA, left atrium; RV, right ventricle; LVOT, left ventricular outflow tract; PV, pulmonary valve; RA, right atrium; RVOT, right ventricular outflow tract

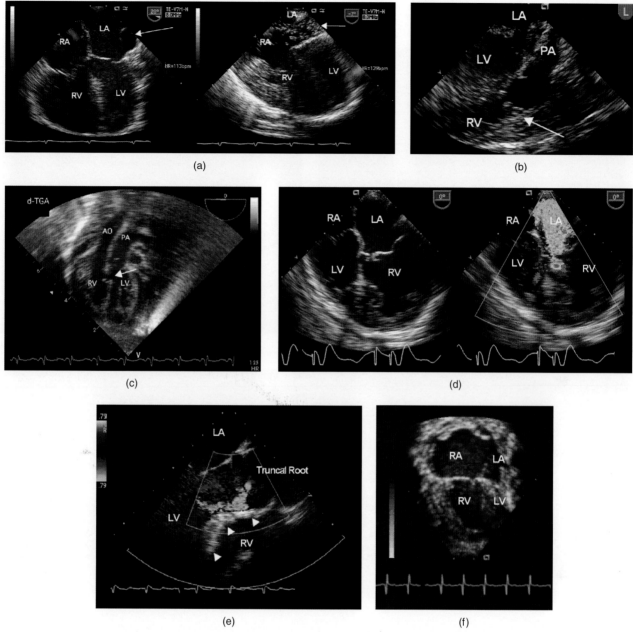

Plate 11.3 Representative echocardiographic images of congenital heart defects. (a) Left superior vena cava to the coronary sinus: *left* panel displays a dilated coronary sinus in short axis (*arrow*) in the four-chamber view. *Right* panel depicts contrast echocardiogram with agitated injection into a left arm vein. Microbubbles are seen along the long axis of the coronary sinus entering the right atrium. (b) Tetralogy of Fallot: long-axis view of infant with tetralogy of Fallot displaying severe infundibular obstruction (*arrow*). The size of the pulmonary annulus in this infant is within normal range and mild valvar stenosis is present. (c) *d*-Transposition of the great arteries: the discordant ventriculoarterial connection can be seen in this transgastric view of a neonate with *d*-transposition. An associated perimembranous VSD is noted (*arrow*). (d) Ventricular inversion (*l*-Transposition of the great arteries): *left* panel displays four-chamber view in a patient with ventricular inversion. The discordant atrioventricular connection is shown, as the left atrium empties into a trabeculated right ventricle, on the left. Apical (Ebstein-like) displacement of the left-sided tricuspid valve is present. The *right* panel demonstrates a large tricuspid regurgitant jet. (e) Truncus arteriosus (postoperative): color flow Doppler interrogation in the aortic long-axis view displays a jet of truncal (neoaortic) regurgitation impacting the VSD patch (*arrows*) in patient post-truncus arteriosus repair. (f) Hypoplastic left heart syndrome: Four-chamber view of infant with hypoplastic left heart syndrome. The image demonstrates an essentially nonexistent left ventricle, dilated right atrium, hypertrophied right ventricle, and large atrial communication. AO, aorta; LA, left atrium; LV, left ventricle; PA, main pulmonary artery; RA, right atrium; RV, right ventricle; VSD, ventricular septal defect

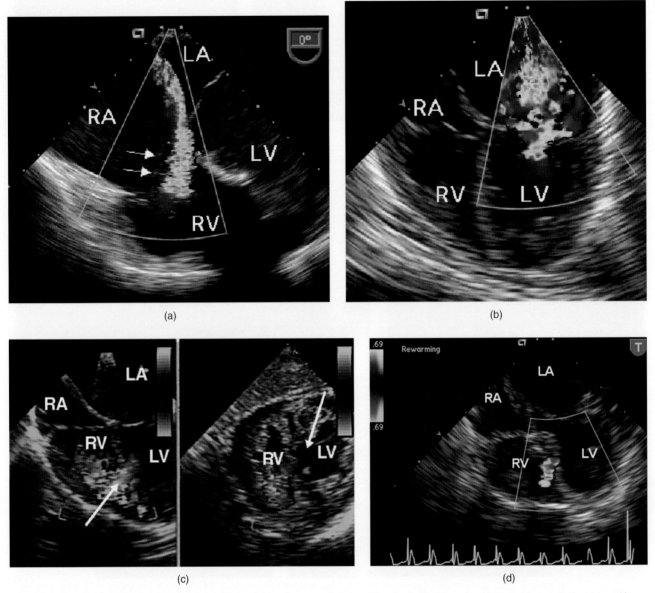

Plate 11.4 Echocardiographic images of congenital heart defects demonstrating the utility of color flow Doppler. (a) Tricuspid regurgitation: tricuspid regurgitant jet (*arrows*) coursing along the atrial septum in a patient with annular dilation and elevated right ventricular pressures. (b) Mitral regurgitation: broad jet of mitral regurgitation in infant with congenital mitral valve disease. (c) Large mid-muscular defect: color Doppler interrogation in the four-chamber (*left* panel) and short-axis views (*right* panel) demonstrating left-to-right shunting across a large mid-muscular VSD (marked by *arrows*). (d) Residual ventricular septal defect: a mid-muscular VSD is identified by color Doppler while on cardiopulmonary bypass during the warming period after patch closure of perimembranous VSD. LA, left atrium; LV, left ventricle; RA, right atrium; RV, right ventricle; VSD, ventricular septal defect

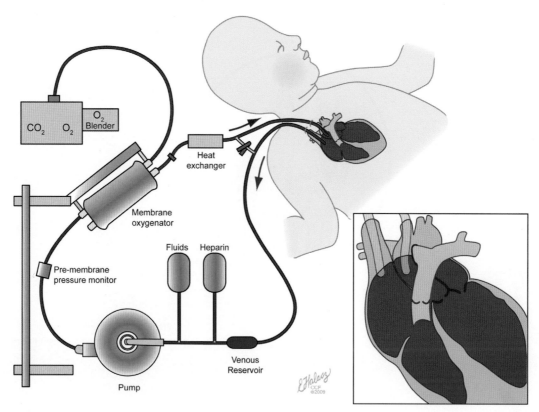

Plate 30.1 ECMO circuit showing the different components

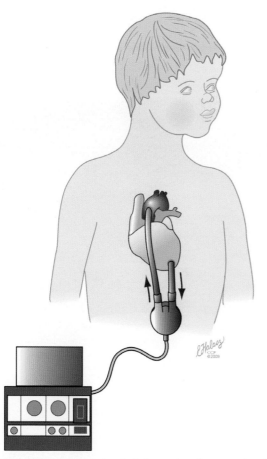

Plate 30.2 VAD circuit displaying the inflow and outflow cannulae, the assist device, and the control console

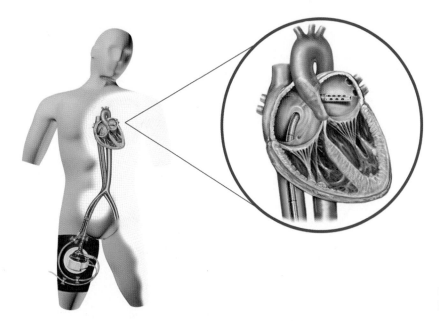

Plate 30.3 TandemHeart showing the magnified inflow cannula across the interatrial septum

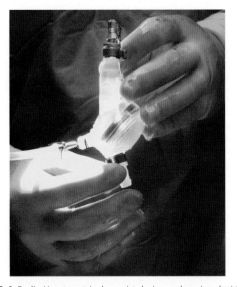

Plate 30.4 Berlin Heart ventricular assist device undergoing deairing by the surgeon before implantation

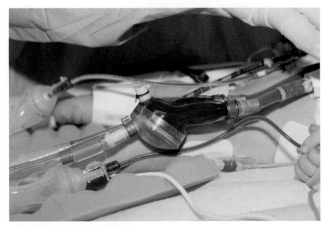

Plate 30.5 Berlin Heart ventricular assist device displaying the inflow and outflow cannulae as well as the pneumatically driven membrane pump

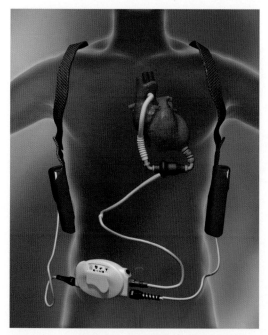

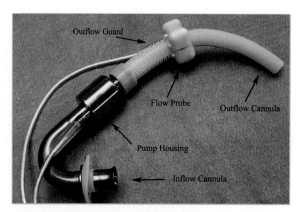

Plate 30.7 MicroMed DeBakey VAD Child

Plate 30.6 Heart Mate II displaying the device, the external console, and the battery pack for ambulation

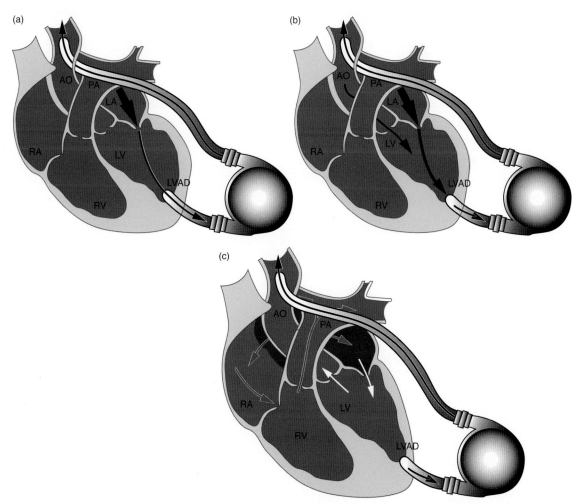

Plate 30.8 Valvular and nonvalvular conditions that affect ventricular assist device function detected by transesophageal echocardiography: (a) mitral stenosis, RV (b) aortic insufficiency, and (c) patent foramen ovale. AO, aorta; PA, pulmonary artery; RA, right atrium; LA, left atrium; RV, right ventricle; LV, left ventricle

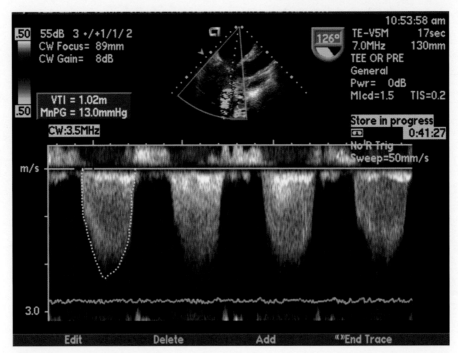

Plate 30.9 Continuous-wave Doppler interrogation of the inflow cannula of a Heart Mate ventricular assist device. In this mid-esophageal long-axis view at 120°, the cannula is oriented toward the intraventricular septum, causing turbulent blood flow with a peak velocity of >2.3 m/s and a mean gradient of 13 mm Hg

27. Creazzo TL, Godt RE, Leatherbury L, et al. (1998) Role of cardiac neural crest cells in cardiovascular development. Annu Rev Physiol 60:267–286.

28. Streeter GL (1951) Developmental Horizons in Human Embryos: Description of Age Groups XI to XXIII. Carnegie Institute, Washington, DC.

29. Kirby ML, Gale TF, Stewart DE (1983) Neural crest cells contribute to normal aorticopulmonary septation. Science 220:1059–1061.

30. Kirby ML (1987) Cardiac morphogenesis—recent research advances. Pediatr Res 21:219–224.

31. Bergwerff M, Verberne ME, DeRuiter MC, et al. (1998) Neural crest cell contribution to the developing circulatory system: implications for vascular morphology? Circ Res 82:221–231.

32. Van Mierop LH, Kutsche LM (1986) Cardiovascular anomalies in DiGeorge syndrome and importance of neural crest as a possible pathogenetic factor. Am J Cardiol 58:133–137.

33. Clark EB, Nakazawa M, Takao A (2000) Etiology and Morphogenesis of Congenital Heart Disease: Twenty Years of Progress in Genetics and Developmental Biology. Futura Publishing, New York.

34. Edwards JE (1948) Anomalies of the derivatives of the aortic arch system. Med Clin North Am 32:925–949.

35. Bogers AJ, Gittenberger-de Groot AC, Poelmann RE, et al. (1989) Development of the origin of the coronary arteries, a matter of ingrowth or outgrowth? Anat Embryol (Berl) 180:437–441.

36. Aikawa E, Kawano J (1982) Formation of coronary arteries sprouting from the primitive aortic sinus wall of the chick embryo. Experientia 38:816–818.

37. Conte G, Pellegrini A (1984) On the development of the coronary arteries in human embryos, stages 14–19. Anat Embryol (Berl) 169:209–218.

38. Hutchins GM, Kessler-Hanna A, Moore GW (1988) Development of the coronary arteries in the embryonic human heart. Circulation 77:1250–1257.

39. Vrancken Peeters MP, Gittenberger-de Groot AC, Mentink MM, et al. (1997) Differences in development of coronary arteries and veins. Cardiovasc Res 36:101–110.

40. Fineman JR, Soifer SJ (1998) The fetal and neonatal circulations. In: Chnag AC, Hanley FL, Wernovsky G, Wessel DL (eds) Pediatric Cardiac Intensive Care. Williams and Wilkins, Baltimore, pp. 17–24.

41. Rudolph AM (2001) Congenital Diseases of the Heart; Clinical–Physiological Considerations. Futura Publishing, Armonk, New York.

42. Rudolph AM (1970) The changes in the circulation after birth. Their importance in congenital heart disease. Circulation 41:343–359.

43. Stanger P, Rudolph AM, Edwards JE (1977) Cardiac malpositions. An overview based on study of sixty-five necropsy specimens. Circulation 56:159–172.

44. Porter CJ, Edwards WD (2008) Atrial septal defects. In: Allen HD, Driscoll DJ, Shaddy RE, Feltes TF (eds) Moss and Adams' Heart Disease in Infants, Children and Adolescents: Including the Fetus and Young Adult, 7th edn. Lippincott Williams & Wilkins, Philadelphia, pp. 632–645.

45. Wenink AC, Zevallos JC (1988) Developmental aspects of atrioventricular septal defects. Int J Cardiol 18:65–78.

46. Cetta F, Minich LL, Edwards WD, et al. (2008) Atrioventricular septal defects. In: Allen HD, Driscoll DJ, Shaddy RE, Feltes TF (eds) Moss and Adams' Heart Disease in Infants, Children and Adolescents: Including the Fetus and Young Adult, 7th edn. Lippincott Williams & Wilkins, Philadelphia, pp. 646–667.

47. Perry LW, NeilL CA, Ferencz C (1993) Infants with congenital heart disease: the cases. In: Ferencz C, Loffredo CA, Rubin J, Magee CC (eds) Epidemiology of Congenital Heart Disease: The Baltimore–Washington Infant Study 1981–1989. Futura Publishing, New York, pp. 33–61.

48. Epstein ML (2008) Tricuspid atresia, stenosis, and regurgitation. In: Allen HD, Driscoll DJ, Shaddy RE, Feltes TF (eds) Moss and Adams' Heart Disease in Infants, Children and Adolescents: Including the Fetus and Young Adult, 7th edn. Lippincott Williams & Wilkins, Philadelphia, pp. 817–834.

49. McDaniel NL, Gutgesell HP (2008) Ventricular septal defects. In: Allen HD, Driscoll DJ, Shaddy RE, Feltes TF (eds) Moss and Adams' Heart Disease in Infants, Children and Adolescents: Including the Fetus and Young Adult, 7th edn. Lippincott Williams & Wilkins, Philadelphia, pp. 667–682.

50. Bartelings MM, Gittenberger-de Groot AC (1989) The outflow tract of the heart–embryologic and morphologic correlations. Int J Cardiol 22:289–300.

51. Bartelings MM, Gittenberger-de Groot AC (1991) Morphogenetic considerations on congenital malformations of the outflow tract. Part 2: complete transposition of the great arteries and double outlet right ventricle. Int J Cardiol 33:5–26.

52. Kirby ML, Waldo KL (1990) Role of neural crest in congenital heart disease. Circulation 82:332–340.

53. Kirby ML, Waldo KL (1995) Neural crest and cardiovascular patterning. Circ Res 77:211–215.

54. Cabalka AK, Edwards W, Dearani JA (2008) Truncus arteriosus. In: Allen HD, Driscoll DJ, Shaddy RE, Feltes TF (eds) Moss and Adams' Heart Disease in Infants, Children and Adolescents: Including the Fetus and Young Adult, 7th edn. Lippincott Williams & Wilkins, Philadelphia, pp. 911–922.

55. Wernovsky G (2008) Transposition of the great arteries. In: Allen HD, Driscoll DJ, Shaddy RE, Feltes TF (eds) Moss and Adams' Heart Disease in Infants, Children and Adolescents: Including the Fetus and Young Adult, 7th edn. Lippincott Williams & Wilkins, Philadelphia, pp. 1038–1087.

56. Siwik ES, Erenberg FG, Zahka KG, et al. (2008) Tetralogy of Fallot. In: Allen HD, Driscoll DJ, Shaddy RE, Feltes TF (eds) Moss and Adams' Heart Disease in Infants, Children and Adolescents: Including the Fetus and Young Adult, 7th edn. Lippincott Williams & Wilkins, Philadelphia, pp. 888–910.

57. Moore P, Brook M, Heymann MA (2008) Patent ductus arteriosus and aortopulmonary window. In: Allen HD, Driscoll DJ, Shaddy RE, Feltes TF (eds) Moss and Adams' Heart Disease in Infants, Children and Adolescents: Including the Fetus and Young Adult, 7th edn. Lippincott Williams & Wilkins, Philadelphia, pp. 683–702.

58. Weinberg PM (2008) Aortic Arch Anomalies. In: Allen HD, Driscoll DJ, Shaddy RE, Feltes TF (eds) Moss and Adams'

Heart Disease in Infants, Children and Adolescents: Including the Fetus and Young Adult, 7th edn. Lippincott Williams & Wilkins, Philadelphia, pp. 730–760.

59. Epstein ML (2000) Vascular rings and slings. In: Moller JH, Hoffman JE (eds) Pediatric Cardiovascular Medicine, 1st edn. Churchill Livingstone, Philadelphia, p. 643.

60. Matherne GP, Lim DS (2008) Congenital anomalies of the coronal vessels and the aortic root. In: Allen HD, Driscoll DJ, Shaddy RE, Feltes TF (eds) Moss and Adams' Heart Disease in Infants, Children and Adolescents: Including the Fetus and Young Adult, 7th edn. Lippincott Williams & Wilkins, Philadelphia, pp. 702–715.

61. Geva T, Van Praagh S (2008) Anomalous systemic venous connections. In: Allen HD, Driscoll DJ, Shaddy RE, Feltes TF (eds) Moss and Adams' Heart Disease in Infants, Children and Adolescents: Including the Fetus and Young Adult, 7th edn. Lippincott Williams & Wilkins, Philadelphia, pp. 792–817.

62. Franklin RC, Jacobs JP, Krogmann ON, et al. (2008) Nomenclature for congenital and paediatric cardiac disease: histori-cal perspectives and The International Pediatric and Congenital Cardiac Code. Cardiol Young 18 (Suppl 2):70–80.

63. Shinebourne EA, Macartney FJ, Anderson RH (1976) Sequential chamber localization—logical approach to diagnosis in congenital heart disease. Br Heart J 38:327–340.

64. Tynan MJ, Becker AE, Macartney FJ, et al. (1979) Nomenclature and classification of congenital heart disease. Br Heart J 41:544–553.

65. Anderson RH, Becker AE, Freedom RM, et al. (1984) Sequential segmental analysis of congenital heart disease. Pediatr Cardiol 5:281–287.

66. Van Praagh R (1984) The segmental approach clarified. Cardiovasc Intervent Radiol 7:320–325.

67. Sharma S, Devine W, Anderson RH, et al. (1988) The determination of atrial arrangement by examination of appendage morphology in 1842 heart specimens. Br Heart J 60:227–231.

68. de la Cruz MV, Nadal-Ginard B (1972) Rules for the diagnosis of visceral situs, truncoconal morphologies, and ventricular inversions. Am Heart J 84:19–32.

5 Physiology and molecular biology of the developing circulation

Dean B. Andropoulos, M.D., M.H.C.M.
Texas Children's Hospital, Baylor College of Medicine, Houston, Texas, USA

Introduction

The circulatory system in congenital heart disease continually changes and develops in response to both normal and pathologic stimuli. Response to anesthetic and surgical interventions must be understood in this framework, and is often radically different from the usual, expected pediatric and adult situations with a "normal" cardiovascular system. This chapter reviews developmental changes of the cardiovascular system from fetal life through adulthood, both in the normal and pathophysiologic states associated with congenital heart disease. Not much is known about the development of the normal and diseased human heart. Much of the information discussed in this chapter is derived from animal models, and undoubtedly new information will be discovered as human myocardial tissue is studied.

Anesthesia for Congenital Heart Disease 2nd edition. Edited by Dean Andropoulos, Stephen Stayer, Isobel Russell and Emad Mossad. © 2010 Blackwell Publishing.

Development from fetus to neonate

Circulatory pathways

The fetus receives oxygenated and nutrient-rich blood from the placenta via the umbilical vein, and ejects desaturated blood through the umbilical arteries to the placenta, and thus the placenta, not the lung, serves as the organ of respiration. Blood flow thus largely bypasses the lungs in utero, accounting for only about 7% of the fetal combined ventricular output [1]. Pulmonary vascular resistance is high, and the lungs collapsed and filled with amniotic fluid. This is the basis for the fetal circulation, which is a parallel circulation, rather than the series circulation seen postnatally. Three fetal circulatory shunts exist to carry better-oxygenated blood from the umbilical vein to the systemic circulation: the ductus venosus, ductus arteriosus, and foramen ovale (Figure 5.1a). Approximately 50% of the umbilical venous blood, with an oxygen tension of about 30–35 mm Hg, passes through the ductus venosus, and then into the right atrium. There it streams preferentially across the foramen ovale, guided

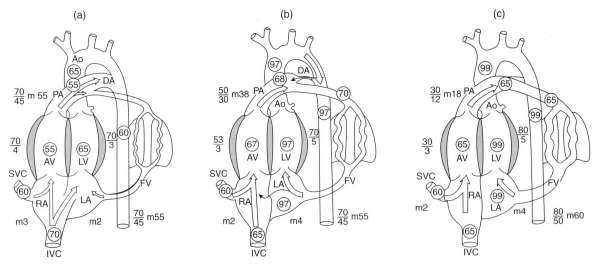

Figure 5.1 Transition from fetal to mature circulation. (a) Fetal circulation. (b) Transitional circulation. (c) Mature circulation. Circled numbers are oxygen saturations, uncircled numbers are pressures in mm Hg. M, mean pressure; RV, right ventricle; LV, left ventricle; RA, right atrium; LA, left atrium; DA, ductus arteriosus; Ao, aorta; PA, pulmonary artery; SVC, superior vena cava; IVC, inferior vena cava; PV, pulmonary vein (Reproduced with permission from Reference [2])

by the valves of the sinus venosus and Chiari network into the left atrium. Thus, the brain and upper body preferentially receive this relatively well-oxygenated blood, which accounts for 20–30% of the combined ventricular output. Blood returning in the inferior vena cava represents about 70% of the total venous return to the heart, and two-thirds of this deoxygenated blood passes into the right atrium and ventricle. About 90% of the blood flows through the ductus arteriosus to supply the lower fetal body.

After birth, there is a dramatic fall in pulmonary vascular resistance and increase in pulmonary blood flow, with inflation and oxygenation of the lungs (Figure 5.2). The placental circulation is removed, and all of these changes lead to closure of the ductus venosus, constriction of the ductus arteriosus, and reversal of pressure gradients in the left and right atria, leading to closure of the foramen ovale. This leads to a state called the transitional circulation (Figure 5.1b), characterized by high pulmonary artery pressures and resistance (much lower than in utero, however), and a small amount of left-to-right flow through the ductus arteriosus. This is a labile state, and failure to maintain lower pulmonary vascular resistance can rapidly lead to reversion to fetal circulatory pathways, and right-to-left shunting at the ductus arteriosus and foramen ovale. This maintenance of fetal circulatory pathways is necessary for survival in many congenital heart diseases, particularly those dependent on a patent ductus arteriosus for all or a significant portion of systemic or pulmonary blood flow, or atresia of atrioventricular valves. Maintenance of ductal patency with PGE_1 is crucial in these lesions. In two-ventricle heart with large intracardiac shunts, maintenance of the fetal circulation leads to right-to-left shunting at the foramen and ductal levels, and thus hypoxia.

Conversion to the mature circulation (Figure 5.1c) in the normal heart occurs over a period of several weeks, as pulmonary vascular resistance falls further, and the ductus arteriosus closes permanently by thrombosis, intimal proliferation, and fibrosis. Factors favoring the transition from fetal to mature circulation include normal oxygen

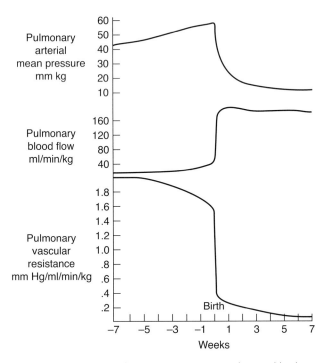

Figure 5.2 Changes in pulmonary artery pressure, pulmonary blood flow, and pulmonary vascular resistance in the lamb after birth (Reproduced with permission from Reference [2])

tensions and physical expansion of the lungs, normal pH, nitric oxide (NO), and prostacyclin. Factors favoring reversion to fetal circulation include low oxygen tension, acidotic pH, lung collapse, and inflammatory mediators (leukotrienes, thromoboxane A2, platelet activating factor) as seen in sepsis and other related conditions, and endothelin A receptor activators [3].

Myocardial contractility

The fetal myocardium is characterized by poorly organized cellular arrangements, and fewer myofibrils with a random orientation, in contrast to the parallel, well-organized myofibrillar arrangement of the adult myocardium [4] (see below). Fetal hearts develop less tension per gram than adult hearts because of increased water content and fewer contractile elements. Calcium cycling and excitation contraction coupling are also very different, with poorly organized T-tubules and immature sarcoplasmic reticulum (SR), leading to more dependence on free cytosolic ionized calcium for normal contractility. Despite this immature state, the fetal heart can increase its stroke volume in a limited fashion up to left atrial pressures of 10–12 mm Hg according to the Frank–Starling relationship, as long as afterload (i.e., arterial pressure) is kept low [5]. These features continue throughout the neonatal and early infancy period.

Development from neonate to older infant and child

At birth the neonatal heart must suddenly change from a parallel circulation to a series circulation, and the left ventricle in particular must adapt immediately to dramatically increased preload from blood returning from the lungs, and increased afterload as the placental circulation is removed. The very high oxygen consumption of the newborn necessitates a high cardiac output for the first few months of life. However, animal models have demonstrated that the fetal and newborn myocardium develops less tension in response to increasing preload (sarcomere length), and that cardiac output increases less to the same degree of volume loading [6,7] (Figure 5.3). Resting tension, however, is greater in the newborn compared to the mature heart. This information suggests that the newborn heart is operating near the top of its Frank–Starling curve, and that there is less reserve in response to both increased afterload and preload. This observation is borne out clinically in newborns after complex heart surgery, who are often intolerant of even small increases in left atrial pressure or mean arterial pressure. The newborn myocardium also has only a limited ability to increase its inotropic state in response to exogenous catecholamines, and is much more dependent on heart rate to maintain cardiac output than is the mature heart. One reason for this is the high levels

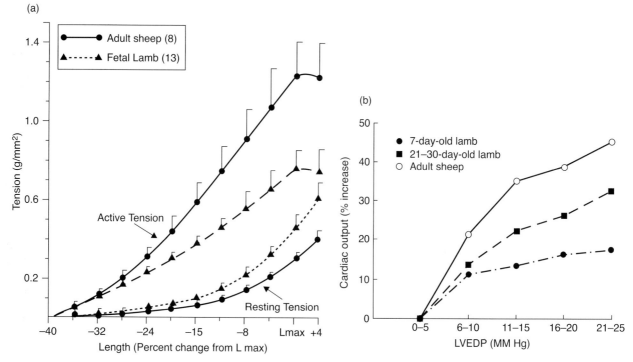

Figure 5.3 (a) Isometric resting and active length–tension relationships in fetal and adult lamb cardiac muscle strips (Reproduced with permission from —Reference [6]). (b) Response to volume load of normal saline at 5 ml/kg/min, at constant heart rate. LVEDP, left ventricular end-diastolic pressure (Reproduced with permission from Reference [7])

of circulating endogenous catecholamines that appear after birth, necessary to make the transition to extrauterine life [8]. As these levels decrease in the weeks after birth, contractile reserve increases.

The neonatal myocardium is less compliant than the mature myocardium, with increased resting tension as noted above, and a significantly greater increase in ventricular pressure with volume loading [9]. This implies that diastolic function of the neonatal heart is also impaired compared to the mature heart [10]. The myofibrils of the newborn heart also appear to have a greater sensitivity to calcium, developing a greater tension than adult myofibrils when exposed to the same free Ca^{++} concentration in vitro [11].

It must again be emphasized that nearly all of this data was obtained from animal models, and although the information appears to agree with what is observed clinically, there exists a need for noninvasive studies of normal human hearts from the neonatal period through adulthood to confirm these impressions of cardiac development.

Gene expression in cardiac development

Recent progress has been made in understanding the genetic aspects of human cardiac development, and in contrast to the physiologic studies which are almost exclusively performed in animal models, small amounts of human cardiac tissue obtained from biopsy or autopsy specimens can used for these be studies. Some aspects of these developmental changes will be reviewed.

Myosin is the major protein component of the thick filaments of the cardiac myofibril, and differences in the expression of this protein may play a significant role in myocardial contractility. Chromosome 14 has the genetic material responsible for producing the myosin heavy chain that makes up the backbone of the thick filaments, and two major isoforms, the α and β, exist. The β isoform predominates and does not change significantly with maturation [12]. The myosin light chain has multiple isoforms, and the relative proportions of these isoforms changes with development, and also in response to pressure loading of the heart. The isoforms that predominate in the newborn myocardium appear to confer a greater sensitivity to Ca^{++} than those seen in the mature heart [13] and may contribute to the increased sensitivity of the neonatal myocardium to Ca^{++}.

Troponin I, C, and T are critical proteins that bind Ca^{++} and regulate the interaction between myosin and actin, directly affect the force of contraction. Troponin C, the Ca^{++} binding portion of the troponin moiety, does not change with development. Troponin I, however, has two major isoforms: a slow skeletal muscle type that predominates in the heart in fetal and neonatal life and the cardiac isoform, which is the only isoform expressed in the mature

heart [14]. Only the cardiac (mature) isoform responds to β-adrenergic stimulation, producing a faster twitch development and greater twitch tension. However, contractility in the neonatal myofibrils containing the immature myosin light chain isoform is more resistant to acidosis. Four isoforms of troponin T are expressed in the fetal and neonatal heart, but only one in the mature heart. These isoforms exhibit different levels of ATPase activity and Ca^{++} sensitivity (see below), with greater ATPase activity and Ca^{++} sensitivity seen in the immature forms [11] Tropomyosin [15] has two and actin [16] has three isoforms that are expressed in different proportions as developmental changes occur, but the functional significance of these changes has yet to be elucidated.

The extracellular matrix of the heart is important in translating the force generated from shortening of sarcomere length to the cardiac chambers, resulting in stroke volume. The major components of the extracellular matrix are collagen types I and II, glycoproteins, and proteoglycans and the expression of these elements changes with development. The neonatal heart has a higher content of both total and type I collagen (which is stiffer and less compliant than type III collagen) when compared to the total protein content of the heart [17]. The collagen to total protein ratio reaches mature levels by about 5 months of life. This change, along with greater water content of the immature myocardium, may partially explain the diminished diastolic function. Also this relative lack of contractile elements reduces the ability of the neonatal myocardium to increase its inotropic state. A network of collagen-based connections, called the weave network, develops rapidly after birth connecting myocytes and capillaries and allowing greater functional integrity to develop in response to the greater afterload stress on the heart [18]. This development of the extracellular matrix appears to be complete by approximately 6 months of age, and results in a much more efficient transfer of force generated by sarcomere shortening to the cardiac chambers (Figure 5.4).

The cardiac myocytes have receptors on the outside of their sarcolemmal membranes called integrins. These receptors are specific for collagen and fibronectin, and cause the attachment of the extracellular matrix to the myocytes, allowing force transduction to occur [19]. Collagen and vinculin, another cytoskeletal protein, are attached to the sarcomere at the Z disk. The integrins have two subunits, an α and β, which express several isoforms, the relative proportions of which change during development to those that afford greater adherence of the cytoskeletal proteins to the myocytes, resulting in greater structural integrity.

Some enzymes are affected by the loading conditions of the heart. Protein kinase C (PKC) is an enzyme with a major role in transmembrane signal transduction through phosphorylation of a number of downstream intracellular

(a)   (b)

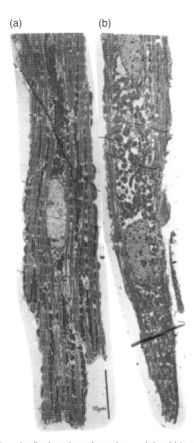

Figure 5.4 Longitudinal sections through an adult rabbit cardiac myocyte (a), and a 3-week-old rabbit cardiac myocyte (b). Note the differences between myofibril organization and structure as well as cell size (Reproduced with permission from Reference [11])

components [20]. There are six isoforms of this enzyme, and the relative percentages of each isoform are not affected during development. However, in aortic stenosis producing left ventricular hypertrophy, all isoforms except PKC-β are dramatically uprgeulated, and in dilated cardiomyopathy there is a dramatic upregulation of PKC-β. Phosphodiesterase (PDE) is an enzyme involved in the termination of the action of cyclic AMP, which regulates the contractile state of the myocardium (see below). Expression of the isoform PDE-5 is dramatically increased in the hypertrophied human right ventricle in patients with pulmonary hypertension, and inhibition of this enzyme improves ventricular contractility [21].

New information is available about the molecular and cellular basis for normal cardiac development and the causes of congenital heart disease [22]. A missense mutation in the myocardial protein actin has been discovered to be the cause of isolated secundum ASD in some patients [23]. Pleuripotent cardiac progenitor cells reside in the human neonatal myocardium in relatively high numbers during the first month of life [24]. This knowledge has given rise to the exciting notion that

these stem cells could potentially be used to facilitate recovery from cardiac morbidity or to enhance surgical repair.

The preceding short review is meant to give the reader an idea of some of the aspects of the molecular biology of the developing circulation. The explosion of new information in this area, and especially new data from human tissue, will lead to a more thorough understanding of the pathophysiology of disease states and suggest avenues for future treatment. For a more complete treatment of this area, the reader is referred to several excellent reviews [25–27].

Innervation of the heart

Clinical observations in newborn infants have led to the hypothesis that the sympathetic innervation and control of the cardiovascular system is incomplete in the newborn infant compared to older children and adults, and that the parasympathetic innervation is intact [4]. Examples of this include the frequency of bradycardia in the newborn in response to a number of stimuli, including vagal, and vagotonic agents, and the relative lack of sensitivity in the newborn to sympathomimetic agents. Histological studies in animal models have demonstrated incomplete sympathetic innervation in the neonatal heart when compared to the adult, but no differences in the number or density of parasympathetic nerves [28,29].

Autonomic cardiovascular control of cardiac activity can be evaluated by measuring heart rate variability in response to both respiration, and to beat-to-beat variability in systolic blood pressure [30]. The sympathetic and parasympathetic input into sinoatrial node activity contribute to heart rate variability changes with greater heart rate variability resulting from greater parasympathetic input into sinoatrial node activity [31]. Studies using these methodologies for normal infants during sleep suggest that the parasympathetic predominance gradually diminishes until approximately 6 months of age, coinciding with greater sympathetic innervation of the heart similar to adult levels [32].

Development from child to adult

Beyond the transition period from fetal to newborn life and into the first few months of postnatal life, there is not much human or animal information concerning the exact nature and extent of cardiac development at the cellular level. Most studies compare newborn or fetal to adult animals [33]. Cardiac chamber development is assumed to be influenced by blood flow [34]. Large flow or volume load in a ventricle results in ventricular enlargement. Small competent atrioventricular valves, as in tricuspid stenosis, result in lower blood flow and a small ventricle. Increases in myocardial mass with normal growth, as well as in ventricular outflow obstruction, are mainly due to hypertrophy of myocytes. Late gestational increases in blood cortisol are responsible for this growth pattern, and there is concern that antenatal glucocorticoids to induce lung maturity may inhibit cardiac myocyte proliferation. In the human infant, it is assumed that the cellular elements of the cardiac myocyte, i.e., adrenergic receptors, intracellular receptors and signaling, calcium cycling and regulation, and interaction of the contractile proteins, are similar to that in the adult by approximately 6 months of age. Similarly, cardiac depression by volatile agents is greater in the newborn changing to adult levels by approximately 6 months of age [35].

Normal values for physiologic variables by age

It is useful for the anesthesiologist to be aware of normal ranges for physiologic variables in premature and full-term newborns of all sizes and in infants and children of all ages (Figure 5.5). Obviously, acceptable ranges for these variables are highly dependent on the individual patient's pathophysiology, but the wide range of "normal" values may reassure the practitioner to accept "low" blood pressure, e.g., if other indices of cardiac function and tissue oxygen delivery are acceptable.

Myocardial sequelae of longstanding congenital heart disease

Hypertrophy of the cardiac chambers is a common response to a number of different chronic pathophysiologic states. Wall thickness increases though hypertrophy of the cardiac myocytes and noncontractile elements. The hypertrophy reduces wall stress in the dilated heart, but also serves to reduce ventricular function, particularly diastolic function. This reduction in function serves to reduce myocardial oxygen consumption in response to a wide variety of chronic stresses, both in pressure and volume overloaded ventricles [38].

Pressure overload hypertrophy results in altered gene expression in the cardiomyocyte. Myosin isoform expression (see below) changes from the faster reacting α-myosin to the slower β-myosin, reducing myocardial function [39]. Integrin-linked kinase expression is increased in patients with hypertrophic cardiomyopathy and induces hypertrophy in an animal model [40]. Altered expression or mutations of other genes that regulate production of cardiac cytoskeletal proteins, such as dystrophin, occur in patients with end-stage cardiomyopathy [41,42].

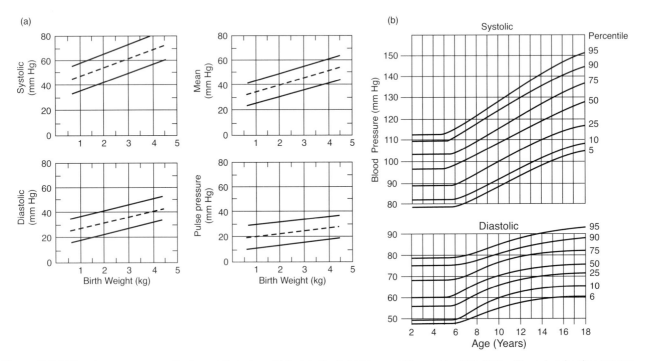

Figure 5.5 (a) Blood pressure measured in the umbilical artery of infants in the first 12 hours of life weighing 600–4200 g (Reproduced with permission from Reference [36]). (b) Blood pressure percentiles, age 2–18 years (Reproduced with permission from Reference [37])

Cardiomyocyte receptor function in normal and diseased hearts

The adrenergic receptor

The adrenergic receptors (ARs) are a part of a large superfamily of receptors that mediate their biological responses through the coupling of a specific guanine nucleotide regulatory protein or G protein [43]. This superfamily of receptors shares a common structural motif, characterized by seven hydrophobic domains spanning the lipid bilayer. The seven domains are attached by three internal loops and three external loops between the amine terminus and the cytoplasmic carboxy terminus. The function of this receptor family is dependent on a specific agonist (or ligand) binding to the receptor, which causes a conformational change in the receptor. This structural change permits the interaction between the intracellular portion of the receptor and guanine nucleotide regulatory protein (or G protein). This interaction also referred to as coupling, inevitably links the activated receptor to a specific biological response. The regulation of the biological response is initiated by the specificity of the receptor for a particular extracellular agonist and the coupling of a specific G protein to that activated receptor.

Once an extracellular ligand (or agonist) is specifically recognized by a cell surface receptor, the receptor goes through a conformational changes that exposes a specific region of the receptor complex to the intracellular side of the plasma membrane [44] (Figure 5.6). This confirmation change triggers the interaction of the G protein with the amino acids of the third intracellular loop of the receptor and hence leading to G protein activation. There are three different G proteins: stimulatory G protein (G_s), inhibitory G protein (G_i) and the G_q. Under normal conditions, all of the β receptors interact with the G_s, the $\alpha 1$ interacts with G_q and $\alpha 2$ interacts with G_i. Each G protein is a heterotrimer made up of three subunits: α, β, and γ. The activation of the G protein-coupled receptor causes an exchange of bound guanosine diphosphate (GDP) for guanosine triphosphate (GTP) within the α subunit and initiates the disassociation of the $\beta-\gamma$ subunit from the α subunit. The GTP-activated α subunit modulates the activity of a specific effector enzyme within a specific signaling pathway by catalyzing the hydrolysis of GTP to GDP and inorganic phosphate. This causes the transference of a high-energy phosphate group to an enzyme and in turn causes the deactivation of the α subunit. This process will eventually lead to the deactivation of the α subunit and the reassociation with the $\beta-\gamma$ complex. This cycle is continuously repeated until the agonist becomes unbound from the receptor. Downstream of enzyme activation, the production of a second messenger regulates the biological response.

AR have been subdivided into two groups of receptors on the basis of the results of binding studies using a series of selective agonists and antagonists. In 1948 Alquist used the difference in rank orders of potency of a series of agonist to separate the ARs into two principal receptor groups, the α and β receptor group [45]. These findings have been confirmed repeatedly with the development of drugs that function to selectively antagonize the α receptor with no

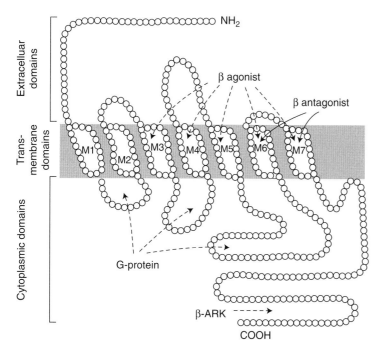

Figure 5.6 Molecular structure of the β-adrenergic receptor, demonstrating its three domains. The transmembrane domains serve as ligand-binding pockets for agonists (dashed arrows) and antagonists (solid arrows). The cytoplasmic domains interact with G proteins and β-adrenergic receptor kinases (Reproduced with permission from Reference [43])

effect on the β receptor. Soon after the distinction between the α and β receptor type was known, it became more evident that the separation of α and β receptors was not sufficient to explain pharmacological studies using rank order of potency for an antagonist, differing from an agonist because it blocks the biological response. With the advent of radioligand-labeled antagonists and new molecular cloning techniques examining receptor gene expression, it became clear that the two principal receptor groups could be further subdivided into additional subtypes.

To date, within the β-adrenergic group four different subtypes have been identified: β_1, β_2, β_3, and β_4. Pharmacologically β_1 and β_2 are differentiated by their affinities to different catecholamines: epinephrine, norepinephrine, and isoproterenol. β_1 has similar affinity for epinephrine and norepinephrine, while β_2 has a higher affinity for epinephrine than to norepinephrine. Both β_1 and β_2 have the same affinity for isoproterenol. The β_3 and β_4 receptors have minor roles in cardiovascular function and will not be further discussed.

The expression and distribution of each subtype is highly dependent on the organ, which adds another level of specificity. Distribution of a particular receptor in two different tissue types may result in two different functions. When examining cardiovascular response to adrenergic stimulation, the β_1 receptor is predominantly expressed in heart tissue. The stimulation of the receptor subtype leads to both inotropic and chronotropic effects on cardiac function, resulting in an increase in the myocardial contractile force and a shortening of contractile timing, respectively. While β_2 can also be found in the heart, it is mostly expressed in vascular smooth muscle tissue. The distribution and function relevance of this receptor subtype in the heart is controversial and may change with alterations in cardiac function. The percentage of β_2 receptors in the nonfailing heart averages about 20% in the ventricle [46] and 30% in the atrium. The percentage of $\beta_1:\beta_2$ receptors is approximately 75:25% in the ventricles of younger hearts [47,48].

Each signaling pathway is specific to each AR. Once the agonist binds to the β_1 receptor causing the coupling of the G protein, the G protein α-subunit becomes activated followed by an increase in adenylate cyclase (AC) activity, which induces the conversion of ATP to cAMP. The second messenger, cAMP, phosporylates protein kinase A (or PKA). The function of a kinase is to phosphorylate other target proteins, which initiates a biological response. PKA phosporylates many effector proteins and the phosphorylation of each functions to increase the concentration of intracellular calcium.

The β_2 receptor has also been shown to function through the cAMP signaling pathway causing the activation of PKA, but not nearly to the extent of β_1 in cardiomyocytes [49]. The response of this stimulation appears to have a larger effect on smooth muscle, e.g., the vascular smooth muscle. In this tissue type, the stimulation of β_2 and the subsequent increase in cAMP promotes the vasodilation of vascular smooth muscle and may lead to alterations in blood pressure. In these tissues, the effect of β_1 stimulation appears to be minimal, due to lack of β_1 receptors in the smooth muscle.

Similar to the β receptor, the α receptors can be pharmacologically subdivided into α_1 and α_2. The α receptor is distributed in most vascular smooth muscle and to a lesser extent in the heart. The α_2 receptor has been found in some vascular smooth muscle; however, its major functional importance is as a presynaptic receptor in the central and peripheral nervous systems. The use of molecular techniques has identified three additional subtypes of the α_1 receptor (α_{1A}, α_{1B}, and α_{1D}) and three additional subtypes of the α_2 receptor [43]. Binding of an agonist to an α_1 receptor in the heart or vascular smooth muscle results in activation of the G_q subunit of the G protein, which activates of phospholipase C (see below), producing diacylglycerol and inostol-1,4,5-triphosphate, which releases Ca^{++} from the SR and increases vascular smooth muscle tone or cardiac contractility. A schematic classification of ARs incorporating recent knowledge of molecular pharmacology and signal transduction is presented in Figure 5.7 [43].

The AR concentration in cardiac tissue is very small and measured as fentomoles per milligram of protein. However, the response to stimulation of the receptor is greatly amplified by the signal that occurs downstream of the receptor. In rat ventricular myocytes, the ratio between the β receptors and the next two downstream signaling components (β receptor: G protein: AC) is 1:200:3 [50]. This demonstrates how a large response can be initiated by the activation of a small number of receptors. In addition, it also shows that the rate-limiting component that ultimately regulates intracellular production of cAMP is receptor density and the enzyme concentration of AC.

Developmental changes in adrenergic receptor signaling

Information concerning changes in AR function during the transition from neonatal to more mature myocardial development is limited to a few animal studies. As noted above, the neonatal heart has a limited inotropic response to catecholamine administration.

β-AR density is higher in the ventricular myocardium of neonatal versus adult rabbits, but the inotropic response to the same concentration of isoproterenol is significantly greater in adult tissue [51]. In the neonatal rat, the mechanism of β-adrenergic-mediated increase in contractility is entirely due to β_2 stimulation, whereas in the adult rat it is due solely to β_1 receptor activation. Coupling of the β_2

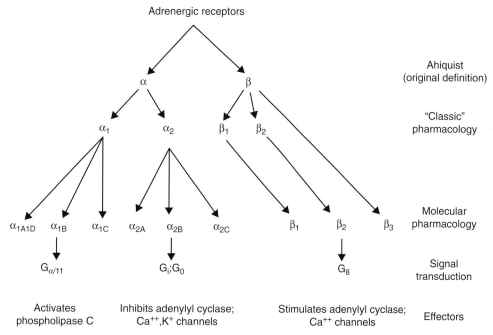

Figure 5.7 A modern schematic classification of adrenergic receptors (Reproduced with permission from Reference [43])

receptor to G_i protein action is apparently defective in the neonatal rat, because the ratio of G_i to G_s subunits is much higher in the neonate. The relative proportion of β_1 and β_2 receptors is the same in neonatal versus adult hearts (17% β_2), and approximates the ratio measured in children with simple acyanotic congenital heart disease, which is about 22% [52].

There is animal and human evidence that α-AR-mediated chronotropic and inotropic effects on the cardiac myocyte change with development. In the neonatal animal model, α stimulation produces positive inotropic and chronotropic effects, whereas in the adult it produces negative effects [53, 54]. The chronotropic response to α_1 stimulation diminished with increasing age in children being evaluated for autonomic dysfunction after vagal and sympathetic blockade [55].

Calcium cycling in the normal heart

Calcium assumes a central role in the process of myocardial contraction and relaxation, serving as the second messenger between depolarization of the cardiac myocyte, and its contraction mediated by the actin–myosin system. Calcium's role in this excitation–contraction coupling in the normal mature heart will be reviewed briefly before discussion of developmental changes and changes with heart failure [56].

Cardiac muscle cell contraction depends on an increase in intracellular Ca^{++} above a certain threshold, and relaxation ensues when intracellular Ca^{++} falls below this

threshold. Two major regions of Ca^{++} flux occur: across the sarcolemmal membrane (slow response), and release from internal stores: the SR (rapid release and reuptake) [57] (Figure 5.8). The primary site of entry of Ca^{++} through the sarcolemmal membrane is through the L-type, or low-voltage-dependent Ca^{++} channels, which occurs in two types: a low-threshold, rapidly inactivating channel, and a higher threshold, more slowly inactivating channel [59]. Depolarization of the sarcolemmal membrane triggers opening of these channels, resulting in the release of large amount of Ca^{++} from the SR, the major internal Ca^{++} storage organelle. Ca^{++} entry through the slowly inactivating channels serves to fill the SR with adequate Ca^{++} stores. Removal of Ca^{++} from the cytoplasm to the exterior of the cell occurs via two major mechanisms: the sodium–calcium (NaO–Ca^{++}) exchanger, and the calcium ATPase pump. The NaO–Ca^{++} exchanger usually serves to exchange three sodium ions (moving into the cell) for one Ca^{++} (moving out of the cell), although the reverse action as well as a 1:1 exchange is possible [60]. The Ca^{++}-ATPase pump actively transports Ca^{++} (in a 1:1 Ca^{++}-ATP ratio) out of the cell in an energy-dependent high-affinity but low-capacity manner [61]. The affinity of the sarcolemmal Ca^{++}-ATPase pump is enhanced by calmodulin, binder of free cytoplasmic Ca^{++}. Although the calcium movement through the sarcolemma plays an important role in balancing internal and external Ca^{++} concentrations and in supplying Ca^{++} to replenish SR Ca^{++} stores, and in initiating the Ca^{++}-induced release of Ca^{++} from the SR, it is important to recognize that the

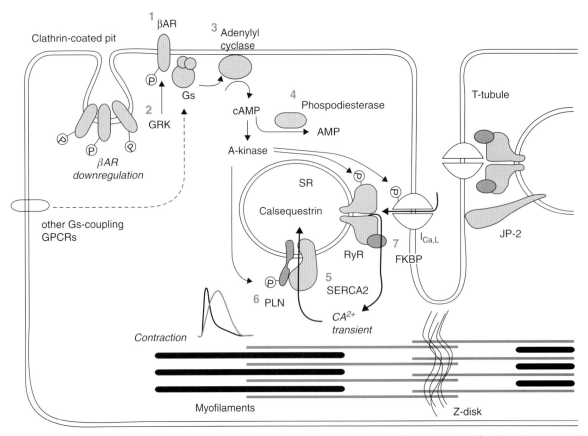

Figure 5.8 Calcium cycling and its relationship to the β-adrenergic receptor system and myocyte myofilaments. See text for discussion. βAR, β-adrenergic receptor; G_s, stimulatory G protein; GRK, G-receptor kinase; cAMP, cyclic AMP; A-kinase, protein kinase A; SR, sarcoplasmic reticulum; RyR, ryanodine receptor; SERCA2, sarcoplasmic reticulum Ca^{++}-ATPase; PLN, phospholamban; $I_{Ca,L}$, L-type Ca^{++} channel; FKBP, FK-506 binding protein; JP-2, junctophilin-2; GPCR, G protein-coupling receptor. Encircled P represents sites of phosphorylation by the various kinases. Numbers 1 through 7 represent targets for pharmacologic therapy in cardiac failure (Reproduced with permission from Reference [58])

amount of Ca^{++} flux is far less than across the SR, the far more important mechanism for excitation–contraction coupling in the mature heart [62]. The sarcolemmal Ca^{++} flux mechanisms play a much more important role in the excitation–contraction coupling of the neonatal (immature) heart.

The massive release and reuptake of Ca^{++} responsible for activation and deactivation of the actin–myosin complex and cardiocyte contraction and relaxation occurs at the level of the SR. The SR is a closed, intracellular membranous network that is intimately related to the myofilaments responsible for contraction [63] (Figure 5.9). The SR is connected to the sarcolemmal membrane via the transverse tubule (T tubule) system. Depolarization of the sarcolemmal membrane results in transfer of charge down the T tubules to the SR, resulting in the opening of SR Ca^{++} channels and the release of large amounts of Ca^{++} into the cyotoplasm where it can then bind to troponin and initiate the actin–myosin interaction. The SR is divided into longitudinal SR and terminal cisternae; the latter connect to the T tubules. The terminal cisternae are primarily

involved in the release of Ca^{++}, and the longitudinal SR in its reuptake [65].

The primary Ca^{++} release mechanism of the SR is the ligand-gated Ca^{++} release channels (also known as the ryanodine receptors) that bind to the drug ryanodine. The channels are activated by two primary mechanisms: depolarization via the T tubules, and binding of intracellular Ca^{++} itself; the predominance of one mechanism over the other differs in cardiac versus skeletal muscle. The close proximity of the L-type sarcolemmal Ca^{++} channels in the T tubules to the ligand-gated Ca^{++} release channels allows the depolarization to rapidly allow Ca^{++} into the cell and open the SR Ca^{++} channels. These ligand-gated Ca^{++} release channels close when the cytosolic Ca^{++} concentration increases; normally it opens at 0.6 μM Ca^{++} and closes at 3.0 μM Ca^{++} [57].

The reuptake and sequestration of Ca^{++} leads to relaxation of the cardiac myocyte and is an active transport mechanism, primarily involving hydrolysis of ATP by the SR Ca^{++}-ATPase (SERCA), located in the longitudinal SR [66]. It binds two Ca^{++} ions with high affinity and rapidly

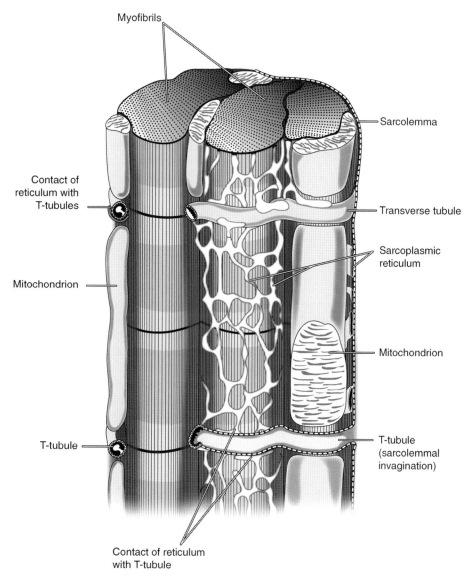

Figure 5.9 Normal, mature cardiac myocyte structure (Reproduced with permission from Reference [64])

transports them to the inside of the SR. This transport system differs from the sarcolemmal membrane: it has higher affinity, allows for more rapid transport, and is not sensitive to calmodulin. Ca^{++} is stored in the SR by calsequestrin, a high-capacity, low-affinity protein that acts as a Ca^{++} sink.

There are two other proteins with essential roles in the regulation of Ca^{++} flux: phospholamban and calmodulin [67,68]. Phospholamban is associated with the SERCA and can be phosphorylated by at least four different protein kinases (see above): cAMP-dependent, Ca^{++}/calmodulin dependent, cGMP dependent, or PKC. When phosphorylated, phospholamban increases the affinity of the SERCA for Ca^{++}, facilitating Ca^{++} flux back into the SR, thus affecting the inotropic and lusitropic state of the heart. Phos-

pholamban plays an important role in the β-adrenergic-mediated increase in inotropic state of the heart. Calmodulin is a Ca^{++} storage protein with four binding sites, found in the cytoplasm, which interacts with the sarcolemmal Ca^{++}-ATPase (increasing its affinity for Ca^{++}) and the SR ligand-gated Ca^{++} release channel (inhibits its activity at optimal cytoplasmic Ca^{++}) and binds to the Ca^{++}/calmodulin-dependent protein kinase [68].

The increase in intracellular cytoplasmic Ca^{++} initiates the contractile process. Myosin is the major component of the thick filaments, which make up the microscopic structure of the myofibril, and its interaction with actin (the major component of the thin filaments) provides the mechanical basis of cardiac muscle cell contraction [69]. Actin and myosin make up approximately 80% of

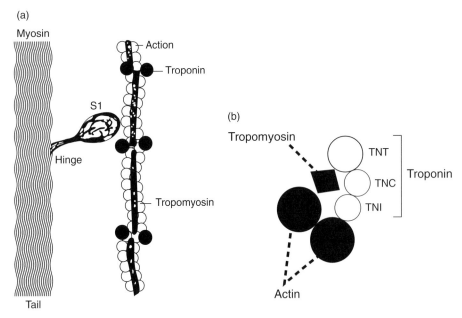

Figure 5.10 (a) Single thick and thin filament showing the S1 cross bridge and hinge mechanism. (b) Relationship of actin to tropomyosin and the three troponin subunits. See text for explanation (Reproduced with permission from Reference [70])

the contractile apparatus, and are arranged in a parallel, longitudinal fashion, projecting from a Z-line or band (Figure 5.10) to form the basic contractile unit called the sarcomere. A three-dimensional lattice consisting of interdigitated thick and thin filaments in a hexagonal array with three thin filaments in close proximity to each thick filaments is formed. The actin and myosin are linked by projections on the myosin protein called S1 cross-bridges, which bind to actin and, via an energy-dependent hinge-like mechanism, produce the sliding filament cross-bridge action that is thought to produce sarcomere shortening and lengthening. The lattice is held together by connecting proteins such as titin, nebulin, and α-actinin [71]. The actin–myosin interaction is initiated when Ca^{++} binds to troponin, a protein closely connected to actin that consists of three subunits: a Ca^{++}-binding subunit (TNC), a tropomyosin-binding unit (TNT), and an inhibitory subunit (TNI). TNC can bind up to four Ca^{++} ions, and this produces a conformational change on the thin filament, which allows the S1 myosin head cross-bridges to attach [72]. This also changes the TNI subunit's conformation, and allows tropomyosin, another protein integral in filament interaction, to move aside and expose the binding sites on actin, allowing the strong binding to the S1 cross-bridges. With Ca^{++} present, actin causes myosin ATPase to hydrolyze one ATP molecule, providing energy that results in the S1 myosin head pulling on the thin filament, resulting in sarcomere shortening. Troponin C is the most important aspect of the regulation of cardiocyte contraction, and has a steep response curve to local levels of Ca^{++}.

The reuptake of Ca^{++} into the SR causes Ca^{++} levels to rapidly decline and the inhibitory form of the troponin, tropomyosin, actin complex returns, resulting in the reversal of the cross-bridge binding and thus sarcomere relaxation.

Besides calcium, many other regulatory mechanisms exist to influence the interaction and sensitivity of Ca^{++} binding to troponin. These mechanisms include β-adrenergic stimulation, thyroid hormone, and phosphorylation by cAMP-dependent protein kinases.

Developmental changes in calcium cycling

Several aspects of the excitation–contraction system are different in the immature heart. The T tubule is not fully formed [73] and the SR has less storage capacity and less structural organization [74], less mRNA expression [74, 75], and less responsiveness to chemical blockade [76, 77]. The inhibitory subunit of troponin (TNI) changes from a predominately cAMP insensitive form to a cAMP responsive form by 9 months of age, an additional factor contributing to the increased responsiveness seen with β-adrenergic stimulation after the neonatal period [78]. All of this information has led to the theory that the neonatal cardiac myocyte is more dependent on free cytosolic Ca^{++} fluxes than is the mature heart, and more susceptible to blockade of the L-type Ca^{++} sarcolemmal channels as a mechanism of myocardial depression. The latter is thought to be the mechanism producing greater myocardial depression observed with halothane in

Table 5.1 Summary of major differences between neonatal and mature hearts

	Neonatal	Mature
Physiology		
Contractility	Limited	Normal
Heart rate dependence	High	Low
Contractile reserve	Low	High
Afterload tolerance	Low	Higher
Preload tolerance	Limited	Better
Ventricular interdependence	Significant	Less
Ca^{++} cycling		
Predominant site of Ca^{++} flux	Sarcolemma	Sarcoplasmic reticulum
Dependence on normal iCa^{++}	High	Lower
Circulating catecholamines	High	Lower
Adrenergic receptors	Downregulated insensitive $\beta2$, a1 predominant	Normal $\beta1$ predominant
Innervation	Parasympathetic predominates; sympathetic incomplete	Complete
Cytoskeleton	High collagen and Water content	Lower collagen and water content
Cellular elements	Incomplete SR, Disorganized myofibrils	Mature SR Organized myofibrils

neonatal rat models compared with sevoflurane, and the same phenomenon seen clinically [79]. A summary of the major differences in cardiac development and function between the neonatal and mature heart is presented in Table 5.1.

Thyroid hormone

Triiodothyronine (T3) has a critical role both in the development of the cardiovascular system and also in acute regulation and performance. Normal T3 levels are essential for normal maturation and development of the heart through expression of genes responsible for the production of the cardiac contractile proteins, elements of the calcium cycling apparatus, and development and density of β-ARs [80]. There are cell nucleus-mediated effects from exogenous T3 that occur from an increase in protein synthesis and require at least 8 hours to develop. These include an upregulation of β-ARs, increase in cardiac contractile protein synthesis, increase in mitochondrial density, volume, and respiration, increase in SERCA m RNA, and changes in myosin heavy chain isoforms. However, there are acute effects of T3 on cardiac myocytes that occur in minutes from interactions with specific sarcolemmal receptors, and include stimulation of L-type Ca^{++} pump activity, stimulation of SR Ca^{++}- ATPase activity, increased protein kinase activity, and decrease in phospholamban [81]. Cardiac surgery and cardiopulmonary

bypass interfere with the conversion of thyroxine (T4) to T3, and serum levels decrease significantly after cardiac surgery in infants and children [82]. T3 infusions improve myocardial function in children after cardiac surgery and reduce intensive care unit stay [83].

Regulation of vascular tone in systemic and pulmonary circulations

The regulation of vascular tone is an important consideration in the understanding and treatment of congenital heart disease. Both the systemic and pulmonary circulations have complex systems to maintain a delicate balance between vasodilating and vasoconstricting mediators in normal patients. Abnormal responses may develop which lead to pulmonary or systemic hypertension, or conversely vasodilation. A schematic representation of some of these mediators is shown in Figure 5.11. To some extent, the control mechanisms reviewed are present in both the systemic and pulmonary circulations; however, certain mechanisms are more important in one circulation. For example, the endothelial-mediated systems (NO–cGMP pathways, etc.) predominate in the pulmonary circulation (low-resistance circulation), whereas the phospholipase systems predominate in the systemic circulation (high-resistance circulation).

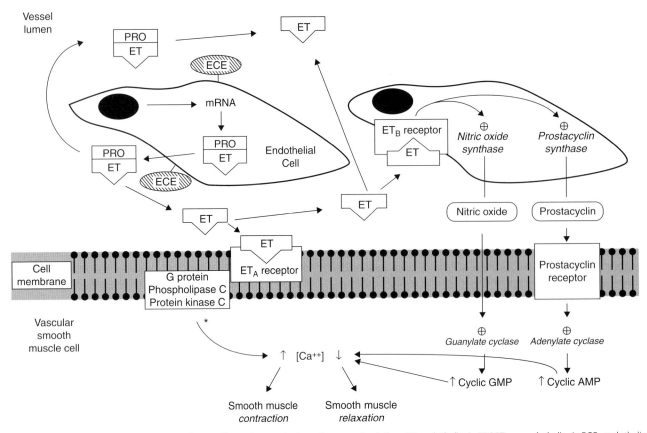

Figure 5.11 Schematic of some major mediators of vascular tone in the pulmonary circulation. ET, endothelin-1; PROET, proendothelin-1; ECE, endothelin converting enzyme. See text for explanation (Reproduced with permission from Reference [84])

Pulmonary circulation

Vasoactive metabolites of arachidonic acid, called eicosanoids, are produced in cell membranes. Eicosanoids metabolized via the lipoxygenase pathway will form leukotrienes, and those metabolized via the cyclooxygenase pathway form the prostaglandins. Important vasodilating prostaglandins include PGE$_1$, which also promotes and maintains patency of the ductus arteriosus. Prostacyclin, PGI$_2$, is a potent pulmonary vasodilator [85]. Prostaglandins act in vascular smooth muscle of the systemic and pulmonary circulations by binding to receptors in the smooth muscle cell membrane, activating AC and increasing cAMP concentrations, which lead to lower Ca^{++} levels and a reduction of vascular tone. Thromboxane A2 is a potent leukotriene that has the opposite effects of the prostaglandins, producing vasoconstriction and platelet aggregation. Imbalance in this system caused by chronic hypoxia can lead to chronic pulmonary hypertension.

NO is an endothelium-derived relaxant factor that causes relaxation of vascular smooth muscle cells after diffusing into the cell and activating guanylate cyclase, increasing the concentration of cGMP, leading to a reduction in the local concentration of Ca^{++} and thus reducing vascular tone [86]. Calcium sensitive potassium channels contribute to the vasodilatation caused by NO via a cGMP-dependent protein kinase [87]. NO is formed from L-arginine by NO synthase and is almost immediately inactivated by binding to hemoglobin. PDE V breaks down cGMP, so the PDE-inhibiting drugs, like sildenafil, potentiate NO-mediated vasodilation [88].

Endothelins are powerful endothelium-derived vasoactive peptides, and endothelin-1 (ET-1) is the best characterized. ET-1 is produced from proedothelin-1 by endothelin-converting enzymes in the endothelial cells of systemic and pulmonary vasculature. Increased pressure, shear stress, and hypoxia can lead to increased production of ET-1 in the pulmonary circulation. Two ET-1 receptors, ETA and ETB, mediate effects on smooth muscle vascular tone [89]. The ETA receptor is found on the smooth muscle cell membrane and mediates vasoconstriction, while the ETB receptor is located on the endothelial cell itself, and results in increased NO synthase activity, producing vasodilation. The primary activity of ET-1 appears to be to stimulate the ETA receptor, and indeed increased levels of ET-1 are found in many pulmonary hypertensive states such as Eisenmenger syndrome and primary pulmonary hypertension [90].

Systemic circulation

There are multiple levels of control over the peripheral circulation. Neural control by the sympathetic and parasympathetic nervous systems is produced from stimulation of receptors on the afferent limb such as stretch receptors within the walls of the heart, and baroreceptors in the walls of arteries, such as the aortic arch and carotid sinuses. Stretch in the arterial wall stimulates the baroreceptors producing vasodilation and heart rate slowing mediated by the vasomotor centers of the medulla [91]. Atrial stretch receptors inhibit secretion of vasopressin from the hypothalamus. The efferent limb of the autonomic nervous system consists of sympathetic and parasympathetic nerve fibers. The sympathetic nerves can be divided into vasoconstrictor and vasodilator fibers. When stimulated, the vasoconstrictor fibers release norepinephrine activating α-ARs and producing vasoconstriction. The vasodilator fibers release acetylcholine or epinephrine, and are mainly present in skeletal muscle. Parasympathetic fibers are vital in control of heart rate and function, but have only a minor role in controlling the peripheral circulation [92].

Hormonal control and receptor-mediated intracellular signaling are other important mechanisms. Norepinephrine primarily stimulates peripheral α receptors and causes vasoconstriction. It is secreted by the adrenal medulla and by sympathetic nerves in proximity to the systemic blood vessels. Epinephrine is also secreted by the adrenal medulla, but its primary action is to stimulate the β_2 receptors in the peripheral circulation, causing vasodilation through cAMP-mediated reductions in intracellular Ca^{++} concentrations.

Angiotensin II is produced by activation of the renin–angiotensin–aldosterone axis in response to reduced flow and pressure sensed by the juxtaglomerular apparatus in the kidney. Renin produces angiotensin I by cleaving angiotensinogen, and angiotensin II is produced when angiotensin I passes through the lung by angiotensin-converting enzyme. Angiotensin II is a potent vasoconstrictor and also induces the hypothalamus to secrete vasopressin (antidiuretic hormone), which also has vasoconstrictor properties.

Atrial natriuretic factor (ANF) is released from atrial myocytes in response to stretch (elevation of right or left atrial pressure) on the atrium. ANF has vasodilatory and cardioinhibitory effects, and sodium retention from decreased tubular reabsorption of sodium in the kidney [93]. B-type natriuretic peptide (BNP) is released by ventricular myocardium, also in response to stretch, and causes an increase in cGMP, leading to vasodilatation in both arterial and venous systems. In addition, it increases urinary sodium and water excretion [94].

Second messenger systems affect the activation of receptors on systemic vascular cell membranes leading to changes in vascular tone. The phosphoinositide signaling system is the common pathway for many of these agonists [91] (Figure 5.12). Membrane kinases phosphorylate phosphatidylinositol, which is an inositol lipid located mainly in the inner lamella of the plasma membrane, producing phosphatidylinositol 4,5 biphosphate. The second messenger, inositol 1,4,5-triphosphate, is produced from this compound by the action of the enzyme phospolipase C (PLC) [95]. The sequence begins with the binding of an agonist, such as angiotensin II, vasopressin, norepinephrine, or endothelin to a receptor with seven membrane spanning domains. This receptor is linked to activated G_q protein subunit, which in turn stimulates phosphatidylinositol-specific phospholipase C (PI-PLC) to produce inositol 1,4,5,-triphosphate, which acts to cause release of Ca^{++} from the SR, activating the actin–myosin system in the smooth muscle cells, producing vasoconstriction. Another second messenger, 1,2-diacylglycerol, is also produced, which goes on to activate PKC, which in turn has a role in mitogenesis and thus proliferation of smooth muscle cells. There are many isozymes of phospholipase C; the form implicated in this series of events is the PLCβ form. The PLCγ isoform is activated when cell growth factors such as platelet-derived growth factor bind to their receptors on the cell surface and active tyrosine kinases. This results in the production of phosphatidylinositol 3,4,5-triphosphate, which is also implicated in mitogenesis.

Vasodilatation of the systemic circulation results from the formation of NO by nitrovasodilators, or by activation of β_2-ARs in the peripheral vasculature, both of which result in the activation of guanylate cyclase and the production of cGMP, which reduces intracellular Ca^{++} concentrations, producing vasodilation [96].

The vascular beds in various peripheral tissues differ in the amount of local metabolic control of vascular tone. For example, pH has much more influence on the pulmonary circuit, with low pH leading to vasoconstriction and higher pH leading to vasodilatation, than in the vascular tone of other tissues. Local CO_2 concentration is much more important to central nervous system vasculature, with high levels leading to vasodilatation. Decrease in oxygen tension will often lead to vasodilatation, as adenosine is released in response to the decreased oxygen delivery; however, decreased oxygen tension increases tone

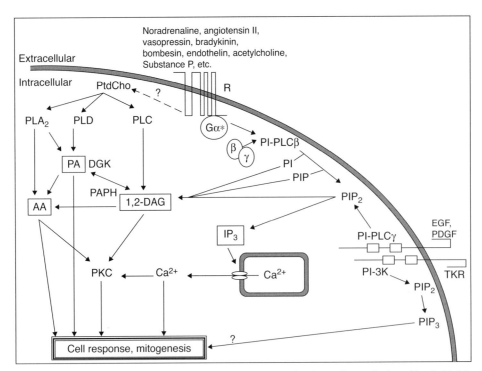

Figure 5.12 Phospholipase C system. Diagram summarizing the major receptor-activated pathways for production of inositol 1,4,5-triphosphate (IP3) and 1,2-diacyglycerol (1,2-DAG). The binding of an agonist to a receptor R with seven membrane-spanning domains results in the activation of the phosphatidylinositol-specific phospholipase Cβ (PI-PLCβ), whereas the stimulation of tyrosine kinase receptors (TKR) by polypeptide growth factors will activate phosphatidylinositol-specific phospholipase Cγ (PI-PLCγ). Both pathways will result in the hydrolysis of phosphatidylinositol 4,5-biphosphate (PIP2) and the formation of IP3 and 1,2-DAG. In addition, agonists that act on the heterotrimeric receptors may stimulate phosphatidylcholine (PtdCho) hydrolysis, and activation of tyrosine kinase receptors will stimulate the production of phosphatidylinositol 3,4,5-triphosphate (PIP3). DGK, diacylglyceral kinase; PAPH, phosphatidic acid phosphohydrolase; Gα^*, activated G protein subunit; β, β subunits, PLD, phospholipase D; PKC, protein kinase C; PI-3K, phosphatidylinositol 3-kinase; PI, phosphatidylinositol; PIP, phosphatidylinositol 4-phosphate; EGF, epidermal growth factor; PDGF, platelet-derived growth factor; PLA2, phospholipase A2; AA, arachidonic acid (Reproduced with permission from. —Reference [91])

in the pulmonary circulation. Autoregulation, or maintaining relatively constant blood flow over a wide range arterial pressures, predominates in the cerebral circulation but is not as critical in other tissue beds. Autoregulation and CO_2 responsiveness are both blunted in the fetal and immature brain [97].

Receptor signaling in myocardial dysfunction, congenital heart disease, and heart failure

A discussion of receptor signaling and calcium cycling in myocardial dysfunction is useful to serve as the basis for understanding many of the therapies discussed later in this text, and this section focuses on receptor physiology and calcium flux in three settings: acute myocardial dysfunction as seen after cardiac surgery and cardiopulmonary bypass, changes seen as responses to chronic cyanotic heart disease, and those seen with chronic congestive heart failure and cardiomyopathy.

Receptor signaling in acute myocardial dysfunction

Acute myocardial dysfunction, such as that sometimes seen after cardiopulmonary bypass, is often treated with catecholamines. These drugs are sometimes ineffective, especially when used in escalating doses. In children, the number and subtype distribution of β-ARs in atrial tissue is not affected from cardiac surgery with bypass; however, the activation of AC by isoproterenol is significantly reduced after bypass [98]. There is an uncoupling of β receptors from the G_s protein-AC complex. Densensitization to moderate or high doses of catecholamines may occur after only a few minutes of administration, because of increased cAMP concentrations results in uncoupling from the G_s protein [99].

After only a few minutes of high dose catecholamine administration may result in inactivation of the phosphorylated ARs from sequestration. These receptors can be sequestered by endocytosis, in a process involving a protein called β-arrestin, which binds to the receptor and a

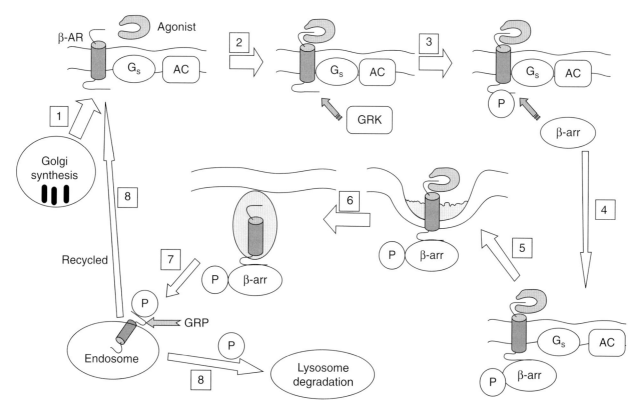

Figure 5.13 Desensitization and downregulation of the β-adrenoreceptor (β-AR). 1, agonist binding; 2, phosphorylation of the β-AR by G protein-coupled receptor kinases (GRK); 3, β-arrestin binds the to the GRK-phosphorylated β-AR, which is bound to the G_s protein. The receptor is then sequestrated to the endosomal compartment (4–7), to be dephosphorylated, and then either recycled back to the sarcolemma (8), or translocated to lysosomes for further degradation (8). AC, adenylate cyclase; GRP, G protein-coupled receptor phosphatase; P, inorganic phsohate groups; β-arr, β-arrestin (Reproduced with permission from —Reference [44])

sarcolemmal protein called clathrin (Figure 5.13). These sequestered receptors may either be recycled back to the cell membrane surface, or be destroyed by lysosomes [100]. This permanent destruction and degradation of receptors occurs after hours of exposure to catecholamines, and is accompanied by decreased mRNA and receptor protein synthesis, resulting in prolonged decrease in AR concentrations, which is reversed by decreasing exogenous catecholamines, but only as fast as new receptors can be synthesized.

Neonatal hearts may exhibit a different response to the acute or prolonged administration of catecholamines. Instead of desensitization, neonatal animal models demonstrate an enhanced β-AR response, accompanied by an increase in AC activity [101]. Desensitization as described above occurs later in development. The exact translation of these data to humans is not clear.

Treatment with catecholamines may also increase the concentration of G_i protein subunits, decreasing the sensitivity of the β-AR. This relative decrease in the ratio of G_s to G_i protein subunits has been demonstrated in rat and dog models [102, 103]. Another possible mechanism

of catecholamine-induced desensitization of the neonatal myocyte was demonstrated in a rat model, where prolonged exposure to norepinephrine caused an initial increase in functional L-type Ca^{++} channels on the sarcolemmal membrane. Continued exposure caused a decrease in L-type Ca^{++} channel mRNA to 50% of control values [104]. SR Ca^{++}-ATPase concentrations are reduced with chronic norepinephrine administration in the dog [105]. Finally, exposing adult or neonatal rat myocytes to high concentrations of catecholamines for 24 hours leads to increased apoptosis of myocardial cells, a genetically programmed energy-dependent mechanism for cell death and removal [106, 107]. This effect was mediated through β-ARs in the adult model, and α receptors in the neonatal model.

All of these studies provide the theoretical basis for the argument that administration of catecholamines to patients with acute myocardial dysfunction should be limited in dose and duration. Obviously, this is difficult to accomplish in the setting of weaning a hemodynamically unstable patient from cardiopulmonary bypass. Strategies that may limit catecholamine dose include administering low doses of catecholamines together with PDE inhibitors, as well as adding corticosteroids, triiodothyronine, and vasopressin [108].

Receptor signaling in congenital heart disease

In the past decade, there is some new information available concerning AR signaling in patients with congenital heart disease. A study of 71 infants and children undergoing cardiac surgery used tissue from the right atrial appendage to study β-AR density, distribution of β_1 and β_2 receptor subtypes, and coupling to AC [109]. This study found that patients with severe or poorly compensated acyanotic (e.g., congestive heart failure) or cyanotic (e.g., severe cyanosis) had significantly reduced β-AR densities. Outside of the newborn period, this downregulation was β_1 selective, but in newborns with critical aortic stenosis or transposition of the great arteries, there was additional significant downregulation of the β_2 subtype. In tetralogy of Fallot patients, those treated with propranolol had a significant increase in the number and density of β-ARs, when compared with untreated patients. β-AR downregulation correlated with increased circulating norepinephrine levels. Finally, in severely affected patients, AC activity was reduced, demonstrating a partial decoupling, as noted above. Other studies have determined that symptomatic tetralogy of Fallot patients, i.e., those with cyanotic spells, have a significantly greater number of β-ARs in their right ventricular outflow tract muscle, and their AC activity was greater when compared to patients without cyanotic spells [110]. α1-ARs are also affected by congenital heart disease. A study of atrial tissue excised at surgery in 17 children evaluated α- versus β-AR stimulation with pharmacologic agents. The α component was responsible for 0–44% of the inotropic response, and β stimulation for 56–100% of the response, with the degree of right ventricular hypertrophy and pressure load correlating with the amount of a stimulation found [111].

Receptor signaling in congestive heart failure and cardiomyopathy

Like adults with heart failure, children with congestive heart failure due to chronic left-to-right shunting and volume overload of the heart have elevated levels of circulating norepinephrine. This leads to a downregulation in β-AR density [112]. The degree of elevation of pulmonary artery pressure and amount of left-to-right shunting correlates with the plasma catecholamine levels, and is inversely correlated with β-AR density. All of these abnormalities return to normal levels after corrective surgery. The degree of receptor downregulation in congestive heart failure correlates with postoperative morbidity in infants and children. Children with an intensive care unit stay of greater than 7 days or those who died during the early postoperative period (9 of the 26) had significantly less β_1 and β_2 mRNA gene expression than those who had better outcomes [113]. In addition, the children receiving propranolol for treatment of their congestive heart failure had higher β-AR mRNA levels and tended to have improved outcomes. Finally, children with dilated cardiomyopathy also have a reduced response to catecholamines with one study showing no significant increase in ejection fraction during dobutamine stress test, with infusion of dobutamine at 5 and then 10 mcg/kg/min [114].

The preceding has been a brief discussion of receptor signaling in pediatric heart disease. This emerging field has many implications for treatment strategies, and the reader is referred to excellent reviews for more detail information on this subject [115].

Myocardial preconditioning

Myocardial preconditioning refers to the finding that repeated, brief exposures of the myocardium to ischemia, volatile anesthetics, or other stresses induces a protective effect to a later (i.e., 12–24 hours), more prolonged, ischemic insult resulting in decreased myocardial infarction size, and improved myocardial function after the insult [116]. Chronic cyanosis also induces a similar protective effect in the myocardium, although the effect size is smaller and more long lasting, i.e., beyond 24 hours. The mechanisms of myocardial preconditioning are complex, but are thought to involve release of various neurohormonal agents and peptides such as adenosine, bradykinin, and NO via a cGMP-dependent mechanism, which then triggers a series of signal transduction events within the cardiomyocyte that confer a "memory" effect that protects the myocardium from future ischemic insults. The signal transduction effects include PKC, tyrosine kinases, mitogen-activated protein kinases, glycogen synthase kinase 3β, and other enzymes [117]. This series of events allows activation of mitochondrial and sacrolemmal K_{ATP} channels, which leads to the preconditioning by elusive mechanisms. One recently discovered candidate for this end effector is the mitochondrial permeability transition pore (MPTP) [117]. This is a nonspecific channel that spans both mitochondrial membranes, and when opened for a prolonged period, a dissipation of mitochondrial electrical potential, inhibition of ATP synthesis, and ultimately mitochondrial swelling, rupture, failure of cellular energy metabolism, and cell death. Agents and stimuli that confer myocardial preconditioning have been found to keep the MPTP closed, thus possibly elucidating further the subcellular mechanisms involved.

Several recent pediatric cardiac surgery studies have been published elucidating the potential effects of myocardial preconditioning, which could have the beneficial effect of ameliorating the myocardial stunning effect seen in operations on infants with long aortic cross clamp times [118]. In a study of 90 infants randomized to sevoflurane, propofol, or midazolam anesthesia for maintenance, plus a sufentanil infusion for analgesia, patients receiving sevoflurane had a very strong trend toward lower troponin T concentrations in the first 24 hours after surgery, potentially signifying less myocardial injury due to the prebypass exposure to sevoflurane [119]. In a novel variation of myocardial preconditioning, remote ischemic preconditioning (RIPC) produced by inflating a blood pressure cuff on a lower extremity to produce a 5-minute period of limb ischemia, for four cycles before cardiopulmonary bypass, was studied in 37 children undergoing cardiac surgery. Patients who underwent RIPC had lower peak troponin I levels (17 vs 22 mcg/L, $p = 0.04$), and lower inotrope score in the RIPC group at both 3 and 6 hours postbypass [120]. This interesting phenomenon of RIPC may work through modulation of the inflammatory response through some as yet unknown humoral mechanism. This entire area of myocardial preconditioning, whether ischemic, anesthetic induced, remote, or other variations, is an important area of future study that may well have several translations into clinical care.

References

1. Rudolph AM (1985) Distribution and regulation of blood flow in the fetal and neonatal lamb. Circ Res 57:811–821.
2. Rudolph AM (1974) Congenital Diseases of the Heart. Year Book Medical Publishers, Chicago.
3. Fineman JR, Soifer SJ, Heymann MA (1995) Regulation of pulmonary vascular tone in the perinatal period. Annu Rev Physiol 57:115–134.
4. Baum VC, Palmisano BW (1997) The immature heart and anesthesia. Anesthesiology 87:1529–1548.
5. Hawkins J, Van Hare GF, Schmidt KG, et al. (1989) Effects of increasing afterload on left ventricular output in fetal lambs. Cir Res 65:127.
6. Friedman WF (1972) The intrinsic physiologic properties of the developing heart. Prog Cardiovasc Dis 15:87–111.
7. Friedman WF, George BL (1985) Treatment of congestive heart failure by altering loading conditions of the heart. J Pediatr 106:697–706.
8. Eliot RJ, Lam R, Leake RD, et al. (1980) Plasma catecholamine concentrations in infants at birth and during the first 48 hours of life. J Pediatr 96:311.
9. Romero T, Covell U, Friedman WF (1972) A comparison of pressure–volume relations of the fetal, newborn, and adult heart. Am J Physiol 222:1285.
10. Teitel DF, Sisd D, Chin T, et al. (1985) Developmental changes in myocardial contractile reserve in the lamb. Pediatr Res 19:948.
11. Nassar R, Malouf NN, Kelly MB, et al. (1991) Force–pCa relation and troponin T isoforms of rabbit myocardium. Circ Res 69:1470–1475.
12. Cummins P, Lambert SJ (1986) Myosin transitions in the bovine and human heart. A developmental and anatomical study of heavy and light chain subunits in the atrium and ventricle. Circ Res 58:846–858.
13. Morano I, Bachle-Stolz C, Katus A, Ruegg JC (1988) Increased calcium sensitivity of chemically skinned human atria by myosin light chain kinase. Basic Res Cardiol 83:35–39.
14. Bodor GS, Oakeley AE, Allen PD, et al. (1992) Troponin I in fetal and normal and failing adult human hearts. Circulation 86 (Suppl I):842.
15. Swynghdauw B (1986) Developmental and functional adaptation of contractile proteins in cardiac and skeletal muscles. Physiol Rev 66:701–771.
16. Boheler KR, Carrier L, de la Bastie D, et al. (1991) Skeletal actin mRNA increases in the human heart during ontogenic development and is the major isoform of control and failing adult hearts. J Clin Invest 88:323–330.
17. Marijianowski MM, Van Der Loos CM, Mohrschladt MF, Becker AE (1994) The neonatal heart has a relatively high content of total collagen and type I collagen, an condition that may explain the less compliant state. J Am Coll Cardiol 23:1204–1208.
18. Borg TK (1982) Development of the connective tissue network in the neonatal hamster heart. Anat Rec 165:435–444.
19. Terracio L, Rubin K, Gullberg D, et al. (1991) Expression of collagen binding integrins during cardiac development and hypertrophy. Circ Res 68:734–744.
20. Simonis G, Briem SK, Schoen SP, et al. (2007) Protein kinase C in the human heart: differential regulation of the isoforms in aortic stenosis or dilated cardiomyopathy. Mol Cell Biochem 305:103–111.
21. Nagendran J, Archer SL, Soliman D, et al. (2007) Phosphodiesterase type 5 is highly expressed in the hypertrophied human right ventricle, and acute inhibition of phosphodiesterase type 5 improves contractility. Circulation 116:238–248.
22. Sander TL, Klinkner DB, Tomita-Mitchell A, Mitchell ME (2006) Molecular and cellular basis of congenital heart disease. Pediatr Clin North Am 53:989–1009.
23. Matsson H, Eason J, Bookwalter CS, et al. (2008) Alpha-cardiac actin mutations produce atrial septal defects. Hum Mol Genet 17:256–265.
24. Amir G, Ma X, Reddy VM, et al. (2008) Dynamics of human myocardial progenitor cell populations in the neonatal period. Ann Thorac Surg 86:1311–1320.
25. Towbin JA, Bowles NE (2001) Molecular genetics of left ventricular dysfunction. Curr Mol Med 1:81–90.
26. Towbin JA, Bowles NE (2002) Molecular diagnosis of myocardial disease. Expert Rev Mol Diagn 2:587–602.
27. Dees E, Baldwin HS (2002) New frontiers in molecular pediatric cardiology. Curr Opin Pediatr 14:627–633.
28. Friedman WF, Pool PE, Jacobowitz D, et al. (1968) Sympathetic innervation of the developing rabbit heart. Biochemical and histochemical comparisons of fetal, neonatal, and adult myocardium. Circ Res 23:25–32.

29. Jacobowitz D, Koelle GB (1965) Histochemical correlations of acetylcholinesterase and catecholamines in postganglionic autonomic nerves of the cat, rabbit and guinea pig. J Pharmacol Exp Ther 148:225–237.

30. Pagani M, Montano N, Porta A, et al. (1997) Relationship between spectral components of cardiovascular variabilities and direct measures of sympathetic nerve activity in humans. Circulation 95:1441–1448.

31. Constant I, Dubois M, Piat V, et al. (1999) Changes in electroencephalogram and autonomic cardiovascular activity during induction of anesthesia with sevoflurane compared with halothane in children. Anesthesiology 91:1604–1615.

32. Katona PG, Frasz A, Egbert J (1980) Maturation of cardiac control in full-term and preterm infants during sleep. Early Hum Dev 4:145–159.

33. Fabiato A, Fabiato F (1978) Calcium induced release of calcium from the sarcoplasmic reticulum of skinned cells from adult human, dog, cat, rabbit, rat and from heart and from fetal and newborn rat ventricles. Ann N Y Acad Sci 307:491–499.

34. Rudolph AM (2000) Myocardial growth before and after birth: clinical implications. Acta Pediatr 89:129–133.

35. Friesen RH, Wurl JL, Charlton GA (2000) Haemodynamic depression by halothane is age-related in paediatric patients. Paediatr Anaesth 10:267–272.

36. Versmold HT, Kitterman JA, Phibbs RH, et al. (1981) Aortic blood pressure during the first 12 hours of life in infants with birth weight 610 to 4,220 grams. Pediatrics 67:607–613.

37. Blumenthal SC (1977) Report of the task force on blood pressure control in children. Pediatrics 59 (Suppl):794–820.

38. Spann JF Jr, Covell JW, Eckberg DL, et al. (1972) Contractile performance of the hypertrophied and chronically failing cat ventricle. Am J Physiol 223:1150–1157.

39. Izumo S, Lompre AM, Matsuoka R, et al. (1987) Myosin heavy chain messenger RNA and protein isoform transitions during cardiac hypertrophy. J Clin Invest 79:970–977.

40. Lu H, Fedak PW, Dai X, et al. (2006) Integrin-linked kinase expression is elevated in human cardiac hypertrophy and induces hypertrophy in transgenic mice. Circulation 114:2271–2279.

41. Vatta M, Stetson SJ, Perez-Verdia A, et al. (2002) Molecular remodeling of dystrophin in patients with end-stage cardiomyopathies and reversal in patients on assistance-device therapy. Lancet 359:936–941.

42. Feng J, Yan J, Buzin CH, et al. (2002) Mutations in the dystrophin gene are associated with sporadic dilated cardiomyopathy. Mol Genet Metab 77:119–126.

43. Moss J, Renz CL (2000) The autonomic nervous system. In: Miller RD (ed) Anesthesia, 5th edn. Churchill Livingstone, Philadelphia, pp. 523–577.

44. Booker PD (2002) Pharmacological support for children with myocardial dysfunction. Paediatr Anaesth 12:5–25.

45. Ahlquist RP (1948) A study of the adrenotropic receptors. Am J Physiol 153:586–600.

46. Bristow MR, Ginsburg R, Umans V, et al. (1986) Beta 1- and beta 2-adrenergic-receptor subpopulations in nonfailing and failing human ventricular myocardium: coupling of both receptor subtypes to muscle contraction and selective beta 1-receptor down-regulation in heart failure. Circ Res 59:297–309.

47. Kozlik R, Kramer HH, Wicht H, et al. (1991) Myocardial beta-adrenoceptor density and the distribution of beta 1- and beta 2-adrenoceptor subpopulations in children with congenital heart disease. Eur J Pediatr 150:388–394.

48. Sun LS, Du F, Quaegebeur JM (1997) Right ventricular infundibular beta-adrenoceptor complex in tetralogy of Fallot patients. Pediatr Res 42:12–16.

49. Xiao RP, Cheng H, Zhou YY, et al. (1999) Recent advances in cardiac beta(2)-adrenergic signal transduction. Circ Res 85:1092–1100.

50. Post SR, Hilal-Dandan R, Urasawa K, et al. (1995) Quantification of signaling components and amplification in the beta-adrenergic-receptor-adenylate cyclase pathway in isolated adult rat ventricular myocytes. Biochem J 311 (Pt 1):75–80.

51. Sun LS (1999) Regulation of myocardial beta-adrenergic receptor function in adult and neonatal rabbits. Bil Neonate 76:181–192.

52. Kozlik R, Kramer HH, Wicht H, et al. (1991) Myocardial beta-adrenoreceptor density and the distribution of beta 1- and beta 2-adrenoceptor subpopulations in children with congenital heart disease. Eur J Pediatr 150:388–394.

53. Tanaka H, Manita S, Matsuda T, et al. (1995) Sustained negative inotropism mediated by alpha-adrenoreceptors in adult mouse myocasdia: developmental conversion from positive response in the neonate. Br J Pharmacol 114:673–677.

54. Sun LS, Rybin VO, Steinberg SF, Robinson RB (1998) Characterization of the alpha-1 adrenergic chronotropic response in neuropeptide Y-treated cardiomyocytes. Eur J Pharmacol 349:377–381.

55. Tanaka H, Takenaka Y, Yamaguchi H, et al. (2001) Evidence of alpha-adrenoceptor-mediated chronotropic action in children. Pediatr Cardiol 22:40–43.

56. Tate CA, Taffet GE, Fisher DJ, Hyek MF (1998) Excitation–contraction coupling: control of normal myocardial cellular calcium movements. In: Garson A, Bricker JT, Fisher DJ, Neish SR (eds) The Science and Practice of Pediatric Cardiology, 2nd edn. Williams & Wilkins, Baltimore, pp. 171–180.

57. Fabiato A (1981) Myoplasmic free calcium concentration reached during the twitch on an intact isolated cardiac cell and during calcium-induced release of calcium from the sarcoplasmic reticulum of a skinned cardiac cell from the adult rat or rabbit ventricle. J Gen Physiol 78:457.

58. Hoshijima M, Chien KR (2002) Mixed signals in heart failure: cancer rules. J Clin Invest 109:849–855.

59. Bean BP (1985) Two kinds of calcium channels in canine atrial cells: difference in kinetic, selectivity, and pharmacology. J Gen Physiol 86:1.

60. Eisner DA, Lederer WJ (1985) Na–Ca exchange: stoichiometry and electrogenicity. Am J Physiol 248:C189.

61. Caroni P, Carafoli E (1981) The Ca^{++}-pumping ATPase of heart sarcolemma. J Biol Chem 256:3263.

62. Fabiato A (1985) Time and calcium independence of activation and inactivation of calcium-induced release of calcium from the sacroplasmic reticulum of a skinned cardiac Purkinje cell. J Gen Physiol 85:247.

63. Van Winkle WB (1986) The structure of striated muscle sarcoplasmic reticulum. In: Entman M, Van Winkle WB (eds) Sarcoplasmic Reticulum in Muscle Physiology. CRC Press, Boca Raton, Florida, pp. 1–20.

64. Bloom W, Fawcett DW (1968) A Textbook of Histology. WB Saunders, Philadelphia, p. 293.

65. Jones LR, Seler SM, Van Winkle WB (1986) Regional differences in sarcoplasmic reticulum function. In: Entman M, Van Winkle WB (eds) Sarcoplasmic Reticulum in Muscle Physiology. CRC Press, Boca Raton, Florida, pp. 21–30.

66. Levitsky DO, Benevolensky DS, Levchenko TS, et al. (1981) Calcium-binding rate and capacity of cardiac sarcoplascmic reticulum. J Mol Cell Cardiol 13:785.

67. Jorgensen AO, Jones LR (1986) Localization of phospholamban in slow but not fast canine skeletal muscle fibers. J Biol Chem 261:3775.

68. Walsh KB, Cheng Q (2004) Intracellular Ca(2+) regulates responsiveness of cardiac L-type Ca(2+) current to protein kinase A: role of calmodulin. Am J Physiol Heart Circ Physiol 286:H186–H194.

69. Murray J, Weber A (1974) The cooperative action of muscle proteins. Sci Am 230:59–71.

70. Michael LH (1998) Cardiac contractile proteins in the normal heart: the contractile process and its regulation. In: Garson A, Bricker JT, Fisher DJ, Neish SR (eds) The Science and Practice of Pediatric Cardiology, 2nd edn. Williams & Wilkins, Baltimore, p. 182.

71. Goldstein M, Michael L, Schroeter J, et al. (1987) Z band dynamics as a function of sarcomere length and the contractile state of muscle. FASEB J 1:133–142.

72. Noble M, Pollack G (1977) Molecular mechanisms of contraction. Cir Res 40:333–342.

73. Chen F, Mottino G, Klitzner TS, et al. (1995) Distribution of the Na^+/Ca^{++} exchange protein in developing rabbit myocytes. Am J Physiol 268:C1126–C1132.

74. Nakanishi T, Seguchi M, Takao A (1988) Development of the myocardial contractile system. Experientia 44:936–944.

75. Mahony L, Jones LR (1986) Developmental changes in cardiac sarcoplasmic reticulum in sheep. J Biol Chem 261:15257–15265.

76. Maylie JG (1982) Excitation–contraction coupling in neonatal and adult myocardium of cat. Am J Physiol 242:H834–H843.

77. Klitzner TS, Chen FH, Raven RR, et al. (1991) Calcium current and tension generation in immature mammalian myocardium: effects of diltiazem. J Mol Cell Cardiol 23:807–815.

78. Sasse S, Brand N, Kypreanou P, et al. (1993) Troponin I gene expression during human cardiac development and in end-stage heart failure. Cir Res 72:932–938.

79. Prakash YS, Seckin I, Hunter IW, et al. (2002) Mechanisms underlying greater sensitivity of neonatal cardiac muscle to volatile anesthetics. Anesthesiology 96:893–906.

80. Davis PJ, Davis FB (1993) Acute cellular actions of thyroid hormone and myocardial function. Ann Thorac Surg 56:S16–S23.

81. Novotny J, Bourova L, Malkova O, et al. (1999) G proteins, β-adrenoceptors, and β-adrenergic responsiveness in immature and adult rat ventricular myocardium: influence of neonatal hypo- and hyperthyroidism. J Mol Cell Cardiol 31:761–772.

82. Mitchell IM, Pollock JC, Jamieson MP, et al. (1992) The effects of cardiopulmonary bypass on thyroid function in infants weighing less than five kilograms. J Thorac Cardiovasc Surg 103:800–805.

83. Bettendorf M, Schmidt KG, Grulich-Henn J, et al. (2000) Tri-iodothyronine treatment in children after cardiac surgery: a double-blind, randomized, placebo-controlled study. Lancet 356:529–534.

84. Haynes WG, Webb DJ (1993) The endothelin family of peptides: local hormones with diverse roles in health and disease? Clin Sci (Lond) 84:485–500.

85. Christman BW, McPherson CD, Newman JH, et al. (1992) An imbalance between the excretion of thromboxane and prostacyclin metabolites in pulmonary hypertension. N Engl J Med 327:70–75.

86. Palmer RM, Ferrige AG, Moncada S (1987) Nitric oxide release accounts for the biological activity of endothelium-derived relaxing factor. Nature 327:524–526.

87. Archer SL, Huang JM, Hampl V, et al. (1994) Nitric oxide and cGMP cause vasorelaxation by activation of a charybdotoxin-sensitive K channel by cGMP-dependent protein kinase. Proc Natl Acad Sci USA 91:7583–7587.

88. Atz AM, Wessel DL (1999) Sildenafil ameliorates effects of inhaled nitric oxide withdrawal. Anesthesiology 91:307–310.

89. Yanagisawa M, Kurihara H, Kimura S, et al. (1988) A novel potent vasoconstrictor peptide produced by vascular endothelial cells. Nature 332:411–415.

90. Cacoub P, Dorent R, Maistre G, et al. (1993) Endothelin-1 in primary pulmonary hypertension and the Eisenmenger syndrome. Am J Cardiol 71:448–450.

91. Izzard AS, Ohanian J, Tulip JR, Heagerty AM (2002) The structure and function of the systemic circulation. In: Anderson RH, Baker EJ, Macartney F, Tigby ML, Shinebourne EA, Tynan M (eds) Paediatric Cardiology, 2nd edn. Churchill Livingstone, London, pp. 95–109.

92. Ebert TJ, Stowe DF (1996) Neural and endothelial control of the peripheral circulation-implications for anesthesia: part I, neural control of the peripheral vasculature. J Cardiothorac Vasc Anesth 10:147–158.

93. Athanassopoulos G, Cokkinos DV (1991) Atrial natriuretic factor. Prog Cardiovasc Dis 33:313–328.

94. deLemos JA, McGuire DK, Drazner MH (2003) B-type natriuretic peptide in cardiovascular disease. Lancet 362:316–322.

95. Katan M, Williams RL (1997) Phosphoinositide-specific phospholipase C: structural basis for catalysis and regulatory interactions. Semin Cell Dev Biol 8:287–296.

96. Moncada S, Higgs A (1993) The L-arginine:nitric oxide pathway. N Engl J Med 329; 2002–2012.

97. Szymonowicz W, Walker AM, Cussen L, et al. (1988) Developmental changes in regional cerebral blood flow in fetal and newborn lambs. Am J Physiol 254:H52–H58.

98. Schranz D, Droege A, Broede A, et al. (1993) Uncoupling of human cardiac beta-adrenergic receptors during

cardiopulmonary bypass with cardioplegic arrest. Circulation 87:422–426.

99. Smiley RM, Kwatra MM, Schwinn DA (1998) New developments in cardiovascular adrenergic receptor pharmacology: molecular mechanisms and clinical relevance. J Cardiothorac Vasc Anesth 12:80–95.

100. Garcia-Sainz HA, Vazquez-Prado J, Carmen-Medina L (2000) α1-adrenoceptors: function and phosphorylation. Eur J Pharmacol 389:1–12.

101. Zeiders JL, Seidler FJ, Slotkin TA (1999) Agonist-induced sensitization of β-adrenoceptor signaling in neonatal rat heart: expression and catalytic activity of adenylyl cylcase. J Pharmacol Exp Ther 291:503–510.

102. Muller FU, Boheler KR, Eschenhagen T, et al. (1993) Isoprenaline stimulates gene transcription of the inhibitory G protein alpha-subunit G_i alpha-2 in rat heart. Circ Res 72:696–700.

103. Lai LP, Suematsu M, Elam H, Liang CS (1996) Differential changes of myocardial beta-adrenoceptor subtypes and G-proteins in dogs with right-sided congestive heart failure. Eur J Pharmacol 309:201–208.

104. Maki T, Gruver EJ, Davidoff AJ, et al. (1996) Regulation of calcium channel expression in neonatal myocytes by catecholamines. J Clin Invest 97:656–663.

105. Lai LP, Raju VS, Delehanty JM, et al. (1998) Altered sarcoplasmic reticulum Ca^{++}-ATPase gene expression in congestive heart failure: effect of chronic norepinephrine infusion. J Mol Cell Cardiol 30:175–185.

106. Communal C, Singh K, Pimentel DR, Colucci WS (1998) Norepinephrine stimulates apoptosis in adult rat ventricular myocytes by activation of the beta-adrenergic pathway. Circulation 98:1329–1334.

107. Iwai-Kanai E, Hasegawa K, Araki M, et al. (1999) Alpha- and beta-adrenergic pathways differentially regulate cell type-specific apoptosis in rat cardiac myocytes. Circulation 100:305–311.

108. Hoffman TM, Wernovsky G, Atz A, et al. (2003) Efficacy and safety of milrinone in preventing low cardiac output syndrome in infants and children after corrective surgery for congenital heart disease. Circulation 107:996–1002.

109. Kozlik-Feldmann R, Kramer HH, Wicht H, et al. (1993) Distribution of myocardial beta-adrenoceptor subtypes and coupling to the adenylate cyclase in children with congenital heart disease and implications for treatment. J Clin Pharmacol 33:588–595.

110. Sun LS, Du F, Quagebeur JM (1997) Right ventricular infundibular beta-adrenoceptor complex in Tetralogy of Fallot patients. Pediatr Res 42:12–16.

111. Borthne K, Haga P, Langslet A, et al. (1995) Endogenous norepinephrine stimulates both alpha 1- and beta adreoceptors in myocardium from with congenital heart defects. J Mol Cell Cardiol 27:693–699.

112. Wu JR, Chang HR, Chen SS, Huang TY (1996) Circulating noradrenaline and beta-adrenergic receptors in children with congestive heart failure. Acta Paediatr 85:923–927.

113. Buchhorn R, Huylpke-Wette M, Ruschewski W, et al. (2002) Beta-receptor downregulation in congenital heart disease: a risk factor for complications after surgical repair? Ann Thorac Surg 73:610–613.

114. Zeng H, Li W, Li Y, et al. (1999) Evaluation of cardiac beta-adrenergic receptor function in children by dobutamine stress echocardiography. Chin Med J 112:623–626.

115. Schwartz SM, Duffy JY, Pearl JM, Nelson DP (2001) Cellular and molecular aspects of myocardial dysfunction. Crit Care Med 29:S214–S219.

116. Baker JE (2004) Oxidative stress and adaptation of the infant heart to hypoxia and ischemia. Antioxid Redox Signal 6:423–429.

117. Baines CP (2007) The mitochondrial permeability transition pore as a target of cardioprotective signaling. Am J Physiol Heart Circ Physiol 293:H903–H904.

118. Booker PD (1998) Myocardial stunning in the neonate. Br J Anaesth 80:371–383.

119. Malagon I, Hogenbirk K, van Pelt J, et al. (2005) Effect of three different anaesthetic agents on the postoperative production of cardiac troponin T in paediatric cardiac surgery. Br J Anaesth 94:805–809.

120. Cheung MM, Kharbanda RK, Konstantinov IE, et al. (2006) Randomized controlled trial of the effects of remote ischemic preconditioning on children undergoing cardiac surgery: first clinical application in humans. J Am Coll Cardiol 47:2277–2282.

6 Anesthetic agents and their cardiovascular effects

Dean B. Andropoulos, M.D., M.H.C.M.
Texas Children's Hospital, Baylor College of Medicine, Houston, Texas, USA

Introduction

A wide variety of anesthetic regimens are used for patients with congenital heart disease (CHD) undergoing cardiac or noncardiac surgery, procedures in the cardiac catheterization laboratory, or other diagnostic or therapeutic procures such as magnetic resonance imaging. The goal of all of these regimens is to produce general anesthesia or adequate sedation, while preserving systemic cardiac output and oxygen delivery. Many of these patients have limited cardiac reserve, and if a cardiac arrest or other adverse cardiac event occurs, successful resuscitation is less frequent than in patients with normal hearts [1]. Thus, intelligent selection of regimen and dosage, with the patient's unique pathophysiology in mind, along with anesthetic requirements for the particular procedure they are undergoing, is essential. This chapter reviews the effects on hemodynamics and myocardial contractility of anesthetic agents and muscle relaxants commonly used for patients with CHD.

Anesthesia for Congenital Heart Disease 2nd edition. Edited by Dean Andropoulos, Stephen Stayer, Isobel Russell and Emad Mossad.
© 2010 Blackwell Publishing.

Volatile agents

In vitro studies of effects on contractility in isolated adult human atrial fibers indicate that direct myocardial contractility depression is greatest with halothane and that sevoflurane is equal to isoflurane and desflurane [2] (Figure 6.1). These studies of myocardium reveal that differences among these agents occur primarily from differing effects on calcium flux through L-type Ca^{++} channels, both trans-sarcolemmal, and in the sarcoplasmic reticulum (SR). Halothane reduces Ca^{++} flux through the sarcolemma more than isoflurane, with the net result that there is less intracellular Ca^{++} available to bind to the troponin-actin-myosin complex which produces myocyte contraction. Another mechanism of myocardial depression is that halothane, but not isoflurane, directly activates ryanodine-sensitive SR Ca^{++} channels, thereby reducing Ca^{++} storage in the SR and making less available for release during contraction. The effects of sevoflurane and desflurane on Ca^{++} flux are similar to isoflurane [2].

It is important to note that infants from the newborn period up to an age of approximately 6 months exhibit an exaggerated degree of depression of myocardial contractility and blood pressure in response to all volatile agents, but especially halothane [3] (Figure 6.2). This is

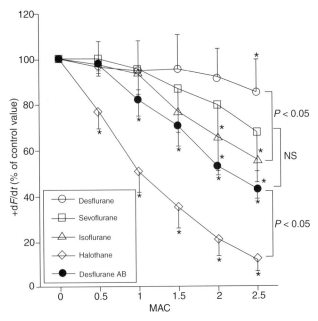

Figure 6.1 Force of contraction over time ($+dF/dt$) of isolated adult human atrial trabeculae in response to 0–2.5 minimum alveolar concentration (MAC) anesthetics. Desflurane AB = desflurane in the presence of α- and β-receptor blockade. Halothane depresses contractility significantly more than all other agents at every MAC (Reproduced with permission from Reference [2])

likely due to the immaturity of the Ca^{++} release and reuptake system, necessitating higher levels of free cytosolic Ca^{++} to be available to bind to the troponin–actin–myosin complex to produce myocyte contraction [5]. Recent evidence supports this theory. Sevoflurane, and to a greater extent, halothane, interfere with both L-type Ca^{++} channel and Na^+–Ca^{++} exchanger Ca^{++} flux at the plasmalemmal membrane more in neonatal than adult rat myocytes [6]. The volatile anesthetics interfered with Ca^{++} release from the SR more in adult rat myocytes. This information provides a mechanism for what is commonly observed clinically.

The effects of volatile agents on systemic vascular resistance (SVR) as measured by arterial blood pressure differ between agents. Ca^{++} flux in the smooth muscles of arterioles is reduced by all of these agents, resulting in less resting tone and thus lower blood pressure and vascular resistance. Halothane exhibits the most pronounced reduction of blood pressure, due to the combination of reduction in arterial tone, as well as the more pronounced depression of myocardial contractility. Isoflurane and sevoflurane lower blood pressure primarily through reduction in SVR [7].

Halothane has not been available in the USA since 2005, and sevoflurane has largely replaced this agent in the rest of the world for induction and maintenance of anesthesia. The Pediatric Perioperative Cardiac Arrest Registry data demonstrated a decrease in anesthetic medication-related cardiac arrests from 37% of the total in 1994–1997 to 18% in 1998–2004; this was primarily attributed to the increasingly infrequent use of halothane leading to fewer arrests, particularly in young infants [8].

In patients with CHD, several studies have been performed comparing new agents to halothane. A study using transthoracic echocardiography comparing halothane, isoflurane, and sevoflurane [7] in 54 children with two-ventricle CHD (Table 6.1) reported that 1 and 1.5 minimum alveolar concentration (MAC) halothane caused significant myocardial depression, resulting in a decline in mean arterial pressure (MAP: decline of 22 and 35%), ejection fraction (EF: decline of 15 and 20%) and cardiac output (CO: 17 and 21%), respectively, in patients 1 month to 13 years undergoing cardiac surgery. Sevoflurane maintained both CO and heart rate (HR), and had less profound hypotensive (MAP decrease 13 and 20% at 1 and 1.5 MAC) and negative inotropic (EF preserved at 1 MAC, 11% decrease at 1.5 MAC) effects compared with halothane. Isoflurane, in concentrations as high as 1.5 MAC, preserved CO and EF, had less suppression of MAP (22 and 25%) than halothane, increased HR (17 and 20%) and decreased systemic vascular resistance (SVR: 20 and 22%).

The effects of these agents on pulmonary (Qp) and systemic (Qs) blood flow in 30 biventricular patients and left-to-right shunts has also been assessed. Halothane, isoflurane, and sevoflurane did not change Qp:Qs as measured by echocardiography [9]. Russell et al. [10] compared halothane with sevoflurane in the prebypass period in 180 children with a variety of cardiac diagnoses, including 14 with single-ventricle physiology, and 40 with tetralogy of Fallot. The incidence of significant hypotension, bradycardia, and arrhythmia requiring drug treatment with atropine, phenylephrine, epinephrine, or ephedrine was higher with halothane (two events per patient vs one). Serum lactate also increased slightly with halothane.

Patients with a single functional ventricle comprise an increasing proportion of patients undergoing anesthetics for both cardiac and noncardiac surgery, and studies of hemodynamic effects of anesthetic agents are limited. Ikemba et al. [11] studied 30 infants with a single functional ventricle immediately before their bidirectional cavopulmonary connection, randomized to receive sevoflurane at 1 and 1.5 MAC, or fentanyl/midazolam at equivalent doses. Myocardial performance index (MPI), a transthoracic echocardiographic measurement of ventricular function that can be applied to single ventricle patients, was not changed with any of these regimens when compared to baseline, indicating that either sevoflurane or fentanyl/midazolam can be used in this population to maintain hemodynamic stability.

In normal children, desflurane commonly produces tachycardia and hypertension during the induction phase, followed by a slight reduction in HR and systolic blood

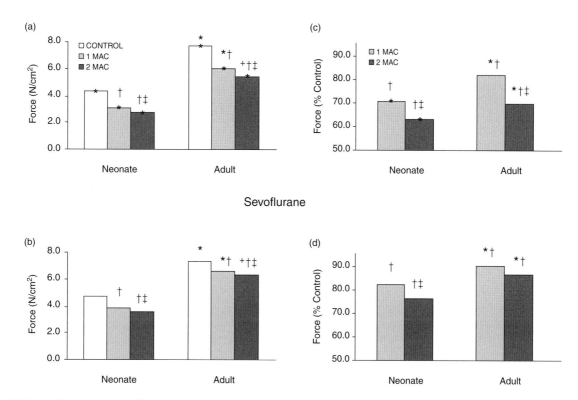

Figure 6.2 Force of contraction (N/cm²) in neonatal versus adult rat ventricular trabecular muscle. Baseline force of contraction is greater in adult tissue, and both halothane and sevoflurane depress contractility more in the neonatal than adult ventricular muscle. Halothane depresses contractility to a greater extent in both age groups. Parts (a) and (b) report raw data, (c) and (d) express results as a percentage of baseline contractility (Reproduced with permission from Reference [4])

Table 6.1 Hemodynamic changes in response to four anesthetic regimens in 54 children with congenital heart disease with two ventricles

		Measured and calculated hemodynamic and echocardiographic variables							
Agent	**MAC**	**HR (beats/min)**	**MAP (mmHg)**	**EF (%)**	**SF (%)**	**SVI (mL/m²)**	**LVEDVI (mL/m²)**	**CI (L/min¹/m²)**	**SVRI (dyn s/cm⁵/m²)**
Halothane	0	129 ± 22	77 ± 15	63 ± 9	40 ± 5	36 ± 16	44 ± 19	4.49 ± 1.87	1425 ± 622
	1	130 ± 19	$60 \pm 11^{*}$	$54 \pm 12^{*}$	$32 \pm 7^{*\dagger}$	$28 \pm 11^{*}$	38 ± 14	3.47 ± 1.17	1331 ± 529
	1.5	129 ± 17	$49 \pm 12^{*}$	$50 \pm 13^{*}$	$30 \pm 8^{*\dagger}$	$26 \pm 11^{*}$	39 ± 12	$3.34 \pm 1.36^{*}$	$1132 \pm 503^{*}$
Sevoflurane	0	123 ± 32	67 ± 8	68 ± 11	44 ± 7	56 ± 41	37 ± 15	6.91 ± 4.32	1014 ± 653
	1	126 ± 26	$58 \pm 13^{*}$	62 ± 9	39 ± 7	52 ± 31	36 ± 18	6.59 ± 4.04	883 ± 592
	1.5	128 ± 25	$58 \pm 13^{*}$	$58 \pm 10^{*}$	39 ± 9	46 ± 26	35 ± 14	5.78 ± 3.06	782 ± 390
Isoflurane	0	112 ± 27	69 ± 12	63 ± 7	39 ± 5	46 ± 2	46 ± 24	4.96 ± 2.74	1377 ± 809
	1	$125 \pm 16^{*}$	$54 \pm 9^{*}$	62 ± 8	37 ± 4	39 ± 17	40 ± 17	4.82 ± 2.20	$1022 \pm 601^{*}$
	1.5	$128 \pm 13^{*}$	$50 \pm 9^{*}$	59 ± 9	36 ± 5	39 ± 17	42 ± 19	4.59 ± 2.12	$950 \pm 513^{*}$
Fentanyl–midazolam	0	$106 \pm 22^{\ddagger}$	66 ± 8	63 ± 6	40 ± 6	46 ± 34	54 ± 25	5.16 ± 4.39	1261 ± 644
	1	$87 \pm 19^{*\S}$	$59 \pm 11^{*}$	60 ± 7	39 ± 5	42 ± 30	47 ± 25	$3.79 \pm 3.05^{*}$	1540 ± 806
	1.5	$82 \pm 18^{*\S}$	$56 \pm 11^{*}$	59 ± 7	38 ± 7	43 ± 30	52 ± 24	$3.67 \pm 2.99^{*}$	1559 ± 875

All values are mean $\pm$ SD.

$^{*}P < 0.05$, one-way analysis of variance, different from 0 minimum alveolar concentration (MAC) within the same anesthetic group. $^{\dagger}P < 0.05$, two-way analysis of variance, halothane versus sevoflurane and fentanyl–midazolam at 1 and 1.5 MAC. $^{\ddagger}P < 0.05$, two-way analysis of variance, fentanyl–midazolam versus halothane at 0 MAC. $^{\S}P < 0.05$, two-way analysis of variance, fentanyl–midazolam versus halothane, sevoflurane, and isoflurane at 1.0 and 1.5 MAC. CI, systemic cardiac index; EF, ejection fraction; HR, heart rate; LVEDVI, left ventricular end-diastolic volume index; MAP, mean arterial pressure; SF, shortening fraction; SVI, stroke volume index; SVRI, systemic vascular resistance index.

Source: Reprinted with permission from Reference [7].

pressure during steady state at 1 MAC anesthetic level [12,13]. There are no reports of its hemodynamic profile in patients with CHD. In a study of 47 children, mean age 12.8 years, undergoing electrophysiological study for supraventricular tachycardia (SVT), desflurane allowed induction of the SVT in all patients, and demonstrated no clinically important differences in any electrophysiologic measurement, compared to a fentanyl-based anesthetic [14]. The arrhythmogenic potential of desflurane has been demonstrated to be similar to that of isoflurane [15].

Six to twelve percent of patients exposed to sevoflurane develop arrhythmias, mostly atrial or junctional [16,17]. A study performed in infants, mean age 7.5 months, found sevoflurane induction caused a 20% incidence of junctional bradycardia (less than 80 beats/min). Isoflurane, when utilized in children for electrophysiologic studies and radiofrequency ablation for SVT, does not affect sinoatrial or atrioventricular node conduction, and all arrhythmias were easily induced [18]. There are case reports of sevoflurane causing torsade de pointes in children with congenital long QT syndrome; this effect may be due to the increase in HR often seen with induction of anesthesia with this agent [19].

Few studies to date have addressed the effects of the different anesthetics on an important group of pediatric patients with heart disease: patients with cardiomyopathy or significantly decreased systolic ventricular function. Diastolic function with halothane and isoflurane has been studied in animal models of cardiomyopathy [20,21]. The two agents differ with halothane producing negative lusitropic effects, while isoflurane conserves or may even improve diastolic function. There are no reports of diastolic function in response to anesthetic agents in patients with CHD.

Nitrous oxide

Despite its ubiquitous use as an adjunct to anesthetic induction and maintenance in patients with CHD, information regarding the effect of nitrous oxide on hemodynamics in patients with CHD is very limited. Its use may be relatively contraindicated where increased FiO2 is indicated, or where enlargement of enclosed air collections is possible, such as in any intracardiac or intrathoracic surgery. Reports of increased pulmonary vascular resistance (PVR), sympathetic stimulation, or significantly decreased cardiac output in response to N2O in adult patients have not been substantiated in children with or without cardiac disease [22,23].

In infants and small children with normal hearts, Murray et al. found that the addition of 30 and 60% N2O to 1 MAC halothane or isoflurane resulted in a decreased HR and cardiac index, without changing EF and stroke volume measured echocardiographically [24]. These authors also demonstrated that when 0.6 MAC halothane or isoflurane was substituted for 60% N2O during 0.9 MAC isoflurane or halothane anesthesia, HR, MAP, and cardiac index were unchanged [25].

In 14 patients with CHD recovering from surgery, Hickey et al. [26] administered 50% N2O and observed a decrease of 9% in HR, 12% in MAP, and 13% in systemic cardiac index. However, mean pulmonary artery pressure and PVR were not significantly changed in these well-ventilated patients with a PaCO2 of 34–35, and pH of 7.47–7.49, even in patients with elevated PVR at baseline. This single report represents the total number of patients with CHD in which N2O administration has been carefully studied. Despite this paucity of information, extensive clinical experience has demonstrated N2O to be safe and effective, particularly as an adjunct to inhaled induction of anesthesia for congenital heart surgery.

Opioids and benzodiazepines

Fentanyl and sufentanil have been studied as a sole anesthetic in patients with CHD. Hickey and Hansen et al. [27–30] provided the basis for this technique with a series of studies in neonates and infants younger than 1 year undergoing complex repairs ranging from the Norwood operation to complete repair of biventricular lesions. Fentanyl doses of 50–75 mcg/kg, and sufentanil doses of 5–40 mcg/kg, administered with pancuronium 0.1–0.15 mg/kg, provided excellent hemodynamic stability with minimal changes in HR and blood pressure throughout the surgery. The increase in pulmonary artery pressure and resistance in response to suctioning in infants recovering from cardiac surgery was eliminated with 25 mcg/kg fentanyl. Moore et al. [31] demonstrated that 5, 10, or 20 mcg/kg sufentanil in children 4–12 years of age had no effect on EF as measured by echocardiography, in patients undergoing repair of biventricular lesions. Increases in HR, blood pressure, and stress hormones were more effectively blunted by the higher doses. Glenski et al. [32] reported M-mode echocardiographic measures of contractility, blood pressure, and HR response using fentanyl (at 100 mcg/kg), or sufentanil (at 20 mcg/kg) in children 6 months to 9 years of age. Measurements were made at three different times: after a premedication with morphine and scopolamine, after induction, and after tracheal intubation. These opioids decreased both EF and shortening fraction after induction, but they returned to or above baseline after intubation.

Midazolam is often added to fentanyl anesthesia to provide sedation and amnesia, as a substitute for low-dose volatile anesthetic agent, particularly in hemodynamically unstable patients and young infants, where the myocardial depressant effects of volatile agents are more pronounced. Fentanyl and midazolam combinations have been studied in two different clinically utilized dose regimens to simulate 1 and 1.5 MAC of volatile agents (fentanyl 8–18 mcg bolus followed by 1.7–4.3 mcg/kg/h infusion and then repeat bolus at 50% of the original doses followed by increase of infusion by 50%, depending on age; midazolam 0.29 mg/kg bolus followed by 139 mcg/kg/h infusion and then repeat bolus 50% of the original dose, followed by increase in infusion of 50% for all ages) for induction and the prebypass period in congenital heart surgery in biventricular patients [7]. Vecuronium was used for muscle relaxation in order to isolate the effects of the other two agents on hemodynamics. Measurements of cardiac output and contractility were made by echocardiography. Fentanyl/midazolam caused a significant decrease (22%) in cardiac output despite preservation of contractility. That was predominantly due to a decrease in HR. Coadministration of a vagolytic agent such as atropine [33] or pancuronium would likely preserve cardiac output. The added effect of midazolam on echocardiographic indices of contractility has not been previously reported; however, increased inotropic support requirements have been documented in infants undergoing cardiac surgery with the addition of midazolam bolus totaling 0.3 mg/kg, and infusion of 0.1 mg/kg/h intraoperatively [34].

The stress response to major cardiac surgery in infants and children has been the subject of considerable interest. Anand and Hickey et al. [35] reported the use of high-dose sufentanil at a total mean dose of 37 mcg/kg as a sole anesthetic for complex neonatal surgery. The sufentanil was continued by infusion for 24 hours postoperatively. This regimen was compared to halothane plus morphine (mean dose of 0.35 mg/kg) intraoperatively, followed by intermittent morphine and diazepam postoperatively. Stress response, as measured by changes in adrenal hormones, cortisol, glucose, and lactate was significantly reduced in the sufentanil group, and mortality and major complications such as sepsis and necrotizing enterocolitis were also significantly reduced. A more recent study from the same institution of 45 infants averaging 3 months of age undergoing biventricular repair was reported [34]. A fentanyl total dose 100 mcg/kg, either given as intermittent boluses of 25 mcg/kg, or as boluses plus infusion, either with or without midazolam, all regimens resulted in a significant endocrine stress response to cardiac surgery. Despite this, outcome was excellent in all groups, with no adverse outcomes related to the anesthetic technique or to stress response. The sole hemodynamic difference between the regimens was a lower MAP during cooling on bypass in the group who received midazolam. Finally, Duncan et al. [36] reported a dose–response study of 2, 25, 50, 100, and 150 mcg/kg fentanyl before bypass in 40 children averaging 13 months and 8.5 kg. The 2 mcg/kg group had significant increases in prebypass norepinephrine, glucose, and cortisol, and significantly higher HR and blood pressure than all other groups. Twenty-five mcg/kg or higher doses eliminated changes in these parameters for the duration of the surgery. It is difficult to interpret the significance of these stress–response studies because they evaluated by different age groups and lesions. Also, there was more than one decade between reports with as improvements in surgical, bypass, and postoperative management. If any group of patients had benefited from attenuation of the stress response, it would appear to be neonatal patients undergoing complex surgery.

Remifentanil is a synthetic ultra-short acting narcotic agent metabolized by plasma esterases with half-life 3–5 minutes that is independent of the duration of infusion [37]. It is particularly useful for short noncardiac procedures with intense stimulation where narcotic-based anesthesia and its hemodynamic stability would be desirable, yet where rapid emergence is also important. Donmez [38, 39] reported a series of 55 children undergoing cardiac catheterization with a remifentanil infusion of 0.1 mcg/kg/min. This regimen maintained excellent cardiovascular stability, with minimal changes in HR, blood pressure, or oxygen saturation. Fifty-eight percent of patients required additional sedation with midazolam or ketamine. Apnea was infrequent, and time to recovery score of 5 (10 point scale) was only 2–4 minutes. Patients undergoing long cardiac catheterization procedures could potentially benefit from this agent. Its use has been reported for atrial septal defect repair, where patients are extubated in the operating room [40]. It apparently does not bind to the cardiopulmonary bypass circuit [41], and its clearance in children before and after cardiopulmonary bypass appears to be predictable within a narrow range, making it a potentially useful agent for "fast track" anesthesia and early extubation for simple surgical procedures. Freisen et al. compared remifentanil 0.3–0.7 mcg/kg/min to fentanyl 15 mcg/kg, both with isoflurane and pancuronium, in fast track pediatric cardiac operations (ASD and VSD repairs), and found that HR was significantly slower in the operating room in the remifentanil group, but there was no difference in time to extubation, analgesic requirements in ICU, nausea/vomiting or hypertension in ICU, or in ICU length of stay [42] (Table 6.2). Akpek et al. compared higher dose remifentanil, 2 mcg/kg load and 2 mcg/kg/min maintenance infusion, with fentanyl 20 mcg/kg load and 20 mcg/kg/h infusion in 33 infants with pulmonary hypertension undergoing surgery for repair of left-to-right shunting defects. Both groups had a midazolam infusion. There were no clinically important differences in hemodynamic, respiratory, or oxygen saturation parameters between groups, and no difference in clinical outcomes [43]. Thus, despite some theoretical advantages due to its pharmacokinetic profile, few clinically

Table 6.2 Patient characteristics and outcomes in children receiving either remifentanil or fentanyl for fast-track cardiac anesthesia

	Remifentanil	Fentanyl
Age (years)	4.3 ± 3.6	3.6 ± 3.9
Weight (kg)	17.4 ± 10.0	16.2 ± 13.8
Induction		
Blood pressure decrease > 25% (n)	10	8
Heart rate decrease > 30% (n)*	17	8
Incision/sternotomy		
Blood pressure increase > 25% (n)	1	2
Heart rate increase > 30% (n)	5	5
Base excess pre-CPB	2.1 ± 1.2	2.8 ± 2.1
Extubation in OR (n)	15	18
Time to extubation (min)	54 ± 94	34 ± 72
Reintubation (n)	0	0
Postoperative fentanyl ($\mu g \cdot kg^{-1} \cdot 12\ h^{-1}$)	4.8 ± 3.5	5.9 ± 3.6
Nitroprusside use (n)	14	13
Ondansetron use (n)	10	5
Duration in PICU (h)	25 ± 10	33 ± 11

Data are means ± SD or number of subjects. $n = 25$ in each group. CPB, cardiopulmonary bypass; OR, operating room; PICU, paediatric intensive care unit. Groups are significantly different ($P < 0.02$).

Source: Reproduced with permission from Reference [42].

significant differences between remifentanil and fentanyl exist.

Propofol

Propofol has become a popular agent for sedation and general anesthesia for cardiac catheterization procedures and for postoperative ICU sedation to facilitate early tracheal extubation. In plasma concentrations found in routine clinical use, propofol has minimal negative inoptropic effects in isolated animal cardiac preparations [44], or in human adult atrial muscle strips [45].

In children with normal hearts on induction, propofol consistently decreases systolic and MAP by 5–25%

[46], without changing HR. There has been one published study using echocardiography to assess myocardial contractility and cardiac output in infants with normal hearts induced with propofol [46]. The shortening fraction or cardiac index was not changed, SVR decreased by 14 and 27% at 1 and 5 minutes after induction. Load independent measures of contractility (stress–velocity index and stress–shortening index) decreased significantly from baseline at 5 minutes after induction with propofol.

Williams et al. [47] measured the hemodynamic effects of propofol in 31 patients 3 months to 12 years at a dose of 50–200 mcg/kg/min undergoing cardiac catheterization (Figure 6.3). They found that propofol significantly decreased MAP and SVR; however, systemic cardiac output, HR, and mean pulmonary artery pressure, as well as PVR, did not change. In patients with cardiac shunts, the net result was a significant increase in the right-to-left shunt, a decrease in the left-to-right shunt, and decreased Qp:Qs, resulting in a statistically significant decrease in PaO_2 and SaO_2, as well as reversal of the shunt from left to right to right to left in two patients. In another study of patients undergoing cardiac catheterization, Lebovic et al. [48] demonstrated that patients could experience a 20% decrease in HR or MAP. Recently, combining propofol infusion with ketamine infusion for cardiac catheterization procedures has demonstrated less change in MAP, preservation of baseline HR, and little effect on recovery time [49].

Zestos et al. [50] studied patients undergoing congenital heart surgery with cardiopulmonary bypass who were selected for early extubation in the ICU ($n = 26$). A propofol infusion at 50 mcg/kg/min was begun after cardiopulmonary bypass, and compared to a placebo control group who received intralipid. The infusions were discontinued upon leaving the operating room, and morphine was given as needed for pain. Both the time to tracheal extubation (33 vs 63 minutes) and the number of morphine doses (1 vs 2.3) were significantly less in the propofol group. No hemodynamic depression was observed in this study. Another recent study with a similar protocol for propofol

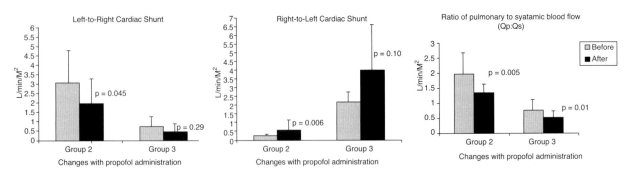

Figure 6.3 Changes in intracardiac shunting in response to propofol induction and infusion in children undergoing cardiac catheterization. Group 2: patients with net left to right cardiac shunting, Group 3: patients with net right to left cardiac shunting. Qp:Qs decreased significantly in both groups (Reproduced with permission from Reference [47])

infusion after weaning from bypass demonstrated that 70% of children undergoing simple and complex surgery were extubated within 9 hours of ICU admission [51].

Propofol has no significant effect on sinoatrial or atrioventricular node conduction, or on the ability to induce SVT, and therefore is desirable as a primary agent during electrophysiologic studies and radiofrequency ablation [18,52]. However, ectopic atrial tachycardia may be suppressed by propofol [53].

Although propofol is very useful for cardiac catheterization, short, stimulating procedures, and short-term sedation after cardiac surgery, its long-term use as an ICU sedative is contraindicated, with several reports of otherwise unexplained metabolic acidosis and myocardial failure after long-term (>48 h), high-dose use in pediatric patients [54,55]. The mechanism of this cardiovascular collapse is postulated to be due to disruption of fatty acid oxidation caused by impaired entry of long-chain acylcarnitine esters into the mitochondria and failure of the mitochondrial respiratory chain [56].

In summary, propofol can be utilized in patients with adequate cardiovascular reserve who can tolerate a mild decrease in contractility and HR, and a decrease in SVR. Propofol may cause an increased intracardiac right-to-left shunt, and reversal of shunt in some patients (i.e., acyanotic tetralogy of Fallot), and thus hemodynamic data obtained in the cardiac catheterization laboratory should be interpreted accordingly.

Ketamine

The general anesthetic and analgesic effects of ketamine are thought to be mediated by its interaction with N-methyl-D-aspartate receptors in the brain [57]. It increases HR, blood pressure, and cardiac output through CNS-mediated sympathomimetic stimulation and inhibition of the reuptake of catecholamines. It has been shown that ketamine is a direct myocardial depressant when studied in isolated myocyte preparations [58], and in adult human failing atrial and ventricular muscle trabeculae [59] (Figure 6.4). The direct myocardial depression caused by ketamine may be unmasked when administered to patients whose sympathomimetic responses are already maximally stimulated from cardiomyopathy, or other condition leading to poor myocardial reserve, because further increase in catecholamine release is limited. Similarly, if the patient is chronically receiving β-adrenergic agonists, catecholamine receptors may be downregulated, resulting in a diminished response to endogenously generated catecholamines, again allowing the myocardial depressant effects of ketamine to predominate.

The mechanism of myocardial depression is by inhibition of L-type voltage-dependent Ca^{++} channels in the

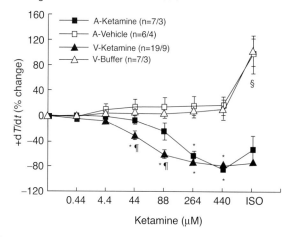

Failing aterial and ventricular muscle

Figure 6.4 Developed tension over time (dT/dt) in cardiac muscle trabeculae in explanted hearts from adults undergoing cardiac transplantation in response to increasing ketamine concentrations. The upper limit of clinical concentration is 44 μM after 2 mg/kg induction dose. A, atrial muscle; V, ventricular muscle. Vehicle, control solution without ketamine; buffer, Krebs–Henseleit buffer control. Numbers in parentheses represent numbers of muscle strips/number of patients, respectively. Iso, change with addition of 1 μM isoproterenol (Reproduced with permission from Reference [59])

sarcolemmal membrane. An increased extracellular Ca^{++} concentration may enhance this effect [58]. This direct myocardial depression effect is greater than that produced by etomidate [45]. In a patient with end-stage cardiomyopathy awaiting heart transplant, hemodynamic collapse occurred after the induction of anesthesia with ketamine [60]. In a study of ketamine versus sufentanil for induction of anesthesia in patients undergoing cardiac transplant, whose average EF was 14% and who were all receiving inotropes and vasodilators preoperatively, it was found that ketamine increased MAP, central venous pressure, and pulmonary artery pressure significantly, and decreased stroke volume index and left ventricular stroke work index [61]. Cardiac index decreased slightly but not to a statistically significant degree. SVR and HR were higher. The sum total of the hemodynamic effects of ketamine induction in these patients was less myocardial work at the expense of a higher myocardial wall tension. Sufentanil induction did not change any of these parameters from baseline.

Other well-recognized untoward effects associated with ketamine use do not differ among patients with CHD. These include emergence reactions, excessive salivation, and an increase in cerebral metabolism, intracranial pressure, cerebral blood flow, and cerebral oxygen consumption [57].

Despite adverse effects of ketamine that are delineated above, this drug has been a mainstay of induction of

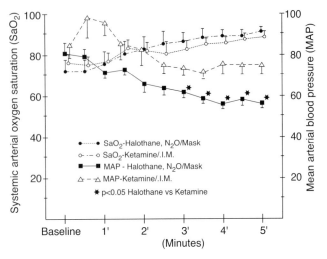

Figure 6.5 Oxygen saturation and MAP in response to induction with intramuscular ketamine versus halothane in patients with right to left cardiac shunting, most of whom had tetralogy of Fallot (Reproduced with permission from Reference [64])

general anesthesia in patients with CHD [62, 63]. It can be administered IV or IM; and it will reliably maintain HR, blood pressure, and systemic cardiac output at an induction dose of 1–2 mg/kg IV, or 5–10 mg/kg IM, and a maintenance dose of 1–5 mg/kg/h in patients with a variety of CHDs, including tetralogy of Fallot [64, 65] (Figure 6.5). The question about exacerbation of pulmonary hypertension has been addressed in two important studies. Morray et al. [66] demonstrated that in cardiac catheterization patients, 2 mg/kg ketamine caused a minimal (<10%) increase in mean pulmonary artery pressure, and ratio of pulmonary to SVR (Rp:Rs), with no change in direction of shunting or Qp:Qs. Hickey et al. [28] studied postoperative cardiac surgery patients with normal PaCO2 and demonstrated that ketamine 2 mg/kg had no effect on pulmonary artery pressure or calculated PVR, in patients with either normal or elevated baseline PVR. Williams et al. reported that ketamine 2 mg/kg load followed by an infusion of 10 mcg/kg/min did not change PVR at all in 15 children with severe pulmonary hypertension, when breathing spontaneously with a baseline of 0.5 MAC sevoflurane [67] (Figure 6.6).

Ketamine, supplemented with small doses of midazolam and/or morphine, has been used for interventional cardiac catheterization procedures [68] and for postoperative analgesia after cardiac surgery in children. Hemodynamic stability has been excellent, with few complications. The most notable adverse effect was transient apnea in 10% of spontaneously breathing newborns undergoing balloon atrial septostomy in the catheterization laboratory.

Intramuscular induction of anesthesia may be achieved with ketamine 5 mg/kg, succinylcholine 4 mg/kg, and atropine 20 mcg/kg mixed in the same syringe. This regimen is useful for small patients who present to the operating room without IV access in whom the inhalational induction of anesthesia may produce undesirable hemodynamic effects. Endotracheal intubation can usually be achieved in 3–5 minutes, and attention can be turned to establishing intravenous access with the airway secure and a stable hemodynamic state.

In summary, ketamine is an attractive choice for IV or IM induction of anesthesia in patients with CHD with good or moderately limited hemodynamic reserve, including those with pulmonary hypertension or cyanosis.

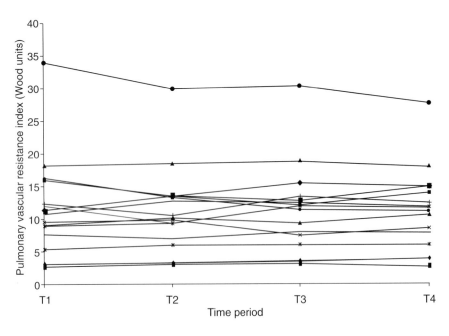

Figure 6.6 Pulmonary vascular resistance changes in 15 children with pulmonary hypertension undergoing cardiac catheterization, in response to ketamine 2 mg/kg IV, followed by an infusion of 10 mcg/kg/min while breathing spontaneously with a baseline of 0.5 MAC sevoflurane. T1, baseline before ketamine; T2, 5 minutes after ketamine load; T3, 10 minutes after ketamine load; T4, 15 minutes after ketamine load (Reproduced with permission from Reference [67])

However, care must be taken in patients with severely limited cardiac reserve and depressed myocardial contractility. Such patients may be chronically receiving β-adrenergic or similar agents, or their own endogenous sympathomimetic system is maximally stimulated because of a low cardiac output state. The myocardial depressant properties of ketamine may be unmasked and lead to hemodynamic compromise.

Etomidate

Etomidate is an imidazole derivative introduced into clinical practice in 1972. It is thought to produce its hypnotic effects (without analgesia) by interaction with γ-aminobutyric acid receptors [57]. Besides having a desirable lack of effect on hemodynamics, etomidate reduces cerebral blood flow and cerebral metabolic rate for oxygen consumption (30–50%) and intracranial pressure. It has little effect on ventilation, does not release histamine, and does not change airway smooth muscle tone. Of all the available IV induction agents, etomidate consistently demonstrates the smallest amount of direct myocardial depression in several in vitro models. Two well-designed studies using adult human atrial and ventricular tissue demonstrated no effect of etomidate on myocardial contractility in concentrations seen in clinical use (Figure 6.7).

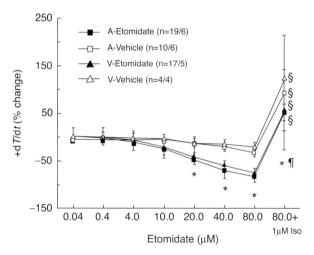

Failing atrial and ventricular muscle

Figure 6.7 Developed tension over time (d*T*/d*t*) in cardiac muscle trabeculae in explanted hearts from adults undergoing cardiac transplantation in response to increasing etomidate concentrations. The upper limit of clinical concentration is 4 μM. A, atrial muscle; V, ventricular muscle. Vehicle, 35% propylene glycol, in which etomidate is solubilized. Numbers in parentheses represent numbers of muscle strips/number of patients, respectively. Iso, change with addition of 1 μM isoproterenol (Reproduced with permission from Reference [69])

In the same model, ketamine showed slight, and thiopental strong, negative inotropic effects in clinical concentration ranges. This was true even in abnormal myocardial samples of ventricular tissue taken from hearts removed for cardiac transplantation [45,69]. In a study of right ventricular tissue excised from infants and children during tetralogy of Fallot repair, etomidate did not change contractility in the clinical concentration range in an in vitro tissue bath study, but did blunt responsiveness to isoproterenol at high concentrations, raising the possibility that the pediatric myocardium may respond differently after etomidate [70].

All of these beneficial effects of etomidate are offset by a number of undesirable effects. Etomidate is water insoluble and thus is formulated in propylene glycol, and commonly produces pain on injection, which may be ameliorated by pretreatment with lidocaine, and 1:1 dilution with sterile water. A new etomidate formulation dissolving the drug in a fat emulsion of medium- and long-chain triglycerides virtually eliminates pain on injection in children [71]. Myoclonic movement, hiccoughs, and nausea and vomiting are frequent [57]. It should be noted that, as in adults, a single dose of etomidate used for induction in pediatric patients undergoing cardiac surgery with cardiopulmonary bypass suppresses the usual increase in plasma cortisol levels by inhibiting 11-β-hydroxylase, the enzyme that converts 11-deoxycortisol to cortisol [39]. Cortisol levels returned to normal 24 hours later.

There are few published reports of the hemodynamic effects of etomidate in children with CHD. Twenty patients with a variety of congenital defects were studied in the cardiac catheterization laboratory. These authors found that etomidate at 0.3 mg/kg bolus followed by an infusion of 26 mcg/kg/min had similar effects as ketamine 4 mg/kg followed by an infusion of 83 mcg/kg/min, namely a slight increase in HR but no change in MAP during induction or the 60-minute infusion [72]. Sarkhar et al. [73] studied etomidate bolus 0.3 mg/kg in 12 children undergoing cardiac catheterization for device closure of ASD, or radiofrequency ablation of atrial arrhythmias. There were no significant changes in any hemodynamic parameter, including HR, MAP, filling pressures, vascular resistances, Qp:Qs, or mixed venous oxygen saturation. A case report of stable hemodynamics in a pediatric patient with end-stage cardiomyopathy receiving a second anesthetic 4 weeks after cardiovascular collapse with ketamine induction (see above) demonstrates the utility of the drug in this population [60]. Etomidate has been utilized for induction of anesthesia in adults with congenital cardiac conditions such as ruptured aneurysm of the sinus of Valsalva, and cesarean section in a patient with uncorrected coronary artery to pulmonary artery fistula, and has been demonstrated to be devoid of cardiovascular effects in these patients [74,75].

Thus, it would appear that etomidate is best utilized in patients with the most limited cardiac reserve. It seems to be particularly useful in teenagers or adults with poorly compensated palliated CHD presenting for cardiac transplantation or revision of previous surgeries.

Dexmedetomidine

Dexmedetomidine is a recently introduced intravenous agent that is an imidazole derivative, and a highly selective α2-adrenergic receptor agonist (1620:1 α_2 to α_1 activity vs 220:1 for clonidine). Dexmedetomidine thus is a centrally acting agent that produces sedation, and a dose-dependent decrease in HR and MAP by decreasing CNS sympathetic nervous system activity. It also potentiates opioid effects, and thus is potentially suitable for use both during and after pediatric cardiac surgery, as a component of a general anesthetic, and as a sedative/analgesic agent in the ICU. Usual dose for sedation is 0.2–0.7 mcg/kg/h; a loading dose of 0.5–1 mcg/kg given over 10 minutes can be utilized if desired. It has minimal effect on respiration, and its clearance of 0.013 L/kg/min, volume of distribution of 1.0 L/kg and terminal half-life of 1.8 hours in children, are similar to adult values [76]. Because it is an imidazole derivative, it has the potential for adrenal suppression with prolonged use.

Dexmedetomidine has been studied as an adjunct agent in general anesthesia for pediatric cardiac surgery. In a study by Mukhtar et al., dexmedetomidine 0.5 mcg/kg load followed by 0.5 mcg/kg/h infusion, with an isoflurane–fentanyl–midazolam anesthetic, significantly reduced HR, MAP, and cortisol, blood glucose, and serum catecholamine response in children aged 1–6 years undergoing cardiac surgery with bypass, when compared to the baseline anesthetic [77].

Dexmedetomidine has been studied for postoperative sedation after pediatric cardiac surgery. Chrysostomu et al. studied 38 pediatric patients after two-ventricle repair with cardiopulmonary bypass. Thirty-three of 38 were extubated, and average age was 8 years; dexmedetomidine infusion rate varied from 0.1 to 0.75 mcg/kg/h (mean 0.3), and desired sedation was achieved in 93% and analgesia in 83% of patients, respectively. There was no respiratory depression, but hypotension was observed in 15% of patients [78]. Dexmedetomidine has also been described as useful in weaning opioid-tolerant cardiac surgery patients relatively quickly with no hemodynamic side effects [79]. Dexmedetomidine as a sole sedative agent for pediatric cardiac catheterization was studied by Munro et al. in 20 children [80]. A loading dose of 1 mcg/kg was followed by an infusion of 1 mcg/kg/h, and propofol boluses were given for movement or increasing bispectral index value. 60% of patients required propofol boluses,

and there was a slight decrease in MAP but not in HR, and no patient experienced airway obstruction or respiratory depression. Dexmedetomidine plus ketamine has been compared to dexmedetomidine plus propofol for pediatric cardiac catheterization in 44 patients [81]. There was no difference in sedation scores or respiratory parameters, HR was slower in the dexmedetomidine group, and MAP was not different. Recovery time was significantly longer in the dexmedetomidine group versus the propofol group.

It is important to note that dexmedetomidine frequently causes bradycardia and thus may not be suitable as a sedative for electrophysiologic studies. In 12 children undergoing EP studies, Hammer et al. found that dexmedetomidine 1 mcg/kg load, followed by 0.7 mcg/kg/h infusion for 20 minutes decreased HR by 15–20%, but more importantly depressed sinus node recovery times, sinus node automaticity, and increased atrioventricular nodal block cycle lengths and PR interval [81] (Table 6.3).

Dexmedetomidine is thus a potentially useful agent as an adjunct to general anesthesia, a postoperative sedative, and an adjunct sedative for cardiac catheterization (non-electrophysiologic studies) in pediatric cardiac surgery patients. The patient must be able to tolerate the predictable

Table 6.3 Electrophysiologic variables at baseline and after a 20-minute infusion of dexmedetomidine

	Baseline	DEX	P
Surface ECG intervals			
SCL	606 ± 140 ms	788 ± 165 ms	<0.01
PR	144 ± 19 ms	162 ± 17 ms	<0.01
QRS	76 ± 11 ms	79 ± 13 ms	NS
QTc	394 ± 9 ms	424 ± 9 ms	<0.01
Sinus automaticity			
CSNRT	212 ± 179 ms	293 ± 180 ms	<0.01
Atrial muscle properties			
AERP	207 ± 31 ms	208 ± 17 ms	NS
AV nodal properties			
AH interval	73 ± 14 ms	82 ± 12 ms	<0.01
AVNBCL	352 ± 87 ms	436 ± 105 ms	<0.01
AVNERP	310 ± 85 ms	360 ± 88 ms	<0.02
VABCL	372 ± 111 ms	460 ± 134 ms	<0.01
His Purkinje properties			
HV interval	40 ± 7 ms	40 ± 6 ms	NS
Ventricular muscle properties			
VERP	220 ± 22 ms	230 ± 19 ms	0.06

ECG, electrocardiogram; SCL, sinus cycle length; PR, PR interval; QRS, QRS duration; QTC, corrected QT interval; CSNRT, corrected sinus node recovery time; AERP, atrial effective refractory period; AH interval, atrial–His interval; AVNBCL, AV node block cycle length; AVNERP, AV node effective refractory period; VABCL, ventriculo-atrial block cycle length; HV interval, His-ventricular interval; VERP, ventricular effective refractory period.
Source: Reproduced with permission from Reference [82].

decrease in HR, and frequent decrease in MAP associated with dexmedetomidine.

Special conditions effecting anesthetic pharmacokinetics and pharmocodynamics in congenital cardiac anesthesia

Intracardiac shunts

The presence of a right-to-left intracardiac shunt decreases the rate of rise of the concentration of inhaled anesthetic in the arterial blood, as a portion of the systemic cardiac output bypasses the lungs and then dilutes the anesthetic concentration in the systemic arterial blood [83]. The anesthetic concentration in the blood thus never equals the exhaled concentration. Huntington et al. [83] studied six children with right-to-left shunts from a fenestrated Fontan operation whose average pulmonary to systemic blood flow ratio was 0.58. These patients achieved an arterial anesthetic concentration (Fa) of only 55% of inspired halothane concentration (Fi) after 15 minutes during washin of 0.8% halothane. After closure of the right-to-left shunt (occlusion of Fontan fenestration in the cardiac catheterization laboratory), the arterial concentration of halothane equaled the inspired concentration. This difference between Fa and Fi is greater during induction or washout; and greater with less soluble drugs such as sevoflurane, desflurane, and nitrous oxide, than with less soluble drugs such as halothane.

In the face of significant right-to-left intracardiac shunting, intravenous agents given by bolus may pass directly into the left side of the heart with less dilution by systemic venous blood and passage through the pulmonary vascular system. This may result in transient high arterial, brain, and cardiac concentrations of drugs such as lidocaine [84]. Intravenous induction agents and muscle relaxants may also achieve sufficient arterial and brain concentrations more rapidly with right-to-left intracardiac shunts [85].

Left-to-right intracardiac shunts have little effect on the speed of induction with inhaled anesthetic agents [86]. The recirculation of blood through the lungs results in increased uptake of anesthetic and in a higher blood anesthetic concentration in the pulmonary capillaries, which in capillary blood, reducing anesthetic uptake. The two effects cancel each other. Only in the case of severe congestive heart failure from left-to-right shunt, with significant interstitial and alveolar edema, would left to right intracardiac shunting be expected to slow inhalation induction, from the combined effects of diffusion limitation and ventilation–perfusion mismatch resulting alveolar dead space ventilation in which no new anesthetic agent is taken up.

Cardiopulmonary bypass

The onset of cardiopulmonary bypass affects plasma levels of intravenous drugs by a number of different mechanisms [87]. Hemodilution of the patient's blood volume by a factor of 50–300%, depending of the size of the patient and the priming volume of the circuit, causes an immediate reduction in plasma levels. Many drugs also bind to the membrane oxygenator and other components of the bypass circuit, resulting in a further decrease in plasma levels. This effect is variable and is dependent on the drug, the type of bypass circuit used (i.e., silicone vs. polypropylene), the age and size of the patient, and the plasma and bypass prime albumin concentrations. Hypothermia slows the metabolism of all drugs by reducing the rate of reaction of all enzymes involved in drug metabolism, whether they are in the liver (cytochrome P450 system), kidney, or plasma. Rewarming significantly increases the rate of metabolism of intravenous agents.

A constant, stable fentanyl plasma level [88] can be achieved in most children through the administration of a loading dose of 30–50 mcg/kg followed by an infusion of 0.15–0.3 mcg/kg/min. Plasma fentanyl levels decrease by 70–75% immediately upon institution of cardiopulmonary bypass with a silicone membrane oxygenator. After cooling to 18–25°C, fentanyl metabolism decreases considerably and free drug concentrations change very little, even without added drug [89]. Metabolism then increases and drug levels decline in the plasma as rewarming proceeds. Data concerning common anesthetic adjuvants such as midazolam suggest similar changes in plasma concentrations [87]. Thus, without supplementation of intravenous agents such as fentanyl and midazolam, either just before or at the initiation of bypass, there is an increased risk of awareness. A similar risk would appear to be true during the final phases of the rewarming period. Indeed, this concept is borne out by recent studies using bispectral index (see below) as an indicator of depth of sedation in children undergoing bypass with mild hypothermia [90]. Modified ultrafiltration has been reported to double the plasma fentanyl concentrations in a study of five neonates and infants, from 12.4 to 27.5 ng/mL [91].

Neuromuscular blocking agents have an enhanced effect during hypothermic bypass [87], both from decreased metabolism and clearance, and because of the effects of hypothermia to potentiate the pharmocodynamic effects of the drugs at the neuromuscular junction. These effects rapidly reverse themselves during rewarming. These drugs have a small volume of distribution and thus few tissue stores from which to re-equilibrate plasma levels. Thus, plasma levels would be expected to decline in proportion to the hemodilution factor of the pump prime, subject to changes in protein binding. This may be offset by reductions in the patient's plasma volume on bypass due to vasoconstriction. The action of these drugs in response to bypass is accordingly more variable than other commonly used intravenous anesthetic agents. There is limited pediatric information available. Monitoring of neuromuscular blockade with a twitch monitor is recommended if early reversal is desired.

Volatile agents may be used during bypass to supplement anesthetic depth, or as vasodilators. Isoflurane is most commonly utilized at a concentration of 0.5–2% inspired into the sweep gas of the bypass circuit. Multiple adult studies have demonstrated the effectiveness and relatively rapid washin of this agent [87]. However, pediatric data is limited, and because sweep gas flow rates are often less than 1 L/min, uptake is probably much slower and it cannot be assumed that the desired blood anesthetic level is rapidly reached when volatile anesthetic agents are administered through the bypass circuit to infants and small children. Washout of volatile agents is also slower at low sweep gas rates, and volatile agents should be discontinued early during the rewarming period to avoid the myocardial depressant effects of these agents while attempting to wean the patient from bypass.

Hypothermia

Studies performed on animal models reveal hypothermia reduces MAC of volatile anesthetics [92]. Liu et al. [93] studied the MAC of isoflurane in 33 children with left-to-right intracardiac shunts at 37, 34, or 31°C. They found MAC was reduced by 28% at 31°C when compared to normothermia, indicating a decrease in MAC of approximately 5% per degree centigrade cooling. Bispectral index value (BIS) has been demonstrated to correlate strongly with temperature during mild hypothermic bypass in children [94], providing supporting evidence that hypothermia alone provides general anesthesia.

Monitoring anesthetic depth and awareness

Until recently, the only means available to the clinician to monitor anesthetic depth and assess the risk of awareness was through a general knowledge of the pharmacokinetic and pharmacodynamic properties of anesthetics, along with measurement of the end-tidal anesthetic concentrations and clinical signs of depth of anesthesia. The clinical signs of inadequate anesthesia in the paralyzed cardiac surgical patient include autonomic signs such as papillary dilation, tearing, and tachycardia/hypertension. These signs are often unreliable, given the hemodynamic derangements common in this population, manipulation by the surgeon causing activation of baroreceptor reflex re-

sponses, and the use of vasoactive and chronotropic drugs, or drugs that block the autonomic response. Recently the bispectral index, a highly processed electroencephalogram, has become available [90,94–96]. Available pediatric data suggest that this modality correlates with end-tidal levels of volatile anesthetics and with MAC awake levels, with better correlation in children over 1–2 years of age, although interpatient variability is significant [90]. Studies in both infants and older children undergoing congenital heart surgery with cardiopulmonary bypass, demonstrate that the index (a dimensionless number 0–100) decreases with lower nasopharyngeal temperature, and increases during the rewarming phase. However, BIS did not correlate with hemodynamic, metabolic, or hormonal indices of light anesthesia. The BIS has been demonstrated to be more sensitive to changes in the levels of volatile anesthetics and propofol, and less sensitive to narcotics and benzodiazepines. In our experience, we commonly find that BIS increases during rewarming on bypass to levels in the range for risk of awareness despite large doses of fentanyl and midazolam. Pediatric studies of BIS during cardiac surgery are limited, and larger prospective studies are needed to demonstrate the validity and utility of device. In general pediatric anesthesia, recent evidence supports a correlation with the BIS and other EEG-based monitors with the depth of anesthesia in older children, best with teenagers, but evidence for use of these devices in infants and young children is lacking [97].

Neuromuscular blocking agents and antagonists

Succinylcholine

Succinylcholine is rarely indicated for anesthesia for CHD because of its association with the development of malignant hyperthermia, hyperkalemic cardiac arrest, and bradycardia after intravenous bolus administration. Succinylcholine will produce a more rapid onset of muscle relaxation than nondeporlarizing muscle relaxants [98], and generally its use is limited to full-stomach emergency indications, i.e., cardiac transplant, to treat laryngospasm, and as part of an intramuscular induction.

Infants and children frequently exhibit bradycardia, nodal rhythm, ventricular premature beats, and rarely, asystole, after intravenous dosing of 1–2 mg/kg without atropine pretreatment. The frequency of all of these arrhythmias increases with a second dose. A dose of 4 mg/kg given intramuscularly, either alone, or with atropine 20 mcg/kg, and ketamine 5–10 mg/kg in the same syringe, rarely causes bradycardia [99].

Pancuronium

Pancuronium is frequently used in doses of 0.1–0.3 mg/kg for initial relaxation for CHD [100] and is particularly desirable in many small infants and young children because of the vagolytic and mild sympathomimetic effects, which preserve or increase HR, especially in the face of concomitant bradycardia from high-dose narcotic anesthesia.

Vecuronium

Vecuronium is devoid of cardiovascular effects in children [101]. It is a useful agent when increases in HR are undesirable, e.g., hypertrophic cardiomyopathy. When no uncertainties about ability to manage the airway are evident, it is a useful alternate to succinylcholine in a dose of 0.3–0.4 mg/kg for modified rapid sequence induction.

Rocuronium

Rocuronium is a moderately rapid onset intermediate duration nondepolarizing neuromuscular blocker that is useful at a dose of 0.6–1.2 mg/kg IV. At the upper dose ranges, it is an acceptable substitute for succinylcholine for modified rapid sequence induction. Cardiovascular effects are minimal, however, because it causes pain on injection, or because it is a weak vagolytic medication, an increase in HR is often observed after injection. This agent may be utilized for intramuscular administration in doses of 1.8–2 mg/kg, and when injected into the deltoid will produce suitable intubating conditions in 3–4 minutes [102].

Atracurium and cisatracurium

These agents are nonorgan dependent for elimination and are attractive choices in the face of significant hepatic and renal dysfunction. Atracurium at high dosages frequently causes histamine release, resulting in hypotension when injected rapidly [98], making it undesirable for many patients with CHD. Cisatracurium is a stereoisomer of atracurium, also degraded by Hoffmann elimination, dose not release histamine, and like vecuronium, is devoid of cardiovascular effects even when administered rapidly [103].

Antagonists

The muscarinic effects of neostigmine must be blocked by atropine or glycopyrrolate to prevent potentially serious decreases in HR. Because the onset of cardiovascular effects of neostigmine and glycopyrrolate are similar, a most useful regimen is to utilize neostigmine and glycopyrrolate in the same syringe in a 5:1 ratio of neostigmine:glycopyrrolate (i.e., 75 mcg/kg:15 mcg/kg) injected slowly to minimize the small risk of arrhythmia with neostigmine. Despite longstanding use of neostigmine for reversal of neuromuscular blockade, it may cause bradycardia or cardiac arrest, even if administered with appropriate anticholinergic agents. Sawasdiwipachai et al. report a case of a 1-year-old who suffered a cardiac arrest 2 weeks after a heart transplant, after a myocardial biopsy, and reversal of cisatracurium neuromuscular blockade with 70 mcg/kg neostigmine, and glycopyrrolate 0.014 mcg/kg [104]. Acute cardiac rejection and an abnormal conduction system were postulated as causes in this infant. Sugammadex, a new agent that can reverse neuromuscular blockade by competitive displacement of nondepolarizing neuromuscular blocking agents from the acetylcholine receptor, has been reported to prolong QTc interval in some adult patients, and so its potential for safer reversal requires further investigation [105].

References

1. Lewis JK, Minter MG, Eshelman SJ, Witte MK (1983) Outcome of pediatric resuscitation. Ann Emerg Med 12:297–299.
2. Hanouz JL, Massetti M, Guesne G (2000) In vitro effects of desflurane, sevoflurane, isoflurane, and halothane in isolated human right atria. Anesthesiology 92:116–124.
3. Friesen RH, Wurl JL, Charlton GA (2000) Haemodynamic depression by halothane is age-related in paediatric patients. Paediatr Anaesth 10:267–272.
4. Prakash YS, Cody MJ, Hannon JD, et al. (2000) Comparison of volatile anesthetic effects on actin-myosin crossbridge cycling in neonatal vs. adult cardiac muscle. Anesthesiology 92:1114–1125.
5. Baum VC, Palmisano B (1997) The immature heart and anesthesia. Anesthesiology 87:1529–1548.
6. Prakash YS, Seckin I, Hunter LW, Sieck GC (2002) Mechanisms underlying greater sensitivity of neonatal cardiac muscle to volatile anesthetics. Anesthesiology 96:893–906.
7. Rivenes SM, Lewin MB, Stayer SA, et al. (2001) Cardiovascular effects of sevoflurane, isoflurane, halothane, and fentanyl-midazolam in children with congenital heart disease: an echocardiographic study of myocardial contractility and hemodynamics. Anesthesiology 94:223–229.
8. Bhananker SM, Ramamoorthy C, Geiduschek JM, et al. (2007) Anesthesia-related cardiac arrest in children: update from the Pediatric Perioperative Cardiac Arrest Registry. Anesth Analg 105:344–350.
9. Laird TH, Stayer SA, Rivenes SM, et al. (2002) Pulmonary-to-systemic blood flow ratio effects of sevoflurane, isoflurane, halothane, and fentanyl/midazolam with 100% oxygen in children with congenital heart disease. Anesth Analg 95:1200–1206.
10. Russell IA, Miller-Hance WC, Gregory G, et al. (2001) The safety and efficacy of sevoflurane anesthesia in infants and children with congenital heart disease. Anesth Analg 92:1152–1158.

Skipped 1 image

Skipped 1 image

Skipped 1 image

Skipped 1 image

Skipped 1 image

Skipped 1 image

Skipped 1 image

Skipped 1 image

Skipped 1 image

Skipped 1 image

Skipped 1 image

Skipped 1 image

Skipped 1 image

Skipped 1 image

Skipped 1 image

Skipped 1 image

Skipped 1 image

Skipped 1 image

Skipped 1 image

Skipped 1 image

Skipped 1 image

11. Ikemba CM, Su JT, Stayer SA, et al. (2004) Myocardial performance index with sevoflurane-pancuronium versus fentanyl-midazolam-pancuronium in infants with a functional single ventricle. Anesthesiology 101:1298–1305.

12. Taylor RH, Lerman J (1992) Induction, maintenance and recovery characteristics of desflurane in infants and children. Can J Anaesth 39:6–13.

13. Zwass MS, Fisher DM, Welborn LG, et al. (1992) Induction and maintenance characteristics of anesthesia with desflurane and nitrous oxide in infants and children. Anesthesiology 76:373–378.

14. Schaffer MS, Snyder AM, Morrison JE (2000) An assessment of desflurane for use during cardiac electrophysiological study and radiofrequency ablation of supraventricular dysrhythmias in children. Paediatr Anaesth 10:155–159.

15. Moore MA, Weiskopf RB, Eger EI, et al. (1993) Arrhythmogenic doses of epinephrine are similar during desflurane or isoflurane anesthesia in humans. Anesthesiology 79:943–997.

16. Blayney MR, Malins AF, Cooper GM (1999) Cardiac arrhythmias in children during outpatient general anaesthesia for dentistry: a prospective randomised trial. Lancet 354:1864–1866.

17. Viitanen H, Baer G, Koivu H, Annila P (1999) The hemodynamic and Holter-electrocardiogram changes during halothane and sevoflurane anesthesia for adenoidectomy in children aged one to three years. Anesth Analg 89:1423–1425.

18. Lavoie J, Walsh EP, Burrows FA, et al. (1995) Effects of propofol or isoflurane anesthesia on cardiac conduction in children undergoing radiofrequency catheter ablation for tachydysrhythmias. Anesthesiology 82:884–887.

19. Saussine M, Massad I, Raczka F, et al. (2006) Torsade de points during sevoflurane anesthesia in a child with congenital long QT syndrome. Paediatr Anaesth 16:63–65.

20. Vivien B, Hanouz JL, Gueugniaud PY, et al. (1997) Myocardial effects of halothane and isoflurane in hamsters with hypertrophic cardiomyopathy. Anesthesiology 87:1406–1416.

21. Pagel PS, Lowe D, Hettrick DA, et al. (1996) Isoflurane, but not halothane, improves indices of diastolic performance in dogs with rapid ventricular, pacing-induced cardiomyopathy. Anesthesiology 85:644–654.

22. Schulte-Sasse U, Hess W, Tarnow J (1982) Pulmonary vascular responses to nitrous oxide in patients with normal and high pulmonary vascular resistance. Anesthesiology 57:9–13.

23. Hilgenberg JC, McCammon RL, Stoelting RK (1980) Pulmonary and systemic vascular responses to nitrous oxide in patients with mitral stenosis and pulmonary hypertension. Anesth Analg 59:323–326.

24. Murray DJ, Forbes RB, Dull DL, Mahoney LT (1991) Hemodynamic responses to nitrous oxide during inhalation anesthesia in pediatric patients. J Clin Anesth 3:14–19.

25. Murray D, Forbes R, Murphy K, Mahoney L (1988) Nitrous oxide: cardiovascular effects in infants and small children during halothane and isoflurane anesthesia. Anesth Analg 67:1059–1064.

26. Hickey PR, Hansen DD, Strafford M, et al. (1986) Pulmonary and systemic hemodynamic effects of nitrous oxide in infants with normal and elevated pulmonary vascular resistance. Anesthesiology 65:374–378.

27. Hickey PR, Hansen DD (1984) Fentanyl- and sufentanil-oxygen-pancuronium anesthesia for cardiac surgery in infants. Anesth Analg 63:117–124.

28. Hickey PR, Hansen DD, Cramolini GM, et al. (1985) Pulmonary and systemic hemodynamic responses to ketamine in infants with normal and elevated pulmonary vascular resistance. Anesthesiology 62:287–293.

29. Hickey PR, Hansen DD, Wessel DL, et al. (1985) Blunting of stress responses in the pulmonary circulation of infants by fentanyl. Anesth Analg 64:1137–1142.

30. Hansen DD, Hickey PR (1986) Anesthesia for hypoplastic left heart syndrome: use of high-dose fentanyl in 30 neonates. Anesth Analg 65:127–132.

31. Moore RA, Yang SS, McNicholas KW, et al. (1985) Hemodynamic and anesthetic effects of sufentanil as the sole anesthetic for pediatric cardiovascular surgery. Anesthesiology 62:725–731.

32. Glenski JA, Friesen RH, Berglund NL, Henry DB (1988) Comparison of the hemodynamic and echocardiographic effects of sufentanil, fentanyl, isoflurane and halothane for pediatric cardiovascular surgery. J Cardiothorac Anesth 2:147–155 (Abstract).

33. McAuliffe G, Bissonnette B, Cavalle-Garrido T, Boutin C (1997) Heart rate and cardiac output after atropine in anaesthetised infants and children. Can J Anaesth 44:154–159.

34. Gruber EM, Laussen PC, Casta A, et al. (2001) Stress response in infants undergoing cardiac surgery: a randomized study of fentanyl bolus, fentanyl infusion, and fentanyl-midazolam infusion. Anesth Analg 92:882–890.

35. Anand KJ, Hickey PR (1992) Halothane-morphine compared with high-dose sufentanil for anesthesia and postoperative analgesia in neonatal cardiac surgery. N Engl J Med 326:1–9.

36. Duncan HP, Cloote A, Weir PM, et al. (2000) Reducing stress responses in the pre-bypass phase of open heart surgery in infants and young children: a comparison of different fentanyl doses. Br J Anaesth 84:556–564.

37. Bailey PL, Egan TD, Stanley TH (2000) Intravenous opioid anesthetics. In: Miller RD (ed) Anesthesia, 5th edn. Churchill-Livingstone, Philadelphia, pp. 273–376.

38. Donmez A, Kizilkan A, Berksun H, et al. (2001) One center's experience with remifentanil infusions for pediatric cardiac catheterization. J Cardiothorac Vasc Anesth 15:736–739.

39. Donmez A, Kaya H, Haberal A, et al. (1998) The effect of etomidate induction on plasma cortisol levels in children undergoing cardiac surgery. J Cardiothorac Vasc Anesth 12:182–185.

40. Davis PJ, Wilson AS, Siewers RD, et al. (1999) The effects of cardiopulmonary bypass on remifentanil kinetics in children undergoing atrial septal defect repair. Anesth Analg 89:904–908.

41. Davis DA, Spurrier EA, Healy RM, et al. (2001) Remifentanil blood concentrations in infants undergoing congenital heart surgery. Anesth Analg 92:SCA 124 (Abstract).

42. Friesen RH, Veit AS, Archibald DJ, Campanini RS (2003) A comparison of remifentanil and fentanyl for fast track paediatric cardiac anaesthesia. Paediatr Anaesth 13:122–125.
43. Akpek EA, Erkaya C, Donmez A, et al. (2005) Remifentanil use in children undergoing congenital heart surgery for left-to-right shunt lesions. J Cardiothorac Vasc Anesth 19:60–66.
44. Suzer O, Suzer A, Aykac Z, Ozuner Z (1998) Direct cardiac effects in isolated perfused rat hearts measured at increasing concentrations of morphine, alfentanil, fentanyl, ketamine, etomidate, thiopentone, midazolam and propofol. Eur J Anaesthesiol 15:480–485.
45. Gelissen HP, Epema AH, Henning RH, et al. (1996) Inotropic effects of propofol, thiopental, midazolam, etomidate, and ketamine on isolated human atrial muscle. Anesthesiology 84:397–403.
46. Wodey E, Chonow L, Beneux X, et al. (1999) Haemodynamic effects of propofol vs thiopental in infants: an echocardiographic study. Br J Anaesth 82:516–520.
47. Williams GD, Jones TK, Hanson KA, Morray JP (1999) The hemodynamic effects of propofol in children with congenital heart disease. Anesth Analg 89:1411–1416.
48. Lebovic S, Reich DL, Steinberg LG, et al. (1992) Comparison of propofol versus ketamine for anesthesia in pediatric patients undergoing cardiac catheterization. Anesth Analg 74:490–494.
49. Akin A, Esmaoglu A, Guler G, et al. (2005) Propofol and propofol-ketamine in pediatric patients undergoing cardiac catheterization. Pediatr Cardiol 26:553–557.
50. Zestos MM, Walter HL, Cauldwell CB, et al. (1998) The efficacy of propofol sedation in children after pediatric open heart surgery. Anesthesiology 89:A1315 (Abstract).
51. Cray SH, Holtby HM, Kartha VM, et al. (2001) Early tracheal extubation after paediatric cardiac surgery: the use of propofol to supplement low-dose opioid anaesthesia. Paediatr Anaesth 11:465–471.
52. Sharpe MD, Dobkowski WB, Murkin JM, et al. (1995) Propofol has no direct effect on sinoatrial node function or on normal atrioventricular and accessory pathway conduction in Wolff-Parkinson-White syndrome during alfentanil/midazolam anesthesia. Anesthesiology 82:888–895.
53. Lai LP, Lin JL, Wu MH, et al. (1999) Usefulness of intravenous propofol anesthesia for radiofrequency catheter ablation in patients with tachyarrhythmias: infeasibility for pediatric patients with ectopic atrial tachycardia. Pacing Clin Electrophysiol 22:1358–1364.
54. Cray SH, Robinson BH, Cox PN (1998) Lactic acidemia and bradyarrhythmia in a child sedated with propofol. Crit Care Med 26:2087–2092.
55. Bray RJ (1998) Propofol infusion syndrome in children. Paediatr Anaesth 8:491–499.
56. Wysowski DK, Pollock ML (2006) Reports of death with use of propofol (Diprivan) for nonprocedural (long-term) sedation and literature review. Anesthesiology 105:1047–1051.
57. Reves JG, Glass PSA, Lubarsky DA (2000) Nonbarbiturate intravenous anesthetics. In: Miller RD (ed) Anesthesia, 5th edn. Churchill-Livingstone, Philadelphia, pp. 228–272.
58. Kudoh A, Matsuki A (1999) Ketamine inhibits inositol 1,4,5-trisphosphate production depending on the extracellular Ca^{2+} concentration in neonatal rat cardiomyocytes. Anesth Analg 89:1417–1422.
59. Sprung J, Schuetz SM, Stewart RW, Moravec CS (1998) Effects of ketamine on the contractility of failing and nonfailing human heart muscles in vitro. Anesthesiology 88:1202–1210.
60. Schechter WS, Kim C, Martinez M, et al. (1995) Anaesthetic induction in a child with end-stage cardiomyopathy. Can J Anaesth 42:404–408.
61. Gutzke GE, Shah KB, Glisson SN, et al. (1989) Cardiac transplantation: a prospective comparison of ketamine and sufentanil for anesthetic induction. J Cardiothorac Anesth 3:389–395.
62. Levin RM, Seleny FL, Streczyn MV (1975) Ketamine-pancuronium-narcotic technic for cardiovascular surgery in infants—a comparative study. Anesth Analg 54:800–805.
63. Radnay PA, Hollinger I, Santi A, Nagashima H (1976) Ketamine for pediatric cardiac anesthesia. Anaesthesist 25:259–265.
64. Greeley WJ, Bushman GA, Davis DP, Reves JG (1986) Comparative effects of halothane and ketamine on systemic arterial oxygen saturation in children with cyanotic heart disease. Anesthesiology 65:666–668.
65. Tugrul M, Camci E, Pembeci K, et al. (2000) Ketamine infusion versus isoflurane for the maintenance of anesthesia in the prebypass period in children with tetralogy of Fallot. J Cardiothorac Vasc Anesth 14:557–561.
66. Morray JP, Lynn AM, Stamm SJ, et al. (1984) Hemodynamic effects of ketamine in children with congenital heart disease. Anesth Analg 63:895–899.
67. Williams GD, Philip BM, Chu LF, et al. (2007) Ketamine does not increase pulmonary vascular resistance in children with pulmonary hypertension undergoing sevoflurane anesthesia and spontaneous ventilation. Anesth Analg 105:1578–1584.
68. Singh A, Girotra S, Mehta Y, et al. (2000) Total intravenous anesthesia with ketamine for pediatric interventional cardiac procedures. J Cardiothorac Vasc Anesth 14:36–39.
69. Sprung J, Ogletree-Hughes ML, Moravec CS (2000) The effects of etomidate on the contractility of failing and nonfailing human heart muscle. Anesth Analg 91:68–75.
70. Ogletree ML, Eapen JA, East DL, et al. (2004) The in vitro effect of etomidate on the contractility of ventricular muscles from pediatric hearts with congenital heart disease. Anesthesiology 101:A1451 (Abstract).
71. Nyman Y, von Hofsten K, Palm C, et al. (2006) Etomidate-Lipuro® is associated with considerably less injection pain in children compared with propofol with added lidocaine. Br J Anaesth 97:536–539.
72. Nguyen NK, Magnier S, Georget G, et al. (1991) Anesthesia for heart catheterization in children. Comparison of 3 techniques. Ann Fr Anesth Reanim 10:522–528.
73. Sarkar M, Laussen PC, Zurakowski D, et al. (2005) Hemodynamic responses to etomidate on induction of anesthesia in pediatric patients. Anesth Analg 101:645–650.
74. Amar D, Komer CA (1993) Anesthetic implications of a ruptured aneurysm of the sinus of Valsalva. J Cardiothorac Vasc Anesth 7:730–733.

75. Tay SM, Ong BC, Tan SA (1999) Cesarean section in a mother with uncorrected congenital coronary to pulmonary artery fistula. Can J Anaesth 46:368–371.

76. Petroz GC, Sikich N, James M, et al. (2006) A phase I, two-center study of the pharmacokinetics and pharmacodynamics of dexmedetomidine in children. Anesthesiology 105:1098–1110.

77. Mukhtar AM, Obayah EM, Hassona AM (2006) The use of dexmedetomidine in pediatric cardiac surgery. Anesth Analg 103:52–56.

78. Chrysostomou C, Di Filippo S, Manrique AM, et al. (2006) Use of dexmedetomidine in children after cardiac and thoracic surgery. Pediatr Crit Care Med 7:126–131.

79. Finkel JC, Johnson YJ, Quezado ZM (2005) The use of dexmedetomidine to facilitate acute discontinuation of opioids after cardiac transplantation in children. Crit Care Med 33:2110–2112.

80. Munro HM, Tirotta CF, Felix DE, et al. (2007) Initial experience with dexmedetomidine for diagnostic and interventional cardiac catheterization in children. Paediatr Anaesth 17:109–112.

81. Tosun Z, Akin A, Guler G, et al. (2006) Dexmedetomidine-ketamine and propofol-ketamine combinations for anesthesia in spontaneously breathing pediatric patients undergoing cardiac catheterization. J Cardiothorac Vasc Anesth 20:515–519.

82. Hammer GB, Drover DR, Cao H, et al. (2008) The effects of dexmedetomidine on cardiac electrophysiology in children. Anesth Analg 106:79–83.

83. Huntington JH, Malviya S, Voepel-Lewis T, et al. (1999) The effect of a right-to-left intracardiac shunt on the rate of rise of arterial and end-tidal halothane in children. Anesth Analg 88:759–762.

84. Bokesch PM, Castaneda AR, Ziemer G, Wilson JM (1987) The influence of a right-to-left cardiac shunt on lidocaine pharmacokinetics. Anesthesiology 67:739–744.

85. Gozal Y, Mints B, Drenger B (2002) Time course of neuromuscular blockade with rocuronium in children with intracardiac shunts. J Cardiothorac Vasc Anesth 16:737–738.

86. Tanner GE, Angers DG, Barash PG, et al. (1985) Effect of left-to-right, mixed left-to-right, and right-to-left shunts on inhalational anesthetic induction in children: a computer model. Anesth Analg 64:101–107.

87. Hall RI (2000) Changes in pharmacokinetics and pharmacodynamics of drugs administered during cardiopulmonary bypass. In: Gravlee GP, Davis RF, Kurusz M, Utley JR (eds) Cardiopulmonary Bypass: Principles and Practice, 2nd edn. Lippincott Williams & Wilkins, Philadelphia, pp. 265–302.

88. Koren G, Crean P, Klein J, et al. (1984) Sequestration of fentanyl by the cardiopulmonary bypass (CPB). Eur J Clin Pharmacol 27:51–56.

89. Koren G, Barker C, Goresky G, et al. (1987) The influence of hypothermia on the disposition of fentanyl–human and animal studies. Eur J Clin Pharmacol 32:373–376.

90. Laussen PC, Murphy JA, Zurakowski D, et al. (2001) Bispectral index monitoring in children undergoing mild hypothermic cardiopulmonary bypass. Paediatr Anaesth 11:567–573.

91. Taenzer AH, Groom R, Quinn RD (2005) Fentanyl plasma levels after modified ultrafiltration in infant heart surgery. J Extra Corpor Technol 37:369–372.

92. Antognini JF (1993) Hypothermia eliminates isoflurane requirements at 20 degrees C. Anesthesiology 78:1152–1156.

93. Liu M, Hu X, Liu J (2001) The effect of hypothermia on isoflurane MAC in children. Anesthesiology 94:429–432.

94. Kussman BD, Gruber EM, Zurakowski D, et al. (2001) Bispectral index monitoring during infant cardiac surgery: relationship of BIS to the stress response and plasma fentanyl levels. Paediatr Anaesth 11:663–669.

95. Davidson AJ, McCann ME, Devavaram P, et al. (2001) The differences in the bispectral index between infants and children during emergence from anesthesia after circumcision surgery. Anesth Analg 93:326–330.

96. Rosen DA, Rosen KR, Steelman RJ, et al. (1999) Is the BIS monitor vital in children undergoing cardiothoracic surgery? Anesthesiology 91:A1244 (Abstract).

97. Davidson AJ (2007) Monitoring the anesthetic depth in children—an update. Curr Opin Anaesthesiol 20:236–243.

98. Fisher DM (1999) Neuromuscular blocking agents in paediatric anaesthesia. Br J Anaesth 83:58–64.

99. Hannallah RS, Oh TH, McGill WA, Epstein BS (1986) Changes in heart rate and rhythm after intramuscular succinylcholine with or without atropine in anesthetized children. Anesth Analg 65:1329–1332.

100. Lucero VM, Lerman J, Burrows FA (1987) Onset of neuromuscular blockade with pancuronium in children with congenital heart disease. Anesth Analg 66:788–790.

101. Sloan MH, Lerman J, Bissonnette B (1991) Pharmacodynamics of high-dose vecuronium in children during balanced anesthesia. Anesthesiology 74:656–659.

102. Reynolds LM, Lau M, Brown R, et al. (1996) Intramuscular rocuronium in infants and children. Dose-ranging and tracheal intubating conditions. Anesthesiology 85:231–239.

103. Taivainen T, Meakin GH, Meretoja OA, et al. (2000) The safety and efficacy of cisatracurium 0.15 mg.kg(-1) during nitrous oxide-opioid anaesthesia in infants and children. Anaesthesia 55:1047–1051.

104. Sawasdiwipachai P, Laussen PC, McGowan FX, et al. (2007) Cardiac arrest after neuromuscular blockade reversal in a heart transplant infant. Anesthesiology 107:664–665.

105. Pühringer FK, Rex C, Sielenkämper AW, et al. (2008) Reversal of profound, high-dose rocuronium-induced neuromuscular blockade by sugammadex at two different time points: an international, multicenter, randomized, dose-finding, safety assessor-blinded, phase II trial. Anesthesiology 109:188–197.

7 Cardiopulmonary bypass

Ralph Gertler, M.D.
Institute of Anesthesiology and Intensive Care, German Heart Centre of the State of Bavaria and the Technical University Munich, Munich, Germany

Dean B. Andropoulos, M.D.
Texas Children's Hospital, Baylor College of Medicine, Houston, Texas, USA

Introduction

In 1954 Lillehei first reported the effective use of extracorporeal circulation in repair of congenital heart disease (CHD) using cross circulation with the patient's parent functioning as the oxygenator. Over fifty-five years ago, on May 6, 1953 John H. Gibbon Jr for the first time successfully performed open-heart surgery using cardiopulmonary bypasses (CPBs) for the closure of a large atrial septal defect. The heart–lung machine, consisting of a simple oxygenator in conjunction with roller pumps, took over the function of the heart and lungs for the duration of

Anesthesia for Congenital Heart Disease 2nd edition. Edited by Dean Andropoulos, Stephen Stayer, Isobel Russell and Emad Mossad.
© 2010 Blackwell Publishing.

26 minutes. The machine worked properly during the total bypass time of 45 minutes, apart from some fibrin formation on the oxygenator due to inadequate anticoagulation [1]. Gibbons success stood at the end of approximately 20 years of developing a heart–lung machine. In a 1937 publication, Gibbon published his first results of an experimental CPB in cats. In 1939 the former president of the American Association of Thoracic Surgeons, Leo Eloesser, said during a discussion following a lecture by Gibbons that his presentation reminded him of the seemingly impossible, fantastic stories of the novel writer Jules Verne that later often became reality [2]. In a series of 19 consecutive bypass uses in dogs, at least 12 of the animals could survive.

The idea of perfusion with artificially produced circulating arterial blood came not from Gibbon. The idea was first documented in 1812 inspired by the French physiologist César Julien-Jean Le Gallois. In his monograph "Expériences sur le principe de la vie" he described experiments to define the relationship of respiratory, nervous system, and blood circulation. On August 9, 1951 Dogliotti and Constantini in Turin for the first time used a partial bypass on humans [3]. When a patient whose condition during the surgical removal of a large mediastinal tumor drastically deteriorated, a heart–lung machine was used to maintain the perfusion for 20 minutes and the patient was stabilized.

Johan Willem Kolff observed on March 16, 1943 during the clinical use of an artificial dialyzer that oxygen was quickly absorbed by a cellulose membrane. This observation was the basis for the later development of membrane oxygenators. Later Kolff could present the first membrane oxygenator at the first Congress of the American Society for Artificial Internal Organs on June 5, 1955 [4]. The first commercial oxygenators came available in the 1960s and cardiac surgery techniques took off at that point.

Subsequent attempts to use the heart–lung machine to help correct congenital heart defects were hindered by high morbidity and mortality rates until Barratt-Boyes and Castaneda started using hypothermic circulatory arrest in the late 1960s and early 1970s. With the introduction of CPB, new anesthetic challenges arose and were described by Dr Arthur Keats and his colleagues at Texas Children's Hospital. Surgical progress continued, new procedures were devised, and anesthetic care became steadily more sophisticated. Less than two decades later pediatric cardiac surgery and anesthesia have progressed to providing multistage palliation for infants with single ventricle physiology. Today CPB is an elementary piece of daily pediatric cardiac anesthesia practice. The maturation of neonatal CPB over the last 50 years has undoubtedly been the most critical advance leading to improved outcomes in pediatric cardiac surgery.

Extracorporeal perfusion in newborn, infants, and children is in many aspects different from the adult patient. This is caused by the underlying physiologic changes as well as the different pathophysiology secondary to shunt physiology.

In this chapter we take a look at the equipment with a primary focus on pediatric bypass and further look at the effects of CPB on different organ systems. However, the emphasis of the chapter is to examine specific management issues that occur in daily practice. Further details on specific technical issues can be found in excellent extensive textbooks on the topic [5].

The cardiopulmonary bypass circuit

Major differences need to be considered when dealing with the pediatric patient on CPB (Table 7.1). These include the degree of hemodilution, flow rates and perfusion pressure, temperature, cannulation, prime and blood gas management, ultrafiltration, hemodynamic management, and in certain cases the presence of aortopulmonary collaterals.

Hemodilution

Recent efforts to minimize circuit volumes have led to the development of smaller circuit elements. However, there continues to be a gross degree of hemodilution realized in the neonatal patient. This can be as much as 3–15 times the amount of hemodilution seen in an adult. For example, in a 3-kg child, given 85 cc/kg, an EBV (estimated blood volume) of 255 cc contrasts to an average circuit prime volume of 300–400 cc. Thus, a prime:EBV ratio can exceed >2–3:1, or >100–150% of a neonate's blood volume.

Table 7.1 Differences between adult and pediatric cardiopulmonary bypass

Parameter	Adult	Pediatrics
Temperature	Rarely below 32°C	Commonly 18–20°C
Deep hypothermic cardiocirculatory arrest (DHCA)	Rare	Common for Arch repair (HLHS, IAA)
Pump prime	Crystalloids	Blood components and albumin
Dilution	25–33%	Up to 200%
Perfusion pressure	50–80 mm Hg	30–50 mm Hg
Flow rates	2.5 L/min/m² or 50–65 cc/kg/min	0–250 cc/kg/min
pH Management	Alpha-stat	pH-Stat
Hypoglycemia	Rare, only in hepatic injury	Common due to low hepatic glycogen stores
Hyperglycemia	Frequent, increases mortality	Less common, may be protective
Cannulation techniques	Standardized, mostly ascending aorta and single stage venous cannula	Variable, including ductus, aorta, main pulmonary artery; mostly bicaval venous cannulation
Ultrafiltration	Rare	Standard modified ultrafiltration or conventional ultrafiltration

In the average adult circuit only a 25–33% dilution rate is realized. This degree of dilution necessitates the addition of donor blood up to a body weight of approximately 10 kg to maintain an adequate hematocrit for optimal oxygen delivery on bypass.

Perfusion pressures

Perfusion pressures in the neonate can be quite low, <30 mm Hg. This is often due to the lack of reactivity of the neonatal vasculature or presence of a shunt like a PDA. With meticulous management of blood gases, hematocrit, temperature, and flow rates, there should be no indication for the use of vasoconstricting agents to maintain an ideal blood pressure.

Flow rates

The flow ranges for neonates are quite variable and wide. Flows range from 0 to 200 cc/kg/min. Deep hypothermic circulatory arrest (DHCA) is one end of the spectrum, contrasted with high metabolic demands, vent return, circuit shunts, or patient collaterals, all of which contribute to the necessity of high flow rates on the other end. This can often exceed a cardiac index of 3 L/min/m^2. The flow rates are calculated on the basis of weight, but the perfusionist must adapt flows according to the individual case and demands.

Blood gas management

It is our current practice to employ pH-stat management on all cases in which temperatures are taken to hypothermic levels. In this temperature-corrected strategy, the P_{CO_2} remains unchanged from 37°C (40 mm Hg). This strategy allows for cerebral vasodilation and more even cooling. The reflective P_{CO_2} ranges at 37°C can be >80–100 mm Hg.

Cannulation

Whether CABG or valve operations, standard or femoral, adult cannulation techniques are quite predictable. The larger vessels accommodate the necessary cannulae, causing rare anatomic distortion with cannula placement. Usually one or two cannulae are used, with femoral cannulation available as an alternative choice if needed.

In neonatal and pediatric practice, the choices in decision making are variable. Anatomic limitations can occur or the size may be prohibitive to flow requirements. One, two, or three cannulae may be needed, such as in the presence of a persistent left superior vena cava without a bridging vein. Unlike the adult patient, femoral cannulation as an alternative is not an option below 15–20 kg. The perfusionist and surgeon must have good communication for cannulation techniques to match flow requirements.

Aortopulmonary collaterals

Uncommon in adults, but rather common in patients with chronic cyanosis with decreased pulmonary blood flow, aortopulmonary collaterals can be a challenge. Flow rates are frequently affected and temperatures may need to be lowered substantially to accommodate the field. Flows may need to be decreased in conjunction with the use of vasodilating agents. Phentolamine 0.1 mg/kg and nitroglycerine are the drugs of choice during cooling and rewarming, titrated to effect. Phenylephrine is contraindicated and would only enhance collateral flow.

Temperature ranges

As a very basic comparison, there is a trend to conducting adult cases at tepid or normothermic temperatures while many neonatal cases are utilizing very cold temperatures with or without DHCA. The perfusion considerations are multiple and this topic is discussed in a separate section on hypothermia and deep hypothermic cardiocirculatory arrest.

Glucose management

It is of utmost importance to maintain euglycemia in the neonate. Although there are increased glycogen stores in the neonatal myocardium, there are low hepatic glycogen stores. Exogenous glucose may be necessary in the early neonatal period to maintain normal glucose levels.

Perfusion considerations on CPB are directed at efforts to maintain normal glucose levels such as washing packed cells or minimizing glucose content in cardioplegia or IV fluids. When glucose levels are greater than 300 mg/dL a saline hemodilutional washout with the hemoconcentrator is utilized. Frequent monitoring is recommended. Levels should be maintained at approximately 150 mg/dL just prior to DHCA.

Hyperglycemia worsens neurological injury as elevated glucose levels result in increased anaerobic metabolism of glucose and increased lactic acidosis. This leads to further depletion of ATP. Hypoglycemia alone can be treated, but coupled with hypothermia, cerebral blood flow may be compromised by altering autoregulation. This can be further exacerbated with hyperventilation as what may occur in weaning a patient with pulmonary hypertension from CPB.

Equipment

One circuit size for the adult patients at a given institution can adequately provide flows for patients from 50 kg and more. Most pediatric centers employ two or three circuits on the basis of the patient weight, procedure, and flow requirements.

Ultrafiltration

Utilization of ultrafiltration in some form whether it be conventional or modified is seen on >90% of our neonatal and pediatric cases. Several system modifications may be necessary to allow for these options.

Basic bypass circuit setup

A basic bypass circuit (Figure 7.1) consists of a venous reservoir, a oxygenator/heat exchanger unit, roller pumps for perfusion, suction, and cardioplegia and the connecting tubing, cannulae, as well as monitoring and alarm devices. Major differences exist between adult and pedi-

atric CPB, stemming from anatomic, metabolic, and physiologic differences in these two groups of patients (Table 7.1). Much progress has been made in miniaturization of circuits and components. Current technology allows a total priming volume as low as 122 cc for a neonatal circuit setup [6].

Cannulation and tubing

The selection of cannulas occurs on the basis of flow requirements and the anatomic relations. Single stage venous cannulation is rare and selective upper and lower vena cava cannulation plus an additional cannulation of a left persistent vena cava is routine. Particular care must be observed during inferior vena cava cannulation as

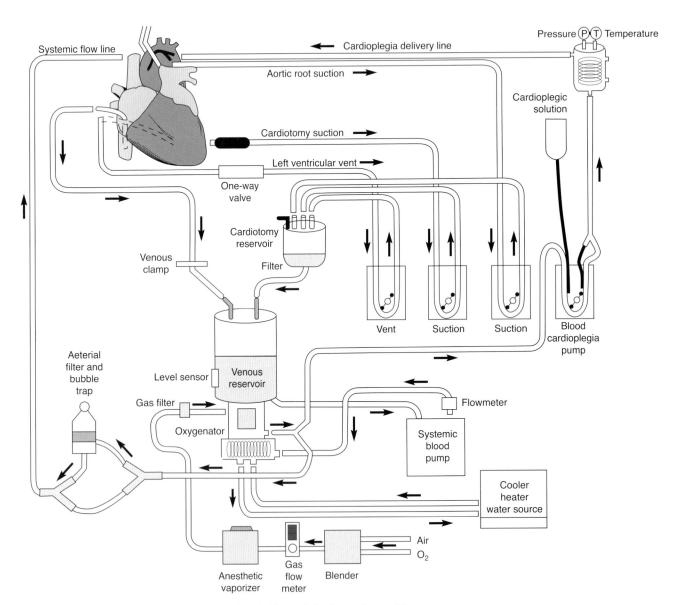

Figure 7.1 Cardiopulmonary bypass circuit (Reproduced with permission from Reference [5])

malplacement into one of the liver veins or obstruction can easily happen.

In daily clinical practice, the amount of systemic venous return on CPB is directly correlated to the amount of the pump flow and vice versa. Venous drainage is often limited by the small size of the cannula and tubing as well as individual characteristics, circuit used, and the use of accessory systems. Generally venous drainage is obtained by gravity, placing the venous reservoir of the CPB circuit about 30 cm lower than the heart level; in this way a negative pressure equivalent to about 20–25 mm Hg is obtained. This is adequate for the vast majority of adult patients undergoing conventional procedures. In pediatric patients, however, where relatively small-size cannulas and tubing of the venous circuit are used to reduce the pump priming, additional systems need to be used to artificially increase the venous drainage provided by gravity only. The system most often used is vacuum-assisted venous return. In this system a constant vacuum (up to 80 mm Hg) is created in the airtight venous reservoir, allowing more blood to be drained from the patient via the venous line. This system allows the performance of surgical procedures on CPB even in small infants without the need of large-size venous tubing and, therefore, without increasing the volume of the pump priming [7]. The major potential limit in the clinical application of this system is the high risk of generating gaseous microemboli in the venous circuit. If the arterial pump is stopped for various reasons and the vacuum source is left on the venous reservoir, microbubble transgression can occur from the gas compartment to the liquid compartment of the oxygenator, creating another source of gaseous microemboli as soon as the arterial pump is turned on again [8].

Arterial cannulation is usually via the ascending aorta. Exceptions, however, are frequent in the newborn with malformation of the ascending aorta (e.g., interrupted aortic arch and hypoplastic left heart syndrome). In that case scenario the ductus is primarily cannulated to maintain body perfusion on bypass and the pulmonary arteries are snared to prevent runoff until an anatomic correction takes place.

The clinician must also be aware that femoral cannulation is not feasible in small children <15 kg because of the small vessel size. Thus, on redo operations, this method of establishing CPB is usually not an option and careful dissection of the chest must take place.

The aortic cannula represents the smallest diameter in the pediatric CPB circuit. The tubing on the other hand is responsible for the tremendous foreign surface and priming volume. The clever selection of tubing dimensions can reduce the volume effectively (Tables 7.2 and 7.3). If, for example, you consider a 3.5 kg newborn with an approximate blood volume of 300 cc, the addition of a sucker line with a $\frac{1}{4}$ in. diameter and a total length of 250 cm would

Table 7.2 Cardiopulmonary bypass tubing volumes

Tubing diameter (in.)	Volume per meter length
$\frac{1}{2}$	126
$\frac{3}{8}$	71
$\frac{1}{4}$	33
$\frac{3}{16}$	18

take up approximately $\frac{1}{3}$ of the patient's blood volume (82.5 mL) before reaching the reservoir.

Malposition of cannulas is particularly problematic in pediatric perfusion. Systemic perfusion may be adversely impacted when placement of either venous or arterial cannulas is not ideal. If venous obstruction occurs, the consequences are magnified because of low perfusion pressures. If the inferior vena cava cannula causes venous obstruction in the splanchnic bed, increased hydrostatic pressure causes ascites, and reduced perfusion pressure results in significant renal, hepatic, and gastrointestinal (GI) dysfunction. Obstruction of the superior vena cava will produce an increase in intracranial pressure and result in decreased cerebral perfusion pressure and cerebral edema. It is possible to see preferential flow to one side of the cerebral circulation or down the distal aorta (Figure 7.2). Transcranial Doppler monitoring of cerebral flow velocity or cerebral oximetry is likely to provide an early warning of altered flow patterns caused by cannula misplacement [9]. Cooling patterns showing rectal cooling preceding tympanic membrane cooling may suggest a disproportionate amount of pump flow being directed away from the cerebral circulation [10].

Pumps

The two pumps most commonly used for CPB are roller pumps and centrifugal pumps. Roller pumps have the advantages of simplicity, low cost, ease and reliability of flow calculation, and the ability to pump against high resistance without reducing flow. Disadvantages include the need to assess occlusiveness, spallation of the inner tubing surface that potentially produces particulate arterial emboli, capability for pumping large volumes of air, and ability to create large positive and negative pressures. Centrifugal pumps offer the advantage of lesser air

Table 7.3 Cardiopulmonary bypass tubing sizes

Patient weight	Arterial and venous tubing sizes
$\frac{3}{16}$ in. arterial line, $\frac{1}{4}$ in. venous line	<10 kg
$\frac{1}{4}$ in. arterial line, $\frac{3}{8}$ in. venous line	<20 kg
$\frac{3}{8}$ in. arterial line, $\frac{3}{8}$ in. venous line	<50 kg

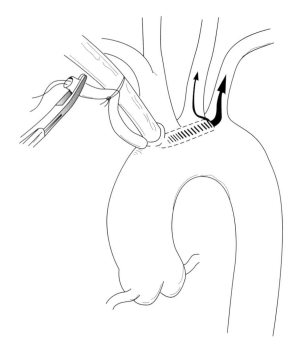

Figure 7.2 Position of the aortic cannula high up in the ascending aorta. This cannulation technique is helpful for arch repair or any surgery involving the ascending aorta. Particular attention needs to be observed to avoid preferential perfusion of the left cranium (Reproduced with permission from Reference [9])

pumping capabilities, lesser abilities to create large positive and negative pressures, less blood trauma, and virtually no spallation. Disadvantages include higher cost, the lack of occlusiveness (creating the possibility of accidental patient exsanguination), and afterload-dependent flow requiring constant flow measurement. In the setting of short-term CPB for cardiac surgery, it remains uncertain whether the selection of a certain pump over another has clinical significance.

Oxygenator

The efficiency of gas exchange in the natural lung is mainly attributable to the large surface area generated by the airway and circulatory networks and the low resistance to diffusion. These same features are essential to the design of an efficient artificial lung. Other necessary features of an ideal oxygenator include minimal trauma to blood, thromboresistance, minimal reaction with blood components, minimal generation of gaseous microemboli, ability to maintain performance over long periods, low prime volume, consistent physical properties, reliability, ease of use, and low cost. The efficiency of the membrane oxygenator is two to three times less than the efficiency of the natural lung at rest, and about eight times less than the natural lung under conditions of maximal exercise. The primary limiting factor to efficient gas exchange in membrane oxygenators appears to be blood phase resistance to both O_2 and CO_2 diffusion. A second factor that has limited the use of microporous membranes in situations of long-term extracorporeal support is the progressive decrease in gas exchange function. The most common microporous membrane oxygenator design nowadays is the hollow-fiber type in which the membrane is formed into fibers that are bundled or woven together. The fibers are 200–250 μm in diameter, 10–15 cm long, and the membrane thickness is 25–50 μm. Although the existence of micropores in the membrane significantly increased the gas exchange of membrane oxygenators, long-term use results in the progressive wetting of the surface, plasma leakage through the pores, and subsequent deterioration of membrane performance.

Priming

Bypass priming is adapted to the particular requirements of the patient. The composition, however, is often a matter of opinion and differences are as wide as the number of pediatric heart centers. Consensus probably only consists upon the question of reduction of volumes to a minimum to reduce transfusion requirements and dilutional effects of the patient.

Despite recent advances in technology, the majority of neonates and infants still require perioperative transfusion of homologous blood components. The lower the body weight of the patient, the more foreign blood products need to be added to the prime. To maintain colloid osmotic pressure and a minimal amount of coagulation factors, albumin and FFP (fresh frozen plasma) are added. The level of ionized calcium is adjusted since all blood products contain significant amounts of citrate. This can lead to acute hypocalcemia and cardiac arrest going on bypass. In addition, added erythrocyte concentrates should be as fresh as possible (<3–5 days old) to avoid hyperkalemia and hyperlactemia as side effects. The reasons for this suggestion are that the level of 2,3-DPG in stored red blood cells decreases, metabolic load increases (potassium and lactate levels by the end of the 2nd day are up to 7–25 mmol/L [11]), and the risk of complications going on bypass is higher. The risk is particularly high in infants <5 kg if the prime contains irradiated blood [12]. If the red blood cells in the prime are older than 5 days, a prime blood gas should be checked and corrected. Circulating and filtrating the prime for 20 minutes alleviates most of these problems. Alternatively, processing packed red blood cells via a cell saver is reasonable and may add additional benefits like the avoidance of hyperglycemia, high citrate levels, and hyperkalemia [13]. Also, lactate levels are reduced and microaggregates bigger than 20 μm are eliminated. Care must be taken to avoid using normal saline as a washing solution since a hyperchloremic

Table 7.4 Patient blood volumes by weight

Weight (kg)	Blood volume (cc/kg)
<10	85
10–20	80
20–30	75
30–50	70
>50	65

metabolic acidosis can be induced in newborns and infants. In addition, the use of cell-saving devices during pediatric cardiac surgery provides another mean of reducing foreign blood exposure [14].

Packed red blood cell requirements can be calculated on the basis of weight and starting hematocrit. The drop in hematocrit is calculated as:

$$\text{Delta-Hct} = \frac{\text{Hct-Pat} \times \text{BV-Pat}}{\text{BV-Pat} + \text{PV}}$$

where BV-Pat = blood volume patient (see Table 7.4) and PV = priming volume

The transfusion requirement is calculated as:

$$\begin{aligned}\text{PRBC (ml)} = {} & \text{Hct-desired} \times (\text{BV-Pat} + \text{PV}) \\ & - \frac{(\text{BV-Pat} \times \text{Hct-Pat})}{60\%},\end{aligned} \quad (7.1)$$

whereby 60% is the average hematocrit of stored packed red blood cells.

In newborn, a goal hematocrit on pump of 30% is maintained. Older patients or special circumstances (e.g., severe hypoxia) may require adjustments to a lower limit of around 25% or higher than 30% (severe hypoxia), even though both limits are controversial. Historically, many centers permitted marked hemodilution on CPB to avoid transfusion. Recent studies question this approach and provide evidence of improved neurological function when higher hematocrits are maintained during CPB. A randomized controlled clinical study in infants undergoing CPB demonstrated adverse perioperative and developmental outcomes with hemodilution [15]. This issue remains controversial, although the clinical data in support of higher hematocrits of at least 25% are compelling [16,17]. Also hemostasis may be improved by higher hematocrit levels.

Management of pediatric cardiopulmonary bypass

Stages of cardiopulmonary bypass

Cardiac cases using CPB can be divided into several basic phases: prebypass period and anticoagulation, bypass pe-

riod with initial cooling, cross-clamping and myocardial protection, reperfusion of the heart, separation from CPB, modified ultrafiltration and haemostasis, and lastly, chest closure and transfer to the ICU.

Prebypass period

The prebypass period begins with surgical incision and lasts through initial dissection and preparation for cannulation. During this period transesophageal echocardiography (TEE) is performed to confirm the diagnosis and establish a basis for postbypass comparison. Baseline activated clotting time values are obtained and metabolic abnormalities corrected. Cannulation of the great vessels just prior to CPB can often precipitate arrhythmias, hypotension, and arterial desaturation, especially in small infants and children. Hemodynamic stability is maintained by cautious fluid administration and small boluses of vasopressors, as necessary. If the aortic cannula is already in place, it is common practice to coordinate the administration of volume between the anesthesiologist and perfusionist while the surgeon completes cannulation.

Anticoagulation and hemostatic management

Development of the coagulation system is incomplete at birth and continues in the postnatal period until the age of about 6 months. This increases the risk of bleeding disproportionately in the neonatal and infant group up to 1 year or approximately 8 kg of weight [18–20]. Cyanotic infants may be particularly impaired secondary to polycythemia, lower fibrinogen levels, low platelet count and abnormal platelet function [21], decreased concentrations of factors V, VII, and VIII, and increased fibrinolysis [22,23].

Of particular importance is the role of antithrombin III (ATIII) levels that do not reach adult values until 3–6 months. This low level of ATIII may reduce the ability of heparin to provide anticoagulation adequate to prevent thrombin generation during CPB in infants [24] and may require an initial heparin dose of 400 IU/kg and higher. It has also recently been shown that in infants with CHD levels of other thrombin inhibitors are depressed compared with healthy infants. This may partially explain the high levels of thrombin generation during infant CPB.

The coagulopathy induced by CPB affects children more profoundly than adults. There are many factors implicated including hemodilution, contact activation, and initiation of a systemic inflammatory response.

Despite large doses of heparin during CPB, heparin does not block thrombin generation but partially inhibits thrombin after it is produced. Thrombin is continuously generated and a consumptive coagulopathy is initiated [25,26]. The lower potential of newborn plasma to generate thrombin might in part downregulate thrombin markers during CPB. This, however, does not seem significant enough to completely prevent the subsequent reperfusion-induced thrombin peak [27]. Thromboelastography has actually shown that neonates and infants develop faster and stronger clots than adults [28]. In addition, acquired coagulation defects in 58% of noncyanotic and 71% of cyanotic infants have been reported [29–31]. If thrombin formation could be completely inhibited during CPB, the consumption of coagulation proteins and platelets could largely be prevented.

Initial heparin doses range from a 300–400 IU/kg bolus before cannulation, 200–400 IU/kg in the circuit, and 50–100 IU/kg ongoing administration every 30–120 minutes. Heparin's peak therapeutic effect occurs within 2 minutes. CPB may delay the peak effect by 10–20 minutes from hypothermia or hemodilution. Plasma binds 95% of heparin with some uptake by the extracellular fluid, alveolar macrophages, splenic/hepatic endothelial cells, and vascular smooth muscle. The plasma half-life is dose dependent, i.e., 126 ± 24 minutes at a dose of 400 IU/kg versus 93 ± 6 minutes at a dose of 200 IU/kg [32]. Heparin is metabolized by the reticuloendothelial system and eliminated by the kidneys. Hypothermia and renal impairment, but not hepatic impairment, delay elimination. A roughly linear relationship exists between heparin dose and the activated clotting time (ACT) if certain criteria are maintained [33], namely normal ATIII and factor XII activities, normothermia, near normal platelet function, a platelet count greater than 50,000, and fibrinogen concentration greater than 100 mg/dL. However, in children the correlation is rather poor [34]. An ACT is measured before heparinization and repeated a minimum of 3 minutes after giving heparin. CPB is not initiated until an adequate ACT or heparin level is confirmed.

Given the variability in the ACT, heparin concentration can also be measured directly. A two-point (straight line) dose–response curve assists in judging how much additional heparin to administer. Acceptable levels during CPB are 2–4 U/mL, in the newborn population up to 6 U/mL. This regimen increased required heparin doses on CPB, but results in lower protamine doses and less blood loss [35].

The optimum method of assessing adequate anticoagulation during CPB in children has thus not yet been defined and much work is still required in this area.

The use of heparin-coated biocompatible perfusion circuits is probably useful in reducing the degree of activation of the coagulation system in children [36,37], but rather expensive and has not gained wide acceptance.

The optimal ACT for CPB is controversial. Although the minimum recommended ACT is 400 seconds, others recommend 480 seconds [33], since heparin only partially inhibits thrombin formation. This is done to minimize the consumptive coagulopathy that may result from barely

adequate anticoagulation. Failure to achieve a satisfactory ACT may be due to inadequate heparin or to low concentrations of antithrombin III, or "heparin resistance." Increases in acute phase reactant proteins such as factor VIII and fibrinogen commonly shorten the APTT and may appear as heparin resistance.

If 500 IU/kg of heparin fail to achieve an adequate ACT, ATIII deficiency becomes more likely and fresh frozen plasma or recombinant ATIII [32] (30 IU/kg) is necessary to increase antithrombin concentration.

Initiation of cardiopulmonary bypass and flow requirements

After heparinization and cannulation, CPB is started by opening the venous outflow cannula to the reservoir. Slow decompression of the heart and maintaining a minimal output of the beating heart reduces the drop in blood pressure due to the hemodilution. Based on weight or body surface area, a flow requirement is calculated. The cardiac index is approximately 25–50% greater than that of an adult. For newborns, a flow of 2.6–3.2 L/ min/m^2 is recommended and for infants 2.4–2.6 L/min/m^2 is sufficient. If normothermic CPB is chosen, flow rates in the range of 3.0–3.5 L/min/m^2 are required [38]. This can be reduced during hypothermia (Figure 7.3). Infants have a much more compliant vasculature, which results in lower perfusion pressures on CPB. Causes for severe hypotension after initiation of bypass can be the presence of hemodynamically relevant shunts, e.g., major aortopulmonary collateral arteries (MAPCAs) or an open ductus that both lead to a circulatory steal in the systemic circulation, requiring higher flows and possibly early control by the surgeon. Increased bronchial and noncoronary collateral flow draining into the left atrium can be a particular problem,

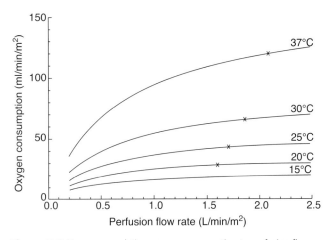

Figure 7.3 Nomogram relating oxygen consumption to perfusion flow rate and temperature. Crosses indicate the clinical flow rates used by Kirklin and Barrett-Boyes (Reproduced with permission from Reference [39])

especially in cyanotic children, with a resultant significant negative impact on myocardial protection during periods of aortic cross-clamping.

The adequacy of perfusion is monitored by the usual parameters. These are mean arterial pressure, the online measurement of mixed venous saturation, pH, base excess, and the regular testing of blood for heparin levels and lactate and other indices of end organ perfusion (e.g., urine output, somatic and cerebral oxygenation values [NIRS, for example]).

Cooling and temperature management

Systemic cooling is utilized for nearly every case. Hypothermia is classified as mild (30–36°C), moderate (22–30°C), or deep (17–22°C). In general, lower temperatures are used for more complex operations that carry a greater potential for requiring periods of low-flow bypass or circulatory arrest. Cooling is primarily achieved through the heat exchanger in the bypass circuit.

Infants have a high ratio of surface area to body weight. Infants also have an immature thermal autoregulatory center. Because of these factors, wide fluctuations in body temperature easily occur. Warming and cooling on bypass occur much more readily. If the clinician is not careful, cooling can occur too rapidly, and deep brain structures may become dangerously cold. There is some evidence to suggest that cooling too rapidly is deleterious to neurological function. Thus, it is important to cool slowly, evenly, and completely, and most investigators recommend at least 20 minutes of cooling if circulatory arrest is used [40]. The opposite is also true. It is very easy to warm too rapidly and for hyperthermic overshoot to occur. Recent data suggest that hyperthermia can be very damaging, and temperature differences of even 1 or 2°C are highly significant [41]. Special bypass techniques (see below) have been developed to avoid the necessity of using DHCA, and may also be performed during this time.

Aortic cross-clamping, myocardial ischemia, and protection

Repair of most congenital heart lesions is becoming more feasible. Perioperative myocardial damage remains the most common cause of morbidity and mortality after successful surgical repair. Thus, effective myocardial protection assumes an even greater role than in the adult since perioperative insults are less well tolerated and more difficult to treat. Neonatal hearts may be difficult to protect because of immaturity, cyanosis, hypertrophy of the right ventricle, complex coronary artery pattern, and duration of ischemia to achieve a good repair.

The neonatal heart is ultrastructurally immature. Myofibrils are arranged in a disorderly fashion and have a smaller percentage of contractile proteins than do those in the adult (30% vs 60%) [42]. The immature heart shows fewer mature mitochondria and a lower oxidative capacity [43]. Control of myocardial contractility in infants depends more on adrenal function and circulating catecholamines than on direct autonomic influences. There are also differences in myocardial calcium metabolism. In the mature myocardium, the sarcoplasmic reticulum is the predominant source of calcium ion for excitation–contraction coupling, but the sarcoplasmic reticulum is poorly developed in the immature heart. Because the neonatal myocardial cell is deficient in T-tubules, it is incapable of internal release and reuptake of calcium for contraction and instead depends heavily on transmembrane calcium transport for myocardial contraction. These differences in calcium handling by the cell provide some explanation for the clinical observation that newborns require greater serum ionized calcium levels for optimal myocardial contractility. Experimental evidence suggests that the newborn myocardium tolerates ischemia and reperfusion better than the adult heart. However, in practice, pediatric patients undergoing cardiac surgery have a greater incidence of low cardiac output postoperatively than do adults. The discrepancy between the experimental evidence and the clinical experience may relate to the cardiac anomalies involved. Ventricular hypertrophy and cyanosis are common, and the hypertrophied heart have been found to have decreased subendocardial blood flow [44] and lower concentrations of high-energy phosphates before arrest. Chronic cyanosis has been associated with a decreased threshold for anaerobic metabolism during stress [45], diminished myocardial reserve [46], asynchronous left ventricular wall motion [47], and downregulation of beta-adrenergic receptors [48]. Reoxygenation injury with release of oxygen radicals upon initiation of CPB can further exacerbate the preexisting injury [49]. The abrupt increase in oxygen levels on bypass in chronically hypoxic infants leads to the loss of antioxidant reserve capacity and subsequent loss of myocardial function. Preventive measures include leukodepletion of blood prime, use of inline arterial filters and normoxic management (PO_2 80–100) initiating bypass. Over the course of 10–20 minutes, FIO_2 can be increased to obtain PO_2 levels in the usual 100–150 mm Hg range. Since blood is fully oxygenated at such levels, further increases in oxygen levels only confer minimal increases in the oxygen content of blood.

Finally, many congenital cardiac procedures require incision of the ventricular muscle, which markedly changes the geometry of the chamber and induces focal edema.

The cornerstone of myocardial protection in pediatric cardiac surgery is hypothermia. Systemic hypothermia to some degree is used in nearly all congenital cardiac repairs. It is particularly important in cyanotic infants with increased noncoronary collateral flow to the heart.

Myocardial protection can be problematic in these cases because of cardioplegia washout and rewarming of the myocardium. Because systemic hypothermia allows reduced flow rates, it decreases myocardial collateral flow. Blood cardioplegia is often used in adults, but its advantages may be lost in infants undergoing deep hypothermia. However, if greater cardioplegic temperatures are used (warm cardioplegia), there is a clear advantage to the use of blood cardioplegia [50]. The optimal electrolyte composition of cardioplegia for pediatric patients is controversial. There is great institutional variation among solutions used. A certain amount of calcium is necessary in the solution to prevent severe injury that may result from calcium paradox [51]. However, excessive amounts are deleterious. The addition of magnesium, a natural calcium antagonist, may solve this dilemma. Increasing magnesium levels has been shown to improve postoperative rhythm stability and reduce calcium-induced mitochondrial dysfunction during reperfusion. Thus, in the absence of magnesium enrichment, hypocalcemic cardioplegia results in adequate myocardial protection in stressed hypoxic hearts. Magnesium was particularly beneficial during normocalcemic cardioplegia solution [52].

Induction and maintenance of cardioplegic cardiac arrest

During induction, some institutions use warm blood cardioplegia with amino acid supplementation in stressed, hypoxic hearts to recover the intracellular energy stores before arrest [53]. This results in complete preservation of myocardial function, particularly in the chronic, hypoxic heart that might become ischemic under situations of stress.

After aortic cross-clamping and sequestration of the coronary circulation, cardioplegia is generally administered in an antegrade fashion into the aortic root. Since the neonatal heart lacks stenotic lesions, adequate distribution is not an issue. Perfusion pressures should be in the normal range of diastolic blood pressures and should not be higher than 30–50 mm Hg. Higher pressures can lead to myocardial edema, particularly in the neonatal hypoxic heart [54]. The need for multidose cardioplegia in infants is controversial [55]. There is some evidence that multidose cardioplegia may actually lead to poorer structural and functional recovery [56]. It was postulated that this worsened injury may be an effect of increased permeability of the immature microvasculature, resulting in myocardial edema.

Myocardial collaterals are more important in neonatal hearts and can quickly lead to rewarming of the myocardium. Profound hypothermia or the reduction of flow can only provide limited additional protection, since other vital organs can be compromised (brain, kidney). Periodic reapplication of cardioplegia at 10–20 minutes intervals counteracts noncoronary collateral washout.

Reperfusion

Reperfusion is considered the phase when the coronaries are reperfused with regular systemic blood flow after cross-clamp removal and the patient is fully warmed. This time is probably an important time in the course of cardioplegic arrest, since many mechanisms of cellular damage are completed during this phase. Optimally normal sinus rhythm and myocardial contractility are restored during this time, while the patient is slowly rewarmed. In adults, reperfusion with warm blood before unclamping the aorta improved metabolic and functional recovery. Substrate enriched reperfusion with the amino acids aspartate and glutamate, however, results in full recovery of function in infants [57]. Depending on the total ischemic time of the heart (equal to the cross-clamp time), the heart requires time to restore the ATP storages in the myocardium. In general, 10–15 minutes are considered the minimum time requirement. For longer cross-clamp times, 25% of the time is considered appropriate as reperfusion time at our institution. The release of the cross-clamp often leads to a drop in blood pressure due to the higher release of metabolic waste from the heart compared to the adult. This should not be adjusted by the application of calcium at this point to reduce the immediate reperfusion injury. Calcium gluconate 10–20 mg/kg can be added immediately before separating from bypass to correct the slight hypocalcemic state of CPB and improve myocardial contractility but should be avoided during the first 15 minutes of reperfusion of the heart. Additional doses of calcium are added to maintain slightly elevated levels of ionized calcium after bypass in neonates and infants, particularly since calcium and other electrolytes are lost quickly through the use of modified ultrafiltration and the infusion of citrate-rich blood products.

Separation from cardiopulmonary bypass and postbypass phase

During rewarming surgery is completed, inotropic and vasoactive agents are started, and ventilation commences after thorough suctioning. Hemofiltration and blood transfusion are used to achieve the desired hematocrit. Transducer are rezeroed and leveled. Left atrial and/or pulmonary artery (PA) monitoring lines, if indicated, are placed at this time, as are temporary atrial and ventricular pacing wires. If the patient is incompletely rewarmed before separation from CPB, a significant afterdrop with precipitous postbypass reduction in core body temperature can occur. This would lead to vasoconstriction, shivering, increased oxygen consumption, and acidosis. However, postischemic hyperthermia can lead to delayed neuronal cell death [58]. Mild degrees of hypothermia and certainly the avoidance of hyperthermia are essential in the perioperative period [59]. In the pediatric patient group, rectal temperature mostly reflects peripheral temperature. Several endpoints have been proposed like nasopharyngeal temperatures greater than 35.0°C, bladder temperature greater than 36.2°C [60], or skin temperatures greater than 30°C [61]. We use an endpoint of 35.5°C rectal temperature, which is supported by the literature [62].

Finally, a blood gas is checked before weaning to optimize electrolytes and hematocrit. Once the patient is ventilated, warm and in a stable rhythm as well as all post-CPB requirements are met, weaning is initiated by slowly decreasing venous return. Arterial perfusion is continued until the appropriate filling is reached. If all parameters are stable, modified ultrafiltration is started. The heart is observed carefully during this process to avoid overfilling or recognize right heart failure early on. Also, radial artery pressures may not be accurate following CPB and tends to underestimate both the systolic and mean central aortic pressure. A questionable pressure should be confirmed with central aortic pressure. A pulse oximeter waveform appearing immediately after termination of CPB is a sign of good peripheral perfusion and adequate rewarming. There might be a larger arterial–alveolar gradient between end-tidal carbon dioxide and arterial carbon dioxide tension at the end of bypass due to ventilation perfusion mismatch. A rapidly increasing height of capnogram is a sure sign of good cardiac output during the termination of CPB.

Conventional ultrafiltration and modified ultrafiltration

The application of the CPB machine in children leads more often to a significant capillary leak than in adults. This is caused by the relative larger foreign surface exposure and the inflammatory response.

Hemofiltration has been defined as ultrafiltration with the return of replacement fluids for the losses. In contrast, ultrafiltration simply removes fluid from the body through a convective process involving filtration across membranes. Conventional ultrafiltration (CUF) on bypass or modified ultrafiltration (MUF) at the end of the bypass run both lead to positive effects on the amount of proinflammatory cytokines and a reduction of total interstitial body water after extracorporeal circulation. CUF or MUF are therefore standard elements of today's pediatric perfusion systems. The most effective and easiest seems to be the MUF, first described by Naik and Elliott [63,64]. In this case, the bypass circuit is modified and the flow reversed at the end of CPB before protamine is given. Blood from the aortic cannula is guided through a hemofilter

Table 7.5 Effects of modified ultrafiltration (MUF)

PVR, PAP	Decreases due to oxygenation and warming
Stroke volume, CO	LV stroke volume increases secondary to improved pulmonary blood flow
SVR, blood pressure	Increases due to the reduction of vasoactive substances (interleukines, bradykinin, etc.)
Hemoglobin, Hematocrit	Increases due to hemoconcentration
Interstitial body and lung water	Decreases secondary to water removal
Improved gas exchange [65]	Improved V/Q mismatch

PVR, pulmonary vascular resistance; PAP, pulmonary artery pressure; CO, cardiac output; SVR, systemic vascular resistance; V/Q, ventilation/perfusion.
Source: Reproduced with permission from Reference [66].

(blood flow rate of 100–300 mL/min) and back to the right atrium after warming and oxygenating the blood. The ultrafilter pump is run at 10–30 mL/kg/min, with a vacuum on the ultrafilter. Replacement volume is taken from the reservoir as necessary. There are different ways of deciding when to stop filtering; some just use a cutoff time of 15–20 minutes and others stop when the circuit volume has become diluted or when the desired hematocrit is reached. Frequently, the surgeon's patience is the limiting factor. Filtering also will be stopped if the patient becomes unstable. Multiple beneficial effects can be observed (see Table 7.5); particularly important are the increase in hematocrit, the reduction of cytokines, improved myocardial perfusion, and a reduction in pulmonary vascular resistance (PVR) with improvement of right heart function. A steal phenomenon has been described by excessive flow rates diverting blood from the aorta to the filter, leading to cerebral and systemic deoxygenation. Disadvantages are a delay in heparin reversal and decannulation of approximately 10–20 minutes as well as the possibility of hemodynamic instability, if preload is not adequately maintained by the perfusionist. However, surgical hemostasis can be carried out during this time period. The combination with zero balance ultrafiltration on bypass can eliminate additional unnecessary volume from cardioplegia or irrigation. The use of filtration during CPB (conventional, dilutional, or zero balance ultrafiltration) also removes inflammatory mediators and vasoactive substances [67]. Studies [66] have shown that compared with control patients, patients who have modified ultrafiltration after bypass have substantially less increase in total body water, have less interleukin-8 and complement in their bloodstream [68,69], require less blood transfusion [70,71], show improved coagulation factors [72,73] and faster recovery of systolic blood pressure [63], pulmonary function [74], and cerebral metabolic activity [75]. Modified ultrafiltration performed after CPB reverses hemodilution and decreases tissue edema and thereby accelerates postoperative recovery [76].

Failure to separate from cardiopulmonary bypass

Occasionally, despite escalating inotropic support, a child is unable to maintain adequate cardiac output and systemic oxygen delivery and therefore a return to CPB must be considered. Immediate TEE evaluation should be investigated for the possibility of residual defects that require surgical attention. If no further surgical intervention is warranted, the source of the difficulty in weaning from CPB should be sought and other therapies must be considered. Is the hematocrit level adequate for this child? Too much hemodilution can lead to decreased systemic vascular resistance. The ideal hematocrit depends on the pathology and probably in the range of 35–45% for complex repairs. Is the vascular resistance too low? In children with low systemic vascular resistance who are either nonresponsive to catecholamine infusions or who are experiencing adverse effects due to catecholamine therapy, arginine vasopressin has been shown to be a potent vasoconstrictor, with infusions resulting in increased mean arterial pressures and decreased catecholamine dependence. Its use in children appears promising when cardiac function is adequate [77,78]. Fixed doses of 0.01-0.04 U/kg/h of vasopressin are used. Exposure to endotoxin and cytokines as on CPB can trigger a de novo synthesis of the inducible, calcium-dependent isoform of nitric oxide synthase. Methylene blue inhibits this process by decreasing intracellular cyclic guanosine monophosphate concentrations through guanylate cyclase inhibition, thus blocking its vasodilator properties. It increases arterial pressure, systemic vascular resistance, and left ventricular stroke work, but does not increase cardiac output, oxygen delivery, or oxygen consumption. Methylene blue in a dose of 2 mg/kg followed by 1 mg/kg/h has been used successfully in the setting of perioperative vasoplegia in adults [79], neonatal sepsis [80], and in a case report of infective endocarditis in a 10-year-old girl [81]. Side effects are rare in doses <2 mg/kg, but pulmonary hypertension and other side effects can occur with repeat doses [82]. Is the right heart failing? Pulmonary hypertension with resultant right heart failure may occur post-CPB, either as a result of long-standing increases in PA pressures or PVR, now exacerbated by the effects of CPB, or as a result of acute increases in PA pressures or PVR secondary to protamine administration. Management has been challenging, as intravenous medications often affect both systemic and pulmonary vascular pressures. Selective pulmonary vasodilatation became possible with the introduction of inhaled nitric oxide (iNO), an endothelium-derived va-

sodilator that is rapidly deactivated by hemoglobin [83]. Several groups of patients have been shown to potentially benefit from iNO administration post-CPB [84,85]. Patients with single ventricle physiology undergoing total cavopulmonary anastomosis (Fontan procedure) with elevated PVR post-CPB, as well as children with elevated pulmonary venous pressures secondary to total anomalous pulmonary venous connection or congenital mitral stenosis, frequently show improvement with administration of iNO. For patients on iNO, caution should be exercised when transporting from the operating room to the intensive care unit in order to avoid interruption of therapy, as rebound pulmonary hypertension and rapid clinical deterioration may occur. Other options to lower PVR include sildenafil 0.5 mg/kg through a nasogastric tube [86] or nebulized prostacyclin [87]. In the event that severe left or right ventricular dysfunction persists in the absence of residual anatomic defects that can be surgically corrected, consideration may be given to continued mechanical support of the circulation. Currently, immediate pediatric options for mechanical circulatory support are extracorporeal membrane oxygenation in neonates, infants, and children. It is most useful when recovery of ventricular function is expected within 24–72 hours, or when cardiopulmonary support is unavoidable.

Heparin reversal and transfusion management

During modified ultrafiltration, cardiac function and the quality of the surgical repair are assessed via TEE, and if found to be satisfactory, protamine is administered to neutralize residual heparin after finishing the filtration process. In small infants and palliated anatomies, the goal hematocrit coming off bypass should be around 40%. This improves hemodynamic stability and allows immediate correction of coagulation disorders by infusion of blood products.

One to 1.5 mg/kg of protamine is given for each 100 units of the initial heparin dose to antagonize its effect. This assumes that any further doses are given to maintain a heparin level and prevents overdosing of protamine with its associated effects on platelet function (reduction of the interaction of GPIb receptor interaction with vWF) [88]. If the ACT is still elevated or prime blood is given back to the patient an additional 25% of the initial dose of protamine is added and the ACT rechecked. However, particularly in infants, the administration of protamine and the persistent treatment of a suspected incomplete heparin reversal should not distract and delay the treatment of other commonly associated postbypass coagulopathies like thrombocytopenia, platelet dysfunction, and other coagulation factor deficiencies [89–92]. A randomized study of 26 infants and children compared heparin reversal using standard 1 mg/1 mg ratio of total administered heparin for patients in one group and of the individualized residual bypass heparin concentration in the other group. They found that individualized management of anticoagulation and its reversal results in less activation of the coagulation cascade, less fibrinolysis, and reduced blood loss and need for transfusions [35]. After $^1/_3$–$^1/_2$ of the planned protamine dose is administered, blood from the surgical field must not be returned to the cardiotomy reservoir to avoid circuit thrombosis in case it is necessary to go back on bypass. An ACT or heparin level confirms adequate heparin neutralization. More protamine (0.5–1 mg/kg) can be given if either test remains prolonged and bleeding is a problem. Hypotensive protamine reactions can occur when protamine complexes with heparin because complement is released. This is much less common in children than adults. Hypotension can be attenuated by adding calcium (2 mg/1 mg protamine). Pediatric protamine reactions are rare occurring in 1.7–2.8% of patients undergoing CPB [93]. Life-threatening reactions to protamine represent true allergic reactions. Protamine reactions are treated with calcium chloride, volume resuscitation, adrenaline, norepinephrine, and other inotropic support as required. For severe reactions, it may be necessary to readminister heparin and resume CPB.

Haemostatic management can be guided by thrombelastography. Newer devices allow a full "point of care" functional assessment of the coagulation within 10–15 minutes [94].

Antifibrinolytic therapy

Bleeding is more common in pediatric cardiac surgery patients than in adults. Both qualitative and quantitative abnormalities in coagulation proteins have significant functional sequelae, which influence the hematologic responses to CPB. CHD itself has long been associated with coagulation abnormalities, including platelet abnormalities and fibrinolysis. There is extensive published research on the use of aprotinin and lysine analog antifibrinolytics to modify the adverse effects of CPB in adults, but for pediatrics, their dose and effects is much less clear.

Two agents are currently available to modify the haemostatic response to CPB: ε-aminocaproic acid (EACA) and tranexamic acid. Aprotinin, an established esterase inhibitor, has been withdrawn from the market due to safety concerns in adult patients and will only be discussed briefly.

ε-Aminocaproic acid and tranexamic acid

Both EACA and TA appear effective in reducing bleeding and transfusion in cyanotic patients, provided an adequate dose is administered. Their efficacy in other high-risk and mixed populations is not as well established. Contrary to aprotinin, they seem to lack significant clinical anti-inflammatory efficiency beyond their effects on coagulation [95,96]. Suppression of excessive plasmin activity may play an important role in the generation of proinflammatory cytokines during and after CPB [97]. For an excellent review in detail please refer to a recent review by Eaton [98].

Aprotinin

Aprotinin is a nonspecific serine protease inhibitor derived from bovine lung. Aprotinin is believed to exert its effects through inhibition of kallikrein and plasmin, with decreased hemostatic activation, inhibition of fibrinolysis, and preservation of platelet function. Kallikrein is part of the contact activation that accelerates the activation of the hemostatic, inflammatory, and fibrinolytic systems during CPB. Aprotinin appears to decrease bleeding and transfusion requirements in specific circumstances. The study by Mossinger et al. [99] illustrates the potential of aprotinin in pediatric heart surgery. Sixty patients weighing <10 kg undergoing primary corrective congenital heart surgery with CPB were enrolled. Aprotinin dosing was based on published pharmacokinetic data [100]. Aprotinin-treated patients had less blood loss and were less likely to be transfused with red blood cells and cryoprecipitate. A more recent meta-analysis of aprotinin in pediatric cardiac surgery found a 33% reduction in the proportion of children receiving blood transfusions [101].

In addition, aprotinin suppressed thrombin activation, inhibited D-dimer production, and improved postoperative PO_2/FIO_2 ratios [99]. Mechanical ventilation time in treated patients was less than half that of controls. Interestingly, the authors failed to show a difference in multiple biochemical measures of the inflammatory response, including interleukin (IL)-6, IL-8, and IL-10. Complement C3 was lower in treated patients only at 4 and 24 hours postoperatively. These findings were not seen in a small trial on neonates where aprotinin had no effect on outcome variables [102]. Concerns about the safety of aprotinin have been raised in the recent past mostly related to one of three areas: thrombosis, renal effects, and anaphylaxis [103–114].

Dosing

Aprotinin
Aprotinin dosing studies suggest that a continuous infusion is necessary to maintain effective plasma levels on CPB; an initial loading dose should be at least 30,000 KIU/kg, and the pump prime dose should be based on

the volume of the pump, rather than the weight of the patient.

Tranexamic acid

Chauhan et al. [115], in a dose-ranging study of TA published in 2004, found the most effective dosing scheme of the four studied to be a 10 mg/kg load, 10 mg/kg in the pump prime, and 10 mg/kg after protamine.

Epsilon aminocaproic acid

Based on a pharmacokinetic study [116], the initial loading dose is 75 mg/kg, a pump priming dose of 75 mg/kg followed by an infusion of 75 mg/kg/h to establish and maintain a therapeutic plasma concentration (130 mcg/mL) in 95% of patients.

Rapid IV injection of TA or EACA may cause hypotension. We infuse loading doses over approximately 20 minutes.

Comparison studies of antifibrinolytics

With the considerable variability among studies of the three drugs under consideration in terms of design, dose, and outcomes, it is difficult to draw any conclusions about relative efficacy from the literature. There are a few published comparison studies. Chauhan et al. [117] compared low-dose aprotinin, EACA, and the combination in 300 cyanotic patients undergoing cardiac surgery. There was no difference between EACA-treated and aprotinin-treated patients in any measured variable. The same group compared TA and EACA in a placebo-controlled study of 150 patients with cyanotic CHD [115]. Both drugs were superior to placebo, but there were no significant differences between the treated groups with respect to 24-hour blood loss, transfusion or reexploration rate. Finally, the effect of aprotinin and TA was compared in 100 children, evenly divided into four groups: placebo, TA, aprotinin, and a combination of the two drugs [118]. Again, all treatment groups faired better than placebo in 24-hour blood loss and transfusion, with no significant differences among the three treated groups. Thus, the limited comparative evidence would suggest that the three drugs are equivalent in efficacy for reduction of bleeding and transfusion, at least with the doses and patients studied, and there is little or no advantage to combination therapy.

In summary, evidence supports the efficacy of the lysine analog antifibrinolytics and aprotinin to decrease bleeding and transfusion in pediatric patients undergoing cardiac surgery involving CPB. This benefit is likely to be more significant in high-risk groups, such as cyanotic patients, newborn, complex surgery, and reoperations. The safety profile of these drugs is not fully understood and requires further research in the future.

Effects of cardiopulmonary bypass on organ systems

CPB -induced systemic inflammatory response syndrome (SIRS) is a host response to the exposure of blood components to the foreign surface of the CPB circuit and initiation of the complement cascade. Although the lungs are often the primary organ targeted, SIRS after CPB may be severe enough to affect all other end-organ functions. Currently, there are a number of strategies being employed targeting prevention of SIRS and multisystem organ failure including the use of corticosteroids, protease inhibitors, thromboxane inhibitors or antagonist, prostacyclins, complement inhibitors, and cytokine inhibitors including monoclonal antibodies and IL-1 receptor antagonist.

A study in children by Bronicki et al. [119] used a single dose of dexamethasone before CPB in 29 patients. They found an eightfold decrease in IL-6 levels and a greater than threefold decrease in tumor necrosis factor-α levels after CPB. They also found that complement component C3a and absolute neutrophil count were not affected by dexamethasone. Limiting to all studies using steroids was the lack of effect on outcome [120]. For further details on mechanism and treatment refer to Chapter 8.

Neurological injury and protection

Brain injury in children with CHD has been documented before and after surgery for CHD. Some complications appear soon after the operation, such as seizures, stroke, and coma, whereas others appear long after the operation, such as cognitive deficits and psychomotor delay. Radiological and pathological studies have described a spectrum of brain lesions after pediatric cardiac surgery, located mainly in the neocortex, periventricular white matter, and basal ganglia, corresponding to the neurological deficits seen clinically [121, 122]. These subtle defects manifest as a developmental signature that includes cognitive and intellectual impairment, attention and executive function deficits, visual–spatial and visual–motor skill deficiencies, speech and language delays, and behavioral difficulties. The spectrum of lesions is consistent with hypoxic–ischemic injury, contrary to mostly embolic events in the adult population. When this injury occurs—before, during, or after the operation—remains uncertain. Adverse neurological outcomes after neonatal cardiac surgery are multifactorial and related to both fixed and modifiable mechanisms. Fixed factors include known genetic syndromes, structural central nervous system malformations (incidence of up to 29% in hypoplastic left heart syndrome [122]), multiple surgeries (leading to multiple insults), blood flow patterns in utero, preoperative cerebral hypoxia, embolic events occurring

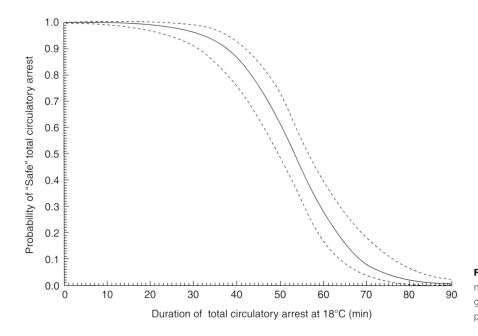

Figure 7.4 At 18°C, the likelihood of neurological injury becomes exponentially greater beyond 45 minutes (Reproduced with permission from Reference [39])

during the balloon atrial septostomy procedure [123], socioeconomic status, and poorly defined genetic predisposition. Potentially modifiable factors include preoperative hypoxia–ischemia, intraoperative use of DHCA, and postoperative cardiopulmonary derangements are clearly valuable toward improving neurological outcomes. Some interventions that may limit brain injury from DHCA include preoperative steroids and aprotinin, hyperoxygenation before DHCA, allowing at least 20 minutes of cooling duration to ensure adequate cerebral protection, packing the head in ice, intermittent cerebral perfusion between 15 and 20-minute periods of DHCA (Figure 7.4), and modified ultrafiltration after CPB. Other modifiable factors of CPB management include optimal flow at all temperatures [124,125], the avoidance of extreme hemodilution [16] and emboli [126], pH-stat management [127], and modulation of the inflammatory response by the use of ultrafiltration and steroids [119]. Whereas myocardial protection and systemic oxygen delivery is continuously monitored during neonatal CPB, adequate cerebral perfusion has traditionally been evaluated by surrogate markers such as perfusion pressure, mixed venous oxygen saturation, or base deficit and lactate levels. However, there are now real-time intraoperative cerebral monitoring devices available for clinical use, the potential benefits of which are becoming recognized (Figure 7.5). The most widely used technologies include near-infrared spectroscopy (NIRS), transcranial Doppler (TCD), raw and processed electroencephalography (EEG), and serum measurement of S100B protein. Online technologies allow immediate interventions upon interruption of optimal cerebral flow and may improve outcome [129]. Improved strategies to prevent injury in these arenas are much needed [130].

Pulmonary effects

Postbypass lung injury may be a result of ischemic reperfusion injury or may be associated with the systemic inflammatory response caused by extracorporeal circulation [131]. Alveolar injury is also associated with cyclic closing and opening of alveoli with shear injury to the alveolar–capillary interface causing increased permeability and pulmonary edema with a significant pulmonary inflammatory reaction [132]. Postoperative pulmonary dysfunction after CPB is possibly caused by a decrease in total lung capacity, functional residual capacity, atelectasis, pulmonary edema, increased inspiratory oxygen, and ventilation–perfusion mismatch [133]. Administration of 100% oxygen during CPB may lead to absorption atelectasis and oxygen toxicity. Lung injury could be prevented in a piglet model using continuous pulmonary perfusion on CPB [134]. In a study by Pizov et al. [135],

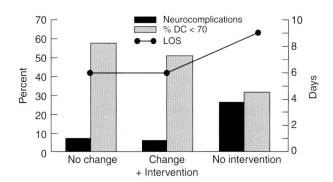

Figure 7.5 Effect of Neuromonitoring on outcome. %DC < 7d, percentage discharged from the hospital in <7 days; LOS, length of stay (Reproduced and adapted with permission from Reference [128])

lung function improved later postoperatively in patients ventilated with 100% oxygen during CPB. Several studies have looked at modes of ventilation on bypass and their effects. Continued ventilation throughout CPB has been linked to superior postoperative respiratory function in certain clinical scenarios, possibly due to attenuation of the ischemia–reperfusion injury, but has yet to gain wider acceptance. Maintaining ventilation and PA perfusion during CPB have shown some benefits in limiting pulmonary platelet and neutrophil sequestration, and attenuating thromboxane B_2 response after CPB [136, 137]. To date, the evidence favoring continuous ventilation alone during CPB on cardiopulmonary function is inconsistent, with most studies showing no benefit [138]. At our institution, we prefer continued ventilation at low tidal volumes, room air, and low PEEP settings in patients undergoing simple procedures without cross-clamping like a RV–conduit exchange, etc. (if tolerated by the surgeon). In more complex cases, we start ventilation after thorough pulmonary toilet and suctioning with a recruitment maneuver. This is usually done in the context of de-airing and aortic clamp removal. Afterward, we continue ventilation at low settings with approximately 2 cc/kg and a PEEP setting of 5–8 cm H_2O with an FIO_2 of 0.21. Full ventilation is resumed right before weaning from bypass, usually in a pressure-regulated, volume-controlled mode to maintain minute ventilation with stable tidal volumes. The pressure limit is carefully watched and set 5 cm H_2O above the upper inspiratory pressure.

Renal, hepatic, and gastrointestinal effects

Little is known about the epidemiology and risk factors for the development of acute renal failure (ARF) in children post-CPB for cardiac surgery. The incidence of acute renal insufficiency complicating open-heart surgery in children is high, approximating 11–17% [139, 140]. Low cardiac output was a significant predictor of developing a renal injury. This is often related to the complexity of the operation. On one hand, better and more sophisticated surgical and CPB techniques are available. On the other hand, children with more complicated cardiac lesions requiring longer CPB time are operated on today. There is also evidence that the neonatal kidney is more vulnerable to conditions of hemodynamic stress, with loss of autoregulation leading to blood pressure-dependent renal blood flow and ischemia-induced renal injury. All of these conditions render the neonate more prone to complications of ischemia than the older infant or child. Renal replacement therapy is required in 1.6–7.7% of patients. In children, the mortality rate in those requiring dialysis following CPB is reported to range from 46 to 67%. However, renal failure is often temporary. Among those who recover, 93–100% of survivors of renal replacement

therapy after CPB surgery have normal renal function at discharge from hospital [141, 142]. Peritoneal dialysis is a safe and effective treatment for children after CPB surgery and should be initiated early in the course of acute renal injury [143–146].

Several investigations provide evidence that intestinal organ function is altered during CPB. Splanchnic, but not systemic, oxygen extraction increases during normothermic, nonpulsatile CPB. Splanchnic blood flow is not significantly affected by normothermic or hypothermic CPB at normal pump flows compared with the prebypass condition [147, 148]. The increase in splanchnic oxygen extraction during hypothermia indicating a splanchnic oxygen supply/demand mismatch, was therefore most likely caused by a decrease in splanchnic oxygen delivery, in turn caused by a decrease in hemoglobin concentration secondary to hemodilution. The splanchnic region might be more susceptible to a decrease in oxygen delivery by hemodilution, compared to other organs. Normothermic CPB leads to a loss of GI barrier function independent of the duration of CPB. Current data indicate that intestinal mucosal autoregulation is maintained during CPB within the pressure range of 50–75 mm Hg [149]. Improving pump flow rather than infusing vasoconstrictive drugs to increase aortic pressure can improve both splanchnic and renal perfusion [150] and improve the postoperative course in children [151]. Although GI complications may have a low incidence (0.3–3%), they are associated with a high mortality (13–63%) [152, 153]. Several risk factors (e.g., use of vasopressors, preexisting comorbidities, perioperative hypotensive episodes, and valve surgery) have been evaluated for the development of alterations in GI organ function. Liver dysfunction rarely occurs after CPB.

Endocrine and metabolic response to cardiopulmonary bypass

In children, hypoalbuminaemia and hyperchloraemia are the predominant acid–base abnormalities after CPB, whereas lactic acidosis and wide ion gap acidosis are rare [154]. Hyperchloraemia following CPB appears to be a benign phenomenon. By contrast, hypoalbuminaemia, an alkalinizing force, was associated with a prolonged requirement for intensive care.

Special cardiopulmonary bypass management issues

Warm cardiopulmonary bypass

Hypothermic CPB associated with cold myocardial protection is commonly used for neonatal cardiac surgery. The rationale is to protect the brain in case of failure

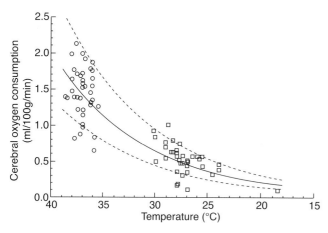

Figure 7.6 Relation between cerebral oxygen consumption and nasopharyngeal temperature during CPB at 2 L/min/m² (Reproduced with permission from Reference [39])

of oxygen delivery (Figure 7.6). In addition, hypothermic bypass helps complete cold myocardial protection by delaying myocardial rewarming and maintaining a low metabolic state. There is a growing body of evidence demonstrating that hypothermia also induces deleterious effects, which may culminate in organ dysfunctions. The price to pay for the benefits of hypothermia are impaired haemostasis [155], microcirculatory dysfunction, capillary leakage, parenchymal oxygen delivery, endotoxin release, disturbed glucose metabolism [156], or myocardial contractility [157]. Hypothermia delays recovery of mechanical function of the myocardium and reduces basal metabolism. This reduction has only a minimal impact on oxygen need. Less known is the deleterious effect of hypothermia on the myocardium. Reactivity of the microcirculation seems to be impaired after deep hypothermia and possibly also many cellular functions. Lungs are very sensitive to CPB, and hypothermia could increase the capillary leakage more than normothermia by inducing microcirculatory dysfunction and impairing endothelial responses [158]. By reducing oxygen demand, hypothermia is effective in protecting the brain, but it impairs vasomotor and cerebral oxygen regulation [159], alters energetic metabolism [160], and increases intracranial pressure and rewarming may induce neurological injury [161]. Furthermore, the protective effect of hypothermia on the inflammatory reaction and neurological recovery may have been previously exaggerated [162]. The inflammatory reaction induced by CPB seems to be delayed rather than diminished by hypothermia [163]. Finally, in DHCA, long-term follow-up has shown impaired neurodevelopmental outcome [164]. Therefore, normothermic CPB, already commonly used in adult cardiac surgery, has been promoted and progressively extended into pediatric practice [165]. Good results have been achieved with normothermic by-

pass for even complex operations like the arterial switch operation [166, 167].

Normothermia in pediatric cardiac surgery is not the only characteristic of normothermic CPB. Other factors to be considered are flow and hematocrit. The flow generally used for mild hypothermic CPB is 2.0–2.4 L/min/m² (Figure 7.3). In normothermic CPB, pump flow is maintained throughout the procedure at 3.0–3.5 L/min/m². In terms of hemodilution on CPB, hematocrit is maintained above 30% during the procedure, with 40% by the end of CPB for normothermic CPB. Thus, normothermic CPB is better characterized by "normothermic, high-flow, high-hematocrit CPB" [38].

Deep hypothermic circulatory arrest

Hypothermia was used early on to improve intracardiac surgical exposure. Bigelow was the first to show in 1950 that hypothermia decreases the metabolic rate (Figure 7.6) [168]. It decreases blood loss [165], provides myocardial protection [169], and, most of all, is neuroprotective [170]. This mostly relates to the decrease in the metabolic rate by 64% by cooling from 37 to 27°C. Also, at a given temperature the amount of gas in solution increases proportional to the decrease in temperature (ideal gas law). In CPB, this translates to cooling the patient not only to lower metabolic rate but also to obtain a higher solubility of oxygen in blood and tissues. Pearl et al. [171] were able to show that the use of hyperoxia with a pH-strategy led to the least production of acids during 60 minutes of deep hypothermic cardiocirculatory arrest. This is probably related to increased tissue oxygen loading prearrest.

Disadvantages of hypothermia include disruption of cerebral autoregulation (Figure 7.7), prolongation of CPB, and a greater tendency toward postoperative bleeding

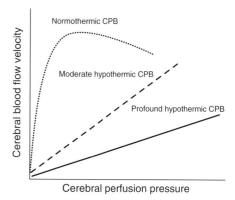

Figure 7.7 Representation of the relationship of cerebral blood flow velocity (CBFV) and cerebral perfusion pressure (CPP) during different temperatures of cardiopulmonary bypass conduct (Reproduced and adapted from Reference [159])

[172]. Postoperative recovery, however, is not prolonged by hypothermia [173]. Also, the wound infection rate does not seem to be influenced by hypothermic bypass [174]. Hypothermia during cardiac surgery only gained widespread use after the development of a heat exchanger that could be integrated into the CPB machine [175].

DHCA involves cooling the patient's body temperature to 17–18°C, stopping the bypass machine, draining the blood from the patient into the venous reservoir, and removing the cannulas from the heart. After the first reports of DHCA in the 1960s, this technique gained popularity in the 1970s and 1980s, because of the perfectly bloodless field it provided. This facilitated complex intracardiac and aortic repairs in newborns and small infants [176] as well as reduced edema. However, it soon became evident that DHCA was associated with neurological morbidity. Choreoathetosis, seizures, coma, and hemiparesis were all noted, especially with prolonged (>60 minutes) DHCA [177]. Clinical and experimental evidence suggest that deep hypothermic cardiocirculatory arrest preferentially damages the basal ganglia, which control tone and movement. The main input of the basal ganglia is the striatum, a highly dopaminergic region of the brain. Increases in free dopamine levels as an indicator of brain damage and cell disruption occur earlier in prolonged deep hypothermic cardiocirculatory arrest versus low-flow bypass strategies [178] and about 15 minutes earlier using alpha-stat versus pH-stat management [179]. It is interesting to note that the incidence of these acute morbidities seemed to increase when alpha-stat management became the accepted standard in many centers. Long-term adverse neurodevelopmental outcomes have also been associated with long periods of DHCA, including abnormalities in mental development, and in fine and gross motor skills. The Boston Circulatory Arrest Study is a remarkable achievement in which 180 newborns undergoing the arterial switch operation from 1988–1992 were studied, with follow-up now complete to age 8 years [180]. The CPB protocol in those years included alpha-stat management, routine hemodilution to a hematocrit of 20%, and the absence of an arterial filter on the CPB circuit. A DHCA time of greater than 41 minutes was associated with a significant increase in long-term neurological problems (Figure 7.4). Although the 41-minute cutoff is now a well-accepted number in congenital heart surgery, multiple changes have subsequently been made to bypass protocols. Results from animal experiments utilizing a neonatal piglet model of DHCA, as well as data from the Boston Circulatory Arrest Study, lead to the following recommendations for increasing the patient's safety margin when utilizing DHCA:

- Hematocrit of 25–30% should be the target [181].
- Systemic hypothermia should be achieved slowly, over no less than 20 minutes (Figure 7.8) [182].

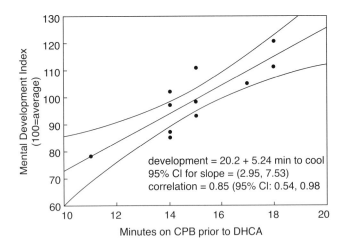

Figure 7.8 Cognitive development of children following early repair of transposition of the great arteries using deep hypothermic circulatory arrest (Reproduced with permission from Reference [40])

- pH-stat blood gas management should be used, at least for cooling, to improve tissue oxygen loading and more even cerebral cooling (Figure 7.9) [183,184].
- Core body temperatures of 17–18°C should be utilized, and ice bags should be applied to the head [185].
- Hyperoxia right before arrest improves tissue oxygen loading [171].
- DHCA should be divided into periods of no longer than 20 minutes, allowing a reperfusion period of at least 2 minutes between each segment of DHCA, to improve neurological outcome [186].
- Low-flow CPB (at greater than 40–50 mL/kg/min) offers greater cerebral protection than DHCA [187]; selective cerebral perfusion may be better than low flow CPB (see below).

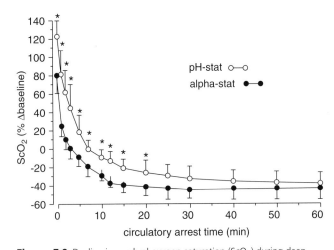

Figure 7.9 Decline in cerebral oxygen saturation (ScO₂) during deep hypothermic circulatory arrest in piglets (Reproduced with permission from Reference [183])

- Cold reperfusion of the brain after deep hypothermic cardiocirculatory arrest for 5–10 minutes may be beneficial to restore cerebral autoregulation and washout accumulated metabolites before adding the metabolic burden of rewarming to the brain [188].
- Normoxemia should be maintained to decrease exacerbation of brain injury after DHCA [189].

Neurological monitoring is useful in the individual patient to aid in determining the safe duration of deep hypothermic cardiocirculatory arrest (Figure 7.5) [183,190].

Although there are situations where DHCA must be utilized, many surgeons are avoiding it whenever possible, minimizing its duration and dividing the periods of its use, or using alternate methods, such as selective cerebral perfusion.

Selective antegrade cerebral perfusion

In order to avoid the use of DHCA, several novel CPB techniques have been developed over the past 5 years to allow perfusion of only the brain during critical periods of surgery, such as aortic reconstruction during the Norwood operation, interrupted aortic arch (IAA) repair with VSD, coarctation with VSD, or cases requiring the Damus–Kaye–Stansel procedure [191,192]. These techniques are collectively referred to as selective cerebral perfusion. Many different techniques have been described on the basis of the primary description by Pigula [191]. Regional low-flow cerebral perfusion (RLFP) is one variation in which a small Goretex® graft of 3–4 mm is sewn onto the innominate artery prior to initiation of CPB, and is then used as the aortic cannula during CPB. Other options include a high cannulation technique of the innominate artery [193]. During aortic reconstruction snares are placed around the brachiocephalic vessels and CPB flow is decreased, with only the brain receiving perfusion via the right carotid artery during this period. In this way, a bloodless operative field can be achieved, just as if DHCA was being performed, yet the brain is still receiving blood flow and oxygen, increasing protection from hypoxic ischemic brain injury. Another potential advantage of this technique is seen in newborns who frequently have extensive arterial collaterals between the proximal branches of the aorta and the lower body via the internal mammary and long thoracic arteries. In this instance, the use of selective cerebral perfusion also provides minimal blood flow to the lower body, protecting renal, hepatic, and GI systems from hypoxic damage as well [194]. Despite these theoretical advantages, and a study demonstrating that selective cerebral perfusion does provide oxygenated blood flow to both cerebral hemispheres [195], long-term outcome studies are still missing to proof that it is superior to standard techniques of deep hypothermic cardiocircula-

tory arrest. Preliminary results are promising and support the notion of improved cerebral protection [193,196].

Neurological monitoring has been used to aid in determining how much flow is necessary during RLFP [195]. Approximately 40–50% of full flow is used (starting at 40 mL/kg/min) and adjusted according to brain saturation and/or transcranial Doppler measurements, maintaining baseline saturation in the range before the onset of RLFP (90–95% range). Average flows during RLPF reach around 64 mL/kg/min to maintain baseline flow and pressure to overcome vessel resistances and capillary opening pressures [196,197]. Flows <40 mL/kg/min over time are unable to maintain oxygen saturation greater than 40% after deep hypothermic cardiocirculatory arrest [198]. If the left regional saturation rSo_2 falls to more than 10% below the right, flow is increased further assuming that the circle of Willis could be variant or incomplete since all flow to the left has to cross the circle. If a left radial arterial line or a femoral arterial line/umbilical artery catheter is in place, abdominal perfusion pressures of ~12 mm Hg correlating to radial artery pressures of 25–30 mm Hg are maintained [194].

Blood gas management: pH-stat versus alpha-stat

Some degree of hypothermia is utilized for nearly every cardiac operation in order to slow the metabolism and oxygen consumption of all organs, particularly the brain and heart [199]. During cooling, the carbon dioxide contained in blood becomes more soluble and its partial pressure decreases. The $PaCO_2$ sensed by the body therefore decreases as body temperature decreases, with the result that at a core temperature of 17–18°C, if pH and $PaCO_2$ have not been corrected for temperature, the body is experiencing a pH of about 7.6 and $PaCO_2$ of 15–18 mm Hg [200]. This very low $PaCO_2$ causes cerebral vasoconstriction, particularly during the cooling phase of bypass, which in turn leads to lower cerebral blood flow, less efficient brain cooling, and consequently less cerebral protection at a given temperature [183]. Since blood samples are heated to 37°C prior to measurement of pH, $PaCO_2$, and PaO_2, the use of pH-stat management indicates that blood gases are being corrected for the patient's actual body temperature by increasing the $PaCO_2$ on bypass as it is measured at 37°C, so that the body experiences a $PaCO_2$ of approximately 40 and a pH of 7.4 at all temperatures. Conversely, alpha-stat management means not correcting the blood gases for temperature, as if the patient's blood was always at 37°C, with the goal of pH 7.4 and $PaCO_2$ 40. In the early days of CPB, pH-stat was utilized to preserve cerebral blood flow [200]. Randomized controlled studies in the 1970s and 1980s on adults undergoing CPB confirmed that acute, post-CPB neurological problems were worsened with the use of pH-stat management [201]. Alpha-stat management was therefore adopted for both adult and pediatric CPB. However, recent animal studies in a neonatal piglet model have challenged this conclusion, proving that neurological outcome, both behavioral and neuropathological, is significantly worse when alpha-stat management is used [183, 184].

Advantages of pH-stat CPB have been shown to include:
- A decreased brain metabolic rate [202]
- An increased rate of brain cooling and reperfusion [203], thereby providing better protection through more even and faster cooling and rewarming secondary to increased CBF [203, 204].
- Molecular effects of altered arterial PO_2 and pH including changes in cerebral oxygenation and brain enzyme activity as well as decreased brain electrical activity [204–206].
- pH-Stat also improves oxygen delivery through decreased oxyhemoglobin affinity [207] by counteracting the pH and hypothermia associated leftward shift in the oxyhemoglobin dissociation curve.
- Increased cortical oxygenation before arrest (through hypercapnic capillary vasodilation [208]) and decreased oxygen metabolic rate providing slower deoxygenation compared to alpha-stat management (10 vs 7 minutes) (Figure 7.9) [183]. Cortical anoxia occurs at 36 minutes versus 24 minutes for alpha-stat management, a margin of safety of 50%.

In cyanotic infants with aortopulmonary collaterals, pH-stat management results in significantly improved brain oxygenation as measured by near-infrared cerebral oximetry [209]. A retrospective study of 16 patients revealed worse neurodevelopmental outcomes with alpha-stat management [181]. In a randomized prospective trial of pH versus alpha-stat management in 182 infants <9 months of age, there was a strong trend toward improved outcomes with pH-stat management, including earlier return of EEG activity, fewer seizures, and improved psychomotor development index were observed [128]. Bellinger et al. [210] in their landmark study examined the effects of alpha-stat and pH-stat on developmental and neurological outcomes after deep hypothermic CPB in infants. Psychomotor Development Index scores of 110 patients did not differ significantly between the groups ($p = 0.97$). Bellinger concluded that the use of alpha-stat or pH-stat strategy is not consistently associated with improved or impaired early neurodevelopmental outcomes in infants undergoing deep hypothermic CPB [210].

One reason for the differing results between pediatric and adult studies is that the increased cerebral blood flow produced by pH-stat management leads to a greater number of cerebral emboli in adults. Emboli occur much less frequently in children, and the primary etiology of neurological injury from CPB in pediatric patients is hypoxic–ischemic [211]. Thus, the increased cerebral blood flow observed on CPB with pH-stat management lessens this risk in children. Interestingly, this putative mechanism has been recently challenged by a study involving a controlled microembolic load and DHCA in pigs that revealed that pH-stat was still associated with improved outcomes when compared with alpha-stat [212]. Recent studies have also revealed a decrease in peak postoperative troponin levels, reduced ventilator dependence, and reduced ICU stays with pH-stat versus alpha-stat [213].

Currently, the preferred technique in adults is the alpha-stat method because it is believed that cell function and autoregulation is better preserved by maintaining neutral pH according to the temperature of the cell. In pediatric cardiac surgery, however, unlike the adults, pH-stat enhances cerebral and systemic protection during deep hypothermic cardiocirculatory arrest. Most congenital heart surgery programs have reverted to pH-stat management. This necessitates careful attention to $PaCO_2$ during all phases of bypass, potentially reducing the sweep gas flow to decrease the efficiency of CO_2 removal, and often adding inspired CO_2 to the sweep gas of the bypass circuit, particularly in small infants.

Complications and safety

The most frequent causes of death or injury related to CPB mishaps have been arterial embolism and consumptive coagulopathies. Other life-threatening events include clots in the extracorporeal circuit, inadequate pressures and flows, aortic dissections, separation of extracorporeal lines, drug administration errors, protamine administration during CPB, heparin overdose, transfusion reactions, negative pressure complications (principally air entrainment), electrical failure, and failure to provide gas exchange. The incidence of fatal accidents is in the range of 1 in 1000 to 1 in 1800 procedures. Near misses or incidents occur in approximately 1 in 300 cases.

Prebypass checklists, vigilance on the part of all members of the team, and the use of standard perfusion monitors and devices will minimize catastrophes.

The most common problems in pediatric practice are inadequate pressures or flow from either poor venous return (most often due to placement) or problems at the arterial site (malposition of the aortic cannula, e.g., in the innominate artery with preferential perfusion of the right carotid; dissection or hematoma).

Most situations can be controlled by rapid recognition, correction or–in rare cases–separation from bypass and restoration of normal circulation, unless the aorta has been ruptured. A great deal of suspicion and good communication amongst the team is vital in that aspect.

Table 7.6 Checklist for cardiopulmonary bypass management

Before CPB

1. Check temperature, maintain normothermia during induction and preparation
2. Assure adequate noninvasive and invasive monitoring: blood pressure, EKG, pulse-oximetry, stethoscope, central venous line, arterial line
3. Positioning
4. Deepening of anesthetic level
5. Discuss management on bypass with perfusionist including prime composition
6. Antifibrinolytics and steroids, as indicated
7. Heparin 300–400 U/kg before arterial cannulation
8. Check ACT > 400 s; if insufficient, give 100 U/kg extra heparin
9. Supplement anesthetics on initiation of bypass

During CPB

1. Stop ventilation and drips when full flow is reached
2. Inspect head perfusion and venous backflow
3. Evaluate quality of perfusion (perfusion pressure, CVP, diuresis, ABG, temperature gradient, neuro-monitoring, upper body congestion)
4. "2-minute rule of perfusion": full flow cardiopulmonary bypass for 2 min and then ABG before cooling or cross-clamping

During repair

1. Prepare for separation:
   a. Drips (inotropic drugs, calcium)
   b. Pacemaker
   c. Preorder blood products (fibrinogen or cryoprecipitate, platelets, FFP, PRBC)
   d. Prepare protamine (precautions to prevent inadvertent administration)
2. Set and control temperature and rewarming (heating blanket, room temperature)
3. Zero and level transducers
4. Redose anesthetics, if noncontinuous
5. Check ABG in preparation for discontinuation of CPB, correct abnormalities
6. Suction and ventilate

After CPB

1. Separate when
   a. Rectal temperature > 35.5°C
   b. Stable rhythm or pace maker stimulation
   c. Heart well contracting
   d. Fully ventilated
   e. Enough reperfusion time passed
2. Fine tune blood pressure, consider direct BP measurement at the aortic cannula for hypotension. Volume ± drips
3. Strongly consider MUF for 10–15 min
4. Check ABG
5. Evaluate TEE for residual defects during modified ultrafiltration
6. Protamine 1–1.5 mg/100 IU heparin
7. Check ACT, ABG
8. Consider coagulation monitoring in high risk patients and redo operations
9. Chest closure, recheck ABG.
10. Transport to the ICU, report to the receiving team

FFP, fresh frozen plasma; CVP, central venous pressure; PRBC, packed red blood cells; ABG, arterial blood gas; MUF, modified ultrafiltration; TEE, transesophageal echocardiography; ACT, activated clotting time.

Conclusions

In summary, pediatric CPB is challenging as it extends the spectrum of extracorporeal circulation in many aspects. Familiarity with differences to adult bypass circuits and management is of utmost importance and the team consisting of cardiac surgeon, perfusionist, and anesthesiologist have to work very close to reach the goal of good perfusion practice. The results, however, of this hard work are rewarding and enable many children a better perspective and life expectancy. A checklist approach allows the novice to improve quickly (see Table 7.6).

References

1. Gibbon JH (1954) Application of a mechanical heart and lung apparatus to cardiac surgery. Minn Med 37:171–185.
2. Shumacker HJ (1982) John Heysham Gibbon Jr. September 29, 1903—February 5, 1973. Biographical Memoirs 53:213–247.
3. Dogliotti AM Costantini A (1951) First case of the human use of an apparatus for extracorporeal blood circulation. Minerva Chir 6:657–659.
4. Kolff WJ (1955) The artificial coil lung. ASAIO J 1:39–42.
5. Hessel EA, Hill AG (2000) Circuitry and cannulation techniques. In: Gravlee GP, Davis RF, Kursz M, Utley JR (eds) Cardiopulmonary Bypass: Principles and Practice. Lippincott, Williams & Wilkins, Philadelphia, pp. 69–97.
6. Charette K, Hirata Y, Bograd A, et al. (2007) 180 ml and less: cardiopulmonary bypass techniques to minimize hemodilution for neonates and small infants. Perfusion 22:327–331.
7. Darling E, Kaemmer D, Lawson S, et al. (1998) Experimental use of an ultra-low prime neonatal cardiopulmonary bypass circuit utilizing vacuum-assisted venous drainage. ASAIO J 30:184–189.
8. Davila RM, Rawles T, Mack MJ (2001) Venoarterial air embolus: a complication of vacuum-assisted venous drainage. Ann Thorac Surg 71:1369–1371.
9. Gottlieb EA, Fraser CD, Jr., Andropoulos DB, Diaz LK (2006) Bilateral monitoring of cerebral oxygen saturation results in recognition of aortic cannula malposition during pediatric congenital heart surgery. Paediatr Anaesth 16:787–789.
10. Kern FH, Jonas RA, Mayer JE, Jr., et al. (1992) Temperature monitoring during CPB in infants: does it predict efficient brain cooling? Ann Thorac Surg 54:749–754.
11. Smith HM, Farrow SJ, Ackerman JD, et al. (2008) Cardiac arrests associated with hyperkalemia during red blood cell transfusion: a case series. Anesth Analg 106:1062–1069.
12. Vohra HA, Adluri K, Willets R, et al. (2007) Changes in potassium concentration and haematocrit associated with cardiopulmonary bypass in paediatric cardiac surgery. Perfusion 22:87–92.
13. Swindell CG, Barker TA, McGuirk SP, et al. (2007) Washing of irradiated red blood cells prevents hyperkalaemia during cardiopulmonary bypass in neonates and infants undergoing surgery for complex congenital heart disease. Eur J Cardiothorac Surg 31:659–664.
14. Golab HD, Takkenberg JJ, van Gerner-Weelink GL, et al. (2007) Effects of cardiopulmonary bypass circuit reduction and residual volume salvage on allogeneic transfusion requirements in infants undergoing cardiac surgery. Interact Cardiovasc Thorac Surg 6:335–339.
15. Newburger JW, Jonas RA, Wernovsky G, et al. (1993) A comparison of the perioperative neurologic effects of hypothermic circulatory arrest versus low-flow cardiopulmonary bypass in infant heart surgery. N Engl J Med 329:1057–1064.
16. Newburger JW, Jonas RA, Soul J, et al. (2008) Randomized trial of hematocrit 25% versus 35% during hypothermic cardiopulmonary bypass in infant heart surgery. J Thorac Cardiovasc Surg 135:347–354.
17. Wypij D, Jonas RA, Bellinger DC, et al. (2008) The effect of hematocrit during hypothermic cardiopulmonary bypass in infant heart surgery: results from the combined Boston hematocrit trials. J Thorac Cardiovasc Surg 135:355–360.
18. Williams GD, Bratton SL, Ramamoorthy C (1999) Factors associated with blood loss and blood product transfusions: a multivariate analysis in children after open-heart surgery. Anesth Analg 89:57–64.
19. Williams GD, Bratton SL, Riley EC, Ramamoorthy C (1998) Association between age and blood loss in children undergoing open heart operations. Ann Thorac Surg 66:870–875.
20. Andrew M, Paes B, Johnston M (1990) Development of the hemostatic system in the neonate and young infant. Am J Pediatr Hematol Oncol 12:95–104.
21. Mauer HM, McCue CM, Caul J, Still WJ (1972) Impairment in platelet aggregation in congenital heart disease. Blood 40:207–216.
22. Williams GD, Bratton SL, Nielsen NJ, Ramamoorthy C (1998) Fibrinolysis in pediatric patients undergoing cardiopulmonary bypass. J Cardiothorac Vasc Anesth 12:633–638.
23. Kern FH, Morana NJ, Sears JJ, Hickey PR (1992) Coagulation defects in neonates during cardiopulmonary bypass. Ann Thorac Surg 54:541–546.
24. Chan AK, Leaker M, Burrows FA, et al. (1997) Coagulation and fibrinolytic profile of paediatric patients undergoing cardiopulmonary bypass. Thromb Haemost 77:270–277.
25. Boisclair MD, Lane DA, Philippou H, et al. (1993) Thrombin production, inactivation and expression during open heart surgery measured by assays for activation fragments including a new ELISA for prothrombin fragment F1 + 2. Thromb Haemost 70:253–258.
26. Brister SJ, Ofosu FA, Buchanan MR (1993) Thrombin generation during cardiac surgery: is heparin the ideal anticoagulant? Thromb Haemost 70:259–262.
27. Langstrom S, Rautiainen P, Mildh L, et al. (2008) Thrombin regulation in neonates undergoing cardiopulmonary bypass. Thromb Haemost 99:791–792.
28. Miller BE, Bailey JM, Mancuso TJ, et al. (1997) Functional maturity of the coagulation system in children: an evaluation using thrombelastography. Anesth Analg 84:745–748.
29. Rinder CS, Gaal D, Student LA, Smith BR (1994) Platelet-leukocyte activation and modulation of adhesion receptors in pediatric patients with congenital heart disease undergoing cardiopulmonary bypass. J Thorac Cardiovasc Surg 107:280–288.
30. Henriksson P, Varendh G, Lundstrom NR (1979) Haemostatic defects in cyanotic congenital heart disease. Br Heart J 41:23–27.
31. Osthaus WA, Boethig D, Johanning K, et al. (2008) Whole blood coagulation measured by modified thrombelastography (ROTEM) is impaired in infants with congenital heart diseases. Blood Coagul Fibrinolysis 19:220–225.
32. Hirsh J, Raschke R, Warkentin TE, et al. (1995) Heparin: mechanism of action, pharmacokinetics, dosing

considerations, monitoring, efficacy, and safety. Chest 108 (4 Suppl):258S–275S.

33. Bull BS, Huse WM, Brauer FS, Korpman RA (1975) Heparin therapy during extracorporeal circulation. II. The use of a dose-response curve to individualize heparin and protamine dosage. J Thorac Cardiovasc Surg 69:685–689.

34. Culliford AT, Gitel SN, Starr N, et al. (1981) Lack of correlation between activated clotting time and plasma heparin during cardiopulmonary bypass. Ann Surg 193:105–111.

35. Codispoti M, Ludlam CA, Simpson D, Mankad PS (2001) Individualized heparin and protamine management in infants and children undergoing cardiac operations. Ann Thorac Surg 71:922–927.

36. Jensen E, Andreasson S, Bengtsson A, et al. (2004) Changes in hemostasis during pediatric heart surgery: impact of a biocompatible heparin-coated perfusion system. Ann Thorac Surg 77:962–967.

37. Jensen E, Andreasson S, Bengtsson A, et al. (2003) Influence of two different perfusion systems on inflammatory response in pediatric heart surgery. Ann Throac Surg 75:919–925.

38. Corno AF (2007) Normal temperature and flow: are the "physiological" values so scary? Eur J Cardiothorac Surg 31:756–757.

39. Kirklin JW, Barrett-Boyes BG (1993) Hypothermia, circulatory arrest, and cardiopulmonary bypass. In: Kirklin JW, Barrett-Boyes BG (eds) Cardiac Surgery, 2nd edn. Churchill Livingstone, New York, p. 91.

40. Bellinger DC, Wernovsky G, Rappaport LA, et al. (1991) Cognitive development of children following early repair of transposition of the great arteries using deep hypothermic circulatory arrest. Pediatrics 87:701–707.

41. Mora CT, Henson MB, Weintraub WS, et al. (1996) The effect of temperature management during cardiopulmonary bypass on neurologic and neuropsychologic outcomes in patients undergoing coronary revascularization. J Thorac Cardiovasc Surg 112:514–522.

42. Friedman WF (1972) The intrinsic physiologic properties of the developing heart. Prog Cardiovasc Dis 15:87–111.

43. Klitzner TS (1991) Maturational changes in excitation–contraction coupling in mammalian myocardium. J Am Coll Cardiol 17:218–225.

44. Attarian DE, Jones RN, Currie WD, et al. (1981) Characteristics of chronic left ventricular hypertrophy induced by subcoronary valvular aortic stenosis. I. Myocardial blood flow and metabolism. J Thorac Cardiovasc Surg 81:382–388.

45. Graham TP, Jr., Erath HG, Jr., Boucek RJ, Jr., Boerth RC (1980) Left ventricular function in cyanotic congenital heart disease. Am J Cardiol 45:1231–1236.

46. Barragry TP, Blatchford JW, Tuna IC, et al. (1987) Left ventricular dysfunction in a canine model of chronic cyanosis. Surgery 102:362–370.

47. Visner MS, Arentzen CE, Ring WS, Anderson RW (1981) Left ventricular dynamic geometry and diastolic mechanics in a model of chronic cyanosis and right ventricular pressure overload. J Thorac Cardiovasc Surg 81:347–357.

48. Bernstein D, Voss E, Huang S, et al. (1990) Differential regulation of right and left ventricular beta-adrenergic receptors

in newborn lambs with experimental cyanotic heart disease. J Clin Invest 85:68–74.

49. Ihnken K, Morita K, Buckberg GD, et al. (1995) Reduction of reoxygenation injury and nitric oxide production in the cyanotic immature heart by controlling pO_2. Eur J Cardiothorac Surg 9:410–418.

50. Magovern GJ, Jr., Flaherty JT, Gott VL, et al. (1982) Failure of blood cardioplegia to protect myocardium at lower temperatures. Circulation 66 (2 Pt 2):I60–I67.

51. Pearl JM, Laks H, Drinkwater DC, et al. (1993) Normocalcemic blood or crystalloid cardioplegia provides better neonatal myocardial protection than does low-calcium cardioplegia. J Thorac Cardiovasc Surg 105:201–206.

52. Kronon M, Bolling KS, Allen BS, et al. (1997) The relationship between calcium and magnesium in pediatric myocardial protection. J Thorac Cardiovasc Surg 114:1010–1019.

53. Kronon MT, Allen BS, Bolling KS, et al. (2000) The role of cardioplegia induction temperature and amino acid enrichment in neonatal myocardial protection. Ann Thorac Surg 70:756–764.

54. Kronon M, Bolling KS, Allen BS, et al. (1998) The importance of cardioplegic infusion pressure in neonatal myocardial protection. Ann Thorac Surg 66:1358–1364.

55. DeLeon SY, Idriss FS, Ilbawi MN, et al. (1988) Comparison of single versus multidose blood cardioplegia in arterial switch procedures. Ann Thorac Surg 45:548–553.

56. Sawa Y, Matsuda H, Shimazaki Y, et al. (1989) Comparison of single dose versus multiple dose crystalloid cardioplegia in neonate. Experimental study with neonatal rabbits from birth to 2 days of age. J Thorac Cardiovasc Surg 97:229–234.

57. Kronon MT, Allen BS, Rahman S, et al. (2000) Reducing postischemic reperfusion damage in neonates using a terminal warm substrate-enriched blood cardioplegic reperfusate. Ann Thorac Surg 70:765–770.

58. Chopp M, Chen H, Dereski MO, Garcia JH (1991) Mild hypothermic intervention after graded ischemic stress in rats. Stroke 22:37–43.

59. Shum-Tim D, Nagashima M, Shinoka T, et al. (1998) Postischemic hyperthermia exacerbates neurologic injury after deep hypothermic circulatory arrest. J Thorac Cardiovasc Surg 116:780–792.

60. Muravchick S, Conrad DP, Vargas A (1980) Peripheral temperature monitoring during cardiopulmonary bypass operation. Ann Thorac Surg 29:36–41.

61. Ramsay JG, Ralley FE, Whalley DG, et al. (1985) Site of temperature monitoring and prediction of afterdrop after open heart surgery. Can Anaesth Soc J 32:607–612.

62. Kim WG, Yang JH (2005) End-point temperature of rewarming after hypothermic cardiopulmonary bypass in pediatric patients. Artif Organs 29:876–879.

63. Naik SK, Knight A, Elliott M (1991) A prospective randomized study of a modified technique of ultrafiltration during pediatric open-heart surgery. Circulation 84 (5 Suppl):III422–III431.

64. Naik SK, Knight A, Elliott MJ (1991) A successful modification of ultrafiltration for cardiopulmonary bypass in children. Perfusion 6:41–50.

65. Aeba R, Katogi T, Omoto T, et al. (2000) Modified ultrafiltration improves carbon dioxide removal after cardiopulmonary bypass in infants. Artif Organs 24: 300–304.

66. Elliott MJ (1993) Ultrafiltration and modified ultrafiltration in pediatric open heart operations. Ann Thorac Surg 56:1518–1522.

67. Yndgaard S, Andersen LW, Andersen C, et al. (2000) The effect of modified ultrafiltration on the amount of circulating endotoxins in children undergoing cardiopulmonary bypass. J Cardiothorac Vasc Anesth 14:399–401.

68. Wang MJ, Chiu IS, Hsu CM, et al. (1996) Efficacy of ultrafiltration in removing inflammatory mediators during pediatric cardiac operations. Ann Thorac Surg 61:651–656.

69. Journois D, Pouard P, Greeley WJ, et al. (1994) Hemofiltration during cardiopulmonary bypass in pediatric cardiac surgery. Effects on hemostasis, cytokines, and complement components. Anesthesiology 81:1181–1189.

70. Daggett CW, Lodge AJ, Scarborough JE, et al. (1998) Modified ultrafiltration versus conventional ultrafiltration: a randomized prospective study in neonatal piglets. J Thorac Cardiovasc Surg 115:336–341.

71. Draaisma AM, Hazekamp MG, Frank M, et al. (1997) Modified ultrafiltration after cardiopulmonary bypass in pediatric cardiac surgery. Ann Thorac Surg 64:521–525.

72. Ootaki Y, Yamaguchi M, Oshima Y, et al. (2002) Effects of modified ultrafiltration on coagulation factors in pediatric cardiac surgery. Surg Today 32:203–206.

73. Friesen RH, Campbell DN, Clarke DR, Tornabene MA (1997) Modified ultrafiltration attenuates dilutional coagulopathy in pediatric open heart operations. Ann Thorac Surg 64:1787–1789.

74. Mahmoud AB, Burhani MS, Hannef AA, et al. (2005) Effect of modified ultrafiltration on pulmonary function after cardiopulmonary bypass. Chest 128:3447–3453.

75. Skaryak LA, Kirshbom PM, DiBernardo LR, et al. (1995) Modified ultrafiltration improves cerebral metabolic recovery after circulatory arrest. J Thorac Cardiovasc Surg 109:744–751.

76. Sever K, Tansel T, Basaran M, et al. (2004) The benefits of continuous ultrafiltration in pediatric cardiac surgery. Scand Cardiovasc J 38:307–311.

77. Lechner E, Dickerson HA, Fraser CD, Jr., Chang AC (2004) Vasodilatory shock after surgery for aortic valve endocarditis: use of low-dose vasopressin. Pediatr Cardiol 25: 558–561.

78. Liedel JL, Meadow W, Nachman J, et al. (2002) Use of vasopressin in refractory hypotension in children with vasodilatory shock: five cases and a review of the literature. Pediatr Crit Care Med 3:15–18.

79. Grayling M, Deakin CD (2003) Methylene blue during cardiopulmonary bypass to treat refractory hypotension in septic endocarditis. J Thorac Cardiovasc Surg 125:426–427.

80. Driscoll W, Thurin S, Carrion V, et al. (1996) Effect of methylene blue on refractory neonatal hypotension. J Pediatr 129:904–908.

81. Taylor K, Holtby H (2005) Methylene blue revisited: management of hypotension in a pediatric patient with bacterial endocarditis. J Thorac Cardiovasc Surg 130:566.

82. Zhang H, Rogiers P, Preiser JC, et al. (1995) Effects of methylene blue on oxygen availability and regional blood flow during endotoxic shock. Crit Care Med 23:1711–1721.

83. Pepke-Zaba J, Higenbottam TW, et al. (1991) Inhaled nitric oxide as a cause of selective pulmonary vasodilatation in pulmonary hypertension. Lancet 338 (8776):1173–1174.

84. Journois D, Pouard P, Mauriat P, et al. (1994) Inhaled nitric oxide as a therapy for pulmonary hypertension after operations for congenital heart defects. J Thorac Cardiovasc Surg 107:1129–1135.

85. Russell IA, Zwass MS, Fineman JR, et al. (1998) The effects of inhaled nitric oxide on postoperative pulmonary hypertension in infants and children undergoing surgical repair of congenital heart disease. Anesth Analg 87:46–51.

86. Raja SG, Macarthur KJ, Pollock JC (2006) Is sildenafil effective for treating pulmonary hypertension after pediatric heart surgery? Interact Cardiovasc Thorac Surg 5:52–54.

87. Wittwer T, Pethig K, Struber M, et al. (2001) Aerosolized iloprost for severe pulmonary hypertension as a bridge to heart transplantation. Ann Thorac Surg 71:1004–1006.

88. Barstad RM, Stephens RW, Hamers MJ, Sakariassen KS (2000) Protamine sulphate inhibits platelet membrane glycoprotein Ib-von Willebrand factor activity. Thromb Haemost 83:334–337.

89. Gibson BE, Todd A, Roberts I, et al. (2004) Transfusion guidelines for neonates and older children. Br J Haematol 124:433–453.

90. McCall MM, Blackwell MM, Smyre JT, et al. (2004) Fresh frozen plasma in the pediatric pump prime: a prospective, randomized trial. Ann Thorac Surg 77:983–987.

91. Ereth MH, Nuttall GA, Klindworth JT, et al. (1997) Does the platelet-activated clotting test (HemoSTATUS) predict blood loss and platelet dysfunction associated with cardiopulmonary bypass? Anesth Analg 85:259–264.

92. Razon Y, Erez E, Vidne B, et al. (2005) Recombinant factor VIIa (NovoSeven) as a hemostatic agent after surgery for congenital heart disease. Paediatr Anaesth 15:235–240.

93. Seifert HA, Jobes DR, Ten Have T, et al. (2003) Adverse events after protamine administration following cardiopulmonary bypass in infants and children. Anesth Analg 97:383–389.

94. Reinhofer M, Brauer M, Franke U, et al. (2008) The value of rotation thromboelastometry to monitor disturbed perioperative haemostasis and bleeding risk in patients with cardiopulmonary bypass. Blood Coagul Fibrinolysis 19:212–219.

95. Reid RW, Zimmerman AA, Laussen PC, et al. (1997) The efficacy of tranexamic acid versus placebo in decreasing blood loss in pediatric patients undergoing repeat cardiac surgery. Anesth Analg 84:990–996.

96. McClure PD, Izsak J (1974) The use of epsilon-aminocaproic acid to reduce bleeding during cardiac bypass in children with congenital heart disease. Anesthesiology 40:604–608.

97. Greilich PE, Brouse CF, Whitten CW, et al. (2003) Antifibrinolytic therapy during cardiopulmonary bypass reduces

proinflammatory cytokine levels: a randomized, double-blind, placebo-controlled study of epsilon-aminocaproic acid and aprotinin. J Thorac Cardiovasc Surg 126:1498–1503.

98. Eaton MP (2008) Antifibrinolytic therapy in surgery for congenital heart disease. Anesth Analg 106:1087–1100.

99. Mossinger H, Dietrich W, Braun SL, et al. (2003) High-dose aprotinin reduces activation of hemostasis, allogeneic blood requirement, and duration of postoperative ventilation in pediatric cardiac surgery. Ann Thorac Surg 75:430–437.

100. Mossinger H, Dietrich W (1998) Activation of hemostasis during cardiopulmonary bypass and pediatric aprotinin dosage. Ann Thorac Surg 65 (6 Suppl):S45–S50.

101. Arnold DM, Fergusson DA, Chan AK, et al. (2006) Avoiding transfusions in children undergoing cardiac surgery: a meta-analysis of randomized trials of aprotinin. Anesth Analg 102:731–737.

102. Williams G, Ramamoorthy C, Pentcheva K, et al. (2008) A randomized, controlled trial of aprotinin in neonates undergoing open-heart surgery. Pediatr Anesth 18:812–819.

103. Moore RA, McNicholas KW, Naidech H, et al. (1985) Clinically silent venous thrombosis following internal and external jugular central venous cannulation in pediatric cardiac patients. Anesthesiology 62:640–643.

104. Jaquiss RD, Ghanayem NS, Zacharisen MC, et al. (2002) Safety of aprotinin use and re-use in pediatric cardiothoracic surgery. Circulation 106 (12 Suppl 1):I90–I94.

105. Seto S, Kher V, Scicli AG, et al. (1983) The effect of aprotinin (a serine protease inhibitor) on renal function and renin release. Hypertension 5:893–899.

106. Mangano DT, Tudor IC, Dietzel C (2006) The risk associated with aprotinin in cardiac surgery. N Engl J Med 354:353–365.

107. Karkouti K, Beattie WS, Dattilo KM, et al. (2006) A propensity score case-control comparison of aprotinin and tranexamic acid in high-transfusion-risk cardiac surgery. Transfusion 46:327–338.

108. Fergusson DA, Hebert PC, Mazer CD, et al. (2008) A comparison of aprotinin and lysine analogues in high-risk cardiac surgery. N Engl J Med 358:2319–2331.

109. Szekely A, Sapi E, Breuer T, et al. (2008) Aprotinin and renal dysfunction after pediatric cardiac surgery. Paediatr Anaesth 18:151–159.

110. Dietrich W (1998) Incidence of hypersensitivity reactions. Ann Thorac Surg 65 (6 Suppl):S60–S64.

111. Dietrich W, Ebell A, Busley R, Boulesteix AL (2007) Aprotinin and anaphylaxis: analysis of 12,403 exposures to aprotinin in cardiac surgery. Ann Thorac Surg 84:1144–1150.

112. Dietrich W, Spath P, Ebell A, Richter JA (1997) Prevalence of anaphylactic reactions to aprotinin: analysis of two hundred forty-eight reexposures to aprotinin in heart operations. J Thorac Cardiovasc Surg 113:194–201.

113. Dietrich W, Spath P, Zuhlsdorf M, et al. (2001) Anaphylactic reactions to aprotinin reexposure in cardiac surgery: relation to antiaprotinin immunoglobulin G and E antibodies. Anesthesiology 95:64–71.

114. Adkins B (2005) Neonatal T cell function. J Pediatr Gastroenterol Nutr 40 (Suppl 1):S5–S7.

115. Chauhan S, Das SN, Bisoi A, et al. (2004) Comparison of epsilon aminocaproic acid and tranexamic acid in pediatric cardiac surgery. J Thorac Cardiovasc Surg 18:141–143.

116. Ririe DG, James RL, O'Brien JJ, et al. (2002) The pharmacokinetics of epsilon-aminocaproic acid in children undergoing surgical repair of congenital heart defects. Anesth Analg 94:44–49.

117. Chauhan S, Kumar BA, Rao BH, et al. (2000) Efficacy of aprotinin, epsilon aminocaproic acid, or combination in cyanotic heart disease. Ann Thorac Surg 70:1308–1312.

118. Bulutcu FS, Ozbek U, Polat B, et al. (2005) Which may be effective to reduce blood loss after cardiac operations in cyanotic children: tranexamic acid, aprotinin or a combination? Paediatr Anaesth 15:41–46.

119. Bronicki RA, Backer CL, Baden HP, et al. (2000) Dexamethasone reduces the inflammatory response to cardiopulmonary bypass in children. Ann Thorac Surg 69:1490–1495.

120. Sobieski MA, Graham JD, Pappas PS, et al. (2008) Reducing the effects of the systemic inflammatory response to cardiopulmonary bypass: can single dose steroids blunt systemic inflammatory response syndrome? ASAIO J 54:203–206.

121. McConnell JR, Fleming WH, Chu WK, et al. (1990) Magnetic resonance imaging of the brain in infants and children before and after cardiac surgery. A prospective study. Am J Dis Child 144:374–378.

122. Glauser TA, Rorke LB, Weinberg PM, Clancy RR (1990) Congenital brain anomalies associated with the hypoplastic left heart syndrome. Pediatrics 85:984–990.

123. McQuillen PS, Hamrick SE, Perez MJ, et al. (2006) Balloon atrial septostomy is associated with preoperative stroke in neonates with transposition of the great arteries. Circulation 113:280–285.

124. Karl TR, Hall S, Ford G, et al. (2004) Arterial switch with full-flow cardiopulmonary bypass and limited circulatory arrest: neurodevelopmental outcome. J Thorac Cardiovasc Surg 127:213–222.

125. Jonas RA (2005) The effect of extracorporeal life support on the brain: cardiopulmonary bypass. Semin Perinatol 29:51–57.

126. Svenarud P, Persson M, Van Der Linden J (2004) Effect of CO_2 insufflation on the number and behavior of air microemboli in open-heart surgery: a randomized clinical trial. Circulation 109:1127–1132.

127. du Plessis AJ, Jonas RA, Wypij D, et al. (1997) Perioperative effects of alpha-stat versus pH-stat strategies for deep hypothermic cardiopulmonary bypass in infants. J Thorac Cardiovasc Surg 114:991–1000.

128. Austin EH, Edmonds HL, Auden SM, et al. (1997) Benefit of neurophysiologic monitoring for pediatric cardiac surgery. J Thorac Cardiovasc Surg 114:707–717.

129. Nelson DP, Andropoulos DB, Fraser CD, Jr. (2008) Perioperative neuroprotective strategies. Semin Thorac Cardiovasc Surg Pediatr Card Surg Annu 49–56.

130. McKenzie ED, Andropoulos DB, DiBardino D, Fraser CD, Jr. (2005) Congenital heart surgery 2005: the brain: it's the heart of the matter. Am J Surg 190:289–294.

131. von Ungern-Sternberg BS, Petak F, Saudan S, et al. (2007) Effect of cardiopulmonary bypass and aortic clamping on functional residual capacity and ventilation distribution in children. J Thorac Cardiovasc Surg 134:1193–1198.

132. Ranieri VM, Suter PM, Tortorella C, et al. (1999) Effect of mechanical ventilation on inflammatory mediators in patients with acute respiratory distress syndrome: a randomized controlled trial. JAMA 282:54–61.

133. Hachenberg T, Tenling A, Nystrom SO, et al. (1994) Ventilation-perfusion inequality in patients undergoing cardiac surgery. Anesthesiology 80:509–519.

134. Zheng JH, Xu ZW, Wang W, et al. (2004) Lung perfusion with oxygenated blood during aortic clamping prevents lung injury. Asian Cardiovasc Thorac Ann 12:58–60.

135. Pizov R, Weiss YG, Oppenheim-Eden A, et al. (2000) High oxygen concentration exacerbates cardiopulmonary bypass-induced lung injury. J Cardiothorac Vasc Anesth 14:519–523.

136. Friedman M, Sellke FW, Wang SY, et al. (1994) Parameters of pulmonary injury after total or partial cardiopulmonary bypass. Circulation 90 (5 Pt 2):II262–II268.

137. de Perrot M, Liu M, Waddell TK, Keshavjee S (2003) Ischemia-reperfusion-induced lung injury. Am J Respir Crit Care Med 167:490–511.

138. Ng CS, Wan S, Yim AP, Arifi AA (2002) Pulmonary dysfunction after cardiac surgery. Chest 121:1269–1277.

139. Skippen PW, Krahn GE (2005) Acute renal failure in children undergoing cardiopulmonary bypass. Crit Care Resusc 7:286–291.

140. Kist-van Holthe tot Echten JE, Goedvolk CA, Doornaar MB, et al. (2001) Acute renal insufficiency and renal replacement therapy after pediatric cardiopulmonary bypass surgery. Pediatr Cardiol 22:321–326.

141. Giuffre RM, Tam KH, Williams WW, Freedom RM (1992) Acute renal failure complicating pediatric cardiac surgery: a comparison of survivors and nonsurvivors following acute peritoneal dialysis. Pediatr Cardiol 13:208–213.

142. Shaw NJ, Brocklebank JT, Dickinson DF, et al. (1991) Long-term outcome for children with acute renal failure following cardiac surgery. Int J Cardiol 31:161–165.

143. Werner HA, Wensley DF, Lirenman DS, LeBlanc JG (1997) Peritoneal dialysis in children after cardiopulmonary bypass. J Thorac Cardiovasc Surg 113:64–68.

144. Pedersen KR, Hjortdal VE, Christensen S, et al. (2008) Clinical outcome in children with acute renal failure treated with peritoneal dialysis after surgery for congenital heart disease. Kidney Int 108:S81–S86.

145. Sorof JM, Stromberg D, Brewer ED, et al. (1999) Early initiation of peritoneal dialysis after surgical repair of congenital heart disease. Pediatr Nephrol 13:641–645.

146. Bokesch PM, Kapural MB, Mossad EB, et al. (2000) Do peritoneal catheters remove pro-inflammatory cytokines after cardiopulmonary bypass in neonates? Ann Thorac Surg 70:639–643.

147. Mathie RT, Ohri SK, Batten JJ, et al. (1997) Hepatic blood flow during cardiopulmonary bypass operations: the effect of temperature and pulsatility. J Thorac Cardiovasc Surg 114:292–293.

148. Ohri SK, Bowles CW, Mathie RT, et al. (1997) Effect of cardiopulmonary bypass perfusion protocols on gut tissue oxygenation and blood flow. Ann Thorac Surg 64:163–170.

149. Nygren A, Thoren A, Houltz E, Ricksten SE (2006) Autoregulation of human jejunal mucosal perfusion during cardiopulmonary bypass. Anesth Analg 102:1617–1622.

150. Bastien O, Piriou V, Aouifi A, et al. (2000) Relative importance of flow versus pressure in splanchnic perfusion during cardiopulmonary bypass in rabbits. Anesthesiology 92:457–464.

151. Sato K, Watanabe H, Sogawa M, et al. (2006) Vasoconstrictor administration during cardiopulmonary bypass affects acid–base balance in infants and children. Artif Organs 30:101–105.

152. Allen KB, Salam AA, Lumsden AB (1992) Acute mesenteric ischemia after cardiopulmonary bypass. J Vasc Surg 16:391–395.

153. Ott MJ, Buchman TG, Baumgartner WA (1995) Postoperative abdominal complications in cardiopulmonary bypass patients: a case-controlled study. Ann Thorac Surg 59:1210–1213.

154. Hatherill M, Salie S, Waggie Z, et al. (2005) Hyperchloraemic metabolic acidosis following open cardiac surgery. Arch Dis Child 90:1288–1292.

155. Boldt J, Knothe C, Welters I, et al. (1996) Normothermic versus hypothermic cardiopulmonary bypass: do changes in coagulation differ? Ann Thorac Surg 62:130–135.

156. Pigula FA, Siewers RD, Nemoto EM (2001) Hypothermic cardiopulmonary bypass alters oxygen/glucose uptake in the pediatric brain. J Thorac Cardiovasc Surg 121:366–373.

157. Lewis ME, Al-Khalidi AH, Townend JN, et al. (2002) The effects of hypothermia on human left ventricular contractile function during cardiac surgery. J Am Coll Cardiol 39:102–108.

158. Yamada S (2004) Impaired endothelial responses in patients with deep hypothermic cardiopulmonary bypass. Kurume Med J 51:1–7.

159. Hillier SC, Burrows FA, Bissonnette B, Taylor RH (1991) Cerebral hemodynamics in neonates and infants undergoing cardiopulmonary bypass and profound hypothermic circulatory arrest: assessment by transcranial Doppler sonography. Anesth Analg 72:723–728.

160. Bissonnette B, Pellerin L, Ravussin P, et al. (1999) Deep hypothermia and rewarming alters glutamate levels and glycogen content in cultured astrocytes. Anesthesiology 91:1763–1769.

161. Bissonnette B, Holtby HM, Davis AJ, et al. (2000) Cerebral hyperthermia in children after cardiopulmonary bypass. Anesthesiology 93:611–618.

162. Lindholm L, Bengtsson A, Hansdottir V, et al. (2003) Regional oxygenation and systemic inflammatory response during cardiopulmonary bypass: influence of temperature and blood flow variations. J Cardiothorac Vasc Anesth 17:182–187.

163. Caputo M, Bays S, Rogers CA, et al. (2005) Randomized comparison between normothermic and hypothermic cardiopulmonary bypass in pediatric open-heart surgery. Ann Thorac Surg 80:982–988.

164. Hovels-Gurich HH, Seghaye MC, Schnitker R, et al. (2002) Long-term neurodevelopmental outcomes in school-aged children after neonatal arterial switch operation. J Thorac Cardiovasc Surg 124:448–458.

165. Rasmussen LS, Sztuk F, Christiansen M, Elliott MJ (2001) Normothermic versus hypothermic cardiopulmonary bypass during repair of congenital heart disease. J Cardiothorac Vasc Anesth 15:563–566.

166. Durandy Y, Hulin S, Lecompte Y (2002) Normothermic cardiopulmonary bypass in pediatric surgery. J Thorac Cardiovasc Surg 123:194.

167. Pouard P, Mauriat P, Ek F, et al. (2006) Normothermic cardiopulmonary bypass and myocardial cardioplegic protection for neonatal arterial switch operation. Eur J Cardiothorac Surg 30:695–699.

168. Bigelow WG, Lindsay WK, Greenwood WF (1950) Hypothermia; its possible role in cardiac surgery: an investigation of factors governing survival in dogs at low body temperatures. Ann Surg 132:849–866.

169. Kuniyoshi Y, Koja K, Miyagi K, et al. (2003) Myocardial protective effect of hypothermia during extracorporeal circulation—by quantitative measurement of myocardial oxygen consumption. Ann Thorac Cardiovasc Surg 9: 155–162.

170. Croughwell N, Smith LR, Quill T, et al. (1992) The effect of temperature on cerebral metabolism and blood flow in adults during cardiopulmonary bypass. J Thorac Cardiovasc Surg 103:549–554.

171. Pearl JM, Thomas DW, Grist G, et al. (2000) Hyperoxia for management of acid-base status during deep hypothermia with circulatory arrest. Ann Thorac Surg 270:751–755.

172. Felfernig M, Blaicher A, Kettner SC, et al. (2001) Effects of temperature on partial thromboplastin time in heparinized plasma in vitro. Eur J Anaesthesiol 18:467–470.

173. Birdi I, Regragui I, Izzat MB, et al. (1997) Influence of normothermic systemic perfusion during coronary artery bypass operations: a randomized prospective study. J Thorac Cardiovasc Surg 114:475–481.

174. Naylor CD, Lichtenstein SV, Fremes SE et al. (1994) Randomised trial of normothermic versus hypothermic coronary bypass surgery. The Warm Heart Investigators. Lancet 343 (8897):559–563.

175. Sealy WC, Brown IW, Jr., Young WG, et al. (1959) Hypothermia and extracorporeal circulation for open heart surgery: its simplification with a heat exchanger for rapid cooling and rewarming. Ann Surg 150:627–639.

176. Barratt-Boyes BG, Simpson M, Neutze JM (1971) Intracardiac surgery in neonates and infants using deep hypothermia with surface cooling and limited cardiopulmonary bypass. Circulation 43 (5 Suppl):I25–I30.

177. Wong PC, Barlow CF, Hickey PR, et al. (1992) Factors associated with choreoathetosis after cardiopulmonary bypass in children with congenital heart disease. Circulation 86 (5 Suppl):II118–II126.

178. Pastuszko P, Liu H, Mendoza-Paredes A, et al. (2007) Brain oxygen and metabolism is dependent on the rate of low-flow cardiopulmonary bypass following circulatory arrest in newborn piglets. Eur J Cardiothorac Surg 31: 899–905.

179. Markowitz SD, Mendoza-Paredes A, Liu H, et al. (2007) Response of brain oxygenation and metabolism to deep hypothermic circulatory arrest in newborn piglets: comparison of pH-stat and alpha-stat strategies. Ann Thorac Surg 84:170–176.

180. Wypij D, Newburger JW, Rappaport LA, et al. (2003) The effect of duration of deep hypothermic circulatory arrest in infant heart surgery on late neurodevelopment: the Boston Circulatory Arrest Trial. J Thorac Cardiovasc Surg 126:1397–1403.

181. Jonas RA, Bellinger DC, Rappaport LA, et al. (1993) Relation of pH strategy and developmental outcome after hypothermic circulatory arrest. J Thorac Cardiovasc Surg 106: 362–368.

182. Bellinger DC WG, Rappaport LA (2003) Rapid cooling of infants on cardiopulmonary bypass adversely affects later cognitive function. Circulation 78:II358.

183. Kurth CD, O'Rourke MM, O'Hara IB (1998) Comparison of pH-stat and alpha-stat cardiopulmonary bypass on cerebral oxygenation and blood flow in relation to hypothermic circulatory arrest in piglets. Anesthesiology 89:110–118.

184. Priestley MA, Golden JA, O'Hara IB, et al. (2001) Comparison of neurologic outcome after deep hypothermic circulatory arrest with alpha-stat and pH-stat cardiopulmonary bypass in newborn pigs. J Thorac Cardiovasc Surg 121:336–343.

185. Brooker RF, Zvara DA, Velvis H, Prielipp RC (1997) Topical ice slurry prevents brain rewarming during deep hypothermic circulatory arrest in newborn sheep. J Cardiothorac Vasc Anesth 11:591–594.

186. Langley SM, Chai PJ, Miller SE, et al. (1999) Intermittent perfusion protects the brain during deep hypothermic circulatory arrest. Ann Thorac Surg 68:4–12.

187. Hickey PR (1998) Neurologic sequelae associated with deep hypothermic circulatory arrest. Ann Thorac Surg 65 (6 Suppl):S65–S69.

188. Rodriguez RA, Austin EH, 3rd, Audenaert SM. (1995) Postbypass effects of delayed rewarming on cerebral blood flow velocities in infants after total circulatory arrest. J Thorac Cardiovasc Surg 110:1686–1690.

189. Tsui SS, Schultz JM, Shen I, Ungerleider RM (2004) Postoperative hypoxemia exacerbates potential brain injury after deep hypothermic circulatory arrest. Ann Thorac Surg 78:188–196.

190. Sakamoto T, Hatsuoka S, Stock UA, et al. (2001) Prediction of safe duration of hypothermic circulatory arrest by near-infrared spectroscopy. J Thorac Cardiovasc Surg 122:339–350.

191. Pigula FA, Nemoto EM, Griffith BP, Siewers RD (2000) Regional low-flow perfusion provides cerebral circulatory support during neonatal aortic arch reconstruction. J Thorac Cardiovasc Surg 119:331–339.

192. Tchervenkov CI, Korkola SJ, Shum-Tim D, et al. (2001) Neonatal aortic arch reconstruction avoiding circulatory

arrest and direct arch vessel cannulation. Ann Thorac Surg 72:1615–1620.

193. Malhotra SP, Hanley FL (2008) Routine continuous perfusion for aortic arch reconstruction in the neonate. Semin Thorac Cardiovasc Surg Pediatr Card Surg Annu 57–60.

194. Pigula FA, Gandhi SK, Siewers RD, et al. (2001) Regional low-flow perfusion provides somatic circulatory support during neonatal aortic arch surgery. Ann Thorac Surg 72:401–406.

195. Andropoulos DB, Stayer SA, McKenzie ED, Fraser CD, Jr. (2003) Regional low-flow perfusion provides comparable blood flow and oxygenation to both cerebral hemispheres during neonatal aortic arch reconstruction. J Thorac Cardiovasc Surg 126:1712–1717.

196. Fraser CD, Jr., Andropoulos DB (2008) Principles of antegrade cerebral perfusion during arch reconstruction in newborns/infants. Semin Thorac Cardiovasc Surg Pediatr Card Surg Annu 61–68.

197. Burrows FA, Bissonnette B (1993) Cerebral blood flow velocity patterns during cardiac surgery utilizing profound hypothermia with low-flow cardiopulmonary bypass or circulatory arrest in neonates and infants. Can J Anaesth 40:298–307.

198. Amir G, Ramamoorthy C, Riemer RK, et al. (2006) Visual light spectroscopy reflects flow-related changes in brain oxygenation during regional low-flow perfusion and deep hypothermic circulatory arrest. J Thorac Cardiovasc Surg 132:1307–1313.

199. Greeley WJ, Kern FH, Ungerleider RM, et al. (1991) The effect of hypothermic cardiopulmonary bypass and total circulatory arrest on cerebral metabolism in neonates, infants, and children. J Thorac Cardiovasc Surg 101:783–794.

200. Swan H (1984) The importance of acid-base management for cardiac and cerebral preservation during open heart operations. Surg Gynecol Obstet 158:391–414.

201. Patel RL, Turtle MR, Chambers DJ, et al. (1996) Alpha-stat acid-base regulation during cardiopulmonary bypass improves neuropsychologic outcome in patients undergoing coronary artery bypass grafting. J Thorac Cardiovasc Surg 111:1267–1279.

202. Hindman BJ, Dexter F, Cutkomp J, Smith T (1995) pH-stat management reduces the cerebral metabolic rate for oxygen during profound hypothermia (17 degrees C). A study during cardiopulmonary bypass in rabbits. Anesthesiology 82:983–995.

203. Aoki M, Nomura F, Stromski ME, et al. (1993) Effects of pH on brain energetics after hypothermic circulatory arrest. Ann Thorac Surg 55:1093–1103.

204. Hiramatsu T, Miura T, Forbess JM, et al. (1995) pH strategies and cerebral energetics before and after circulatory arrest. J Thorac Cardiovasc Surg 109:948–957.

205. Miller AL, Corddry DH (1981) Brain carbohydrate metabolism in developing rats during hypercapnia. J Neurochem 36:1202–1210.

206. Yoshioka H, Miyake H, Smith DS, et al. (1995) Effects of hypercapnia on ECoG and oxidative metabolism in neonatal dog brain. J Appl Physiol 78:2272–2278.

207. Callaghan PB, Lister J, Paton BC, Swan H (1961) Effect of varying carbon dioxide tensions on the oxyhemoglobin dissociation curves under hypothermic conditions. Ann Surg 154:903–910.

208. Duelli R, Kuschinsky W (1993) Changes in brain capillary diameter during hypocapnia and hypercapnia. J Cereb Blood Flow Metab 13:1025–1028.

209. Sakamoto T, Kurosawa H, Shin'oka T, et al. (2004) The influence of pH strategy on cerebral and collateral circulation during hypothermic cardiopulmonary bypass in cyanotic patients with heart disease: results of a randomized trial and real-time monitoring. J Thorac Cardiovasc Surg 127:12–19.

210. Bellinger DC, Wypij D, du Plessis AJ, et al. (2001) Developmental and neurologic effects of alpha-stat versus pH-stat strategies for deep hypothermic cardiopulmonary bypass in infants. J Thorac Cardiovasc Surg 121:374–383.

211. Scallan MJ. (2003) Brain injury in children with congenital heart disease. Paediatr Anaesth 13:284–293.

212. Dahlbacka S, Heikkinen J, Kaakinen T, et al. (2005) pH-stat versus alpha-stat acid-base management strategy during hypothermic circulatory arrest combined with embolic brain injury. Ann Thorac Surg 79:1316–1325.

213. Nagy ZL, Collins M, Sharpe T, et al. (2003) Effect of two different bypass techniques on the serum troponin-T levels in newborns and children: does pH-Stat provide better protection? Circulation 108:577–582.

8

The inflammatory response and its modification

Emad B. Mossad, M.D.
Texas Children's Hospital, Baylor College of Medicine, Houston, Texas, USA

Elumalai Appachi, M.D.
Cleveland Clinic, Cleveland, Ohio, USA

Nature's reaction to every injury, whether physical, chemical, or bacterial, is inflammation, or in other words, congestion with its resulting benefits.

—E.H. Beckman, M.D.,
Southern Minnesota Medical
association, Saint Mary's
Hospital, Mayo Clinic, August
1907

Introduction

The normal human response to an abnormal allergen or environment is the triggering of a defense mechanism, mediated through a humoral or cellular immune response. This is no more obvious than the response of the body to cardiopulmonary bypass (CPB) and the abnormal environment of extracorporeal circulation (ECC) [1].

Despite significant advances in cardiac surgery in the past 50 years, and major strides in improving the outcome of congenital cardiac defect repair, CPB remains an inte-

gral part of most operations. Cardiac surgery continues to carry an inherent risk of triggering a cascade of reactions leading to the systemic inflammatory response syndrome (SIRS), and manifested as multisystem organ failure, especially in small infants and children [2,3].

Clinically, the inflammatory response is manifested as reduced pulmonary function, with decreased compliance, worsening oxygenation, and prolonged need for postoperative mechanical ventilation. Cardiovascular dysfunction, requiring inotropic support, and occasionally the use of mechanical assist devices, occurs in more than 50% of children following cardiac surgery. In addition, 3–7% of children experience renal and hepatic dysfunction, in some series neurological morbidity occurs in up to 30% of patients, and a high percentage have significant tissue edema and weight gain [4].

Mechanisms of activation

The inflammatory response is triggered with the initiation of CPB, from contact of blood with the nonendothelial surface of ECC, activating the coagulation and complement cascades. Other triggers of inflammation include

Anesthesia for Congenital Heart Disease 2nd edition. Edited by Dean Andropoulos, Stephen Stayer, Isobel Russell and Emad Mossad.
© 2010 Blackwell Publishing.

Table 8.1 Inflammatory triggers and mediators on cardiopulmonary bypass

Complement	C3a, C5a, C5b-9
Leukocyte and adhesion molecules	CD11b/CD 18, E-selectin, ICAM-1, Integrins
Arachidonic acid metabolites	Thromboxane A2, prostaglandins
Endotoxin	
Cytokines	TNF-α, IL-6, IL-8, IL-10
Platelet Activating factor (PAF)	
Nitric Oxide (NO)	
Endothelins	Endothelin-1
Oxygen free radicals	Superoxide anion, singlet oxygen, hydroxyl radicals, hydrogen peroxide
Procalcitonin	PCT

bowel hypoperfusion with endotoxemia, and organ ischemia and reperfusion injury with release of the aortic cross-clamp and termination of bypass. Multiple triggers, mediators and effectors interact to initiate, propagate, and maintain the inflammatory response and produce end-organ damage (Table 8.1).

Blood contact with the artificial surface activates the intrinsic coagulation pathway (increased factor XIIa), as well as the extrinsic pathway (factor VII contact with tissue factor). Despite the use of high-dose systemic heparin, and maintaining an adequate activated clotting time (ACT > 480 s), markers of thrombin generation (prothrombin F_{1+2}, fibrinopeptide A) increase with the progression of bypass. The fibrinolytic system is also activated, with increased kallikrein, bradykinin, and tissue plasminogen activator (tPA) [5].

The complement system is a series of 19 functionally linked plasma proteins that, once activated, interact to effect humoral immunity and inflammatory response. The complement proteins generally are inactive until activated by antigen–antibody complex (classical pathway) or by infectious organisms (alternate pathway). The main event in complement activation is the generation of C3a and C3b from C3 by the action of C3 convertases, and increased C5a (neutrophil attractant) at the onset of bypass [6]. The classic pathway is activated at the end of bypass by the protamine–heparin complex and increased C4a concentration. The end result is release of activated anaphylotoxins (C3a, C4a, and C5a) that in turn cause histamine release, increased vascular permeability, and neutrophil activation. C5a is the most potent of the anaphylotoxins, acts directly on the endothelial cells, stimulating contraction, vascular leak, and exocytosis. The combined effect of actions of C5a, C3a, and C4a on mast cells, endothelial cells, and neutrophils determines the inflammatory response at the site of complement activation, and thus the degree of

organ damage. In a group of 29 children undergoing cardiac surgery, Seghaye [7] showed a significant increase in C3a and C5a at the initiation of CPB, significant transpulmonary neutropenia, and correlation between the degree of complement activation with postoperative morbidity. The elevation of C3a and C5a is proportional to the duration of CPB and increasing age of patients. Infants have a more pronounced increase in C3a and C5a when compared to neonates [8].

The initiation of CPB is associated with decreased gastric mucosal pH, intestinal hypoperfusion, and increased permeability. The absorption of ingested monosaccharides (L-rhamnose), dependent on transcellular transport, is decreased during and following CPB, due to intestinal cellular edema. Meanwhile, paracellular transport and urinary excretion of disaccharides (cellobiose) is increased up to the third postoperative day [9].

Levels of circulating endotoxin and the need for inotropic support correlate with increased intestinal mucosal permeability. The severity of necrotizing enterocolitis (NEC) in newborns correlates with the amount of endotoxin and mediators of inflammation (proinflammatory interleukins IL-1β and IL-8) in the circulation [10]. The lipopolysaccharide (LPS) bacterial outer membrane of gram negative organisms, and circulating endotoxin, bind to macrophages and monocytes, initiating release of mediators of inflammation.

Procalcitonin (PCT) is a 13 kDa propeptide of calcitonin. Endotoxemia, gram-positive infections, sepsis, and ECC are major triggers for PCT induction. Other stimuli include major surgery, severe trauma, and burns. In states of shock, increased PCT levels have been detected together with other signs and markers of systemic inflammation, such as fever, elevated leukocyte count, and cytokine release. PCT is more sensitive than C-reactive protein (CRP) and other markers in the early diagnosis of severe sepsis, and the onset of systemic inflammatory response with multisystem organ failure following cardiac surgery [11]. Serum PCT concentrations increase significantly in children immediately following CPB, peaked in the first day, and returned to baseline by fifth postoperative day [12]. Peak plasma concentrations of >5 ng/mL correlated with APACHE II scores, onset of postoperative cardiac failure, and other complications. Plasma concentration also differentiated survivors from nonsurvivors (>15 ng/mL) in adult and pediatric cardiac surgery [13] (Figure 8.1).

The final trigger to the inflammatory cascade is the ischemia–reperfusion injury that occurs with unclamping the aorta, discontinuing CPB, and resuming pulsatile perfusion. Both in clinical observations [14] and experimental models [15] of ischemia and reperfusion, there is significant increase in neutrophil count, plasma granulocyte elastase, serum IL-6 and IL-8, associated with pulmonary

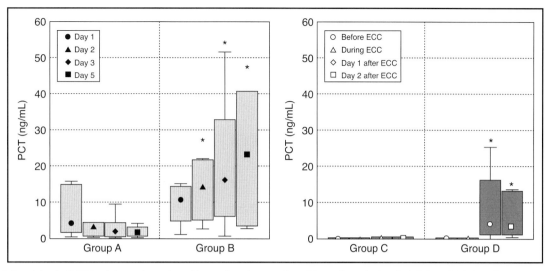

Figure 8.1 Procalcitonin (PCT) levels in septic survivors (Group A) and nonsurvivors (Group B) on the 1st, 2nd, 3rd, and 5th day of treatment and in patients who underwent cardiac operations and recovered uneventfully (Group C) or had significant postoperative complications (Group D) (Adapted and reproduced with permission from Reference [13])

leukocyte sequestration, myocardial and cerebral neutrophil infiltration, and organ dysfunction.

Pathophysiology of the inflammatory response

Following activation by surface contact, complement, endotoxemia, and reperfusion, the inflammatory response is mediated by expression and secretion of tumor necrosis factor-alpha (TNF-α), various cytokines and arachidonic acid metabolites [16].

Macrophages and monocytes, which are already primed by C5a, release TNF-α (also known as cachexin due to its prominent presence in cachexia of chronic illness) in response to stimulation by endotoxin. Plasma levels of TNF-α have been shown to increase during and after CPB with a bimodal peak at 2 and 18–24 hours postoperatively [17]. TNF-α release is the initial event in the release of further pro- and anti-inflammatory cytokines (Figure 8.2) [18]. TNF-α acts on mononuclear phagocytes, and on the vascular endothelium, to stimulate secretion of a cascade of pro- and anti-inflammatory cytokines that share many biologic activities.

Cytokines are polypeptide or glycopeptide hormones of low molecular weight (5–28 kDa) that are produced by various cell types. They mediate and regulate the immune and inflammatory response to external stimuli, and facilitate the communication between leukocytes (hence the name "interleukins" or IL). The cell types producing cytokines include macrophages, monocytes, lymphocytes, and endothelial cells. Cytokines are not stored as preformed molecules, and their synthesis is initiated by

new gene transcription. Once synthesized, cytokines are rapidly secreted, resulting in a burst of serum cytokine release. Cytokines often influence the synthesis and release of other cytokines, leading to a cascade-like increase of their plasma concentrations in a series of successive waves. Positive and negative regulatory mechanisms mediate the biological effects and concentration of the various cytokines. The wave of release begins with an increase in serum TNF-α, followed by release of several proinflammatory (interleukins IL-1β, IL-6, and IL-8) and anti-inflammatory (IL-10) cytokines.

TNF-α, C3a, and C5a stimulate macrophage and monocyte IL-1β production and release. IL-1β levels have been to shown to increase after CPB and reach its peak levels at 24 hours postoperatively. IL-1β also activates neutrophils and endothelial cells to cause adhesion between them. IL-1β stimulates the production of IL-6 and IL-8 and thus plays a central role in the inflammatory process. It has been shown to cause decreased myocardial β-adrenergic receptor (BAR) response to catecholamine stimulation. It also causes fever by the production of prostaglandin E_2 in the hypothalamus, thus known as the endogenous pyrogen.

IL-6 is produced by various cell types, including macrophages, monocytes, endothelial cells, lymphocytes, and fibroblasts in response to TNF-α. It is known as the acute phase interleukin. The acute phase response consists of fever, leucocytosis, altered vascular permeability, decreased synthesis of albumin, and increased synthesis of acute phase proteins, like CRP by the liver. IL-6 levels peak 3–6 hours after CPB and correlate with postoperative organ dysfunction. In one study, plasma IL-6 levels in children undergoing ventricular septal defect repair

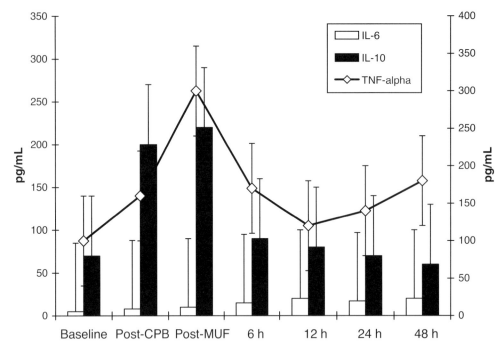

Figure 8.2 Pro-inflammatory and anti-inflammatory cytokine responses to cardiopulmonary bypass in children. TNF, Tumor necrosis factor; IL, Interleukin; MUF, modified ultrafiltration (Reproduced with permission from Reference [18])

(105 ± 12 pg/mL) were significantly lower than levels in patients who underwent complex surgical repairs (220 ± 25 pg/mL) [17]. Elevated levels of IL-6 after bypass may be related to the severity of the preoperative condition, the duration of CPB, or myocardial compromise postoperatively. IL-6 seems to be the best indicator of outcome after sepsis or CPB-induced multiorgan failure.

IL-8 is the chemokine that attracts neutrophils to the site of inflammation. The same cell types that produce other cytokines also produce IL-8, through stimulation by endotoxin and TNF-α. Levels of IL-8 begin to rise at rewarming, and peak at 1–3 hours after CPB, and are present after 24 hours. IL-8 attracts neutrophils to the site of inflammation and causes upregulation of adhesion molecules necessary for neutrophil adhesion to endothelial cells. It also stimulates neutrophils to release oxygen-free radicals and proteolytic enzymes that enhance endothelial damage.

Another group of pro-inflammatory cytokines, the β-chemokines monocyte chemoattractant protein (MCP-1), is significantly increased following CPB, and correlates with duration of bypass, longer surgical time, and increased need for inotropes [19].

IL-10 is an anti-inflammatory cytokine as opposed to IL-6 and IL-8, which are pro-inflammatory cytokines. IL-10 levels also increase and peak around 3 hours after CPB (Figure 8.2). IL-10 provides its anti-inflammatory effect by directly inhibiting the release of pro-inflammatory cytokines from neutrophils and macrophages. IL-10 stimulates the release of IL-1 receptor antagonist and TNF

soluble receptors 1 and 2, both of which exert anti-inflammatory effects [20].

Interestingly IL-6 stimulates the release of IL-10 by macrophages, endothelial cells, and monocytes. Interaction between pro- and anti-inflammatory cytokines likely determines the severity of the inflammatory response and multiorgan dysfunction following CPB in children [21].

There are conflicting reports regarding the time of release, the degree of increase in plasma levels, and the relative ratio between pro- and anti-inflammatory cytokines in the literature. These discrepancies may stem from the source of sampling (arterial or venous blood), the timing of when blood is sampled, and the various of measurement techniques (enzyme-linked immunosorbent assay, radioimmunoassay, or in vitro cell cytotoxicity assay). However, it is clear that the initial response is a release of TNF-α with an early and late peak, followed by a series of waves of interleukin release.

Interactions and ratios between pro- and anti-inflammatory cytokines likely determine the severity of the inflammatory response and multiorgan dysfunction following CPB in children. In a study of 24 neonates with hypoplastic left heart syndrome (HLHS) undergoing stage-1 repair, and 21 with d-TGA undergoing arterial switch repair, there was a significant increase in pro- and anti-inflammatory cytokines postoperatively. Neonates with HLHS had an activated inflammatory response before CPB, which remained significant in the postoperative period. Accelerated interleukin expression and an abnormal cytokine balance (lower IL-10/IL-6 ratio) correlate with longer time to extubation, longer ICU length of stay, and increased peritoneal fluid drainage [22].

Other important mediators of inflammation are the leukotrienes, arachidonic acid metabolites, endothelin, and oxygen-free radicals. The leukotrienes and arachidonic acid metabolites are humoral inflammatory mediators produced by macrophages, neutrophils, and monocytes after stimulation by C5a and IL-8. Leukotriene B_4 causes chemotaxis, release of proteolytic enzymes, and generation of oxygen-free radicals from neutrophils. Other leukotrienes cause arteriolar constriction and induce a profound increase in vascular permeability. Thromboxane A_2 and prostaglandins are arachidonic acid metabolites. Thromboxane A_2 has strong vasoconstrictor and platelet aggregating properties. Thromboxane A_2 has been shown to cause myocardial dysfunction and pulmonary hypertension after CPB in animal models. Prostaglandins ($PGE_{1\ and\ 2}$ and prostacyclin) on the other hand have vasodilating and anti-platelet aggregating properties, and therefore counter balance the effect of thromboxane A_2 [23].

Endothelin-1 (ET-1) is a 21-amino acid polypeptide produced primarily by vascular endothelial cells in the systemic and pulmonary circulations, and is a potent vasoconstrictor [24]. ET-1 participates in several biologic activities, including vascular smooth muscle proliferation, fibrosis, cardiac and vascular hypertrophy, and inflammation. ET-1 is released from the endothelial cells, and is a potent vasoconstrictor. It thus regulates arterial blood pressure and influences cardiac output [25]. Increased levels of ET-1 have been demonstrated in patients who develop pulmonary hypertension. Elevated levels of ET-1 occur after CPB and correlate with postoperative renal dysfunction. ET-1 release after CPB may also cause myocardial ischemia and the development of pulmonary edema.

These mediators of the inflammatory response (TNF-α, interleukins IL-1β, IL-6, and IL-8, and arachidonic acid metabolites) modulate the response of the body to the inflammatory trigger of bypass through neutrophil–endothelial adhesion, BAR downregulation, and inducible nitric oxide synthase (iNOS) production.

Once activated, neutrophils adhere to endothelial cells, and eventually migrate out of the vessel wall into the tissues (Figure 8.3). There are specific adhesion molecules on the surface of neutrophils and endothelial cells [26]. These molecules include selectins (present on leukocytes, *L-selectin*, endothelial cell, *E-selectin*, and platelets,

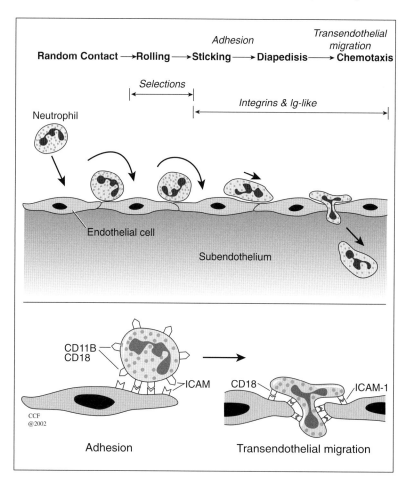

Figure 8.3 Neutrophil adhesion, diapedesis, transendothelial migration, and chemotaxis (see text for explanation)

P-selectin), integrins (neutrophil only), and the immunoglobulin superfamily (endothelial cells only) [27,29]. One study found that atrial and skeletal muscle E-selectin mRNA levels increase significantly following CPB in children. ELAM-1 (endothelial leukocyte adhesion molecule-1) presents on the endothelial surface after stimulation of TNF-α or IL-1, and plays a key role in the binding of neutrophils to endothelium.

The integrins are receptors responsible for cellular interactions and have α and β subunits. The β_2 subunit of integrins facilitates the adhesion of neutrophils to other cells and also plays a key role in the inflammatory response. The common β_2 subunit is called CD18 and the α subunits are called CD11a, CD11b, and CD11c. Upregulated CD11b expression on neutrophils likely contributes to neutrophil sequestration in the heart and lungs after bypass.

The immunoglobulin superfamily of receptors includes ICAM-1 and ICAM-2 (intercellular adhesion molecule-1 and 2); the expression of these molecules on the endothelial surface is induced by C5a, TNF-α, IL-1β, or endotoxin. Plasma concentrations of soluble adhesion molecules increase significantly after CPB in cyanotic children, in younger patients, and with longer bypass times [28] IL-8 promotes neutrophil interaction with ICAM-1 receptors on the endothelial cells and neutrophil migration to the extravascular tissues.

The neutrophils extend pseudopods that probe for the path of least resistance at the interendothelial junctions. Increased vascularity, blood stasis, and endothelial injury allow the neutrophils to crawl between the endothelial cells. The proteolytic enzymes from the neutrophil granules digest the basement membrane to allow migration to subendothelial tissues. Once in the subendothelial space, neutrophils cause tissue injury by releasing proteases, elastases, toxic oxygen radicals, and arachidonic acid metabolites. The released elastase causes damage to endothelial cells, underlying basement membrane, subendothelial matrix, and parenchyma of various organs, and plasma levels are significantly elevated after CPB.

Platelets activation during CPB occurs from the action of C5a and also by platelet-activating factor (PAF) secreted by endothelial cells, which leads to the expression of platelet P-selectin. Platelets attached to the vascular endothelium play an important role in neutrophil adhesion and transmigration by attracting more neutrophils to the endothelium from the expression of P-selectin [29,30].

Endothelial cells are responsible for the permeability barrier through which the exchange of substances takes place by transcytosis. The endothelium also promotes structural changes of the blood vessel in response to a local change in environment. The vascular endothelium is exposed to various inflammatory stimuli including endotoxin, cytokines, and the physical injury of surgical trauma. These stimuli cause a disruption of the barrier function, vasoconstriction, abnormal coagulation, leukocyte adhesion, smooth muscle proliferation, and release of more mediators of inflammation like cytokines released from the cytoplasmic vacuoles called Weibel–Palade bodies.

Another mechanism by which the inflammatory response is mediated is through BAR downregulation. Discontinuation of CPB is a critical event, often associated with transient myocardial dysfunction, requiring increasing inotropic support. Canine transmyocardial left ventricular biopsies reveal the density of BAR to be significantly decreased following bypass [31]. The response of BAR in the myocardium or bronchial smooth muscles to nonselective β-agonists (isoproterenol), or selective β_2-agonists (zinterol), is impaired following CPB. The decreased density, and desensitization of BAR, is reproducible with TNF-α exposure, and correlates with the post-CPB increase in serum cytokines [32].

The endothelium-derived relaxing factor, nitric oxide is a natural regulator of vasomotor tone and blood flow to organs. Under normal conditions picomolar concentrations of NO are formed in the circulation through the effect of constitutive nitric oxide synthase (cNOS). However, at the start of CPB, hemodilution, nonpulsatile flow, and circuit contact activate endothelial iNOS, to produce excessive (nanomolar) concentrations of NO. NO will modulate vasodilation, neutrophil adhesion, and tissue injury by TNF-α, cytokines, and other mediators of inflammation [33].

The negative inotropic effect of TNF-α on isolated papillary muscle contraction was blocked in the presence of *N*-monomethyl-L-arginine (L-NMMA), a specific NOS inhibitor. The concentration-dependent, reversible myocardial depression of TNF-α reappears with the addition of L-arginine [34]. Neuronal apoptosis following hypothermic circulatory arrest, especially in the hippocampus and neocortex, is significantly reduced by neuronal NOS inhibition [35]. NO regulates P-selectin expression, neutrophil adhesion and sequestration on CPB, and further propagation of the bypass-induced inflammatory response [36].

Clinical effects of the inflammatory response

Complications following CPB due to the systemic inflammatory response remain common and obvious, despite significant improvement in equipment, material, and the conduct of surgery. Following prolonged surgery, children may present to the intensive care unit with marked whole-body edema and multiple organ failure, especially those patients who require greater pharmacologic and mechanical support (Figure 8.4).

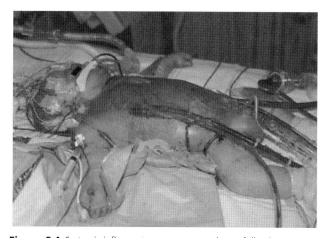

Figure 8.4 Systemic inflammatory response syndrome following extracorporeal circulation, leading to multisystem organ failure in a neonate with congenital heart disease.

High fever, thrombocytopenia, cardiorespiratory insufficiency, and failure of one or more vital organ systems occur in more than 3.5% of children after open-heart surgery [37].

One study found 13/24 neonates developed capillary leak syndrome (CLS), which was associated with higher complement (C5a) and cytokine (TNF-α) levels postoperatively (Figure 8.5). Plasma albumin fell significantly, and histamine release during CPB was more pronounced in patients with CLS [38].

There is strong association between triggering the inflammatory response, and the development of coagulopathy following bypass. An inverse correlation is present between in vitro platelet aggregation and plasma IL-1β or IL-6 levels. Cytokines are important mediators of disseminated intravascular coagulopathy, fibrinolysis, and bleeding associated with CPB and sepsis [39]. Cardiac surgery still consumes more than 20% of the nation's blood supply, and almost 80% of all transfusions are used in only 15% of patients, who commonly show other signs of multisystem organ failure and systemic inflammatory response.

Myocardial dysfunction requiring inotropic support is common in the immediate postoperative period. The severity of cardiac depression appears to be associated with the extent of stimulation of the inflammatory response. In adults presenting for myocardial revascularization on CPB, a bimodal increase in TNF-α and IL-6 is noted postoperatively that is proportional to the duration of cross-clamp. Left ventricular wall motion abnormalities, episodes of myocardial ischemia, and inotropic requirements correlate with cytokine expression [40]. Cardiac index and systemic vascular resistance are inversely related, while pulmonary capillary wedge pressure is directly related to IL-6 increase postoperatively [40,41]. Preoperative depression of cardiac function appears to predispose the patient to develop an accentuated inflammatory response, with a significant increase in post-pump cytokines in patients with ejection fraction less than 0.45 preoperatively, compared to those with normal cardiac function [41].

Myocardial damage appears to occur up to the fourth postoperative day in children following repair of congenital heart defects, and the changes in serum troponin, creatine kinase, and PCT correlate with the increases in markers of inflammation [42].

The pulmonary injury following CPB is one of the major causes of morbidity after cardiac surgery in children, and is sometimes referred to as "pump-lung." Pulmonary edema, microatelectasis, increased alveolar–arterial oxygen gradient (A-aO$_2$ gradient), and increased pulmonary vascular resistance are observed postoperatively. Duration of CPB in children correlates with decreases in surfactant, transpulmonary neutropenia, and neutrophil lung sequestration. Granulocyte adhesion molecule expression (CD11b/CD18, MCP-1), and increase in serum IL-8, correlates with a deterioration in oxygenation in children after surgery [43]. Serum and alveolar epithelial IL-6 increase

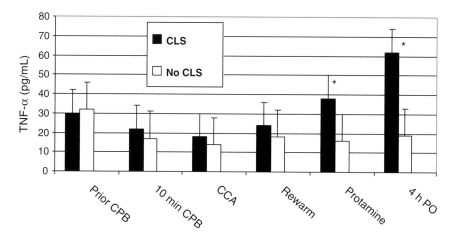

Figure 8.5 Course of TNF-α before, during, and after CPB in neonates with (*black*), and without (*white*) capillary leak syndrome (CLS). CCA, complete circulatory arrest; PO, postoperatively ($^* = p < 0.05$) (Adapted and reproduced with permission from Reference [38])

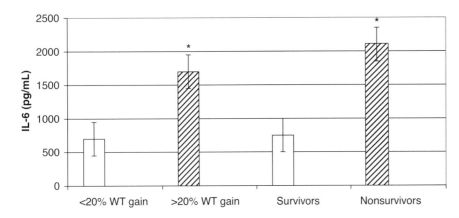

Figure 8.6 Relation of serum IL-6 levels to fluid retention and survival in children at 2 hours following CPB ($* = p < 0.05$) (Adapted and reproduced with permission from Reference [44])

significantly following CPB in children, and correlate with intraoperative blood transfusion, fluid gain, pediatric risk of mortality score (PRISM), and survival (Figure 8.6) [44].

Neurological injury occurs frequently in children following repair of congenital heart disease, with gross deficits (strokes, seizures) found in 3%, and psychomotor, and neurodevelopment dysfunction found in more than 30% of children. Despite a relation between adhesion molecules, TNF-α, and cognitive dysfunction in other disease states, these markers of systemic inflammatory response showed no relationship with neurological outcome at 5-day and 3-month performance tests [45]. However, other studies have shown an association between markers of neurological injury (S-100β and neuron-specific enolase) and the severity of septic shock and other systemic inflammatory states [46, 47].

The risk of acute renal failure (2.7%) and gastrointestinal complications (1%) in children following CPB is associated with triggering the inflammatory response [48, 49]. In patients with severe end-stage cardiomyopathy, 5/16 developed fulminant hepatic failure despite adequate hemodynamic support by a left ventricular assist device. Markers of inflammation (CRP, IL-6, and IL-8) were significantly increased in patients who developed hepatic dysfunction [50].

Modification of the inflammatory response

Multiple treatment modalities and interventions are used in an attempt to limit the generation and extent of inflammation after bypass and avoid organ dysfunction [51]. One obvious method to decrease the triggering of inflammation is to avoid CPB, and currently over 16% of coronary artery bypass graft surgeries are performed without bypass. However, the use of CPB remains essential for all intracardiac repairs of congenital heart defects. Thus, the interventions designed to limit the inflammatory response

to CPB include (1) preoperative therapies (intestinal decontamination, presurgical inotropes, and anesthetics), (2) modifications of circuit biocompatibility (heparin-coating, pulsatile flow, prime solution), (3) changes in CPB conduct (temperature, leukocyte depletion, and hemofiltration), and (4) pharmacological interventions (steroids, aprotinin, and monoclonal antibodies). These treatment modalities are commonly used in concert, to treat the multifaceted inflammatory response to bypass (Figure 8.7).

Digestive decontamination

Endotoxemia in children with congenital heart disease is present in 40% of patients preoperatively, and 96% following CPB. Plasma levels of IL-6, disturbed hemodynamics, and mortality are higher in children with more significant endotoxemia [52]. The use of selective digestive decontamination (polymyxin E, tobramycin, and amphotericin B) for 72 hours preoperatively reduces gut content of enterobacteria, and lowers endotoxin and cytokine concentrations postbypass [53]. However, there are no data on changes in clinical outcome as a result of adequate digestive decontamination.

Inotropic support

Perioperative administration of low-dose milrinone improves splanchnic perfusion on CPB, thus limiting intestinal mucosal ischemia and injury, thereby decreasing translocation of intestinal flora and endotoxemia. The use of milrinone 0.5 mcg/kg/min improves gastric intramucosal acidosis, reduces hepatic venous return, and reduces postoperative IL-6 [54].

Prime solution and blood transfusion

The use of plasma expanders and the maintenance of colloidal osmotic pressure in prime solution limits activation of the alternative and common complement pathways [55]. In many centers, fresh whole blood is used

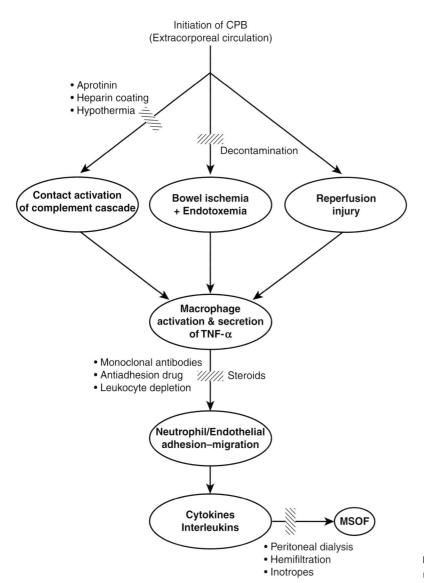

Figure 8.7 Treatment options of the inflammatory response to cardiopulmonary bypass

for priming the CPB circuit in neonates and infants in an attempt to limit the inflammatory response, myocardial injury, and coagulopathy in these patients. However, in a single center, randomized, double-blind control study, the use of fresh whole blood (<48 hours) failed to present any advantage to those infants when compared to reconstituted blood. In fact, children who received fresh whole blood had longer durations of mechanical ventilation, intensive care unit length of stay, increased cumulative fluid balance, and more prominent markers of inflammation postoperatively [56].

Despite allogeneic blood transfusion causing more immunosuppression than autologous blood [57], exposure to any transfusion, especially platelet concentrates, leads to significant increase in markers of inflammation (C3a, C5a, TNF-α, and IL-6) [58]. The magnitude of the interleukin response to CPB correlates with blood transfusion and du-

ration of bypass [59]. The number and age of transfused units has a significant impact on short- and long-term outcome following cardiac surgery. In a study comparing patients who received newer blood versus older blood (median storage duration 11 days vs 20 days), Koch and colleagues [60] showed a significant increase in intubation >72 hours, renal failure and sepsis with older blood (4% vs 2.8% with newer blood, $p = 0.01$), and a cumulative effect with the number of transfused units. In-hospital mortality, and mortality at 1-year follow-up, was also lower with newer blood (7.4% vs 11%, $p < 0.001$).

Oxygenators and perfusion mechanics

Compared to bubble oxygenators, the use of membrane oxygenators in pediatric cardiac surgery is associated with better cardiac performance, better postoperative pulmonary compliance, and decreased shunt fraction, free hemoglobin, blood loss, postoperative pyrexia, and length of hospitalization. When extracorporeal perfusion lasts more than 2 hours, membrane oxygenators reduce the release of granulocyte adhesion molecules, lactoferrin, myeloperoxide, and proinflammatory cytokines [61,62].

The use of nonpulsatile flow is associated with a progressive increase in systemic vascular resistance, decreased tissue oxygen consumption, metabolic acidosis, and the expression of inflammatory markers. Pulsatile perfusion (although less popular), and nonocclusive centrifugal pumps can be used during pediatric CPB, and may limit complement activation, and reduce the inflammatory response [63,64].

Temperature control

The use of hypothermic CPB appears to offer a protective effect from the inflammatory response. One study compared maintaining a core temperature of 28°C versus 36°C, and found markers of inflammation to be significantly reduced [65]. In an in vitro pediatric CPB circuit preparation, neutrophil activation and upregulation of adhesion molecules were significantly increased on normothermic (35°C) compared to hypothermic (17°C) bypass [66]. Even though a predominance of literature supports the concept that moderate or deep hypothermic bypass attenuates the inflammatory response and decreases histological organ damage [67], some investigators have shown no difference in those markers with changing temperature [68,69]. In a study of 30 children with body weight <10 kg, only minor differences in cytokines and inflammatory markers were detected between those with moderate (25°C) or mild (32°C) hypothermia. Duration of aortic cross-clamp and CPB time had a more significant impact on the inflammatory response than the temperature at which bypass was conducted [70].

Heparin-coated circuits

The use of a heparin-coated (HC) or bonded extracorporeal circuit reduces heparin requirements during cardiac operations, and improves oxygen tension (HC 597.2 ± 31.2 vs control 220.5 ± 42.3 mm Hg), and pulmonary vascular resistance (HC 408.6 ± 69.4 vs control 1159.8 ± 202.4 dyne s/cm^5) 2 hours after CPB [71]. Heparin bonding of the entire circuit, or the oxygenator (which forms >80% of the circuit surface area in children), significantly reduces postoperative central hyperthermia and respiratory index. Plasma levels of terminal complement complexes, and expression of neutrophil adhesion molecules and serum cytokines are markedly reduced in children managed with HC circuits [72–74]. Two different processes of coating circuits with heparin have been described. The Carmeda

process (Medtronic, Inc., Minneapolis, MN) deposits a polymer coating on the circuit-surface, followed by covalently bonding heparin fragments to that coating. The Duraflo II process (Baxter Healthcare Corp., Irvine, CA) modifies the physicochemical properties of unfractionated heparin with a binding agent, giving it a high affinity for synthetic surfaces [75]. Although Carmeda equipment appears more effective in reducing complement activation, both methods were similar in blunting the expression of cytokines and the inflammatory response.

Leukocyte depletion

The use of a blood cell separator can limit the triggering of the inflammatory response and its deleterious effects. Leukocyte and platelet depletion (LPD) decrease leukocyte and platelet counts; and serum elastase, thromboxane, and thrombin–antithrombin III complex (TAT) are also lowered. This therapy leads to higher arterial oxygen tension and a lower respiratory index, improved maximum stroke work index, and use of lower catecholamine doses [76,77].

Conventional and modified ultrafiltration

The hemodilution effects of CPB are pronounced in children due to the disproportionately large priming volume and surface area of the circuit. Hemoconcentration applies a hydrostatic pressure gradient to a semipermeable membrane, removing excess water, low-molecular-weight substances, and inflammatory mediators. The filter can be used during rewarming, and placed between the oxygenator and the venous reservoir, conventional ultrafiltraion (CUF), typically performed during bypass, or after CPB, it is placed between the arterial cannula and the right atrium, modified ultrafiltraion (MUF). The suction pressure should not exceed 200 mm Hg, removing fluid at a rate <50 mL/k/min. Both methods are effective in reducing proinflammatory cytokines, complement activation (C3a, C5a), and weight gain [78,79].

Cytokine removal strategies using CUF or MUF are limited to the intraoperative period, and are unable to limit the inflammatory response due to reperfusion injury in the postoperative period. The use of a Tenckhoff catheter for removal of peritoneal fluid was shown to remove significant amounts of IL-6 and IL-8, and may be beneficial in improving the pro- to anti-inflammatory (IL-6/IL-10) serum cytokine balance [80].

Intravenous anesthetics

The use of intravenous anesthetics to modulate the inflammatory response to CPB is an interesting and evolving area of investigation. The effect of pharmacologic concentrations of intravenous anesthetics on the expression of leukocyte adhesion molecules and release of cytokines has been studied in a cultured whole blood sample, incubated with LPS endotoxin [81]. Compared to control, the LPS-stimulated TNF-α response was inhibited by thiopentone (12.8%) and ketamine (46.4%), augmented by propofol (172.3%), and unchanged with midazolam or fentanyl.

Aprotinin

Aprotinin reduces endotoxin activation of the plasma kallikrein–kinin and complement system [82]. Aprotinin is a serine protease inhibitor commonly used in adult and pediatric cardiac surgery to decrease blood loss and transfusion requirements. Aprotinin shortens sternal closure times, decreases 24-hour chest tube drainage, transfusion of packed red blood cells and platelets, and overall hospital expense in children with cyanotic heart disease [83,84]. Aprotinin is an expensive medication, with known risk of anaphylaxis. Exposure to topical aprotinin in fibrin sealant, resulted in developing aprotinin-specific immunoglobulin E and G in 8–39% of children [85]. However, only aprotinin blocks kallikrein and plasmin, thus preventing contact activation, the release of cytokines, and the inflammatory response to CPB. Aprotinin decreases leukocyte accumulation, and suppresses expression of inflammatory genes as P-selectin and ICAM following myocardial ischemia and reperfusion. In a rat model of ischemia/reperfusion, aprotinin inhibited differential inflammatory protein expression, myocyte apoptosis and myocardial injury [86]. In a bronchial epithelial cell line, aprotinin blocks the expression of iNOS and the production of injurious concentrations of NO in response to cell stimulation with TNF-α and other cytokines [87,88]. In a recent review of randomized control studies of antifibrinolytic use in pediatric cardiac surgery, aprotinin was the only agent effective in decreasing blood loss and transfusion requirements, while blunting reperfusion myocardial injury and decreasing transpulmonary pressure gradients and pulmonary hypertension following bidirectional cavopulmonary shunts and Fontan operations [89]. The efficacy of aprotinin varies between studies, probably due to a significant variability in dosing regimen between centers.

Recent studies have identified the risk of aprotinin in adults undergoing coronary revascularization. In a large scale observational study of 4374 patients, Mangano et al. [90] identified 100% increased risk of renal failure requiring dialysis, 55% increased risk of myocardial infarction or heart failure, and 81% increased risk of stroke postoperatively in adults receiving aprotinin compared to other antifibrinolytic agents. However, similar reviews of pediatric patients identified no increased risk of renal, neurological, or myocardial injury in cohorts of children receiving aprotinin compared to placebo or other agents [91,92].

Corticosteroids

The beneficial effects of steroid administration before CPB to attenuate the "post-pump syndrome" have long been investigated. Earlier studies focused on the hemodynamic effects methylprednisolone (MPSS at 10–30 mg/kg) or Dexamethasone (DXM at 1–6 mg/kg). Both glucocorticoids increased cardiac index, reduced peripheral vascular resistance, and improved microcirculation and visceral perfusion [93]. Steroid use has an equal, and even a synergistic effect with other agents, such as aprotinin, in blunting the inflammatory response. MPSS improved oxygenation, cardiac index, and cytokine balance following CPB, when added to high-dose aprotinin [94,95].

Several investigations have shown that steroid pretreatment modulates different aspects of the inflammatory response, and the most recent studies are summarized in Table 8.2 [96–107]. Steroids blunt the endotoxin-mediated increases in CD11b/CD18, and neutrophil surface adhesion receptor expression [94]. They reduce the expression of proinflammatory cytokines, and LPS-stimulated production of IL-1β and TNF-α by macrophages. MPSS has been shown to block the upregulation of neutrophil integrin adhesion receptors, and preserve chemotactic properties, as well attenuate complement activation with protamine administration [97]. DXM decreases proinflammatory cytokines, and expression of ELAM-1, and ICAM-1 adhesion receptors [98]. The net results of steroid pretreatment appear to include improvement in hemodynamics, pulmonary mechanics, and recovery of cerebral perfusion and metabolism following deep hypothermic circulatory arrest [97,98,102]. Steroids cause attenuation of capillary leak and weight gain, and reduce postoperative pyrexia, through limiting the inflammatory response.

In a survey of national and international pediatric cardiac centers, Checchia et al. [108] reported a 97% frequency of steroid use among centers caring for a total of >11,000 children annually (35/36 responders). Most centers used MPSS (30 mg/kg) or DXM (1 mg/kg) but varied in timing of dose either preoperatively (18 centers), in the prime (11 centers) or using multiple doses (6 centers). The type, timing, and dose of steroid used are controversial, and may explain the discrepancy in outcome of some studies. Administration of steroids 1–8 hours prior to incision appears to have a stronger impact on cytokines and acute phase-reactants (CRP) than does the same dosage used in the pump-prime [96,101]. The administration of MPSS 20–30 mg/kg prior to surgical incision significantly improved the anti- to proinflammatory cytokine balance, and

Table 8.2 Recent randomized evaluations of steroid effect on inflammatory response to cardiopulmonary bypass [96–107]

Study	Steroid use: type, dose, and time	Subjects	Biochemical markers	Clinical effects
Butler J (1996) [96]	MPSS 10 mg/kg Pump prime	24 children	↓ IL-6, CRP	↓ postoperative fever
Lodge AJ (1999) [97]	MPSS 30 mg/k 8 h and 1.5 h preop versus pump prime	18 neonatal piglets		↑ compliance ↓ A-a gradient, PVR, fluid gain
Bronicki (2000) [98]	DXM 1 mg/k 1 h prior to CPB	29 children	↓ IL-6, TNF-α ↔ C3a, neutrophil count	↓ rectal temp. ↓ A-a gradient ↓ mechanical ventilation
Mossad E (2000) [99]	MPSS 20 or 30 mg/k prior to incision	47 infants	↓ IL-6, IL-8 ↑ IL-10	↓ PD drainage
Langley S (2000) [100]	MPSS 30 mg/k IM 8 h and 2 h preop	16 neonatal piglets on DHCA		↑ recovery of regional and global CBF and CMRO$_2$
Volk T (2001) [101]	MPSS 15 mg/k preoperative	39 adults	↓ IL-1β, IL-6, IL-8, TNF-α response to LPS. ↑ IL-10	
Mott AR (2001) [102]	MPSS 1 mg/k × 4 doses Preop and 24 h postop	246 children		↑ risk of PPS
Varan B (2002) [103]	MPSS 2 or 30 mg/kg pre-CPB	30 children	No difference in IL-6/IL-8, CRP	No difference in Temperature, mechanical ventilation
Shum-Tim D (2003) [104]	MPSS 30 mg/kg 4 h preop, pump prime versus placebo	18 neonatal piglets	↓ IL-6, ↑COP only with preop dose	↓ weight gain, markers of brain injury only with preop dose
Schroeder VA (2003) [105]	MPSS 30 mg/kg pre and intraop versus intraop	29 children	↓myocardial mRNA expression, IL-6, ↓ΔA-VO2	↓fluid gain ↑intubation time
Gessler P (2005) [106]	MPSS 30 mg/kg to prime circuit versus placebo	50 infants	No difference in markers IL-8 correlate with CPB duration	No difference in oxygenation index, inotrope use
Santos AR (2007) [107]	Inhaled steroids (Budesonide) @ end CPB, 6 and 12 h versus placebo	32 infants	No effect on bronchoalveolar IL-6/8	No effect on lung compliance or oxygenation index

MPSS, methylprednisolone sodium succinate; TNF, tumor necrosis factor; IL, interleukins; CRP, C-reactive protein; DXM, dexamethasone; A-a gradient, alveolar-to-arterial oxygen gradient; PVR, pulmonary vascular resistance; Ig, immunoglobulin; PD, peritoneal dialysis; CBF, cerebral blood flow; CMRO$_2$, cerebral oxygen metabolic rate; DHCA, deep hypothermic circulatory arrest; LPS, lipopolysaccharide; PPS, post-pericardiotomy syndrome.

maintained a favorable postoperative clinical outcome (Figure 8.8) [99].

Side effects of steroid use must be considered and include hyperglycemia, immunosuppersion due to T-cell dysfunction, impaired wound healing, prolonged mechanical ventilation, peptic ulcer, suppression of the pituitary–adrenal axis, salt and water retention, and hypokalemia. Those side effects should be evaluated, managed effectively, balancing the benefit to the risk of steroid use [109].

Anticytokine and monoclonal antibodies

Experimental studies have shown a benefit for strategies to block cytokines in sepsis-like syndromes, using soluble TNF-α receptors and neutralizing factors, and IL-1β receptor antagonists [110]. Inhibition of neutrophil adhesion using monoclonal antibodies and anti-selectins leads to improved recovery of ventricular function, myocardial oxygen consumption, and attenuates myocardial neutrophil proliferation following cold cardioplegic ischemia

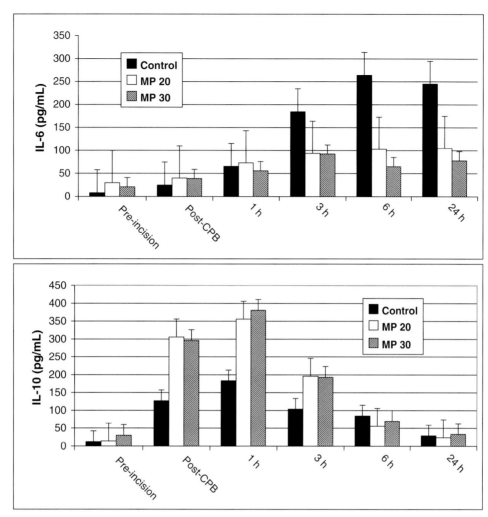

Figure 8.8 Serum IL-6 (a) and IL-10 (b) concentrations before and after cardiopulmonary bypass (CPB): control (no steroids), MP 20 (methylprednisolone 20 mg/kg), MP 30 (methylprednisolone 30mg/kg) ($^* = p < 0.05$) (Reproduced with permission from Reference [99])

[111–113]. Clinical studies have shown the safety and efficacy of a humanized, recombinant, single chain antibody specific for human C5 in limiting the inflammatory response to bypass. Patients receiving 1–2 mg/kg intravenously of the complement inhibitor preoperatively had effective inhibition of the proinflammatory complement byproducts (sC5b-9), and reduced surface adhesion molecules (CD11b/CD18) [114]. Those patients had a 40% reduction in myocardial injury, improved scores on a mini-mental state examination, and a significant reduction in blood loss. There is ongoing investigation in this area, especially in children, to identify antiadhesion molecules and cytokine inhibitors that limit the response of the body to the stress of bypass.

The inflammatory response to CPB is a cascade of events, with multiple triggers, mediators and modulators, culminating in end-organ injury, and poor outcome. The treatment modalities to this inflammatory response need to be preemptive, multifaceted and used in combination

to prevent the response, blunt its degree of expression, or limit the severity of organ dysfunction [94,115]. In one study, the use of four anti-inflammatory strategies (MPSS, aprotinin, leukocyte depletion, or HC circuit) effectively attenuated markers of the inflammatory response to ECC, and decreased mortality to 2.3%, compared to a 5.7% risk stratification predicted mortality of the population studied [115].

Unanswered questions

Although the etiology of the systemic inflammatory response in cardiac surgery appears to be related to the contact-activation and exposure to the extracorporeal circuit, markers of inflammation have been detected in operations done without bypass. The combined stress of surgical trauma, vascular injury, and anesthesia may contribute significantly to the CPB-induced inflammatory response. In children operated upon with and without CPB, the activation of the alternate complement pathway, cytokines, and adhesion molecule expression were seen in both groups (C3d: 8.16 ± 3.6 vs 4.12 ± 1.43 mg/L, peak IL-6: 164.4 vs 277.8 pg/mL, ICAM-1: 241 ± 35 vs 325 ± 29 pg/mL, E-selectin: 56.1 ± 32.8 vs 42.4 ± 17.7 pg/mL, CPB vs no CPB, respectively) [116].

Avoiding bypass will not completely eliminate the risk of triggering the inflammatory response to surgical stress [117]. In a series of 43 patients undergoing coronary artery bypass grafting on or off-pump, avoiding CPB did not prevent the acute phase inflammatory response [118]. Both groups had significant microalbuminuria and increased CRP postoperatively. Oxygenation index (A-aO$_2$ gradient and shunt fraction) worsened postoperatively with or without exposure to ECC.

The response to surgical stress and CPB varies significantly between patients, with a wide range of cytokine release and adhesion molecule expression, in response to the same triggers. The patient's preoperative cardiac function appears to contribute to the extent of inflammatory response. Patients with severe end-stage heart failure have elevated serum TNF-α levels, which correlate with their New York Heart Association status and degree of ventricular dysfunction. The proinflammatory cytokines play an important role in the pathogenesis of heart failure, but may also be triggered and released in the circulation from poor visceral perfusion [119]. The increase in serum IL-6 and TNF-α was more pronounced in patients with depressed preoperative cardiac function and lower ejection fraction [41]. The impact of preoperative diagnosis and condition is evident in the extent of inflammatory response of neonates with HLHS compared to other lesions both before and after surgical interventions [120].

Similar to other disease states, the inflammatory response may have a spectrum of genetic expression responsible for the variability in response to the stimulus of CPB [121]. The expression of adhesion molecules in response to transient cerebral ischemia can be genetically modulated, and this presents a new target site for therapy of postischemic reperfusion injury [122].

Treatment modalities to the inflammatory response may have side effects that supercede their benefits. Glucocorticoids cause postoperative hyperglycemia, and may aggravate ischemic neuronal damage. Despite effective suppression of the complement and interleukin response, DXM increased the size of cerebral infarct by 10-fold using a middle cerebral artery occlusion model [123]. There is evidence that steroids may worsen neurological outcomes in neonatal patients following a 42-day tapering course of steroids in ventilator-dependent low-birth-weight infants. One-year follow-up showed a significant increase in intracranial abnormalities, and a greater risk of developing cerebral palsy [124].

The synergistic immunosuppression caused by high-dose MPSS and CPB (suppression of IL-2 helper T-cell function, and increased natural killer cells) may be detrimental [97]. The use of preoperative digestive decontamination, leukocyte depletion, and steroids may also increase the risk for postoperative infection.

Finally, stimulation of the inflammatory response is a complex process necessary for wound healing and immune defense. Therefore, the goal of any therapy must not be the complete suppression of the inflammatory response to CPB. In fact, despite an abolished complement and adhesion-molecule response to CPB in a complement-deficient animal model, bypass-associated lung injury still occurs [125]. Patients with leukocyte adhesion deficiency syndrome (LADS I&II), manifest absence of cell surface expression adhesion molecules, and have a significant risk of recurrent bacterial infections, skin lesions with impaired pus formation, and delayed wound healing. Replacement therapy with granulocyte–macrophage colony-stimulating factor increases cytokine and integrin expression, and improves their clinical condition [126].

The inflammatory response is a natural defense mechanism that protects the body from foreign antigens and limits their injury to a local site. However, when the stimulus is excessive, the response becomes exaggerated and harmful, and requires multimodal therapy to limit end-organ injury, but not abolish it completely [127].

References

1. Royston D (1997) The inflammatory response and extracorporeal circulation. J Cardiothorac Vasc Anesth 11:341–354.
2. Hall RI, Smith MS, Rocker G (1997) The systemic inflammatory response to cardiopulmonary bypass: pathophysiology, therapeutics and pharmacologic considerations. Anesth Analg 85:766–782.
3. Wan S, LeClerc JL, Vincent JL (1997) Inflammatory response to cardiopulmonary bypass: mechanisms involved and possible therapeutic strategies. Chest 112:676–692.
4. Brix-Christensen V (2001) The systemic inflammatory response after cardiac surgery with cardiopulmonary bypass in children. Acta Anaesthesiol Scand 45:671–679.
5. Hsu LC (1997) Biocompatability in cardiopulmonary bypass. J Cardiothorac Vasc Anesth 11:376–382.
6. Chenoweth DE, Cooper SW, Hugli TE, et al. (1981) Complement activation during cardiopulmonary bypass: evidence for generation of C3a and C5a anaphylatoxins. N Engl J Med 304:497–503.
7. Seghaye MC, Duchateau J, Grabitz RG, et al. (1993) Complement activation during cardiopulmonary bypass in infants and children. Relation to postoperative multiple system organ failure. J Thorac Cardiovasc Surg 106:978–987.
8. Sonntag J, Dahnert I, Stiller B, et al. Complement activation during cardiovascular operations in infants. Ann Thorac Surg 65:525–531.

9. Oudemans-vanStraaten HM, Jansen PGM, Hoek FJ, et al. (1996) Intestinal permeability, circulating endotoxin, and postoperative systemic responses in cardiac surgery patients. J Cardiothorac Vasc Anesth 10:187–194.

10. Edelson MB, Bagwell CE, Rozycki HJ (1999) Circulating pro-and counter-inflammatory cytokine levels and severity in necrotizing enterocolitis. Pediatrics 103:765–771.

11. Brunkhorst FM, Wegscheider K, Forycki ZF, et al. (2000) Procalcitonin for early diagnosis and differentiation of SIRS, sepsis, severe sepsis and septic shock. Intensive Care Med 26 (Suppl 2):S148–S152.

12. Arkader R, Troster EJ, Abellan DM, et al. (2004) Procalcitonin and C-reactive proten kinetics in postoperative pediatric cardiac surgical patients. J Cardiothorac Vasc Anesth 18:160–165.

13. Adamik B, Kubler-Kielb J, Golebiowska B, et al. (2000) Effect of sepsis and cardiac surgery with cardiopulmonary bypass on plasma level of nitric oxide metabolites, neopterin, and procalcitonin: correlation with mortality and postoperative complications. Intensive Care Med 26:1259–1267.

14. Kawamura T, Wakusawa R, Okada K, et al. (1993) Elevation of cytokines during open heart surgery with cardiopulmonary bypass: participation of interleukin 8 and 6 in reperfusion injury. Can J Anaesth 40:1016–1021.

15. Benjelloun N, Renolleau S, Represa A, et al. (1999) Inflammatory responses in cerebral cortex after ischemia in the P7 neonatal rat. Stroke 30:1916–1924.

16. Khabar KS, ElBarbary MA, Khouqeer F, et al. (1997) Circulating endotoxin and cytokines after cardiopulmonary bypass; differential correlation with duration of bypass and systemic inflammatory response/multiple organ dysfunction syndromes. Clinic Immunol Immunopathol 85:97–103.

17. Duval EL, Kavelaars A, Veenhuizen L, et al. (1999) Pro- and anti-inflammatory cytokine patterns during and after cardiac surgery in young children. Euro J Pediatr 158:387–393.

18. Chew MS, Brandslund I, Brix-Christensen V, et al. (2001) Tissue injury and the inflammatory response to pediatric cardiac surgery with cardiopulmonary bypass: a descriptive study. Anesthesiology 94:745–753.

19. Lotan D, Zilberman D, Dagan O, et al. (2001) β-Chemokine secretion patterns in relation to clinical course and outcome in children after cardiopulmonary bypass: continuing search to abrogate systemic inflammatory response. Ann Thorac Surg 71:233–237.

20. Madhok AB, Ojamaa K, Haridas V, et al. (2006) Cytokine response in children undergoing surgery for congenital heart disease. Pediatr Cardiol 27:408–413.

21. Hovels-Gurich HH, Schumacher K, Vazquez-Jimenez JF, et al. (2002) Cytokine balance in infants undergoing cardiac operation. Ann Thorac Surg 73:601–609.

22. Appachi E, Mossad E, Mee RBB, et al. (2007) Perioperative serum interleukins in neonates with hypoplastic left heart syndrome and transposition of the great arteries. J Cardiothorac Vasc Anesth 21:184–190.

23. Friedman M, Wang SY, Sellke FW, et al. (1995) Pulmonary injury after total or partial cardiopulmonary bypass by thromboxane synthesis inhibition. Ann Thorac Surg 59:598–603.

24. Beghetti M, Black SM, Fineman JR (2005) Endothelin-1 in congenital heart disease. Pediatr Res 57:16R–20R.

25. Kageyama K, Hashimoto S, Nakajima Y, et al. (2007) The change of plasma Endothelin-1 levels before and after surgery with or without Down syndrome. Pediatr Anesth 17:1071–1077.

26. Springer TA (1990) Adhesion receptors of the immune system. Nature 346:425–434.

27. Kilbridge PM, Mayer JE, Newburger JW, et al. (1994) Induction of intercellular adhesion molecule-1 and E-selectin mRNA in heart and skeletal muscle of pediatric patients undergoing cardiopulmonary bypass. J Thorac Cardiovasc Surg 107:1183–1192.

28. Blume ED, Nelson DP, Gauvreau K, et al. (1997) Soluble adhesion molecules in infants and children undergoing cardiopulmonary bypass. Circulation 96 (Suppl 1) II352–II357.

29. Asimakopoulos G, Taylor KM (1998) Effects of cardiopulmonary bypass on leukocyte and endothelial adhesion molecules. Ann Thorac Surg 66:2135–2144.

30. Lotan D, Prince T, Dagan O, et al. (2001) Soluble P-selectin and the postoperative course following cardiopulmonary bypass in children. Paediatr Anaesth 1:303–308.

31. Schwinn DA, Leone BJ, Spahn DR, et al. (1991) Desensitization of myocardial β-adrenergic receptors during cardiopulmonary bypass. Evidence for early uncoupling and late downregulation. Circulation 84:2559–2567.

32. Emala CW, Kuhl J, Hungerford CL, et al. (1997) TNF-α inhibits isoproterenol-stimulated adenylyl cyclase activity in cultured airway smooth muscle cells. Am J Physiol 272:L644–L650.

33. Brett SJ, Quinlan GJ, Mitchell J, et al. (1998) Production of nitric oxide during surgery involving cardiopulmonary bypass. Crit Care Med 26:272–278.

34. Finkel MS, Oddis CV, Jacob TD, et al. (1992) Negative inotropic effects of cytokines on the heart mediated by nitric oxide. Science 257:387–389.

35. Tseng EE, Brock MV, Lange MS, et al. (1997) Neuronal nitric oxide synthase inhibition reduces neuronal apoptosis after hypothermic circulatory arrest. Ann Thorac Surg 64:1639–1647.

36. Hayashi Y, Sawa Y, Nishimura M, et al. (2000) P-selectin participates in cardiopulmonary bypass-induced inflammatory response in association with nitric oxide and peroxynitrite production. J Thorac Cardiovasc Surg 120:558–565.

37. Kozik DJ, Tweddell JS (2006) Characterizing the inflammatory response to cardiopulmonary bypass in children. Ann Thorac Surg 81:S2347–S2354.

38. Seghaye MC, Grabitz RG, Duchateau J, et al. (1996) Inflammatory reaction and capillary leak syndrome related to cardiopulmonary bypass in neonates undergoing cardiac operations. J Thorac Cardiovasc Surg 112:687–697.

39. Marshall JC (2001) Inflammation, coagulopathy, and the pathogenesis of multiple organ dysfunction syndrome. Crit Care Med 29 (7 Suppl):S99–S106.

40. Hennein HA, Ebba H, Rodriguez JL, et al. (1994) Relationship of the proinflammatory cytokines to myocardial ischemia and dysfunction after uncomplicated coronary revascularization. J Thorac Cardiovasc Surg 108:626–635.

41. Deng MC, Dasch B, Erren M, et al. (1996) Impact of left ventricular dysfunction on cytokines, hemodynamics and outcome in bypass grafting. Ann Thorac Surg 62:184–190.

42. Hammer S, Loeff M, Reichenspurner H, et al. (2001) Effect of cardiopulmonary bypass on myocardial function, damage and inflammation after cardiac surgery in newborns and children. Thorac Cardiovasc Surg 49:349–354.

43. Gilliland HE, Armstrong MA, McMurray TJ (1999) The inflammatory response to pediatric cardiac surgery: correlation of granulocyte adhesion molecule expression with postoperative oxygenation. Anesth Analg 89:1188–1191.

44. Hauser GJ, Ben-Ari J, Colvin MP, et al. (1998) Interleukin-6 levels in serum and lung lavage fluid of children undergoing open heart surgery correlate with postoperative morbidity. Intensive Care Med 24:481–486.

45. Westaby S, Saatvedt K, White S, et al. Is there a relationship between cognitive dysfunction and systemic inflammatory response after cardiopulmonary bypass? Ann Thorac Surg 71:667–672.

46. Nguyen DN, Spapen H, Su F, et al. (2006) Elevated serum levels of S-100β protein and neuron-specific enolase are associated with brain injury in patients with severe sepsis and septic shock. Crit Care Med 34:1967–1974.

47. Hsu AA, Fenton K, Weistein S, et al. (2008) Neurologic injury markers in children with septic shock. Pediatr Crit Care Med 9:245–251.

48. Picca S, Principato F, Mazerra E, et al. (1995) Risks of acute renal failure after cardiopulmonary bypass surgery in children: a retrospective 10-year case-control study. Nephrol Dial Transplant 10:630–636.

49. Halm HA (1996) Acute gastrointestinal complications after cardiac surgery. Am J Crit Care 5:109–120.

50. Masai T, Sawa Y, Ohtake S, et al. (2002) Hepatic dysfunction after left ventricular mechanical assist in patients with end-stage heart failure: role of inflammatory response and hepatic microcirculation. Ann Thorac Surg 73:549–555.

51. Hennein HA (2001) Inflammation after cardiopulmonary bypass: therapy for the postpump syndrome. Semin Cardiothorac Vasc Anesth 5:236–255.

52. Lequier LL, Nikaidoh H, Leonard SR, et al. (2000) Preoperative and postoperative endotoxemia in children with congenital heart disease. Chest 117:1706–1712.

53. Martinez-Pellus AE, Merino P, Bru M, et al. (1997) Endogenous endotoxemia of intestinal origin during cardiopulmonary bypass. Role of type of flow and protective effect of selective digestive decontamination. Intensive Care Med 23:1251–1257.

54. Mollhoff T, Loick HM, Van Aken H, et al. (1999) Milrinone modulates endotoxemia, systemic inflammation, and subsequent acute phase response after cardiopulmonary bypass. Anesthesiology 90:72–80.

55. Bonser RS, Dave JR, Davies ET, et al. (1990) Reduction of complement activation during bypass by prime manipulation. Ann Thorac Surg 49:279–283.

56. Mou SS, Giroir BP, Molitor-Kirsch E, et al. (2004) Fresh whole blood versus reconstituted blood for pump priming in heart surgery in infants. N Engl J Med 351:1635–1644.

57. Avall A, Hyllner M, Bengtson JP, et al. (1997) Postoperative inflammatory response after autologous and allogeneic blood transfusion. Anesthesiology 87:511–516.

58. Muylle L, Joos M, Wouters E, et al. (1993) Increased tumor necrosis factor α (TNFα), Interleukin-1, and interleukin-6 (IL-6) levels in the plasma of stored platelet concentrates: relationship between TNFα and IL-6 levels and febrile transfusion reactions. Transfusion 33:195–199.

59. Whitten CW, Hill GE, Ivy R, et al. (1998) Does the duration of cardiopulmonary bypass or aortic cross-clamp, in the absence of blood/or blood product administration, influence the IL-6 response to cardiac surgery? Anesth Analg 86:28–33.

60. Koch CG, Li L, Sessler DI, et al. (2008) Duration of red cell storage and complications after cardiac surgery. N Engl J Med 358:1229–1239.

61. Nilsson L, Tyden H, Johansson O, et al. (1990) Bubble and membrane oxygenators-comparison of postoperative organ dysfunction with special reference to inflammatory activity. Scand J Thorac Cardiovasc Surg 24:59–64.

62. Gillinov AM, Bator JM, Zehr KJ, et al. (1993) Neutrophil adhesion molecule expression during cardiopulmonary bypass with bubble and membrane oxygenators. Ann Thorac Surg 56:847–853.

63. Ashraf SS, Tian Y, Cowan D, et al. (1997) Proinflammatory cytokine release during pediatric cardiopulmonary bypass: influence of centrifugal and roller pumps. J Thorac Cardiovasc Anesth 11:718–722.

64. Hornick P, Taylor K (1997) Pulsatile and nonpulsatile perfusion: the continuing controversy. J Cardiothorac Vasc Anesth 11:310–315.

65. Menasche P, Haydar S, Peynet J, et al. (1994) A potential mechanism of vasodilation after warm heart surgery. The temperature-dependent release of cytokines. J Thorac Cardiovasc Surg 107:293–299.

66. El Habbal MH, Carter H, Smith LJ, et al. (1995) Neutrophil activation in pediatric extracorporeal circuits: effect of circulation and temperature variation. Cardiovasc Res 29:102–107.

67. Qing M, Vazquez-Jimenez JF, Klosterhalfen B, et al. (2001) Influence of temperature during cardiopulmonary bypass on leukocyte activation, cytokine balance, and postoperative organ dysfunction. Shock 15:372–377.

68. Frering B, Philip I, Dehoux M, et al. (1994) Circulating cytokines in patients undergoing normothermic cardiopulmonary bypass. J Thorac Cardiovasc Surg 108:636–641.

69. Birdi I, Caputo M, Underwood M, et al. (1999) The effects of cardiopulmonary bypass temperature on inflammatory response following cardiopulmonary bypass. Eur J Cardiothorac Surg 16:540–545.

70. Eggum R, Ueland T, Mollnes T, et al. (2008) Effect of perfusion temperature on the inflammatory response during pediatric cardiac surgery. Ann Thorac Surg 85:611–617.

71. Redmond JM, Gillinov AM, Stuart RS, et al. (1993) Heparin-coated bypass circuits reduce pulmonary injury. Ann Thorac Surg 56:474–479.

72. Ashraf S, Tian Y, Cowan D, et al. (1997) Release of proinflammatory cytokines during pediatric cardiopulmonary

bypass: heparin-bonded versus nonbonded oxygenators. Ann Thorac Surg 64:1790–1794.

73. Schreurs HH, Wijers MJ, Gu YJ, et al. (1998) Heparin-coated bypass circuits: inflammatory response in pediatric cardiac operations. Ann Thorac Surg 66:166–171.

74. Ozawa T, Yoshihara K, Koyama N, et al. (2000) Clinical efficacy of heparin-bonded bypass circuits related to cytokine responses in children. Ann Thorac Surg 69:584–590.

75. Baufreton C, Moczar M, Intrator L, et al. (1998) Inflammatory response to cardiopulmonary bypass using two different types of heparin-coated extracorporeal circuits. Perfusion 13:419–427.

76. Morioka K, Muraoka R, Chiba Y, et al. (1996) Leukocyte and platelet depletion with a blood cell separator: effects on lung injury after cardiac surgery with cardiopulmonary bypass. J Thorac Cardiovasc Surg 111:45–54.

77. Chiba Y, Morioka K, Muraoka R, et al. (1998) Effects of depletion of leukocytes and platelets on cardiac dysfunction after cardiopulmonary bypass. Ann Thorac Surg 65:107–114.

78. Journois D, Pouard P, Greeley WJ, et al. (1994) Hemofiltration during cardiopulmonary bypass in pediatric cardiac surgery. Effects on hemostasis, cytokines, and complement components. Anesthesiology 81:1181–1189.

79. Hennein HA, Kiziltepe U, Barst S, et al. (1999) Venovenous modified ultrafiltration after cardiopulmonary bypass in children: a prospective randomized study. J Thorac Cardiovasc Surg 117:496–505.

80. Bokesch PM, Kapural MB, Mossad EB, et al. (2000) Do peritoneal catheters remove proinflammatory cytokines after cardiopulmonary bypass in neonates? Ann Thorac Surg 70:639–643.

81. Larsen B, Hoff G, Wilhelm W, et al. (1998) Effects of intravenous anesthetics on spontaneous and endotoxin-stimulated cytokine response in cultured human whole blood. Anesthesiology 89:1218–1227.

82. Trapnell JE, Rigby CC, Talbot CH, et al. (1974) A controlled trial of trasylol in the treatment of acute pancreatitis. Br J Surg 61:177–182.

83. Chauhan S, Kumar BA, Rao BH, et al. (2000) Efficacy of aprotinin, epsilon aminocaproic acid, or combination in cyanotic heart disease. Ann Thorac Surg 70:1308–1312.

84. Miller BE, Tosone SR, Tam VK, et al. (1998) Hematologic and economic impact of aprotinin in reoperative pediatric cardiac operations. Ann Thorac Surg 66:535–541.

85. Scheule AM, Beierlein W, Wendel HP, et al. (1998) Fibrin sealant, aprotinin, and immune response in children undergoing operations for congenital heart disease. J Thorac Cardiovasc Surg 115:883–889.

86. Buerke M, Pruefer D, Sankat D, et al. (2007) Effects of Aprotinin on Gene expression and protein synthesis after ischemia and reperfusion in rats. Circulation 116 (Suppl I):I-121–I-126.

87. Hill Ge, Taylor JA, Robbins RA (1997) Differing effects of aprotinin and epsilon aminocaproic acid on cytokine-induced inducible nitric oxide synthase expression. Ann Thorac Surg 63:74–77.

88. Mojcik CF, Levy JH (2001) Aprotinin and the systemic inflammatory response after cardiopulmonary bypass. Ann Thorac Surg 71:745–754.

89. Eaton MP (2008) Antifibrinolytic therapy in surgery for congenital heart disease. Anesth Analg 106:1087–1100.

90. Mangano DT, Tudor IC, Dietzel C (2006) The risk associated with Aprotinin in cardiac surgery. N Engl J Med 354:353–365.

91. Backer CL, Kelle AM, Stewart RD, et al. (2007) Aprotinin is safe in pediatric patients undergoing cardiac surgery. J Thorac Cardiovasc Surg 134:1421–1428.

92. Szekely A, Sapi E, Breuer T, et al. (2008) Aprotinin and renal dysfunction after pediatric cardiac surgery. Pediatr Anesth 18:151–159.

93. Niazi Z, Flodin P, Joyce L, et al. (1979) Effects of glucocorticoids in patients undergoing coronary artery bypass surgery. Chest 76:262–268.

94. Hill GE, Alonso A, Spurzem JR, et al. (1995) Aprotinin and methylprednisolone equally blunt cardiopulmonary bypass-induced inflammation in humans. J Thorac Cardiovasc Surg 110:1658–1662.

95. Tassani P, Richter JA, Barankay A, et al. (1999) Does high-dose methylprednisolone in aprotinin-treated patients attenuate the systemic inflammatory response during coronary artery bypass grafting procedures? J Cardiothorac Vasc Anesth 13:165–172.

96. Butler J, Pathi VL, Paton RD, et al. (1996) Acute-phase responses to cardiopulmonary bypass in children weighing less than 10 kilograms. Ann Thorac Surg 62:538–542.

97. Lodge AJ, Chai PJ, William-Daggett C, et al. (1999) Methylprednisolone reduces the inflammatory response to cardiopulmonary bypass in neonatal piglets: timing of dose is important. J Thorac Cardiovasc Surg 117:515–522.

98. Bronicki RA, Backer CL, Baden HP, et al. (2000) Dexamethasone reduces the inflammatory response to cardiopulmonary bypass in children. Ann Thorac Surg 69:1490–1495.

99. Mossad E, Appachi E, Kapural M, et al. (2000) Effects of methylprednisolone on the inflammatory response to cardiopulmonary bypass in children. Anesth Analg 90:SCA 28.

100. Langley SM, Chai PJ, Jaggers JJ, et al. (2000) Preoperative high dose methylprednisolone attenuates the cerebral response to deep hypothermic circulatory arrest. Eur J Cardiothorac Surg 17:279–286.

101. Volk T, Schmutzler M, Engelhardt L, et al. (2001) Influence of aminosteroid and glucocorticoid treatment on inflammation and immune function during cardiopulmonary bypass. Crit Care Med 29:2137–2142.

102. Mott AR, Fraser CD, Kusnoor AV, et al. (2001) The effect of short-term prophylactic methylprednisolone on the incidence and severity of postpericardiotomy syndrome in children undergoing cardiac surgery with cardiopulmonary bypass. J Am Coll Cardiol 37:1700–1706.

103. Varan B, Tokel K, Mercan S, et al. (2002) Systemic inflammatory response related to cardiopulmonary bypass and its

modification by methylprednisolone: high dose versus low dose. Pediatr Cardiol 23:437–441.

104. Shum-Tim D, Tchervenkov CL, Laliberte E, et al. (2003) Timing of steroid treatment is important for cerebral protection during cardiopulmonary bypass and circulatory arrest: minimal protection of pump prime methylprednisolone. Eur J Cardiothorac Surg 24:125–132.

105. Schroeder VA, Pearl JM, Schwartz SM, et al. (2003) Combined steroid treatment for congenital heart surgery improves oxygen delivery and reduces postbypass inflammatory mediator expression. Circulation 107:2823–2828.

106. Gessler P, Hohl V, Carrel T, et al. (2005) Administration of steroids in pediatric cardiac surgery: impact on clinical outcome and systemic inflammatory response. Pediatr Cardiol 26:595–600.

107. Santos AR, Heidemann SM, Walters III HL, et al. (2007) Effect of inhaled corticosteroid on pulmonary injury and inflammatory mediator production after cardiopulmonary bypass in children. Pediatr Crit Care Med 8:465–469.

108. Checchia PA, Bronicki RA, Costello JM, et al. (2005) Steroid use before pediatric cardiac operations using cardiopulmonary bypass: An international survey of 36 centers. Pediatr Crit Care Med 6:442–445.

109. Morariu AM, Loef BG, Aarts LPJ, et al. (2005) Dexamethason: benefits and prejudice for patients undergoing coronary artery bypass grafting: a study on myocardial, pulmonary, renal, intestinal and hepatic injury. Chest 128:2677–2687.

110. Dinarello CA, Gelfand JA, Wolff SM (1993) Anticytokine strategies in the treatment of systemic inflammatory response. JAMA 269:1829–1835.

111. Gillinov AM, Redmond JM, Zehr KJ, et al. (1994) Inhibition of neutrophil adhesion during cardiopulmonary bypass. Ann Thorac Surg 57:126–133.

112. Muira T, Nelson DP, Schermerhorn ML, et al. (1996) Blockade of selectin-mediated leukocyte adhesion improves postischemic function in lamb hearts. Ann Thorac Surg 62:1295–1300.

113. Nagashima M, Shin'oka T, Nollert G, et al. (1998) Effects of a monoclonal antibody to P-selectin on recovery of neonatal lamb hearts after cold cardioplegic ischemia. Circulation 98 (Suppl II):II391–II397.

114. Fitch JCK, Rollins S, Matis L, et al. (1999) Pharmacology and biologic efficacy of a recombinant, humanized, single chain antibody C5 complement inhibitor in patients undergoing coronary artery bypass graft surgery with cardiopulmonary bypass. Circulation 100:2499–2506.

115. Gott JP, Cooper WA, Schmidt FE, et al. (1998) Modifying risk for extracorporeal circulation: trial of four antiinflammatory strategies. Ann Thorac Surg 66:747–754.

116. Tarnok A, Hambsch J, Emmrich F, et al. (1999) Complement activation, cytokines, and adhesion molecules in children undergoing cardiac surgery with or without cardiopulmonary bypass. Pediatr Cardiol 20:113–125.

117. Ascione R, Lloyd CT, Underwood MJ, et al. (2000) Inflammatory response after coronary revascularization with or without cardiopulmonary bypass. Ann Thorac Surg 69:1198–1204.

118. Harmoinen A, Kaukinen L, Porkkala T, et al. (2006) Off-pump surgery does not eliminate microalbuminuria or other markers of systemic inflammatory response to coronary artery bypass surgery. Scand Cardiovasc J 40:110–116.

119. Kapadia S, Dibbs Z, Kurrelmeyer K, et al. (1998) The role of cytokines in the failing heart. Cardiol Clin 16:645–656.

120. Appachi E, Mossad E, Mee RBB, et al. (2007) Perioperative serum interleukins in neonates with hypoplastic left heart syndrome and transposition of the great arteries. J Cardiothorac Vasc Anesth 21:184–190.

121. Rao AK, Sheth S, Kaplan R (1997) Inherited hypercoagulable states. Vasc Med 2:313–320.

122. Feuerstein GZ, Wang X, Barone FC (1997) Inflammatory gene expression in cerebral ischemia and trauma: potential new therapeutic targets. Ann N Y Acad Sci 825:179–193.

123. Tsubota S, Adachi N, Chen J, et al. (1999) Dexamethasone changes brain monoamine metabolism and aggravates ischemic neuronal damage in rats. Anesthesiology 90:515–523.

124. O'Shea TM, Kothadia JM, Klinepeter KL, et al. (1999) Randomized placebo-controlled trial of a 42-day tapering course of dexamethasone to reduce the duration of ventilator dependency in very low birth weight infants: outcome of study participants at 1-year adjusted age. Pediatrics 104:15–21.

125. Gillinov AM, Redmond JM, Winkelstein JA, et al. (1994) Complement and neutrophil activation during cardiopulmonary bypass: a study in the complement-deficient dog. Ann Thorac Surg 57:345–352.

126. Williams MA, Withington S, Newland AC, et al. (1998) Monocyte anergy in septic shock is associated with a predilection to apoptosis and is reversed by granulocyte-macrophage colony-stimulating factor ex-vivo. J Infect Dis 178:1421–1433.

127. Miles MP. (2008) How do we solve the puzzle of unintended consequences of inflammation? Systematically. J Appl Physiol 105:1023–1025.

2 Monitoring

9 Vascular access and monitoring

Dean B. Andropoulos, M.D., M.H.C.M.
Texas Children's Hospital, Baylor College of Medicine, Houston, TX, USA

Introduction

Hemodynamic assessment and treatment through invasive access to the circulation is crucial for every patient undergoing surgery for congenital cardiac disease. Secure, reliable venous and arterial access is necessary for accurate beat-to-beat monitoring of pressures and waveforms, and frequent sampling for blood gases, hematocrit, coagulation studies, and metabolic parameters. In this manner pathophysiologic processes associated with the patient's underlying disease or the surgical procedure can be detected and treated as early as possible, with the goal of lessening morbidity. Central venous access is critical to directly infuse vasoactive medications and to deliver bolus drugs to achieve the desired hemodynamic effects in as short a time as possible. Large bore peripheral

Anesthesia for Congenital Heart Disease 2nd edition. Edited by
Dean Andropoulos, Stephen Stayer, Isobel Russell and Emad Mossad.
© 2010 Blackwell Publishing.

venous access is important to infuse crystalloids, colloids, and blood products with minimal resistance to flow. All of these procedures may be technically difficult, time consuming, and have significant morbidity, especially in newborns or small infants who comprise an increasingly large portion of the patients presenting for surgery. Meticulous attention to the details of vascular access by the pediatric cardiac anesthesiologist can maximize the benefits and minimize the risks to the patient. This chapter reviews the techniques of vascular access in congenital cardiac surgery patients, emphasizing newer imaging modalities to guide successful placement, and strategies to avoid complications.

Venous access

Peripheral veins

Any visible peripheral vein, and many that are not visible, may be utilized for peripheral venous access. One strategy in pediatric cardiac patients is to cannulate a small superficial vein on the hand or foot with a small catheter (24 or 22 ga) before induction, or during inhalation induction of anesthesia to facilitate the early administration of muscle relaxants and provide expeditious airway management. Later, with the airway secure and with an immobile patient, larger bore peripheral venous access can be achieved. Recommended sizes are 22 ga 1″ catheters for infants newborn through 6 months, 20 ga 1.25″ catheters for 6 months to 3 years, 18 ga 1.5″ for 3–12 years, and 16 or 14 ga 2″ catheters for teenage or adult patients. Resistance to fluid flow predicted by Poiseuille's law is proportional to the length of the catheter and the viscosity of the fluid, and inversely proportional to the fourth power of the catheter radius. When rapidly infusing the more viscous colloids or packed red blood cells, it is important to use a large bore, short catheter in a large peripheral vein. Central venous catheters (CVCs) are usually less desirable for this use due to their smaller lumens and much longer lengths.

Any unusual resistance to infusion through a peripheral intravenous catheter must be immediately investigated. If the catheter is inaccessible, immediately change to a functioning catheter to avoid extravasation. Caustic or vasoactive substances, e.g., calcium chloride, dopamine, and epinephrine, should not be injected through peripheral veins unless no other alternative exists. Because of the risk of extravasation and tissue necrosis, such drugs should all be injected centrally.

The saphenous vein at the ankle is large and in a constant anatomic position in patients of all ages. It can usually be cannulated even if it cannot be seen or palpated. A recommended technique is to apply a tourniquet below the knee, prepare the site antiseptically, and extend the ankle at the medial malleolus with one hand while puncturing the skin at a shallow angle of 10–30° with an angiocatheter 0.5–1 cm anterior and 1 cm inferior to the medial malleolus. Advance the catheter slowly in the groove between the malleolus and the tibialis tendon until blood return through the needle is established. Advance the needle and catheter together several millimeters, then advance the catheter over the needle into the vein with the index finger of the same hand that made the skin puncture, while maintaining extension of the ankle so that the saphenous vein is tethered straight in its course, to minimize the possibility of puncturing the posterior wall due to kinking of the vein. If the vein can be entered but the catheter will not advance its full length into the vein, a small flexible guidewire of 0.015″ or 0.018″ may be used to assist in cannulation of the saphenous or any other peripheral vein [1]. Other large peripheral veins may be found in infants and children on the dorsum of the hand, at the wrist superficial to the radial head, as branches of the cephalic or brachial venous system in the antecubital fossa, or on the dorsolateral aspect of the foot. The latter site is especially prominent in many newborns.

The external jugular vein is almost always visible in infants and children undergoing cardiac surgery, and is often enlarged and easily cannulated due to elevated right heart pressures. A recommended technique is to choose the larger external jugular vein, place a small rolled towel under the shoulders and place the patient in 30° Trendelenburg position, prepare the site antiseptically, and have an assistant compress the vein gently with pressure just above the clavicle to further distend it. Rotation of the head 45–90° away from the side of cannulation and slight extension of the neck and traction of the skin over the vein with one hand will tether the vein into a straighter course to facilitate successful cannulation. The vein is punctured high in its visible course with an angiocatheter attached to a syringe filled with heparinized saline, and with the needle bent upward 10–20° to facilitate the very flat, superficial angle of incidence necessary to cannulate the vein without puncturing its back wall. With constant, gentle aspiration of the syringe, the vein is entered and catheter advanced into the vein. Short peripheral catheters of the same size as recommended above should be used. A catheter advanced too far into the venous plexus beneath the clavicle will often exhibit resistance to the free, gravity driven, flow of fluid, and traction or withdrawal of the catheter a few millimeters may be necessary. External jugular catheters are often difficult to secure to the skin on the neck, and suturing them in place is recommended. This will enhance stability postoperatively as the patient begins moving. One advantage of using the external jugular vein for a peripheral venous catheter is that it is easily accessible under the surgical drapes, and can be frequently monitored for extravasation or kinking of the catheter, which is more common with this site than with the other commonly used peripheral veins.

Umbilical vein

The umbilical vein in the fetus is a conduit to carry oxygenated and detoxified blood from the placenta, through the abdominal wall, the liver, and patent ductus venosus to the inferior vena cava (IVC) and the right atrium (RA) [2] (Figure 9.1). This vessel can usually be cannulated at the umbilical stump for the first 3–5 days of postnatal life. Passage into the IVC depends on the patency of the ductus venosus, which often exists for the first few days, just as the ductus arteriosus. Sterile technique without a guidewire is used to pass the catheter blindly a premeasured distance. If no resistance to passage is met and free blood return is achieved, the catheter tip is usually in the high IVC or RA, and functions as a CVC. Catheter tip position must be determined by radiography as soon as possible to determine if it is through the ductus venosus

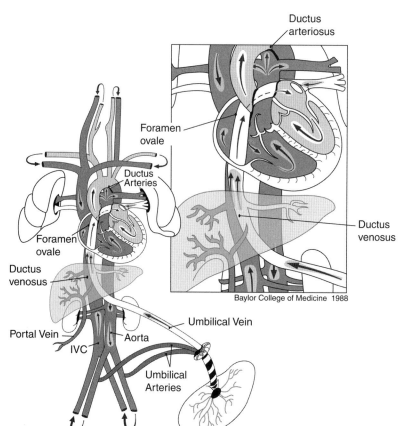

Baylor College of Medicine 1988

Figure 9.1 The fetal circulation. A catheter placed in the umbilical vein should have its tip through the ductus venosus into the inferior vena cava at or near its junction with the right atrium. The tip of an umbilical artery catheter should lie at the level of the third lumbar vertebral body, between the origin of the renal arteries and the bifurcation of the aorta (Used with permission from Reference [2])

into the IVC or the RA. Often the ductus venosus is not patent, and the catheter tip passes into branches of the hepatic veins, and is visible in the liver radiographically. In this location, the catheter must not be used except for emergencies. Central venous pressure (CVP) monitoring is inaccurate in this position, and portal vein thrombosis, liver, and intestinal necrosis can occur with the infusion of hyperosmolar or vasoactive drugs such as sodium bicarbonate and dopamine. An alternative site for central access must be chosen.

Recently, 5 Fr double and triple-lumen umbilical venous catheters (UVC) have become available [3,4]. The multiple lumens allow concomitant CVP monitoring, vasoactive infusions, and a large 18 ga lumen for volume infusion. If a single-lumen 5 Fr UVC is present preoperatively, it can be exchanged in the operating room for a triple-lumen catheter using a 70–80 cm long, 0.018″ or 0.021″ guidewire.

Every neonate with cardiac disease for whom surgery is planned in the first two weeks of life should have a multilumen UVC placed as soon as possible, before the ductus venosus closes. The umbilical vein is a central venous access site that is easily cannulated, will not be available for subsequent interventions, and will reduce the time required for vascular access in the operating room. Most importantly, other sites will be spared, i.e., femoral,

jugular, and subclavian veins will not be exposed to the risk of thrombosis and permanent occlusion. This complication in the neonate carries a high rate of morbidity and mortality. UVC cannulation is especially important for patients with planned multiple interventions such as single-ventricle patients, who often require at least two cardiac catheterizations and two additional surgeries. A UVC can be left in place for as long as 14 days if no complications are suspected. When the umbilical vein is utilized, transthoracic right atrial catheters with their attendant risks of bleeding and pericardial or pleural effusions may be avoided.

Percutaneous central venous access

Percutaneous central venous access is the standard approach in many cardiac surgery programs [5]. We recommend using a double-lumen central line of the smallest acceptable size for percutaneous CVC placement. For all sites, either audio Doppler or two-dimensional ultrasound is used to facilitate insertion. The larger distal lumen is used for CVP monitoring and drug injection, and the smaller proximal lumen for vasoactive infusions. The smallest available double-lumen catheter is currently 4 Fr in size. Superior vena cava (SVC) catheters should be used

PART 2 Monitoring

Table 9.1 Recommended central venous catheter sizes and lengths

Patient weight (kg)	Internal Jugular/ subclavian vein	Femoral vein
<10	4 Fr, 2 lumen, 8 cm	4 Fr, 2 lumen, 12 cm
10–30	4 Fr, 2 lumen, 12 cm	4 Fr, 2 lumen, 12–15 cm
30–50	5 Fr, 2 lumen, 12–15 cm	5 Fr, 2 lumen, 15 cm
50–70	7 Fr, 2 lumen, 15 cm	7 Fr, 2 lumen, 20 cm
>70	8 Fr, 2 lumen, 16 cm	8 Fr, 2 lumen 20 cm

with caution or not at all in patients weighing less than 4 kg because of the increased risk of thrombosis (see section on "Complications of Vascular Access"). Recommended sizes and lengths are shown in Table 9.1.

Sterile technique using gown and wide draping leads to a "cleaner" insertion technique with fewer infectious complications [6]. In cardiac patients, the left side SVC lines should generally be avoided. The risk of erosion/perforation is greater, and 5–15% of patients with congenital cardiac disease have a persistent left SVC, which most often drains to either coronary sinus or the left atrium, neither of which is a desirable location for a catheter tip. So, if left-sided line placement is contemplated, ascertain by echo/cath report presence of left SVC. If this is not known, choose an alternate site, i.e., femoral or intracardiac.

The following general discussion of the Seldinger technique in pediatric patients can be applied to all percutaneous vascular access sites, either venous or arterial. The Seldinger technique is used for all percutaneous central venous cannulations. After wide sterile skin preparation with iodine or chlorhexidine-based solution, wide draping is carried out, preferably with a clear, fluid impermeable adhesive aperture drape so that the underlying anatomy is clearly visible. Slow, controlled, careful needle manipulation, especially in small infants, must be emphasized. The slight movement in or out of only 1 mm or less may be enough to prevent passage of the guidewire. It is very important to have the guidewire prepared to insert and immediately accessible when the vein is entered, so the anesthesiologist does not have to look away from the puncture site to reach for the wire on a distant tray, often resulting in enough movement of the needle to prevent successful guidewire passage. After the desired vein is entered, the needle position is fixed by stabilizing it against the patient's body with the heel of nondominant hand, and the guidewire is carefully advanced into the RA. The resistance to wire passage should be minimal. Experienced operators learn to recognize the "feel" of a guidewire passing successfully. If any resistance is encountered, the wire must be carefully withdrawn, and another approach made if the needle is still in the vessel, ascertained by free aspiration of blood. Forcing a guidewire in the face of resistance

can lead to significant complications. The electrocardiogram (ECG) should be carefully observed as the guidewire is slowly advanced. Premature atrial contractions (PACs) are usually observed as the first guidewire-induced dysrhythmia, signifying atrial location. If no PACs are observed, the operator should suspect that the guidewire is not in the atrium. If ventricular extrasystoles are the first observed dysrhythmia, especially if they are multifocal in nature, the wire is very likely in an artery, and the left ventricle has been entered retrograde. The wire must be withdrawn immediately, or the position ascertained by imaging, e.g., transesophageal echocardiography (TEE). In difficult or questionable cases, TEE may be utilized to visualize the guidewire, and this is strongly recommended before the passage of a vessel dilator or the catheter. After guidewire passage, a very small skin incision with a #11 scalpel is made. Finally, careful dilation and catheter passage follows. The dilators in the prepackaged CVC kits are often one size larger than the catheter, i.e., 5 Fr dilator for 4 Fr catheter. This may be undesirable for small infants, and either passage of the catheter without dilation, or use of a dilator the same size as the catheter is preferable to make the smallest possible hole in the vein to minimize bleeding and trauma to the vessel wall, both of which may lead to an increased incidence of thrombosis or vascular insufficiency. Meticulous attention must be paid to blood loss in small infants during catheterization procedures, with direct compression of bleeding puncture sites using the heel of the nondominant hand, while threading dilators, catheters, etc. Use of an assistant may be necessary in difficult catheterizations. After passage of the catheter to the desired depth, it is secured with sutures and a dressing. If more than 1 cm of catheter is outside the patient, additional suturing or catheter holding devices are necessary.

Internal jugular vein

The right internal jugular vein (IJV) is the most common site chosen for central venous access in pediatric cardiac surgery. It is large, and runs in close proximity superficial to the carotid artery along most of its length. The primary advantage of using the IJV is that it provides a direct route to RA, and thus a high rate of optimal catheter positioning if the vessel can be cannulated. Various studies report only a 0–2% incidence of catheter tip outside the thorax, in contrast to the subclavian route [7,8]. The primary disadvantage comes from difficulty in cannulation in small infants, who have large heads and short necks, and thus difficulty in obtaining the shallow angle of approach necessary to access the vessel. Also some series report a 10–15% incidence of carotid artery puncture in infants and ultrasound studies of neck vessel anatomy reveal the partial or complete overlap of the IJV anterior to the carotid artery [8]. This site is also not comfortable

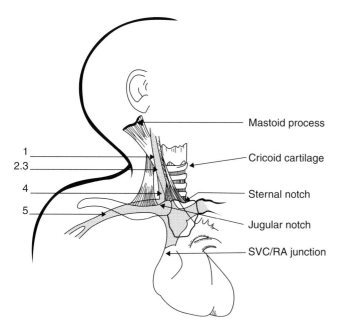

Figure 9.2 Sites for central venous cannulation of the superior vena cava. 1: high approach, midway between mastoid process and sternal notch; 2,3: middle approach using apex of muscular triangle or cricoid cartilage; 4: low approach using jugular notch; 5: lateral approach to subclavian venipuncture (Used with permission from Reference [12])

for some awake infants, and tip migration may be significant with turning the head or flexion/extension of the neck [9]. All insertion techniques involve placing a small roll under the shoulders, using steep Trendelenburg position, and rotating the head no more than 45° to the left. Greater rotation will produce more overlap of the IJV and carotid artery, and increase the risk of carotid puncture [10]. Recent studies have demonstrated that liver compression and simulated Valsalva maneuver also increase the diameter of the IJV, possibly increasing the success rate of cannulation [11].

There are numerous approaches to the IJV, some of which are described here (Figure 9.2):

1 Muscular "Triangle" method: puncture at top of junction where the sternal and clavicular heads of the sternomastoid muscle meet, lateral to carotid impulse, directing the needle at ipsilateral nipple. These landmarks are often not well defined in infants.

2 Puncture exactly halfway along a line between the mastoid process and the sternal notch, just lateral to the carotid impulse.

3 Use the cricoid ring as a landmark, and puncture just lateral to carotid impulse.

4 Jugular notch technique: puncture just lateral to carotid impulse, just above the jugular notch on medial clavicle—a low approach.

An ultrasound technique (see below) should be used to clearly identify the course of the vessel and to detect any

significant overlap with the carotid artery. There is no need to use a finder needle for small catheters, where access needle is 20 ga or smaller. Surface landmarks are often inaccurate for estimating the correct depth of insertion for SVC lines, i.e., locating the tip midway between the sternal notch and nipple. (See discussion below for method to ascertain the correct placement for all sites.)

Subclavian vein

The subclavian vein is positioned immediately behind the medial third of the clavicle [13, 14]. Advantages of this route include the subclavian vein's relatively constant position in all ages in reference to surface landmarks, stability and less tip migration with patient movement, and comfort for the awake patient [15, 16]. Disadvantages include an incidence of pneumothorax, especially with an inexperienced operator, and an occasional inability to dilate the space between the clavicle and first rib. Also in 5–20% of patient, subclavian catheters will enter the contralateral brachiocephalic vein or ipsilateral IJV, instead of the SVC [17].

Technique: a small rolled towel is positioned vertically between the scapulae, steep Trendelenburg position used, and the arms are restrained in neutral position at the patient's sides. This position maximizes the length of subclavian vein overlapping the clavicle, and moves the vein anterior, bringing it in close proximity to the posterior surface of the clavicle [11]. The right subclavian vein should always be the first choice (see below). Turn the head toward the side being punctured (i.e., toward right for right-sided line). This position will compress the IJV on that side and prevent the guidewire from entering it, especially in infants [18], which may lead to complications such as dural sinus thrombosis [19]. It will not, however, prevent the guidewire from crossing the midline and entering the contralateral brachiocephalic vein [18]. The needle is bent upward in mid shaft at a 10–20° angle to assure a very shallow course. In our experience, the puncture site that is most successful is 1–2 cm lateral to the midpoint of the clavicle [11], directly lateral from the sternal notch, with the needle directed at the sternal notch. Contact the clavicle first to assure shallow angle of incidence to minimize the risk of pneumothorax. Then, the needle is "walked" carefully underneath the clavicle and advanced slowly with constant aspiration until blood return is achieved. Advancing the needle only during expiration is recommended to minimize the risk of pneumothorax. Having an assistant manually ventilate the patient will facilitate this process. If not successful, the needle is withdrawn slowly with gentle aspiration, because about 50% of infant subclavian veins are cannulated during withdrawal due to compression or kinking of the vein during needle advancement. Slow, controlled, careful needle manipulation, especially in small infants, must be emphasized. After the vein is entered, advance the guidewire; there should be no resistance. Look for PACs, sometimes only one or two, as a sign that the wire is in the heart. If no dysrhythmias are seen, withdraw the wire, rotate it 90° clockwise, and advance it again until PACs are seen. Use a dilator (be very careful not to advance it too far, only far enough to expand the space between the clavicle and first rib) and pass the catheter to the desired depth using one of the guidelines noted below.

Complications during subclavian catheterization occur when a needle angle of incidence is too cephalad, resulting in arterial puncture, or too posterior, resulting in pneumothorax. If the needle course remains shallow, just underneath the clavicle, and directed straight horizontally at the sternal notch, complications are rare. Advancing the needle too far in infants may result in puncture of the trachea.

External jugular vein

Advantages of this approach are its superficial location and thus low risk of arterial puncture. Disadvantage is that the younger the patient, the less likely the guidewire will pass into the atrium; the success rate is less than 50% if the patient is younger than 1 year, and only 59% in patients younger than 5 years [20,21]. Positioning is the same as the internal jugular approach, the vein is punctured high in its course, and the guidewire is passed. Often it can be observed turning medially toward the SVC. If no resistance is felt, and PACs are seen, or guidewire is visualized on the TEE, then passage has been successful. Because of the low success rate of central cannulation from the external jugular vein approach, our practice is to use the IJV first in all patients.

Femoral vein

The femoral vein has long been used for central venous catheterization in pediatric patients, with no greater infection or other complication rate compared to other sites [22,23]. This is the site of choice for single ventricle patients through the first 6 months of life, because of the increased thrombosis risk with the use of other sites in this population. A successful cavopulmonary connection will depend on a patent SVC circulation to provide over half of their pulmonary blood flow. Thus, SVC thrombosis will lead to inadequate drainage from the upper half of the body to the pulmonary circulation and cause SVC syndrome. The left side is preferred because it avoids the cardiologists' favorite site, the right femoral vein. The single ventricle patient will receive multiple interventions, e.g., catheterizations and surgeries, so preserving vascular patency is extremely important.

Technique: the patient is positioned with a rolled towel under the hips for moderate extension. The puncture site should be 1–2 cm inferior to the inguinal ligament (line from the anterior superior iliac spine to the symphysis pubis), and 0.5–1 cm medial to the femoral artery impulse, with the needle directed at the umbilicus. Ultrasound guidance (see below) is important for the greatest chance for first pass, atraumatic placement. The guidewire is passed, ensuring no resistance. A vessel dilator is used and then the catheter is passed all the way to the hub to position the tip in the mid-IVC. It is important to puncture the vessel well below the inguinal ligament, to minimize the risk of unrecognized retroperitoneal bleeding. Bleeding below the inguinal ligament is easily recognized and treated with direct pressure.

Several studies have conclusively demonstrated that in the absence of increased intra-abdominal pressure or IVC obstruction, mean CVP as measured in the IVC below the diaphragm is identical to that measured in the RA in patients with and without congenital heart disease [24–28]. The only caveat is in the patient with interrupted IVC with azygous vein continuation into the SVC, a condition commonly encountered in patients with the heterotaxy syndromes. The equivalence of IVC and right atrial pressures under these conditions has not been evaluated, but the catheter can be used as any other central line for infusion of drugs and fluids.

Direct transthoracic intracardiac vascular access

These are catheters placed by the surgeon directly into the right or left atrial appendages or upper pulmonary vein and threaded into the left atrium, secured by a purse-string suture [29]. Pulmonary artery (PA) catheters are placed high in the right ventricular outflow tract, through the pulmonary valve, or into the main PA. Some institutions employ continuous mixed venous oxygen saturation monitoring with PA catheters [30]. Transthoracic catheters are usually placed during rewarming on cardiopulmonary bypass. They may be used for pressure monitoring or vasoactive drug infusion. Advantages of this approach include saving time before bypass because percutaneous central lines are not placed, tip location is assured by direct vision, and vessel injury from percutaneous catheters is avoided. Disadvantages are that no central access is available before bypass, which may be important for unstable patients, and there is a low risk of cardiac tamponade when these catheters are removed. For this reason, many institutions do not remove the mediastinal drainage tube postoperatively until the intracardiac lines are removed, or wait 3–5 days, to minimize the risk of bleeding. This limits the lifespan of these lines and may leave the patient without adequate venous access, or may delay discharge from the intensive care unit or hospital while waiting to remove these catheters.

A left atrial catheter is frequently utilized when a degree of postoperative left ventricular dysfunction is anticipated, as in complex newborn surgery such as the arterial switch operation, or after mitral valve surgery. PA catheters are utilized in the face of known significant preoperative and anticipated postoperative pulmonary hypertension, i.e., obstructed total anomalous pulmonary venous return, some complete atrioventricular canal patients, or patients with severe mitral valve disease.

In the largest series reported detailing the use and complications of transthoracic catheters, there was overall a 0.6% incidence of serious complications, defined as significant bleeding or catheter retention out of 6690 transthoracic catheters. This risk was greatest for PA catheters (1.07% with three severe cardiac tamponade and 1 death out of 1680 catheters), followed by left atrial catheters, and then right atrial catheters [29]. More recent reports give similar results, documenting a higher risk of bleeding with platelet count <50,000/L, and a 0.6% incidence of atrial thrombus in out of 523 catheters [31]. To date there are no outcome studies comparing the transthoracic and percutaneous catheters.

Continuous SVC oxygen saturation monitoring after the Norwood operation for hypoplastic left heart syndrome

Continuous monitoring of mixed venous saturation (SvO_2) in the SVC using near infrared oximetric catheters has recently been demonstrated to be very useful in postbypass management of neonates undergoing the Norwood operation for hypoplastic left heart syndrome [32]. Therapy is directed at maintaining SvO_2 at 50% or greater, and when this goal is achieved as part of an overall management strategy, 30-day survival has been greater than 95% in recent reports. $SvO_2 < 30\%$ confers a significant risk of anaerobic metabolism and increased risk for poor outcome.

These catheters are placed by the surgeon transthoracically during rewarming, a short distance into the SVC. They remain in place for 2–5 days, and are removed similar to other transthoracic catheters. Complication rate, e.g., bleeding or thrombosis, has been zero in the series reported thus far.

Tunneled Broviac type percutaneous or intracardiac lines

In patients with difficult venous access who are anticipated to have a prolonged postoperative course, tunneled silicone catheters may be used to ensure necessary access. These can be placed percutaneously in standard fashion,

i.e., in subclavian, jugular, or femoral veins, by cutdown, or placed transthoracically into the RA, as with a standard transthoracic catheter, but with a subcutaneous tunnel placing the skin exit site several centimeters from the chest wall entry site. These catheters often necessitate an additional anesthetic for removal, but in certain patients are cost effective, and preserve other access sites for future interventions, and are less thrombogenic than standard polyurethane transthoracic catheters [33].

Ascertainment of correct position of central venous catheters

Correct placement of CVCs is essential to prevent complications (see below), and to give accurate intravascular pressure information. The tip of a CVC should lie in the SVC, parallel to the vein wall, to minimize the perforation risk. Many authorities recommend placement in the upper half of the SVC, where the tip will be above the pericardial reflection in most patients, thus minimizing the risk of tamponade if perforation occurs [34]. In small patients, the SVC is often short, i.e., 4–5 cm total length, and the pericardium is usually opened during cardiac surgery in these patients, providing drainage in case of perforation. In addition, the risk of arrhythmias is present as well with a catheter positioned in the RA. Various methods to determine correct placement are discussed below.

Radiography

The chest radiograph is considered the gold standard for correct placement, but obtaining and processing a chest radiograph is time consuming, costly, and usually not necessary in the operating room. A chest radiograph should be obtained immediately postoperatively (Figure 9.3), position of intravascular catheters ascertained and adjustments made by the anesthesiologist if necessary. It is important to note that an anteroposterior radiograph may miss malposition in one of several ways. The most common is for an SVC catheter to be directed posteriorly down the azygous vein, which may not be detected by anteroposterior radiograph alone. Ideally, the tip of the catheter should be parallel to the SVC wall, in the mid-SVC, but in any case it should be above the SVC–RA junction. The position of the pericardial reflection is variable in infants and young children, and radiographic landmarks such as the carina to ascertain tip placement above the pericardial reflection are not reliable [35].

Transesophageal echocardiography

TEE is used for many congenital heart operations. Catheter tips and guidewires are easily imaged with TEE (Figure 9.4), and one study using TEE-guided CVC placement demonstrated a 100% success rate for correct

(a)   (b)

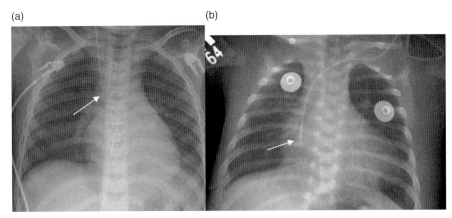

Figure 9.3 (a) Postoperative chest radiograph with the tip of a right internal jugular vein catheter in proper position in the mid-superior vena cava (*arrow*). (b) Tip of catheter malpositioned, deep in the right atrium (*arrow*)

placement in the SVC when TEE was used, versus 86% when surface anatomical landmarks were used in infants and children undergoing congenital heart surgery [17]. The TEE probe is placed before CVC attempts are made, and the SVC–right atrial junction in the 90° plane is imaged. When the vessel is punctured and the guidewire passed, it should be visualized passing from the SVC into the RA. Then the catheter is passed to its full length, the guidewire removed, and the tip of the CVC identified. Flushing the CVC with saline creates an easily visible stream of contrast that identifies the tip. The CVC is then pulled back until it is above the RA, in the distal SVC 1–2 cm above the crista terminalis. Using this technique, immediate, accurate confirmation of placement is obtained before final securing, and before the surgery. The proximal SVC, which is more than 2 cm above the RA, is difficult to image using TEE, so this method is most accurate in placing CVC in the distal SVC. Also, the commonly accepted radiographic SVC–RA junction is often higher than the SVC–RA junction noted by TEE [17].

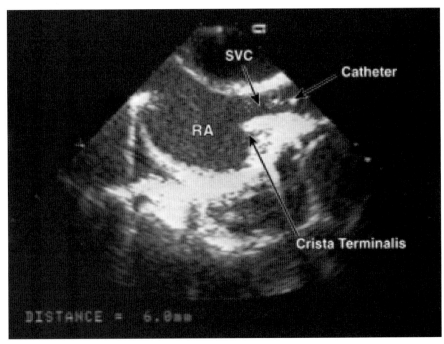

Figure 9.4 Transesophageal echocardiographic image of the superior vena cava (SVC)–right atrial (RA) junction in sagittal plane in an infant. The tip of the right internal jugular catheter is in the SVC, 6 mm above the RA (Used with permission from Reference [17])

Electrocardiographically guided placement

The intravascular ECG may be used in children to guide correct CVC placement [32,36,37]. Either a 0.9 or 3% saline-filled lumen with special ECG adaptor, or a guidewire within the lumen attached to a sterile alligator clip and leadwire substituted for the right arm surface ECG lead may be used. Entry of the catheter tip into the RA is signified by the sudden appearance of a P atriale, an exaggerated, large, upright P wave. The catheter tip is then pulled back 1–2 cm into the desired position in the SVC. Success rate for proper placement in the reported studies has been 80–90%, but there have been no controlled studies in children comparing this method to other methods. This method also requires special equipment not always available.

Height- and weight-based formulae

A recent large study of CVC placement in infants and children undergoing congenital heart surgery developed formulae for correct insertion depth on the basis of height and weight [12] (Table 9.2). CVC were inserted in the right internal jugular or subclavian vein and the postoperative radiograph studies were used to determine the tip position in reference to the SVC–RA junction. The length of catheter inside the patient was added to this distance to determine the position of the SVC–RA junction, and formulae developed that would predict placement above the RA, in the SVC 97.5% of the time (95% confidence interval 96–99%). All catheter tips predicted to be in the atrium using this data would be high in the RA within 1 cm of the SVC–RA junction, minimizing any perforation risk. The formulae are simple and easily implemented because

Table 9.2 Recommended length of superior vena cava central venous catheter (CVC) insertion in pediatric patients on the basis of weight: right-sided internal jugular or subclavian

Patient weight (kg)	Length of CVC insertion (cm)
2–2.9	4
3–4.9	5
5–6.9	6
7–9.9	7
10–12.9	8
13–19.9	9
20–29.9	10
30–39.9	11
40–49.9	12
50–59.9	13
60–69.9	14
70–79.9	15
80 and above	16

weight and height are known on all patients undergoing cardiac surgery.

For patients with height less than 100 cm: (Height ÷ 10) − 1 cm is the correct insertion distance, i.e., a 75 cm patient would have the catheter secured at 6.5 cm for either the internal jugular or the subclavian route.

For patients with height 100 cm or greater: (Height ÷ 10) − 2 cm is the correct distance. The caveats to this seemingly useful technique are that for the IJV, the puncture site was high, exactly midway between the mastoid process and the sternal notch; and for the subclavian, a puncture site 1–2 cm lateral to the midpoint of the clavicle. If different puncture sites are utilized, the operator must adjust the formulae accordingly. Also, the formulae have not yet been evaluated for accuracy in a prospective fashion.

Percutaneously inserted central catheters

Percutaneously inserted central catheters (PICC) have been utilized in the neonatal nursery for more than a decade, and have become standard practice for ill newborns expected to require prolonged venous access. The complication rate for these catheters is very low, and they are usually relatively easy to insert into the central circulation via the antecubital, saphenous, scalp, hand, axillary, or wrist veins, when placed by experienced, skilled personnel. Such personnel include nurses [38] or physicians placing them at the bedside, or in the interventional radiology suite [39] with ultrasound and fluoroscopic guidance. The key to successful placement is early access, before all large visible superficial veins are injured from attempts at peripheral intravenous placements. For this reason, the PICC line is optimally placed in the critically ill newborn with congenital heart disease in the first 12–24 hours after admission. Like all CVCs, they occasionally cause complications such as perforation of the atrium, or embolization of a portion of the catheter [40]. The infection rate is very low.

Technique: a suitable vein should be identified. The branches of the basilic vein on the medial half of the antecubital fossa offer the highest success rate because of the large size and direct continuation with the axillary and subclavian veins. The cephalic vein tributaries can also be used, but are less likely to pass into the axillary vein. Other sites, e.g., the saphenous, hand, and scalp veins, are cannulated as for a peripheral intravenous catheter. The site is prepared and draped, and appropriate local anesthesia and/or intravenous analgesia are administered. The vein is entered using a large breakaway needle or angiocatheter, and a 2 Fr nonstyleted silicone catheter flushed with heparinized saline is passed with forceps a distance measured from the entry site to the SVC–RA junction. Continued easy passage without resistance and continuous ability to aspirate blood signify proper placement. A radiograph, with injection of diluted contrast if needed, should be obtained prior to use. Proper catheter tip position is in the SVC or IVC, not in the RA. Occasionally, the PICC line will not pass centrally, i.e., into the intrathoracic portion of the subclavian vein or further, or into the IVC. In this case, it should be considered no differently than a peripheral venous line. For central PICC lines, any centrally delivered medication or fluid may be used, i.e., parenteral nutrition, dopamine, CaCl, etc. The 2 Fr PICC lines are too small for rapid fluid boluses or blood products, therefore inadequate as the sole prebypass access for cardiac surgery. Recently, 3 Fr soft polyurethane double-lumen PICC lines, with two 22 g lumens, have become available, which can be placed using modified Seldinger technique, with a central vein placement rate of 66% [41]. Alternatively, 3 Fr PICC lines, placed with the aid of ultrasound and fluoroscopic guidance with a guidewire in the interventional radiology suite, may be used in newborns with caution, especially in the SVC position, because of the risk of thrombosis [42]. In older infants and children, these larger catheters are preferred. Tan et al. [43] reported a series of 124 such catheters in cardiac surgical neonates, noting a low thrombosis rate of 1.6%, and a low infection rate of 3.6 per 1000 catheter days, with a median onset of 37 days; thus these catheters can be extremely useful in this population.

Arterial access

Tables 9.3 and 9.4 display recommended catheter sizes for arterial access on the basis of site and patient weight.

Radial artery

This is the preferred location in the newborn if umbilical artery line is not possible or needs to be replaced, and in virtually all other patients. Placement on the same side of an existing or planned systemic to PA shunt is avoided, e.g., a right-sided modified Blalock–Taussig shunt.

Technique: The wrist is extended slightly with rolled gauze, the fingers taped loosely to an armboard, with the thumb taped separately in extension to tether skin sur-

Table 9.3 Recommended arterial catheter sizes: radial, dorsalis pedis (DP), posterior tibial (PT), brachial arteries

Weight (kg)	Radial/DP/PT arteries (g)	Brachial artery (g)
<2	24	Not recommended
2–5	22	24
5–30	22	22
>30	20	22

Table 9.4 Recommended arterial catheter sizes: femoral, axillary arteries

Weight (kg)	Femoral/axillary arteries
<10	2.5 Fr, 5 cm long
10–50	3 Fr, 8 cm long
>50	4 Fr, 12 cm long

DP, dorsalis pedis; PT, posterior tibial.

face over the radial artery (Figure 9.5. An angiocatheter flushed with heparinized saline is used to increase the rapidity of flashback of blood into the hub of the needle after aseptic preparation. The skin is punctured at a 15–20° angle at the proximal wrist crease at the point of maximal impulse of the artery. Palpation is the usual method of identifying the artery, but audio Doppler localization can be helpful if the pulse is weak. Lighter planes of anesthesia provide stronger pulses and increase the success rate of cannulation. The first attempt, before any hematoma formation, always yields the greatest chance for success, so the operator should optimize conditions, e.g., positioning, lighting, and identification of the vessel. Puncture of the artery with the needle is signified by brisk flashback. The needle and catheter are then advanced 1–2 mm into the artery, and an attempt is made to thread the catheter primarily over the needle its full length into the artery. Threading should have minimal resistance and is signified by the continuing flow of blood into hub of needle. If threading is not successful, the needle is replaced carefully in the angiocatheter, and the needle and catheter can be passed through the back wall of artery. Then the needle is removed, and a 0.015″ guidewire with flexible tip can be used to assist threading of catheter. The catheter is pulled back very slowly, and when vigorous arterial back flow occurs, the guidewire is passed, and the catheter threaded over the guidewire into the artery [44]. Minimal resistance signifies successful threading. If unsuccessful, further attempts may be made at the same site, or at slightly more proximal sites to avoid areas of arterial spasm, thrombosis, or dissection. The circulation distal to the catheter should be assessed by inspection of color and capillary refill time of fingertips and nail beds, and quality of signal from a pulse oximeter probe. A recommended technique for securing the catheter is with a clear adhesive dressing and transparent tape so that the insertion site and hub of the catheter are visible at all times.

Femoral artery

The superficial femoral artery is a large vessel that is easily accessible in almost all patients [45], and is a logical second choice when radial arterial access is not available. In infants, especially patients with Trisomy 21, transient

(a)

(b)

(d)

(c)

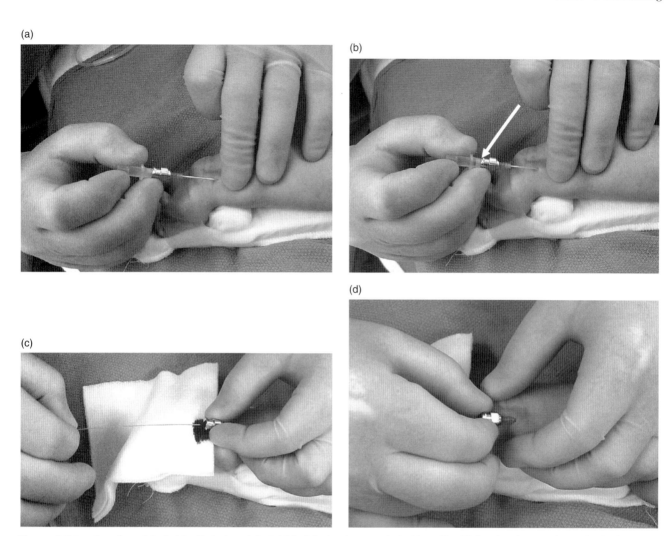

Figure 9.5 Insertion of a radial arterial catheter in an infant. (a) Radial artery is approached with a saline-filled angiocatheter, at the proximal wrist crease. (b) Rapid flashback of arterial blood (arrow) is noted with arterial puncture using liquid stylet technique. (c) A 0.015″ guidewire is inserted and threaded into the artery. (d) The angiocatheter is threaded over the guidewire

arterial insufficiency develops in up to 25% of patients after arterial catheterization when 20 ga (3 Fr) catheters are used [45]. For this reason, in the author's institution, the smallest commercially available catheter, 2.5 Fr (equal to 21 ga) is used in patients weighing less than 10 kg (see Table 9.4).

Technique: A small towel is placed under the patient's hips to extend the leg slightly to neutral position. Slight external rotation, with the knees restrained by taping to the operating room bed fixes adequate position. After sterile prep and drape, the course of the superficial femoral artery is palpated and punctured 1–2 cm inferior to the inguinal ligament, to avoid puncturing the artery above the pelvic rim, where a retroperitoneal hematoma could develop. If the pulse is weak, as in the case of aortic arch obstruction, use of audio Doppler effectively identifies the course of the vessel. The puncture technique varies,

and may include direct puncture with an angiocatheter, or Seldinger technique using the needle in the commercially supplied kit, or a 21 ga butterfly needle with the extension tubing removed. All of the above are flushed with heparinized normal saline to increase the rapidity of flashback. A small flexible guidewire, 0.015″ or 0.018″, is used. It is normally possible to thread a polyethylene catheter over the guidewire without making a skin incision, and under no circumstances is dilating the tract and artery with a dilator recommended, which could cause arterial spasm, dissection, or bleeding around the catheter if the puncture site is large. The catheter is secured by suturing around the entry site of catheter and wings around the hub. Distal perfusion is immediately assessed, and a pulse oximeter probe is placed on the foot for continuous monitoring and early warning of arterial perfusion problems.

Brachial artery

The brachial artery has been successfully used for monitoring for cardiac surgery in children, but using this site for arterial monitoring should generally be avoided because it has poor collateral circulation compared to the radial, femoral, and axillary arteries. Theoretically, there should be a higher incidence of arterial insufficiency with this site, but a study by Schindler et al. of 386 brachial artery catheters in infants and children undergoing cardiac surgery documented no permanent ischemic damage, and only 3 temporary arterial occlusions, when 22 and 24 g catheters were used [46]. It should only be used in situations when there are limited other options, e.g., a right upper extremity arterial line is required to monitor pressure during cross-clamping for repair of coarctation of the aorta, or during bypass for aortic arch hypoplasia or interruption.

Technique: a 24 ga catheter should be used in patients under 5 kg. The arm is restrained in neutral position on an armboard, and the arterial impulse is palpated above the elbow crease, well above the bifurcation into radial and ulnar arteries. Cannulation proceeds as for the radial artery. Meticulous attention to distal perfusion must be paid at all times, and the catheter removed for any signs of ischemia. Pulse oximeter monitoring of distal pulses will provide early detection of perfusion problems. The catheter should be removed or replaced with a catheter in a site with better collateral circulation as soon as possible after the repair.

Axillary artery

The axillary artery is large and well collateralized, and several series in critically ill children have demonstrated this to be a viable option with a low complication rate when other sites are not accessible [47, 48]. However, given the potential morbidity of an ischemic arm and hand, and the theoretical problem of intrathoracic bleeding, this puncture site should be considered a site of last resort when there are limited options.

Technique: the arm is abducted 90°, and extended slightly at the shoulder to expose the artery. The artery is palpated high in the axilla, and punctured using an angiocatheter, then exchanged over a guidewire for a longer catheter, or by primary Seldinger technique. A catheter that is too short (e.g., 22 ga 1 in. long) will often be pulled out of the vessel with shoulder extension. Therefore, the shortest recommended catheter is 5 cm long (see Table 9.4.) Careful attention must be paid to distal perfusion, as with the brachial artery. Tip position should be ascertained by chest radiograph, and should not lie deeper than the first rib. The proximity to the brachiocephalic vessels makes it imperative that the catheter be flushed very gently by hand after blood draws, and that no air bubbles or clots ever be introduced, because of the risk of retrograde cerebral embolization.

Umbilical artery

The umbilical artery is accessible for the first few days of life, and is the site of choice for newborns requiring surgery in the first week of life (Figure 9.1). Complication rate is lower with the catheter tip placed in the high position, i.e., above the diaphragm, versus low tip position, i.e., at the level of the third lumbar vertebra [49]. The catheter can be left in place for 7–10 days. A relationship to intestinal ischemia and necrotizing colitis has been demonstrated [50], and enteral feeding with an umbilical artery catheter in place is controversial [51]. Umbilical catheters are most commonly inserted by the neonatal staff in the delivery room or neonatal ICU shortly after birth. Technique involves cutting off the umbilical stump with an umbilical tape encircling the base to provide hemostasis, dilating the umbilical artery, and blindly passing a 3.5 Fr catheter a distance based on weight, then assessing position as soon as possible radiographically. Lower extremity emboli, vascular insufficiency, and renal artery thrombosis have all been described [52]; however, the overall risk is low and this site is highly desirable because it is a large central artery yielding accurate pressure monitoring [53] during all phases of the surgery, and preserves access for future interventions.

Temporal artery

The superficial temporal artery at the level just above the zygomatic arch is large and easily accessible in newborns, particularly the premature infant. It was widely used in the 1970s in neonatal nurseries [54], but rapidly fell out of favor with the realization that significant complications, e.g., retrograde cerebral emboli, were disturbingly common [55, 56]. It should only be used when a brachiocephalic pressure must be measured for the surgery in the face of an aberrant subclavian artery, so that the only way to measure pressure during cross-clamping or on bypass is via direct aortic pressure, or temporal artery pressure. Examples are coarctation of the aorta, aortic arch interruption or hypoplasia, with aberrant right subclavian artery that arises distal to the area of aortic obstruction [57]. The catheter must be used only during the case, blood drawing and flushing should be minimized, and it must be removed as soon as possible after the repair.

Technique: a 24 g catheter is used for newborns. The artery is palpated just anterosuperior to the tragus of the ear, just superior to the zygomatic arch. A very superficial angle of approach, i.e., 10–15°, is used, and the artery is cannulated the same as described for the radial artery.

Dorsalis pedis/posterior tibial arteries

Superficial foot arteries should not be used for bypass cases, because of the well-known peripheral vasoconstriction, and vasomotor instability in the early postbypass period, which is more pronounced with these arteries than with the radial artery. It is frequently not possible to obtain an accurate arterial pressure waveform in the early post-bypass period. These arteries may be used for nonbypass cases, and in the intensive care unit.

Technique: dorsalis pedis—the foot is plantar flexed slightly to straighten the course of the artery, which is palpated between the second and third metatarsal. A superficial course is taken and the artery cannulated. Posterior tibial—the foot is dorsiflexed to expose the artery between the medial malleolus and the Achilles tendon. The artery is often deep to the puncture site, so a steeper angle of incidence is required.

Ulnar artery

The ulnar artery should only be used as a last resort in a desperate situation when other options are not available, because its use is only considered when radial artery attempts have been unsuccessful or thrombosed by past interventions. There is a high risk of ischemia of the hand if both the radial and ulnar artery perfusion is significantly compromised. Despite this, one series of 18 ulnar artery catheters in critically ill infants and children had an ischemia rate not different from radial and femoral artery catheters of 5.6% [58].

Arterial cutdown

Cutdown of the radial artery is a reliable and often efficient method to establish access for congenital heart surgery. Some centers use this method as the first and primary method of securing arterial access, while others only resort to it when all other attempts fail. Despite the speed and ease of access for a cutdown, available literature indicates a higher rate of bleeding at the site, infection, failure, distal ischemia, and long-term vessel occlusion compared to percutaneous techniques [59,60]. It is for these reasons that the authors' institution uses cutdowns only when percutaneous methods have failed.

Technique: the arm is positioned as for percutaneous radial catheterization. After surgical preparation and draping, an incision is made at the proximal wrist crease between the styloid process and the flexor carpi radialis tendon, either parallel or perpendicular to the artery. Sharp and blunt dissection is carried out until the artery is identified, and it is isolated with a heavy silk suture, vessel loop, or right angle forceps. It is no longer considered necessary to ligate the artery distally to prevent bleeding, and

in fact the artery may remain patent after a cutdown if not ligated distally. The simplest and very effective technique is to cannulate the exposed artery directly with an angio-catheter, in the same manner as for percutaneous radial artery catheter placement. The catheter is then sutured to the skin at its hub, and the incision closed with nylon sutures on either side of the catheter. Removal entails cutting the suture at the hub of the catheter, removing the catheter, and applying pressure for a few minutes until any bleeding stops. The remaining skin sutures can be removed at a later date.

Percutaneous pulmonary artery catheterization

Percutaneous PA catheterization has a limited role in congenital heart surgery for several reasons. The small size of many patients precludes placement of adequate-sized sheaths and catheters, and most patients have intracardiac shunting, invalidating results of standard thermodilution cardiac output measurements and confusing mixed venous oxygen saturation (SvO_2) measurements. In addition, frequent need for right-sided intracardiac surgery makes PA catheterization undesirable. Thus, when PA pressure or SvO_2 monitoring is indicated, transthoracic PA lines are the most common method in congenital heart surgery.

The most common indications for percutaneous PA catheterization in congenital heart surgery are in patients over 6 months of age able to accept a 5 or 6 Fr introducer sheath in the femoral or IJV. Patients having surgery on left heart structures who do not have intracardiac shunting, who are at risk for left ventricular dysfunction or pulmonary hypertension, may benefit from the information available. Examples include aortic surgery, aortic valve repair or replacement, subaortic resection or myomectomy for hypertrophic cardiomyopathy, and mitral valve repair or replacement.

Technique [61]: an oximetric catheter is recommended. Commercially available models are 5.5 Fr or 8.5 Fr, and thus require a 6 Fr or 9 Fr sheath, respectively. The 5.5 Fr catheter should be used in patients under 50 kg, and the 8.5 Fr in patients over 50 kg. The sheath is placed into the internal jugular, femoral, or subclavian veins as described above. The preferred sites of insertion are (1) right internal jugular, (2) left subclavian, and (3) femoral vein because of the direct path and curvature of the catheter. If an oximetric catheter is used, it is calibrated prior to insertion. The balloon integrity should be tested before insertion by inflating the recommended volume of air or CO_2, and the sterility sleeve is inserted before placement. The PA and CVP ports are connected, flushed, and calibrated before insertion. The PA catheter is inserted 10–15 cm with the balloon deflated, depending on patient size. The balloon is inflated, and the catheter advanced slowly toward the tricuspid valve, whose position is indicated by enlarging V waves on the CVP trace. The catheter is advanced through the tricuspid valve by advancing during diastole until the characteristic right ventricular trace is visible, with no dicrotic notch, and a diastolic pressure of 0–5 mm Hg. Then, the catheter is advanced carefully through the pulmonary valve during systole, until the characteristic PA tracing is visible, with a dicrotic notch and higher diastolic pressure. The catheter is then advanced gently until the pulmonary capillary wedge pressure tracing is obtained, at which time the balloon is deflated so the PA tracing rapidly returns. Difficulty with advancing through the pulmonary valve may be assisted by counterclockwise rotation of the catheter while advancing, positioning the patient right side down and giving a fluid bolus, or by using TEE to visualize the tip and guide subsequent attempts [62]. The catheter must not be left in the wedge position except during brief periods because of the risk of PA rupture and lung ischemia distal to the catheter. During bypass, the catheter can be pulled back several centimeters to reduce the risk of perforation on bypass.

Information obtainable with a PA catheter: RA, PA, PCWP pressures. In the absence of mitral valve stenosis or pulmonary venous or arterial hypertension, PA diastolic pressure ≈ PCWP ≈ LAP ≈ left ventricular end-diastolic pressure (LVEDP). LVEDP is proportional to left ventricular end-diastolic volume, the classic measure of preload [63]. Despite the presence of pulmonary hyper-

tension or residual mitral stenosis (diagnosed with postoperative TEE), information from the PA catheter can still be used to direct therapy.

Cardiac index may be measured by standard thermodilution methods, with care taken to input the correct calculation constant into the monitor software according to the catheter size and length, and volume and temperature of injectate. The average of three consecutive injections made in rapid succession at the same point in the respiratory cycle, i.e., expiration, will optimize conditions to achieve an accurate measurement during steady state conditions. Vascular resistances and stroke volume can also be calculated, using the formulae in Table 9.5 [63, 64].

Hemodynamic data represents only half of the information available from an oximetric PA catheter. The other half consists of oxygen delivery and consumption measurements and calculations, which may also be used to guide therapy in the critically ill patient with low cardiac output syndrome [63, 64] (Table 9.6). They require either measurement of mixed venous and systemic arterial saturations from blood samples from the tip of the PA catheter and arterial line (measured by co-oximetry, not calculated), or substitution of these values with SvO_2 from the oximetric catheter (a valid assumption if properly calibrated), and pulse oximeter value instead of measured systemic saturation. There are data from adult and pediatric critical care literature suggesting that the ability to increase and maximize both oxygen delivery and consumption may improve outcome, and is a predictor of survival from critical illness, including postoperative cardiac surgery [65–68].

Table 9.5 Derived hemodynamic parameters

Formula	Normal values		
	Adult	Infant	Child
$CI = \dfrac{CO}{BSA}$	2.8–4.2 L/min/m²	2–4 L/min/m²	3–4 L/min/m²
$SVI = \dfrac{SV}{BSA}$	30–65 mL/beat/m²	40–75 mL/beat/m²	40–70 mL/beat/m²
$LVSWI = \dfrac{1.36(MAP - PCWP) \times SVI}{100}$	45–60 g m/m²	20–40 g m/m²	30–50 g m/m²
$RVSWI = \dfrac{1.36(PAP - CVP) \times SI}{100}$	5–10 g m/m²	5–11 g m/m²	5–10 g m/m²
$SVRI = \dfrac{(MAP - CVP) \times 80}{CI}$	1500–2400 dyne s/cm⁻⁵ m²	900–1200 dyne s/cm⁻⁵ m²	1300–1800 dyne s/cm⁻⁵ m²
$PVRI = \dfrac{(PAP - PCWP) \times 80}{CI}$	250–400 dyne s/cm⁻⁵ m²	<200 dyne s/cm⁻⁵ m²	<200 dyne s/cm⁻⁵ m²

CI, cardiac index; CO, thermodilution cardiac output; BSA, body surface area; SV, stroke volume; SVI, stroke volume index; LVSWI, left ventricular stroke work index; MAP, mean arterial pressure; PCWP, pulmonary capillary wedge pressure; CVP, central venous pressure; PAP, pulmonary arterial pressure; RVSWI, right ventricular stroke work index; SVRI, systemic vascular resistance index; PVRI, pulmonary vascular resistance index.

Table 9.6 Derived oxygen delivery/consumption parameters

Formula	Normal values		
	Adult	Infant	Child
Arterial O$_2$ content $CaO_2 = (1.39HbSaO_2) + (0.0031PaO_2)$	18–20 mL/dL	15–18 mL/dL	16–18 mL/dL
Mixed venous O$_2$ content $CvO_2 = (1.39HbSvO_2) + (0.0031PvO_2)$	13–16 mL/dL	11–14 mL/dL	12–14 mL/dL
Arteriovenous O$_2$ content difference $avDO_2 = CaO_2 - CvO_2$	4–5.5 mL/dL	4–7 mL/dL	4–6 mL/dL
Pulmonary capillary O$_2$ content $CcO_2 = (1.39HbScO_2) + (0.0031PcO_2)$	19–21 mL/dL	16–19 mL/dL	17–19 mL/dL
Pulmonary shunt fraction $Qs/Qt = 100(Cco_2 - Cao_2)/(Cco_2 - Cvo_2)$	2–8%	2–8%	2–8%
O$_2$ delivery index $Do_2I = 10COCao_2/BSA$	450–640 mL/min/m^2	450–750 mL/min/m^2	450–700 mL/min/m^2
O$_2$ consumption index $Vo_2I = 10 CO(Cao_2 - Cvo_2)$	85–170 mL/min/m^2	150–200 mL/min/m^2	140–190 mL/min/m^2

Hb, hemoglobin; Sao$_2$, measured arterial oxygen saturation; Pao$_2$, partial pressure of oxygen in arterial blood; Svo$_2$, measured mixed venous oxygen saturation; Pvo$_2$, partial pressure of oxygen in mixed venous blood; Sco$_2$, measured pulmonary capillary oxygen saturation; Pco$_2$, partial pressure of oxygen in pulmonary capillary blood; Qs, pulmonary shunt blood flow; Qt, total pulmonary blood flow.

Ultrasound guidance for vascular access in congenital heart surgery

Numerous studies demonstrate that ultrasound guidance, either two-dimensional visual ultrasound [69] or audio Doppler ultrasound, improves the outcome of central venous cannulation, in both children and adults [70,71]. Use of these methods leads to fewer attempts, decreased insertion time, fewer unintended arterial punctures, and fewer unintended arterial catheter placements. The consensus of many experts in the field of vascular access is that use of these guidance techniques should be considered standard of care.

A 9.2 MHz pencil-thin audio Doppler probe can be gas sterilized and reused. The probe is applied to the site, and the course of the artery and vein are ascertained by their characteristic audio profiles—high-pitched, intermittent, systolic flow for the artery, and a low-pitched, continuous venous hum for the vein. The probe is centered over the loudest signal, perpendicular to the skin surface, and the vessel is punctured exactly in the axis of the center of the probe. A "pop" followed by the continuous sound of blood aspiration can often be heard when the vessel is entered. The guidewire, dilator, and catheter are then passed as above. A variation of the audio Doppler technique is a device with the Doppler probe within the needle [72]. However, these needles are expensive, direct comparison has not shown them to be superior to visual ultrasound for cannulation, and because the lumen of the needle is partially occluded with the Doppler probe, flashback of blood is slow and unreliable.

Two-dimensional echocardiography, either in the form of commercially available devices for CVC cannulation only (Sonosite®) or surface probes on standard echocardiography machines, can be used to image large vessels (Figure 9.6a). The color Doppler feature on the latter may be particularly useful to identify desired vessels during difficult vascular access. The IJV is the most frequently accessed vessel with ultrasound, and it is visualized superficial to and lateral to the carotid artery. The IJV is also easily compressible with the probe and is gently pulsatile, while the carotid artery is round, difficult to compress with probe pressure, and very pulsatile (Figure 9.6b). The probe is held directly over the desired vessel, with the goal of puncturing it exactly in the midline. The needle can be seen indenting and then puncturing the vessel during correct placement (Figure 9.6c).

Visual ultrasound is particularly useful to clarify the anatomy after several previous attempts have been made. One can identify the vessel in the midst of a hematoma that has formed, or recognize overlap of the artery and vein. Once the vessel has been punctured and the guidewire passed, the ultrasound can be used to visualize the guidewire in the lumen of the vessel by scanning closer to the heart. Ultrasound methods are described most often for the IJV, but are also useful for the femoral and subclavian veins. Pirotte et al. described a novel ultrasound technique for subclavian vein access in infants and

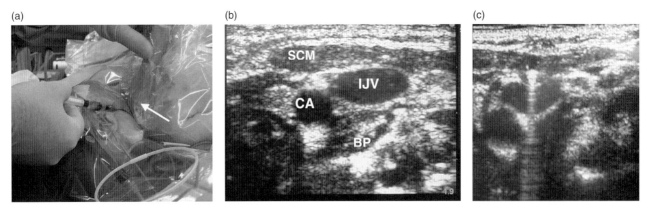

Figure 9.6 (a) Ultrasound-guided puncture of the internal jugular vein in an infant. Arrow denotes 13 MHz pediatric probe. (b) Two-dimensional ultrasound view of the right internal jugular vein and carotid artery in an infant. CA, carotid artery; IJV, internal jugular vein; SCM, sternocleidomastoid muscle; BP, brachial plexus. (c) Needle just prior to puncture of the right IJV.

children, using supraclavicular imaging for placement of infraclavicular catheters, with a success rate of 100% (84% first attempt) in 25 patients 2.2–27 kg [73] (Figure 9.7). It should also be noted that real time ultrasonographic visualization of needle insertion, vessel puncture, and guidewire passage of the IJV in infants results in fewer attempts and faster cannulation than merely marking the skin after ultrasound visualization followed by blind puncture of the vessel [74].

Audio Doppler can be used to assist in the cannulation of any artery, and is particularly useful when pulses are diminished from previous attempts, hypotension, or vasospasm. Visual ultrasound can also be used to cannulate radial arteries, and Schwemmer et al. found that this technique resulted in a 100% success rate, versus 80% for the traditional palpation method; and also resulted in higher success rate on the first attempt, and lower number of attempts [75].

Interpretation of intravascular pressure waveforms

The normal systemic arterial pressure waveform changes with progression distally from the central arterial circulation, e.g., ascending aorta, distally to abdominal aorta and femoral arteries, and then to the peripheral arterial such as the radial and dorsalis pedis/posterior tibial arteries [63] (Figure 9.8). In general, the more central sites will produce less peaked systolic pressure waves with slightly lower systolic pressure readings. The dicrotic notch is pronounced in the central arteries. With distal progression, pulse wave amplification will produce a higher peaked systolic pressure wave with a slightly higher systolic pressure. This is most pronounced in the arteries of the foot, where the systolic pressure may be 5–15 mm Hg higher than the ascending aorta. The mean and diastolic pressures change very little with progression. This concept is very important in interpreting arterial pressure tracings. The postbypass arterial tracing is frequently dampened with catheters in small distal arteries, e.g., radial or foot arteries [76]. This usually resolves within a few minutes after bypass. For particularly long and difficult operations with long bypass and cross-clamp times, it may be useful to place catheters in larger arteries, e.g., femoral or umbilical, or to measure the pressure directly in the aortic root immediately after bypass to ascertain an accurate arterial pressure.

The arterial pressure tracing can yield more information than simply the systolic and diastolic blood pressures [77, 78]. The slope of the upstroke of the pressure wave may be an indicator of systemic ventricular contractility, i.e., the steeper the upslope, the better the contractility. Significant reductions in contractility flatten the upslope. The position of the dicrotic notch may give an indication of peripheral vascular resistance. In infants, the normal dicrotic notch is in the upper half of the pressure wave. With low peripheral resistance, as in arterial runoff through a patent ductus arteriosus, the dicrotic notch is lower on the descending limb of the waveform, due to diastolic runoff into the PA, resulting in a relatively longer period of ventricular systole. The area under the curve of the systolic portion of the arterial tracing increases with increased stroke volume. Finally, a hypovolemic patient will often exhibit more pronounced respiratory variation during positive pressure ventilation, as the stoke volume decreases when positive pressure impedes an already limited venous return (Figure 9.9). Computerized pulse-contour analysis of the arterial pressure waveform has been used to measure stroke volume (see section on "new techniques in pediatric intravascular monitoring").

Mechanical and electronic components of the intravascular pressure measurement system are important considerations when interpreting waveforms [63]. The shortest

(a)

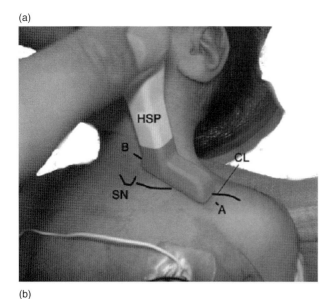

(b)

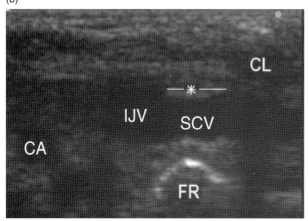

(c)

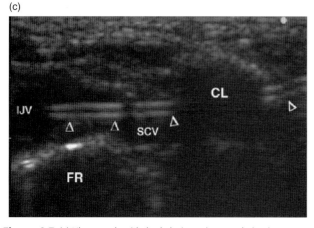

Figure 9.7 (a) Ultrasound-guided subclavian vein cannulation in an infant. (a) Surface landmarks and 10 MHz 2.5-cm linear hockey stick probe (HSP), positioned to obtain supraclavicular view. (b) Longitudinal axis of insonation to visualize vein; CL, clavicle; SN, sternal notch; A, skin puncture site; B, sonographic anatomy of subclavian vein. SCV, subclavian vein; IJV, internal jugular vein; CA, carotid artery; FR, first rib; * length of subclavian vein visualized. (c) Subclavian catheter after placement. Arrowheads are course of catheter (Used with permission from Reference [73])

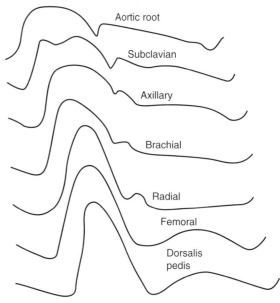

Figure 9.8 Progression of the arterial pressure tracing from the root of the aorta to more peripheral arteries. Pulse wave amplification produces a higher systolic peak and slightly lower diastolic pressure in the smaller distal arteries, especially the dorsalis pedis (Used with permission from Reference [63])

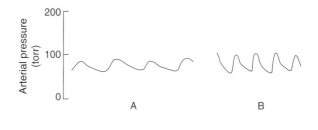

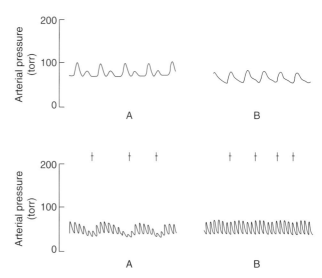

Figure 9.9 Top panel: the arterial pressure tracing with depressed (A), and normal (B) myocardial contractility. Middle panel: Low (A) and normal (B) systemic vascular resistance. Lower panel: hypovolemia (A), and normovolemia (B); arrows represent positive-pressure ventilations (Used with permission from Reference [77])

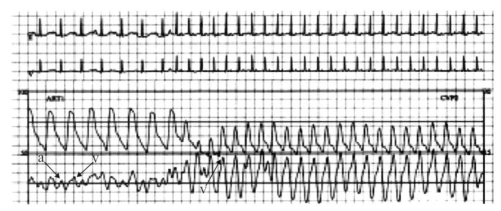

Figure 9.10 ECG demonstrating normal sinus rhythm the first third of the panel, with onset of supraventricular tachycardia. Note the arterial pressure tracing with a 12–15 torr decrease in systolic pressure, and the loss of the A wave on the central venous pressure tracing, with the appearance of large V waves with a systolic pressure increase from 10 to 16 mm Hg

possible large bore, stiff plastic tubing should be used. Minimizing the number of stopcocks and connections will also improve the fidelity of the transmitted pressure wave. Thorough flushing before use to produce a bubble- and clot-free fluid path is critical. Periodic recalibration at the right atrial level is important to account for "drift" in the transducer setting. When ringing or overdamping is recognized, some monitor models offer adjustment of electronic filter frequency. The routine setting should be 12 Hz. If the arterial tracing is underdamped, e.g., overshoot producing an artificially high spike as the systolic pressure, filter frequency may be decreased as low as 3 Hz to compensate. Conversely, if overdamped, the filter frequency may be increased to as high as 40 Hz. Mechanical devices (Rose, Accudynamics, Sorenson Research, Salt Lake City, UT) may also be inserted to change the resonance frequency and/or damping factor of the system. Under no circumstances should a bubble be intentionally introduced into the system to produce increased damping effect. Appropriateness of resonance frequency may be tested by flushing the system from a pressurized bag of heparinized saline, stopping suddenly, and observing the number and amplitude of oscillations required to return to baseline waveform. Proper damping is signified by one oscillation below, and one above the mean before return to normal waveform [79,80].

Failure of arterial pressure monitoring systems is always possible during congenital heart surgery, due to mechanical problems such as kinking or clotting of the catheter. Spasm of the artery is more common than in adults, and the artery may be compressed, such as aberrant right subclavian compression from a TEE probe, or compression of an axillary artery from a sternal retractor. A backup oscillometric blood pressure cuff should always be present. In addition, a reasonable precaution is to have the groins prepped into the field so the surgeon can place a catheter in the femoral artery percutaneously or by cut-down.

Central venous, right and left atrial waveforms

Normal atrial (i.e., central venous) pressure waveforms consist of the A, C, and V waves corresponding to atrial contraction, closure of the tricuspid or mitral valves, and ventricular contraction. Normal right atrial A wave pressure is lower than V wave pressure, which is usually less than 10 mm Hg. Changes from the normal tracing can give important information about the hemodynamic status and cardiac rhythm of the patient. For example, when atrioventricular synchrony is lost, as in junctional ectopic tachycardia or supraventicular tachycardia, the A wave disappears, and the V wave enlarges considerably, reflecting backward transmission of ventricular pressure through an ineffectively emptied atrium (Figure 9.10). Determining the cardiac rhythm from the ECG is often difficult at rapid heart rates because the P wave of the ECG is indiscernible. The left or right atrial waveform can give crucial added information in this situation, clearly retaining the A wave in cases of sinus tachycardia. Competency of the AV valves can also be assessed from the atrial tracing. Mitral or tricuspid regurgitation will produce a large V wave on the left atrial tracing. It is often very useful to record the vascular pressure tracings in sinus rhythm at baseline for later comparison.

New techniques in pediatric intravascular monitoring

Cardiac output monitoring

Because traditional percutaneous, balloon-tipped PA catheterization is limited in small children, and those with intracardiac shunting, several other recent methods to measure cardiac output and oxygen delivery in patients with congenital heart disease have been applied. Lithium

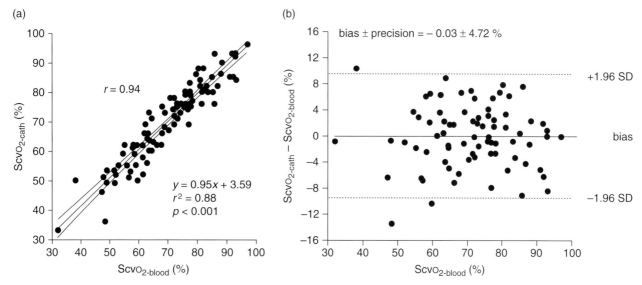

Figure 9.11 Central venous oxyhemoglobin saturation ($ScvO_2$) in the superior vena cava, comparing blood co-oximetry to fiberoptic reflectance spectroscopy. (a) Correlation between catheter ($ScvO_{2\text{-cath}}$ %) and blood co-oximetry ($ScvO_{2\text{-blood}}$ %). (b) Bland–Altman plot of bias and precision between the two methods (Used with permission from Reference [84])

dilution cardiac output (LiDCO) uses a standard central line in the SVC or even a peripheral IV catheter, and a special femoral artery catheter equipped with a lithium-detecting electrode. A dilute solution of lithium chloride is injected into the vein, and arterial blood is withdrawn into the lithium electrode. The cardiac index is related to the area under the curve of the change of lithium concentration. This method has been demonstrated to have reasonable correlation with thermodilution cardiac output in children after congenital heart surgery. In a study of 48 measurements in 17 patients 2.6–34 kg, correlation between LiDCO and thermodilution cardiac output was good ($r^2 = 0.96$, mean bias was -0.1 ± 0.31 L/min/m^2) [81].

Transpulmonary thermodilution cardiac output uses a similar principle as LiDCO, with temperature as the indicator instead of lithium concentration. Cold saline is injected into a CVC, and via a thermistor placed in a femoral artery, a time temperature curve is derived, which correlates reasonably well with standard thermodilution cardiac output as measured by a standard PA catheter [82]. Both lithium and any thermodilution method are limited to patients without any intracardiac shunting, significantly restricting their use in congenital heart disease.

Yet another newer method is pulse contour analysis of the arterial waveform (PiCCO), which relates the contour and area under the curve to the stroke volume, and thus the cardiac output. This continuous method is periodically calibrated using the transpulmonary thermodilution cardiac output as described above (again making the method

invalid with intracardiac shunting), and demonstrates a good correlation with transpulmonary thermodilution in a recent study of 24 pediatric patients after cardiac surgery ($r^2 = 0.86$, mean bias 0.05 ± 0.4 L/min/m^2) [83].

Central venous oxygen saturation monitoring

Monitoring of intravascular oxyhemoglobin saturation using reflectance catheters has been used in the umbilical artery, PA, and adult-sized CVCs for a number of years, but only recently have standard pediatric-sized 4 and 5 Fr, double- and triple-lumen CVCs become available for routine use to measure central venous oxygen saturation ($ScvO_2$) in pediatric patients. In 16 pediatric patients undergoing cardiac surgery, Liakopoulos et al. demonstrated good correlation between $ScvO_2$ as measured with the catheter, versus blood co-oximetry ($r^2 = 0.88$, bias $-0.03 \pm 4.72\%$) [84] (Figure 9.11). The advantage of this method is that it is an accurate measure of oxygen delivery that is independent of intracardiac shunting, and thus may have better utility in the congenital heart disease patient.

Complications of vascular access

Thrombosis

This is the single most frequent complication, especially among infants. Central venous thrombosis secondary to vascular access develops in 5.8% of neonatal patients, which is 10 times that of older patients, and accounts for 40–50% of central venous thromboses after congenital heart surgery [85]. The frequency significantly decreases in patients over 6 months of age. Factors that contribute to the risk of thrombosis include (1) large bore catheters in small vessels, i.e., larger than 4 Fr in small infants, (2) duration of cannulation exceeding 7 days, (3) venous stasis due to extreme fluid restriction or low cardiac output, (4) infusion of high osmolarity fluids, i.e., concentrated dextrose in parenteral nutrition fluids, and (5) hypercoagulable states [86]. Other risk factors for thrombosis include protein C resistance due to factor V Leiden mutation, prothrombin mutations, and methylenetetrahydrofolate reductase mutations [87]. In addition, elevated preoperative C reactive protein [88], and arterial catheterization with the use of vasoconstrictors such as norepinephrine, vasopressin, or terlipressin [89]. Immediate consequences of SVC thrombosis include SVC syndrome [90] with increased intracranial pressure, and chylothorax from ineffective drainage of the thoracic duct into the SVC. IVC thrombus leads to ascites, renal and intestinal dysfunction, and edema of the lower abdomen and extremities. The patient must be assessed carefully for signs of thrombosis, and suspicion of thrombosis should be evaluated by ultrasound examination. Treatment modalities include removing the catheter, heparinization, thrombolytic agents such as tissue plasminogen activator and urokinase [91, 92], antithrombin III replacement [93, 94], and surgical thrombectomy. Mortality from SVC thrombosis is reported as high as 33% and therefore critical to try to prevent this complication, preferably by avoiding SVC catheters in patients under 4 kg. Thrombosis also leads to a higher rate of infection [95, 96]. Heparin-bonded catheters may decrease the rate of thrombosis and do not increase risk of bleeding [95,97]. They may also lead to a lower rate of catheter colonization and infection [98]. However, it is currently not possible to bond both heparin and antibiotics to the same catheter. In patients with occlusion of central veins from previous catheters, magnetic resonance venography may be useful in identifying patent veins for future interventions [99].

Thrombosis or dissection of an artery is a serious complication that must be treated immediately. Immediately after arterial catheter placement, it is important to inspect the distal extremity, comparing it to the other extremity and palpate distal pulses. Placement of a pulse oximeter probe distal to the catheter serves as a continuous monitor and early warning of vascular insufficiency. Transient compromise to perfusion immediately after catheter placement due to arterial spasm, or during low output states may be observed. However, when extremity perfusion is significantly compromised treatment by removal of the catheter, use of vasodilators, warming the extremity, heparin, thrombolytics, surgical consultation for thrombectomy, or surgical reconstruction is indicated [100].

Malposition/perforation

CVC tips should not lie in the RA. Adult and pediatric studies have consistently demonstrated a higher rate of heart and great vessel perforation with associated cardiac tamponade when catheter tips are in the atrium [33,101–105]. Perforation is also less common with right-sided lines, e.g., right IJ or subclavian, because the catheter tip is parallel to the vein wall. The catheter tip of left-sided lines is frequently at a 45–90° angle of incidence to the SVC or atrium, and mechanical models demonstrate that this position is more likely to lead to great vessel perforation [106]. Finally, 5–10% of patients with congenital heart disease have a left SVC [105], which most often drains into the coronary sinus or left atrium and both of these sites are undesirable locations for a catheter tip [107]. Thus the ideal position of a CVC is in the mid-SVC with the tip parallel to the vein wall (Figures 9.2 and 9.4). Soft polyurethane or silicone catheters are also much less likely to perforate than stiffer polyethylene catheters [106]. Perforation is recognized by inability to consistently aspirate blood, an abnormal waveform, and signs and symptoms of pericardial tamponade or hemothorax. Treatment involves aspiration of all the blood possible through the catheter and establishing alternate access, intravascular volume replacement, and drainage of the pericardial or pleural blood, by needle, tube, or surgical exploration.

Many authorities recommend positioning the tip of the catheter in the superior half of the SVC, above the pericardial reflection. This recommendation is based on the theoretical concept that if there is a perforation, cardiac tamponade will not be produced, and also the catheter tip will be above the SVC bypass cannula and thus yield accurate CVP measurements on bypass [108]. There are several problems with this approach in congenital heart surgery, particularly in small patients. First the SVC is often only 4–5 cm long, leaving little room for error in placement. It is preferable to have the catheter slightly too deep in the SVC, because this will lead to accurate pressure measurements and proper infusions of drugs and fluids. When a multilumen catheter is positioned too high, a proximal port may not be intravascular, leading to extravasation of important or caustic drugs and fluids [109]. In addition, the pericardium is usually opened in congenital heart surgery, and drained postoperatively, rendering placement above the pericardial reflection unnecessary. Many series of catheter placements in children document that the IJ route results in tip placement in the SVC or RA 98–100% of the time, whereas the subclavian route has a 5–15% incidence of catheter malposition, i.e., across the midline in the contralateral brachiocephalic vein or up the ipsilateral IJV.

Despite numerous previous reports of cardiac perforation by CVCs, and the publication of studies documenting height- and weight-based formulae for depth of insertion of SVC catheters in infants [37], reports of cardiac perforation resulting in death or necessitating surgical exploration by sternotomy continue to occur [110].

When IVC catheters are used, accurate CVP measurements are obtained whether above or below the diaphragm usually. UVC catheters should be above the level of the diaphragm at the IVC–RA junction, but not in the RA [111] to ensure passage through the ductus venosus and parallel position to the IVC wall [112]. In a series of 128 portal vein thromboses in neonates, 73% of them had a UVC and in half of these the UVC was malpositioned; this constituted a major risk factor for poor outcome [113].

A recently described complication from femoral venous catheters is inadvertent placement in the lumbar venous plexus, which may result in paraplegia from epidural hematoma or infusion of vasoconstrictive substances [114, 115]. Catheterization of the lumbar venous plexus usually occurs when there is partial or total occlusion of the IVC from previous interventions, and the guidewire passes posteriorly through collateral circulation into the lumbar plexus. This malposition may be suspected during insertion when resistance to catheter passage is encountered or the catheter will not thread its entire length. An anteroposterior radiograph reveals an abnormal catheter course, often appearing to be more lateral than normal. A lateral radiograph will definitely diagnose such malposition where the catheter tip passes posterior to the vertebral bodies. The catheter must be removed immediately and the patient assessed for neurological deficit if this malposition is discovered. Retroperitoneal hematoma from perforation of the femoroiliac vessels from catheter or guidewire can also occur [116].

Inadvertent arterial puncture can nearly always be prevented by the use of an ultrasound guidance system for CVC placement (see above). However, if this complication occurs, the following general principles are useful: after needle puncture if there is any question about whether the vessel is an artery, remove the needle immediately, elevate the area, and hold firm pressure for 5–10 minutes. A small bore needle puncture of the carotid or femoral artery, e.g., 20 ga or smaller, is not usually an indication to cancel surgery. If a larger hole is created in the artery, i.e., a dilator and the catheter have been placed, pressure transduction can be used to confirm location. In this case, a discussion with the surgeon must ensue. Normally, the catheter can be removed, and pressure held without consequences unless a very large catheter was used, e.g., introducer sheath or large bore CVP catheter, in that case surgical exploration and repair should be undertaken. In most cases of elective cardiac surgery, it is prudent to postpone the case if a large hole has been made in the artery. The case can usually be safely performed 24 hours later if no bleeding has occurred. In emergency or urgent cases that must proceed despite a large hole in the artery, the neck or groin should be prepped into the field for exploration if excessive bleeding or hematoma formation occurs.

Pneumothorax

This complication is most frequent with the subclavian approach, but also may occur with the internal jugular approach, especially with the low puncture sites, e.g., jugular notch approach. To avoid this complication with the subclavian approach, it is important to advance the needle only during expiration. A very shallow approach with the needle directed just posterior to the clavicle and at the sternal notch is also important. For the IJV, a higher puncture site, and limiting the caudad advancement of the needle to stop above the clavicle will usually prevent this complication [117].

Continuous aspiration should be performed as the needle is advanced using a saline-filled syringe. If air is aspirated as the needle advanced attempts at venipuncture should stop immediately, and careful monitoring for compromise of ventilation and hemodynamics should ensue. A chest radiograph should be obtained if the start of surgery is not imminent to make the diagnosis, and pleural drainage by needle, catheter, or tube should be undertaken if indicated. After sternotomy, the pleura can be opened on that side during sternotomy if pneumothorax is diagnosed or suspected.

Infection

Catheter-related sepsis results in significant morbidity, some mortality, prolongation of ICU stay, and increased expense. The incidence of arterial catheter-related infection is low. A study of 340 arterial catheters in children revealed a 2.3% incidence of local site infection, and 0.6% catheter sepsis [118]. There is strong evidence that several strategies may be employed to reduce this complication [119]. The first is the use of full barrier precautions, e.g., sterile gown, mask, gloves, and careful septic technique during insertion [6]. Second, chlorhexidine has been shown to be superior to other antiseptic solutions. Finally, antibiotic bonding to the resin of the catheter will reduce infection [120]. This can be done in several ways, i.e., antibiotics already embedded in the resin (minocycline/rifampin or chlorhexidine/silver sulfadiazine), or applied at the time of insertion by soaking the outer and inner surfaces of the catheter in a negatively charged antibiotic at 100 mg/mL concentration such as vancomycin, cefazolin, or other cephalosporins. Antibiotic is slowly released from the catheter, delaying and reducing colonization and reducing the incidence of catheter sepsis. The increased cost per catheter is about $20, but one episode of catheter sepsis is estimated to cost $14,000 in

1995 [120]. In a study of antibiotic impregnated catheters in 225 critically ill children, minocycline–rifampin-coated catheters delayed the onset of infection in those patients who were infected to 18 days, from 5 days in nonantibiotic catheters [121]. CVCs indwelling more than 5–7 days have an increased incidence of colonization and sepsis [122], as well as vessel thrombosis. Suspicion of catheter sepsis should be followed by peripheral blood culture, and blood culture from the central line. The catheter should be removed when possible and the tip cultured. Institute antibiotic therapy empirically tailored to the most common institution-specific pathogens, and provide coverage for *Staphylococcus epidermidis*, which continues to be a common pathogen in catheter-related sepsis. A comprehensive, systematic intervention program to prevent central line associated bloodstream infections in a very busy cardiac ICU, including insertion, access, and maintenance protocols, and a protocol for timely removal of central lines, reduced the infection rate from 7.8 infections per 1000 catheter days to 2.3 infections per 1000 catheter days [123].

Arrhythmias

Other complications associated with vascular access procedures include arrhythmias. Ectopic atrial tachycardia, in particular, has been associated with a catheter tip in the RA [124,125]. Atrial fibrillation has also been associated with CVC placement [126]. More commonly, arrhythmias occur with the passage of the guidewire [127], and include isolated PACs, supraventricular tachycardia, and if the guidewire is advanced into the right ventricle, premature ventricular contractions, and even ventricular tachycardia or fibrillation. Complete heart block has also been described during guidewire passage in small infants [128]. Great care must be taken when passing the guidewire to stop advancing it when significant arrhythmias are encountered, and when advancing the catheter over the wire to retract the wire as the catheter is advanced. Patients particularly at risk for significant arrhythmia are those with known history of arrhythmia, and also those with significant right ventricular hypertrophy.

Systemic air embolus

Systemic air embolus is a constant threat for patients with central or peripheral venous catheters and intracardiac shunting [129], particularly two ventricle patients with right-to-left shunting, and single ventricle patients in infancy who have obligate mixing of systemic and pulmonary venous return in the systemic ventricle. Air may lodge in the coronary arteries (especially the right) PA, or cerebral vessels, leading to potentially serious complications. Observation of the transesophageal echocardiogram or transcranial Doppler ultrasound as used for neurological monitoring reveals rapid passage of any introduced systemic venous air into the aorta and cerebral circulation. For this reason, meticulous attention must be paid to prevent introduction of air into the systemic venous circulation as much as possible. Precautions include thorough de-airing of all intravenous infusions before connection to the patient, de-airing of continuous flush central venous lines, air filters on continuous infusions, and careful technique when injecting drugs and fluids. The latter involves holding any syringe upright, flushing fluid from the proximal intravenous tubing into it, and aspirating and tapping the syringe first before injecting so that any air is trapped at the superior aspect of the syringe. Constant vigilance of all infusions, and use of TEE as a monitor for intracardiac air and the transcranial Doppler for systemic arterial air may reduce the risk of significant air embolus.

Other complications

Thoracic duct injury, chylothorax [130], brachial plexus injury, cervical dural puncture [131], phrenic nerve injury [132], vertebral arteriovenous fistula [133], Horner syndrome [134], and tracheal puncture have also been described. These complications can essentially be eliminated with skilled personnel using ultrasound-guided techniques to accurately identify the location of the vessel.

Finally, embolization of catheter or guidewire fragments sheared off during difficult insertion procedures occur occasionally [20]. Never withdraw a guidewire or catheter through a needle if any resistance is encountered. If resistance is encountered, the guidewire and needle, or catheter and needle, must be withdrawn completely from the vessel together as a unit.

Conclusions

Vascular access is a critical issue for every patient undergoing congenital heart surgery. Each team of practitioners develops their own approach to vascular access, and no one approach, i.e., transthoracic versus percutaneous CVCs, or percutaneous versus cutdown radial artery access, has been demonstrated to be superior to any other. Complication rates, time for insertion, and expense are significant factors. Application of the principles of safe insertion, particularly a strategy to preserve access sites in small single ventricle patients, ultrasound guidance of catheter placement, and the use of antibiotic impregnated catheters will improve the outcome of vascular access procedures.

References

1. Steward DJ (1999) Venous cannulation in small infants: a simple method to improve success. Anesthesiology 90:930–931.
2. Parellada JA, Guest AL (1998) Fetal circulation and changes occurring at birth. In: Garson A, Bricker JT, McNamara DG (eds) The Science and Practice of Pediatric Cardiology. Williams & Wilkins, Baltimore, pp. 349–358.
3. Pinheiro JM, Fisher MA (1992) Use of a triple-lumen catheter for umbilical venous access in the neonate. J Pediatr 120:624–626.
4. Khilnani P, Goldstein B, Todres ID (1991) Double lumen umbilical venous catheters in critically ill neonates: a randomized prospective study. Crit Care Med 19:1348–1351.
5. Mitto P, Barankay A, Spath P, et al. (1992) Central venous catheterization in infants and children with congenital heart diseases: experiences with 500 consecutive catheter placements. Pediatr Cardiol 13:14–19.
6. Raad II, Hohn DC, Gilbreath BJ (1994) Prevention of central venous catheter-related infections by using maximal sterile barrier precautions during insertion. Infect Control Hosp Epidemiol 15:231–238.
7. Hayashi Y, Uchida O, Takaki O (1992) Internal jugular vein catheterization in infants undergoing cardiovascular surgery: an analysis of the factors influencing successful catheterization. Anesth Analg 74:688–693.
8. Mallinson C, Bennett J, Hodgson P, Petros AJ (1999) Position of the internal jugular vein in children: a study of the anatomy using ultrasonography. Paediatr Anaesth 9:111–114.
9. Fischer GW, Scherz RG (1973) Neck vein catheters and pericardial tamponade. Pediatrics 52:868–871.
10. Sulek CA, Gravenstein N, Blackshear RH, Weiss L (1996) Head rotation during internal jugular vein cannulation and the risk of carotid artery puncture. Anesth Analg 82:125–128.
11. Verghese ST, Nath A, Zenger D, et al. (2002) The effects of the simulated Valsalva maneuver, liver compression, and/or Trendelenburg position on the cross-sectional area of the internal jugular vein in infants and young children. Anesth Analg 94:250–254.
12. Andropoulos DB, Bent ST, Skjonsby B, Stayer SA (2001) The optimal length of insertion of central venous catheters for pediatric patients. Anesth Analg 93:883–886.
13. Tan BK, Hong SW, Huang MH, Lee ST (2000) Anatomic basis of safe percutaneous subclavian venous catheterization. J Trauma 48:82–86.
14. Tripathi M, Tripathi M (1996) Subclavian vein cannulation: an approach with definite landmarks. Ann Thorac Surg 61:238–240.
15. Venkataraman ST, Orr RA, Thompson AE (1988) Percutaneous infraclavicular subclavian vein catheterization in critically ill infants and children. J Pediatr 113:480–485.
16. Finck C, Smith S, Jackson R, Wagner C (2002) Percutaneous subclavian central venous catheterization in children younger than one year of age. Am Surg 68:401–404.
17. Andropoulos DB, Stayer SA, Bent ST (1999) A controlled study of transesophageal echocardiography to guide central venous catheter placement in congenital heart surgery patients. Anesth Analg 89:65–70.
18. Jung CW, Bahk JH, Kim MW, et al. (2002) Head position for facilitating the superior vena caval placement of catheters during right subclavian approach in children. Crit Care Med 30:297–299.
19. Fuenfer MM, Georgeson KE, Cain WS (1998) Etiology and retrieval of retained central venous catheter fragments within the heart and great vessels of infants and children. J Pediatr Surg 33:454–456.
20. Nicolson SC, Sweeney MF, Moore RA, Jobes DR (1985) Comparison of internal and external jugular cannulation of the central circulation in the pediatric patient. Crit Care Med 13:747–749.
21. Taylor EA, Mowbray MJ, McLellan I (1992) Central venous access in children via the external jugular vein. Anaesthesia 47:265–266.
22. Stenzel JP, Green TP, Fuhrman BP, et al. (1989) Percutaneous femoral venous catheterizations: a prospective study of complications. J Pediatr 114:411–415.
23. Venkataraman ST, Thompson AE, Orr RA (1997) Femoral vascular catheterization in critically ill infants and children. Clin Pediatr (Phila) 36:311–319.
24. Reda Z, Houri S, Davis AL, Baum VC (1995) Effect of airway pressure on inferior vena cava pressure as a measure of central venous pressure in children. J Pediatr 126:961–965.
25. Lloyd TR, Donnerstein RL, Berg RA (1992) Accuracy of central venous pressure measurement from the abdominal inferior vena cava. Pediatrics 89:506–508.
26. Yung M, Butt W (1995) Inferior vena cava pressure as an estimate of central venous pressure. J Paediatr Child Health 31:399–402.
27. Litmanovitch M, Hon H, Luyt DK, et al. (1995) Comparison of central venous pressure measurements in the intrathoracic and the intra-abdominal vena cava in critically ill children. Anaesthesia 50:407–410.
28. Chait HI, Kuhn MA, Baum VC (1994) Inferior vena caval pressure reliably predicts right atrial pressure in pediatric cardiac surgical patients. Crit Care Med 22:219–224.
29. Gold JP, Jonas RA, Lang P, et al. (1986) Transthoracic intracardiac monitoring lines in pediatric surgical patients: a ten-year experience. Ann Thorac Surg 42:185–191.
30. Schranz D, Schmitt S, Oelert H (1989) Continuous monitoring of mixed venous oxygen saturation in infants after cardiac surgery. Intensive Care Med 15:228–232.
31. Flori HR, Johnson LD, Hanley FL, Fineman JR (2000) Transthoracic intracardiac catheters in pediatric patients recovering from congenital heart defect surgery: associated complications and outcomes. Crit Care Med 28:2997–3001.
32. Hoffman MA, Langer JC, Pearl RH (1988) Central venous catheters—no X-rays needed: a prospective study in 50 consecutive infants and children. J Pediatr Surg 23:1201–1203.
33. Linder LE, Curelaru I, Gustavsson B, et al. (1984) Material thrombogenicity in central venous catheterization: a comparison between soft, antebrachial catheters of silicone elastomer and polyurethane. J Parenter Enteral Nutr 8:399–406.

34. Lovell M, Baines D (2000) Fatal complication from central venous cannulation in a paediatric liver transplant patient. Paediatr Anaesth 10:661–664.

35. Inagawa G, Ka K, Tanaka Y, et al. (2007) The carina is not a landmark for central venous catheter placement in neonates. Paediatr Anaesth 17:968–971.

36. Simon L, Teboul A, Gwinner N, et al. (1999) Central venous catheter placement in children: evaluation of electrocardiography using J-wire. Paediatr Anaesth 9:501–504.

37. Parigi GB, Verga G (1997) Accurate placement of central venous catheters in pediatric patients using endocavitary electrocardiography: reassessment of a personal technique. J Pediatr Surg 32:1226–1228.

38. BeVier PA, Rice CE (1994) Initiating a pediatric peripherally inserted central catheter and midline catheter program. J Intraven Nurs 17:201–205.

39. Tseng M, Sadler D, Wong J (2001) Radiologic placement of central venous catheters: rates of success and immediate complications in 3412 cases. Can Assoc Radiol J 52:379–384.

40. Khilnani P, Toce S, Reddy R (1990) Mechanical complications from very small percutaneous central venous Silastic catheters. Crit Care Med 18:1477–1478.

41. Bueno TM, Diz AI, Cervera PQ, et al. (2008) Peripheral insertion of double-lumen central venous catheter using the Seldinger technique in newborns. J Perinatol 28:282–286.

42. Foo R, Fujii A, Harris JA, et al. (2001) Complications in tunneled CVL versus PICC lines in very low birth weight infants. J Perinatol 21:525–530.

43. Tan LH, Hess B, Diaz LK, et al. (2007) Survey of the use of peripherally-inserted central venous catheters in neonates with critical congenital cardiac disease. Cardiol Young 17:196–201.

44. Yeldirim V, Ozal E, Cosar A, et al. (2006) Direct versus guidewire-assisted pediatric radial artery cannulation technique. J Cardiothorac Vasc Anesth 20:48–50.

45. Glenski JA, Beynen FM, Brady J (1987) A prospective evaluation of femoral artery monitoring in pediatric patients. Anesthesiology 66:227–229.

46. Schindler E, Kowald B, Suess H, et al. (2005) Catheterization of the radial or brachial artery in infants and children. Paediatr Anaesth 15:677–682.

47. Lawless S, Orr R (1989) Axillary arterial monitoring of pediatric patients. Pediatrics 84:273–275.

48. Greenwald BM, Notterman DA, DeBruin WJ, McCready M (1990) Percutaneous axillary artery catheterization in critically ill infants and children. J Pediatr 117:442–444.

49. Barrington KJ (2000) Umbilical artery catheters in the newborn: effect of position of the catheter tip. Cochrane Database Syst Rev 2:CD000505.

50. Joshi VV, Draper DA, Bates RD, III (1975) Neonatal necrotizing enterocolitis. Occurrence secondary to thrombosis of abdominal aorta following umbilical arterial catheterization. Arch Pathol 99:540–543.

51. Chase MC (1999) Feeding with an umbilical arterial line. Neonatal Netw 18:51–52.

52. O'Neill JA, Jr., Neblett WW, III, Born ML (1981) Management of major thromboembolic complications of umbilical artery catheters. J Pediatr Surg 16:972–978.

53. Butt WW, Whyte H (1984) Blood pressure monitoring in neonates: comparison of umbilical and peripheral artery catheter measurements. J Pediatr 105:630–632.

54. Prian GW (1977) Temporal artery catheterization for arterial access in the high risk newborn. Surgery 82:734–737.

55. Bull MJ, Schreiner RL, Garg BP, et al. (1980) Neurologic complications following temporal artery catheterization. J Pediatr 96:1071–1073.

56. Prian GW (1977) Complications and sequelae of temporal artery catheterization in the high-risk newborn. J Pediatr Surg 12:829–835.

57. Brown BR (1976) Intraoperative monitoring of left temporal and right radial arterial pressures during aortic-arch surgery. Anesthesiology 44:62–64.

58. Kahler AC, Mirza F (2002) Alternative arterial catheterization site using the ulnar artery in critically ill pediatric patients. Pediat Crit Care Med 3:370–374.

59. McIntosh BB, Dulchavsky SA (1992) Peripheral vascular cutdown. Crit Care Clin 8:807–818.

60. Souza N, Carvalho AC, Carvalho WB, et al. (2000) Complications of arterial catheterization in children. Rev Assoc Med Bras 46:39–46.

61. Introna RP, Martin DC, Pruett JK, et al. (1990) Percutaneous pulmonary artery catheterization in pediatric cardiovascular anesthesia: insertion techniques and use. Anesth Analg 70:562–566.

62. Rimensberger PC, Beghetti M (1999) Pulmonary artery catheter placement under transoesophageal echocardiography guidance. Paediatr Anaesth 9:167–170.

63. Reich D.L, Moskowitz DM, Kaplan JA (1999) Hemodynamic monitoring. In: Kaplan JA, Reich DL, Konstadt SN (eds) Cardiac Anesthesia. W.B. Saunders, Philadelphia, pp. 321–358.

64. Vargo TA (1998) Catheterization hemodynamic measurements. In: Garson A, Bricker JT, McNamara DG (eds) The Science and Practice of Pediatric Cardiology. Williams & Wilkins, Baltimore, pp. 961–993.

65. Bishop MH, Shoemaker WC, Appel PL (1995) Prospective, randomized trial of survivor values of cardiac index, oxygen delivery, and oxygen consumption as resuscitation endpoints in severe trauma. J Trauma 38:780–787.

66. Velmahos GC, Demetriades D, Shoemaker WC (2000) Endpoints of resuscitation of critically injured patients: normal or supranormal? A prospective randomized trial. Ann Surg 232:409–418.

67. Buheitel G, Scharf J, Hofbeck M, Singer H (1994) Estimation of cardiac index by means of the arterial and the mixed venous oxygen content and pulmonary oxygen uptake determination in the early post-operative period following surgery of congenital heart disease. Intensive Care Med 20:500–503.

68. Rossi AF, Seiden HS, Gross RP, Griepp RB (1999) Oxygen transport in critically ill infants after congenital heart operations. Ann Thorac Surg 67:739–744.

69. Verghese ST, McGill WA, Patel RI, et al. (1999) Ultrasound-guided internal jugular venous cannulation in infants: a prospective comparison with the traditional palpation method. Anesthesiology 91:71–77.

70. Randolph AG, Cook DJ, Gonzales CA, Pribble CG (1996) Ultrasound guidance for placement of central venous catheters: a meta-analysis of the literature. Crit Care Med 24:2053–2058.

71. Etheridge SP, Berry JM, Krabill KA, Braunlin EA (1995) Echocardiographic-guided internal jugular venous cannulation in children with heart disease. Arch Pediatr Adolesc Med 149:77–80.

72. Verghese ST, McGill WA, Patel RI, et al. (2000) Comparison of three techniques for internal jugular vein cannulation in infants. Paediatr Anaesth 10:505–511.

73. Pirotte T, Veyckemans F. (2007) Ultrasound-guided subclavian vein cannulation in infants and children: a novel approach. Br J Anaesth 98:509–514.

74. Hosokawa K, Shime N, Kato Y, et al. (2007) A randomized trial of ultrasound image-based skin surface marking versus real-time ultrasound-guided internal jugular vein catheterization in infants. Anesthesiology 107:720–804.

75. Schwemmer U, Arzet HA, Trautner H, et al. (2006) Ultrasound-guided arterial cannulation improves success rate. Eur J Anaesthesiol 23:476–480.

76. Gallagher JD, Moore RA, McNicholas KW, Jose AB (1985) Comparison of radial and femoral arterial blood pressures in children after cardiopulmonary bypass. J Clin Monit 1:168–171.

77. Gregory GA (2002) Monitoring during surgery. In: Gregory GA (ed). Pediatric Anesthesia. Churchill Livingstone, New York, pp. 249–265.

78. Mahajan A, Shabanie A, Turner, J (2002) Pulse contour analysis of cardiac output monitoring in congenital heart surgery. Anesthesiology 97:A488 (Abstract).

79. Francke A, Wachsmuth H (2000) How accurate is invasive blood pressure determination with fluid-filled pressure line systems? Anaesthesiol Reanim 25:46–54.

80. Allan MW, Gray WM, Asbury AJ (1988) Measurement of arterial pressure using catheter-transducer systems. Improvement using the Accudynamic. Br J Anaesth 60:413–418.

81. Linton RA, Jonas MM, Tibby SM, et al. (2000) Cardiac output measured by lithium dilution and transpulmonary thermodilution in patients in a paediatric intensive care unit. Int Care Med 26:1507–1511.

82. Pauli C, Fakler U, Genz T, et al. (2002) Cardiac output determination in children; equivalence of the transpulmonary thermodilution method to the direct Fick principle. Intensive Care Med 28:947–952.

83. Fakler U, Pauli C, Balling G, et al. (2007) Cardiac index monitoring by pulse contour analysis and thermodilution after pediatric cardiac surgery. J Thorac Cardiovasc Surg 133:224–228.

84. Liakopoulos OJ, Ho JK, Yezbick A, et al. (2007) An experimental and clinical evaluation of a novel central venous catheter with integrated oximetry for pediatric patients undergoing cardiac surgery. Anesth Analg 105:1598–1604.

85. Petaja J, Lundstrom U, Sairanen H, et al. (1996) Central venous thrombosis after cardiac operations in children. J Thorac Cardiovasc Surg 112:883–889.

86. Nowak-Gottl U, Kotthoff S, Hagemeyer E (2001) Interaction of fibrinolysis and prothrombotic risk factors in neonates, infants and children with and without thromboembolism and underlying cardiac disease: a prospective study. Thromb Res 103:93–101.

87. Alioglu B, Avci Z, Tokel K, et al. (2008) Thrombosis in children with cardiac pathology: analysis of acquired and inherited risk factors. Blood Coagul Fibrinolysis 19:294–304.

88. Cholette JM, Rubenstein JS, Alfieris GM, et al. (2007) Elevated risk of thrombosis in neonates undergoing initial palliative cardiac surgery. Ann Thorac Surg 84:1320–1325.

89. Borrego R, Lopez-Herce J, Mencia S, et al. (2006) Severe ischemia of the lower limb and of the intestine associated with systemic vasoconstrictor therapy and femoral arterial catheterization. Pediatr Crit Care Med 7:267–269.

90. Raszka WV, Jr., Smith FR, Pratt SR (1989) Superior vena cava syndrome in infants. Clin Pediatr 28:195–198.

91. Leaker M, Massicotte MP, Brooker LA, Andrew M (1996) Thrombolytic therapy in pediatric patients: a comprehensive review of the literature. Thromb Haemost 76:132–134.

92. Gupta AA, Leaker M, Andrew M, et al. (2001) Safety and outcomes of thrombolysis with tissue plasminogen activator for treatment of intravascular thrombosis in children. J Pediatr 139:682–688.

93. Andrew M, Michelson AD, Bovill E, et al. (1998) Guidelines for antithrombotic therapy in pediatric patients. J Pediatr 132:575–588.

94. Petaja J, Peltola K, Rautiainen P (1999) Disappearance of symptomatic venous thrombosis after neonatal cardiac operations during antithrombin III substitution. J Thorac Cardiovasc Surg 118:955–956.

95. Krafte-Jacobs B, Sivit CJ, Mejia R, Pollack MM (1995) Catheter-related thrombosis in critically ill children: comparison of catheters with and without heparin bonding. J Pediatr 126:50–54.

96. Raad II, Luna M, Khalil SA, et al. (1994) The relationship between the thrombotic and infectious complications of central venous catheters. JAMA 271:1014–1016.

97. Pierce CM, Wade A, Mok Q (2000) Heparin-bonded central venous lines reduce thrombotic and infective complications in critically ill children. Intensive Care Med 26:967–672.

98. Shah PS, Shah N (2007) Heparin-bonded catheters for prolonging the patency of central venous catheters in children. Cochrane Database Syst Rev 4:CD005983.

99. Shankar KR, Abernethy LJ, Das KS (2002) Magnetic resonance venography in assessing venous patency after multiple venous catheters. J Pediatr Surg 37:175–179.

100. Flanigan DP, Keifer TJ, Schuler JJ, et al. (1983) Experience with Iatrogenic pediatric vascular injuries. Incidence, etiology, management, and results. Ann Surg 198:430–442.

101. Collier PE, Goodman GB (1995) Cardiac tamponade caused by central venous catheter perforation of the heart: a preventable complication. J Am Coll Surg 181:459–463.

102. Fukuda H, Kasuda H, Shimizu R (1993) Right ventricular perforation and cardiac tamponade caused by a central venous catheter. Masui 42:280–283.

103. van Engelenburg KC, Festen C (1998) Cardiac tamponade: a rare but life-threatening complication of central venous catheters in children. J Pediatr Surg 33:1822–1824.

104. Cherng YG, Cheng YJ, Chen TG, et al. (1994) Cardiac tamponade in an infant. A rare complication of central venous catheterisation. Anaesthesia 49:1052–1054.

105. Lonnqvist PA, Olsson GL (1991) Persistent left superior vena cava—an unusual location of central venous catheters in children. Intensive Care Med 17:497–500.

106. Gravenstein N, Blackshear RH (1991) In vitro evaluation of relative perforating potential of central venous catheters: comparison of materials, selected models, number of lumens, and angles of incidence to simulated membrane. J Clin Monit 7:1–6.

107. Suarez-Penaranda JM, Rico-Boquete R, Munoz JI, et al. (2000) Unexpected sudden death from coronary sinus thrombosis. An unusual complication of central venous catheterization. J Forensic Sci 45:920–922.

108. Hayashi Y, Maruyama K, Takaki O, et al. (1995) Optimal placement of CVP catheter in paediatric cardiac patients. Can J Anaesth 42:479–482.

109. Bolton DT (1997) Extravasation associated with a multilumen central catheter. Anaesthesia 52:1119.

110. Wang CC, Chen YW, Wu ET, et al. (2007) Identification and management of cardiac perforation by a double lumen catheter in an infant. Paediatr Anaesth 17:500–501.

111. Sigda M, Speights C, Thigpen J (1992) Pericardial tamponade due to umbilical venous catheterization. Neonatal Netw 11:7–9.

112. Raval NC, Gonzalez E, Bhat AM, et al. (1995) Umbilical venous catheters: evaluation of radiographs to determine position and associated complications of malpositioned umbilical venous catheters. Am J Perinatol 12:201–204.

113. Morag I, Epelman M, Daneman A, et al. (2006) Portal vein thrombosis in the neonate: risk factors, course, and outcome. J Pediatr 148:735–739.

114. Lavandosky G, Gomez R, Montes J (1996) Potentially lethal misplacement of femoral central venous catheters. Crit Care Med 24:893–896.

115. Zenker M, Rupprecht T, Hofbeck M, et al. (2000) Paravertebral and intraspinal malposition of transfemoral central venous catheters in newborns. J Pediatr 136:837–840.

116. Bodhey NK, Gupta AK, Sreedhar R, et al. (2006) Retroperitoneal hematoma: an unusual complication after femoral vein cannulation. J Cardiothorac Vasc Anes 20:859–861.

117. Maruyama K, Hayashi Y, Ohnishi Y, Kuro M (1995) How deep may we insert the cannulation needle for catheterization of the internal jugular vein in pediatric patients undergoing cardiovascular surgery? Anesth Analg 81:883–884.

118. Furfaro S, Gauthier M, Lacroix J, et al. (1991) Arterial catheter-related infections in children. A 1-year cohort analysis. Am J Dis Child 145:1037–1043.

119. O'Grady NP, Alexander M, Dellinger EP (2002) Guidelines for the prevention of intravascular catheter-related infections. The Hospital Infection Control Practices Advisory Committee, Center for Disease Control and Prevention, U.S. Pediatrics 110:e51.

120. Raad I, Darouiche R, Dupuis J (1997) Central venous catheters coated with minocycline and rifampin for the prevention of catheter-related colonization and bloodstream infections: a randomized, double-blind trial. The Texas Medical Center Catheter Study Group. Ann Intern Med 127:267–274.

121. Chelliah A, Heydon KH, Zaoutis TE, et al. (2007) Observational trial of antibiotic-coated central venous catheters in critically ill pediatric patients. Pediatr Infect Dis J 26:816–820.

122. Damen J, Van der Tweel, I (1988) Positive tip cultures and related risk factors associated with intravascular catheterization in pediatric cardiac patients. Crit Care Med 16:221–228.

123. Costello JM, Morrow DF, Graham DA, et al. (2008) Systematic intervention to reduce central line associated bloodstream infection rates in a pediatric cardiac intensive care unit. Pediatrics 121:915–923.

124. Lin MH, Young ML, Wang NK, Shen CT (2001) Central venous catheter-induced atrial ectopic tachycardia with reverse alternating Wenckebach periods. J Formos Med Assoc 100:50–52.

125. Conwell JA, Cocalis MW, Erickson LC (1993) EAT to the beat: "ectopic" atrial tachycardia caused by catheter whip. Lancet 342:740.

126. Baines D (2000) Persistent atrial fibrillation following central venous cannulation. Paediatr Anaesth 10:454–455.

127. Lee TY, Sung CS, Chu YC, et al. (1996) Incidence and risk factors of guidewire-induced arrhythmia during internal jugular venous catheterization: comparison of marked and plain J-wires. J Clin Anesth 8:348–351.

128. Cephus CE, Mott AR, Kertesz NJ, et al. (2007) Transient complete atrioventricular block after placement of a central venous catheter in a neonate. Pediatr Crit Care Med 8:64–66.

129. Morello FP, Donaldson JS, Saker MC, Norman JT (1999) Air embolism during tunneled central catheter placement performed without general anesthesia in children: a potentially serious complication. J Vasc Interv Radiol 10:781–784.

130. Kurekci E, Kaye R, Koehler M (1998) Chylothorax and chylopericardium: a complication of a central venous catheter. J Pediatr 132:1064–1066.

131. Miyamoto Y, Kinouchi K, Hiramatsu K, Kitamura S (1996) Cervical dural puncture in a neonate: a rare complication of internal jugular venipuncture. Anesthesiology 84:1239–1242.

132. Williams JH, Hunter JE, Kanto WP, Jr., Bhatia J (1995) Hemidiaphragmatic paralysis as a complication of central venous catheterization in a neonate. J Perinatol 15:386–388.

133. van Tets WF, van Dullemen HM, Tjan GT, van Berge HD (1992) Vertebral arteriovenous fistula caused by puncture of the internal jugular vein. Eur J Surg 158:627–628.

134. Zeligowsky A, Szold A, Seror D, et al. (1991) Horner syndrome: a rare complication of internal jugular vein cannulation. J Parenter Enteral Nutr 15:199.

10 Neurological monitoring and outcome

Chandra Ramamoorthy, M.B., B.S.; F.F.A. (UK)
Lucile Packard Children's Hospital, Stanford University School of Medicine, Stanford, California, USA

Dean B. Andropoulos, M.D.
Texas Children's Hospital, Baylor College of Medicine, Houston, Texas, USA

Introduction

The incidence of acute neurological complications following heart surgery in children ranged from 6 to 25% in reports from the 1980s to 1990s [1,2]. A more recent retrospective report of a series of 706 children undergoing heart surgery found that 2.3% had acute neurological complications [3]. Unlike adults, who undergo heart surgery with cardiopulmonary bypass (CPB) where acute postoperative neurological sequelae are largely embolic in nature [4], in children the etiology of neurological dysfunction is due to hypoxia/ischemia [5,6]. Techniques such as deep hypothermic circulatory arrest (DHCA) and low-flow bypass, which have allowed successful correction of complex cardiac defects in neonates and infants, may themselves contribute to neurological damage in this vulnerable population [7,8]. Furthermore, bypass circuitry and the conduct of CPB, the management of arterial blood gas (ABG)—α-stat (not correcting ABG for temperature) versus pH-stat (correcting ABG for temperature), hematocrit on bypass, and rate and extent of cooling and

rewarming are all important contributors to potential brain dysfunction after CPB [6,9].

Reducing the frequency and severity of CNS insults should improve neurological outcome. However, central nervous malformations in patients with congenital heart disease are more common [5], specifically those with hypoplastic left heart syndrome [10] where brain dysgenesis may approach 30%. Magnetic resonance imaging (MRI) studies of term newborns with congenital heart disease and no other identified genetic syndromes reveal a 20–40% incidence of white matter injury prior to surgical intervention. These white matter insults are similar to that reported in preterm newborns, suggesting abnormal in utero brain development [11]. In addition, children with chromosomal defects, particularly those with microdeletions of chromosome 22, have a higher incidence of central nervous system abnormalities [12], as do neonates with coarctation of aorta [13]. Hence these developmental brain disturbances add to the acquired brain injury in the perioperative setting.

During CPB, vital organs other than the brain have been routinely monitored. Any strategy for cerebral rescue from perioperative brain insults must rely on a neurological monitoring system that is easy, reliable, and reproducibly detects adverse events. Despite the existence of several modalities of brain monitoring, neurological monitoring remains in its infancy and has not become the standard of

Anesthesia for Congenital Heart Disease 2nd edition. Edited by
Dean Andropoulos, Stephen Stayer, Isobel Russell and Emad Mossad.
© 2010 Blackwell Publishing.

care. In this chapter, we review cerebral physiology during cardiac surgery in children, the current modalities for neurological monitoring and their limitations, evidence that neurological monitoring improves neurological outcome, and finally strategies for improving neurological outcome.

Cerebral physiology during cardiac surgery

The experimental basis for understanding neurophysiology in infants and children undergoing cardiac surgery involving CPB with DHCA comes largely from a series of landmark clinical studies undertaken in the late 1980s through mid-1990s by Greeley, Kern, Ungerleider, and colleagues [14–18]. These investigators measured cerebral blood flow (CBF) by the xenon clearance method in patients during hypothermic CPB and calculated cerebral oxygen extraction by measuring oxygen saturation in the arterial blood (inflow) and in the jugular venous bulb (outflow). Under deep hypothermic conditions, CBF is significantly reduced, but there is an exponentially greater reduction in cerebral metabolic rate ($CMRO_2$) (Figure 10.1).

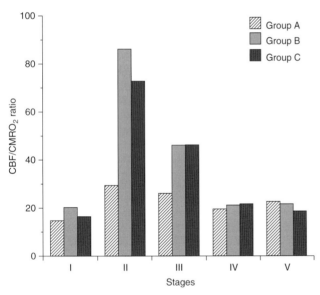

Figure 10.1 Cerebral blood flow (CBF)/cerebral metabolic rate for oxygen ($CMRO_2$) ratio during cardiac surgery in 46 pediatric patients aged 1 day to 14 years. Stage I: before cardiopulmonary bypass (CPB); Stage II: stable hypothermic conditions at 5 minutes; Stage III: stable hypothermic conditions at 25 minutes or just after deep hypothermic circulatory arrest (DHCA); Stage IV: rewarmed on CPB; Stage V: after CPB. Group A was cooled to 28°C without DHCA, Group B was cooled to 18°C without DHCA, and Group C cooled to 18°C with DHCA. There is a significant increase in CBF/$CMRO_2$ during deep hypothermic condition, favoring perfusion over CBF; flow/metabolism coupling is present at other times (Reproduced with permission from Reference [16]

Hence a state of luxury perfusion exists with an excess of flow relative to oxygen consumption. The temperature coefficient, or Q10, is the ratio of $CMRO_2$ at two temperatures separated by 10°C, and demonstrates an exponential decrease in $CMRO_2$. In neonates, infants, and children, the Q10 is 3.65, meaning $CMRO_2$ decreases by 3.65 times from baseline at 37° to 27°, and if cooled to 17°, $CMRO_2$ will decrease 3.65 times from the level found at 27°C. Based on these data, the investigators derived a "safe" duration of DHCA at various temperatures. This was estimated to be 11–19 minutes at 28°C and 39–65 minutes at 18°C. This calculation of a safe duration of circulatory arrest is similar to that seen in a clinical outcome study [19], and these studies confirm that hypothermia is an important factor for neuroprotection.

In patients undergoing circulatory arrest, both CBF and $CMRO_2$ remain decreased after rewarming, and following separation from CPB. The decreased CBF may be due to higher cerebral vascular resistance [20], and can be ameliorated with a 10-minute period of cold full-flow reperfusion before rewarming [21].

The rate and manner of cooling also have significant effects on cerebral oxygenation during CPB [18]. Kern et al. exposed infants to two different cooling strategies, aggressive or gradual, finding that gradual cooling more effectively reduced cerebral metabolism; however, there was considerable patient variability.

Another important factor is the question of pressure–flow autoregulation during hypothermic bypass [22]. Using transcranial Doppler ultrasound (TCD), 25 infants were studied during bypass using normothermia (36–37°C), moderate hypothermia (23–25°C), or profound hypothermia (14–20°C). CBF velocity was measured over a wide range of cerebral perfusion pressures (CPPs), ranging from 6 to 90 mm Hg. Cerebral pressure–flow autoregulation was preserved during normothermic bypass, with CBF increasing linearly until a CPP of 40 mm Hg and then leveling off. In contrast, during both moderate and profound hypothermia, flow became pressure passive, increasing linearly with pressure as high as 60 mm Hg.

Even though hypothermia leads to a loss of cerebral autoregulation, the CBF response to changes in arterial carbon dioxide tension is preserved in children [15]. Hence blood gas management (α-stat or pH-stat) during CPB significantly affects CBF and may have an impact on neurological outcome [23,24]. Both in vivo and ex vivo studies have demonstrated that pH-stat strategy results in greater CBF, greater efficiency and uniformity of brain cooling, and higher brain oxyhemoglobin saturation and less reduced cytochrome aa3 signifying more O_2 at the mitochondrial level [25–27].

Finally, using α-stat management and a xenon washout technique, Kern et al. [17] demonstrated that at moderate and deep hypothermia, reductions of bypass flow by

Table 10.1 Minimal cardiopulmonary bypass flow rates based on data of Kern et al.

Temperature (°C)	CMRO$_2$ (mL/100 g/min)	Predicted MPFR (mL/kg/min)
37	1.480	100
32	0.823	56
30	0.654	44
28	0.513	34
25	0.362	24
20	0.201	14
18	0.159	11
15	0.112	8

CMRO$_2$, cerebral metabolic rate for oxygen; MPFR, minimal predicted flow rate.
Source: Reproduced with permission from Reference [15].

35–45% do not change CBF and CMRO$_2$. When flow was reduced by 45–70%, a significant decrease in CBF and CMRO$_2$ resulted, associated with an increase in oxygen extraction. Even at lower flows, CBF and CMRO$_2$ decreased significantly, but oxygen extraction did not increase, suggesting an excess of flow over metabolic needs. Based on these measurements, the authors derived predicted minimal acceptable pump flow rates at various temperatures for the average pediatric patient (Table 10.1). Their prediction was validated in neonates undergoing the arterial switch operation at 18°C, who required pump flows of 10–20 mL/kg/min to maintain CBF measured by TCD [28].

Neurological monitoring during congenital heart surgery

Electroencephalographic technologies

The standard electroencephalogram (EEG) employing between 2 and 16 channels has been utilized in congenital heart surgery [29]. It is a rough guide of anesthetic depth, and can document electrocerebral silence before DHCA [30]. EEG is affected by several factors including anesthetic agents, temperature, and CPB. Impracticalities of the use of an intraoperative EEG include electrical signal interference, complexity of placement, and interpretation. Newer devices using processed EEG technology are more user friendly and have been extensively reviewed [31, 32]. The value of perioperative EEG monitoring in congenital heart surgery is unclear. For example, hypoplastic left heart syndrome neonates frequently have a normal perioperative EEG yet frequently demonstrate abnormalities of pre- and postoperative brain MRI suggestive of ischemia [33].

The Bispectral (BIS) Index monitor (Aspect Medical Systems, Nantick, MA) is currently promoted to guide the depth of anesthesia. BIS sensor electrodes are applied to the forehead and temple producing a frontal–temporal montage, which connects to a processing unit. The device is easy to use, electrodes are easy to place, and the monitor requires no calibration or warm up time. Via a proprietary algorithm of Aspect Corporation, BIS uses Fourier transformation and bispectral analysis of a one-channel processed EEG pattern to compute a single number, the BIS Index [34]. This index ranges from 0 (isoelectric EEG) to 100 (awake) with mean awake values in the 90–100 range in adults, infants, and children [35]. Depth of sedation is difficult to predict using BIS scores due to significant individual variability and anesthetic agent [36]. For BIS to be effective as a monitor of the depth of anesthesia, one would have to know exact BIS values for each anesthetic administered for an individual patient, thus reducing its value [37]. BIS can be used to recognize EEG burst suppression, or electrical silence, which could be useful during DHCA. The monitor displays a real-time EEG waveform, but is subject to motion artifact, EMG activity and radiofrequency interference from electrical equipment in the operating room. Little or no data exists in children on the use of other EEG devices such as the Physiometrix®, Narcotrend®, or Cerebral Function Monitor® [31]. During CPB, hemodilution and hypothermia alter pharmacokinetics and pharmacodynamics, which can lead to awareness under anesthesia. The overall incidence of awareness in adults undergoing cardiac surgery varies from 1.1 [37] to 23%, which is more than in general surgical procedures [38, 39]. The incidence of awareness under general anesthesia is similar in children [40]. Although there are no documented reports of awareness under anesthesia in children undergoing heart surgery, BIS monitoring may still be useful to detect a level of awareness.

In a cohort of children undergoing open-heart surgery with an anesthetic tailored for "fast-tracking," BIS scores increased during rewarming, a period considered at risk for awareness under anesthesia [41]. However in this study, and in a similar study in infants younger than 1 year [42], BIS did not correlate with stress hormone levels, a surrogate for light levels of anesthesia, nor with plasma fentanyl levels. At present, there is little evidence to support the use of BIS in neonates and infants undergoing anesthesia and therefore the value of BIS to assess burst suppression during DHCA is in further doubt. This is due to the different sleep–arousal patterns in this subset.

Monitors of cerebral oxygenation

Jugular venous bulb oximetry

Jugular bulb venous oximetry (SjvO$_2$) has been utilized in children with congenital heart disease since the late 1980s. It is considered the gold standard for the assessment of global cerebral oxygenation against which all noninvasive measurements are compared. The catheter can be placed by retrograde cannulation of the right internal jugular vein, with or without fluoroscopic confirmation of catheter tip placement [17]. Alternatively, the catheter can be placed by the surgeon after the heart and great vessels are exposed, by cannulating the superior vena cava (SVC) retrograde and advancing it into the jugular venous bulb [43]. $SjvO_2$ can be measured continuously with an oximetric catheter [44], or intermittent sampling for direct measurement of oxygen saturation. The drawbacks of this method include the invasive and time-consuming nature of retrograde internal jugular vein cannulation rendering it primarily a research tool. Noninvasive monitoring of cerebral oxygen saturation (rSO_2) is more practical.

Near-infrared spectroscopy

Near-infrared spectroscopy (NIRS) is a noninvasive optical technique used to monitor brain tissue oxygenation. Most devices utilize 2–4 wavelengths of infrared light at 700–1000 nm, where oxygenated and deoxygenated hemoglobin (Hb) have distinct absorption spectra [45–47]. Commercially available devices measure the concentration of oxy- and deoxyhemoglobin, using variants of the Beer–Lambert equation: $\log(I/I_0) = \varepsilon_\lambda LC$ Where I_0 is the intensity of light before passing through the tissue, I is the intensity of light after passing through the tissue, and the ratio of I/I_0 is absorption. Absorption of the near-infrared light depends on the optical path length (L), the concentration of the chromophore in that path (C), and

the molar absorptivity of the chromophore at the specific wavelength used (ε_λ).

Cerebral oximetry assumes that 75% of the cerebral blood volume in the light path is venous, and 25% is arterial. This 75:25 ratio is derived from theoretical anatomical models. Watzman et al. [48] attempted to verify this index in children with congenital heart disease by measuring jugular venous bulb saturation and arterial saturation, and comparing it to cerebral saturation measured with frequency-domain near-infrared spectroscopy. The actual ratio in patients varied widely, but averaged 85:15.

In the various models of cerebral oximeters currently on the market, the sensor electrode is placed on the forehead (Figure 10.2) below the hairline. A light-emitting diode or laser emits infrared light, which passes through a "banana-shaped" tissue volume in the frontal cerebral cortex, to two or three detectors placed 3–5 cm from the emitter. By using different sensing optodes and multiple wavelengths, extracranial and intracranial Hb absorption can be separated. Narrow arcs of light travel across skin and skull but do not penetrate the cerebral cortex. Deep arcs of light cross skin, skull, dura, and cortex. Subtracting the two absorptions measured, shallow from the deep, leaves absorption that is due to intracerebral chromophores, and this processing renders the cerebral specificity of the oximeter. However, the accuracy of NIRS is confounded by the light scattering that alters the optical path length and the available commercial clinical devices solve this problem differently.

Three cerebral oximeters are currently available: the INVOS, NIRO 500, and the Foresight. Of the three, the pediatric model of Somanetics INVOS system

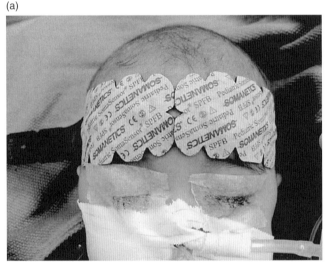

(a)

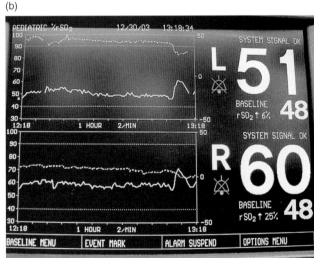

(b)

Figure 10.2 (a) Bilateral near-infrared spectroscopy (NIRS) probes. (b) Screen of NIRS monitor. Regional cerebral oxygen saturation (rSO_2) trend for left and right cerebral hemispheres, before bypass in neonate undergoing Norwood procedure is seen on left of screen. Current rSO_2 on the right, with baseline values, and relative change from baseline displayed under current rSO_2

(Somanetics, Inc., Troy, MI) (INVOS 5100) is in most common use and is designed for patients 4–40 kg and uses a different algorithm that takes into account the thinner skull and extracranial tissues compared to the adult [49]. More recently a neonatal probe has become available which is easier to apply as it conforms well to their forehead shape. This device is US Food and Drug Administration (FDA) approved for use in children and adults as a trend only monitor. It is compact, easy to use, and requires little warm up. The INVOS processor displays a numerical value at the measured regional rSO_2. The rSO_2 is reported as a percentage on a scale from 15 to 95%. A cerebral blood volume index (Crbvi) can also be calculated, representing the total Hb in the light path, which may be used as an estimate of cerebral blood volume; however, this is not an FDA-approved application for clinical use but only for research purposes.

The NIRO 500 (Hamamatsu Photonics, Hamamatsu, Japan) uses four wavelengths of light that allows for the determination of cytochrome aa3 concentration [50]. It uses spatially resolved spectrophotometry to calculate absolute concentrations of oxygenated and total Hb, rather than as saturations and reports a tissue oxygenation index (TOI). This device may be more accurate than the INVOS system due to the increased number of wavelengths of light; however, it is not FDA approved for use in the USA.

A more recent FDA-approved device is the Foresight monitor (Casmed, Branford, CT). This device also uses four wavelengths of light: 690, 778, 800, and 850 nm. The purpose of the additional wavelengths is to better discriminate non-Hb sources of infrared absorption, which may lead to a more accurate calculation of oxygenated and total Hb concentrations [51]. The Foresight monitor reports the percentage of oxygenated Hb to total Hb as a cerebral tissue oxygen saturation ($SCTO_2$). The three currently available probes are designed for patients weighing from 2.5 to 8 kg, 8 to 40 kg, and >40 kg.

Comparison between these commercial devices reveals differences in measured values thus making direct data comparisons difficult [46]. However, regardless of the device used, it is important to remember that all devices measure combined arterial and venous blood oxygen saturation, and cannot be assumed to be identical to $SjvO_2$. Maneuvers to increase arterial oxygen saturation, i.e., increasing FIO_2, will increase cerebral oxygenation as measured by these devices, but the $SjvO_2$ may remain unchanged.

The Foresight device is still relatively new and comparison data with the INVOS is not available. However, the Foresight monitor may predict a more accurate value for the true brain saturation compared to the INVOS monitor that will make between patient comparisons easier.

In an attempt to validate the noninvasive measurement of rSO_2 in children with congenital heart disease, $SjvO_2$ and rSO_2 have been compared. In 40 infants and children [52] undergoing congenital heart surgery or cardiac catheterization, the correlation for paired measurements was inconclusive except for infants younger than 1 year. In 30 patients undergoing cardiac catheterization, an improved correlation $r = 0.93$ was found [53], and there is a linear correlation between changes in arterial CO_2 and cerebral saturation. All of these experimental data lead to the appealing idea that NIRS can be used to direct therapy and influence outcome in congenital heart surgery.

Clinical data in pediatric cardiac surgery

These can be divided into preoperative, intraoperative, and postoperative. These studies for the most part are observational and long-term neurocognitive follow-up data is limited. Baseline preoperative rSO_2 as measured by a frequency-domain oximeter varies with cardiac lesion [47]. The baseline cerebral saturation is about 70% in acyanotic patients without large left-to-right intracardiac shunts breathing room air. On room air, rSO_2 for cyanotic patients is usually 40–60%; hypoplastic left heart syndrome (HLHS) patients receiving <21% FIO_2 preoperatively have lower rSO_2, averaging 53%, versus those receiving FIO_2 0.21 and 3% inspired CO_2, where rSO_2 averages 68% [54].

Changes in cerebral oxygenation have been characterized during CPB in children with or without DHCA [55] (Figure 10.3). rSO_2 predictably decreases during DHCA to a nadir approximately 60–70% below baseline values obtained prebypass [55] and the nadir is reached at about 40 minutes, after which there is no further decrease. At this point, it appears that the brain does not continue the uptake of oxygen and interestingly this time period appears to correlate with clinical and experimental studies suggesting that 45 minutes is the safe duration for circulatory arrest [16,19]. The DHCA initiation at higher temperature results in a faster fall in rSO_2 reaching the nadir sooner [56]. Reperfusion immediately results in an increase in rSO_2 levels seen at full bypass flow before DHCA.

In clinical use of NIRS monitors, low rSO_2 is often defined as a decrease of more than 20% in relative value from a baseline established preinduction on room air, or after induction on room air with normal $PaCO_2$ values (i.e., if baseline rSO_2 is 60%, a decrease to below 48% is considered an indication for treatment). rSO_2 less than 50% is also often treated, with the assumption as noted above that prolonged low rSO_2 may eventually lead to hypoxic ischemic brain injury. Treatment involves increasing oxygen delivery to the brain, or decreasing oxygen consumption. One approach to treatment is displayed in Table 10.2.

The question often arises whether bilateral cerebral hemisphere NIRS monitoring is necessary. In a study of 20 patients undergoing ACP via the right innominate artery, half of the patients had a left–right difference of >10% [57].

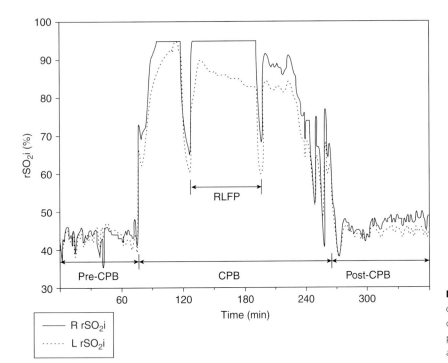

Figure 10.3 Typical changes in regional cerebral oxygen saturation (rSO$_2$) during cardiac surgery with cardiopulmonary bypass, regional cerebral low-flow perfusion (RLFP), and deep hypothermic circulatory arrest

In 60 neonates undergoing surgery with conventional bypass, only 10% had greater than 10% difference between left and right sides at baseline, and this difference persistent in only one patient [58]. Based on these data, bilateral monitoring is probably necessary only when special CPB techniques are used for aortic arch reconstruction, or when anatomical variants, i.e., bilateral SVC or abnormalities of the brachiocephalic vessels, are present.

Table 10.2 Treatment algorithm for low cerebral oxygen saturation (rSO$_2$) [108]

1. Establish baseline rSO$_2$ on FiO$_2$ 0.21, PaCO$_2$ 40 mm Hg, stable baseline hemodynamics, prebypass if possible
2. Treat decreased rSO$_2$ of >20% relative value below baseline, or <50% absolute value
3. Pre/postbypass (in order of ease/rapidity to institute)
   a. Increase FiO$_2$
   b. Increase PaCO$_2$
   c. Increase cardiac output/O$_2$ delivery with volume infusions, inotropic support, vasodilators, etc.
   d. Increase depth of anesthesia
   e. Decrease temperature
   f. Increase hemoglobin
4. During CPB
   a. Increase CPB flow and/or mean arterial pressure
   b. Increase PaCO$_2$
   c. Increase FiO$_2$
   d. Decrease temperature
   e. Increase hemoglobin
   f. Check aortic and venous cannula positioning

This is our routine practice at Texas Children's Hospital where on occasion we have noted an acute unilateral decrease in cerebral saturation with clamping the innominate artery in preparation for antegrade cerebral circulation. In this situation, we assume that the circle of Willis in not sufficiently patent to provide adequate cerebral perfusion through one carotid artery and have changed the cannulation technique.

Relationships between low cerebral saturation (rSO$_2$) and adverse neurological outcome

Cerebral oximetry reflects a balance between oxygen delivery and oxygen consumption by the brain (CMrO$_2$). The cerebral oxygen content will therefore be affected both by the arterial saturation of Hb and the Hb concentration. There then must exist a cerebral saturation value, ischemic threshold, below which brain injury is likely due to oxygen deprivation as demand outstrips the supply. In a neonatal piglet study using frequency domain NIRS [59], Kurth et al. showed that cerebral lactate levels rose at NIRS values of 44% or lower; major EEG changes occurred when the cerebral saturation declined to 37%, with reductions in cerebral ATP levels when oximetry readings were 33% or lower. This concept was confirmed in another neonatal piglet model using hypoxic gas mixtures showing that rSO$_2$ > 40% did not change EEG or brain pathology obtained 72 hours later; rSO$_2$ 30–40% produced no EEG changes, but at 72 hours there were ischemic neuronal changes in the hippocampus, and mitochondrial injury occurred. At rSO$_2$ < 30%, there was circulatory failure,

EEG amplitude decreased, and there was vacuolization of neurons and severe mitochondrial injury [60]. Finally in a similar piglet model, the hypoxic–ischemic cerebral saturation–time threshold for brain injury found rSO_2 of 35% for 2 hours or more produced brain injury [61]. In general, most clinical studies use either 20% below established baseline or an oximetry reading of 45–50% for the threshold for treatment based on evidence of new MRI lesions or clinical exam that brain injury is more likely to develop under these circumstances.

This threshold was validated recently in a group of neonates undergoing preoperative, intra-, and postoperative rSO_2 monitoring; prolonged low rSO_2 (>180 min with $rSO_2 \leq 45\%$) was associated with the presence of new ischemic lesions on postoperative MRI when compared to the presurgical study. Therefore, both the extent of decreased cerebral saturation (ischemic threshold) and the time spent below this ischemic threshold are important in predicting the development of new postoperative brain injury by MRI [33].

There is additional clinical evidence suggesting that low cerebral saturations correlate with adverse neurological outcome. A study of 26 infants and children undergoing surgery utilizing DHCA [62], three patients had acute neurological changes: seizures in one and prolonged coma in two; all of whom manifest low rSO_2. In these three patients, the increase in rSO_2 was much less after the onset of CPB and the duration of cooling before DHCA shorter. In a retrospective study of multimodality neurological monitoring in 250 infants and children undergoing cardiac surgery with bypass [29], relative cerebral oxygen desaturation of more than 20% below prebypass baseline resulted in abnormal events in 58% of patients. If left untreated, 26% of these patients had adverse postoperative neurological events.

In a study of 16 patients undergoing neonatal cardiac surgery, with NIRS monitoring and pre- and postoperative brain MRI, 6 patients developed a new postoperative brain injury; these patients had a lower rSO_2 during aortic cross-clamp period versus those without new brain injury (48% vs 57%, $p = 0.008$) [63]. In a recent study of 44 neonates undergoing the Norwood operation, who were tested at age 4–5 using a visual–motor integration (VMI) test, the first 34 patients did not have NIRS monitoring, and the last 10 did have NIRS monitoring with a strict treatment protocol for low rSO_2 values <50%. No patients with NIRS monitoring had a VMI score < 85 (normal is 100) versus 6% without NIRS monitoring. Mean rSO_2 in the perioperative period was associated with VMI score, with no patient with mean $rSO_2 \geq 55$ having VMI less than 96 [64].

Animal models that use NIRS can also act as a guide to the safe duration of DHCA. In a study of piglets, the time of the nadir of rSO_2 values during DHCA correlated with neurological outcome: a longer period without apparent oxygen uptake by the brain correlated with a greater chance of adverse neurological outcome. The maximum safe duration without brain oxygen uptake at 17°C was 30 minutes [27]. In another piglet model, NIRS was used to detect cerebral desaturation when the SVC was partially or totally occluded [65]. This has clinical relevance because cerebral desaturation from decreased CBF velocity may develop in small infants undergoing bicaval cannulation, who frequently have SVC obstruction, or in patients undergoing cavopulmonary anastomosis, where the SVC is partially occluded during the operation [66].

Another potential benefit of routine NIRS monitoring is to avert the rare but very real and devastating potential neurological disaster from cannulation problems, where rSO_2 declines dramatically from cannula malposition and cerebral arterial or venous obstruction, yet all other bypass parameters are normal [67,68].

Thus, far most studies on cerebral oximetry are observational and descriptive and the value of NIRS is difficult to definitively establish when evaluating the brain of neonates and children. Prospective randomized trials are confounded by the duration of follow-up that is required and the multifactorial etiology contributing to adverse neurological outcomes. Even though very large studies of changes in outcome through the use of pulse oximetry have never clearly demonstrated benefit, we would not practice without it [69]. Similarly, in the authors' opinion cerebral oximetry is an invaluable tool in monitoring and managing children during undergoing congenital heart surgery.

Transcranial Doppler ultrasound

Transcranial Doppler ultrasound (TCD) is a sensitive, real-time monitor of CBF velocity and emboli during congenital heart surgery. Currently available instruments utilize pulsed-wave ultrasound at 2 Mhz frequency, which is range-gated, emits a power of 100 mW, and has a sample volume length of up to 15 mm. A display of the frequency spectrum of Doppler signals is easily interpreted, and peak systolic and mean flow velocities, in cm/s, are displayed, as well as a pulsatility index that is equal to the peak velocity minus the end-diastolic velocity divided by the mean velocity.

The most consistent and reproducible technique for clinical use in patients of all ages is to monitor the middle cerebral artery (MCA) through the temporal window, which can usually be found just above the zygoma and just anterior to the tragus of the ear [70]. Several transducer probes are available, ranging from very small disc probes suitable for infants and children to larger, heavier probes for adolescents and adults. The depth of the sample volume and angle of insonation is adjusted until the bifurcation of the MCA and the anterior cerebral artery (ACA) are detected. This is heralded by a maximal antegrade signal (positive deflection, toward the transducer) from the MCA, accompanied by retrograde flow (negative deflection, away from the transducer) of the same or very similar velocity and waveform, as the MCA flow. The same location should be monitored for an individual patient. Insonation at the MCA–ACA bifurcation also offers the advantage of minimizing interpatient variability. In addition, the MCA supplies the largest volume of tissue of any of the basal cerebral arteries [71]. In infants, an alternative site for monitoring is through the anterior fontanelle, using a hand-held pencil-type probe, placing the probe over the lateral edge of the fontanelle, and aiming caudally, at a greater depth than for the temporal window.

TCD has been used extensively in pediatric cardiac surgical research to examine cerebral physiology in response to CPB, hypothermia, low-flow bypass, regional low-flow perfusion to the brain, and circulatory arrest. Hillier et al. [72] used TCD to study cerebrovascular hemodynamics during hypothermic bypass with DHCA in 10 infants finding that CBF velocity did not return to baseline levels after DHCA. Calculated cerebral vascular resistance (mean arterial pressure – central venous pressure/CBFV) was increased immediately after DHCA, and remained so until the end of bypass. The observed decrease in CBFV during cooling was thought to be due to decreased metabolic demand by the brain and thus less blood flow, although α-stat strategy was used. This could be explained by relative cerebral vasoconstriction during cooling in smaller arterioles downstream to the MCA and ACA, since these large arteries do not change their caliber in response to changes in Pa_{CO_2} [73]. TCD of the MCA through the temporal window was used to describe the cerebral pressure–flow velocity relationship during hypothermic bypass in 25 infants younger than 9 months. CBFV was examined over a wide range of CPPs (varying from 6 to 90 mm Hg), and at three temperatures: normothermia (36–37°C), moderate hypothermia (23–25°C), and profound hypothermia (14–20°C). Cerebral pressure flow autoregulation was preserved at normothermia, partially affected at moderate hypothermia, and totally lost at profound hypothermia; results which agree with previous research done using xenon to quantitate CBF [14].

TCD has also been utilized to determine the threshold of detectable cerebral perfusion during low-flow CPB. Zimmerman et al. [28] studied 28 neonates undergoing the arterial switch operation with α-stat pH management. At 14–15°C, the pump flow was sequentially reduced to 0 mL/kg/min. All patients had detectable CBF down to 20 mL/kg/min, while one had no perfusion at 20 mL/kg/min, and eight had none at 10 mL/kg/min, leading the authors to conclude that 30 mL/kg/min was the minimum acceptable flow in this population. Finally, Andropoulos et al. [74] used TCD of the MCA to deter-

mine the level of bypass flow necessary during regional low-flow perfusion for neonatal aortic arch reconstruction. They studied 34 neonates undergoing the Norwood operation or aortic arch advancement and established a baseline mean CBFV (22 cm/s) under full-flow bypass (150 mL/kg/min) using pH-stat management at 17–22°C. They then used TCD to determine how much bypass flow was necessary to match this value, finding that a mean of 63 mL/kg/min was necessary.

Cerebral emboli are a frequent threat during open-heart surgery in children. Emboli are easily detected by TCD, although this is subject to artifacts such as electrocautery and physical contact with the ultrasound transducer [75]. The number of emboli detected in the carotid artery during pediatric congenital heart surgery did not appear to correlate with acute postoperative neurological deficits [75]. However, acute drops in CBF detected by TCD can allow for adjustment of aortic or SVC cannulae, which may avert neurological disaster [66].

Temperature monitoring

Hypothermia remains the cornerstone of brain protection for ischemic injury. Cerebral hyperthermia frequently develops after congenital heart surgery with CPB. The metabolic rate and oxygen consumption of neurons is raised during a period when O_2 delivery may be compromised from decreased CO. This places vulnerable watershed areas or partially damaged neurons at risk for permanent cell death [76]. Bissonnette et al. [77] measured temperatures in the jugular bulb (JBVT), tympanic membrane, lower esophagus, and rectum during and after surgery in 15 infants and showed that the JBVT temperature continued to rise for at least 6 hours postoperatively when the study ended. The authors found that the commonly monitored rectal temperature does not reflect brain temperature in the perioperative period. Other investigators also confirm and show that the nasopharyngeal, not tympanic, temperature best reflects brain temperature [76]. Although Cotrell et al. were unable to show a causal relation between postoperative temperature and neurocognitive outcomes in several hundred infants undergoing cardiac surgery with bypass [78], more recently in a multicenter trial of total body hypothermia for neonatal asphyxia, the treatment group had reduced risk of death and moderate–severe disability compared to controls [79,80].

Since hypothermia is considered a major factor in the systemic inflammatory response to CPB, European centers report neonatal surgery with either total body normothermia or selective cerebral hypothermia [81,82]. The long-term neurocognitive outcomes from such modalities are unclear at present.

Improving neurological outcome in children undergoing open heart surgery

It is clear that neurological injury in infants and children undergoing congenital heart surgery is multifactorial in origin, and prevention remains the key to avoiding permanent CNS injury. A multilayer strategy for detection and prevention of neurological abnormalities in the perioperative period is presented.

Preoperative care

The principles of maintaining adequate cardiac output and oxygen delivery to the brain are critically important in the immediate preoperative period. Appropriate inotropic support, ventilation strategies, avoiding hyperthermia, blood transfusion, or prompt balloon atrial septostomy when indicated will stabilize patients and improve oxygen delivery. In some centers, 40–50% of patients presenting for cardiac surgery in the newborn period have their defects diagnosed prenatally. Whenever possible, delivery should occur in a center experienced in the care of newborns with congenital heart disease, and immediate appropriate care instituted.

When patients with HLHS are diagnosed prenatally and delivered in a referral center, acute neurological complications are reduced versus those without prenatal diagnosis and delivered in an outlying hospital [83]. Neurological examination, cranial ultrasound, computed tomography scan, and MRI have detected abnormalities related to preoperative hypoxic–ischemic injury, or malformations, including those associated with chromosomal abnormalities [84–86].

Management of cardiopulmonary bypass

pH-stat versus α-stat blood gas management

pH-stat management corrects blood gas values for temperature during CPB allowing for greater CBF during hypothermia, greater oxygen delivery, and more even distribution of flood flow. The oxyhemoglobin dissociation curve is shifted to the right, facilitating unloading of oxygen [87]. In animal models of DHCA, neurological outcome is improved when pH-stat is used. In humans (infants), this has been more difficult to demonstrate, although there are trends toward a lower death rate [24], fewer seizures, and greater hemodynamic stability. Long-term neurological follow-up to 4 years of age does not demonstrate a difference if pH versus α-stat is used [87].

Low-flow bypass versus DHCA

DHCA, particularly if prolonged over 30–45 minutes, is associated with a higher incidence of neurological complications. One hundred eighty patients younger than 3 months undergoing repair of transposition of the great arteries were randomized to low-flow CPB versus DHCA in a landmark study at Boston Children's Hospital [7]. There was a higher incidence of seizures and elevated brain creatine kinase in the DHCA group. Seizures became more common after 30 minutes of DHCA. At 1-year follow-up, a significant relationship was found between the duration of circulatory arrest and psychomotor development [88]. At 4 years, the DHCA patients fared worse on examination of fine motor function. At 8 years, patients receiving DHCA with a cut point of 41 minutes fared worse on overall performance in mental and psychomotor tasks, with some subtests showing worse results at shorter DHCA times [19]. These studies provide evidence that low-flow bypass is superior to DHCA in prevention of neurological injury.

Regional cerebral perfusion

Until recently, neonatal aortic reconstruction surgery was believed to require DHCA. The Norwood palliation for hypoplastic left heart syndrome and aortic arch advancement for repair of the interrupted or severely hypoplastic aortic arch are the most common examples. In recent years, novel perfusion techniques, such as regional cerebral perfusion [89], have been developed. Using this technique, the brain is perfused during the aortic reconstruction through a Goretex graft sewn into the base of the innominate artery, or through special small aortic cannulae advanced into the innominate artery (Figure 10.4). Neurological monitoring [74] has demonstrated adequate CBF and oxygenation using this technique. Utilizing this technique, DHCA to the brain can be limited to less than 10 minutes for the Norwood palliation, or eliminated altogether. This approach has theoretical advantages, and improved neurological outcome is expected. Recently in a group of newborns who underwent the Norwood procedure using either DHCA or ACP showed no differences in neurocognitive outcome at 1 year of age [90]. However, ACP flow rates in this study were only 25 mL/kg/min, and were not adjusted through the use of cerebral oximetry or TCD monitoring, and this flow rate has been shown to be inadequate in some patients [91,92].

Rate of cooling and rewarming on bypass

There is evidence that in some patients brain metabolism is not adequately suppressed during rapid cooling to deep hypothermic levels. In a study of infants undergoing

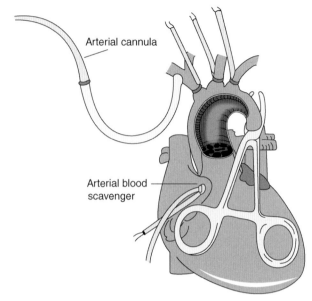

Figure 10.4 Regional cerebral perfusion for the Norwood Stage I palliation for hypoplastic left heart syndrome. Arterial inflow for bypass is provided by a small polytetrafluoroethylene graft sewn to the right innominate artery. Instead of deep hypothermic circulatory arrest, flow is provided to the brain at low rates, while the brachiocephalic vessels and descending thoracic aorta are snared, providing a bloodless operating field (Reproduced with permission from Reference [89])

cooling to 15°C, 6 of 17 had low jugular venous bulb saturation when this temperature was achieved, suggesting ongoing oxygen consumption that outstripped delivery of oxygen to the brain [43]. Uneven or inefficient cooling of the brain may lead to neurological deficits. Cooling less than 20 minutes is associated with lower developmental scores among newborns undergoing the arterial switch operation using DHCA [93], and the risk of developing choreoathetosis is related to shorter periods of cooling [94].

Hemodilution strategy

Traditionally, we have thought that the hematocrit should be reduced to approximately 20% during deep hypothermia to offset the increase in viscosity from cooling. Recently, this hypothesis has been challenged and found that patients have improved developmental scores using a target hematocrit of 30 provides versus 20 [27]. Combining the results of two hematocrit trials at Boston Children's Hospital evaluated the neurodevelopmental outcomes of 271 infants at age 1 year, and found that the Psychomotor Development Index increased linearly with hematocrit up to 23.5%. The Mental Development Index did not exhibit an association with hematocrit. The overall conclusion of this analysis was that although a hematocrit of 24% or higher improved outcome in these studies, but because

the effects of hemodilution vary considerably according to age, perfusion strategy, pH management, and other variables, that no one universally safe hemodilution level exists [95].

Neuroprotectant agents

At the current time, there is little evidence that any pharmacological intervention has the potential to improve neurological outcome in children undergoing congenital heart surgery. Corticosteroids, barbiturates, phenytoin, and aprotinin have been postulated to offer some degree of neuroprotection, but there is no current evidence to support this. One study in newborns has suggested that allopurinol may improve early outcome after congenital heart surgery [96]. Halogenated anesthetic agents used in the bypass circuit, particularly desflurane show promise in a neonatal pig model [97]. Other agents, such as erythropoietin, which has been found to protect the brain against hypoxic–ischemic insults in a variety of animal models, may have promise in neonatal cardiac surgery [98].

Glucose management

In the Boston circulatory arrest study [7], hyperglycemia was not associated with worse neurological outcome and does not appear to be a risk factor for children; in fact the probability of a perioperative seizure in the newborn is—two to three times greater with a serum glucose less than 100 mg/dL versus glucose greater than 200 mg/dL [99]. In a study of 188 neonates and infants younger than 6 months undergoing surgery with CPB, mean ICU admission glucose was 328 mg/dL, maximum was 340 mg/dL, and 89% of patients had at least one value >200 mg/dL. Hyperglycemia was not associated with lower neurodevelopment scores at 1 year of age [100]. There is no consensus in the pediatric cardiac literature as to optimal glucose management and whether a tight glucose control should even be attempted.

Postoperative management

The immediate postoperative period is likely a time of greatest perioperative risk for the development of a neurological insult. Cardiac output and brain oxygen delivery must be optimized at a time when the myocardium is recovering from the insult of ischemia and the options of increasing delivery with bypass or reducing brain oxygen consumption with active cooling are limited. Tweddel et al. have shown an improvement in survival and in neurological outcome from careful monitoring of superior vena caval saturation among patients after the Norwood procedure, and treating low SvO_2 [101]. Ungerleider et al. have promoted the use of postoperative mechanical

(a)

(b)

(c)

(d)

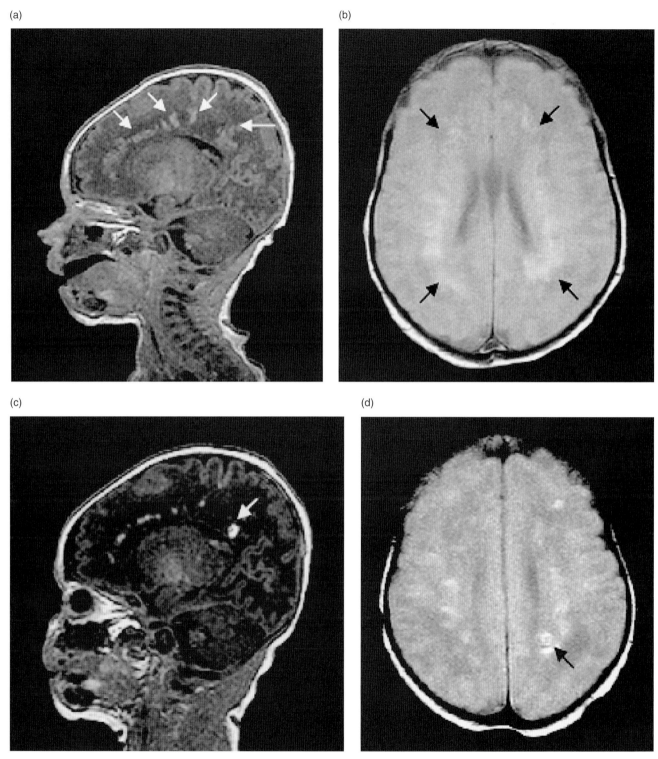

Figure 10.5 (a) Preoperative sagittal T1-weighted MR image of a 35-week gestational age infant with hypoplastic left heart syndrome. Significant white matter injury (WMI) is present in the periventricular areas (arrows). (b) Preoperative axial proton-density T2-weighted image. Again note extensive WMI (arrows). (c) 7-day postoperative T1 sagittal MRI after Norwood Stage I palliation. Note slight improvement to WMI, but new intraparenchymal/intraventricular hemorrhage and infarction in the atrium near the body of the left lateral ventricle (arrow). (d) Proton-density T2-weighted image. Again note WMI and new hemorrhage (arrow)

circulatory support for Norwood patients in order to ensure continued oxygen delivery to the brain [102]. Deep sedation and avoidance of hyperthermia will reduce brain oxygen consumption, but this has not been proven to reduce the risk of neurological injury. Consideration should be given to monitoring of rSO_2 in certain high-risk patients. This approach also awaits prospective study of effectiveness in preventing adverse neurological outcomes.

Neurological outcomes in the modern era

Long-term neurodevelopmental abnormalities are found in 21–69% of school-aged children undergoing complex cardiac surgery as infants in the late 1980s and in the 1990s [103]. More recently, Tabbutt et al., in reporting the 1 year neurodevlopmental outcomes in infants with HLHS, noted that 65% had abnormal neuromuscular examination and almost half had severe psychomotor delay [104]. A particularly important finding is that many of these patients do not have gross neurological deficits, but have learning disabilities, problems with fine motor control, and attention-deficit hyperactivity disorder. In a study of 109 school-aged children who underwent neonatal cardiac surgery from 1992 to 1997, 49% were receiving remedial school services, and 30% met criteria for attention-deficit hyperactivity disorder [105]. In 61 neonatal arterial switch patients whose surgery was done in 1996–2003, with a full-flow pH-stat bypass technique with limited DHCA use, neurodevelopmental outcome at age 5 years was better than in previous eras, with a full scale IQ of 97, with verbal intelligence 97, motor score of 96, and VMI score of 95 (population norm is 100 on all tests). However, 26% of children had some speech or language difficulty, and 11% had a learning disability [106]. Traditional trials of perioperative interventions designed to improve neurodevelopmental status require at least 5 years to assess the outcome. Studies of premature infants have found that brain MRI changes correlate well with neurodevelopmental outcome and are an acceptable surrogate to judge the early results of interventions [107] (Figure 10.5). We recently reported a study of 69 neonates undergoing complex cardiac surgery in 2005–2008 with a high-flow, high-hematocrit CPB strategy, and cerebral oxymetry monitoring using a treatment protocol for low rSO_2. The incidence of new brain MRI injury 7 days postoperatively was 36%, and new white matter injury 15%, with a low severity of injury [108]. Neurodevelopmental outcome will be assessed on these patients through 5 years of age to determine if this perfusion and monitoring strategy not only improves MRI findings but truly improves outcome.

Conclusions

As the mortality rate for all congenital heart surgery trends downward toward 1–2% in most large centers, attention has increasingly turned to other morbidities affecting quality of life, none of which is more important than neurological outcome. Neurological morbidity is clearly decreasing as well, but remains a troubling problem. Basic science and clinical outcome studies have been performed in the past 15 years, but more outcome data is required. Despite clinical and experimental evidence that DHCA is detrimental to neurological outcome, widespread use continues, and not restricted to newborn surgery. Comparative studies with novel techniques such as regional low-flow cerebral perfusion, and neuroprotectant agents, with long-term neurological follow-up, need to be performed in order to address this question. Noninvasive monitors now available for cerebral oxygenation, blood flow, and EEG—do they improve outcome? Will newer technologies, i.e., frequency-domain spectrophotometers for measurement of cerebral oxygenation, prove to be more accurate? These questions will need to be addressed as we strive to improve the quality of life for our patients.

References

1. Fallon P, Aparicio JM, Elliott MJ, Kirkham FJ (1995) Incidence of neurological complications of surgery for congenital heart disease. Arch Dis Child 72:418–422.
2. Ferry PC (1987) Neurologic sequelae of cardiac surgery in children. Am J Dis Child 141:309–312.
3. Menache CC, du Plessis AJ, Wessel DL, et al. (2002) Current incidence of acute neurologic complications after open-heart operations in children. Ann Thorac Surg 73:1752–1758.
4. Murkin JM (1999) Commentary. J Thorac Cardiovasc Surg 118:420–421.
5. Kirkham FJ (1998) Recognition and prevention of neurological complications in pediatric cardiac surgery. Pediatr Cardiol 19:331–345.
6. du Plessis AJ (1999) Mechanisms of brain injury during infant cardiac surgery. Semin Pediatr Neuro 6:32–47.
7. Newburger JW, Jonas RA, Wernovsky G (1993) A comparison of the perioperative neurologic effects of hypothermic circulatory arrest versus low-flow cardiopulmonary bypass in infant heart surgery. N Engl J Med 329:1057–1064.
8. Bellinger DC, Jonas RA, Rappaport LA (1995) Developmental and neurologic status of children after heart surgery with hypothermic circulatory arrest or low-flow cardiopulmonary bypass. N Engl J Med 332:549–555.
9. Wypij D, Jonas RA, Bellinger DC, et al. (2008) The effect of hematocrit during hypothermic cardiopulmonary bypass in infant heart surgery: Results from the combined Boston hematocrit trials. J Thorac Cardiovasc Surg 135:355–360.

10. Glauser TA, Rorke LB, Weinberg PM, Clancy RR (1990) Congenital brain anomalies associated with the hypoplastic left heart syndrome. Pediatrics 85:984–990.

11. Miller SP, McQuillen PS, Hamrick S, et al. (2007) Abnormal brain development in newborns with congenital heart disease. N Engl J Med 357:1928–1938.

12. Bingham PM, Zimmerman RA, McDonald-McGinn D, et al. (1997) Enlarged Sylvian fissures in infants with interstitial deletion of chromosome 22q11. Am J Med Genet 74:538–543.

13. Young RS, Liberthson RR, Zalneraitis EL (1982) Cerebral hemorrhage in neonates with coarctation of the aorta. Stroke 13:491–494.

14. Greeley WJ, Ungerleider RM, Kern FH, et al. (1989) Effects of cardiopulmonary bypass on cerebral blood flow in neonates, infants, and children. Circulation 80:I209–I215.

15. Kern FH, Ungerleider RM, Quill TJ (1991) Cerebral blood flow response to changes in arterial carbon dioxide tension during hypothermic cardiopulmonary bypass in children. J Thorac Cardiovasc Surg 101:618–622.

16. Greeley WJ, Kern FH, Ungerleider RM (1991) The effect of hypothermic cardiopulmonary bypass and total circulatory arrest on cerebral metabolism in neonates, infants, and children. J Thorac Cardiovasc Surg 101:783–794.

17. Kern FH, Ungerleider RM, Reves JG (1993) Effect of altering pump flow rate on cerebral blood flow and metabolism in infants and children. Ann Thorac Surg 56:1366–1372.

18. Kern FH, Ungerleider RM, Schulman SR (1995) Comparing two strategies of cardiopulmonary bypass cooling on jugular venous oxygen saturation in neonates and infants. Ann Thorac Surg 60:1198–1202.

19. Wypij D, Newburger JW, Rappaport LA, et al. (2003) The effect of duration of deep hypothermic circulatory arrest in infant heart surgery on late neurodevelopment: the Boston Circulatory Arrest Trial. J Thorac Cardiovasc Surg 126:1397–1403.

20. Jonassen AE, Quaegebeur JM, Young WL (1995) Cerebral blood flow velocity in pediatric patients is reduced after cardiopulmonary bypass with profound hypothermia. J Thorac Cardiovasc Surg 110:934–943.

21. Rodriguez RA, Austin EH, III, Audenaert SM (1995) Postbypass effects of delayed rewarming on cerebral blood flow velocities in infants after total circulatory arrest. J Thorac Cardiovasc Sur 110:1686–1690.

22. Taylor RH, Burrows FA, Bissonnette B (1992) Cerebral pressure-flow velocity relationship during hypothermic cardiopulmonary bypass in neonates and infants. Anesth Analg 74:636–642.

23. Priestley MA, Golden JA, O'Hara IB, et al. (2001) Comparison of neurologic outcome after deep hypothermic circulatory arrest with alpha-stat and pH-stat cardiopulmonary bypass in newborn pigs. J Thorac Cardiovasc Surg 121:336–343.

24. du Plessis AJ, Jonas RA, Wypij D (1997) Perioperative effects of alpha-stat versus pH-stat strategies for deep hypothermic cardiopulmonary bypass in infants. J Thorac Cardiovasc Surg 114:991–1000.

25. Hiramatsu T, Miura T, Forbess JM (1995) pH strategies and cerebral energetics before and after circulatory arrest. J Thorac Cardiovasc Surg 109:948–957.

26. Aoki M, Nomura F, Stromski ME (1993) Effects of pH on brain energetics after hypothermic circulatory arrest. Ann Thorac Surg 55:1093–1103.

27. Sakamoto T, Zurakowski D, Duebener LF (2002) Combination of alpha-stat strategy and hemodilution exacerbates neurologic injury in a survival piglet model with deep hypothermic circulatory arrest. Ann Thorac Surg 73:180–189.

28. Zimmerman AA, Burrows FA, Jonas RA, Hickey PR (1997) The limits of detectable cerebral perfusion by transcranial Doppler sonography in neonates undergoing deep hypothermic low-flow cardiopulmonary bypass. J Thorac Cardiovasc Surg 114:594–600.

29. Austin EH, III, Edmonds HL, Jr., Auden SM (1997) Benefit of neurophysiologic monitoring for pediatric cardiac surgery. J Thorac Cardiovasc Surg 114:707–715, 717.

30. Akiyama T, Kobayashi K, Nakahori T (2001) Electroencephalographic changes and their regional differences during pediatric cardiovascular surgery with hypothermia. Brain Dev 23:115–121.

31. Bowdle TA (2006) Depth of anesthesia monitoring. Anesthesiology Clin 24:793–822.

32. Davidson AJ (2006) Measuring anesthesia in children using the EEG. Paediatr Anaesth 16:374–387.

33. Dent CL, Spaeth JP, Jones BV, et al. (2006) Brain magnetic resonance imaging abnormalities after the Norwood procedure using regional cerebral perfusion. J Thorac Cardiovasc Surg 131:190–197.

34. Sigl JC, Chamoun NG (1994) An introduction to bispectral analysis for the electroencephalogram. J Clin Monit 10:392–404.

35. Denman WT, Swanson EL, Rosow D, et al. (2000) Pediatric evaluation of the bispectral index (BIS) monitor and correlation of BIS with end-tidal sevoflurane concentration in infants and children. Anesth Analg 90:872–877.

36. Ibrahim AE, Taraday JK, Kharasch ED (2001) Bispectral index monitoring during sedation with sevoflurane, midazolam, and propofol. Anesthesiology 95:1151–1159.

37. Phillips AA, McLean RF, Devitt JH, Harrington EM (1993) Recall of intraoperative events after general anaesthesia and cardiopulmonary bypass. Can J Anaesth 40:922–926.

38. Goldmann L, Shah MV, Hebden MW (1987) Memory of cardiac anaesthesia. Psychological sequelae in cardiac patients of intra-operative suggestion and operating room conversation. Anaesthesia 42:596–603.

39. Dowd NP, Cheng DC, Karski JM, et al. (1998) Intraoperative awareness in fast-track cardiac anesthesia. Anesthesiology 89:1068–1073.

40. Davidson AJ, Huang GH, Czarnecki C, et al. (2005) Awareness during anesthesia in children: a prospective cohort study. Anesth Analg 100:653–661.

41. Laussen PC, Murphy JA, Zurakowski D, et al. (2001) Bispectral index monitoring in children undergoing mild hypothermic cardiopulmonary bypass. Paediatr Anaesth 11:567–573.

42. Kussman BD, Gruber EM, Zurakowski D, et al. (2001) Bispectral index monitoring during infant cardiac surgery: relationship of BIS to the stress response and plasma fentanyl levels. Paediatr Anaesth 11:663–669.

43. Kern FH, Jonas RA, Mayer JE, et al. (1992) Temperature monitoring during CPB in infants: does it predict efficient brain cooling? Ann Thorac Surg 54:749–754.

44. Sandstrom K, Nilsson K, Andreasson S, Larsson LE (1995) Jugular bulb temperature compared with non-invasive temperatures and cerebral arteriovenous oxygen saturation differences during open heart surgery. Paediatr Anaesth 9:123–128.

45. Kurth CD, Steven JM, Nicolson SC, et al. (1992) Kinetics of cerebral deoxygenation during deep hypothermic circulatory arrest in neonates. Anesthesiology 77:656–661.

46. Yoshitani K, Kawaguchi M, Tatsumi K, et al. (2002) A comparison of the INVOS 4100 and the NIRO 300 near infrared spectrophotometers. Anesth Analg 94:586–570.

47. Kurth CD, Steven JL, Montenegro LM (2001) Cerebral oxygen saturation before congenital heart surgery. Ann Thorac Surg 72:187–192.

48. Watzman HM, Kurth CD, Montenegro LM, et al. (2000) Arterial and venous contributions to near-infrared cerebral oximetry. Anesthesiology 93:947–953.

49. Dullenkopf A, Frey B, Baenziger O, et al. (2003) Measurement of cerebral oxygenation state in anaesthetized children using the INVOS 5100 cerebral oximeter. Paediatr Anaesth 13:384–391.

50. Grubhofer G, Tonninger W, Keznickl P, et al. (1999) A comparison of the monitors INVOS 3100 and NIRO 500 in detecting changes in cerebral oxygenation. Acta Anaesthesiol Scand 43:470–475.

51. Rais-Bahrami K, Rivera O, Short BL (2006) Validation of a noninvasive neonatal optical cerebral oximeter in venovenous ECMO patients with a cephalad catheter. J Perinatol 26:628–635.

52. Daubeney PE, Pilkington SN, Janke E, et al. (1996) Cerebral oxygenation measured by near-infrared spectroscopy: comparison with jugular bulb oximetry. Ann Thorac Surg 61:930–934.

53. Abdul-Khaliq H, Troitzsch D, Berger F, Lange PE (2000) Regional transcranial oximetry with near infrared spectroscopy (NIRS) in comparison with measuring oxygen saturation in the jugular bulb in infants and children for monitoring cerebral oxygenation. Biomed Tech (Berl) 45:328–332.

54. Ramamoorthy C, Tabbutt S, Kurth CD (2002) Effects of inspired hypoxic and hypercapnic gas mixtures on cerebral oxygen saturation in neonates with univentricular heart defects. Anesthesiology 96:283–288.

55. Kurth CD, Steven JM, Nicolson SC (1995) Cerebral oxygenation during pediatric cardiac surgery using deep hypothermic circulatory arrest. Anesthesiology 82:74–82.

56. Daubeney PE, Smith DC, Pilkington SN (1998) Cerebral oxygenation during paediatric cardiac surgery: identification of vulnerable periods using near infrared spectroscopy. Eur J Cardiothorac Surg 13:370–377.

57. Andropoulos DB, Diaz LK, Stayer SA, et al. (2004) Is bilateral monitoring of cerebral oxygen saturation necessary during neonatal aortic arch reconstruction? Anesth Analg 98:1267–1272.

58. Kussman BD, Wypij D, DiNardo JA, et al. (2005) An evaluation of bilateral monitoring of cerebral oxygen saturation during pediatric cardiac surgery. Anesth Analg 101:1294–1300.

59. Kurth CD, Levy WJ, McCann J (2002) Near-infrared spectroscopy cerebral oxygen saturation thresholds for hypoxia-ischemia in piglets. J Cereb Blood Flow Metab Mar; 22 (3):335–341.

60. Hou X, Ding H, Teng Y, et al. (2007) Research on the relationship between brain anoxia at different regional oxygen saturations and brain damage using near-infrared spectroscopy. Physiol Meas 28:1251–1265.

61. Kurth CD, McCann JC, Wu J, et al. (2009) Cerebral oxygen saturation-time threshold for hypoxic–oschemic injury in piglets. Anesth Analg 108:1268-1277.

62. Kurth CD, Steven JM, Nicolson SC (1995) Cerebral oxygenation during pediatric cardiac surgery using deep hypothermic circulatory arrest. Anesthesiology 82:74–82.

63. McQuillen PS, Barkovich AJ, Hamrick SE, et al. (2007) Temporal and anatomic risk profile of brain injury with neonatal repair of congenital heart defects. Stroke 38 (Part 2):736–741.

64. Hoffman GM, Mussatto KM, Brosig CL, et al. (2008) Cerebral oxygenation and neurodevelopmental outcome in hypoplastic left heart syndrome. Anesthesiology 109:A7 (Abstract).

65. Sakamoto T, Duebener LF, Tayler G, et al. (2002) Obstructed SVC cannula may result in cerebral ischemia which can be detected by near-infrared spectroscopy during CPB. Anesth Analg 93, SCA 82.

66. RA Rodriguez, Cornel G, Splinter WM, et al. (2000) Cerebrovascular effects of aortovenous cannulations for pediatric cardiopulmonary bypass. Ann Thorac Surg 69:1229–1235.

67. Gottlieb EA, Fraser CD, Andropoulos DB, Diaz LK (2006) Bilateral monitoring of cerebral oxygen saturation results in recognition of aortic cannula malposition during pediatric congenital heart surgery. Paediatr Anaesth 16:787–789.

68. Ing RJ, Lawson DS, Jaggers J, et al. (2004) Detection of unintended partial superior vena cava occlusion during a bidirectional cavopulmonary anastomosis. J Cardiothorac Vasc Anesth 18:472–474.

69. Pedersen T, Pedersen BD, Moller AM (2003) Pulse oximetry for perioperative monitoring. Cochrane Database Syst Rev 2:CD002013.

70. Fischer AQ, Truemper EJ (1993) Applications in the neonate and child. In: Bibikian VL, Wechlser LR (eds) Transcranial Doppler Ultrasonography, 2nd edn. Butterworth-Heineman, Oxford, England, pp. 355–375.

71. Truemper EJ, Fischer AQ (1993) Cerebrovascular developmental anatomy and physiology in the infant and child. In: Bibikian VL, Wechsler LR (eds). Transcranial Doppler Ultrasonography, 2nd edn. Butterworth-Heineman, Oxford, England, pp. 281–320.

72. Hillier SC, Burrows FA, Bissonnette B, Taylor RH (1991) Cerebral hemodynamics in neonates and infants undergoing cardiopulmonary bypass and profound hypothermic circulatory arrest: assessment by transcranial Doppler sonography. Anesth Analg 72:723–728.

73. Huber P, Handa J (1967) Effect of contrast material, hypercapnia, hyperventilation, hypertonic glucose and

papaverine on the diameter of the cerebral arteries: angiographic determination in man. Invest Radiol 2:17–32.

74. Andropoulos DB, Stayer SA, McKenzie ED, Fraser CD, Jr. (2003) Novel cerebral physiologic monitoring to guide low-flow cerebral perfusion during neonatal aortic arch reconstruction. J Thorac Cardiovasc Surg 125:491–499.

75. O'Brien JJ, Butterworth J, Hammon JW, et al. (1997) Cerebral emboli during cardiac surgery in children. Anesthesiology 87:1063–1069.

76. Kurth CD, Steven JM (2000) Keeping a cool head. Anesthesiology 93:598–600.

77. Bissonnette B, Holtby HM, Davis AJ, et al. (2000) Cerebral hyperthermia in children after cardiopulmonary bypass. Anesthesiology 93:611–618.

78. Cottrell SM, Morris KP, Davies P, et al. (2004) Early postoperative body temperature and developmental outcome after open heart surgery in infants. Ann Thorac Surg 77:66–71.

79. Shankaran S, Laptook AR, Ehrenkranz RA, et al. (2005) Whole-body hypothermia for neonates with hypoxic–ischemic encephalopathy. N Engl J Med 353:1574–1584.

80. Perlman JM (2006) Summary proceedings from the neurology group on hypoxic–ischemic encephalopathy. Pediatrics 117:S28–S33.

81. Pouard P, Mauriat P, Ek F, et al. (2006) Normothermic cardiopulmonary bypass and myocardial cardioplegic protection for neonatal arterial switch operation. Eur J Cardiothorac Surg 30:695–699.

82. Oppido G, Napoleone CP, Turci S, et al. (2006) Moderately hypothermic cardiopulmonary bypass and low-flow antegrade selective cerebral perfusion for neonatal aortic arch surgery. Ann Thorac Surg 82:2233–2239.

83. Mahle WT, Clancy RR, McGaurn SP, et al. (2001) Impact of prenatal diagnosis on survival and early neurologic morbidity in neonates with the hypoplastic left heart syndrome. Pediatrics 107:1277–1282.

84. Limperopoulos C, Majnemer A, Shevell MI, et al. (1999) Neurologic status of newborns with congenital heart defects before open heart surgery. Pediatrics 103:402–408.

85. McConnell JR, Fleming WH, Chu WK (1990) Magnetic resonance imaging of the brain in infants and children before and after cardiac surgery: a prospective study. Am J Dis Child 144:374–378.

86. van Houten JP, Rothman A, Bejar R (1996) High incidence of cranial ultrasound abnormalities in full-term infants with congenital heart disease. Am J Perinatol 13:47–53.

87. Laussen PC (2002) Optimal blood gas management during deep hypothermic paediatric cardiac surgery: alpha-stat is easy, but pH-stat may be preferable. Paediatr Anaesth 12:199–204.

88. Hickey PR (1998) Neurologic sequelae associated with deep hypothermic circulatory arrest. Ann Thorac Surg 65:S65–S69.

89. Pigula FA, Siewers RD, Nemoto EM (1999) Regional perfusion of the brain during neonatal aortic arch reconstruction. J Thorac Cardiovasc Surg 117:1023–1024.

90. Goldberg CS, Bove EL, Devaney EJ, et al. (2007) A randomized clinical trial of regional cerebral perfusion versus deep hypothermic circulatory arrest: outcomes for infants with functional single ventricle. J Thorac Cardiovasc Surg 133:880–887.

91. Hofer A, Haizenger B, Geiselseider G, et al. (2005) Monitoring of selective antegrade cerebral perfusion using near infrared spectroscopy in neonatal aortic arch surgery. Eur J Anaesthesiol 22:293–298.

92. Fraser CD, Jr., Andropoulos DB (2008) Principles of antegrade cerebral perfusion during arch reconstruction in newborns/infants. Semin Thorac Cardiovasc Surg Pediatr Card Surg Annu 61–68.

93. Bellinger DC, Wernovsky G, Rappaport LA (1991) Cognitive development of children following early repair of transposition of the great arteries using deep hypothermic circulatory arrest. Pediatrics 87:701–707.

94. Wong PC, Barlow CF, Hickey PR (1992) Factors associated with choreoathetosis after cardiopulmonary bypass in children with congenital heart disease. Circulation 86:II118–II126.

95. Wypij D, Jonas RA, Bellinger DC, et al. (2008) The effect of hematocrit during hypothermic cardiopulmonary bypass in infant heart surgery: results from the combined Boston hematocrit trials. J Thorac Cardiovasc Surg 135:355–360.

96. Clancy RR, McGaurn SA, Goin JE (2001) Allopurinol neurocardiac protection trial in infants undergoing heart surgery using deep hypothermic circulatory arrest. Pediatrics 108:61–70.

97. Loepke AW, Priestley MA, Schultz SE, et al. (2002) Desflurane improves neurologic outcome after low-flow cardiopulmonary bypass in newborn pigs. Anesthesiology 97:1521–1527.

98. Nelson DP, Andropoulos DB, Fraser CD Jr. (2008) Perioperative neuroprotective strategies. Semin Thorac Cardiovasc Surg Pediatr Card Surg Annu 49–56.

99. Burrows FA, McGowan FX (1996) Neurodevelopmental consequences of cardiac surgery for congenital heart disease. In: Greeley WI (ed) Perioperative Management of the Patient with Congenital Heart Disease. Williams & Wilkins, Baltimore, pp. 133–174.

100. Ballweg JA, Wernovsky G, Ittenbach RF, et al. (2007) Hyperglycemia after infant cardiac surgery does not adversely impact neurodevelopmental outcome. Ann Thorac Surg 84:2052–2058.

101. Tweddell JS, Ghanayem NS, Mussatto KA, et al. (2007) Mixed venous oxygen saturation monitoring after stage 1 palliation for hypoplastic left heart syndrome. Ann Thorac Surg 84:1301–1310.

102. Giacomuzzi C, Heller E, Mejak B, et al. (2005) Assessing the brain using near-infrared spectroscopy during postoperative ventricular circulatory support. Cardiol Young 15 (Suppl 1):154–158.

103. Wernovsky G (2006) Current insights regarding neurological and developmental abnormalities in children and young adults with complex congenital cardiac disease. Cardiol Young 16 (Suppl 1):92–104.

104. Tabbutt S, Nord AS, Jarvik, GP, et al. (2008) Neurodevelopmental outcomes after staged palliation for hypoplastic left heart syndrome. Pediatrics 121:476–483.

105. Shillingford AJ, Glanzman MM, Ittenbach RF, et al. (2008) Inattention, hyperactivity, and school performance in a population of school-age children with complex congenital heart disease. Pediatrics 121:e759–e767.

106. Neufeld RE, Clark BG, Robertson CM, et al. (2008) Five-year neurocognitive and health outcomes after the neonatal arterial switch operation. J Thorac Cardiovasc Surg 136:1413–1421.

107. Sherlock RL, McQuillen PS, Miller SP (2009) Preventing brain injury in newborns with congenital heart disease: Brain imaging and innovative trial designs. Stroke 40:327–332.

108. Andropoulos DB, Hunter JV, Nelson DP, et al. (2009) Brain MRI injury before and after neonatal cardiac surgery with high-flow bypass and maximized oxygen delivery strategy. J Thorac Cardiovasc Surg in press.

11

Transesophageal echocardiography in congenital heart disease

Isobel A. Russell, M.D., Ph.D.
Moffit-Long Hospitals, University of California, San Francisco, California, USA

Wanda C. Miller-Hance, M.D.
Texas Children's Hospital, Baylor College of Medicine, Houston, Texas, USA

Introduction

The transesophageal approach is an excellent window for imaging intracardiac and vascular structures due to the proximity of the esophagus to the heart and major blood vessels. Initial efforts on using the esophagus as a site of echocardiographic imaging were made in the mid-1970s by Frazin [1]. Since the introduction of transesophageal echocardiography (TEE) to the intraoperative setting in the late 1980s, the utility of this imaging approach has been demonstrated in adult patients in the evaluation of valvular repair, prosthetic valve function, structural heart disease, monitoring of myocardial ischemia and left ventricular preload, as well as during noncardiac surgery [2–12]. As surgical advances in the care of patients with heart dis-

ease have evolved, contributions of TEE are continually demonstrated [13–15]. Transesophageal imaging provides for immediate detection of suboptimal surgical interventions thus improving outcomes, avoiding subsequent reoperations, and reducing morbidity, mortality, and costs [16–18].

Until the early 1990s, intraoperative evaluation of infants and children undergoing interventions for cardiovascular pathology was not feasible via the transesophageal approach because probe sizes were not suitable for examination in this patient group. The subsequent development of miniaturized technology demonstrated that echocardiography could be performed safely in the pediatric population [19–23].

This chapter focuses on TEE for monitoring and evaluation of patients with congenital heart disease (CHD), highlighting the benefits and practice of this imaging approach in the intraoperative setting, particularly in the pediatric age group.

Anesthesia for Congenital Heart Disease 2nd edition. Edited by Dean Andropoulos, Stephen Stayer, Isobel Russell and Emad Mossad.
© 2010 Blackwell Publishing.

History of pediatric intraoperative epicardial echocardiography

In 1989 Ungerleider and colleagues provided one of the first demonstrations of the use of intraoperative echocardiography in congenital heart surgery [24]. Covered transducers were directly applied to the anterior surface of the heart in order to document the adequacy of the surgical repair. This approach "directed specific and efficient repair immediately so that all patients left the operating room with surgically acceptable results." The experience provided strong support for the concept that intraoperative echocardiography could guide specific surgical or anesthetic adjustments in pediatric cardiac surgery and underscored the useful role of epicardial echocardiography of CHD [25–28].

Intraoperative epicardial imaging at the present time is reserved for infants in whom transesophageal probes cannot be used because of size constraints and in patients with contraindications to esophageal instrumentation. Limitations to the epicardial approach relate to limited windows of interrogation, potential for hemodynamic changes, and requirement for participation and experience in cardiovascular imaging by the surgeon.

History of pediatric intraoperative TEE

Cyran et al. described the first successful experience in intraoperative TEE for pediatric patients using an adult-sized probe in children as young as 7.5 years of age [29]. The first probe specifically designed for infants weighing as little as 3 kg was subsequently reported by Kyo and Omoto with the Aloka/Corometrics Company (Japan) [30,31]. This was a single-plane, 5-MHz, 26-element phased array probe with a maximum diameter of 6.8 mm. Reports regarding this device appeared in the early 1990s documenting the accuracy, immediacy, and feasibility of TEE in the assessment of pediatric cardiac surgery [19,21,32,33]. Initial experience demonstrated that TEE had enhanced diagnostic capabilities in some patients over transthoracic echocardiography, and the advantage of accuracy equal to that obtained using epicardial imaging [34,39].

Despite the limitations of TEE, it was shown that when compared to epicardial echocardiography, this approach did not interrupt surgery, caused potential arrhythmias or hypotension, or increased the infection risk [40].

In 1992 clinical investigations began with the introduction of a new high-resolution single-plane TEE probe with continuous wave Doppler capabilities (5.0-MHz phase array, 48-element TEE probe) (Figure 11.1). This new probe produced images superior to those obtained with the previous technology [41]. The subsequent introduction of pediatric biplane probes allowed for examinations using both the transverse (horizontal) plane and the longitudinal (vertical) plane (Figure 11.1) [42–45]. The additional plane of interrogation provided for a more complete examination of the ventricular outflow tracts. Several investigators demonstrated that advancing existing single or biplane probes into the fundus of the stomach could provide a view that favorably imaged the outflow tracts, allowing for quantitative assessment of outflow tact obstructions [46,47]. Accordingly, the transgastric views emerged overcoming some of the limitations of single and biplane imaging.

Multiplane imaging was the last modality to be introduced and it has now been available for pediatric patients (Figure 11.1) for a number of years [48]. A high-resolution minimultiplane TEE probe (5-MHz, 48-element, 9.5–10-mm diameter) presently allows for the acquisition of images in multiple planes over a 180° arc. This has been of particular benefit in the assessment of complex structural heart defects. An even smaller prototype device (micromultiplane TEE probe) with high-resolution capabilities, (7.5-MHz, 48-element, 8.2-mm diameter) developed by General Electric Corporate Research in association with Odelf Corporation (the Netherlands) has been investigated and proposed as an ideal probe in infants under 2 kg [49,50]. Unfortunately, technological limitations related to the small size of the probe have hindered the further development of this device.

Live three-dimensional transesophageal echocardiography (3D-TEE) has recently become available using a matrix array probe [51, 52]. This technology is superior to prior efforts in the field. The current imaging device provides for unique applications in patients over 30 kg in weight. 3D-TEE is increasingly being applied in the perioperative setting [53–56]. Early experience not surprisingly also documents benefits in patients with CHD [57–60]. It is hoped that once these or equivalent devices become available for use in infants and small children, the unique windows afforded by the 3D technology should enhance the acquisition of structural and functional information in the pediatric age group in the operating room and other clinical settings [61].

The catheters designed for intracardiac echocardiography (ICE) have been utilized via the transesopheageal approach as an alternative to standard intraoperative imaging in small infants. Although these devices are not formally marketed for this particular application and several limitations are recognized, they may provide clinically useful information in some cases.

To date, most institutions use a combination of imaging approaches, for the comprehensive evaluation of the pediatric heart. TEE has been a rapidly evolving field and is considered the standard of care by many cardiac surgical

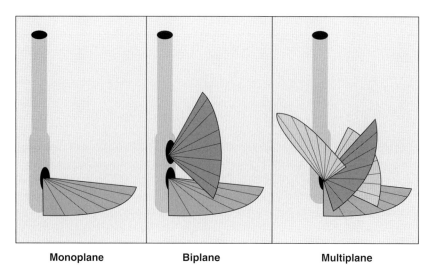

Monoplane   Biplane   Multiplane

Figure 11.1 Transesophageal echocardiographic probes. The *left* panel displays the single plane (monoplane or uniplane probe) that allows for transverse (horizontal) plane imaging. The *middle* panel depicts the biplane device that provides for both transverse and longitudinal (vertical) plane interrogation. The *right* panel displays the multiplane (omniplane) probe that provides for any number of planes to be acquired in a 0–180° arc

centers for intraoperative evaluation of pediatric patients undergoing surgery for congenital and acquired heart disease [62,63].

Indications for TEE

Transthoracic echocardiography provides excellent definition of cardiovascular anatomy in most infants and young children. Therefore, TEE should not be considered a substitute for a complete transthoracic preoperative examination but rather a complimentary imaging modality.

TEE provides diagnostic-quality images in the majority of patients with congenital cardiac anomalies when the transthoracic examination or other studies have not successfully elucidated the necessary clinically relevant information. By overcoming limitations related to poor windows, suboptimal image quality, or lung interference, TEE is able to facilitate morphologic and functional assessment of most structural cardiac defects.

Indications for TEE in children have been proposed by various groups. Initial efforts by the Committee on Standards for Pediatric Transesophageal Echocardiography, Society of Pediatric Echocardiography were published in 1992 [64]. Subsequently, task forces of the American Society of Anesthesiologists and the Society of Cardiovascular Anesthesiologists established practice guidelines for perioperative TEE [65]. Shortly thereafter, the American College of Cardiology (ACC)/American Heart Association (AHA) Task Forces, in collaboration with the American Society of Echocardiography (ASE), proposed recommendations for the clinical application of echocardiography [66]. The ACC/AHA/ASE reconvened in 2003 to update these guidelines [66]. The indications for pediatric intraoperative TEE from the four reports respectively are summarized as follows:

1 Intraoperative and postrepair examinations are indicated when operations are performed on cardiac defects in which there are significant residual abnormalities such as outflow tract obstruction, valve regurgitation, or stenosis or intracardiac communications are anticipated or suspected [64].
2 Most cardiac defects requiring repair under cardiopulmonary bypass are a Category 1 indication for intraoperative TEE, including pre- and postcardiopulmonary imaging (defined as that being supported by the strongest evidence or expert opinion substantiating that TEE is useful in improving clinical outcomes) [65].
3 Monitoring and guidance during cardiothoracic procedures associated with the potential for residual shunts, valvular regurgitation, obstruction, or myocardial dysfunction is a Class I indication (defined as conditions for which there is evidence and/or general agreement that a given procedure or treatment is useful and effective) [66].
4 Surgical repair of most congenital heart lesions that require cardiopulmonary bypass is a Class I indication. The updated guidelines list assessment of residual flow after interruption of a patent ductus arteriosus as a Class IIb indication (conditions for which there is conflicting evidence and/or a divergence of opinion about the usefulness/efficacy of a procedure or treatment). Repair of an uncomplicated secundum atrial septal defect is considered a Class III indication (defined as conditions for which there is evidence and/or general agreement that the procedure/treatment is not useful/effective in some cases may be harmful) [67].

The latest group that has reported on the subject is a task force of the Pediatric Council of the American Society of Echocardiography [68]. In the updated clinical indications for the performance of TEE in pediatric patients with acquired or congenital cardiovascular disease

Table 11.1 Indications for transesophageal echocardiography in the patient with congenital heart disease

Diagnostic indications
  Patient with suspected CHD and nondiagnostic TTE
  Presence of PFO and direction of shunting as possible etiology for stroke
  Evaluation of intra or extracardiac baffles following the Fontan, Senning, or Mustard procedure
  PFO evaluation with agitated saline contrast to determine possible right-to-left shunt, prior to transvenous pacemaker insertion
  Aortic dissection (Marfan syndrome)
  Intracardiac evaluation for vegetation or suspected abscess
  Evaluation for intracardiac thrombus prior to cardioversion for atrial flutter/fibrillation
  Pericardial effusion or cardiac function evaluation and monitoring postoperative patient with open sternum or poor acoustic windows
  Evaluating status of prosthetic valve
Perioperative indications
  Immediate preoperative definition of cardiac anatomy and function
  Postoperative surgical results and function
TEE-guided interventions
  Guidance for placement of ASD or VSD occlusion device
  Guidance for blade or balloon atrial septostomy
  Catheter tip placement for valve perforation and dilation in catheterization laboratory
  Guidance during radiofrequency ablation procedure
  Results of minimally invasive surgical incision or video assisted cardiac procedure

ASD, atrial septal defect; CHD, congenital heart disease; PFO, patent foramen ovale; TTE, transthoracic echocardiography; VSD, ventricular septal defect.
Source: Reproduced with permission from Reference [68].

(group collectively referred to as "the patient with CHD") the following major categories were outlined: diagnostic assessment, perioperative evaluation, and related to interventions. These are expanded upon in Table 11.1. In regards to perioperative indications, the recommendations are for the use of TEE for immediate preoperative definition of cardiac anatomy and function, and postoperative assessment of surgical results, hemodynamic monitoring, and real-time clinical decision making.

Technique for TEE

Equipment

A number of transesophageal probes are commercially available for use in the pediatric age group. The most commonly used echocardiographic platforms in North America include Philips Medical Systems (former Hewlett Packard, Agilent, and ATL Technologies, Andover, MA), Siemens Ultrasound, Mountain View, CA (former Acusson Technologies), and General Electric/Vingmed General Electric Medical Systems Milwaukee, WI. Commonly used TEE probes and their specifications are listed in Table 11.2. Other devices suitable for pediatric use are marketed by several companies in Europe and Asia.

In general, probes are not interchangeable among the various echocardiographic platforms and may not be interchangeable between machines across the same platform.

Probe selection

Although transesophageal probes can be used into tiny neonates, in fact a case report documents safety in a 1.7-kg baby, most centers that routinely utilize TEE consider the use of this approach relatively safe in infants with a weight over 3 kg [69]. The pediatric multiplane probe is suitable for all ages and may be considered in small infants; however, the relatively large and nonflexible tip may present a challenge for insertion, and potentially a higher risk, in the extremely small neonate. There are minimal differences between the actual tip dimensions of current pediatric probes; however, in some neonates the biplane probes may in be easier to insert.

Probe insertion and manipulation can be associated with hemodynamic and/or respiratory compromise therefore vigilance is imperative. In some cases, the arterial blood pressure tracing or pulse oximetry signal may be partially or completely attenuated by probe manipulation (Figure 11.2). Patients with certain pathologies (i.e., anomalous pulmonary venous drainage, vascular rings/slings) may be at higher risk of hemodynamic or respiratory compromise with TEE probe insertion and/or manipulation. They particularly deserve careful assessment of the risk–benefit ratio. In the event of acute hemodynamic or airway changes, the probe should be repositioned or removed immediately.

The superior resolution capabilities of the adult-sized multiplane probes make these devices preferable for children above 15–20 kg. The intracardiac probe (ICE) that

Table 11.2 Transesophageal echocardiographic probes

Transesophageal probes	Tip dimensions (W × H × L, in mm)	Shaft dimensions (W × L, in mm)	Number of elements	Imaging frequencies (MHz)
Philips (Hewlett Packard/Agilent)				
Pediatric biplane	9.3 × 8.8 × 27	8 × 80	64	5.5–7.5
Pediatric multiplane	10.7 × 7.2 × 25.4	7.4 × 70	48	4.0–7.0
Adult multiplane (Omni II)	14.5 × 11.2 × 42	10.5 × 100	64	4.0–7.0
Acuson (Siemens)				
Pediatric biplane (V7B)	9.5 × 8.5 × 31	8.5 × 85	48	5.0–8.0
Pediatric multiplane (V7M)	10.7 × 8 × 36*	7 × 70	48	4.0–8.0
Adult multiplane (V5M)	14.5 × 11.5 × 45	10.5 × 110	64	3.5–7.0
General Electric/Vingmed				
Pediatric multiplane (8T, MPTE)	10.7 × 7.5 × 37.5*	7 × 70	48	3.3–8.0
Adult multiplane (6T/6Tv and 5T/PAMPTE)	14 × 12.5 × 40	10.5 × 110	64	4.4–8.0

*Length of inflexible distal part of probe.

Probe specification information provided by respective companies. Imaging frequencies may vary with specific ultrasound system.

has been used for transesophageal applications in small infants is a 5.5–10 MHz single longitudinal plane device with a diameter of 3.3 mm. The probe has size advantage over standard imaging devices; however, the presence of only a single plane may limit its usefulness [70].

Probe insertion

Prior to transesophageal imaging, several considerations should be entertained. These include a review of relevant clinical information, appraisal of potential contraindications, and informed consent. In addition, it is extremely helpful to review available imaging studies, particularly prior echocardiograms. The standard safety precautions associated with an endoscopic procedure should be followed. Although serious complications during TEE are rare, it should be considered that this is a semi-invasive/invasive procedure that may result in potential risks.

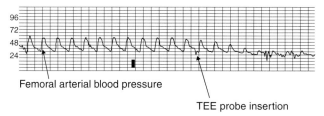

Figure 11.2 Hemodynamic changes in a neonate associated with transesophageal echocardiography (TEE) probe insertion. The graphic illustrates abrupt changes in systemic arterial blood pressure (recorded from a femoral artery line) associated with TEE probe insertion in a neonate with total anomalous pulmonary connection. Hypotension was considered the result of probe compression of the pulmonary venous confluence

In the outpatient setting several options are available for anesthetic care [71]. A combination of oropharyngeal topical anesthesia and intravenous sedation may be considered for the older child, adolescent, or young adult. Small children usually require deep sedation or general anesthesia. Endotracheal intubation is used in most cases; however, a few recent reports document the use of a laryngeal mask airway during limited esophageal instrumentation [72,73].

Standard cardiorespiratory monitoring should include intermittent blood pressure assessments during the procedure, in addition to electrocardiography, pulse oximetry, and capnography. The facilities should be equipped with oxygen and suction capabilities. In addition, drugs and equipment for emergency therapy or cardiopulmonary resuscitation should be readily available.

Patients with CHD may have significant hemodynamic alterations and be marginally compensated; therefore, the judicious, titrated administration of suitable drugs and agents is warranted. In the case of patients with cyanotic heart disease, additional considerations apply. These include potential for paradoxical air embolism during the administration of intravenous fluids or drugs, detrimental effects related to the rapid onset of anxiolytics, anticholinergics and sedatives, and decreases in systemic vascular resistance associated increases in the magnitude of right-to-left shunting resulting in further systemic arterial desaturation.

In the operative setting after induction of general anesthesia and endotracheal intubation, gastric contents may be suctioned to optimize image quality. Some centers prefer nasal rather than oral endotracheal intubation in view of concerns related to the stability of an endotracheal tube during TEE probe manipulation. Regardless of the intubation route, the endotracheal tube should be securely taped to minimize potential displacement.

The lubricated unlocked probe should be advanced gently into esophagus. A forward thrust of the mandible frequently assists in the passage of the probe. On occasion direct guidance of the probe with a gloved finger may be helpful. If significant difficulty is encountered and attempts at probe insertion are unsuccessful, direct visualization of the oropharynx with a laryngoscope may assist in esophageal intubation. The probe should never be advanced if resistance is encountered. Once the transducer is positioned behind the heart, the patient's head can be turned to the side to avoid interference with the surgical procedure during manipulation of the probe.

No data regarding optimal head position during probe insertion in children was available until recently. The traditional recommendation has been for the head to remain in the midline position. A study that evaluated this issue suggests that children under 10 kg in weight should have the head positioned to the side rather than midline during probe insertion. If unsuccessful or difficult with the head in the midline position, the authors recommend turning the head to the side and reattempting probe insertion. The rationale for this investigation relied on the assumption that turning the head to the side closes the ipsilateral pyriform sinus and dilates the contralateral pyriform sinus, theoretically making probe insertion safer and easier [74].

A recent investigation in adult patients documented that rigid laryngoscope-assisted insertion of TEE probes reduces the incidence of oropharyngeal mucosal injury, odynophagia, and the number of insertion attempts [75]. The same may apply to the pediatric age group.

Probe manipulation and imaging planes

The TEE probe can be manipulated in several general directions; advanced or withdrawn, anteflexed or retroflexed, and rotated clockwise or counterclockwise relative to the sagittal plane (Figure 11.3) [76,77]. The current multiplane probe obviates some of the manipulations required in previous single and biplane devices and allows for rotation of the plane (forward and backward).

As general principles of transducer manipulation, in the normally positioned heart, anteflexion brings structures anterior and toward the base of the heart into view, clockwise rotation allows for imaging of rightward structures, and counterclockwise rotation permits viewing of left-sided structures. In the smallest neonates, minimal adjustments in probe position are adequate to change from view to view.

Since both, biplane and multiplane probe-types are currently used in clinical practice in children, the discussion that follows describes the echocardiographic examination using each of these devices. Guidelines have been

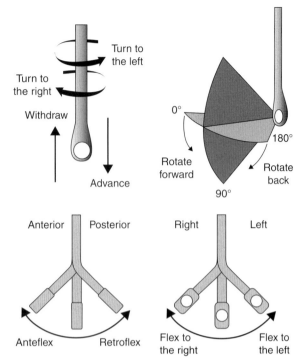

Figure 11.3 Manipulation of the transesophageal echocardiography (TEE) probe during image acquisition. The possible manipulations of the TEE probe are depicted (Reproduced with permission from Reference [77])

published for performing a comprehensive intraoperative multiplane echocardiographic examination [77]. Although these recommendations were established for adult patients, similar principles can be applied to the pediatric patient. All examinations should include careful two-dimensional imaging and spectral and color flow Doppler interrogation. To evaluate for small intracardiac shunts or the presence of specific pathology, contrast injection with agitated saline into a central vein or appropriate peripheral vein may be used. In addition to assisting in the identification of small intracardiac shunts, contrast echocardiography may also be useful in the identification of anomalous systemic venous connections, as seen in patients with persistent drainage of a left superior vena cava into the coronary sinus [78,79].

The basic examination described in the following sections is provided as a reference and assumes levocardia (heart in the left thoracic cavity, apex pointing to the left), visceroatrial situs solitus (stomach to the left, liver to the right, and normal atrial arrangement), and concordant atrioventricular and ventriculoarterial connections. The wide spectrum of structural cardiovascular malformations dictates a modified scheme from the basic examination in many patients. In addition, it is recognized that the views described cannot be obtained in all patients, nor the planes and angles of interrogation will necessarily conform to each patient's unique anatomy.

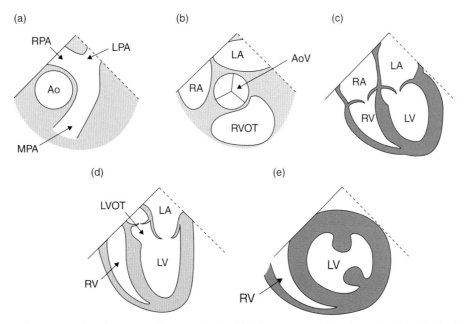

Figure 11.4 Diagrammatic representation of transverse plane examination. (a) Pulmonary artery view: the main and branched pulmonary arteries are depicted in this view, obtained at 0° at the mid-esophageal level. (b) Aortic short-axis view: the aortic valve cusps can be seen in this short-axis view obtained with 30–40° of probe angulation at the base of the heart. (c) Four-chamber view: this view demonstrates the atrial and ventricular chambers and septal structures. This is obtained at 0° at the mid-esophageal level. (d) Five-chamber view: structures demonstrated in this view include the right and left atria, right and left ventricles, and left ventricular outflow tract/aorta. (e) Left ventricular mid-papillary short-axis view: this view provides for short-axis sections of the left ventricle and portions of the right ventricle (obtained at 0–20°). The left ventricular papillary muscles are well demonstrated in this view. This view is particularly helpful in the evaluation of left ventricular systolic function (global and segmental) and the assessment of ventricular filling. Ao, aorta; MPA, main pulmonary artery; RPA, right pulmonary artery; LPA, left pulmonary artery; AoV, aortic valve; RA, right atrium; RVOT, right ventricular outflow tract; LA, left atrium; RV, right ventricle; LV, left ventricle; LVOT, left ventricular outflow tract

Although a specific sequence for the TEE examination cannot be emphasized, it is extremely helpful for each individual to develop his or her own organized approach in order to perform a comprehensive interrogation in an expeditious manner. This examination may be shortened by unique patient conditions or specific circumstances.

Transverse plane examination

After gentle insertion of the probe, the most cranial short-axis view is obtained at the base of the heart (mid-esophagus) from which the probe is anteflexed slightly to display the aorta, main pulmonary artery, and its bifurcation. The proximal branched pulmonary arteries can be imaged in most patients; however, interposition of the left mainstem bronchus makes imaging of the left pulmonary artery somewhat difficult (Figure 11.4a). Advancement of the probe displays the aortic valve in short axis, the proximal ascending aorta, and the origins of the coronary arteries. A 30° rotation of the plane at the level of the base of the heart defines the anatomy of the aortic valve, cusps, commissures, and valve motion throughout the cardiac cycle (Figure 11.4b). Rotation of the probe in counterclockwise fashion from this position displays the left-sided pulmonary veins; clockwise rotation shows the

right pulmonary veins, superior vena cava, and right atrial appendage. Advancing the probe further into the mid-esophagus allows for the four- and five-chamber views to be obtained (Figure 11.4c,d). These display the atrial, atrioventricular, and ventricular septae and atrioventricular valves. Further advancement of the probe in the lower esophagus displays left ventricular short-axis images, seen as multiple cross-sectional views of the left ventricle, mitral valve, papillary muscles (Figure 11.4e). Oblique sections of the right ventricle are obtained by slight probe flexion and/or rotation at this level.

Longitudinal plane examination

The TEE long-axis examination is feasible with biplane or multiplane probes [45,80–83]. Long-axis views of the atrium and large systemic veins (bicaval view), right and left ventricular outflow tracts, and left ventricle can be obtained. With the longitudinal transducer of the biplane probe or clockwise rotation of the multiplane probe at 90° displays the interatrial septum and entrance of the superior and inferior vena cavae into the right atrium (Figure 11.5a). Counterclockwise rotation of the biplane probe or rotation of the multiplane probe to 110–120° provides visualization of the left ventricular outflow tract and ascending

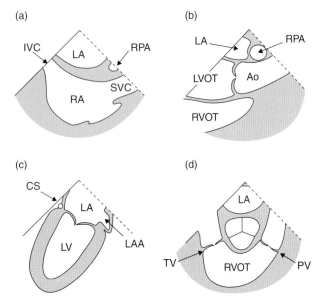

Figure 11.5 Diagrammatic representation of the *longitudinal plane examination*. (a) Bicaval view: the superior and inferior vena cavae are seen as they enter the right atrium. This view (90°) allows for evaluation of the atrial septum in the longitudinal plane. The left atrium is also displayed. The pulmonary veins can be interrogated by minimally rotating the transducer from this reference point. The right pulmonary artery is frequently seen in its short axis. (b) Aortic long-axis view: interrogation from the mid-esophageal window at 110° allows for visualization of the left ventricular outflow tract and aorta in the long axis. (c) Two-chamber view: rotation of the transducer to the left at a 90° angle of interrogation displays the left atrium and left ventricle. The coronary sinus and left atrial appendage are easily identified. (d) Right ventricular inflow-outflow view: this view, obtained by the probe at a 60° angle, provides for images of the tricuspid valve, right ventricular inlet and outlet portions, pulmonary valve, and main pulmonary artery. RA, right atrium; LA, left atrium; RPA, right pulmonary artery; SVC, superior vena cava; IVC, inferior vena cava; LVOT, left ventricular outflow tract; RVOT, right ventricular outflow tract; Ao, aorta; LV, left ventricle; LAA, left atrial appendage; CS, coronary sinus; TV, tricuspid valve; PV, pulmonary valve

aorta (Figure 11.5b). Further counterclockwise rotation of the biplane probe shows portions of the right ventricular outflow tract and main pulmonary artery. The two-chamber view (left atrium and left ventricle) can be obtained with additional counterclockwise probe rotation of the biplane probe or multiplane probe at 90° (Figure 11.5c).

Multiplane examination

In addition to all the planes described above, the multiplane probe allows for additional views to be obtained that may not be feasible with biplane devices. An example of this is the right ventricular inflow and outflow view obtained at 60° (Figure 11.5d) [84]. A significant advantage of multiplane imaging in CHD is that it allows for assess-

ment of structures that do not follow the usual planes of interrogation of the normal heart.

Transgastric examination

The transgastric examination allows for additional two-dimensional and Doppler information to be obtained. This refines the data gathered from the transesophageal windows and in some cases, additional diagnostic details is obtained not possible otherwise. This is of particular benefit when only a single-plane or a biplane probe is available.

The suggested approach to the transgastric exam is as follows: the probe is advanced into the stomach, anteflexed maximally, and positioned anterior to the fundus. When the patient's abdomen is exposed during this maneuver, it is frequently possible to observe the tip of the probe outpouching the abdominal wall. If there is difficulty in achieving the views, the probe is relaxed and withdrawn, then readvanced and withdrawn with maximal anteflexion to ensure adequate probe contact. Anteflexion should not be performed if resistance is encountered. From this position, rotation of the probe to the left with moderate deflection (relaxation of the flexion) provides images of the right ventricular outflow tract and the proximal pulmonary trunk as it courses anteriorly across the surface of the heart (Figure 11.6a); clockwise rotation and slight flexion from this position permits similar evaluation of the left ventricular outflow tract (Figure 11.6b). The flexion of the probe is then increased slightly to define the inlet and outlet components of the ventricular septum as well as the atria and atrioventricular valves (Figure 11.6c). The entrance of the pulmonary veins into the left atrium is demonstrated from this plane, and with rotation of the probe to the right, the venous connections to the right atrium can also be seen. Because the probe is some distance from the heart with a portion of the liver interposed, small movements of the transducer subtend large imaging arcs, permitting examination of the heart from the posterior atrial wall to near the anterior surface of the right ventricle. Once imaging of the outflow tracts is completed, pulsed-, continuous-wave Doppler and color flow mapping are performed. The transgastric approach allows for favorable alignment of the Doppler angle of interrogation with the outflow tracts to optimizing spectral Doppler signals and the assessment of outflow tract gradients.

Sequential segmental morphologic analysis

The variety of cardiac malformations, wide spectrum of anatomic arrangements, and complexity of the defects present significant challenges in the echocardiographic evaluation of CHD, even to the specialists. A segmental approach is indispensable in the transthoracic assessment

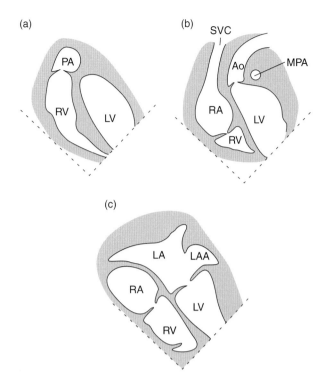

Figure 11.6 Diagrammatic representation the *transgastric exam*. (a) Right ventricular outflow tract view: advancement of the probe into the stomach (at 0°) displays sections of the right ventricular apex and outflow, and proximal aspect of the main pulmonary artery. (b) Left ventricular outflow tract view: probe flexion from the transgastric window reveals the left ventricular outflow tract from a vantage point favorable for spectral Doppler interrogation. (c) Four-chamber view: all cardiac chambers can be displayed from this window, in addition to the interatrial and interventricular septae. The pulmonary veins are frequently seen as they enter the posterior aspect of the left atrium. PA, pulmonary artery; RV, right ventricle; LV, left ventricle; SVC, superior vena cava; RA, right atrium; Ao, aorta; MPA, main pulmonary artery; LV, left ventricle; LAA, left atrial appendage

and should also be extended to the transesophageal examination. Although the segmental anatomy is defined in most patients preoperatively, the suggested practice includes the assessment of atrial arrangement or situs, venous drainage, atrioventricular and ventriculoarterial connections, valvar structures, outflow, great arteries, and septum. This should be combined by the interrogation of flow velocities with Doppler echocardiography.

Evaluation of congenital heart defects by TEE

Preoperative evaluation

The echocardiographic information of relevance in the prebypasss evaluation of the most common lesions is

noted in Table 11.3. Representative images of some of these anomalies are provided in Color Plates 11.1–11.4.

A number of educational resources, including textbooks in pediatric echocardiography and other publications provide comprehensive reviews on transesophageal imaging and hemodynamic assessment in CHD [85–90]. These are suggested as a reference.

Assessment of residual pathology

The postbypass echocardiographic examination requires focus on the specific pathology in question. Guidelines for the postoperative evaluation of common lesions/interventions are suggested in Table 11.4. Problems that may require return to bypass for surgical revision include: residual intracardiac shunts, outflow tract obstructions, and valvular regurgitation.

Assessment of pressure gradients

Doppler measurements predictions by echocardiography rely on the use of the modified Bernoulli equation (peak pressure difference = $4V^2$; Figure 11.7). In our series and others, good correlation has been documented between Doppler estimates of pressure gradients and direct pressure measurements [47,91,92]. It is important to note that preoperative determination of pressure gradients obtained when patients are awake or lightly sedated may differ from those obtained in the operating room under general anesthesia and conditions that may influence ventricular loading conditions and systolic function.

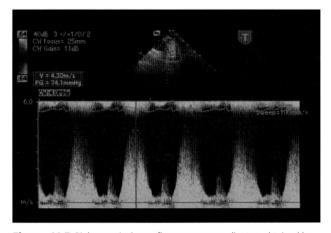

Figure 11.7 Right ventricular outflow pressure gradient as obtained by TEE. Continuous wave Doppler interrogation of the right ventricular outflow tract in a patient following repair of tetralogy of Fallot demonstrates residual obstruction. The peak velocity in this region measures 4.3 meters per second, predicting a right ventricular outflow tract gradient of 74 mm Hg (derived by application of the modified Bernoulli equation or $4V^2$). The patient required return to cardiopulmonary bypass.

Table 11.3 Prebypass echocardiographic data by type of congenital heart defect

Cardiac pathology	Presurgical echocardiographic information of interest
Atrial septal defect	Define location and size of defect Evaluate pulmonary venous drainage Assessment of atrioventricular valve regurgitation Baseline determination of ventricular function
Ventricular septal defect	Define location and size of defect Evaluate for additional intracardiac shunts Investigate for associated pathology (aortic valve herniation/prolapse, aortic regurgitation, subaortic membrane, pulmonary valve stenosis, double-chamber right ventricle, atrioventricular valve regurgitation) Baseline determination of ventricular function
Atrioventricular septal defect	Define location, size, and type of defects Evaluate for additional septal defects Assessment of atrioventricular valve (Rastelli type, atrioventricular valve regurgitation, relation of valvar structures to ventricles, balanced vs dominant type, valvar support apparatus) Interrogation of ventricular outflows (for obstruction) Baseline determination of ventricular function
Aortic stenosis	Evaluate location and severity of obstruction (subvalvar, valvar, supravalvar) Define aortic valve anatomy Evaluate for aortic regurgitation Assess for ventricular hypertrophy and function
Pulmonic stenosis	Evaluate location and severity of obstruction (subvalvar, valvar, supravalvar) Define pulmonary valve anatomy Determine size of pulmonary arteries Evaluate for intracardiac shunts Assess for ventricular hypertrophy and function
Pulmonary/conduit regurgitation	Evaluate severity of regurgitation and possible obstruction Interrogate atrial and ventricular septum for shunts Assess ventricular sizes and function
Tetralogy of Fallot	Define size and location of septal defects Evaluate right ventricular outflow tract (subvalvar, valvar, supravalvar regions) Define morphology, obstruction, gradients Determine size of pulmonary arteries Evaluate aortic valve competence/aortic override Evaluate origin and course of coronary arteries Baseline determination of ventricular function
d-Transposition of the great arteries	Evaluate ventriculoarterial relationships and intracardiac shunts (location, size, flow direction, relation to outflows) Assessment of outflow tract obstruction Evaluate atrioventricular and semilunar valves Evaluate origin and course of coronary arteries Assessment of septal geometry (as an indicator of ventricular pressures) Evaluate ventricular sizes and function
Double outlet right ventricle	Evaluate septal defects (size, shunt direction, location, relation of ventricular septal defect to great arteries) Assess physiology based on anatomic findings (i.e., ventricular septal defect, transposition or Taussig–Bing, tetralogy type) Evaluate great artery relationship (normal, malposed, side by side) Evaluate for outflow obstruction Assess ventricular sizes and function

Table 11.3 (*Continued*)

Cardiac pathology	Presurgical echocardiographic information of interest
Truncus arteriosus	Evaluate septal defects (size, location)
	Evaluate truncal valve (for stenosis/regurgitation)
	Assess origin of the pulmonary arteries (type of truncus), pulmonary blood flow
	Assess ventricular function
Single ventricle	Evaluate morphologic type
	Assess atrioventricular and semilunar valves, inflows, and outflows
	Interrogate for adequacy of interatrial communication if indicated
	Evaluate prior surgical interventions
	Assess ventricular function

Assessment of ventricular filling and function

TEE is extremely useful for examination of factors that directly affect cardiac output such as preload, contractility, and afterload. This modality has also been shown to be a reliable monitor of left ventricular filling changes in pediatric patients. In a study designed to evaluate whether TEE would identify changes in cardiac filling resulting from manipulations of blood volume in children, blood was withdrawn until the systolic blood pressure decreased by 5 and 10 mm Hg [93]. Experienced anesthesiologists–echocardiographers blinded to study events were able to identify with high sensitivity and specificity these mild reductions in blood volume by TEE changes in left ventricular end-diastolic area.

Estimation of ventricular areas and volumes is known to be time consuming and impractical in the operating room setting, representing a potential distraction from patient care for the care provider. Furthermore, significant limitations of this assessment are recognized in structurally abnormal hearts. These factors account for the fact that the routine intraoperative evaluation of ventricular preload mostly takes place through a qualitative assessment.

Several studies have documented the utility of TEE in the evaluation of ejection fraction. Estimation of ejection fraction reached a good correlation ($r = 0.98$) when compared to measures of ejection fraction by transthoracic echocardiography [94]. A comparison made between transthoracic and TEE for assessment of ventricular function in pediatric patients, however, demonstrated poor correlation possibly due to technical limitations [95].

Over the last several years there has been increasing interest in the routine evaluation of diastolic function by echocardiography in both pediatric and adult age groups. Abnormalities of ventricular relaxation and compliance are known to contribute to perioperative morbidity [96–99]. Diastolic dysfunction plays a major role in many congenital and acquired pathologies in the pediatric age group. Unfortunately, the evaluation of diastolic func-

tion in young patients has met several challenges, including the many confounding variables that influence appropriate Doppler assessment and interpretation of findings. These difficulties are further magnified by applying criteria developed for transthoracic echocardiography to the transesophageal approach.

As in the case of adults, segmental wall motion abnormalities as detected by TEE in pediatric patients may be considered a surrogate of compromised myocardial blood flow [100]. In this regard, the use of TEE may be of particular benefit to patients undergoing procedures that involve coronary artery manipulations [101].

Influences of TEE on anesthetic and surgical management

Numerous reports document the benefits of TEE technology in the intraoperative setting as a diagnostic tool and in regards to surgical decision making [21,23,34,42,43,102–110]. Recent publications continue to support the major impact of this modality during surgery for congenital and pediatric acquired heart disease [111,112].

The overall incidence of a change in surgical management with the aid of intraoperative TEE has been reported in the literature is noted to be between 3 and 15% [41,104,108,109,113,114]. Various studies have suggested that preoperative diagnoses can be changed in 3–5% of cases and the return to bypass rate as directed by TEE to be in the 3% range. A report on intraoperative TEE during congenital heart surgery in a wide range of patients (2 days to 85 years) described major impact in 13.8% of the group [113]. This was more frequent during reoperations and in those undergoing valve repairs and complex outflow tract reconstructions.

Several studies have also documented the many contributions of TEE to anesthetic management [115, 116]. Two large investigations that included a large number of congenital cases demonstrated changes in inotropic strategy and volume replacement to be frequent interventions

Table 11.4 Postbypass echocardiographic data by type of congenital heart defect repair or surgical procedure

Cardiac pathology	Evaluate for the following in the postsurgical echocardiographic exam
Atrial septal defect	
Secundum	Residual shunt Atrioventricular valve regurgitation Ventricular function
Sinus venosus	Residual shunt Superior vena cava obstruction Pulmonary venous obstruction (if associated anomalous pulmonary venous return) Ventricular function
Ventricular septal defect	
Perimembranous	Residual shunt (tiny leaks may be acceptable at the edges of the patch) Atrioventricular valve regurgitation, aortic insufficiency Right ventricular pressure can be calculated by using the tricuspid regurgitant jet or residual ventricular septal defect peak velocity Ventricular function
Supracristal, subarterial (doubly committed)	Residual shunt (as above) Residual or new aortic/pulmonary insufficiency compared to prebypass exam Ventricular function
Muscular or Inlet	Residual shunt (as above, tiny/small residual muscular ventricular septal defect may be acceptable Atrioventricular valve regurgitation Ventricular function
Atrioventricular septal defect	
Partial or ostium primum ASD/cleft mitral valve	Residual shunts Residual/new atrioventricular valve regurgitation (mild regurgitation may be acceptable) Mitral inflow obstruction (if mitral cleft closed) Ventricular function
Complete atrioventricular septal defect	Residual atrial or ventricular level shunts Atrioventricular valve stenosis (particularly if annuloplasty or left-sided cleft closure performed) Atrioventricular valve regurgitation Left ventricular outflow tract obstruction Ventricular function
Aortic stenosis (subvalvar, valvar, supravalvar)	Residual outflow obstruction or aortic insufficiency New ventricular septal defect Mitral regurgitation Ventricular function
Ross procedure	Aortic stenosis or insufficiency Right ventricular outflow tract conduit (for stenosis/regurgitation) Global and segmental left ventricular function
Tetralogy of Fallot	Residual ventricular septal defect or unmasked defects Residual right ventricular outflow tract obstruction Pulmonary regurgitation Right ventricular systolic pressure can be assessed by using the tricuspid regurgitant jet Right and left ventricular function
Right ventricular conduit operation	Conduit stenosis or insufficiency Atrioventricular valve competence Ventricular function
Arterial switch operation (Jatene procedure)	Neoaortic and pulmonic anastomoses (for stenosis) Semilunar valve competence Outflow tracts (for obstruction) Atrioventricular valve regurgitation Residual intracardiac shunts Coronary flow Global and segmental left ventricular function

Table 11.4 (*Continued*)

Cardiac pathology	Evaluate for the following in the postsurgical echocardiographic exam
Double outlet right ventricle	Residual intracardiac shunts Outflow tract obstruction Atrioventricular/semilunar valve regurgitation Right ventricular to pulmonary artery conduit function (if applicable) Ventricular function
Truncus arteriosus	Truncal valve (aortic) stenosis and insufficiency Right ventricular to pulmonary conduit (for stenosis or insufficiency) Atrioventricular valve regurgitation Residual ventricular level shunt Estimate right ventricular/pulmonary artery pressures Ventricular function
Fontan or Glenn procedure	Flow in Fontan/Glenn connections Evaluate Fontan fenestration if performed Atrioventricular valve regurgitation Atrial septum for evidence of obstruction (if stenosis/atresia of atrioventricular valve) Ventricular function
Total anomalous pulmonary venous return	Adequacy of pulmonary venous anastomosis Residual atrial level shunt Atrioventricular valve regurgitation Right ventricular/pulmonary artery pressure (can be estimated from tricuspid or pulmonary regurgitant jets) Right and left ventricular function

guided by TEE [116, 117]. Additional benefits of TEE in congenital heart surgery include detection of complications, assessment of the adequacy of cardiac deairing, and guidance during placement of intravascular/intracardiac catheters [118].

Technological advances over recent years include refinement of devices available for mechanical circulatory support in children and increased sophistication of hardware that facilitates surgical interventions. The usefulness of TEE has also been demonstrated in these settings [50,119].

Influences of intraoperative echocardiography on clinical outcomes

There is limited data regarding improvement in clinical outcomes based on intraoperative TEE. Despite the lack of rigorous scientific scrutiny, the experience regarding the contributions of TEE has been so compelling that the technology has been incorporated into clinical practice in many centers.

A prospective study designed to evaluate the efficacy of intraoperative epicardial color flow mapping to predict outcome after surgical repair noted that if patients left the operating room with residual pathology, there was a high rate of reoperation and of early death [120]. Alterations in ventricular function after bypass also resulted in a higher

incidence of early death. Patients with acceptable surgical results, as documented by epicardial echocardiography, had a greater than 90% likelihood of long-term acceptable outcome.

In a series that included 230 patients, if a residual abnormality was detected by TEE and revised, the outcome was excellent in 76% (13 of 17) of patients [121]. Twelve patients were identified who had suboptimal outcomes, 2/12 (16%) had residual defects who may have been amenable to further surgery, and 10 (84%) had final outcomes that were believed to be unrelated to a problem identifiable by TEE. Thus, if immediate revision of a repair was performed, the outcome was improved, and if the patient was left with a residual defect, the outcome was suboptimal.

In addition to the patient benefits afforded by this imaging modality, the cost-effectiveness of routine TEE during congenital and pediatric heart surgery has also been shown [16,122].

TEE in the catheterization laboratory

Over the several decades, transcatheter-based therapies and interventional procedures have become increasingly employed in the nonsurgical management of cardiovascular anomalies. Many of these approaches have extended from the cardiac catheterization laboratory to the operating room (and vice versa) as combined efforts of interventional cardiologists and cardiothoracic surgeons. TEE allows for safer and more effective application of these approaches, decreased in fluoroscopic time, a lesser amount of contrast material administered, and duration of the interventional procedure [123–125].

Studies addressing the role of this imaging modality confirm major contributions. They include (1) acquisition of detailed anatomic and hemodynamic data prior to and during the procedure, (2) real-time evaluation of catheter/device placement across cardiovascular structures, (3) immediate assessment of the results, and (4) monitoring of procedural complications. The refinement in interventional cardiac catheterization techniques coupled with advances in TEE now allow for the high success rate of these procedures and their low incidence of complications.

Miscellaneous issues relevant to the practice of TEE

Contraindications

Conditions associated with increased risk of complications, such as esophageal pathology, severe respiratory decompensation, or inadequate control of the airway, are generally considered to be contraindications to TEE. Additional clinical scenarios that require assessment of risk–benefit ratio for TEE include cervical spine injury or deformity and severe coagulopathy. In the presence of a gastrostomy-feeding tube, the TEE examination is still feasible; however, we defer the transgastric examination. In patients with a known aberrant (retroesophageal) subclavian artery, we suggest placement of the catheter for arterial blood pressure monitoring in an extremity not being supplied by the anomalous vessel, since loss of the arterial pressure tracing may be seen upon esophageal intubation or probe manipulation [126, 127]. Monitoring by pulse oximetry in the extremity supplied by the aberrant vessel may be useful as an indicator of adequate distal bed perfusion. Surgical interventions to address isolated vascular anomalies, such as vascular rings, generally do not benefit significantly from TEE. In these cases, TEE probe insertion can lead to respiratory compromise as the trachea and esophagus are restricted to a confined space by the surrounding vascular structures.

In infants with anomalous pulmonary venous connections, consideration should be given to potential compression of the posterior pulmonary venous confluence by the transesophageal probe resulting in detrimental hemodynamic effects (see Figure 11.2) [128]. A potential approach in this clinical scenario is the introduction of the probe after sternotomy or during the bypass period [129].

Complications

The overall favorable safety profile of TEE has been well documented in the literature [130]. Although a number of complications related to transesophageal instrumentation have been reported, the extensive clinical experience to date indicates that serious complications associated with TEE are rare [131]. This is also the case in the pediatric age group [113,116,117,132].

Most children, including infants, tolerate transesophageal examination well; however, hemodynamics and respiratory parameters must be closely monitored in all patients. Blood pressure changes resulting from aortic compression during probe manipulation may or may not be evident depending on the location of the arterial catheter or oximetric sampling probe. Accordingly, placement of the imaging probe in the intraoperative setting is recommended following arterial line placement.

A few case reports have noted life-threatening hemodynamic deterioration associated with TEE probe insertion/manipulation [133]. Respiratory compromise can also occur in association with probe manipulation, in addition to movement of the endotracheal tube resulting in displacement or tracheal extubation. Capnography may be particularly helpful in the recognition of these complications. If desaturation acutely occurs, correct position of the endotracheal tube must be confirmed immediately and occasionally the TEE probe must be withdrawn. Anytime the probe is withdrawn, the endotracheal tube should be firmly held to prevent inadvertent extubation.

Andropoulos and colleagues examined the impact of TEE on ventilation and hemodynamic variables in small infants undergoing cardiac surgery [134, 135]. No significant changes in several measured parameters of gas exchange and pulmonary mechanics were observed in relation to probe insertion. The investigation noted that hemodynamic complications from TEE, although possible, were rare in this patient group. Although hemodynamic or respiratory alterations can occur in small infants, this data suggest that these are relatively infrequent occurrences and fear of compromise should not prevent use of intraoperative TEE in patients when otherwise indicated.

Esophageal irritation and injury can occur related to intraoperative TEE. A study where flexible esophagoscopy was performed following TEE in infants and children demonstrated frequent mild mucosal injury [136]. Another report documented an 18% incidence of dysphagia among pediatric patients undergoing cardiac operations where TEE was used. Although the lack of a control group in this investigation did not allow for the assessment of the direct effects of TEE, this suggested that the probe was a risk factor in this cohort [137].

A report of an unrecognized esophageal perforation in a small infant during intraoperative TEE underscores the fact that meticulous care must be exercised in the insertion and manipulation of these probes in all patients, but particularly in the critically ill neonate [138]. This report also raises the concern that this occurrence may be higher than previously suspected and recommends that clinicians keep this diagnosis in mind in the presence of crepitus in the neck, subcutaneous emphysema, pneumomediastinum, or retropharyngeal gas or other physical findings that may suggest perforation.

Endocarditis prophylaxis

Although endoscopic procedures may be associated with bacteremia, the overall incidence of bacteremia as a result of upper gastrointestinal endoscopy is considered small [139, 140]. Endocarditis has been reported temporally related to a TEE examination; however, the incidence of positive bacterial blood cultures immediately following TEE has been shown to be extremely low and within the expected rate of false-positive results.

Based on the low likelihood of endocarditis, it was previously considered that routine antibiotic prophylaxis for TEE was unwarranted. It was suggested optional in very high-risk individuals [141]. Recent American Heart Association guidelines, however, do not recommend the administration of antibiotics solely to prevent endocarditis for patients who undergo gastrointestinal tract procedures [142]. Although TEE prophylaxis is not specifically addressed in the recommendations, it would be reasonable to assume that this also applies to upper esophageal instrumentation.

Limitations

It should be acknowledged that the TEE imaging windows are limited by the confines of the esophagus and stomach, restricting transducer mobility and limiting potential for optimal Doppler angle alignment. Other challenges relate to reduced far field imaging and difficulties in the evaluation of some cardiovascular structures. Additional limitations include the fact that the examinations are performed under suboptimal ambient lighting and circumstances that may limit the performance of a comprehensive study.

The literature extensively documents the utility of TEE in congenital heart surgery and in the detection of residual abnormalities that may require immediate revision. However, when decisions regarding return to bypass are undertaken, it should considered that a variety of factors may influence the echocardiographic findings, potentially under or overestimating the hemodynamic severity of the condition in question. These factors include the level of inotropic support, catecholamine state during the immediate bypass period, loading conditions, and functional state of the myocardium. Therefore, the study should be interpreted within this context. Decisions regarding return to bypass also require assessment of the overall risk–benefit ratio and in many instances this represents a clinical judgment not exclusively based on the echocardiographic information, but also influenced by numerous factors.

Training and certification

Guidelines for physician training in TEE were initially published by the American Society of Echocardiography Committee for Physician Training in 1992 [143]. The report indicated that individuals using TEE should have (i) thorough knowledge of cardiac disease and hemodynamic alterations associated with acquired and congenital disorders, (ii) understanding of ultrasonic image formation and Doppler assessment of intracardiac blood flow, and (iii) familiarity with the range of normal structural findings and the echocardiographic manifestations of a large number of cardiac disorders.

Practice guidelines specifically addressing the use of perioperative TEE were first published in 1996 [65]. Subsequently, a task force by the American Society of Echocardiography and Society of Cardiovascular Anesthesiologists suggested guidelines for physician training [144]. Different levels of expertise in echocardiography were recognized in the report and level-specific recommendations for training outlined. The advanced level of training assumed comprehensive cognitive and technical skills to allow for the full potential applications of the TEE technology, in addition to those required for basic level perioperative TEE practice.

It is well recognized that performance and competency in TEE performed in patients with CHD and pediatric acquired heart disease require specialized knowledge, skills, and training. This aspect of TEE practice was considered within the advanced training pathway. Suggested requirements included:

1 Knowledge of CHD (if congenital practice planned, knowledge must be detailed).
2 Detailed knowledge of all other diseases of the heart and great vessels relevant in the perioperative period (if pediatric practice planned, knowledge may be more general than detailed).
3 Detailed knowledge of the techniques, advantages, disadvantages, and potential complications of commonly used cardiac surgical procedures for treatment of acquired and CHD.

In recognition of the unique aspects and evolving applications of TEE in this patient group, the Pediatric

Council of the American Society of Echocardiography has developed recent guidelines [68]. The document outlined essential knowledge base and skills, in addition to requirements for training and maintenance of proficiency. For physicians without formal training in pediatric cardiology or without a focus on TEE, acquisition of medical/echocardiographic knowledge base and practical skills equivalent to those acquired during pediatric cardiology specialty training were suggested, in order for TEE to be performed independently. Recommended skills included knowledge of cardiac anatomy, congenital and acquired cardiac pathology, pathophysiology, differential diagnosis, and alternative diagnostic modalities. Previously, it was strongly recommended that a pediatric cardiologist knowledgeable in TEE participate in the performance and interpretation in studies in infants and young children and those with complex heart disease. Although most recent guidelines do not specifically address this issue, this recommendation appears well-founded.

Given these recommendations and training requirements, it has been asked how should one proceed as an anesthesiologist interested in pediatric TEE or the applications of this technology in patients with CHD. The issue of who should be responsible for the intraoperative TEE interpretation in these patients and the respective roles of perioperative providers regarding TEE has also been addressed [145–149]. Published data indicates that properly trained cardiac anesthesiologists are able to utilize this technology competently resulting in changes in medical and surgical management in a significant number of patients [115,116]. We suggest that one should follow the general guidelines established by the American Society of Anesthesiologists and the Society of Cardiovascular Anesthesiologists as follows: "anesthesiologists with advanced training in perioperative TEE should be able to exploit the full diagnostic potential of TEE in the perioperative period." Because it is essential in many intraoperative applications to obtain a definitive interpretation of the TEE examination at the time of surgery, it is recommended that anesthesiologists actively pursue collaboration with surgeons, cardiologists, or other physicians involved in a patient's care as a team approach.

The Society of Cardiovascular Anesthesiologists has developed a process that recognizes knowledge and proficiency of perioperative TEE [150,151]. This examination is currently administered by the National Board of Echocardiography. The examination focuses on adult heart disease with a small component of CHD in the adult; pediatric TEE has not been addressed.

Quality assurance

All quality assurance programs for echocardiography should consider the following elements: indications for the studies, technical aspects of the examination (performance and archiving), appropriateness of study interpretation, equipment acquisition and maintenance (including probe care), professional communication, education, and billing.

Typically, the examinations are interpreted and reports are completed the same day of the study. Some centers highly encourage ongoing review of the recorded images as a teaching tool and, in particular, retrospective review of the all diagnostic data when significant discrepancies are identified between the interpretation of the studies and surgical findings.

Conclusions

In most centers, TEE is considered the standard of care for intraoperative assessment of congenital heart repairs prior to removal of the bypass hardware and sternal closure [63,152]. This has also become the case for surgical interventions in pediatric patients with acquired heart disease.

Over the years, the transesophageal imaging modality has become a valuable adjunct to surgical, hemodynamic, and anesthetic management. The literature documents the significant perioperative benefits of TEE in these patient populations and the impact in clinical decision making. Diagnoses can be confirmed or altered preoperatively, the surgical plan can be modified, complications can be detected, and the operative procedures can be immediately evaluated and revised if necessary. Contributions to anesthetic care include real-time monitoring of ventricular filling, cardiac function, ensuring adequate cardiac deairing, in addition to optimization of hemodynamic management strategies. The intraoperative transesophageal findings may assist in the formulation of plans for postoperative care.

The overview presented regarding the contributions of TEE to pediatric cardiac surgery and the care of patients with CHD demonstrate the impact of this technology on clinical care and its likely positive influence on outcomes.

References

1. Frazin L, Talano JV, Stephanides L, et al. (1976) Esophageal echocardiography. Circulation 54:102–108.
2. Schluter M, Langenstein BA, Polster J, et al. (1982) Transoesophageal cross-sectional echocardiography with a phased array transducer system. Technique and initial clinical results. Br Heart J 48:67–72.
3. Smith JS, Cahalan MK, Benefiel DJ, et al. (1985) Intraoperative detection of myocardial ischemia in high-risk patients: electrocardiography versus two-dimensional transesophageal echocardiography. Circulation 72:1015–1021.

4. Abel MD, Nishimura RA, Callahan MJ, et al. (1987) Evaluation of intraoperative transesophageal two-dimensional echocardiography. Anesthesiology 66:64–68.
5. De Bruijn PN, Clements FM, Hill R (eds) (1987) Transesophageal Echocardiography. Developments in Critical Care Medicine and Anesthesiology, Vol. 13. Nijhoff, Boston.
6. Goldman ME, Mora F, Guarino T, et al. (1987) Mitral valvuloplasty is superior to valve replacement for preservation of left ventricular function: an intraoperative two-dimensional echocardiographic study. J Am Coll Cardiol 10:568–575.
7. Nellessen U, Schnittger I, Appleton CP, et al. (1988) Transesophageal two-dimensional echocardiography and color Doppler flow velocity mapping in the evaluation of cardiac valve prostheses. Circulation 78:848–855.
8. Leung JM, O'Kelly B, Browner WS, et al. (1989) Prognostic importance of postbypass regional wall-motion abnormalities in patients undergoing coronary artery bypass graft surgery. SPI Research Group. Anesthesiology 71:16–25.
9. Taams MA, Gussenhoven EJ, Cahalan MK, et al. (1989) Transesophageal Doppler color flow imaging in the detection of native and Bjork-Shiley mitral valve regurgitation. J Am Coll Cardiol 13:95–99.
10. Van Den Brink RB, Visser CA, Basart DC, et al. (1989) Comparison of transthoracic and transesophageal color Doppler flow imaging in patients with mechanical prostheses in the mitral valve position. Am J Cardiol 63:1471–1474.
11. Foster GP, Isselbacher EM, Rose GA, et al. (1998) Accurate localization of mitral regurgitant defects using multiplane transesophageal echocardiography. Ann Thorac Surg 65:1025–1031.
12. Hofer CK, Zollinger A, Rak M, et al. (2004) Therapeutic impact of intra-operative transoesophageal echocardiography during noncardiac surgery. Anaesthesia 59:3–9.
13. Applebaum RM, Cutler WM, Bhardwaj N, et al. (1998) Utility of transesophageal echocardiography during port-access minimally invasive cardiac surgery. Am J Cardiol 82:183–188.
14. Shanewise JS, Zaffer R, Martin RP (2002) Intraoperative echocardiography and minimally invasive cardiac surgery. Echocardiography 19:579–582.
15. Pu M, Stephenson ER, Jr., Davidson WR, Jr., et al. (2003) An unexpected surgical complication of ventricular assist device implantation identified by transesophageal echocardiography: a case report. J Am Soc Echocardiogr 16:1194–1197.
16. Benson MJ, Cahalan MK (1995) Cost-benefit analysis of transesophageal echocardiography in cardiac surgery. Echocardiography 12:171–183.
17. Eltzschig HK, Rosenberger P, Loffler M, et al. (2008) Impact of intraoperative transesophageal echocardiography on surgical decisions in 12,566 patients undergoing cardiac surgery. Ann Thorac Surg 85:845–852.
18. Shernan S (2008) Perioperative echocardiography: past, present and future. J Am Soc Echocardiogr 21:25A–26A.
19. Ritter SB (1990) Transesophageal echocardiography in children: new peephole to the heart [comment]. J Am Coll Cardiol 16:447–450.
20. Ritter SB, Thys D (1989) Pediatric transesophageal color flow imaging: smaller probes for smaller hearts. Echocardiography 6:431–440.
21. Stumper OF, Elzenga NJ, Hess J, et al. (1990) Transesophageal echocardiography in children with congenital heart disease: an initial experience. J Am Coll Cardiol 16:433–441.
22. Ritter SB, Hillel Z, Narang J, et al. (1989) Transesophageal real time Doppler flow imaging in congenital heart disease: experience with a new pediatric transducer probe. Dyn Cardiovasc Imag 2:92–96.
23. Lam J, Neirotti RA, Nijveld A, et al. (1991) Transesophageal echocardiography in pediatric patients: preliminary results. J Am Soc Echocardiogr 4:43–50.
24. Ungerleider RM, Kisslo JA, Greeley WJ, et al. (1989) Intraoperative prebypass and postbypass epicardial color flow imaging in the repair of atrioventricular septal defects [see comments]. J Thorac Cardiovasc Surg 98:90–99; discussion 99–100.
25. Ungerleider RM, Kisslo JA, Greeley WJ, et al. (1995) Intraoperative echocardiography during congenital heart operations: experience from 1,000 cases. Ann Thorac Surg 60:S539–S542.
26. Ungerleider RM, Greeley WJ, Sheikh KH, et al. (1990) Routine use of intraoperative epicardial echocardiography and Doppler color flow imaging to guide and evaluate repair of congenital heart lesions. A prospective study. J Thorac Cardiovasc Surg 100:297–309.
27. Gussenhoven EJ, van Herwerden LA, Roelandt J, et al. (1987) Intraoperative two-dimensional echocardiography in congenital heart disease. J Am Coll Cardiol 9:565–572.
28. Papagiannis J, Kanter RJ, Armstrong BE, et al. (1993) Intraoperative epicardial echocardiography during repair of tetralogy of Fallot. J Am Soc Echocardiogr 6:366–373.
29. Cyran SE, Kimball TR, Meyer RA, et al. (1989) Efficacy of intraoperative transesophageal echocardiography in children with congenital heart disease. Am J Cardiol 63:594–598.
30. Kyo S, Koike K, Takanawa E, et al. (1989) Impact of transesophageal Doppler echocardiography on pediatric cardiac surgery. Int J Card Imaging 4:41–42.
31. Omoto T, Kyo S, Matsumura M (1989) Recent technological progress in transesophageal color Doppler flow imaging with special reference to newly developed biplane and pediatric probes. In: Erbel R, Khandheria BK, Brennecke R (eds) Transesophageal Echocardiography: A New Window to the Heart. Springer-Verlag, Berlin, pp. 21–26.
32. Ritter SB (1991) Transesophageal real-time echocardiography in infants and children with congenital heart disease. J Am Coll Cardiol 18:569–580.
33. Ritter SB (1990) Pediatric transesophageal color flow imaging 1990: the long and short of it. Echocardiography 7:713–725.
34. Muhiudeen IA, Roberson DA, Silverman NH, et al. (1990) Intraoperative echocardiography in infants and children with congenital cardiac shunt lesions: transesophageal versus epicardial echocardiography. J Am Coll Cardiol 16:1687–1695.
35. Stumper O, Kaulitz R, Sreeram N, et al. (1990) Intraoperative transesophageal versus epicardial ultrasound in

surgery for congenital heart disease. J Am Soc Echocardiogr 3:392–401.

36. Sreeram N, Stumper OF, Kaulitz R, et al. (1990) Comparative value of transthoracic and transesophageal echocardiography in the assessment of congenital abnormalities of the atrioventricular junction. J Am Coll Cardiol 16:1205–1214.

37. Roberson DA, Muhiudeen IA, Silverman NH, et al. (1991) Intraoperative transesophageal echocardiography of atrioventricular septal defect. J Am Coll Cardiol 18:537–545.

38. Muhiudeen IA, Roberson DA, Silverman NH, et al. (1992) Intraoperative echocardiography for evaluation of congenital heart defects in infants and children [see comments]. Anesthesiology 76:165–172.

39. Wienecke M, Fyfe DA, Kline CH, et al. (1991) Comparison of intraoperative transesophageal echocardiography to epicardial imaging in children undergoing ventricular septal defect repair. J Am Soc Echocardiogr 4:607–614.

40. Roberson DA, Muhiudeen IA, Silverman NH (1990) Transesophageal echocardiography in pediatrics: technique and limitations. Echocardiography 7:699–712.

41. Muhiudeen I, Silverman N (1993) Intraoperative transesophageal echocardiography using high resolution imaging in infants and children with congenital heart disease. Echocardiography 10:599–608.

42. Gentles TL, Rosenfeld HM, Sanders SP, et al. (1994) Pediatric biplane transesophageal echocardiography: preliminary experience. Am Heart J 128:1225–1233.

43. Lam J, Neirotti RA, Lubbers WJ, et al. (1993) Usefulness of biplane transesophageal echocardiography in neonates, infants and children with congenital heart disease [published erratum appears in Am J Cardiol 1994 Mar 15;73 (8):625]. Am J Cardiol 72:699–706.

44. O'Leary PW, Hagler DJ, Seward JB, et al. (1995) Biplane intraoperative transesophageal echocardiography in congenital heart disease. Mayo Clin Proc 70:317–326.

45. Seward JB (1995) Biplane and multiplane transesophageal echocardiography: evaluation of congenital heart disease. Am J Card Imaging 9:129–136.

46. Hoffman P, Stumper O, Rydelwska-Sadowska W, et al. (1993) Transgastric imaging: a valuable addition to the assessment of congenital heart disease by transverse plane transesophageal echocardiography. J Am Soc Echocardiogr 6:35–44.

47. Muhiudeen IA, Silverman NH, Anderson RH (1995) Transesophageal transgastric echocardiography in infants and children: the subcostal view equivalent. J Am Soc Echocardiogr 8:231–244.

48. Sloth E, Hasenkam JM, Sorensen KE, et al. (1996) Pediatric multiplane transesophageal echocardiography in congenital heart disease: new possibilities with a miniaturized probe. J Am Soc Echocardiogr 9:622–628.

49. Shiota T, Lewandowski R, Piel JE, et al. (1999) Micromultiplane transesophageal echocardiographic probe for intraoperative study of congenital heart disease repair in neonates, infants, children, and adults. Am J Cardiol 83:292–295, A7.

50. Scohy TV, Gommers D, Jan ten Harkel AD, et al. (2007) Intraoperative evaluation of micromultiplane transesophageal echocardiographic probe in surgery for congenital heart disease. Eur J Echocardiogr 8:241–246.

51. Hung J, Lang R, Flachskampf F, et al. (2007) 3D echocardiography: a review of the current status and future directions. J Am Soc Echocardiogr 20:213–233.

52. Sugeng L, Shernan SK, Salgo IS, et al. (2008) Live 3-dimensional transesophageal echocardiography initial experience using the fully-sampled matrix array probe. J Am Coll Cardiol 52:446–449.

53. Jungwirth B, Mackensen GB (2008) Real-time 3-dimensional echocardiography in the operating room. Semin Cardiothorac Vasc Anesth 12:248–264.

54. Sugeng L, Shernan SK, Weinert L, et al. (2008) Real-time three-dimensional transesophageal echocardiography in valve disease: comparison with surgical findings and evaluation of prosthetic valves. J Am Soc Echocardiogr 21:1347–1354.

55. Grewal J, Mankad S, Freeman WK, et al. (2009) Real-time three-dimensional transesophageal echocardiography in the intraoperative assessment of mitral valve disease. J Am Soc Echocardiogr 22:34–41.

56. Shernan SK (2009) Intraoperative three-dimensional echocardiography: ready for primetime? J Am Soc Echocardiogr 22:27A-28A.

57. Acar P, Massabuau P, Elbaz M (2008) Real-time 3D transoesophageal echocardiography for guiding Amplatzer septal occluder device deployment in an adult patient with atrial septal defect. Eur J Echocardiogr 9:822–823.

58. Klein AJ, Kim MS, Salcedo E, et al. (2009) The missing leak: a case report of a baffle-leak closure using real-time 3D transoesophageal guidance. Eur J Echocardiogr 10:464–467.

59. Lodato JA, Cao QL, Weinert L, et al. (2009) Feasibility of real-time three-dimensional transoesophageal echocardiography for guidance of percutaneous atrial septal defect closure. Eur J Echocardiogr 10:543–548.

60. Martin-Reyes R, Lopez-Fernandez T, Moreno-Yanguela M, et al. (2009) Role of real-time three-dimensional transoesophageal echocardiography for guiding transcatheter patent foramen ovale closure. Eur J Echocardiogr 10:148–150.

61. Mercer-Rosa L, Seliem MA, Fedec A, et al. (2006) Illustration of the additional value of real-time 3-dimensional echocardiography to conventional transthoracic and transesophageal 2-dimensional echocardiography in imaging muscular ventricular septal defects: does this have any impact on individual patient treatment? J Am Soc Echocardiogr 19:1511–1519.

62. Muhiudeen Russell IA, Miller-Hance WC, Silverman NH (1998) Intraoperative transesophageal echocardiography for pediatric patients with congenital heart disease. Anesth Analg 87:1058–1076.

63. Stevenson JG (2003) Utilization of intraoperative transesophageal echocardiography during repair of congenital cardiac defects: a survey of North American centers. Clin Cardiol 26:132–134.

64. Fyfe DA, Ritter SB, Snider AR, et al. (1992) Guidelines for transesophageal echocardiography in children. J Am Soc Echocardiogr 5:640–644.

65. Task Force on Transesophageal Echocardiography (1996) Practice guidelines for perioperative transesophageal echocardiography. A report by the American Society of Anesthesiologists and the Society of Cardiovascular Anesthesiologists Task Force on Transesophageal Echocardiography. Anesthesiology 84:986–1006.

66. Cheitlin MD, Alpert JS, Armstrong WF, et al. (1997) ACC/AHA guidelines for the Clinical Application of Echocardiography. A report of the American College of Cardiology/American Heart Association Task Force on Practice Guidelines (Committee on Clinical Application of Echocardiography). Developed in collaboration with the American Society of Echocardiography. Circulation 95:1686–1744.

67. Cheitlin MD, Armstrong WF, Aurigemma GP, et al. (2003) ACC/AHA/ASE 2003 guideline update for the clinical application of echocardiography: summary article: a report of the American College of Cardiology/American Heart Association Task Force on Practice Guidelines (ACC/AHA/ASE Committee to Update the 1997 Guidelines for the Clinical Application of Echocardiography). Circulation 108:1146–1162.

68. Ayres NA, Miller-Hance W, Fyfe DA, et al. (2005) Indications and guidelines for performance of transesophageal echocardiography in the patient with pediatric acquired or congenital heart disease: report from the task force of the Pediatric Council of the American Society of Echocardiography. J Am Soc Echocardiogr 18:91–98.

69. Mart CR, Fehr DM, Myers JL, et al. (2003) Intraoperative transesophageal echocardiography in a 1.4-kg infant with complex congenital heart disease. Pediatr Cardiol 24:84–85.

70. Bruce CJ, O'Leary P, Hagler DJ, et al. (2002) Miniaturized transesophageal echocardiography in newborn infants. J Am Soc Echocardiogr 15:791–797.

71. Mart CR, Parrish M, Rosen KL, et al. (2006) Safety and efficacy of sedation with propofol for transoesophageal echocardiography in children in an outpatient setting. Cardiol Young 16:152–156.

72. Hsu JH, Wang CK, Hung CW, et al. (2007) Transesophageal echocardiography and laryngeal mask airway for placement of permanent central venous catheter in cancer patients with radiographically unidentifiable SVC-RA junction: effectiveness and safety. Kaohsiung J Med Sci 23:435–441.

73. Galante D (2008) Transesophageal Doppler probe and proseal laryngeal mask airway. A new technique for probe insertion in pediatric anesthesia [letter]. Anesth Analg 107:348.

74. Mart CR, Rosen KL (2009) Optimal Head Position During Transesophageal Echocardiographic Probe Insertion for Pediatric Patients Weighing Up to 10 kg. Pediatr Cardiol 30:441–446.

75. Na S, Kim CS, Kim JY, et al. (2009) Rigid laryngoscope-assisted insertion of transesophageal echocardiography probe reduces oropharyngeal mucosal injury in anesthetized patients. Anesthesiology 110:38–40.

76. Shanewise JS (2001) Performing a complete transesophageal echocardiographic examination. Anesthesiol Clin North America 19:727–767.

77. Shanewise JS, Cheung AT, Aronson S, et al. (1999) ASE/SCA guidelines for performing a comprehensive intraoperative multiplane transesophageal echocardiography examination: recommendations of the American Society of Echocardiography Council for Intraoperative Echocardiography and the Society of Cardiovascular Anesthesiologists Task Force for Certification in Perioperative Transesophageal Echocardiography. J Am Soc Echocardiogr 12:884–900.

78. Van Hare GF, Silverman NH (1989) Contrast two-dimensional echocardiography in congenital heart disease: techniques, indications and clinical utility. J Am Coll Cardiol 13:673–686.

79. Valdes-Cruz LM, Pieroni DR, Roland JM, et al. (1977) Recognition of residual postoperative shunts by contrast echocardiographic techniques. Circulation 55:148–152.

80. Seward JB, Khandheria BK, Edwards WD, et al. (1990) Biplanar transesophageal echocardiography: anatomic correlations, image orientation, and clinical applications. Mayo Clin Proc 65:1193–1213.

81. Bansal RC, Shakudo M, Shah PM, et al. (1990) Biplane transesophageal echocardiography: technique, image orientation, and preliminary experience in 131 patients. J Am Soc Echocardiogr 3:348–366.

82. Omoto R, Kyo S, Matsumura M, et al. (1992) Evaluation of biplane color Doppler transesophageal echocardiography in 200 consecutive patients. Circulation 85:1237–1247.

83. Seward JB, Khandheria BK, Oh JK, et al. (1988) Transesophageal echocardiography: technique, anatomic correlations, implementation, and clinical applications. Mayo Clin Proc 63:649–680.

84. Seward JB, Khandheria BK, Freeman WK, et al. (1993) Multiplane transesophageal echocardiography: image orientation, examination technique, anatomic correlations, and clinical applications. Mayo Clin Proc 68:523–551.

85. Silverman NH (1993). Pediatric Echocardiography. Williams and Wilkins, Baltimore.

86. Snider AR, Serwer GA, Ritter SB. (1997) Echocardiography in Pediatric Heart Disease. Echocardiography in Pediatric Heart Disease. Mosby-Year Book, Inc, St. Louis, pp. 203–206.

87. Valdes-Cruz LM, Cayre RO (1999). Echocardiographic Diagnosis of Congenital Heart Disease. Lippincot-Raven Publishers, Philadelphia.

88. Stumper O, Sutherland GR (eds) (1994) Transesophageal Echocardiography in Congenital Heart Disease. London, Hodder Headline Group, Boston.

89. Russell IA, Rouine-Rapp K, Stratmann G, et al. (2006) Congenital heart disease in the adult: a review with internet-accessible transesophageal echocardiographic images. Anesth Analg 102:694–723.

90. Sundar S, DiNardo JA (2008) Transesophageal echocardiography in pediatric surgery. Int Anesthesiol Clin 46:137–155.

91. Stevenson JG, Sorensen GK, Gartman DM, et al. (1993) Left ventricular outflow tract obstruction: an indication for intraoperative transesophageal echocardiography. J Am Soc Echocardiogr 6:525–535.

92. Rosenfeld HM, Gentles TL, Wernovsky G, et al. (1998) Utility of intraoperative transesophageal echocardiography in

the assessment of residual cardiac defects. Pediatr Cardiol 19:346–351.

93. Reich DL, Konstadt SN, Nejat M, et al. (1993) Intraoperative transesophageal echocardiography for the detection of cardiac preload changes induced by transfusion and phlebotomy in pediatric patients. Anesthesiology 79:10–15.

94. Doerr HK, Quinones MA, Zoghbi WA (1993) Accurate determination of left ventricular ejection fraction by transesophageal echocardiography with a nonvolumetric method. J Am Soc Echocardiogr 6:476–481.

95. Bailey JM, Shanewise JS, Kikura M, et al. (1995) A comparison of transesophageal and transthoracic echocardiographic assessment of left ventricular function in pediatric patients with congenital heart disease. J Cardiothorac Vasc Anesth 9:665–669.

96. Nishimura RA, Tajik AJ (1997) Evaluation of diastolic filling of left ventricle in health and disease: Doppler echocardiography is the clinician's Rosetta Stone. J Am Coll Cardiol 30:8–18.

97. Schmitz L, Koch H, Bein G, et al. (1998) Left ventricular diastolic function in infants, children, and adolescents. Reference values and analysis of morphologic and physiologic determinants of echocardiographic Doppler flow signals during growth and maturation. J Am Coll Cardiol 32:1441–1448.

98. Bernard F, Denault A, Babin D, et al. (2001) Diastolic dysfunction is predictive of difficult weaning from cardiopulmonary bypass. Anesth Analg 92:291–298.

99. Border WL, Michelfelder EC, Glascock BJ, et al. (2003) Color M-mode and Doppler tissue evaluation of diastolic function in children: simultaneous correlation with invasive indices. J Am Soc Echocardiogr 16:988–994.

100. Balaguru D, Auslender M, Colvin SB, et al. (2000) Intraoperative myocardial ischemia recognized by transesophageal echocardiography monitoring in the pediatric population: a report of 3 cases. J Am Soc Echocardiogr 13:615–618.

101. Rouine-Rapp K, Rouillard KP, Miller-Hance W, et al. (2006) Segmental wall-motion abnormalities after an arterial switch operation indicate ischemia. Anesth Analg 103:1139–1146.

102. Fyfe DA, Kline CH. (1991) Transesophageal echocardiography for congenital heart disease. Echocardiography 8:573–586.

103. Hsu YH, Santulli T, Jr., Wong AL, et al. (1991) Impact of intraoperative echocardiography on surgical management of congenital heart disease. Am J Cardiol 67:1279–1283.

104. Roberson DA, Muhiudeen IA, Cahalan MK, et al. (1991) Intraoperative transesophageal echocardiography of ventricular septal defect. Echocardiography 8:687–697.

105. Stumper O, Kaulitz R, Elzenga NJ, et al. (1991) The value of transesophageal echocardiography in children with congenital heart disease. J Am Soc Echocardiogr 4:164–176.

106. Tee SD, Shiota T, Weintraub R, et al. (1994) Evaluation of ventricular septal defect by transesophageal echocardiography: intraoperative assessment. Am Heart J 127:585–592.

107. Stevenson JG. (1995) Role of intraoperative transesophageal echocardiography during repair of congenital cardiac defects. Acta Paediatr Suppl 410:23–33.

108. Bezold LI, Pignatelli R, Altman CA, et al. (1996) Intraoperative transesophageal echocardiography in congenital heart surgery. The Texas Children's Hospital experience. Tex Heart Inst J 23:108–115.

109. Xu J, Shiota T, Ge S, et al. (1996) Intraoperative transesophageal echocardiography using high-resolution biplane 7.5 MHz probes with continuous-wave Doppler capability in infants and children with tetralogy of Fallot. Am J Cardiol 77:539–542.

110. Bengur AR, Li JS, Herlong JR, et al. (1998) Intraoperative transesophageal echocardiography in congenital heart disease. Semin Thorac Cardiovasc Surg 10:255–264.

111. Kavanaugh-McHugh A, Tobias JD, Doyle T, et al. (2000) Transesophageal echocardiography in pediatric congenital heart disease. Cardiol Rev 8:288–306.

112. Lim DS, Dent JM, Gutgesell HP, et al. (2007) Transesophageal echocardiographic guidance for surgical repair of aortic insufficiency in congenital heart disease. J Am Soc Echocardiogr 20:1080–1085.

113. Randolph GR, Hagler DJ, Connolly HM, et al. (2002) Intraoperative transesophageal echocardiography during surgery for congenital heart defects. J Thorac Cardiovasc Surg 124:1176–1182.

114. Ma XJ, Huang GY, Liang XC, et al. (2007) Transoesophageal echocardiography in monitoring, guiding, and evaluating surgical repair of congenital cardiac malformations in children. Cardiol Young 17:301–306.

115. Yumoto M, Katsuya H (2002) Transesophageal echocardiography for cardiac surgery in children. J Cardiothorac Vasc Anesth 16:587–591.

116. Bettex DA, Schmidlin D, Bernath MA, et al. (2003) Intraoperative transesophageal echocardiography in pediatric congenital cardiac surgery: a two-center observational study. Anesth Analg 97:1275–1282.

117. Sloth E, Pedersen J, Olsen KH, et al. (2001) Transoesophageal echocardiographic monitoring during paediatric cardiac surgery: obtainable information and feasibility in 532 children. Paediatr Anaesth 11:657–662.

118. Andropoulos DB, Stayer SA, Bent ST, et al. (1999) A controlled study of transesophageal echocardiography to guide central venous catheter placement in congenital heart surgery patients. Anesth Analg 89:65–70.

119. Ho AC, Chen CK, Yang MW, et al. (2004) Usefulness of intraoperative transesophageal echocardiography in the assessment of surgical repair of pediatric ventricular septal defects with video-assisted endoscopic techniques in children. Chang Gung Med J 27:646–653.

120. Ungerleider RM, Greeley WJ, Sheikh KH, et al. (1989) The use of intraoperative echo with Doppler color flow imaging to predict outcome after repair of congenital cardiac defects. Ann Surg 210:526–533; discussion 533–534.

121. Stevenson JG, Sorensen GK, Gartman DM, et al. (1993) Transesophageal echocardiography during repair of congenital cardiac defects: identification of residual problems necessitating reoperation. J Am Soc Echocardiogr 6:356–365.

122. Bettex DA, Pretre R, Jenni R, et al. (2005) Cost-effectiveness of routine intraoperative transesophageal

echocardiography in pediatric cardiac surgery: a 10-year experience. Anesth Analg 100:1271–1275.

123. Van Der Velde ME, Sanders SP, Keane JF, et al. (1994) Transesophageal echocardiographic guidance of transcatheter ventricular septal defect closure. J Am Coll Cardiol 23:1660–1665.

124. Van Der Velde ME, Perry SB, Sanders SP (1991) Transesophageal echocardiography with color Doppler during interventional catheterization. Echocardiography 8:721–730.

125. Remadevi KS, Francis E, Kumar RK (2009) Catheter closure of atrial septal defects with deficient inferior vena cava rim under transesophageal echo guidance. Catheter Cardiovasc Interv 73:90–96.

126. Pontus SP, Jr., Frommelt PC (1994) Detection of a previously undiagnosed anomalous subclavian artery during insertion of a transesophageal echocardiography probe. Anesth Analg 78:805–807.

127. Bensky AS, O'Brien JJ, Hammon JW (1995) Transesophageal echo probe compression of an aberrant right subclavian artery. J Am Soc Echocardiogr 8:964–966.

128. Frommelt PC, Stuth EA (1994) Transesophageal echocardiographic in total anomalous pulmonary venous drainage: hypotension caused by compression of the pulmonary venous confluence during probe passage. J Am Soc Echocardiogr 7:652–654.

129. Chang YY, Chang CI, Wang MJ, et al. (2005) The safe use of intraoperative transesophageal echocardiography in the management of total anomalous pulmonary venous connection in newborns and infants: a case series. Paediatr Anaesth 15:939–943.

130. Kallmeyer IJ, Collard CD, Fox JA, et al. (2001) The safety of intraoperative transesophageal echocardiography: a case series of 7200 cardiac surgical patients. Anesth Analg 92:1126–1130.

131. Cote G, Denault A (2008) Transesophageal echocardiography-related complications. Can J Anaesth 55:622–647.

132. Stevenson JG (1999) Incidence of complications in pediatric transesophageal echocardiography: experience in 1650 cases. J Am Soc Echocardiogr 12:527–532.

133. Preisman S, Yusim Y, Mishali D, et al. (2003) Compression of the pulmonary artery during transesophageal echocardiography in a pediatric cardiac patient. Anesth Analg 96:85–87.

134. Andropoulos DB, Stayer SA, Bent ST, et al. (2000) The effects of transesophageal echocardiography on hemodynamic variables in small infants undergoing cardiac surgery. J Cardiothorac Vasc Anesth 14:133–135.

135. Andropoulos DB, Ayres NA, Stayer SA, et al. (2000) The effect of transesophageal echocardiography on ventilation in small infants undergoing cardiac surgery. Anesth Analg 90:47–49.

136. Greene MA, Alexander JA, Knauf DG, et al. (1999) Endoscopic evaluation of the esophagus in infants and children immediately following intraoperative use of transesophageal echocardiography. Chest 116:1247–1250.

137. Kohr LM, Dargan M, Hague A, et al. (2003) The incidence of dysphagia in pediatric patients after open heart procedures with transesophageal echocardiography. Ann Thorac Surg 76:1450–1456.

138. Muhiudeen-Russell IA, Miller-Hance WC, Silverman NH (2001) Unrecognized esophageal perforation in a neonate during transesophageal echocardiography. J Am Soc Echocardiogr 14:747–749.

139. Foster E, Kusumoto FM, Sobol SM, et al. (1990) Streptococcal endocarditis temporally related to transesophageal echocardiography. J Am Soc Echocardiogr 3:424–427.

140. Melendez LJ, Chan KL, Cheung PK, et al. (1991) Incidence of bacteremia in transesophageal echocardiography: a prospective study of 140 consecutive patients. J Am Coll Cardiol 18:1650–1654.

141. Dajani AS, Taubert KA, Wilson W, et al. (1997) Prevention of bacterial endocarditis. Recommendations by the American Heart Association [see comments]. JAMA 277:1794–1801.

142. Wilson W, Taubert KA, Gewitz M, et al. (2007) Prevention of infective endocarditis: guidelines from the American Heart Association: a guideline from the American Heart Association Rheumatic Fever, Endocarditis, and Kawasaki Disease Committee, Council on Cardiovascular Disease in the Young, and the Council on Clinical Cardiology, Council on Cardiovascular Surgery and Anesthesia, and the Quality of Care and Outcomes Research Interdisciplinary Working Group. Circulation 116:1736–1754.

143. Pearlman AS, Gardin JM, Martin RP, et al. (1992) Guidelines for physician training in transesophageal echocardiography: recommendations of the American Society of Echocardiography Committee for Physician Training in Echocardiography. J Am Soc Echocardiogr 5:187–194.

144. Cahalan MK, Abel M, Goldman M, et al. (2002) American Society of Echocardiography and Society of Cardiovascular Anesthesiologists task force guidelines for training in perioperative echocardiography. Anesth Analg 94:1384–1388.

145. Fyfe D (1999) Transesophageal echocardiography guidelines: return to bypass or to bypass the guidelines? J Am Soc Echocardiogr 12:343–344.

146. Russell IM, Silverman NH, Miller-Hance W, et al. (1999) Intraoperative transesophageal echocardiography for infants and children undergoing congenital heart surgery: the role of the anesthesiologist. J Am Soc Echocardiogr 12:1009–1014.

147. Stevenson JG (1999) Adherence to physician training guidelines for pediatric transesophageal echocardiography affects the outcome of patients undergoing repair of congenital cardiac defects. J Am Soc Echocardiogr 12:165–172.

148. Stevenson JG (1999) Performance of intraoperative pediatric transesophageal echocardiography by anesthesiologists and echocardiographers: training and availability are more important than hats. J Am Soc Echocardiogr 12:1013–1014.

149. Fyfe DA (1999) Intraoperative transesophageal echocardiography in children with congenital heart disease: how, not Who! J Am Soc Echocardiogr 12:1011–1013.

150. Aronson S, Thys DM (2001) Training and certification in perioperative transesophageal echocardiography: a historical perspective. Anesth Analg 93:1422–1427.

151. Aronson S, Butler A, Subhiyah R, et al. (2002) Development and analysis of a new certifying examination in perioperative transesophageal echocardiography. Anesth Analg 95:1476–1482.

152. Smallhorn JF (2002) Intraoperative transesophageal echocardiography in congenital heart disease. Echocardiography 19:709–723.

12

Bleeding and coagulation: monitoring and management

Bruce E. Miller, M.D.
Children's Healthcare of Atlanta, Emory University School of Medicine, Atlanta, Georgia, USA

Glyn D. Williams, M.B.Ch.B., F.F.A.
Lucile Packard Children's Hospital, Stanford University School of Medicine, Stanford, California, USA

Introduction

Managing the coagulation system during and after cardiopulmonary bypass (CPB) is an integral part of pediatric cardiac anesthesiology and surgery. This management is becoming more intricate as our understanding of coagulation grows, as surgical procedures on younger children with more complex heart defects are undertaken, and as pharmacologic and technological options expand. In this chapter, we review the coagulation problems that exist in pediatric cardiac patients and discuss the management of post-CPB coagulopathies.

The coagulation pathway

The normal hemostatic mechanism that is triggered after vascular injury involves complex and concurrent interactions between platelets, coagulation proteins, and fibrinolysis. The processes have been described as primary, secondary, and tertiary phases of hemostasis.

Anesthesia for Congenital Heart Disease 2nd edition. Edited by Dean Andropoulos, Stephen Stayer, Isobel Russell and Emad Mossad. © 2010 Blackwell Publishing.

Primary hemostasis reduces bleeding in damaged vessels by inducing vasoconstriction at the site of vessel injury and by initiating platelet adhesion, aggregation, and secretion to form a platelet plug. Platelets adhere to exposed subendothelial tissues via an interaction between von Willebrand factor (vWF) and the glycoprotein (Gp) Ib receptor on platelet surfaces. Platelets subsequently release numerous hemostatic mediators from their granules, change the charge on their surface membranes to form an active surface on which the coagulation proteins interact, and express Gp IIb/IIIa fibrinogen receptors on their surfaces. Fibrinogen subsequently binds to these exposed receptors causing platelets to aggregate to each other (Figure 12.1).

Secondary hemostasis leads to the formation of a fibrin clot by sequentially activating circulating coagulation factors to finally form insoluble fibrin. Our understanding of this secondary hemostasis has evolved from the traditional description of independent "intrinsic" and "extrinsic" coagulation pathways being activated in plasma to a concept of coagulation factors interacting on the surfaces of tissue factor (TF)-bearing cells and activated platelets at the site of vascular injury (Figure 12.2). Secondary hemostasis begins with the activation of factor VII upon its exposure to TF, a transmembrane glycoprotein found in the cells of the subendothelial tissue of damaged blood vessels. The activated factor VII (VIIa) and

205

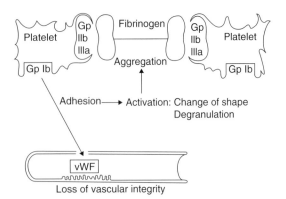

Figure 12.1 Primary hemostasis. Platelet adhesion is mediated via von Willebrand factor (vWF) and platelet receptor GP Ib. Subsequent aggregation is mediated via GP IIb/IIIa receptors (Reproduced with permission from Reference [1])

TF form a complex on these subendothelial cells. The cell-bound VIIa/TF complex then activates factor X (to Xa) and factor IX (to IXa). This sequence of activations was formerly called the "extrinsic pathway" of coagulation because a factor "extrinsic" to the blood, i.e., TF, is required for it to proceed. The newly formed factor Xa complexes with factor Va on the surface of TF-bearing cells and generates small amounts thrombin (IIa) from prothrombin (II). This initially formed small amount of thrombin, while insufficient to initiate fibrin formation, activates platelets and factors V, VIII, and XI [3]. These activated platelets not only participate in the primary hemostasis process but also provide the active surface upon which further coagulation processes occur that result in fibrin formation.

At the same time, the contact of blood with the negatively charged subendothelial tissue of damaged blood vessels activates the contact factors (factors XI and XII,

prekallikrein [PK], and high-molecular-weight kininogen [HMWK]). The result of this activation is enormous and plays roles not only in the coagulation system but also in the related inflammatory response. From the coagulation perspective, however, this activation provides another route of activation of factor XI in addition to that formed by the actions of the cell bound VIIa/TF complex. This coagulation sequence was formerly called the "intrinsic pathway" because all the contact factors are "intrinsic" to the blood.

At this point, activated coagulation factors and activated platelets work together to finally produce fibrin. Factor IXa formed by the actions of both the TF/VIIa complex and factor XIa joins with factor VIIIa on the surface of activated platelets to activate substantial amounts of factor Xa. This factor Xa then joins with factor Va, again on the platelet surfaces, to form the prothrombinase complex that subsequently generates large bursts of thrombin. This thrombin then converts fibrinogen to fibrin clot [3].

Tertiary hemostasis involves fibrin clot maturation and fibrinolysis. Factor XIII is activated to cross-link the fibrin strands. This cross-linked fibrin restores hemostasis in an injured blood vessel by acting as the "mortar" that cements the primary platelet plug. Thrombus is removed by fibrinolysis in order to reestablish normal blood flow through the repaired blood vessel. Circulating plasminogen binds to fibrin within the thrombus. Tissue plasminogen activator (tPA) released from endothelial cells also complexes with fibrin and converts the bound plasminogen to its active form plasmin, leading to the enzymatic degradation of the clot. Further formation of plasmin also occurs as a result of the direct actions of factor XIIa and kallikrein from the contact activation system on plasminogen [4].

The formation and dissolution of a thrombus by these mechanisms is closely regulated by many feedback inhibitors to keep the coagulation process localized to the area of blood vessel injury. Included among these inhibitors are TF pathway inhibitor, antithrombin III, protein C, protein S, thrombin-activatable fibrinolysis inhibitor, plasminogen activator inhibitor, and α_2-antiplasmin [5]. Interactions between coagulation activators and inhibitors contain the coagulation process to the site of blood vessel injury and provide a balance between bleeding and thrombosis.

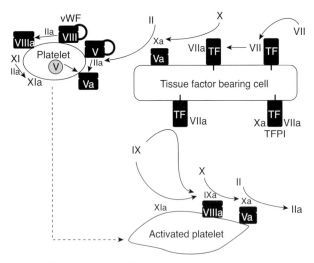

Figure 12.2 Tissue factor-initiated, cell-based hemostasis. TF, tissue factor; vWF, von Willebrand factor; TFPI, tissue factor pathway inhibitor (Reproduced with permission from Reference [2])

Alterations of coagulation in pediatric cardiac patients

Coagulation in children with congenital heart defects is affected by several factors particular to patient age, pathophysiology, and exposure to CPB.

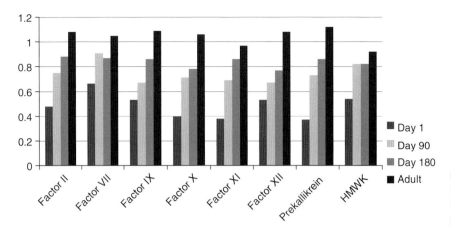

Figure 12.3 Coagulation factor levels during infancy and adulthood. HMWK, high-molecular-weight kininogen (Reproduced with permission and adapted from Reference [6])

Maturational factors

At birth, the coagulation system is immature and continues in a state of maturation throughout the first year of life. Significant deficiencies in levels of the vitamin K-dependent factors (II, VII, IX, and X) and the contact factors (XI, XII, PK, and HMWK) exist at birth. Hepatic immaturity with decreased factor synthesis and accelerated clearance of factors by children's increased basal metabolic rates are cited as causes of these deficiencies [6,7]. Most of these procoagulant factor levels at birth are only 40–50% of those found in adults and do not reach adult levels until after 6 months of age (Figure 12.3). Essentially, all of the inhibitors of coagulation (proteins S and C, heparin cofactor II, and antithrombin III) are also present in low levels during the first year of life and, again, do not attain adult levels until after 6 months of age (Figure 12.4). Only platelet counts and levels of fibrinogen, factors V, VIII, vWF, and XIII are at adult ranges at birth [6]. However, evidence exists that platelet aggregation is impaired [8] and that fibrinogen exists in a dysfunctional "fetal" form in newborns [6,9] even though these factors are not quantitatively deficient.

Despite these quantitative and qualitative deficiencies, the results of most coagulation tests, including prothrombin time (PT) and thrombin clotting time, are within normal adult ranges within a few days after birth [6]. Only the activated partial thromboplastin time (aPTT) is prolonged for a substantial time before falling to adult ranges at about 3 months of age. The maintenance of normal coagulation tests in early infancy suggests a relative balance between procoagulation factors and their inhibitors. If anything, the process tends toward increased coagulability. Thrombotic complications are more common in neonates and thromboelastography (TEG) has shown that neonates and infants actually clot faster and have increased clot strength compared to adults [10]. Despite the maintenance of the functional integrity of the coagulation system in infants, the effect of the maturational deficiencies in their

coagulation systems is that these children have little margin of safety once they encounter the further alterations in hemostasis produced by exposure to CPB.

Influence of congenital cardiac pathophysiology

Baseline coagulation defects have been demonstrated in children with congenital heart defects, although consistent associations between specific cardiac defects and certain hemostatic abnormalities are not evident. Coagulation abnormalities have been reported in 58% of children with noncyanotic defects. Decreased fibrinogen levels and platelet counts, prolonged bleeding times, and fibrinolytic activity were noted, especially in infants. Children with cyanotic defects have been shown to have a 71% incidence of coagulation abnormalities [11], including decreased levels of factors II, VII, IX, and X, defective platelet function, and accelerated fibrinolysis [12–14]. Cyanotic patients with hematocrits greater than 50% have

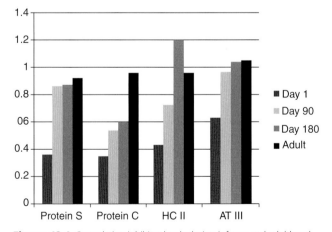

Figure 12.4 Coagulation inhibitor levels during infancy and adulthood. HC II, heparin cofactor II; AT III, antithrombin III (Reproduced with permission a from Reference [6])

been shown to have prolonged PT and aPTT, decreased levels of fibrinogen and factors V and VIII, and thrombocytopenia [15]. The number of hemostatic abnormalities present preoperatively correlates with the severity of the children's polycythemia, and a relationship between the presence of preoperative hemostatic defects in cyanotic children and the severity of postoperative bleeding has been noted [12]. Causes of these abnormalities may include hepatic dysfunction from hypoperfusion or from perfusion with hypoxemic, hyperviscous blood [13].

Interestingly, young children with cyanotic heart defects appear to develop a hypercoagulable state prior to the onset of polycythemia. Evidence for this is seen in the trend for increased levels of platelets, fibrinogen, and factors V and VIII in these children and could help explain findings in the early literature of pulmonary thrombi in infants with cyanotic defects who died before the onset of polycythemia [15].

Coagulation changes induced by CPB

Two consequences of exposure to CPB alter coagulation in pediatric cardiac patients: hemodilution and the nonphysiological activation of contact and TF systems. In the past, priming volumes of the CPB oxygenator and circuit were two to four times the blood volume of neonates and infants, thus producing profound alterations in coagulation factor levels due to hemodilution and causing complex post-CPB coagulopathies. The current trend toward open-heart surgery in very young infants has spurred the development of perfusion equipment with priming volumes only 0.5–1 times the blood volume of the smallest children, thereby reducing the adverse effects of hemodilution. Tubing lengths can be reduced by reconfiguring CPB circuit components and tubing diameters, pumps, filters, reservoirs, and oxygenators have been miniaturized while still providing adequate blood flow and gas exchange.

Upon initiation of bypass, the artificial surfaces of the CPB circuit activate the contact factors (XI, XII, PK, and HMWK). These activated factors trigger not only the coagulation pathway but also the inflammatory response [4]. This inflammatory response causes the expression of TF on monocytes and endothelial cells [16], while aspiration of blood from the surgical field during CPB exposes more TF on cell membranes. Thus, the initiation of CPB triggers the coagulation pathway independent of blood being exposed to a damaged blood vessel. Indeed, thrombin generation during CPB is well documented [17, 18] despite administration of adequate amounts of heparin to prevent catastrophic clotting during CPB.

Concurrently, the fibrinolytic system is also activated as a result of exposure to CPB. Endothelial cells are stimulated to release tPA by thrombin [19], by bradykinin generated during contact activation, and by surgical trauma [20]. tPA converts plasminogen to plasmin, which then initiates fibrinolysis. Factor XIIa and kallikrein from the contact activation system also directly act on plasminogen to generate plasmin [4]. Evidence of fibrinolysis has been documented during CPB in both children and adults [21–23], although this phenomenon quickly resolves after the conclusion of CPB [21,23]. Therefore, both the coagulation and fibrinolytic processes are activated, independent of blood vessel injury, by exposure to CPB. These nonphysiological processes combine to damage platelets and thereby disrupt hemostasis. Indeed, platelet dysfunction after CPB is felt to be the most common etiology for excessive post-CPB bleeding in adults [24]. Post-CPB platelet abnormalities result from several mechanisms (Figure 12.5). Platelet adhesion is decreased due to destruction of Gp Ib receptors by plasmin and the shear stresses encountered during CPB [26]. Platelet aggregation is diminished because platelet activation during CPB by thrombin, plasmin, and fibrin split products (FSPs) depletes platelets of their granules and interferes with their subsequent ability to aggregate to each other. In summary, the primary, secondary, and tertiary phases of normal hemostasis are all affected by exposure to CPB, leading to clinically significant coagulopathies.

Management of CPB-associated coagulation changes

Anticoagulation

Anticoagulation is a coagulation change mandated, rather than produced, by CPB. Because of its instant action and ease of neutralization, heparin is used to achieve this anticoagulation. Heparin's primary action is to inhibit the activity of circulating thrombin by binding to antithrombin III (ATIII) and consequently greatly accelerating ATIII's inhibition of thrombin and other activated coagulation factors. Heparin also inhibits the factor Xa-catalyzed formation of thrombin via an ATIII-independent mechanism [27]. In adults and older children, the increase in activated clotting time (ACT) values in response to heparin administration is proportional to plasma ATIII levels [28]. In neonates and infants, though, there is no correlation between plasma ATIII levels and the ACT response to heparin administration [28,29]. However, when neonates and infants are given a standard weight-based heparin dose, their ACTs are prolonged to values deemed acceptable for the conduct of CPB [28,29]. It may be that other thrombin inhibitors such as heparin cofactor II and α_2-macroglobulin have greater relevance in neonates and infants and brings into question either the importance of

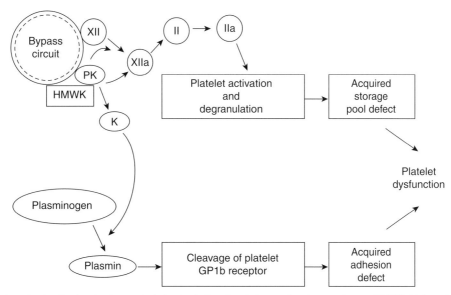

Figure 12.5 Proposed mechanism for the development of platelet dysfunction during cardiopulmonary bypass. HMWK, high-molecular-weight kininogen; K, kallikrein; PK, prekallikrein (Reproduced with permission from Reference [25])

ATIII or the adequacy of ACTs in assessing anticoagulation in these children.

The adequacy of heparinization for CPB can be measured clinically not only by assessing heparin's effect with the ACT but also by measuring its whole blood or plasma level. Neither of these measurements is ideal, though. ACT values are influenced by factors that do not contribute to anticoagulation such as hypothermia and hemodilution [30], both of which are commonly encountered in young children during CPB. Heparin levels, on the other hand, do not take into account the tremendous variability in individual patient responses to heparin. To complicate matters further, ACT values and heparin levels do not correlate in neonates and children during the course of CPB [31].

Ultimately, the adequacy of heparinization is reflected by the level of inhibition of both thrombin generation and thrombin activity during CPB. Less thrombin is generated, less fibrinogen consumed, and less fibrinolysis initiated when children are managed by individualized protocols based on the maintenance of a specified whole blood heparin level as compared to standard heparin dosing protocols based on patient weight and monitored by ACT measurements [32, 33]. While ACT values remained acceptably prolonged by both protocols, heparin levels began to diverge between the two protocols within 60 minutes of the initiation of CPB, falling significantly in the children dosed with the weight-based protocol. The use of the heparin concentration-based protocol resulted in the administration of significantly more heparin and similar or smaller protamine doses to neutralize circulating heparin at the termination of CPB when compared to the weight-based protocol. Additionally, neither 24-hour

postoperative chest tube drainage nor clinical outcome variables were found to differ between the protocols, although one study found a slight increase in the number of donor exposures required by the children dosed according to heparin levels. These data seem to indicate that heparin concentration-based protocols provide a more adequate level of heparinization for children undergoing CPB with little adverse effects.

In practice, though, many more institutions manage intraoperative heparin administration using ACT values rather than heparin level measurements. An ACT is certainly easier and less expensive to obtain. When using only ACT measurements, anesthesiologists and perfusionists should keep in mind that heparin levels have significantly fallen within 1 hour of CPB despite the maintenance of adequate ACT values and should consider the administration of additional heparin if CPB is expected to continue for a substantial period of time.

A potential problem associated with the use of heparin is heparin-induced thrombocytopenia (HIT). The immune-mediated type of this syndrome (type II) can cause limb- and life-threatening vascular thromboses (38–76% incidence), carries a mortality rate of 20–30% [34], and has been reported in adults, children, and even neonates. The pathogenesis involves heparin-induced generation of immunoglobulin G (IgG) that binds multimolecular complexes of heparin and platelet factor 4 (PF4) on platelet surfaces leading to a self-perpetuating cycle of platelet activation, thrombin formation, and further release of PF4 from platelet granules. Endothelial cells and monocytes are also activated by the antiheparin/PF4 IgG resulting in expression of TF and further procoagulant activity [34, 35]. The diagnosis of HIT requires the presence of both clinical and laboratory criteria. Clinical criteria include thrombocytopenia (decrease in platelet count to <150,000/mm^3 or to ≤50% of baseline) with or without venous or arterial thromboses but with the exclusion of other potential causes of thrombocytopenia. Laboratory criteria include positive antigen assays (detect antibodies to heparin/PF4 complexes) and positive functional tests of platelet activation (serotinin release assay) or aggregation [34–36]. Up to 50% of heparin-treated patients develop heparin/PF4 antibodies but only 1–5% patients develop HIT [34]. Therefore, positive laboratory tests alone do not definitively diagnose HIT. However, the tests are sensitive enough that negative results rule out HIT [37]. "Typical-onset HIT" presents 5–10 days after starting a course of heparin, while "rapid-onset HIT" occurs immediately after heparin administration in patients with existing heparin/PF4 antibodies developed from a previous exposure to heparin usually within the past 100 days [35]. Treatment of HIT includes the discontinuation of heparin and the administration of a fast acting, nonheparin anticoagulant such as a direct thrombin inhibitor (lepirudin, argatroban, or bivalirudin) or an antifactor Xa agent (danaparoid or fondaparinux) for at least 1 month [34]. Administration of warfarin, low-molecular-weight heparin, and platelet transfusions are contraindicated during acute HIT [35]. Heparin should continue to be avoided in these patients until assays of heparin/PF4 antibody levels are negative (median of 85 days) [36].

When a patient with a history of type II HIT requires elective cardiac surgery, every effort should be made to postpone the surgery until the heparin/PF4 antibody levels have become negative. At that time, it will be safe to administer heparin for CPB. Fortunately, there is little immune memory in HIT so antibodies are usually not restimulated upon reexposure to heparin and, even if they are, they usually are not regenerated before 5 days after the reexposure [35]. Even so, heparin should not be used during preoperative cardiac catheterization or in flushes for transducer systems or intravenous or intra-arterial catheters. Additionally, heparin-coated catheters and extracorporeal circuit components should be avoided. If postoperative antithrombosis prophylaxis is needed in these patients, a nonheparin anticoagulant should be used [37]. If a patient with a history of type II HIT requires cardiac surgery while heparin/PF4 antibodies are still present, anticoagulation for CPB must be accomplished either by using one of the nonheparin anticoagulants or by administering an antiplatelet agent such as epoprostenol (prostacyclin analogue) or tirofiban (Gp IIb/IIIa inhibitor) in conjunction with heparin [35]. All of these drugs are plagued by a lack of FDA-sanctioned approval for this use, a lack of dosing guideline for pediatric patients, a lack of reversal agents, and a risk of significant postoperative bleeding.

Table 12.1 Consequences of ongoing bleeding

Hemodynamic instability
Cardiac tamponade
Massive transfusion
Hypothermia
Hyperkalemia
Hypocalcemia
Metabolic alkalosis
Dilutional coagulopathy
Cytokine infusion
Respiratory insufficiency
Increased blood donor exposures
Infectious agents
Transfusion reactions
Immunomodulation
Increased morbidity and mortality

Coagulopathies

Aggressive management of the coagulopathies associated with CPB is critical in order to minimize the consequences of ongoing bleeding (Table 12.1). Identification of risk factors and coagulation tests predictive of post-CPB bleeding in children permits adequate preparation for its management. A blood bank service that is able to provide a variety of blood products as well as timely advice is crucial. Preoperative communication with the blood bank staff is mandatory in order to insure the availability of necessary blood products prior to any surgery. Pharmacologic agents known to attenuate or help treat post-CPB coagulopathies should be available as should equipment used in blood conservation techniques such as cell salvage and ultrafiltration. Finally, the potential for late postoperative thrombotic complications should be appreciated in certain subsets of children.

Risk factors

Associations have been found between several patient, laboratory, or surgical characteristics and post-CPB blood loss and transfusion requirements in children. Patient age appears to be the variable with the most significant association. Post-CPB blood loss and blood product administration vary inversely with age. Greater blood loss should be anticipated in children younger than 12 months [38] with neonates being at greatest risk [39]. Body weight less than 8 kg has also been shown to be a predictor of increased post-CPB bleeding [40].

Batteries of preoperative laboratory tests have also been examined to determine their abilities to predict excessive post-CPB bleeding. Few associations have been found. However, a high preoperative hematocrit level (surrogate for cyanotic heart disease), prolonged aPTT, and certain

TEG parameters (reduced α and shear modulus) were associated with 12-hour chest tube drainage in one study of 482 children [41].

Several factors associated with surgical technique also show correlations with post-CPB blood loss and transfusion requirements. In children younger than 1 year, the degree of hypothermia during CPB and the use of deep hypothermic circulatory arrest are significant factors, whereas in children older than 1 year, the duration of CPB, the complexity of the surgical procedure, and repeat sternotomy are significant factors. The surgeon performing the procedure has also been found to be a correlating variable [38].

Coagulation tests

While the presence of a significant coagulopathy at the conclusion of CPB in infants is almost always abundantly clear from the appearance of the surgical field, determining the significance of any ongoing oozing and the causative etiologies of this oozing can be an elusive task after CPB in older children. Multiple coagulation tests obtained during and after CPB have been examined in attempts to identify a test that can be deemed the "gold standard" for delineating significant coagulopathies and children who will bleed excessively after CPB. During CPB, platelet counts and TEG MA values have been found to be associated with postoperative chest tube drainage in children [41]. After CPB and heparin neutralization with protamine, platelet counts, fibrinogen levels, and TEG K, α, and MA values have been found to correlate independently with postoperative chest tube drainage in pediatric patients [40,42]. It seems, therefore, that platelet counts, fibrinogen levels, and TEG parameters provide useful data to help define coagulopathies after CPB in children. Despite these findings, identification of a "gold standard" coagulation test remains elusive.

In adults, algorithms have been established to guide the management of post-CPB coagulopathies and have been based on ACT values, PT, aPTT, platelet counts, fibrinogen levels, and TEG values. Use of these algorithms has resulted in a decrease in postoperative chest tube drainage and blood product usage when compared to therapeutic interventions based solely on clinical judgments of the appearance of the operative field [43,44]. Constructing and testing comparable algorithms for children remains to be accomplished.

In order to use an algorithm to guide the management of post-CPB coagulopathies, the results of coagulation tests must be rapidly available to clinicians. Technology currently exists to allow on-site measurements of whole blood PT, aPTT, and platelet counts in the operating room [43]. Thromboelastograms can be activated with celite, kaolin, or TF to provide rapid data as well

[23,45]. Protamine or heparinase can be used to neutralize heparin in blood samples and thus to allow thromboelastograms to be obtained even during CPB while patients are anticoagulated [22, 23]. After CPB, heparinase-modified TEGs can also be helpful in discerning the contribution of residual circulating heparin to persistently prolonged ACT values after initial protamine administration [46]. Ongoing advancements in technology will probably continue to improve our point-of-care coagulation monitoring capability and thus allow the establishment of practical algorithms to manage post-CPB coagulopathies in children.

Blood product therapy

Whole blood or individual coagulation products can be used to manage post-CPB coagulopathies. Whole blood less than 48 hours old has been shown to better limit post-CPB blood loss in children younger than 2 years undergoing complex surgical procedures when compared to the use of a reconstituted product composed of one unit each of packed RBCs, platelets, and fresh-frozen plasma (FFP) [47]. This improvement in hemostasis was attributed to the presence of better functioning platelets in whole blood. Unfortunately, whole blood less than 48 hours old is not readily available at all pediatric cardiac surgical centers and, when it is, it usually has been stored at 4°C, a factor that significantly depresses platelet function [48]. Additionally, the use of whole blood must be supplemented at times with the transfusion of individual coagulation products to optimally control post-CPB blood loss, especially in younger patients [7].

The transfusion of individual coagulation products is the primary treatment for post-CPB coagulopathies in children in many institutions. The effects of different coagulation products in correcting abnormalities of TEG parameters, platelet counts, and fibrinogen levels after protamine administration in children have been investigated [40]. Since abundant evidence demonstrates that quantitative and qualitative platelet deficiencies [7,24,43,49] exist after CPB, initial treatment of ongoing bleeding after adequate heparin neutralization was with platelet transfusions. Platelet administration substantially improved the TEG parameters in addition to the platelet count. If bleeding continued, cryoprecipitate administration raised fibrinogen levels to normal and significantly further improved TEG parameters, whereas FFP not only failed to increase fibrinogen levels but also worsened all TEG parameters. Patients given platelets followed by FFP had substantially more 24-hour chest tube drainage and required more coagulation products postoperatively than those receiving cryoprecipitate. Therefore, when using component therapy to treat post-CPB coagulopathies in children, platelet transfusion followed by cryoprecipitate, if needed, seems the better approach to restore hemostasis [40].

Recombinant factor VIIa

The use of recombinant factor VIIa (rFVIIa) to help manage post-CPB coagulopathies in children is gaining attention. While rFVIIa is only approved for use in patients with hemophilia A or B who have developed inhibitors to factors VIII or IX and in patients with factor VII deficiency [50], it has been increasingly used outside of these indications to manage bleeding. Administration of rFVIIa enhances the amount of thrombin generation by saturating exposed TF in damaged blood vessel walls and enhances the rate of thrombin generation by stimulating the thrombin burst that occurs on the surfaces of activated platelets adhering to injured vessels [51]. This leads to the formation of clot with a dense fibrin structure that is resistant to premature lysis because of a concomitant increase in activation of the fibrin cross-linker, factor XIII, and of thrombin-activated fibrinolysis inhibitor [5,52]. Although the administration of rFVIIa will enhance thrombin generation even in the presence of low-platelet levels, the transfusion of platelets prior to its administration may improve its effectiveness [5] and the restoration of fibrinogen levels will improve the resulting clot strength [53].

No controlled trials have been performed to justify the use of rFVIIa after CPB in children, but anecdotal reports of its successful use have been reported, even during ECMO. The fact that it is produced using recombinant technology, thus eliminating infectious risks, makes rFVIIa an appealing therapeutic option. However, its significant cost and the lack of an established safety profile limit this appeal. While enhanced thrombin generation after rFVIIa is theoretically limited to sites of vascular injury due to its required interaction with TF and activated adhering platelets, thromboembolic events have been reported after its use [50]. Warnings about the concomitant use of prothrombin-complex concentrates with rFVIIa [54] and the use of rFVIIa in the presence of disseminated intravascular coagulation (DIC) [5] have been issued because of increased thrombotic potential. If administered during ECMO, extra vigilance must be paid to the integrity of the circuit. An increased incidence of acute renal dysfunction has also been noted after rFVIIa administration in adults [55]. For these reasons, many currently advocate the use of rFVIIa as a rescue therapy instead of a primary intervention. Doses ranging from 30 to 500 mcg/kg have been administered to children with 90 mcg/kg being most consistently reported. The half-life of rFVIIa is only 2.5 hours but may be shorter in children because of an increased clearance rate [5,52]. Therefore, repeat doses at 2-hour intervals, if needed, have been advised. Monitoring of coagulation after rFVIIa administration is best accomplished by assessing whole blood coagulation with tests such as the thromboelastogram instead of plasma-based assays like the PT and aPTT [5,56].

Pharmacologic therapies

An even more effective method of combating post-CPB coagulopathies would be their attenuation. Several pharmacologic interventions are used with hopes of accomplishing this goal.

Desmopressin acetate

Desmopressin acetate (1-deamino-8-D-arginine vasopressin [DDAVP]) is a synthetic analogue of the posterior pituitary hormone, vasopressin. Administration of DDAVP has been shown to increase plasma levels of the procoagulant factor VIII:C and of the vWF [49,57]. The vWF plays a major role in mediating platelet adhesion to exposed subendothelium by binding to adhesive Gp Ib receptors on the platelet membrane and to the exposed subendothelial collagen [49]. DDAVP may also improve hemostasis by a direct effect on blood vessel walls to increase platelet adhesiveness and promote platelet spreading at sites of vessel injury [58]. Since DDAVP seems to improve hemostasis by enhancing platelet function and since platelet dysfunction has been incriminated as a cause of post-CPB bleeding, DDAVP has been used in an attempt to curb blood loss after cardiac surgery.

Studies involving the routine prophylactic administration of DDAVP (0.3 μg/kg) to adults undergoing primary coronary artery bypass grafting have shown no reduction in post-CPB blood loss or transfusion requirements [59]. In adults, the use of DDAVP has been shown to be hemostatically beneficial when used during more complex procedures, such as valve replacements or repeat sternotomies [57], or in situations with laboratory documented platelet dysfunction and continued bleeding after CPB [49,60]. Two studies have investigated the prophylactic administration of DDAVP (again 0.3 μg/kg) to children after cardiac surgery, in many cases after complex procedures, and neither has shown a reduction in blood loss or transfusion requirements with this therapy [61,62].

Potential complications following the use of DDAVP could relate to its endocrine functions (vasoconstriction and antidiuretic hormone effects), its activation of tPA, or its augmentation of platelet function and clotting. However, none of these theoretical concerns have been documented in clinical studies.

The routine prophylactic use of DDAVP after CPB in children and adults does not seem to improve hemostasis. Administration of DDAVP to select patients with documented platelet function abnormalities (prolonged bleeding times or decreased TEG MA values) in the face of ongoing bleeding may prove beneficial.

Antifibrinolytics

Epsilon aminocaproic acid (EACA) and tranexamic acid (TA) are the two clinically available antifibrinolytic drugs. Both exert their antifibrinolytic effect most importantly by competitively binding with the lysine binding sites of plasminogen thus altering plasminogen's conformation and preventing plasminogen activators from converting the plasminogen to its active form, plasmin. At significantly higher concentrations, these drugs bind directly to plasmin that has already formed, thus directly inhibiting the plasmin's activity. Both drugs are fairly rapidly excreted by the kidneys virtually intact, although TA boasts a longer half-life. TA is 6–10 times more potent than EACA [63,64].

Both EACA and TA have been shown to inhibit fibrinolytic activity when used prophylactically during CPB [20,65]. Although some postulate that fibrinolysis is not a major contributor to post-CPB bleeding [21–24], a reduction in post-CPB blood loss and transfusion requirements has been demonstrated with the prophylactic use of these drugs in adults [59,64,65]. The contribution of the products of fibrinolysis to the generation of post-CPB platelet dysfunction no doubt plays a role here. Indeed, studies with TA have shown not only that TA preserves platelet function after CPB, but also that the amount of postoperative bleeding correlates with the post-CPB platelet function and not with the occurrence of fibrinolysis [66]. Several investigations focusing on indiscriminant populations of children have revealed no reduction in bleeding or blood product transfusions during the first 24 hours after CPB with the prophylactic use of either EACA or TA [67–69]. However, when analyzed separately, children with cyanosis and children undergoing repeat sternotomies have been found to experience significant reductions in postoperative blood loss and transfusion requirements with the use of one of the antifibrinolytics [67,68,70,71] and thus these populations may provide indications for the use of antifibrinolytics in the pediatric arena.

Multiple dosing regimens have been reported for each of these antifibrinolytics in adult patients and then have been extrapolated to the pediatric population. For EACA, a plasma level of 130 μg/mL is needed to inhibit fibrinolysis [72]. Since EACA that is administered intravenously is rapidly excreted by the kidneys, successful dosing protocols have used a loading dose followed by a continuous infusion. Published pediatric dosing regimens include a loading dose of 75 mg/kg followed by an infusion of 15 mg/kg/h [67] and a loading dose of 150 mg/kg followed by and infusion of 30 mg/kg/h [69]. The higher of these doses was felt by the investigators to be appropriate to achieve the desired plasma levels of 130 μg/mL [69].

Dosing regimens for TA have been analyzed more on a pharmacodynamic basis. Again, most regimens employ a loading dose followed by a continuous infusion because of rapid renal elimination of TA. A dosing protocol using a loading dose of 100 mg/kg after induction followed by another 100 mg/kg dose in the pump prime and an infusion of 10 mg/kg/h has proven beneficial in pediatric patients [70]. It has been emphasized with both antifibrinolytics that since the initiation of fibrinolysis begins with skin incision, administration of these drugs starting prior to skin incision results in significantly more reduction of fibrinolysis, platelet dysfunction, and blood loss than administration after CPB and protamine infusion [66,73].

Much concern has been voiced about potential thrombotic complications after the use of antifibrinolytics; however, none of the previously cited reports found any significant increase in thrombotic or embolic problems in either adults or children. These complications are of more concern when antifibrinolytics are used incorrectly during a hypercoagulable state with compensatory fibrinolysis (DIC) rather than during the primary fibrinolysis that may occur after CPB [74].

Aprotinin

Aprotinin is a nonspecific serum protease inhibitor extracted from bovine lung that has been repeatedly shown to reduce blood loss and transfusion requirements in adults undergoing open-heart surgery [75–77], especially in cases at high risk for post-CPB bleeding [78,79]. Conflicting reports have been published, however, concerning aprotinin's effects on blood loss and transfusion requirements after CPB in children. Much of this conflict has been created by heterogeneity in the age and weights of children receiving aprotinin, in the surgical procedures undertaken on these children, in the transfusion triggers utilized, and in the aprotinin doses used in these children as well as by the poor methodology employed in some studies [80]. A meta-analysis of randomized trials of aprotinin use in pediatric patients has shown a 33% overall reduction in the proportion of children transfused with aprotinin use (56% reduction in children undergoing primary sternotomies) but no significant reduction in volume of blood transfused or in volume of chest tube drainage [80]. Studies in children undergoing repeat sternotomies have documented objective reductions in transfusion requirements, time required for chest closure in the operating room, and ICU and hospital stays resulting in financial savings despite the significant cost of aprotinin [81,82]. Aprotinin's efficacy in neonates undergoing complex open-heart procedures is supported by some but not all studies [83,84]. However, the use of aprotinin during pediatric cardiac surgery gradually became widely accepted clinical practice both in Europe and the USA.

In 2006, two prospective observational studies questioned the safety of aprotinin. These studies associated the use of aprotinin in adults undergoing CPB with a significantly increased risk of postoperative renal dysfunction [85, 86]. No such risk was found with the use of EACA or TA while all three drugs demonstrated similar hemostatic effectiveness. The proposed mechanism for renal dysfunction is aprotinin-induced inhibition of kallikrein at the proximal tubular epithelial cells, thus blocking prostaglandin-mediated dilation of renal afferent arterioles and resulting in decreased deep cortical and medullary perfusion, diminished glomerular filtration rate, and focal tubular necrosis [85]. Additionally, the use of aprotinin was associated with increases in the risks of myocardial infarction, heart failure, and stroke or encephalopathy [85], and an increased 5-year mortality [87] compared with the use of TA. Much discussion has followed the publication of these studies, calling into question the propensity analyses used [88, 89]. Additionally, subsequent similarly conducted work has shown no detrimental influence of the use of aprotinin on post-CPB renal function [90] or the incidence of myocardial infarction or cerebrovascular events [91] in adults. In the pediatric arena, a retrospective review of aprotinin use in children undergoing CPB has found no association with acute renal failure, need for temporary postoperative dialysis, neurological complications, or operative or late mortality [92]. Another retrospective review involving only neonates has similarly shown no increase in post-CPB renal dysfunction [93] and a prospective pediatric study could not demonstrate an independent role for aprotinin in the development of post-CPB renal dysfunction or the need for dialysis [94]. However, the BART study (Blood Conservation Using Antifibrinolytics in a Randomized Trial) showed a 50% increased risk of death within 30 days postoperatively in adults undergoing high-risk cardiac procedures who received aprotinin as opposed to EACA or TA [95]. This finding prompted the early termination of the study and the authors concluded that the use of aprotinin should be precluded in this population of patients. In the meantime, while this issue continues to be debated, the marketing of aprotinin has been suspended worldwide by its manufacturer. Nevertheless, aprotinin is still used in some major pediatric cardiac centers.

Several factors should be kept in mind when administering aprotinin to children. Optimal dosing protocols need to be established to achieve the desired plasma level of 200 KIU/mL in order to inhibit both plasmin and kallikrein. The risk of allergic reactions upon repeat exposures must be remembered [96]. Use of kaolin ACTs or heparin level measurements must be considered to insure safe levels of anticoagulation with the use of aprotinin since aprotinin itself inhibits "intrinsic" coagulation and thus may act synergistically with heparin to prolong celite ACT values [97]. However, it seems likely that aprotinin will never enjoy the wide acceptance that it had during the first 20 years after its introduction to cardiac surgery in 1987 [98].

Table 12.2 Blood conservation techniques

Possible means for reducing allogenic blood transfusions during pediatric cardiac surgery

Management strategy	Neonate	Teenager
Preoperative		
Autologous blood donation	−	+
Erythropoietin, iron	−	+
Plateletpheresis	−	−
Surgery		
Limit hypothermia	+	+
Limit duration of cardiopulmonary bypass	+	+
Avoid circulatory arrest	+	+
Meticulous hemostasis	+	+
Topical sealants	+	+
Anesthesia		
Normothermia after cardiopulmonary bypass	+	+
Transfusion algorithm	+	+
Antifibrinolytic agents	+	+
Acute normovolemic hemodilution	−	?
Anesthetic technique and agents	?	?
Antithrombin III	?	?
FVIIa	+	+
DDAVP	−	−
Cardiopulmonary bypass		
Limit prime volume	+	+
Nonsanguinous prime	?	+
Defined target hematocrit during bypass	+	+
Ultrafiltration	+	+
Cell salvage	+	+
Heparin/protamine titration	+	+
Heparin concentration monitored	?	+
Heparin coated circuit	?	?
Blood substitutes	?	?
Centrifugal pump	−	?
Reinfuse circuit residual fluid	−	−
Postoperative		
Transfusion algorithm	+	+
Reinfuse shed blood	−	?

+, strategy useful in children; ?, strategy possibly useful but benefit unproven in children; −, strategy not useful in children.

Blood conservation

Measures to conserve autologous blood during pediatric open-heart surgery are worthwhile in order to limit the adverse consequences of allogenic blood exposure. Blood conservation is often more successful if multiple measures are employed, but some techniques are less applicable to small children (Table 12.2). Preoperatively, the patient's likelihood of bleeding should be assessed and a blood conservation strategy selected that has a favorable ratio between potential benefit and risk.

Preoperative considerations

Preoperative autologous donation (PAD) is the collection and anticoagulation of whole blood from a patient for anticipated perioperative transfusion. It eliminates the risk of blood-borne infections and incompatibility issues, including graft-versus-host disease, and diminishes immune modulation. The amount of blood collected from a single donation is typically limited to 10% of the child's total blood volume. The rate of donation reactions is 2–5% and increases with decreasing age and weight. Limited venous access and patient stress from multiple procedures are additional concerns and some centers sedate small children during blood donation. PAD is efficacious at reducing allogenic exposure but remains controversial for cardiac surgery because of issues about safety, cost, and the risk of delaying surgery. Suitability of PAD in children with congenital heart disease depends on the anticipated consequences upon a patient's cardiac pathophysiology and is often limited to relatively healthy patients with simple cardiac anomalies. Although typically reserved for older children (>7 years or >40 kg), PAD has been reported useful in infants older than 6 months [99] or >8 kg [100].

Recombinant human erythropoietin alpha (EPO), the primary growth factor for red blood cells, is efficacious at conserving blood when administered to patients donating autologous blood before surgery. Treatment with EPO (100–300 U/kg subcutaneously, prior to each blood donation) increased the amount of autologous blood that could be collected and minimized allogenic blood exposure in children of age range 1.2–14 years [100]. A single dose of EPO without PAD was not efficacious at reducing allogenic transfusions in children [101]. EPO is expensive, invasive, and probably will be limited to children undergoing elective noncomplex cardiac surgery. Platelet count increases with EPO therapy. While this may be an advantage in some cases, it would be a concern in prothrombotic patients, including those with single ventricle physiology.

Intraoperative considerations

The influences of differing anesthesia techniques or agents on bleeding during pediatric cardiac surgery are poorly known. Basic principles would suggest avoidance of high blood pressure and venous congestion. Of interest, patients undergoing unifocalization of aortopulmonary collaterals may be at greater risk for hemorrhage from postoperative liver dysfunction. Intraoperative measures to preserve hepatic blood flow could be worthy of consideration.

Acute normovolemic hemodilution (ANH) is the removal of whole blood from the patient before CPB while maintaining isovolemia by crystalloid or colloid infusion and then infusing the blood after CPB. A study of 32 infants of weight 5–12 kg undergoing noncomplex open-heart surgery found that ANH-treated patients had better postoperative coagulation tests and tended to receive fewer blood products ($p = 0.06$) than controls [102]. The CPB circuit for all patients was primed with homologous red blood cells. Factors influencing selection of patients for ANH include the patient's hemodynamic stability and baseline hematocrit, the type of CPB prime (blood or crystalloid) and the target hematocrit during CPB. ANH may have limited application in small children because the platelets in ANH blood may be insufficient to correct severe post-CPB deficits in platelet number and function.

Platelet-rich plasma can be obtained by plateletpheresis after induction of anesthesia and transfused after CPB. Recent reviews conclude that the current technology is clinically ineffective and plateletpheresis should not be considered for routine use.

Fibrin glue has been used in children undergoing repair of congenital heart defects and is most efficacious in controlling low-pressure venous bleeding. Exposure to topical sealants that contain aprotinin results in an antibody response similar to that observed after intravenous aprotinin administration. When exposed to fibrin glue of bovine origin, patients may develop antibodies against bovine Factor V or X that can then cross-react to inhibit the patients' own Factor V or X.

Perfusion considerations

Although a universally "safe" hemodilution level during CPB cannot be defined because the effects of hemodilution may vary according to diagnosis, age at operation, CPB variables such as pH strategy and flow rate, and other perioperative factors, recent outcome studies indicate that severe hemodilution is harmful. A hematocrit level at the onset of low-flow CPB of approximately 24% or higher was associated with higher Psychomotor Development Index scores and reduced lactate levels in infants undergoing two ventricle repair [103]. Conventional neonatal CPB requires the use of allogeneic blood to prevent unacceptable hemodilution but results in a negative effect on clinical recovery through inflammatory side effects. This would suggest an advantage for eliminating blood use in infant CPB through circuit miniaturization and perfusion techniques [104,106].

Ultrafiltration has been repeatedly demonstrated to be useful during pediatric open-heart surgery. Effects include hemoconcentration of the patient, removal of inflammatory mediators, and an ability to manipulate plasma electrolytes and colloid osmotic pressure. Ultrafiltration reduces the requirement for allogenic blood products by increasing the patient's hematocrit, concentrating coagulation plasma proteins, and modulating the systemic inflammatory response to CPB [107]. Heparin blood concentration increases because it is highly protein bound and hence not filtered [108]. There are several methods of ultrafiltration. A blood-containing CPB prime can be ultrafiltered prior to initiation of CPB; conventional ultrafiltration is performed during CPB; modified ultrafiltration (either arteriovenous or venovenous) occurs after separation from CPB. The amount of ultrafiltrate obtained can be increased by adding fluid to the CPB circuit to maintain isovolemia. It is unclear which of the ultrafiltration variants provides maximal clinical benefit [109].

Blood shed intraoperatively can be collected into an automated centrifuge-based blood salvage instrument that produces a heparin-free suspension of washed, concentrated red blood cells. Likewise, red cells present in the CPB circuit after separation of the patient from CPB can be salvaged. Red cell salvage has been found to be a useful blood conservation technique during pediatric cardiac surgery [110]. Washed red cells lack plasma proteins and will lead to coagulation factor depletion if transfused in large volumes.

Unprocessed residual CPB fluid can be returned to the patient. However, this is not optimal because the fluid has a low hematocrit and contains heparin, fibrinolysis byproducts, and cellular debris. Mediastinal and pleural shed blood can be collected postoperatively and reinfused, but the technique is seldom used in pediatric cardiac surgery. There is concern that reinfused shed blood promotes a coagulopathic state because shed blood not only contains decreased amounts of coagulation factors and increased levels of fibrin degradation products but also stimulates tissue plasminogen activator. Additionally, the hematocrit of shed blood is usually less than 20%.

Summary

Managing the coagulation system is an integral part of pediatric cardiac anesthesiology and surgery. Young children live in a precarious coagulation balance that is quickly disrupted by exposure to CPB. Maintenance of adequate anticoagulation during CPB, appropriate use of coagulation products and pharmacologic therapies, and measures to conserve autologous blood contribute significantly to minimizing or correcting this disruption. Ongoing work in this field continues to enhance our ability to minimize this source of morbidity for children undergoing cardiac surgery.

References

1. Hardy JF, Desroches J (1992) Natural and synthetic antifibrinolytics in cardiac surgery. Can J Anaesth 39:353–365.
2. Monroe DM, Hoffman M, Allen GA, Roberts HR (2000) The factor VII-platelet interplay: effectiveness of recombinant factor VIIa in the treatment of bleeding in severe thrombocytopathia. Semin Thromb Hemost 26:373–377.
3. Hoffman M, Monroe DM, Roberts HR (1998) Activated factor VII activates factors IX and X on the surface of activated platelets: thoughts on the mechanism of action of high-dose activated factor VII. Blood Coagul Fibrinolysis 9 (Suppl):S61–S65.
4. Levy JH (1992) Complement and contact activation. In: Levy JH (ed) Anaphylactic Reactions in Anesthesia and Intensive Care, 2nd edn. Butterworth-Heinemann, Stoneham, pp. 51–62.
5. Midathada MV, Mehta P, Waner M, et al. (2004) Recombinant factor VIIa in the treatment of bleeding. Am J Clin Pathol 121:124–137.
6. Andrew M, Paes B, Johnston M (1990) Development of the hemostatic system in the neonate and young infant. Am J Pediatr Hematol Oncol 12:95–104.
7. Kern FH, Morana NJ, Sears JJ, et al. (1992) Coagulation defects in neonates during cardiopulmonary bypass. Ann Thorac Surg 54:541–546.
8. Mull MM, Hathaway WE (1970) Altered platelet function in newborns. Pediatr Res 4:229–237.
9. Miller BE, Tosone SR, Guzzetta NA, et al. (2004) Fibrinogen in children undergoing cardiac surgery: is it effective? Anesth Analg 99:1341–1346.
10. Miller BE, Bailey JM, Mancuso TJ, et al. (1997) Functional maturity of the coagulation system in children: an evaluation using thrombelastography. Anesth Analg 84:745–748.
11. Kontras SB, Sirak HD, Newton WA, Jr. (1966) Hematologic abnormalities in children with congenital heart disease. JAMA 195:99–103.
12. Ekert H, Gilchrist GS, Stanton R, et al. (1970) Hemostasis in cyanotic congenital heart disease. J Pediatr 76:221–230.
13. Henriksson P, Värendh G, Lundström N (1979) Haemostatic defects in cyanotic congenital heart disease. Br Heart J 41:23–27.
14. Rinder CS, Gaal D, Student LA, et al. (1994) Platelet-leukocyte activation and modulation of adhesion receptors in pediatric patients with congenital heart disease undergoing cardiopulmonary bypass. J Thorac Cardiovasc Surg 107:280–288.
15. Komp DM, Sparrow AW, (1970) Polycythemia in cyanotic heart disease—a study of altered coagulation. J Pediatr 76:231–236.
16. Osterud B, (1995) Cellular interactions in tissue factor expression by blood monocytes. Blood Coagul Fibrinolysis 6:S20–S25.
17. Slaughter TF, LeBleu TH, Douglas JM, Jr., et al. (1994) Characterization of prothrombin activation during cardiac surgery by hemostatic molecular markers. Anesthesiology 80:520–526.
18. Guzzetta NA, Miller BE, Todd K, et al. (2005) An evaluation of the effects of a standard heparin dose on thrombin inhibition during cardiopulmonary bypass in neonates. Anesth Analg 100:1276–1282.
19. Levin EG, Marzec U, Anersone J, et al. (1984) Thrombin stimulates tissue plasminogen activator release from cultured human endothelial cells. J Clin Invest 74:1988–1995.

20. Horrow JC, Hlavacek J, Strong MD, et al. (1990) Prophylactic tranexamic acid decreases bleeding after cardiac operations. J Thorac Cardiovasc Surg 99:70–74.
21. Bentall HH, Allwork SP (1968) Fibrinolysis and bleeding in open-heart surgery. Lancet 1 (7532):4–8.
22. Williams GD, Bratton SL, Nielsen NJ, et al. (1998) Fibrinolysis in pediatric patients undergoing cardiopulmonary bypass. J Cardiothorac Vasc Anesth 12:633–638.
23. Miller BE, Guzzetta NA, Tosone SR, et al. (2000) Rapid evaluation of coagulopathies after cardiopulmonary bypass in children using modified thromboelastography. Anesth Analg 90:1324–1330.
24. Harker LA, Malpass TW, Branson HE, et al. (1980) Mechanism of abnormal bleeding in patients undergoing cardiopulmonary bypass: acquired transient platelet dysfunction associated with selective α-granule release. Blood 56:824–834.
25. Carr ME (1996) Control of perioperative bleeding: pharmacologic agents. In: Wechsler AS (ed) Pharmacologic Management of Perioperative Bleeding. CME Network, Southampton, p. 29.
26. George JN, Pickett EB, Saucerman S, et al. (1986) Platelet surface glycoproteins: studies on resting and activated platelets and platelet membrane microparticles in normal subjects, and observations in patients during adult respiratory distress syndrome and cardiac surgery. J Clin Invest 78:340–348.
27. Hirsh J (1986) Mechanism of action and monitoring of anticoagulants. Semin Thromb Hemost 12:1–11.
28. Dietrich W, Braun S, Spannagl M, et al. (2001) Low preoperative antithrombin activity causes reduced response to heparin in adult but not in infant cardiac-surgical patients. Anesth Analg 92:66–71.
29. Guzzetta NA, Miller BE, Todd K, et al. (2006) Clinical measures of heparin's effect and thrombin inhibitor levels in pediatric patients with congenital heart disease. Anesth Analg 103:1131–1138.
30. Culliford AT, Gitel SN, Starr N, et al. (1981) Lack of correlation between activated clotting time and plasma heparin during cardiopulmonary bypass. Ann Surg 193:105–111.
31. Andrew M (1992) Anticoagulation and thrombolysis in children. Tex Heart Inst J 19:168–177.
32. Codispoti M, Ludlam CA, Simpson D, et al. (2001) Individualized heparin and protamine management in infants and children undergoing cardiac operations. Ann Thorac Surg 71:922–928.
33. Guzzetta NA, Bajaj T, Fazlollah T, et al. (2008) A comparison of heparin management strategies in infants undergoing cardiopulmonary bypass. Anesth Analg 106:419–425.
34. Levy JH, Tanaka KA, Hursting MJ (2007) Reducing thrombotic complications in the perioperative setting: an update on heparin-induced thrombocytopenia. Anesth Analg 105:570–582.
35. Warkentin TE (2003) Heparin-induced thrombocytopenia: pathogenesis and management. Br J Haematol 121:535–555.
36. Warkentin TE, Kelton JG (2001) Temporal aspects of heparin-induced thrombocytopenia. N Engl J Med 344:1286–1292.
37. Warkentin TE, Greinacher A (2003) Heparin-induced thrombocytopenia and cardiac surgery. Ann Thorac Surg 76:638–648.
38. Williams GD, Bratton SL, Ramamoorthy C (1999) Factors associated with blood loss and blood product transfusions: a multivariate analysis in children after open-heart surgery. Anesth Analg 89:57–64.
39. Williams GD, Bratton SL, Riley EC, et al. (1998) Association between age and blood loss in children undergoing open heart operations. Ann Thorac Surg 66:870–876.
40. Miller BE, Mochizuke T, Jerrold JH, et al. (1997) Predicting and treating coagulopathies after cardiopulmonary bypass in children. Anesth Analg 85:1196–1202.
41. Williams GD, Bratton SL, Riley EC, et al. (1999) Coagulation tests during cardiopulmonary bypass correlate with blood loss in children undergoing cardiac surgery. J Cardiothorac Vasc Anesth 13:398–404.
42. Martin P, Horkay F, Rajah SM, et al. (1991) Monitoring of coagulation status using thrombelastography during paediatric open heart surgery. Int J Clin Monit Comput 8:183–187.
43. Despotis GJ, Santoro SA, Spitznagel E, et al. (1994) prospective evaluation and clinical utility of on-site monitoring of coagulation in patients undergoing cardiac operation. J Thorac Cardiovasc Surg 107:271–279.
44. Shore-Lesserson L, Manspeizer HE, DePerio M, et al. (1999) Thromboelastography-guided transfusion algorithm reduces transfusions in complex cardiac surgery. Anesth Analg 88:312–319.
45. Chan KL, Summerhayes RG, Ignjatovic V, et al. (2007) Reference values for kaolin-activated thromboclastography in healthy children. Anesth Analg 105:1610–1613.
46. Tuman KJ, McCarthy RJ, Djuric M, et al. (1994) Evaluation of coagulation during cardiopulmonary bypass with a heparinase-modified thromboelastographic assay. J Cardiothorac Vasc Anesth 8:144–149.
47. Manno CS, Hedbery KW, Kim HC, et al. (1991) Comparison of the hemostatic effects of fresh whole blood, stored whole blood, and components after open heart surgery in children. Blood 77:930–936.
48. Golan M, Modan M, Lavee J, et al. (1990) Transfusion of fresh whole blood stored (4°C) for short period fails to improve platelet aggregation on extracellular matrix and clinical hemostasis after cardiopulmonary bypass. J Thorac Cardiovasc Surg 99:354–360.
49. Czer LSC, Bateman TM, Gray RJ, et al. (1987) Treatment of severe platelet dysfunction and hemorrhage after cardiopulmonary bypass: reduction in blood product usage with desmopressin. J Am Coll Cardiol 9:1139–1147.
50. O'Connell KA, Wood JJ, Wise RP, et al. (2006) Thromboembolic adverse events after use of recombinant human coagulation factor VIIa. JAMA 295:293–298.
51. Hedner U (2000) Recombinant coagulation factor VIIa: from the concept to clinical application in hemophilia treatment in 2000. Semin Thromb Hemost 26:363–366.
52. Hedner U (2004) Dosing with recombinant factor VIIa based on current evidence. Semin Hematol 41:35–39.
53. Tanaka KA, Taketomi T, Szlam F, et al. (2008) Improved clot formation by combined administration of activated factor

VII (NovoSeven®) and fibrinogen (Haemocomplettan® P). Anesth Analg 106:732–738.

54. Veldman A, Neuhaeuser C, Akintuerk H, et al. (2007) rFVIIa in the treatment of persistent hemorrhage in pediatric patients on ECMO following surgery for congenital heart disease. Paediatr Anaesth 17:1176–1181.

55. Karkouti K, Beattie WS, Wijeysundera DN, et al. (2005) Recombinant factor VIIa for intractable blood loss after cardiac surgery: a propensity score-matched case-control analysis. Transfusion 45:26–34.

56. Gabriel DA, Carr M, Roberts HR (2004) Monitoring coagulation and the clinical effects of recombinant factor VIIa. Semin Hematol 41:20–24.

57. Salzman EW, Weinstein MJ, Weintraub RM, et al. (1986) Treatment with desmopressin acetate to reduce blood loss after cardiac surgery: a double-blind randomized trial. N Engl J Med 314:1402–1406.

58. Kentro TB, Lottenberg R, Kitchens CS (1987) Clinical efficacy of desmopressin acetate for hemostatic control in patients with primary platelet disorders undergoing surgery. Am J Hematol 24:215–219.

59. Horrow JC, Van Riper DF, Strong MD, et al. (1991) Hemostatic effects of tranexamic acid and desmopressin during cardiac surgery. Circulation 84:2063–2070.

60. Mongan PD, Hosking MP (1992) The role of desmopressin acetate in patients undergoing coronary artery bypass surgery: a controlled clinical trial with thromboelastographic risk stratification. Anesthesiology 77:38–46.

61. Reynolds LM, Nicolson SC, Jobes DR, et al. (1993) Desmopressin does not decrease bleeding after cardiac operation in young children. J Thorac Cardiovasc Surg 106:954–958.

62. Seear MD, Wadsworth LD, Rogers PC, et al. (1989) The effect of desmopressin acetate (DDAVP) on postoperative blood loss after cardiac operations in children. J Thorac Cardiovasc Surg 98:217–219.

63. Griffin JD, Ellman L (1978) Epsilon-aminocaproic acid (EACA). Semin Thromb Hemost 5:27–40.

64. Øvrum E, Holen E, Abdelnoor M, et al. (1993) Tranexamic acid (Cyklokapron) is not necessary to reduce blood loss after coronary artery bypass operations. J Thorac Cardiovasc Surg 105:78–83.

65. Vander Salm TJ, Kaur S, Lancey RA, et al. (1996) Reduction of bleeding after heart operations through the prophylactic use of epsilon-aminocaproic acid. J Thorac Cardiovasc Surg 112:1098–1107.

66. Soslau G, Horrow J, Brodsky I (1991) Effect of tranexamic acid on platelet ADP during extracorporeal circulation. Am J Hematol 38:113–119.

67. McClure PD, Izsak J (1974) The use of epsilon-aminocaproic acid to reduce bleeding during cardiac bypass in children with congenital heart disease. Anesthesiology 40:604–608.

68. Zonis Z, Seear M, Reichert M, et al. (1996) The effect of preoperative tranexamic acid on blood loss after cardiac operations in children. J Thorac Cardiovasc Surg 111:982–987.

69. Williams GD, Bratton SL, Riley EC, et al. (1999) Efficacy of ε-aminocaproic acid in children undergoing cardiac surgery. J Cardiothorac Vasc Anesth 13:304–308.

70. Reid RW, Zimmerman AA, Laussen PC, et al. (1997) The efficacy of tranexamic acid versus placebo in decreasing blood loss in pediatric patients undergoing repeat cardiac surgery. Anesth Analg 84:990–996.

71. Chauhan S, Das SN, Bisoi A, et al. (2004) Comparison of epsilon aminocaproic acid and tranexamic acid in pediatric cardiac surgery. J Cardiothorac Vasc Anesth 18:141–143.

72. McNicol GP, Fletcher AP, Alkjaersig N, et al. (1962) The absorption, distribution, and excretion of ε-aminocaproic acid following oral or intravenous administration to man. J Lab Clin Med 59:15–24.

73. Daily PO, Lamphere JA, Dembitsky WP, et al. (1994) Effect of prophylactic epsilon-aminocaproic acid on blood loss and transfusion requirements in patients undergoing first-time coronary artery bypass grafting: a randomized, prospective, double-blind study. J Thorac Cardiovasc Surg 108:99–108.

74. Gans H (1966) Thrombogenic properties of epsilon amino caproic acid. Ann Surg 163:175–178.

75. Royston D, Bidstrup BP, Taylor KM, et al. (1987) Effect of aprotinin on need for blood transfusion after repeat open-heart surgery. Lancet 2 (8571):1289–1291.

76. van Oeveren W, Jansen NJG, Bidstrup BP, et al. (1987) Effects of aprotinin on hemostatic mechanisms during cardiopulmonary bypass. Ann Thorac Surg 44:640–645.

77. Levy JH, Pifarre R, Schaff HV, et al. (1995) A multicenter, double-blind, placebo-controlled trial of aprotinin for reducing blood loss and the requirement for donor-blood transfusion in patients undergoing repeat coronary artery bypass grafting. Circulation 92:2236–2244.

78. Bidstrup BP, Royston D, Sapsford RN, et al. (1989) Reduction in blood loss and blood use after cardiopulmonary bypass with high dose aprotinin (Trasylol). J Thorac Cardiovasc Surg 97:364–372.

79. Murkin JM, Lux J, Shannon NA, et al. (1994) Aprotinin significantly decreases bleeding and transfusion requirements in patients receiving aspirin and undergoing cardiac operations. J Thorac Cardiovasc Surg 107:554–561.

80. Arnold DM, Fergusson DA, Chan AKC, et al. (2006) Avoiding transfusions in children undergoing cardiac surgery: a meta-analysis of randomized trials of aprotinin. Anesth Analg 102:731–737.

81. D'Errico CC, Shayevitz JR, Martindale SJ, et al. (1996) The efficacy and cost of aprotinin in children undergoing reoperative open heart surgery. Anesth Analg 83:1193–1199.

82. Miller BE, Tosone SR, Tam VKH, et al. (1998) Hematologic and economic impact of aprotinin in reoperative pediatric cardiac operations. Ann Thorac Surg 66:535–541.

83. Carrel TP, Schwanda M, Vogt PR, et al. (1998) Aprotinin in pediatric cardiac operations: a benefit in complex malformations and with high-dose regimen only. Ann Thorac Surg 66:153–158.

84. Williams GD, Ramamoorthy C, Pentcheva K, et al. (2008) A randomized, controlled trial of aprotinin in neonates undergoing open-heart surgery. Paediatr Anaesth 18 (9):812–819.

85. Mangano DT, Tudor IC, Dietzel C (2006) The risk associated with aprotinin in cardiac surgery. N Engl J Med 354:353–365.

86. Karkouti K, Beattie WS, Dattilo KM, et al. (2006) A propensity score case-control comparison of aprotinin and

tranexamic acid in high-transfusion-risk cardiac surgery. Transfusion 46:327–338.

87. Mangano DT, Miao Y, Vuylsteke A, et al. (2007) Mortality associated with aprotinin during 5 years following coronary artery bypass graft surgery. JAMA 297: 471–479.

88. Body SC, Mazer CD (2006) Pro: aprotinin has a good efficacy and safety profile relative to other alternatives for prevention of bleeding in cardiac surgery. Anesth Analg 103:1354–1359.

89. Levy JH, Ramsay JG, Guyton RA (2006) Aprotinin in cardiac surgery (letter to editor). N Engl J Med 354:1956.

90. Dietrich W, Busley R, Boulesteix AL (2008) Effects of aprotinin dosage on renal function. An analysis of 8,548 cardiac surgical patients treated with different dosages of aprotinin. Anesthesiology 108:189–198.

91. Royston D, Levy JH, Fitch J, et al. (2006) Full-dose aprotinin use in coronary artery bypass graft surgery: an analysis of perioperative pharmacotherapy and patient outcomes. Anesth Analg 103:1082–1088.

92. Backer CL, Kelle AM, Stewart RD, et al. (2007) Aprotinin is safe in pediatric patients undergoing cardiac surgery. J Thorac Cardiovasc Surg 134:1421–1428.

93. Guzzetta NA, Evans FM, Rosenberg ES, et al. (2009) Impact of aprotinin on postoperative renal dysfunction in neonates undergoing cardiopulmonary bypass: a retrospective analysis. Anesth Analg 108:448–455.

94. Székely A, Sápi E, Breuer T, et al. (2008) Aprotinin and renal dysfunction after pediatric cardiac surgery. Paediatr Anaesth 18:151–159.

95. Fergusson DA, Hébert PC, Mazer CD, et al. (2008) A comparison of aprotinin and lysine analogues in high-risk cardiac surgery. N Engl J Med 358:2319–2331.

96. Dietrich W, Ebell A, Busley R, et al. (2007) Aprotinin and anaphylaxis: analysis of 12,403 exposures to aprotinin in cardiac surgery. Ann Thorac Surg 84:1144–1150.

97. de Smet AAEA, Joen MCN, van Oeveren W, et al. (1990) Increased anticoagulation during cardiopulmonary bypass by aprotinin. J Thorac Cardiovasc Surg 100:520–527.

98. Ray WA, Stein CM (2008) The aprotinin story—is BART the final chapter? N Engl J Med 358:2398–2400.

99. Hibino N, Nagashima M, Sato H, et al. (2008) Preoperative autologous blood donation for cardiac surgery in children. Asian Cardiovasc Thorac Ann 16:21–24.

100. Komai H, Naito Y, Okamura Y, et al. (2005) Preliminary study of autologous blood predonation in pediatric open-heart surgery impact of advance infusion of recombinant human erythropoietin. Pediatr Cardiol 26:50–55.

101. Ootaki Y, Yamaguchi M, Yoshimura N, et al. (2007) The efficacy of preoperative administration of a single dose of recombinant human erythropoietin in pediatric cardiac surgery. Heart Surg Forum 10:E115–E119.

102. Friesen RH, Perryman KM, Weigers KR, et al. (2006) A trial of fresh autologous whole blood to treat dilutional coagulopathy following cardiopulmonary bypass in infants. Paediatr Anaesth 16:429–435.

103. Wypij D, Jonas RA, Bellinger DC, et al. (2008) The effect of hematocrit during hypothermic cardiopulmonary bypass in infant heart surgery: results from the combined Boston hematocrit trials. J Thorac Cardiovasc Surg 135:355–360.

104. Hickey E, Karamlou T, You J, et al. (2006) Effects of circuit miniaturization in reducing inflammatory response to infant cardiopulmonary bypass by elimination of allogeneic blood products. Ann Thorac Surg 81:S2367–S2372.

105. Ohuchi K, Hoshi H, Iwasaki Y, et al. (2007) Feasibility of a tiny centrifugal blood pump (TinyPump) for pediatric extracorporeal circulatory support. Artif Organs 31:408–412.

106. Miyaji K, Kohira S, Miyamoto T, et al. (2007) Pediatric cardiac surgery without homologous blood transfusion, using a miniaturized bypass system in infants with lower body weight. J Thorac Cardiovasc Surg 134:284–289.

107. Elliott M (1999) Modified ultrafiltration and open heart surgery in children. Paediatr Anaesth 9:1–5.

108. Williams GD, Ramamoorthy C, Totzek FR, et al. (1997) Comparison of the effects of red cell separation and ultrafiltration on heparin concentration during pediatric open-heart surgery. J Cardiothorac Vasc Anesth 11:840–844.

109. Williams GD, Ramamoorthy C, Chu L, et al. (2006) Modified and conventional ultrafiltration during pediatric cardiac surgery: clinical outcome compared. J Thorac Cardiovasc Surg 132:1291–1298.

110. Cross M (2001) Autotransfusion in cardiac surgery. Perfusion 16:391–400.

3 Preoperative Considerations

13 Preoperative evaluation and preparation*

Emad B. Mossad, M.D. and Javier Joglar, M.D.

Texas Children's Hospital and Baylor College of Medicine, Houston, Texas, USA

Introduction

The comprehensive preoperative evaluation of the patient with congenital heart disease (CHD) is essential for a successful intervention. The anesthesiologist is faced with a challenge of complex anatomic lesions, with different physiologic consequences, with patients who frequently have other system and extracardiac anomalies associated with their cardiac lesion, and with an ever changing

*A portion of the material in this chapter was published previously as Chapter 11: Preoperative Evaluation and Preparation: A Physiologic Approach, by Lydia Cassorla, M.D., in *Anesthesia for Congenital Heart Disease*, 1st edn.

field, new interventions, and management paradigms. The preoperative evaluation requires a multidisciplinary approach, and is best executed in a setting that involves all cardiologists, cardiac surgeons, intensive care specialists, radiologists as well as the anesthesiologist, sharing their skills and knowledge in discussing the patient's condition, the options available, and the best plan to prepare them for an intervention. At our center, as well as many active pediatric cardiac programs, we have a weekly morning conference attended by all disciplines where the data of patients scheduled to undergo procedures during the upcoming week are discussed. Decisions are made regarding additional investigations or information needed and methods to best optimize the patient for the upcoming intervention are examined.

The preoperative period is the anesthesiologist's opportunity to best understand the patient's anatomy and physiologic status, prepare the patient and family for surgery, and establish a safe anesthetic plan.

The focus of this chapter is to discuss the current trends in the care of a child or adult with CHD that affect the preoperative evaluation process, review the terminology and classification of CHD, and examine strategies for risk assessment and stratification in patients with CHD. The chapter evaluates recent advances in preoperative investigations and methods of preparing the patient and family for a cardiac intervention.

Current trends in CHD

The continued evolution in the care of patients with CHD further enforces the need for a careful, comprehensive preoperative assessment and preparation. Current trends include advances in diagnostic tools and technology, early interventions on very small infants, a growing population of adult survivors with CHD, and the creation of new interventions and hybrid approaches to complex cardiac defects.

Demographics

Due to improved diagnosis and outcome, the population of patients with CHD undergoing surgery in the USA is growing. Increasingly, patients survive to adulthood following corrective or palliative surgery, including those with complex structural lesions [1,2]. Anesthesia for noncardiac surgery in patients with CHD is therefore becoming more common in all surgical venues, including outpatient surgery centers and labor and delivery suites. In addition, new mothers with CHD are much more likely to have offspring with cardiac defects than the population at large. A 16% incidence of CHD is reported in the children of women with CHD, irrespective of whether the mother's lesion was unrepaired, palliated, or corrected [3]. This contrasts with an overall incidence of CHD of 0.5–1.2% of live births [4,5]. Immigration brings older children and adults with uncorrected CHD to US medical centers as well.

Diagnostic tools

Diagnostic tools are continually evolving and provide a broad range of preoperative information for assessment. Echocardiography, computerized tomography, and nuclear cardiology now create stunningly detailed images. Fetal diagnosis of CHD is commonplace and has facilitated the coordination of resources at congenital heart surgery centers and improved outcomes [6]. The impact of prenatal diagnosis on outcome was examined in a series of 81 patients with prenatal and 327 with postnatal diagnosis of critical CHD requiring operations in the neonatal period. Prenatal diagnosis resulted in significant improvement in metabolic acidosis and decreased

lactate levels in neonates with left-sided obstructive lesions, and those with ductal-dependent CHD [7]. The anesthesiologist must be able to utilize the information derived from each major diagnostic modality. The potential utility of intraoperative transesophageal echocardiography may also be identified, as small-sized probes permit intraoperative assessment of nearly all pediatric patients.

Surgical and noninvasive approach

Rapid and ongoing evolution of surgery for CHD has had a huge impact on the preoperative preparation required for the pediatric cardiac anesthesiologist. Improved surgical outcomes and a focus upon structural correction in the neonatal period have tremendously increased the number of major procedures performed in the first days and weeks of life. The development of nonsurgical techniques has widened the therapeutic arena to include the interventional cardiac catheterization laboratory as well. Examples include device closure of septal defects, balloon dilation of stenotic valves and vessels, placement of coils and stents, and hybrid interventions. The hybrid approach offers alternative options to neonates with complex lesions, and requires an understanding of the planned procedure by the anesthesiologist for adequate evaluation and preparation [8].

Preoperative stabilization of the neonate

In nearly all cases, the neonate can be stabilized to permit thorough preoperative assessment and preparation of the surgical team. Important therapies include administration of prostaglandin E_1 (PGE_1) to maintain patency of the ductus arteriosus, balloon atrial septostomy to enhance mixing of pulmonary and systemic venous return, and red blood cell transfusion to optimize hemoglobin levels for patients with marginal oxygen transport. Pulmonary vascular resistance (PVR) may be manipulated with alterations of inspired oxygen concentration, carbon dioxide level, and nitric oxide therapy. Inotropic and/or vasodilator support may enhance the ability of the neonatal heart to meet cardiac output demands. In nearly all cases, therefore, the anesthesiologist has time to perform a careful review of the available data and surgical plan.

Surgery on the day of hospital admission

Most elective surgeries and interventional procedures are currently performed on the day of hospital admission for economic reasons. The logistics of the preoperative evaluation of this most challenging group of patients must be carefully coordinated to avoid suboptimal patient assessment or last minute cancellations. Strategies to coordinate the preoperative visit between the various disciplines and guidelines to avoid repetition of examination and investigations are essential to streamline the process without missing pertinent information. In many centers a POCT (preoperative care team) will prepare the patient and family for all cardiac surgical and interventional procedures using a multidisciplinary approach.

Terminology and classification of CHD

Segmental approach to anatomy

In order to understand and communicate information regarding CHD, the anesthesiologist must first make sense of the terminology. The first modern attempt to classify CHD was published in 1936 by Dr Maude E. Abbott [9]. Since that time additional nomenclature published by multiple authors has led to more than one term for many similar conditions and structures. Among others, Lev, Van Praagh, Anderson, and de la Cruz [10–14] have made important contributions in this field. While there is currently no consensus opinion from national or international organizations regarding anatomic terms for CHD, there is a movement to do so. A summary of commonly used terms is presented in Table 13.1.

For practical purposes, it is useful to consider the heart as composed of three types of segments: atria, ventricles, and great arteries [12,15–17]. During normal development, they divide into right- and left-sided structures, each side having characteristic morphologic features. Segments may be described as right- or left-sided to define their location relative to other cardiac structures, or morphologically right or left to describe their anatomic features. Normal anatomy is the standard for defining morphologic features. Therefore, a morphologically right structure is normally right-sided, but may be left-sided, and vice versa [18]. It is essential to describe atrial sidedness or situs, atrioventricular and ventriculoarterial connections, and the apical position in the preoperative evaluation [19,20].

Two variations of transposition of the great arteries illustrate these principles.

Transposition of the great arteries (TGA) = ventriculoarterial discordance:
- TGA with atrioventricular concordance = "complete transposition"

    Pulmonary venous blood passes from left atrium to left ventricle and enters the pulmonary artery. The patient is cyanotic and requires stabilization and surgery in the neonatal period as oxygen transport is dependent upon bidirectional shunting at the atrial and ductal levels.
- TGA with atrioventricular discordance = "corrected transposition"

Pulmonary venous blood passes from left atrium to right ventricle and enters the aorta. In this situation, the two discordant connections balance or "correct" the circulatory abnormality. There is no oxygen desaturation or need for urgent surgery, although the anatomic right ventricle is prone to failure in later life as it is charged with pumping to the systemic circulation.

Classification of CHD

Once familiar with basic anatomic terminology and the segmental approach, one is ready to classify the cardiac pathology. CHD can be classified from an embryologic, anatomic, and a physiologic perspective [21,22]. In most cases, anesthetic management and risks follow from the patient's physiologic state rather than their specific anatomy. In other words, a diverse number of anatomic lesions may lead to a similar physiologic condition and therefore merit similar anesthetic management strategies.

It is more pragmatic, therefore, for the anesthesiologist to group patients based upon the physiologic consequences of their anatomy [23]. This step, which represents the most unique aspect of the preoperative assessment of CHD patients, allows the anesthesiologist to devise a rational anesthetic plan and predict potential intraoperative problems. One criticism of this approach is the fact that the physiologic state of an individual patient may change. For example, an "acyanotic" patient may demonstrate cyanosis if conditions such as PVR or blood pressure change. However, it is precisely the ability of the anesthesiologist to recognize that the physiologic situation has changed, understand the implications in the context of the patient's disease, and respond in a dynamic setting that are the hallmarks of appropriate care. The following pathophysiologic classification is outlined in Table 13.2.

Physiology and compensatory mechanisms

To facilitate the preoperative evaluation, patients may be grouped into acyanotic and cyanotic categories. Acyanotic patients may or may not have left-to-right shunting with augmented pulmonary blood flow. Stabilizing therapies include digoxin and diuretics for patients with systemic or pulmonary congestion, supplemental oxygen and ventilatory support for patients with pulmonary dysfunction, and afterload reduction for those with poor systemic perfusion. Inotropes may be useful to stabilize patients with severe congestive failure. If oxygen transport to the tissues is marginal due to low cardiac output, blood transfusion to increase arterial O_2 content may also be a useful preoperative therapy.

Cyanotic patients have some degree of right-to-left shunt; however, not all have decreased pulmonary blood flow. They may be physiologically grouped according to

Table 13.1 Commonly used anatomic terms for congenital heart disease

Asplenia	Right isomerism, bilateral right sidedness
Balanced ventricles	A pair of ventricles of nearly equal size. Often used to describe the ventricles of a patient with atrioventricular septal defect. Balanced ventricles are more easily separated during surgery to achieve a two-ventricle repair
Bulb	A ventricular structure that gives rise to a great vessel but that has no inlet valve. The orifice connecting it to the other ventricle is a bulbo-ventricular foramen
Concordance	Connection of two structures of identical morphologic sidedness, e.g., morphologically right-to-right, or left-to-left. Used to describe atrioventricular or ventriculoarterial connections. Does not describe position of structures within the body or position with respect to other cardiac structures
Dextrocardia	A right-sided heart, or a heart with a rightward base–apex axis
Discordance	Connection of a morphologically right-sided structure to a morphologically left-sided structure at the atrioventricular or ventriculoarterial level. See concordance
d-Loop ventricles	Looping describes the internal organization of the ventricles. First described by Van Praagh in 1964. "Right-handed" or d-loop is the result of normal looping of the heart in formation. Consistent with the illustration of an imaginary right-hand placed with its palm against the septal surface of the right ventricle, the thumb extending back through the atrioventricular valve toward the atrium, and the fingers extending toward the right ventricular outflow tract and pulmonary valve. With d-looping the left hand would be similarly positioned only for the left ventricle (17)
Dominant ventricle	A ventricle that is much larger than its companion, often a double inlet, or double outlet ventricle or part of an unbalanced atrioventricular septal defect. See unbalanced ventricles
d-Related great vessels	Aortic valve to the right of the pulmonary valve. The normal arrangement is a right-posterior aorta with respect to the pulmonary trunk. (Previously thought to represent ventricular looping, however this is an unreliable marker. Many references have used the term d-transposition, e.g., as synonymous for complete transposition with d-looped ventricles and l-transposition as synonymous with corrected transposition with l-looped ventricles. This is now generally considered incorrect usage of term)
Heterotaxy	An abnormality in left-right arrangement. Includes isomerism syndromes, discordance, and imbalance of morphologically left- and right-sided structures
Levocardia	A left-sided heart, or a heart with a leftward base–apex axis
l-Loop ventricles	Abnormal, "left-handed" ventricular looping. Consistent with the illustration of an imaginary left-hand placed with its palm against the septal surface of the morphologic right ventricle, the thumb extending back through the atrioventricular valve toward the atrium, and the fingers extending toward the right ventricular outflow tract and pulmonary valve. With l-looping the right hand would be similarly positioned only for the morphologic left ventricle. See d-loop ventricles
l-Related great vessels	Aortic valve to the left of the pulmonary valve. (Previously thought to represent l-looped ventricles; however, now known to be an unreliable marker. See d-related great vessels)
Mesocardia	A centrally located heart, or a heart with an inferior base–apex axis
Polysplenia	Left isomerism, bilateral left sidedness
Situs ambiguous	Indeterminate sidedness. Includes isomerism
Situs inversus	Mirror image sidedness with respect to normal with a morphologically right atrium on the left side and a morphologically left atrium on the right side
Situs solitus	Normal sidedness
Straddling valve	Anomalous insertion of atrioventricular valve cords into both sides of the interventricular septum. Severe straddling may preclude a two-ventricular repair

the role of the ductus arteriosus. If either the pulmonary or systemic circulation is dependent upon the ductus, PGE_1 therapy is initiated until surgery is performed. Patients with ductal dependence of the pulmonary blood flow usually have reduced pulmonary blood flow. Those with ductal-dependent systemic blood flow usually have increased pulmonary blood flow and may have limited systemic perfusion. Patients with intracardiac shunting without dependence upon the ductus have variable pulmonary and systemic blood flow and varying degrees of bidirectional shunting. Those with large left-to-right shunts are at risk for acute pulmonary congestion, poor systemic perfusion, and sudden deterioration if interventions such as supplemental oxygen or increased ventilation cause PVR to decline. It is important to identify this category of patients preoperatively as they must be managed very

Table 13.2 Physiologic classification of congenital heart disease

Category	Pulmonary blood flow	Examples
Ductal-dependent lesion with PDA-dependent PBF	Decreased	Pulmonary atresia Tricuspid atresia Severe Ebstein anomaly
Ductal-dependent lesion with PDA-dependent systemic flow	Increased	HLHS Severe preductal coarctation Interrupted aortic arch
Acyanotic CHD with left-to-right shunt	Increased	ASD, VSD, PDA, AVSD, PAPVR
Cyanotic CHD with right-to-left shunt	Decreased	Tetralogy of Fallot Severe PS with an ASD
Mixing lesions	Increased	d-TGA Truncus arteriosus TAPVR Double outlet right ventricle
Obstructive lesions	Normal	Subvalvular or supravalvular stenosis Coarctation Cor-triatriatum

ASD, atrial septal defect; AVSD, atrioventricular septal defect; PAPVR, partial anomalous pulmonary venous return; PBF, pulmonary blood flow; PDA, patent ductus arteriosus; VSD, ventricular septal defect; HLHS, hypoplastic left heart syndrome; d-TGA, transposition of the great arteries; PS, pulmonary stenosis; P/TAPVR, partial/total anomalous pulmonary venous return.

carefully upon transport to the operating room and before cardiopulmonary bypass (CPB).

Arterial desaturation and cyanosis are the result of venous admixture to the systemic circulation, called right-to-left shunting. With normal cardiac anatomy, this occurs most often in the lungs due to alveolar collapse or vascular shunts. In the context of structural heart disease, right-to left shunting is usually accompanied by some element of left-to-right shunting; however, whenever significant arterial oxygen desaturation is present the patient is considered to have cyanotic heart disease. As noted above, when describing a shunt the systemic venous blood is "right" and pulmonary venous blood is "left," regardless of the location or morphologic characteristics of the structures involved.

When venous admixture is significant, the relative volume and saturation of systemic venous and pulmonary venous blood determine arterial saturation. Therefore, systemic arterial saturation will depend to some extent upon factors that determine systemic venous oxygen saturation in addition to the normal determinants of pulmonary venous oxygen saturation. These are outlined in Table 13.3. Arterial saturation will fluctuate with changes in pulmonary function and shunt fraction, but also with changes in hemoglobin, temperature, and cardiac output. If the systemic circulation supplies an important source of pulmonary blood flow, arterial saturation will vary with systemic blood pressure as well. Examples of this situation include patent ductus arteriosus, aortopulmonary collateral vessels, and any prosthetic shunt from the aorta or its branches to the pulmonary artery.

Importance of Qp:Qs

While all patients with cyanotic heart disease have venous admixture, they do not all have decreased pulmonary blood flow. Many are at risk for excess pulmonary blood flow. An important goal of the preoperative assessment is to interpret the patient's arterial saturation in terms of the individual physiology and to estimate a desired value for

Table 13.3 Factors determining SaO_2 with right-to-left shunt

1. Determinants of pulmonary venous oxygen saturation
   a. PAO_2
   b. Gas exchange
   c. Alveolar ventilation
2. Determinants of systemic venous oxygen saturation*
   a. VO_2
   b. Hemoglobin
   c. Cardiac output
   d. Factors affecting the oxyhemoglobin dissociation curve
3. Pulmonary to systemic blood flow ratio (Qp:Qs)*

* Normally, these factors do not play a significant role in determining SaO_2.

SpO$_2$. Optimal saturation for patients with complete mixing of pulmonary and systemic venous return, for example, is not the maximum achievable value. A 1:1 relationship between pulmonary and systemic flow is generally considered optimal, and usually results in arterial oxygen saturation between 75 and 85%. When pulmonary blood flow is limited, incremental increases in the ratio have a relatively large positive effect on arterial saturation. However, when the ratio exceeds 1:1, further increases in pulmonary blood flow have a diminishing effect upon saturation [24]. The benefits of an increased arterial saturation are more than outweighed by the cost of overcirculation to the pulmonary bed. Another way of looking at this problem is that the risk of high output cardiac failure increases while the incremental gains in oxygen content of the blood diminish. This relationship is illustrated in Figure 13.1.

Initial questions for physiologic classification:

- Is the patient cyanotic?
- Is there a left-to-right, right-to-left, or mixed shunt?
- Is either the pulmonary or systemic circulation dependent upon the ductus?
- Is there a pressure or volume overload on any of the cardiac chambers?
- What compensatory mechanisms or stabilizing therapies are in place?
- What is the current degree of cardiopulmonary reserve?
- Is there a risk of deterioration if FIO_2 or ventilation is increased?

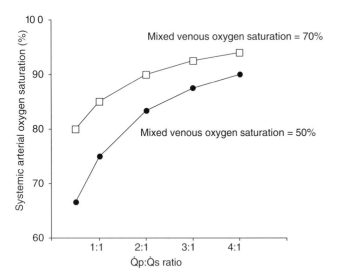

Figure 13.1 The effect of variable Qp:Qs ratio on expected arterial oxygen saturation when systemic and pulmonary venous blood are completely mixed. A pulmonary venous oxygen saturation of 100% is assumed. Note that the incremental increase improvement in systemic arterial saturation diminishes at high Qp:Qs ratios. Two mixed venous saturations are illustrated, 50 and 70%. Mixed venous oxygen saturation will vary with hemoglobin concentration, cardiac output, and oxygen consumption

Preoperative examination and investigations

History and physical examination

A complete medical history and a focused physical examination are performed. Most patients have undergone evaluation by pediatric, pediatric cardiology, and a pediatric cardiac surgery specialist before surgery is scheduled. The anesthesiologist's assessment adds important information in two areas. First, conditions apart from the surgical diagnosis that are of particular interest to anesthetic management may be detected. These include airway abnormalities, bronchospasm, gastroesophageal reflux, and issues pertaining to vascular access. Second, meeting the patient preoperatively provides an opportunity for the anesthesiologist to become familiar with specific details of the physical examination and to form a first-hand impression of the patient's condition and state of reserve. The physical examination should include the measurement of SpO$_2$, blood pressure, and assessment of pulses in all extremities. Previous anesthetic records and operative reports are particularly valuable to answer questions. The side of previous modified Blalock–Taussig shunts should be known prior to induction of anesthesia as arterial pressure may be unreliable in the ipsilateral arm.

CHD is often accompanied by additional defects, many of which are genetic [5,25–27]. In the Baltimore–Washington Infant Heart Study of 1981–1989, nearly 28% of patients had associated anomalies or syndromes [28]. The most common is Down's syndrome (9%); however, a large number of defects are represented. With the growth of genetic science, specific chromosomal etiologies defined with increasing frequency [29].

The evaluation of the airway is an essential component of the preoperative assessment of children with CHD, especially those with chromosomal abnormalities and syndromes. Children with arch obstruction and intracardiac defects have a 27% incidence of airway compression that may become more symptomatic postoperatively following an end-to-side arch reconstruction [30]. Children with Trisomy 21 frequently present for repair of CHD and require a careful evaluation of the atlanto-axial joint to avoid spinal cord compression and injury in the perioperative period [31, 32]. Although many centers have developed algorithms for management strategies in patients with Down's syndrome with suspected spinal cord compression (Figure 13.2), the decisions as to the age of patient to consider and type of study to obtain are not universal [31].

Patients with conotruncal abnormalities, including pulmonary atresia, truncus arteriosus, and interrupted aortic arch, are at an increased risk for chromosome 22q11 deletion, known as velocardiofacial syndrome or DiGeorge syndrome [33]. Hypocalcemia and an absent thymus are

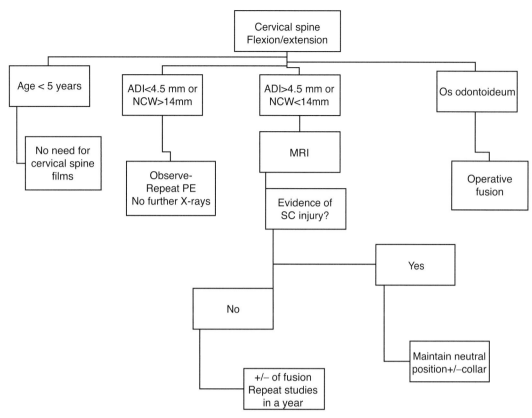

Figure 13.2 Algorithm for the preoperative management and preparation of patients with atlantoaxial sublaxation. ADI, atlanto-dens interval; NCW, neural canal width; PE, physical examination; SC, spinal cord

often demonstrated in this condition. Due to immunologic depression, banked blood products are irradiated to prevent graft versus host disease for patients known to have DiGeorge syndrome and for patients in high risk groups mentioned above. Complete transposition, on the other hand, is usually an isolated cardiac defect without associated anomalies. Vascular anomalies, especially abnormal origin of the subclavian artery, are important to the anesthesiologist, as they may impact the site of optimal monitoring and vascular access. The anesthesiologist must be aware of associated anomalies in CHD patients and assess their pertinence to anesthetic management on a case-by-case basis.

cyanosis appears to be a factor in growth impairment and developmental delay, there is not a direct correlation with degree of hypoxemia. Patients who remain cyanotic after surgery, however, continue to make slower progress [36–38]. Poor growth after birth often results from fatigue during feeding. Other causes of feeding difficulties may also be present. Previous aortic arch surgery (repair of interrupted arch or Norwood reconstruction) may result in esophageal dysfunction. Patients with associated neurological conditions or cleft lip or palate may not feed normally [34]. The anesthesiologist should be especially aware of developmental abnormalities and note any areas that may overlap with potential anesthetic complications.

Growth and development

A relationship between CHD and growth impairment has been documented for decades [34–36]. Infants with more complex lesions are significantly smaller than normal, while those with isolated defects such as atrial septal defect (ASD) and ventricular septal defect (VSD) are generally normal in weight. It is therefore important to assess growth, functional, neurological, and cognitive milestones and note whether they are at or below par. While

Congestive heart failure

Congestive heart failure (CHF) is classically defined as the inability of the heart to meet systemic needs for cardiac output and oxygen transport. In the setting of CHD where primary pump failure is rare, it is usually due to a structural lesion that results in either volume or pressure overload of a ventricle, or both [39, 40]. The term CHF is also used to describe excess pulmonary blood flow without gross inadequacies of systemic flow. This ambiguity sometimes leads to confusion regarding the nature of a problem described as "CHF."

Causes of CHF in infants include volume overload due to large shunts or severe valvular regurgitation, obstructive conditions and cardiac muscle diseases such as endocardial fibroelastosis, and CHF secondary to no cardiac conditions [39]. Patients with systemic right ventricles are particularly at risk. Patients with large shunts typically do not develop heart failure until the PVR falls in the third or fourth week of life, at which time the pulmonary circulation receives a disproportionately high share of blood flow. Rarely, tachy- or bradyarrhythmias may lead to heart failure [41].

Difficulty feeding, excessive perspiration, and poor growth are the most common symptoms of CHF in infants. Findings include cardiomegaly (cardiothoracic ratio >0.5), tachycardia, tachypnea, and pulmonary congestion. Hepatomegaly, a gallop rhythm, pulmonary edema, and vascular collapse may be seen. Respiratory rates of >45 and HR > 150 are suggestive. Mottling and slow capillary refill in the extremities are severe signs. Pharmacologic therapy for CHF includes digoxin, diuretics, afterload reduction, and inotropes for critically ill patients. Supplemental oxygen or respiratory support may be necessary if pulmonary congestion or pulmonary edema is severe [39]. Various methods to grade CHF in children have been studied, with no standard available similar to adult grading systems. Grading of CHF in children must be done preoperatively using child's normal activities, feeding history, and possibly chemical markers as B-type natriuretic peptide [40].

Pulmonary hypertension

The pulmonary circulation is thick-walled and has a high resistance in the fetus. Beginning with the first minutes of life, PVR drops dramatically in response to distension of the vessels with aeration of the lungs, increased $P_{A}O_2$, and multiple endogenous vasodilating factors. The majority of the decrease in PVR is completed by the first 3 weeks of life. Larger pulmonary vessels continue to regress over several months [24]. In patients with CHD, the pressure and resistance of the pulmonary circulation often do not decline normally. Structural disease, depressed pulmonary venous saturation, and excess flow are all potential factors [42].

Systolic pulmonary artery pressures are often estimated by Doppler echocardiography and are measured at cardiac catheterization if anatomically possible. The term "pulmonary hypertension" is ambiguous with regard to etiology. The anesthesiologist must correlate knowledge about pulmonary vascular flow to interpret whether pulmonary hypertension, if present, is due to elevated flow, elevated resistance, or both. If pressure is elevated in proportion to excess flow, one may anticipate a rapid decline in pulmonary pressure when the source of shunt is repaired. Once structural pulmonary vascular changes develop, however, elevations in PVR may be irreversible [43]. Many patients have reactive pulmonary hypertension and demonstrate reduced PVR when exposed to elevated alveolar oxygen concentrations, alkalosis [44], or nitric oxide [43]. For patients scheduled for bidirectional Glenn or Fontan surgeries, the assessment of PVR is a key determinant of eligibility for the procedure, as the pulmonary blood flow will be dependent upon passive flow through the pulmonary circulation [45, 46]. Whenever pulmonary hypertension is present, special attention to the function of the pulmonary ventricle and its valves is merited as well, as secondary changes may have diminished reserve or resulted in cor pulmonale.

Patients with pacemakers

Cardiac pacemakers sense bradycardia, tachycardia, or both. Bradycardia sensing pacemakers are usually placed for sinus node dysfunction or high-grade atrioventricular conduction defects and respond by pacing the selected chambers. Most tachycardia sensing devices today are implantable cardioverter defibrillators (ICDs) and respond by delivering electrical energy aimed at cardioversion. Newer ICDs have bradycardia sensing and pacing capabilities as well. Others may also have the capability to terminate some tachydysrhythmias with rapid pacing, a function that was previously available without ICD capability [47].

Whenever a patient has a permanent pacemaker in place, the indications for pacing, underlying rhythm, device type, and its functional status must be researched preoperatively. This may present a significant challenge, especially with expanding indications for pacing, mobility of patients, and the development of many new and sophisticated devices. In all cases, a preoperative electrocardiogram (ECG) is indicated. If atrial or ventricular pacing is continuous, the underlying rhythm may be unknown without previous medical records. If no pacing is demonstrated, current pacer function may be in question. Consultation with specialists in electrophysiology may be indicated if information is lacking. Electronic interrogation of device settings and reprogramming may be required.

In older models electrocautery may inhibit bradycardia detection and lead to asystole if bradyarhythmia or conduction block is present. Continuous application of an external magnet over bradycardia sensing pacemakers usually reverts function to a fixed rate, asynchronous pacing mode. A decision to reprogram the pacemaker during the perioperative period should be made on a case-by-case basis. It is essential to know if tachycardia sensing is part of the pacemaker capabilities to determine appropriate perioperative management.

All tachycardia sensing capabilities should be disabled prior to surgery, as electrocautery or supraventricular tachyarrhythmias may trigger defibrillation [48, 49]. This may be performed by reprogramming the device or with external application of a magnet. Unfortunately, the action and duration of magnet application to switch off tachycardia sensing differs among major device manufacturers. Regardless of manufacturer, however, an externally applied magnet will not convert bradycardia sensing devices to an asynchronous pacing mode if the device has tachycardia sensing capability as well. The anesthesiologist must therefore carefully assess the need for intraoperative pacing for any patient with a device that has both pacing and ICD capabilities. If the patient relies upon the pacemaker for ventricular pacing, it is prudent to reprogram the device to an asynchronous mode prior to surgery as electrocautery is likely to inhibit sensing of bradycardia and a magnet will have no therapeutic effect. Intraoperative application of external pacing/defibrillator pads is appropriate for all patients with cardiac pacemaker devices.

Preoperative studies

Laboratory studies

Appropriate laboratory studies include CBC, BUN, creatinine, electrolytes, and coagulation studies; a screen for antibodies and a cross-match for appropriate blood products. Unless blood loss or transfusion has recently occurred, an elevated hemoglobin level is a valuable indicator of chronic cyanosis. Diuretic therapy may result in dehydration, hypochloremic metabolic alkalosis, or hypokalemia. Although polycythemic patients may have abnormal coagulation [50, 51], they may also have abnormal coagulation study results if the laboratory is unaware of their hematocrit, as fractional serum volume is reduced and distorts test results. Patients with extremely elevated hemoglobin concentrations (hematocrit >65%) may have poor capillary flow due to hyperviscosity, which can reduce oxygen transport and lead to intravascular coagulation [52, 53]. Guidelines for phlebotomy or rehydration of patients with polycythemia in the preoperative period are necessary to decrease the risk of complications intra- and postoperatively.

Additional studies include serum glucose in infants and critically ill patients and ionized calcium in infants and in patients suspected or known to have DiGeorge syndrome. Blood type and antibody screen is performed in all patients and blood is cross-matched as indicated by patient age, condition, and proposed procedure.

Electrocardiogram

The ECG should be reviewed for signs of abnormal rhythm, conduction, chamber hypertrophy, and as a baseline for postoperative comparison. Its interpretation is complicated by the abnormal position of many structures. ST segment and T wave abnormalities may indicate ventricular strain or ischemia.

Chest radiograph

The clinical relevance of the preoperative chest X-ray to the anesthesiologist is primarily the lung fields and tracheobroncheal tree. Determination of situs may also be assisted by identifying the laterality of the stomach, liver, and their relation to the position of the heart within the thorax. Historically, the chest X-ray has played an important role in the differential diagnosis of many congenital heart lesions. The ability to discern pulmonary vascularity, cardiac size, position, shape, and associated vascular, bronchial and skeletal anomalies are all helpful; however, echocardiography has proven a more powerful and convenient preoperative diagnostic tool [54].

The degree of pulmonary vascular markings and lung water are of principal importance as they may indicate increased pulmonary vascular pressures or congestion. The highest risk category for CHF includes noncyanotic patients with left-to-right shunt, patients with duct-dependent systemic blood flow, and those with mixing lesions and unrestricted pulmonary blood flow. In cyanotic patients, therefore, the pulmonary vasculature will be normal or decreased unless a coexisting left-to-right shunt is present. Cardiomegaly as evidenced by a cardiothoracic ratio > 0.5 is a useful sign of CHF or pericardial effusion in spite of structural lesions and cardiac malposition. Cardiomegaly is usually proportionate to pulmonary arterial vascularity unless coarctation of the aorta or myocardial disease is present [55].

Regional lung disease may also result from CHD. Compression of one or more pulmonary veins or bronchi may result in lobar congestion or hyperinflation. Patients with tetralogy of Fallot with absent pulmonary valve are particularly at risk due to an enlarged pulmonary artery. The anesthesiologist should specifically look at the image of the tracheobronchial tree on the preoperative chest film. Anomalies of situs will include mirror imaging (isomerism) of normal tracheobronchial structures, which may be important if endotracheal intubation is planned. If pulmonary problems occur intraoperatively, advance knowledge of the bronchial anatomy is key to proper interpretation of bronchoscopy findings.

Inspection of the lateral chest film for evidence of reduced space between the sternum and the heart is important for patients undergoing repeat sternotomy. When the retrosternal space is reduced, an increased risk of inadvertent disruption of anterior cardiac or prosthetic structures during surgical dissection through scarred tissue is present. Most commonly the right heart, pulmonary artery, or prosthetic right ventricular outflow conduit is involved. The anesthesia team may wish to tailor their plans regarding intravenous access and blood availability prior to CPB in view of this heightened risk. The surgical and perfusion teams will need to prepare for alternative cannulation sites and the potential for urgent institution of CPB. In selected cases, the surgeon may elect to dissect or cannulate the femoral vessels prior to dissection and sternotomy.

For older patients with coarctation of the aorta, rib notching may be present. This indicates well-developed collateral arterial flow and a reduced risk of ischemia to organs distal to the coarctation site if the aorta is cross-clamped.

Echocardiography

Currently, the anatomic pathology for which congenital heart surgery is scheduled is most often defined by echocardiography. It has proved such a powerful tool that pediatric cardiologists express concern that their auscultatory skill is diminishing due to lack of use. Prior to 1988, nearly all congenital heart surgery patients underwent preoperative cardiac catheterization. Today cardiac catheterization is most often performed to answer remaining physiologic questions following an echocardiographic diagnosis or to further define structures with angiography that are difficult to image with echo. Many patients undergo complete repair of major congenital heart defects without cardiac catheterization [56]. Advantages of echocardiography include its noninvasive nature, relative lack of biologic effects, ample acoustic windows in infants (due to the paucity of bony structures), and the ability to use high-frequency, high-resolution transducers in small patients due to the proximity of cardiac structures to the body surface. Technological advances now permit stunningly clear images that may be transmitted digitally without loss of detail (Figure 13.3). Disadvantages of echocardiography include the inability to obtain absolute rather than relative hemodynamic data, and the high degree of technical skill required to obtain optimal studies and a certain degree of subjective interpretation of spatial relations.

(a)

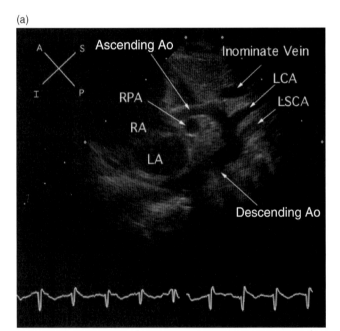

(b)

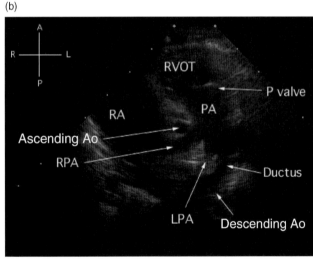

Figure 13.3 (a) Hypoplastic left heart syndrome—aortic arch. "Ductus cut" view. This view is achieved via the suprasternal notch and is useful for imaging the ductus arteriosus, coarctation of the aorta, and other aortic arch anomalies. Note the small ascending aorta compared to the descending component. The innominate artery is not seen as it lies outside the plane of the transducer. The left common carotid and subclavian arteries are clearly visualized as well as the large difference in diameter of the ascending and descending aortic arch components. Note that the size of the right pulmonary artery exceeds that of the ascending aorta. (b) Hypoplastic left heart syndrome—pulmonary artery. Parasternal short-axis view. The pulmonary trunk and branch pulmonary arteries are usually easily visualized with precordial echocardiography. This image demonstrates the large size discrepancy between the ascending aorta and the pulmonary artery as well as a clear view of the ductus connecting to the descending aorta. The right pulmonary artery is better visualized than the left pulmonary artery in this view. PA, pulmonary artery; RPA, right pulmonary artery; LPA, left pulmonary artery; LSCA, left coronary artery; Ao, aorta; LA, left atrium; RA, right atrium; RVOT, right ventricular outflow tract (All images are courtesy of the Pediatric Echocardiography Laboratory at the University of California, San Francisco)

The vast majority of preoperative echocardiographic studies are precordial (transthoracic) rather than transesophageal due to the greater number of available acoustic windows, and the need for general anesthesia in infants and children to facilitate transesophageal studies. It is therefore important for the pediatric cardiac anesthesiologist to become familiar with precordial views and the range of information that can be derived. Normal acoustic windows for precordial echo in infants include suprasternal, parasternal, apical, and subcostal approaches. The plane of the transducer may be oriented in line with the three orthogonal planes of the body: sagittal, coronal, and transverse. More commonly, it is be oriented along the planes of the heart in short axis, or in long axis in the "four-chamber" or "two-chamber" cross-sections. The short and long axis of the heart is normally not in line with the orthogonal planes of the body, however, as the apex is situated to the left and anterior to the base [57,58]. Examples of parasternal short axis and the "ductus cut" views are illustrated in Figure 13.3a,b.

The preoperative assessment of congenital heart surgery patients usually consists of a complete echocardiographic examination including two-dimensional imaging, spectral (pulse and continuous wave) and color Doppler interrogation of cardiac inflow and outflow, as well as imaging of pathologic flow and associated structures of interest. Imaging information is obtained regarding cardiac and great vessel anatomy, as well as myocardial and valvular function. Quantitative echocardiography is useful to calculate shunts, to estimate intracardiac pressures, and to evaluate the severity of myocardial or valvular dysfunction. If tricuspid regurgitation is present, pulmonary arterial systolic pressure can usually be estimated.

Ideally, the anesthesiologist should review the preoperative echo study images for optimal understanding and potential comparison with intraoperative and postoperative echocardiography. As a minimum, all preoperative echocardiogram reports should be available for review and a pediatric echocardiographer should review any studies from outside hospitals to determine the adequacy of the study and interpretation of the pathology [59]. Preoperative echocardiographic assessment should be completed before admission to the operating room and not rely upon an intraoperative transesophageal examination, as the acoustic windows are more limited and physiologic conditions may be significantly altered by general anesthesia and positive pressure ventilation.

Cardiac catheterization

While the indications for cardiac catheterization have decreased in tandem with the rise of other diagnostic modalities, whenever preoperative cardiac catheterization has been performed the anesthesiologist should review the report. It will include measurements of pressure and oxygen saturation from some or all of the cardiac chambers. From these data pressure gradients, systemic and PVRs, and shunts may be quantified. Systemic and pulmonary flow may be calculated as absolute quantities or as a relative ratio. A ratio of greater than one indicates left-to-right shunting, while a ratio of less than one indicates right-to-left shunting. Note that a ratio of close to 1:1 does not by itself rule out bidirectional shunt. The Fick method is used for quantification of pulmonary and systemic flow, using oxygen consumption as the "indicator." While actual O_2 consumption can be measured, it is often estimated from tabled data. Angiography is usually performed to further define any anatomic structures in question [60,61].

Interpretation of data from patients with structural heart disease is a challenge for the beginner; however, the basic principles for measurement and calculation are readily understood. It is useful to follow the sequence of pressures and saturations in a flow-directed pathway to detect evidence of obstruction or shunt. Note that oxygen saturation is normally stable from the right ventricle to the pulmonary artery and from the left atrium to the aorta. Deviations indicate intracardiac shunting. Pressures are normally equal on both sides of the atrioventricular valves at the end of diastole. Peak ventricular systolic pressure normally equals the peak systolic pressure in the corresponding great vessel. Pressure gradients indicate obstruction at or near the valves. Pulmonary venous desaturation may indicate intrapulmonary shunt from lung disease, pulmonary arteriovenous malformation or may result from hypoventilation due to sedation for the procedure. Arterial desaturation indicates right-to-left shunt in the heart, lungs, or the great vessels. Formulae used to calculate flows, shunts, and resistances are presented in Chapter 27 (Table 27.2).

Many patients undergo cardiac catheterization to assess the anatomy and resistance of the pulmonary vasculature. If patients have left-to-right shunting and pulmonary hypertension, interventions in the cardiac catheterization laboratory may be undertaken to assess the reactivity of the pulmonary vasculature. Typically, 100% oxygen or vasodilator therapy including nitric oxide response is utilized while intracardiac and great vessel pressure and saturation measurements are repeated. If the PVR does not decline, the patient may have fixed pulmonary vascular obstructive disease and not benefit from surgical correction.

Pressure and saturation information from cardiac catheterization may be codified in a graphic form for preliminary or final reports. An example is illustrated in Figure 13.4 using normal values. The anesthesiologist should be familiar with the format used for displaying preliminary information at their institution, as formal reports

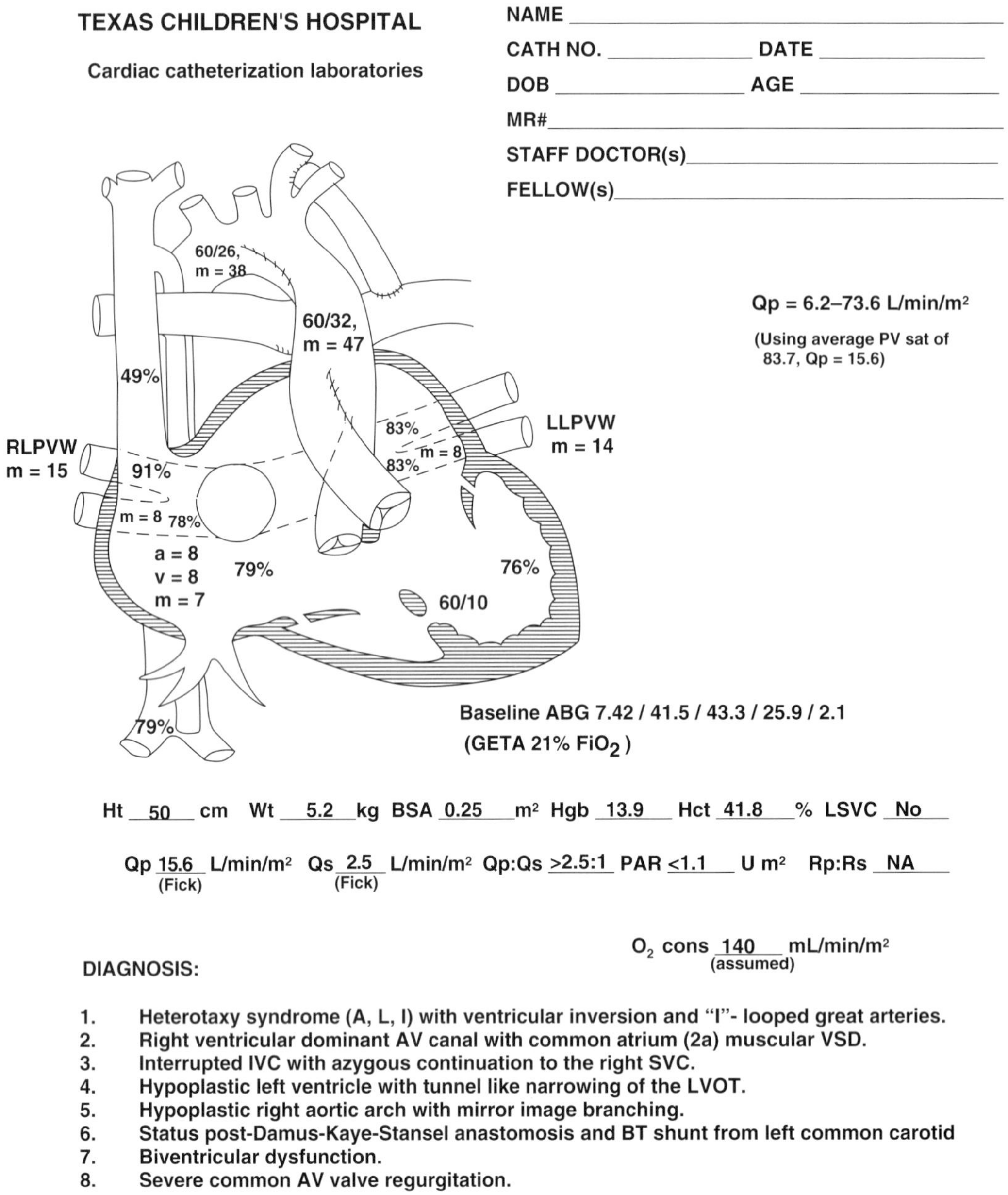

TEXAS CHILDREN'S HOSPITAL

Cardiac catheterization laboratories

NAME _____

CATH NO. _____ DATE _____

DOB _____ AGE _____

MR#_____

STAFF DOCTOR(s)_____

FELLOW(s)_____

$Qp = 6.2–73.6$ L/min/m^2

(Using average PV sat of
83.7, $Qp = 15.6$)

60/26,
m = 38

60/32,
m = 47

49%

83%

LLPVW
m = 14

RLPVW
m = 15

91%

m = 8

83%
83%

m = 8   78%

a = 8
v = 8
m = 7

79%

76%

60/10

79%

Baseline ABG 7.42 / 41.5 / 43.3 / 25.9 / 2.1
(GETA 21% FiO$_2$)

Ht __50__ cm Wt __5.2__ kg BSA _0.25_ m^2 Hgb _13.9_ Hct _41.8_ % LSVC _No_

Qp _15.6_ L/min/m^2 Qs _2.5_ L/min/m^2 Qp:Qs _>2.5:1_ PAR _≤1.1_ U m^2 Rp:Rs _NA_
   (Fick)   (Fick)

O$_2$ cons _140_ mL/min/m^2
      (assumed)

DIAGNOSIS:

1. Heterotaxy syndrome (A, L, I) with ventricular inversion and "I"- looped great arteries.
2. Right ventricular dominant AV canal with common atrium (2a) muscular VSD.
3. Interrupted IVC with azygous continuation to the right SVC.
4. Hypoplastic left ventricle with tunnel like narrowing of the LVOT.
5. Hypoplastic right aortic arch with mirror image branching.
6. Status post-Damus-Kaye-Stansel anastomosis and BT shunt from left common carotid
7. Biventricular dysfunction.
8. Severe common AV valve regurgitation.

Figure 13.4 Cardiac catheterization diagram. Data from a 2-month-old patient with tricuspid and pulmonary atresia are shown. This is a concise, convenient, one-page summary of the patient's anatomy, history, physiology, and catheterization data. It can be stored in paper or digital format and easily projected for surgical case conference. Numbers followed by percentages are measured oxygen saturations; plain numbers are pressure values. a, atrial a-wave pressure; v, atrial v-wave pressure; m, mean pressure; PVWP, pulmonary venous wedge pressure; BT, Blalock–Taussig; ABG, arterial blood gas; BSA, body surface area; LSVC, presence of a left superior vena cava; Qp, pulmonary blood flow; Qs, systemic blood flow; PAR, pulmonary artery vascular resistance; Rp:Rs, ratio of pulmonary to systemic vascular resistance; V̇o$_2$ cons, oxygen consumption

may not be available preoperatively if surgery follows soon after cardiac catheterization.

Magnetic resonance imaging

Improved technology in magnetic resonance imaging (MRI) and magnetic resonance angiography (MRA) has followed the tremendous advances of echocardiography in the diagnosis and assessment of CHD. Application thus far has been predominately for lesions that are difficult to evaluate by echocardiography, such as coarctation of the aorta, branch pulmonary arterial stenosis, pulmonary venous connections, vascular rings, and complex three-dimensional relationships. However, increasingly refined techniques and the ability to perform functional assessment of ejection fraction and regurgitant volumes position

MRI for continued expansion in its role regarding preoperative assessment of CHD patients. Technological advances including fast imaging have enhanced image detail and permitted quantification of shunts, valvular regurgitation, and relative flow to the right and left pulmonary arteries [62–67].

Advantages of MRI over other imaging techniques include the absence of ionizing radiation or contrast agents. The effectiveness of echocardiography also decreases as children grow due to more limited acoustic windows. Therefore, MRI may be an alternative as well as a complementary technique in older children and adults with CHD [68]. MRI is particularly successful for evaluation of some areas that traditionally difficult to assess with echocardiography, such as right ventricular function and pulmonary flow [62,64,66,67,69]. Future perioperative applications include an augmented role in determining the desirability and timing of surgery. For example, the ability to assess right ventricular function may assist in the difficult question of timing for pulmonary valve replacement following initial correction of tetralogy of Fallot [70,71]. Patients considered for the Fontan operation also benefit from assessment of the dimensions of the right and left pulmonary arteries, which is facilitated with MRI [72,73]. Unlike echocardiography, it is rarely performed to establish the primary cardiac diagnosis.

The MRI technique used to generate morphologic images is primarily sliced spin-echo images through the heart and thorax. Imaging slices typically have a thickness of 5 mm with a 1-mm gap between slices. Thinner slices and increased excitation may be used for areas of interest. Compensation for cardiac and respiratory motion is achieved by synchronization with the ECG signal and a sensor on the patient's abdomen. As multiple cardiac cycles are required to complete the image of each slice, the time to complete a study is somewhat dependent upon heart rate. When possible, breath holding or apnea is employed to eliminate respiratory motion. For increased spatial resolution of vascular structures, gadolinium-enhanced MRA is performed. Three-dimensional reconstruction can also be performed using this technology, creating striking images (Figures 13.5 and 13.6). Physiologic information is derived from additional techniques including gated fast gradient-echo sequences and velocity-encoded cine MRI. Blood flow can be calculated from velocity and cross-sectional measurements [62,74]. As experience and technology grow, the role of MRI and MRA in the management of CHD patients is very likely to expand [65,75].

Computerized tomography

While utilized less frequently than MRI, the use of contrast-enhanced conventional or spiral computerized

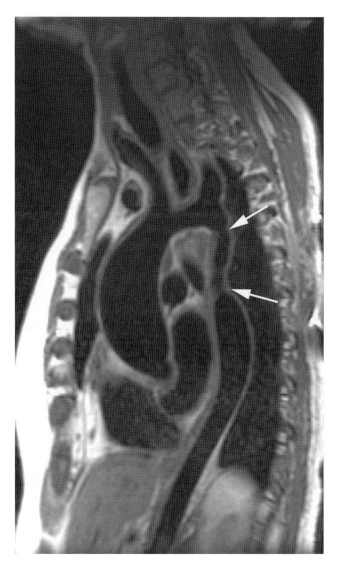

Figure 13.5 Oblique sagittal T1-weighted MRI image of the thorax in a 13-year-old boy shows moderate to severe aortic coarctation (*arrows*). Dilation of the ascending aorta is also present

tomography (CT) imaging has a distinct role in the assessment of CHD patients, particularly those with vascular rings, aortic abnormalities, and pericardial disease [76]. Ultra-fast CT scanning and electron-beam tomography acquire images more quickly than MRI and can be ECG triggered to eliminate motion artifact. Therefore, some pediatric patients may tolerate ultra-fast CT scanning without the sedation that is normally required for more lengthy MRI examinations. When contrast is added to ECG-triggered electron-beam tomographic images, fine resolution permits diagnosis of intracardiac defects, pulmonary vascular anomalies, cardiac muscle mass, and motion [77, 78]. However, the use of ionizing radiation and intravenous contrast remain required in some cases (Figure 13.7).

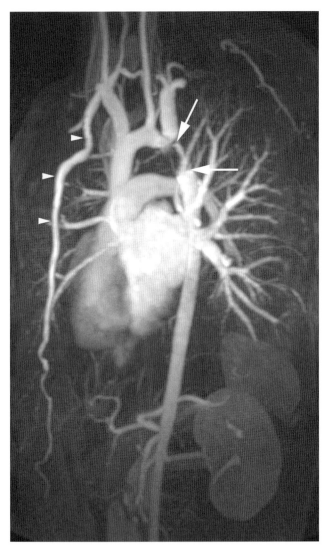

Figure 13.6 Oblique sagittal volume rendered image from a contrast enhanced MRA in a 15-year-old boy study shows severe aortic coarctation (*arrows*) just distal to the origin of the left subclavian artery. Large collateral vessels are seen the posterior superior aspect of the thorax. Enlarged internal mammary arteries are also present (*arrowheads*)

Risk stratification

Determine adequacy of preoperative information

During a busy day caring for critically ill patients, the temptation to accept available preoperative information as complete must be questioned continually. A critical approach is advocated, with an eye out for key information that is not evident. Are the anatomic pathology and the proposed procedure clarified? The indication for surgery, impetus for its timing, and expected outcome for the individual patient must be understood.

How does the proposed surgery fit into the long-term plan? Is the upcoming surgery palliative, corrective, or part of a staged series of procedures? Is it urgent or elective? Only when these questions have been answered can the anesthesiologist determine if the available information is adequate.

Generally, a recent ECG, echocardiogram, chest X-ray, and laboratory examination as outlined above are performed. A summary of information expected in the preoperative assessment is found in Table 13.4. As mentioned, cardiac catheterization is performed less often than in the past due to advances in echocardiography and MRI [56,62,78]. Because many CHD patients are evaluated in outside medical centers prior to surgery, it is particularly helpful to review available information regarding elective cases several days in advance. This provides time to obtain valuable data, reduces unnecessary repetition of tests, and allows for preparation of the patient and the perioperative team.

Risk stratification in adult cardiac patients

The use of preoperative risk assessment methods in adults with heart disease undergoing various procedures has resulted in a wealth of knowledge in this field. In adult

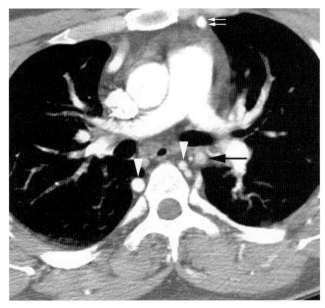

Figure 13.7 Severe aortic coarctation in a 19-year-old male diagnosed with aortic coarctation using narrow collimation contrast enhanced multislice computed tomography. Axial CT image shows severe aortic coarctation. The main pulmonary artery is seen branching into the right and left pulmonary arteries. The ascending aorta is imaged in cross-section alongside the pulmonary artery. In comparison, the *black arrow* indicates the severely narrowed proximal descending thoracic aorta. Enlarged internal mammary arteries (*double white arrows*) and numerous enlarged collateral vessels (*arrowheads*) are also present

Table 13.4 Preoperative assessment

	All cases	As indicated
History and physical exam	X	
Pulse oximetry	X	
Chest X-ray	X	
ECG	X	
CBC, electrolytes, BUN, creatinine	X	
Glucose, calcium		X
Coagulation studies	X	
Blood type and antibody screen	X	
Blood cross-match		X
Echocardiogram: complete 2-D, spectral, and color Doppler study	X	
Cardiac catheterization		X
MRI/MRA		X
Computerized tomography		X

cardiac surgery, risk stratification methods showed increased severity of illness, higher morbidity, as well as early and 1-year mortality in the presence of certain factors. These include older age, emergency procedures, preoperative serum creatinine, left ventricular systolic function, and reoperation. A severity scoring system was studied and validated in a series of 10,000 adult cardiac patients at the Cleveland Clinic [79].

Similar methods were used by the American College of Cardiology and the American Heart Association to develop the practice guidelines for perioperative cardiovascular evaluation for noncardiac surgery [80]. The guidelines identify clinical predictors of increased perioperative risk (MI, CHF, or death) in three categories: major, intermediate, and minor predictors. These guidelines result in a risk stratification of patients undergoing noncardiac surgery into those with high risk (>5%), intermediate (1–5%), and low (<1%) risk for a perioperative event.

In pregnant women with cardiac disease, a risk stratification method has been established, showing increased morbidity to mother and newborn in the presence of cyanosis, cardiac failure, or obstructive lesions [81].

Methods of risk assessment in CHD

Patients with CHD present for preoperative evaluation with a variety of risk factors. A system that integrates these risks can produce a severity scoring system that identifies patients with higher risk, and allow for better preparation and improved outcome for these patients.

Risk factors for these patients may include the presence and degree of cardiac decompensation. Especially in smaller children, it is difficult to grade the degree of heart failure using the adult criteria. Patients with single ven-

tricular physiology have decreased reserve, are volume dependent, and thus have an increased anesthetic risk. In addition, the presence of a single or systemic right ventricle may change the outcome of patients [82].

The type, complexity, and stage of repair of the heart defect will also change the perioperative risk. Additional risks include the extent of desaturation, presence of an obstructive lesion, level of polycythemia, and history of arrhythmias [83]. The number, type, and dose of medications may indicate the degree of decompensation, and may have side effects or interactions with drugs used in the perioperative period.

An example of a severity scoring card is given in Table 13.5, where some of these risks are included, each patient is given a score and result in identifying patients with various degrees of risk. A score of 0–6 is mild risk, 6–14 is moderate risk, and 14–20 is high risk for perioperative complications.

Impact of a risk scoring system

The development of a risk assessment and a scoring card for adults and children undergoing noncardiac surgery can improve the perioperative outcome, decrease mortality and morbidity, and assist in manpower and resource allocation.

Preoperative testing

Similar to adults with other comorbidities, there is a limit to the benefit acquired from escalating number of preoperative tests. The number and invasiveness of tests are decided by the degree of decompensation as well as the extent of surgery planned [84]. A chest X-ray obtained in a patient younger than 30 years, regardless of the extent of surgery, will probably result in minimal beneficial information. Similarly, we should consider the risk for a patient with CHD when deciding on preoperative tests.

Preoperative conditioning

We learn from the vast literature in adult preoperative conditioning that certain interventions can significantly improve the outcome of adults undergoing noncardiac surgery. Simple maneuvers, as smoking cessation for 1 week, starting beta-blockers, statins, aspirin, or even an exercise program, can change the risk for a patient [85]. Can we do the same for patients with CHD? Can we take certain steps to change a high-risk score patient to a lower score? Interventions as lowering preoperative hematocrit, oxygen therapy, use of aspirin, and other anticoagulants shortly preoperatively may change the patient's risk.

Table 13.5 Scoring card for preoperative evaluation of patients with CHD

	0	1	2
CHD	Simple (ASD)	Moderate (ASD + PS)	Complex (tetralogy of Fallot)
CHD	Repaired with no residual	Repaired with residual	Palliated
Obstruction	None	Yes gradient < 40 mm Hg	Yes gradient > 50 mm Hg
Ventricle	Two LV systemic	One LV systemic	One RV systemic
Systemic ventricular dysfunction	Mild	Moderate	Severe
PVR	NL or <2 WU	2–4 WU	>4 WU
SaO_2	>90%	75–90%	<75%
HCT	30–45%	25–30% or 45–60%	<25% or >65%
Arrhythmia	Rare	Atrial	Ventricular
Drugs (anticoagulants, diuretics, digitalis, antiarrhythmics, others)	1	2–3	>3

ASD, atrial septal defect; PS, pulmonary stenosis; CHD, congenital heart disease; PVR, pulmonary vascular resistance

Manpower and resource allocation

The experience of a center can have a significant impact on the outcome of a patient with a certain disease, undergoing a specific type of procedure. This may be due to either the system function as a whole or the presence of individuals with expertise capable of caring for these patients. This fact had been shown in adult cardiology and cardiac surgery (with coronary interventions, bypass grafting, and valvular repair), obstetrical practice (with number of cesarean sections, newborn mortality), and general pediatric surgery.

The same can be experienced in adults and children with CHD undergoing noncardiac surgery. The patients with high preoperative risk score will benefit from a center with large volume of care for these patients, and with the most experienced individuals providing that care in the perioperative period [86,87]. However, patients with low or no risk may be cared for in other settings.

Preparing the patient and family

Patient and family education and informed consent

A detailed discussion of the role of the anesthesiologist in the upcoming surgery is required, incorporating informed consent guidelines. The plans for premedication, monitoring, induction and maintenance of anesthesia, blood transfusion, and postoperative care are discussed. If the patient is old enough to understand, he or she should be included in appropriate sections of this discussion, reassured, and told what to expect. Particular emphasis should be placed on specific instructions. Patients and their families receive a great deal of new information prior to congenital heart surgery. It is a natural time of apprehension for all

concerned. For patients being admitted on the day of surgery, instructions regarding eating and drinking, specific medications, and logistics must be communicated clearly and given to the patient and their family in writing whenever possible.

Fasting, premedication, and preoperative orders

Preoperative fasting

Guidelines for fasting do not differ from other surgeries. Clear liquids are generally considered safe for all patients up to 2 hours prior to surgery, breast milk (unfortified) until 4 hours prior to surgery, and milk, formula, fortified breast milk, or solids up to 6 hours before surgery. Patients with swallowing difficulties, gastroesophageal reflux, abnormal gastric motility, or neurological disease may merit longer fasting times. Special attention is warranted to avoid dehydration in children scheduled for surgery later in the day, particularly those with cyanotic heart disease. If a patient is polycythemic, taking diuretics, or has significant systemic outflow obstruction, consideration should be given to administering intravenous fluid preoperatively as the potential risk of dehydration is increased and the time of surgery may be unpredictable.

Medications

General principles apply regarding administration of regular medications on the day of surgery, and most medications are given. It is especially important to continue inhalers for patients with bronchospasm. Exceptions include diuretics in selected patients, and insulin in diabetic patients. Some experienced clinicians withhold digoxin therapy for 1 day prior to surgery with CPB as it is felt to represent a risk factor for malignant ventricular arrhythmias associated with potassium fluctuations following bypass [39].

Antibiotic prophylaxis for bacterial endocarditis

Prophylactic antibiotics for dental, oral, respiratory tract, gastrointestinal, and genitourinary procedures are indicated in patients with cardiac defects for prevention of endocarditis. Patients who have had congenital heart repairs should also receive antibiotic prophylaxis with the exception of those who have had closure of a secundum ASD, VSD, or patent ductus arteriosus more than 6 months previously. Patients with residual leaks should be treated. The risk of postoperative endocarditis appears to be greatest in patients with prosthetic valves, conduits, and grafts as well as those with tetralogy of Fallot and aortic stenosis. The regimens recommended by the American Heart Association for antibiotic dosage are listed in Chapter 28 [88].

Premedication

The time of separation of the patient from his or her family is particularly stressful for all concerned. Generous premedication is usually helpful to reduce patient anxiety and facilitate separation. If the structural facilities permit induction with family present, this may also be helpful. Cyanosis from cardiac disease is not a general contraindication to premedication [89, 90]. Desaturation due to intracardiac shunt will not be worsened by premedication unless pulmonary blood flow or lung function is affected. The anesthesiologist is generally present during and after premedication. Pulse oximetry may be employed to monitor the effect on saturation with administration and supplemental oxygen should be immediately available. Judicious dosing is warranted in sicker patients, however, as transient decreases in saturation may occur [91] and pulse oximetry is less accurate in lower ranges of saturation [92]. Most patients are admitted on the day of surgery and do not have an intravenous line in place. A variety of medications have been used with success for sedation and anxiolysis in congenital heart surgery patients. General guides are that patients younger than 1 year rarely require premedication, oral medication is preferred to nasal, and injections are universally disliked.

Oral midazolam 0.5–1.0 mg/kg is usually an effective anxiolytic. Generally, no more than 20 mg of midazolam is administered orally. If patients will not take an oral medication, nasal midazolam 0.3 mg/kg can be rapidly injected using a short intravenous catheter or slip-tip syringe. A concentration of 5 mg/cc is recommended to minimize volume, although it is irritating to the nasal mucosa. Rarely, a child or developmentally delayed adult presents a particular challenge with regard to premedication. In such cases, ketamine 4–5 mg/kg with glycopyrrolate 10–20 mcg/kg and midazolam 0.1 mg/kg can be injected intramuscularly. This may also be the agent of choice for induction patients in whom an inhalation induction is deemed risky. Oral ketamine may also be employed in doses of 2–10 mg/kg in combination with midazolam 0.5–1.0 mg/kg [90,93]. Rectal administration of benzodiazepines and barbiturates is also reasonable for patients 1–3 years of age, although not preferable or necessary in the presence of many options through alternate routes.

Preoperative intravenous placement

Older children may express a preference for an intravenous induction of anesthesia. Many have had ample experience with intravenous lines and phlebotomy. Premedication and placement of a topical anesthetic cream is usually helpful, however, as bravery often falters as anxiety mounts on the day of surgery.

Communicate essential findings and plan

Both written and verbal communication is important components of the preparation for surgery. Because a great deal of information is often available for congenital heart surgery patients, an appropriate summary focused upon the pathophysiology and issues pertinent to the anesthetic plan is appropriate. Anatomic findings that impact potential vascular access or monitoring, such as occluded vessels or anomalous origin of the subclavian artery, are valuable parts of this summary. Use of acronyms and names of rare syndromes should be minimized in favor of clear, descriptive terminology. Any important findings in the history or condition of the patient that are not evident in the surgical assessment must be communicated to the surgical team as early as possible, especially if they may impact the readiness of the patient for surgery as planned. When working with such complex patients, it is particularly helpful to speak with preoperatively when questions about the anatomic implications, therapeutic approach, or surgical plan remain.

Summary

The preoperative evaluation of patients prior to congenital heart surgery is a special challenge because of the wide range of potential anatomic and physiologic abnormalities. An interdisciplinary approach to assessment and review of diagnostic studies is optimal for the preparation of the patient and the perioperative team. The pediatric cardiac anesthesiologist requires a working knowledge of pediatric cardiology terminology and commonly used diagnostic modalities to interpret the large amount of patient information that is accumulated for most cases. With these tools, the physiologic consequences of the malformed heart may be appreciated along with the remaining degree of cardiopulmonary reserve.

A system for physiologic classification utilizing non-cyanotic and cyanotic categories with an emphasis on the role of the ductus arteriosus is recommended. Anesthetic strategy follows from the physiologic category and condition of the patient rather than their specific anatomy in most cases. Attention should be paid to compensatory mechanisms and existing therapies as they must be maintained during the preparation for anesthesia and the pre-bypass period.

Patients at particular risk for deterioration at the outset of anesthetic care include those with left-sided obstructive lesions, such as aortic stenosis, and those with excess pulmonary blood flow for whom supplemental oxygen and mechanical ventilation may present new dangers. These individuals must be identified preoperatively and managed accordingly. For most children older than 1 year, including those with cyanosis, routine premedication is appropriate and safe with pulse oximetry and supplemental oxygen available.

References

1. Somerville J (2001) Grown-up congenital heart disease—medical demands look back, look forward 2000. Thorac Cardiovasc Surg 49:21–26.
2. Bedard E, Shore DF, Gatzoulis MA (2008) Adult congenital heart disease: a 2008 review. Br Med Bull 85:151–180.
3. Drenthen W, Pieper GP, Roos-Heselink JW, et al. (2007) Outcome of pregnancy in women with congenital heart disease. J Am Coll Cardiol 49:2303–2311.
4. Hoffman JI (2002) Incidence, mortality and natural history. In: Anderson RH, Barker EJ, Macartney FJ, et al (eds) Paediatric Cardiology, Vol 1. Churchill Livingstone, Edinburgh, pp. 111–121.
5. Reller MD, Strickland MJ, Riehle-Colarusso T, et al. (2008) Prevalence of congenital heart defects in metropolitan Atlanta. J Pediatr 153:807–813.
6. Brick DH, Allan LD (2002) Outcome of prenatally diagnosed congenital heart disease: an update. Pediatr Cardiol 23:449–453.
7. Verheijen PM, Lisowski LA, Stoutenbeek P, et al. (2001) Prenatal diagnosis of congenital heart disease affects preoperative acidosis in the newborn patient. J Thorac Cardiovasc Surg 121:798–803.
8. Galantowicz M, Cheatham JP, Phillips A, et al. (2008) Hybrid approach for hypoplastic left heart syndrome: intermediate results after the learning curve. Ann Thorac Surg 85:2063–2071.
9. Abbott ME (1936) Atlas of Congenital Cardiac Disease. American Heart Association, New York.
10. Lev M (1954) Pathologic diagnosis of positional variations in cardiac chambers in congenital heart disease. Lab Invest 3:71–82.
11. Van Praagh R (1984) Diagnosis of complex congenital heart disease; morphologic-anatomic method and terminology. Cardiovasc Intervent Radiol 7:115–120.
12. Anderson RH, Becker AE, Freedom RM, et al. (1984) Sequential segmental analysis of congenital heart disease. Pediatr Cardiol 5:281–288.
13. de la Cruz MV, Nadal-Ginard B (1972) Rules for the diagnosis of visceral situs, truncoconal morphologies and ventricular inversions. Am Heart J 84:19–32.
14. de la Cruz MV, Barrazueta JR, Arteaga M, et al. (1976) Rules for diagnosis of atrioventricular discordances and spatial identification of ventricles. Br Heart J 38:341–354.
15. Anderson RH, Wilcox BR (1996) How should we optimally describe complex congenitally malformed hearts? Ann Thorac Surg 62:710–716.
16. Edwards WD (2001) Classification and terminology of cardiovascular anomalies. In: Allen HD, Gutgesell HP, Clark EB, Driscoll DJ (eds) Moss and Adams' Heart Disease in Infants, Children, and Adolescents, 6th edn. Lippincott Williams & Wilkins, Philadelphia, pp. 118–142.
17. Van Praagh R (1972) The segmental approach to diagnosis in congenital heart disease. In: Bergsma D (ed) Birth Defects Original Article Series. The National Foundation—March of Dimes, Vol. 7. Williams and Wilkins, Maryland, pp. 4–23.
18. Anderson RH (2002) Anatomy. In: Anderson RH, Barker EJ, Macartney FJ, et al (eds) Paediatric Cardiology. Churchill Livingstone, Edinburgh, pp. 37–55.
19. Edwards WD (1989) Congenital heart disease. In: Schoen FJ (ed) Interventional and Surgical Cardiovascular Pathology; Clinical Correlations and Basic Principles. WB Saunders, Philadelphia, pp. 281–367.
20. Anderson RH (2002) Terminology. In: Anderson RH, Barker EJ, Macartney FJ, et al. (eds) Paediatric Cardiology. Churchill Livingstone, Edinburgh, pp. 19–36.
21. Bargeron LM (1981) Angiography relevant to complicating features. In: Becker AE, Losekoot TG, Marcelletti C, Anderson RH (eds) Paediatric Cardiology, Vol 3. Churchill Livingstone, Edinburgh, pp. 33–47.
22. Rowe RD, Freedom RM, Mehrizi A, et al. (1981) The Neonate With Congenital Heart Disease. Saunders, Philadelphia.
23. Meliones JN, Kern FH, Schulman SR, et al. (1996) Pathophysiological directed approach to congenital heart disease: a perioperative perspective. In: Society of Cardiovascular Anesthesiologists Monograph Perioperative Management of the Patient with Congenital Heart Disease. Williams & Wilkins, Baltimore, pp. 1–42.
24. Rudolph AM (1975) Congenital Diseases of the Heart: Clinical-Physiologic Considerations in Diagnosis and Management. Year Book Medical Publishers, Chicago.
25. Greenwood RD, Rosenthal A, Parisi L, et al. (1975) Extracardiac abnormalities in infants with congenital heart disease. Pediatrics 55:485–492.
26. Neill CA (1987) Congenital cardiac malformations and syndromes. In: Pierpont MEM, Moller JH (eds) The

Genetics of Cardiovascular Disease. Martinus Nijhoff, Boston, pp. 95–112.

27. Clark EB (2001) Etiology of congenital cardiovascular malformations: epidemiology and genetics. In: Allen HD, Gutgesell HP, Clark EB, Driscoll DJ (eds) Moss and Adams' Heart Disease in Infants, Children, and Adolescents, 6th edn. Lippincott Williams & Wilkins, Philadelphia, pp. 64–79.

28. Ferencz C, Rubin JD, Loffredo CA, et al. (1993) Epidemiology of Congenital Heart Disease: the Baltimore–Washington Infant Study 1981–1989. Futura, Mount Kisko.

29. Grech V, Gatt M (1999) Syndromes and malformations associated with congenital heart disease in a population based study. Int J Cardiol 68:151–156.

30. Jhang WK, Park JJ, Seo DM, et al. (2008) Perioperative evaluation of airways in patients with arch obstruction and intracardiac defects. Ann Thorac Surg 85:1753–1758.

31. Litman RS, Zernqast BA, Perkins FM (1995) Preoperative evaluation of the cervical spine in children with Trisomy 21: results of a questionnaire study. Paediatr Anaesth 5:355–361.

32. Song D, Maher CO (2007) Spinal disorders associated with skeletal dysplasias and syndromes. Neurosurg Clin N Am 18:499–514.

33. Ferencz C, Rubin JD, Loffredo CA, et al. (1997) Genetic and Environmental Risk Factors of Major Cardiovascular Malformations: the Baltimore–Washington Infant Study: 1981–1989. Futura, Armonk.

34. Adams FH, Lund GW, Disenhouse RB (1954) Observations on the physique and growth of children with congenital heart disease. J Pediatr 44:674–680.

35. Abad-Sinden A, Sutphen JL (2001) Growth and nutrition. In: Allen HD, Gutgesell HP, Clark EB, Driscoll DJ (eds) Moss and Adams' Heart Disease in Infants, Children, and Adolescents, 6th edn. Lippincott Williams & Wilkins, Philadelphia, pp. 325–326.

36. Limperopoulos C, Majnemer A, Shevell MI, et al. (2002) Predictors of developmental disabilities after open heart surgery in young children with congenital heart defects. J Pediatr 141:51–58.

37. Wray J, Sensky T (2001) Congenital heart disease and cardiac surgery in childhood: effects on cognitive function and academic ability. Heart 85:687–691.

38. Aram DM, Ekelman BL, Ben-Shachar G, et al. (1985) Intelligence and hypoxemia in children with congenital heart disease: fact or artifact? J Am Coll Cardiol 6:889–893.

39. Ross RD, Bollinger RO, Pinsky WW (1992) Grading the severity of congestive heart failure in infants. Pediatr Cardiol 13:72–75.

40. Law YM, Keller BB, Feingold BM, et al. (2005) Usefulness of plasma B-type natriuretic peptide to identify ventricular dysfunction in pediatric and adult patients with congenital heart disease. Am J Cardiol 95:474–478.

41. Izukawa T, Freedom RM (1992) Physical Examination of the cardiovascular system of the neonate. In: Freedom RM, Benson LN, Smallhorn JF (eds) Neonatal Heart Disease. Springer-Verlag, London, pp. 83–89.

42. Fineman JR, Soifer SH, Heymann MA (1995) Regulation of pulmonary vascular tone in the perinatal period. Annu Rev Physiol 57:115–134.

43. Cannon BC, Feltes TF, Fraley JK, et al. (2005) Nitric Oxide in the evaluation of congenital heart disease with pulmonary hypertension: factors related to Nitric Oxide response. Pediatr Cardiol 26:565–569.

44. Rudolph AM, Yuan S (1966) Response of the pulmonary vasculature to hypoxia and H^+ ion concentration changes. J Clin Invest 45:399–411.

45. Nicol ED, Kafka H, Stirrup J, et al. (2008) A simple comprehensive non-invasive cardiovascular assessment in pulmonary arterial hypertension: combined computed tomography pulmonary and coronary angiography. Int J Cardiol August 5 [Epub ahead of print].

46. Mayer JE Jr, Helgason H, Jonas RA, et al. (1986) Extending the limits for modified Fontan procedures. J Thorac Cardiovasc Surg 92:1021–1028.

47. Atlee JL, Bernstein AD (2001) Cardiac rhythm management devices (Part I). Indications, device selection, and function. Anesthesiology 95:1265–1280.

48. Atlee JL, Bernstein AD (2001) Cardiac rhythm management devices (Part II). Perioperative management. Anesthesiology 95:1492–1506.

49. Love BA, Barrett KS, Alexander ME, et al. (2001) Supraventricular arrhythmias in children and young adults with implantable cardioverter defibrillators. J Cardiovasc Electrophysiol 12:1097–1101.

50. Horigome H, Hiramatsy Y, Shigeta O, et al. (2002) Overproduction of platelet microparticles in cyanotic congenital heart disease with polycythemia. J Am Coll Cardiol 39:1072–1077.

51. Mauer HM, McCue CM, Caul J, et al. (1972) Impairment in platelet aggregation in congenital heart disease. Blood 40:207–216.

52. Nihill MR, McNamara DG, Vick RL (1976) The effects of increased blood viscosity on pulmonary vascular resistance. Am Heart J 92:65–72.

53. Thorne SA (1998) Management of polycythaemia in adults with cyanotic congenital heart disease. Heart 79:315–316.

54. Hulett RL, Ovitt TW (2001) The chest roentgenogram. In: Allen HD, Gutgesell HP, Clark EB, Driscoll DJ (eds) Moss and Adams' Heart Disease in Infants, Children, and Adolescents, 6th edn. Lippincott Williams & Wilkins, Philadelphia, pp. 162–170.

55. Higgins CB (1992) Radiography of congenital heart disease. In: Higgins CB (ed) Essentials of Cardiac Radiology and Imaging. Lippincott Co., Philadelphia, pp. 49–90.

56. Tworetzky W, McElhinney DB, Brook MM, et al. (1999) Echocardiographic diagnosis alone for the complete repair of major congenital heart defects. JACC 33:228–233.

57. Silverman NH, Hunter S, Anderson RH, et al. (1983) Anatomical basis of cross sectional echocardiography. Br Heart J 50:421–431.

58. Silverman NH (1993) Echocardiographic Anatomy. In: Silverman NH (ed) Pediatric Echocardiography. Williams & Wilkins, Baltimore, pp. 1–34.

59. Stanger P, Silverman NH, Foster E (1999) Diagnostic accuracy of pediatric echocardiograms performed in adult laboratories. Am J Cardiol 83:908–914.

60. Bridges ND, O'Laughlin MP, Mullins CE, Freed MD (2001) Cardiac catheterization, angiography, and intervention. In: Allen HD, Gutgesell HP, Clark EB, Driscoll DJ (eds) Moss and Adams' Heart Disease in Infants, Children, and Adolescents, 6th edn. Lippincott Williams & Wilkins, Philadelphia, pp. 276–324.

61. Mullins CE, Nihill MR (2000) Cardiac catheterization hemodynamics and intervention. In: Moller JH, Hoffman JE (eds) Pediatric Cardiovascular Medicine. Churchill Livingstone, New York, pp. 203–215.

62. Puchalski MD, Williams RV, Askovich B, et al. (2007) Assessment of right ventricular size and function: echo versus magnetic resonance imaging. Congenit Heart Dis 2:27–31.

63. Pignatelli RH, McMahon CJ, Chung T, et al. (2003) Role of echocardiography versus MRI for the diagnosis of congenital heart disease. Curr Opin Cardiol 18:357–365.

64. Powell AJ, Geva T (2000) Blood flow measurement by magnetic resonance imaging in congenital heart disease. Pediatr Cardiol 21:47–58.

65. Geva T (2002) Future directions of congenital heart disease imaging. Pediatr Cardiol 23:117–121.

66. Marx GR, Geva T (1998) MRI and echocardiography in children: how do they compare. Semin Roentgenol 33:281–292.

67. Geva T, Griel GF, Marshall AC, et al. (2002) Gadolinium-enhanced 3-dimensional magnetic resonance angiography of pulmonary blood supply in patients with complex pulmonary stenosis or atresia: comparison with x-ray angiography. Circulation 106:473–478.

68. Kilner PH (2003) Adult congenital heart disease. In: Higgins CB, De Roos A (eds) Cardiovascular MRI and MRA. Lippincott, Williams & Wilkins, Philadelphia, pp. 353–367.

69. Bove EL, Kavey RE, Byrum CJ, et al. (1985) Improved right ventricular function following late pulmonary valve replacement for residual pulmonary insufficiency or stenosis. J Thorac Cardiovasc Surg 90:50–55.

70. Helbing WA, Bosch HG, Maliepaard C, et al. (1995) Comparison of echocardiographic methods with magnetic resonance imaging for assessment of right ventricular function in children. Am J Cardiol 76:589–594.

71. Thierrien J, Siu SC, McLaughlin PR, et al. (2000) Pulmonary valve replacement in adults late after repair of tetralogy of Fallot: are we operating too late? J Am Coll Cardiol 36:1670–1675.

72. Fontan F, Fernandez G, Costa F, et al. (1989) The size of the pulmonary arteries and the results of the Fontan operation. J Thorac Cardiovasc Surg 98:711–719.

73. Julsrud PR, Ehman RL, Hagler DJ, et al. (1989) Extracardiac vasculature in candidates for Fontan surgery; MR imaging. Radiology 173:503–506.

74. Mohiaddin RH, Pennell DH (1998) MR blood flow measurement. Clinical application in the heart and circulation. Cardiol Clin 16:161–187.

75. Goldin JG, Ratib O, Aberle DR (2000) Contemporary cardiac imaging: an overview. J Thorac Imaging 15:218–229.

76. Arad Y (1998) Electron beam computed tomography for the diagnosis of cardiac disease. S Afr Med J 88:558–563.

77. Leschka S, Oechslin E, Husmann L, et al. (2007) Pre- and postoperative evaluation of congenital heart disease in children and adults with 64-section CT. Radiographics 27:829–846.

78. Haramati LB, Glickstein JS, Issenberg HJ, et al. (2002) MR imaging and CT of vascular anomalies and connections in patients with congenital heart disease: significance in surgical planning. Radiographics 22:337–347, discussion 348–349.

79. Higgins TL, Estafanous FG, Loop FD, et al. (1992) Stratification of morbidity and mortality outcome by preoperative risk factors in coronary artery bypass patients. A clinical severity score. JAMA 267:2344–2348.

80. Eagle KA, Berger P, Hugh C, et al. (2002) ACC/AHA guideline update on perioperative cardiovascular evaluation for noncardiac surgery. Am Coll Cardiol 39:542–553.

81. Siu SC, Sermer M, Colman JM, et al. (2001) Prospective multicenter study of pregnancy outcomes in women with heart disease. Circulation 104:515–521.

82. Piran S, Veldtman G, Siu S, et al. (2002) Heart failure and ventricular dysfunction in patients with single or systemic right ventricles. Circulation 105:1189–1194.

83. Gatzoulis MA, Balaji S, Webber SA, et al. (2000) Risk factors for arrhythmia and sudden cardiac death late after repair of tetralogy of Fallot: a multicentre study. Lancet 356:975–981.

84. Nardella A, Pechet L, Snyder LM (1995) Continuous improvement, quality control, and cost containment in clinical laboratory testing: effects of establishing and implementing guidelines for preoperative tests. Arch Pathol Lab Med 119:518–522.

85. Polderman D, Bax JJ, Kertai MD, et al. (2003) Statins are associated with a reduced incidence of perioperative mortality in patients undergoing major noncardiac vascular surgery. Circulation 107:1848–1851.

86. Kahana M (2001) Pro: only pediatric anesthesiologists should administer anesthetics to pediatric patients undergoing cardiac surgical procedures. J Cardiothorac Vasc Anesth 15:381–383.

87. Chang RK, Klitzner TS (2002) Can regionalization decrease the number of deaths for children who undergo cardiac surgery? A theoretical analysis. Pediatrics 109:173–181.

88. Wilson W, Taubert KA, Gewitz M, et al. (2007) Prevention of infective endocarditis: guidelines from the American Heart Association. Circulation 116:1736–1754.

89. Auden SM, Sobczyk WL, Solinger RE, et al. (2000) Oral ketamine/midazolam is superior to intramuscular meperidine, promethazine, and chlorpromazine for pediatric cardiac catheterization. Anesth Analg 90:299–305.

90. Stow PH, Burrows FA, Lerman J, et al. (1988) Arterial oxygen saturation following premedication in children with cyanotic congenital heart disease. Can J Anaesth 35: 63–66.

91. Schmitt HJ, Schuetz WH, Proeschel, et al. (1993) Accuracy of pulse oximetry in children with cyanotic congenital heart disease. J Cardiothorac Vasc Anesth 7:61–65.

92. Funk W, Jakob W, Riedl T, et al. (2000) Oral preanaesthetic medication for children: double-blind randomized study of a combination of midazolam and ketamine vs. midazolam or ketamine alone. Br J Anaesth 84:335–340.

93. Astuto M, Disma N, Crimi E (2002) Two doses of oral ketamine, given with midazolam, for premedication in children. Minerva Anestesiol 68:593–598.

14 Approach to the fetus, premature, and full-term infant

Kirsten C. Odegard, M.D. and Peter C. Laussen, M.B.B.S.

Children's Hospital, Boston, and Harvard Medical School, Boston, Massachusetts, USA

Introduction

The advances in pediatric cardiology and cardiac surgery over the past 30 years have resulted in a substantial decrease in morbidity and mortality associated with congenital heart disease (CHD). Most congenital heart lesions are now amenable to either anatomical or physiological repair early in infancy. Opinion regarding the optimal timing of corrective surgery for infants with symptomatic CHD regardless of age or weight has undergone radical changes over the last decades. Rather than the previous strategy of initial palliation followed by correction in early childhood, the current approach nowadays include complete repair within days to weeks of birth if feasible. Advances in diagnostic and interventional cardiology, the evolution of surgical techniques and conduct of cardiopulmonary bypass, and refinements in postoperative management have all contributed to the successful strategy of early corrective two-ventricle repair. A further advance in recent years has been the extension of this approach to the premature and low-birth-weight neonate (LBWN). However, the low mortality achieved with two-ventricle repairs has not been the experience in LBWN undergoing palliation for single ventricle defects, such as hypoplastic left heart syndrome (HLHS).

Cardiac surgery in the premature and very-low-birth-weight infants imposes additional challenges for the anesthesiologist. As for any pediatric cardiac procedure, a thorough understanding of the pathophysiology of various defects, the planned surgical procedure, and anticipation of specific postoperative problems are essential. There are additional considerations, however, when providing anesthesia to the premature and LBWN including immaturity of the airway, lungs, cardiovascular system, liver, kidney, and central nervous system makes these infants more susceptible not only to surgical complications but also to anesthetic complications. Finally, as the limits for managing newborns with CHD continue to be extended, an emerging challenge is that of fetal cardiac interventions.

This chapter describes general principles relevant to anesthesia for the newborn, including the premature and the very LBWN with CHD. The impact of sequelae related to prematurity, the outcome of cardiac surgery in the premature and full-term neonate, and new directions with fetal cardiac interventions are discussed.

Approach to treatment in the neonate

Early palliation

In the early experience of cardiac surgery for neonates, particularly those with low birth weight or being

Anesthesia for Congenital Heart Disease 2nd edition. Edited by
Dean Andropoulos, Stephen Stayer, Isobel Russell and Emad Mossad.
© 2010 Blackwell Publishing.

premature, initial palliation or medical management of congenital cardiac defects was preferred with the aim to achieve a certain size prior to repair. This was primarily because of the technical limitations for various surgical repairs and the risks associated with cardiopulmonary bypass. Although the actual "target" size or weight that a neonate should achieve to tolerate successful repair was never well documented, newborns with weight less than 2.0–2.5 kg were considered to be at higher risk.

The aim of palliative procedures is to control pulmonary blood flow sufficiently to allow for growth but without excessive blood flow to the pulmonary circulation and impaired systemic perfusions and volume overload to the systemic ventricle. Nevertheless palliation with a pulmonary artery (PA) band or a modified systemic-to-pulmonary artery shunt such as modified Blalock–Taussig (BT) shunt can be difficult procedures in neonates, and complications even more problematic in LBWN (see Table 14.1). For example, the size of a systemic-to-pulmonary artery shunt can be very difficult to determine and the geometry of the shunt is critical. A relatively large shunt may lead to excessive pulmonary blood flow, congestive heart failure (CHF) and possible pulmonary vascular obstructive disease (PVOD). Conversely, a small shunt leads to inadequate pulmonary blood flow, lower arterial oxygen saturation (SaO_2), possible shunt thrombosis, and distortion or stenosis of pulmonary arteries making further repair even more difficult. Assuming a normal cardiac output, hematocrit, absence of pulmonary venous desaturation, and unrestricted mixing of systemic and pulmonary venous return in the atrium, an ideal SaO_2 between 80 and 85% indicates a relatively balanced circulation with pulmonary to systemic blood flow ratio (Qp:Qs) close to 1:1.

In our experience, a modified BT shunt of 3.5 mm is the optimal size to use in a term neonate greater than 3.0 kg. If a 3.0-mm shunt is used, the risk for sudden thrombosis and acute obstruction in the early postoperative period is increased, even in low-birth-weight newborns; early introduction of anticoagulation with low-dose heparin 10–20 units/kg/h is important once hemostasis has been secured after surgery. A further problem of a small shunt is the likelihood of outgrowing the shunt size causing progressive cyanosis and leading to earlier surgical intervention. Alternatively, if a larger shunt size (i.e., >4.0 mm) is used in a newborn, the excessive pulmonary blood flow may compromise systemic perfusion, cause ventricular volume overload, heart failure, and prolonged postoperative recovery.

Banding of the PA to reduce pulmonary blood flow can also be a difficult palliative procedure. If the band is too tight, severe cyanosis may occur; and if the band is too loose, the increase in pulmonary blood flow will contribute to CHF and possible PVOD. Distortion of the PA secondary to migration of the band may contribute to both proximal and distal artery stenoses and complicate later repair, and can also lead to right ventricular hypertrophy, subaortic stenosis, and pulmonary valve stenosis depending on the relationship of the great arteries to ventricular outflow. Determining the correct size of a band at the time of surgery is difficult. There are no accurate formulas for band size, and the hemodynamic changes at the time of band placement must be closely observed. Ideally, the banded PA will result in an increase in systemic systolic blood pressure of approximately 20%, and depending on the underlying pathology a fall in SaO_2 to around 85% breathing room air. The pressure gradient across the band

Table 14.1 Complications of palliative surgery

	Early complications	Late complications
Systemic-to-pulmonary artery shunt	Excessive pulmonary blood flow Heart failure	Distortion of pulmonary arteries
	Inadequate pulmonary blood flow Cyanosis	Asymmetrical growth of the pulmonary arteries

	Shunt obstruction
	   Thrombus
	   Mechanical
		Pulmonary vascular occlusive disease

Pulmonary Artery Banding	Band too loose: excessive pulmonary blood flow	Complications at band site Distortion and residual stenosis after repair Aneurysm

	Band too tight: inadequate pulmonary blood flow	Complications proximal to band site
		   Right ventricular hypertrophy
		   Subaortic stenosis
		   Pulmonary valve stenosis
		   Complications distal to the band:
		   Pulmonary artery stenosis

can also be directly measured; usually a fall in pressure of approximately 50% proximal to distal across the band is sufficient. Because hemodynamic changes are essential to monitor at the time of PA band placement, it is important to avoid anesthetic techniques that could decrease ventricular function or cardiac output. Therefore, an opioid technique is most often necessary, and extubation delayed until the hemodynamic effect of the band is determined as the patient emerges from anesthesia and starts to wean from mechanical ventilation.

The case for early complete repair

As noted previously, whenever possible, early repair of two ventricle congenital cardiac defect is preferable to limit the consequences of excessive pressure and volume overload to the ventricles and pulmonary circulation, and the potential detrimental effect of chronic hypoxia. The underlying premise is that early repair allows for more normal growth and development.

The considerable advances in cardiac surgery and cardiopulmonary bypass techniques have contributed to a dramatic reduction in the risk for mortality following cardiac surgery in newborns [1–3], but newborns nevertheless remain at risk for end organ injury related to surgery and CPB, particularly neurological injury [4]. Despite this risk, trying to control pulmonary blood flow and volume overload on an immature myocardium with medical management alone is often extremely difficult and unsuccessful.

Further, the problems associated with pulmonary overcirculation, chronic volume, and/or pressure load on the ventricles and cyanosis may substantially affect development and lead to myocardial and pulmonary injury that will affect the outcome from subsequent repairs [4]. It is also likely that the imbalance between pulmonary and systemic blood flow will increase in newborns with a large left-to-right shunt as pulmonary vascular resistance falls in the first few weeks of life and the physiologic nadir in hematocrit is reached. The clinical manifestations of an infant with CHF are shown in Table 14.2. The increased work of breathing and tachypnea secondary to an increase in pulmonary blood flow and total lung water results in an increase in metabolic demand and an increase in the percentage of the total cardiac output directed toward respiratory muscle work (most notably the diaphragm). This essentially diverts cardiac output from other metabolically active functions, in particularly from the splanchnic circulation and absorption of food. The abnormal circulatory physiology is unable to meet metabolic needs and patients fail to thrive.

While it is preferable to correct congenital cardiac defects early in the full-term newborn when possible promote growth and development, this may be difficult to

Table 14.2 Symptoms and signs of congestive heart failure and cardiac failure in a neonate and infant

Low cardiac output
  Tachycardia
  Poor extremity perfusion
  Cardiomegaly
  Hepatomegaly
  Gallop rhythm

Increased respiratory work
  Tachypnea
  Grunting
  Flaring of ala nasi
  Chest wall retraction

Increased metabolic work
  Failure to thrive
  Poor weight gain

achieve in the premature and very LBWN [5–11]. The causes are multifactorial and include technical issues related to small cardiac structures and cannulation for CPB, the immaturity of organ systems (especially the lungs, myocardium, and germinal matrix), increased risk of bleeding from coagulopathy after CPB, and an immature stress response that may increase the risk for infection and promote a catabolic state in newborn with limited nutritional reserves. This directly contributes to an increased mortality risk as well as a longer duration of mechanical ventilation, intensive care, and hospital stay for the premature and LBWN undergoing cardiac surgery.

Outcome

Although the risk for early mortality in neonates undergoing cardiac surgery and CPB may be increased, randomized and prospective studies comparing the morbidity that may occur in neonates with critical lesions who are treated medically in hopes of weight gain, compared to surgical morbidity and mortality have not been performed. Such has been the nature for many of the advances in CHD management.

For example, infants with an increased pulmonary blood flow who undergo delayed surgical intervention often fail to thrive and are at risk for recurrent respiratory infections. Their work of breathing and energy expenditure is significantly increased, and cardiomegaly with hyperinflated lung fields is evident on chest radiograph. Cardiac surgery and CPB may be delayed because of concern for intercurrent infection and the risk for exacerbation or reactivation of inflammatory lung processes, which in turn may cause intrapulmonary shunting and severe hypoxemia, pulmonary hypertension, and prolonged mechanical ventilation. The early repair or palliation of defects to limit pulmonary overcirculation and volume load on the systemic ventricle will often avoid the above complications.

Although the management of neonates in the immediate postoperative period after a two-ventricle repair can be a challenge, the substantial improvements in successful outcomes are such that mortality is no longer a reliable index against which to measure or compare new or alternative treatments in this group of patients. In contrast, this has not been the case for palliative procedures in patients with complex single-ventricle defects, although there has been a steady improvement in survival and longer-term outcome in neonates with single-ventricle disease in recent years.

Limited physiologic reserve

Care of the critically ill neonate requires an appreciation of the special structural and functional features of immature organs. The neonate appears to respond more quickly and extremely to physiologically stressful circumstances; this may be expressed in terms of rapid changes in, for example, pH, lactic acid, glucose, and temperature [12].

The physiology of the preterm and full-term neonate is characterized by a high metabolic rate and O_2 demand (two- to threefold increase compared to adults) that maybe compromised at times of stress because of limited cardiac and respiratory reserve. The myocardium in the neonate is immature with only 30% of the myocardial mass comprising contractile tissue, compared to 60% in mature myocardium. In addition, neonates have a lower velocity of shortening, a diminished length–tension relationship and a reduced ability to respond to afterload stress [13, 14]. Because the compliance of the myocardium is reduced, the stroke volume is relatively fixed and cardiac output is heart-rate dependent, and the Frank–Starling relationship is functional within a narrow range of left ventricular end-diastolic pressure compared to the mature myocardium. The cytoplasmic reticulum and T-tubular system are underdeveloped and the neonatal heart is dependent on the trans-sarcolemmal flux of extracellular calcium to both initiate and sustain contraction. It is important to note that much of this information is derived from animal data. It is not known to what extent prematurity causes an additional detriment in functional myocardial reserve.

Cardiorespiratory interactions are important in neonates and infants. In simple terms, ventricular interdependence refers to a relative increase in ventricular end-diastolic volume and pressure causing a shift of the ventricular septum and diminished diastolic compliance of the opposing ventricle [15]. This effect is particularly prominent in the immature myocardium. Therefore, a volume load from an intracardiac shunt or valve regur-

gitation, and a pressure load from ventricular outflow obstruction or increased vascular resistance, may lead to biventricular dysfunction. For example, in neonates with tetralogy of Fallot and severe outflow obstruction, hypertrophy of the ventricular septum may contribute to diastolic dysfunction of the left ventricle and an increase in end-diastolic pressure. This does not improve immediately after repair in the neonate, as it takes some time for the myocardium to remodel. Therefore, an elevated left atrial pressure is not an unexpected finding after neonatal tetralogy repair. This circumstance may be further exacerbated if there is a persistent volume load to the left ventricle following surgery, such as from a residual ventricle septal defect (VSD).

The mechanical disadvantage of an increased chest wall compliance and reliance on the diaphragm as the main muscle of respiration limits ventilatory capacity in the neonate. The diaphragm and intercostal muscles have fewer Type I muscle fibers, i.e., slow-contracting, high-oxidative fibers for sustained activity, and this contributes to early fatigue when the work of breathing is increased. In the newborn, only 25% of fibers in the diaphragm are Type I, reaching a mature proportion of 55% by 8–9 months of age [16, 17]. Diaphragmatic function may be significantly compromised by raised intra-abdominal pressure, such as from gastric distension, hepatic congestion, and ascites.

The tidal volume of full-term neonates is between 6 and 8 mL/kg and, because of the above mechanical limitations, minute ventilation is respiratory rate dependent. The resting respiratory rate of the newborn infant is between 30 and 40 breaths per minute, which provides the optimal alveolar ventilation to overcome the work of breathing and match the compliance and resistance of the respiratory system. When the work of breathing increases, such as with parenchymal lung disease, airway obstruction, cardiac failure, or increased pulmonary blood flow, a larger proportion of total energy expenditure is required to maintain adequate ventilation. Infants therefore fatigue readily and fail to thrive.

The neonate has a reduced functional residual capacity (FRC) secondary to an increased chest wall compliance (FRC being determined by the balance between chest wall and lung compliance). Closing capacity is also increased in newborns, with airway closure occurring during normal tidal ventilation [18]. Oxygen reserve is therefore reduced, and in conjunction with the increased basal metabolic rate and oxygen consumption two to three times adult levels, neonates and infants are at risk for hypoxemia. However, atelectasis and hypoxemia do not occur in the normal neonate because FRC is maintained by dynamic factors including tachypnea, breath stacking (early inspiration), expiratory breaking (expiratory flow interrupted before zero flow occurs), and from laryngeal breaking (autopositive end-expiratory pressure).

Drug pharmacodynamics and kinetics may be altered in the newborn because of immature hepatic and renal function. In addition to altered drug metabolism, protein binding and clearance, the drug volume of distribution is affected by the increase in total body water of the neonate compared with the older patient. The propensity of the neonatal capillary system to leak fluid out of the intravascular space [19] is especially pronounced in the neonatal lung, in which the pulmonary vascular bed is almost fully recruited at rest and the lymphatic recruitment required to handle increased mean capillary pressures associated with increases in pulmonary blood flow may be unavailable [20].

The glomerular filtration rate is generally low at birth but normalizes quite readily. Urinary sodium excretion increases slowly during the first 2 years of life, and the inability of immature kidneys to concentrate urine and to excrete acute water and sodium loads makes fluid management in neonates and especially preterm infants difficult. Urinary acidification capability is limited in neonates and the bicarbonate threshold reduced. Thus premature infants have decreased serum bicarbonate levels and lower serum pH (a nonanion gap acidosis). Neonates tolerate fluid restriction poorly, so fasting should be kept to a minimum and intravenous fluid started early; however, excessive fluid administration (as after CPB) is also tolerated poorly. In order to induce diuresis in neonates larger doses of furosemide compared to adults are needed. The dosing of drugs, which largely depend on renal excretion, will have to be reduced and if possible the plasma concentration should be closely checked in order to avoid accumulation and side effects.

The caloric requirement for neonates and especially preterm neonates is high (100–150 kcal/kg/24 h) because of metabolic demand. The task of supplying nutrition for growth becomes even more difficult when necessary limits are placed on the total amount of fluid that may be administrated either parentally or by the enteral route in preterm neonates with CHD. Hyperosmolar feedings have been associated with an increased risk of necrotizing enterocolitis (NEC) in the preterm neonate, or to the neonate born at term who has decreased splanchnic blood flow of any cause (e.g., left-sided obstructive lesions) [21].

Systemic inflammatory response to cardiopulmonary bypass

It is well recognized that the exposure of blood elements to the nonendothelial surfaces of the cardiopulmonary bypass circuit, along with ischemic/reperfusion injury, induces a systemic inflammatory response syndrome (SIRS), which includes activation of numerous signaling cascades including compliment, fibrinolytic, proinflammatory cytokine and oxyradical pathways. The effects of the interac-

tions of blood components with the extracorporeal circuit is magnified in neonates due to the large bypass circuit surface area and priming volume relative to patient blood volume.

The inflammatory response is therefore more pronounced in very low-birth-weight and premature newborns, and along with this the clinical manifestations. The immaturity of the stress response, low receptor density and low vascular tone may be additional factors that magnify the clinical features of the SIRS in these patients. The clinical consequences include increased interstitial fluid and generalized capillary leak, and potential multi-organ dysfunction. Total lung water is increased with an associated decrease in lung compliance and increase in A–aO$_2$ gradient. Myocardial edema results in impaired ventricular systolic and diastolic function. A secondary fall in cardiac output by 20–30% is common in neonates in the first 6–12 hours following surgery, contributing to decreased renal function and oliguria [22]. Sternal closure may need to be delayed due to mediastinal edema and associated cardiorespiratory compromise when closure is attempted. Ascites, hepatic ingestion, and bowel edema may affect mechanical ventilation, cause a prolonged ileus, and delay feeding. A coagulopathy post-CPB may contribute to delayed hemostasis.

Over recent years, numerous strategies have evolved to limit the effect of the endothelial injury resulting from the SIRS. Understanding the triggers, timing, and pattern of the complex cascades related to the SIRS is essential to modify or attenuate this response. A variety of anti-inflammatory treatment modalities have been studied including leukocyte depletion, neutrophil adhesion blockade, and heparin coating of the CPB circuit to reduce compliment and leukocyte activation. To date, no single treatment has proven to attenuate the endothelial reaction and clinical response following cardiopulmonary bypass in neonates and infants, which highlights the multifactorial nature of the inflammatory response.

The most important strategy remains limiting both the time spent on bypass and use of deep hypothermic circulatory arrest (DHCA). This is clearly dependent, however, upon surgical expertise, experience, and patient size. For the LBWN, DHCA is often still necessary for complete surgical repair. Deep anesthesia, hypothermia, and corticosteroid administration are bypass strategies that may limit activation of the inflammatory response. Attenuating the stress response, the use of antioxidants such as mannitol and anti-inflammatory agents such as glucocorticoids, altering prime composition to maintain hematocrit and oncotic pressure, and ultrafiltration during rewarming or immediately after bypass are also used to limit the clinical consequences of the inflammatory response.

In addition to activation of stress hormones during cardiopulmonary bypass, triiodothyronine (T$_3$) levels have been demonstrated to be low after cardiolpulmonary bypass, and may remain low for up to 48 hours after surgery, particularly if a sick euthyroid state develops and there is decreased conversion of thyroxine to the active T_3 in peripheral tissues [23]. An increase in glucagon levels, insulin resistance, and steroid administration may contribute to significant hyperglycemia following bypass in neonates. Persistent hyperglycemia may contribute to adverse outcomes and risk for health care acquired infections, but has nor been associated with longer time neurological injury [24]. The use of insulin to achieve tight glycemic control after bypass must be undertaken with caution and frequent measurement of glucose levels is essential because of the risk for unintended hypoglycemia that will cause neurological injury.

Hemofiltration has become a technique commonly used to hemoconcentrate, and possibly remove inflammatory mediators, e.g., complement, endotoxin, and cytokines during or after CPB [25–29]. Hemofiltration techniques include "modified ultrafiltration" (MUF) whereby the patient's blood volume is filtered after completion of bypass, "conventional hemofiltration" whereby both the patient and circuit are filtered during rewarming on bypass, and "zero-balance ultrafiltration" in which high volume ultrafiltration essentially washes the patient and circuit blood volumes during the rewarming process [30]. High flow rates through the ultrafiltration during MUF has been shown to transiently decrease the cerebral circulation in young infants compared with lower blood flow rates, this may be important in newborns after CPB who may have altered cerebral autoregulation [31].

Early clinical experience reported improved systolic and diastolic pressures during filtration, and improved pulmonary function has also been noted with reduction in pulmonary vascular resistance and total lung water [25, 26]. While modified ultrafiltration postbypass has proven to improve early hemodynamic and pulmonary function, the improvement in pulmonary compliance may not be sustained beyond the immediate postultrafiltration period [32]. While these techniques are useful to hemoconcentrate and remove total body water, they do not prevent the inflammatory response. And while it is perhaps modified, this response is nevertheless idiosyncratic; despite all the above maneuvers, some neonates and infants will still manifest significant clinical signs of the SIRS and delayed postoperative recovery [32]. The development of drugs that will prevent the adhesion molecule–endothelial interaction, which is pivotal in the inflammatory response, continues to be pursued in both laboratory and clinical studies.

Peritoneal dialysis has been recommended as a means to treat total body fluid overload, particularly during low-output states following cardiac surgery. Recent studies have reported successful treatment of fluid overload with continuous peritoneal dialysis, without significant morbidity and hemodynamic effects [33, 34]. In addition to decompressing the abdomen, which may in turn improve respiratory mechanics and requirements for mechanical ventilation, peritoneal dialysis also assist with postoperative fluid balance, and may have the potential benefit of removal of proinflammatory cytokines [35].

Neurological injury

Deep hypothermia (<18°C) with either low-flow cardiopulmonary bypass or circulating arrest (CA) may be necessary in selected neonates undergoing cardiac surgery either because of size limitations for cannulation or to facilitate the surgical procedure. The conduct of deep hypothermic or low-flow CPB is critical for optimal myocardial and neurological protection.

In many centers, the practice has shifted away from the use of DHCA if the repair can be satisfactorily accomplished with low−flow techniques [36, 37], or alternate cannulation and cerebral perfusion strategies that allow higher flow bypass at moderate hypothermia. While there may be no optimal "safe" duration of DHCA, the accepted limit has declined over recent years from approximately 60 minutes to the 30-minute range at temperatures <20°C [3, 37]. With improvements in neurological protection over recent years, the incidence of overt injury, i.e., postoperative seizures, has declined substantially. While long-term neurodevelopmental outcome after DHCA in children is still being clarified, this has nevertheless become an important outcome variable when evaluating neurological protection strategies [38].

Neurological injury is an inherent risk for any patient undergoing cardiac surgery and cardiopulmonary bypass. Early in the development of bypass strategies, postoperative seizures were a relatively common occurrence. They were generally self-limiting and did not imply longer-term seizure activity. However, it is now clear that seizures are a manifestation of neurological injury, consistent with the release of excitatory neurotransmitters that produce neuronal injury by N-methyl-D-aspartate receptor-gated calcium channels [39]. Adverse neurological sequelae are multifactorial postbypass and may be secondary to the duration of CPB [40, 41], rate and depth of cooling [42–44], perfusion flow rate [45], duration of circulatory arrest, pH management on bypass [1, 39], hematocrit [2, 46–48], and embolic events. Strategies to optimize cerebral protection during deep hypothermic bypass, with or without circulatory arrest, include a longer duration of cooling (over 20 min), the use of pH-stat strategy of blood gas management during cooling (i.e., addition of CO_2 to the oxygenator), and maintaining a higher hematocrit (>25%) [49–51]. A recent randomized study of hematocrit of 25% versus 35% showed no major benefit or risks overall among infants undergoing two-ventricle repair. It is important to note that developmental outcomes at age 1 year in both randomized groups were below those in the normal population [2], and this finding is consistent with the inherent risk for neurological injury in all neonates undergoing cardiopulmonary bypass. Brain MRI data performed both before and following newborn cardiac surgery and hypothermic bypass demonstrates a disturbing risk for white matter injury and the development of periventricular leukomalacia [52–55]. While the longer-term impact of these injuries are yet to be determined, the risk for brain injury in newborns is clear and supports the use of routine intraoperative neurological monitoring with monitors such as near infra-red spectroscopy, transcranial Doppler assessment of cerebral blood flow velocity, and continuous EEG.

Stress response

In general terms, the "stress response" is a systemic reaction to injury, with hemodynamic, endocrinologic, and immunologic effects (Table 14.3). Stress and adverse postoperative outcome have been linked closely in critically ill newborns and infants. This is not surprising given their precarious balance of limited metabolic reserve and increased resting metabolic rate. Metabolic derangements,

Table 14.3 Systemic response to injury

Autonomic nervous system activation
  Catechol release
  Hypertension, tachycardia, vasoconstriction
Endocrine response
  Anterior Pituitary
   ↑ ACTH, GH
  Posterior Pituitary
   ↑ Vasopressin
  Adrenal Cortex
   ↑ Cortisol, aldosterone
  Pancreas
   ↑ Glucagon
   Insulin resistance
  Thyroid
   ↓ conversion of T_4 to T_3
Metabolic response
  Protein catabolism
  Lipolysis
  Glycogenolysis/gluconeogenesis
  Hyperglycemia
  Salt and water retention
Immunologic responses
  Cytokine production
  Acute phase reaction
  Granulocytosis

such as altered glucose homeostasis, metabolic acidosis, salt and water retention, and a catabolic state contributing to protein breakdown and lipolysis, are commonly seen following major stress in sick neonates and infants [56]. This complex of maladaptive processes may be associated with prolonged mechanical ventilation courses and ICU stay, as well as increased morbidity and mortality.

The neuroendocrine stress response is activated by afferent neuronal impulses from the site of injury, traveling via sensory nerves through the dorsal root of the spinal cord to the medulla and hypothalamus. Anesthesia can therefore have a substantial modulating effect on the neuroendocrine pathways of the stress response by virtue of providing analgesia and loss of consciousness. Outcomes after major surgery in neonates and infants may be improved when the stress response is attenuated. This was initially reported in two controlled, randomized trials comparing N_2O/O_2/curare anesthesia with or without fentanyl in neonates undergoing PDA ligation [12] and with or without halothane in neonates undergoing general surgery [57]. Fentanyl doses as low as 10 mcg/kg may be sufficient for effective baseline anesthesia in neonates, although larger doses are necessary for prolonged anesthesia. A bolus dose of 10–15 mcg/kg has been demonstrated to effectively ameliorate the hemodynamic response to tracheal intubation in neonates [58].

It is important to distinguish between suppression of the endocrine response and attenuation of hemodynamic responses to stress. Because of their direct effects on the myocardium and vascular tone, anesthetic agents can readily suppress the hemodynamic side effects of the endocrine stress response. The same is true when inotropic and vasoactive agents are administered during anesthesia. However, the postoperative consequences of the endocrine stress response, in particular fluid retention and increased catabolism, remain unabated. Relying on hemodynamic variables to assess the level of "stress" is therefore often inaccurate. Metabolic indices such as hyperglycemia and hyperlactatemia are also indirect markers of "stress," particularly as they are influenced by other factors such as fluid administration and cardiac output.

The effect of surgical stress has been particularly evaluated in neonates and infants undergoing cardiac surgery. Wood et al. first demonstrated a substantial increase in epinephrine and norepinephrine levels in response to profound hypothermia and circulatory arrest in infants undergoing cardiac surgery [59]. The hormonal and metabolic response was further characterized by Anand et al. and noted to be more extreme and distinct from that seen in adults [60]. In addition to an increase in catechol, glucagon, endorphin and insulin levels, hyperglycemia, and lactic acidemia persisted into the postoperative period. In an important subsequent study, Anand and Hickey compared a high-dose sufentanil technique with a combined halothane/morphine anesthetic technique in 45 neonates undergoing cardiac surgery and deep hypothermic CPB [61]. They reported a significant attenuation of hormonal and metabolic responses to surgery and bypass in the sufentanil group, with less postoperative morbidity and mortality. A conclusion from these studies supported the notion that reducing the stress response with large-dose opioid anesthesia, and extending this into the immediate postoperative period, was important to reduce the morbidity and mortality associated with congenital heart surgery in neonates.

These studies were performed over a decade ago. During the intervening period, there have been substantial changes in the perioperative management of children with heart disease as well as the management of cardiopulmonary bypass in general; along with these changes, outcomes have considerably improved. Further, it has been well demonstrated that high-dose opioid anesthetic techniques do not consistently block the endocrine stress response to cardiac surgery. To evaluate this further, however, it is necessary to separate prebypass and bypass responses.

Precardiopulmonary bypass

The dose of sufentanil used by Anand and Hickey was extremely high and difficult to translate to the more common practice of fentanyl-based anesthesia. Two more recent studies in neonates, infants, and older children undergoing cardiac surgery have demonstrated attenuation of the *prebypass* endocrine and hemodynamic response to surgical stimulation with a variety of anesthetic techniques. These have included high-dose fentanyl (50 mcg/kg) either by bolus or infusion [62, 63], and high-dose bolus fentanyl (25–150 mcg/kg) with or without low-dose isoflurane [46]. Based on the lack of significant stress responses reported in these studies, it is reasonable to conclude that there was appropriate neuraxial inhibition in these patients and that they were adequately anesthetized during this prebypass phase of surgery. There were no significant postoperative complications (from hemodynamic and pulmonary complications through to awareness) reported in the studies. It is not possible to conclude, however, that one technique is superior to another. No specific dose response between opioid plasma level and level of hormone or metabolic stress response has been established, nor a specific benefit for the method or route of opioid administration, i.e., bolus or continuous infusion.

Cardiopulmonary bypass

The initiation of the endocrine stress response may be from a myriad of causes and the relative contributions are speculative. Besides the surgical stimulus, additional factors include the effects of CPB, i.e., hypothermia, contact activation, hemodilution, and nonpulsatile flow [64–66]. Distinct to the effect of anesthesia in the prebypass phase, anesthesia techniques have *not* been demonstrated to consistently obtund the responses to bypass [61,63,67]. This is primarily because CPB initiates a *second mechanism* for establishing the stress response independent of surgical stimulation, namely the acute phase response and inflammatory cytokine release.

Cytokines are produced from activated leukocytes, fibroblasts, and endothelial cells as an early response to tissue injury and have a major role in mediating immunity and inflammation. Cytokine production reflects the degree of tissue trauma or injury. They stimulate the production of acute phase proteins in the liver (i.e., C-reactive protein, fibrinogen, α_2-macroglobulin, and other antiproteinases), stimulate the adhesion molecule cascade, increase protein catabolism, and augment release of ACTH from the anterior pituitary [68, 69]. In addition to direct tissue injury, exposure of blood to foreign surfaces and the systemic inflammatory response as previously mentioned is also a potent stimulus for cytokine production and, with this, the stress response.

Effect of high-dose opioid anesthesia on stress response

In the early experience of bypass in neonates and infants, the use of high-dose opioid anesthesia to modulate the stress response was perceived to be one of the few clinical strategies available that was associated with the demonstrable improvement in morbidity and mortality [61]. More recently, it has been demonstrated that opioids do not in fact modify the endocrine or metabolic stress response initiated by CPB; despite this, mortality and morbidity continues to remain low. Gruber et al. demonstrated a significant increase in stress hormone levels in infants during CPB compared to prebypass levels, although there was no change in plasma fentanyl concentrations [62].

Whereas the neonate may be more labile to changes in intravascular pressures, pulmonary vascular resistance, and cardiac output than older children, in fact the neonate is quite capable of coping with the acute phase of surgical stress. It is less common now to see neonates in the immediate postbypass period with extensive peripheral edema or anasarca and, along with that, impaired ventricular function, reactive pulmonary hypertension, and substantial alterations in lung compliance and airway resistance. An example of this is the incidence of postoperative pulmonary hypertensive events. Pulmonary hypertensive crisis were more common a decade or more ago in infants who had been exposed to weeks or months of high pulmonary pressure and flow, such as truncus arteriosus, complete atrioventricular canal defects, and transposition of the great arteries with ventricular septal defects. High-dose opioids were an important component of management for patients at risk for pulmonary hypertensive crises; however, this occurs much less frequently nowadays when patients are operated upon at an earlier age and are therefore less likely to have significant or irreversible changes in the pulmonary vascular bed. Therefore, changes in surgical practice, and in particular the timing of surgery, have meant that the longer-term pathophysiologic consequences of various defects are less apparent than what they were 10–20 years ago. A strategy of large-dose opioid anesthesia to blunt the stress response may therefore be a less critical determinant of outcome.

This is not to say, of course, that the high-dose synthetic opioids are not necessary for neonatal cardiac surgery. Synthetic opioids are potent analgesics and provide hemodynamic stability because of their lack of negative inotropic or vasoactive properties. Because of the limited physiologic reserve, the pathophysiology of underlying cardiac defects and the clinical consequences of the systemic inflammatory response to bypass in the neonates, using an anesthetic technique that has minimal hemodynamic side effects, is clearly desirable.

It remains to be determined what the optimal opioid dose should be to ensure an adequate depth of anesthesia. In a retrospective, pharmacodynamic study of fentanyl, Hansen and Hickey demonstrated that 50 mcg/kg of fentanyl was necessary to reduce the potential for sudden ventricular fibrillation in neonates with HLHS prior to CPB [70].

There are many different preferences and techniques for opioid-based anesthesia for cardiac surgery. Our common practice for neonates undergoing cardiac surgery and deep hypothermic CPB is to administer up to 50 mcg/kg of fentanyl prior to sternotomy, and to supplement with low-dose isoflurane titrated to hemodynamic response. During rewarming on CPB, a further 25 mcg/kg of fentanyl is administered, and up to an additional 25 mcg/kg fentanyl post-CPB according to hemodynamic stability and prior to transport to the ICU. The main aim is to provide an anesthetic that maintains hemodynamic stability and allows the anesthesia team to concentrate on all other aspects of the surgery, bypass, and post-CPB care. Sudden changes in hemodynamics before and after bypass may develop secondary to myocardial dysfunction, residual anatomic lesions, loss of sinus rhythm, changes in preload state, variable pulmonary vascular resistance, and alterations in mechanical ventilation to mention a few; using a high-dose opioid anesthesia technique allows the anesthesiologist to focus on an evolving hemodynamic picture without the distraction of side effects from anesthetic drugs.

The risk for cardiac arrest related to pediatric anesthesia in general is increased in newborns and those with the American Society of Anesthesiologists (ASA) physical status greater than 3 [71]. The presence of underlying cardiac disease is an additional risk for cardiac arrest, and in the cardiac operating room the risk for anesthesia-related cardiac arrest was increased 17-fold to 21 per 10,000 anesthetics in a recent large series review [71]. Despite this risk, there was a low mortality associated with cardiac arrest, and this low "failure to rescue" rate is indicative of the preparation and system required to recover patients after an adverse event. It further supports the development of a dedicated cardiac anesthesia team to manage high-risk newborns during cardiac surgery. While it can be difficult to distinguish between factors contributing to cardiac arrest in newborns with underlying cardiac disease, there is an association between altered coronary perfusion and myocardial ischemia and cardiac arrest. Coronary perfusion may be reduced in patients who have uncontrolled or continuous runoff of blood flow from the systemic to pulmonary circulation, and therefore low aortic root diastolic pressure (patients with a diagnosis of truncus arteriosus, patients with a ductus-dependent systemic circulation such as HLHS and interruption of the aortic arch or coarctation with VSD). Patients with altered coronary blood flow, such as those with pulmonary atresia, intact ventricular septum, and a right ventricle-dependent coronary circulation from fistulae, are also at increased risk for ischemia. These patients also have a limited ability to increase coronary blood flow when myocardial oxygen demand is increased, such as secondary to tachycardia, increased contractility, or wall stress in response to a surgical stimulus if there is an inadequate depth of anesthesia to blunt a stress response.

Premature infants and very low-birth-weight neonates

Although the technical aspects of CPB in small neonates are challenging, surgical advances now allow routine corrective repair of complex heart disease in neonates weighing less than 2000 g (LBWN). In our experience, neither gestational age nor patient size precludes successful complete repair of lesions such as tetralogy of Fallot, truncus arteriosus and transposition of the great arteries, and survival for corrective surgery in neonates weighing less than 2000 g may now approach 90% [7,8,10,11,72].

While the successful outcomes of term-newborns undergoing cardiac surgery and CPB is now well established and a standard of care, the continued improved survival of preterm and LBWNs has added a new dimension to management of CHD. In addition to the physiologic limitations previously described for any newborn, compounded by the effects of the underlying cardiac disease and surgical interventions, the complications of prematurity are further considerations. The management of respiratory distress syndrome (RDS), fluid balance, NEC, and intraventricular hemorrhage may be even more difficult in a premature newborn who has CHD. The early repair of specific cardiac defects may be prevented by complications of prematurity. Further, while a technically successful repair may be possible, the longer-term development and hazard function for reintervention in premature and LBWN undergoing cardiac surgery has not been established.

Pulmonary function

The immature airway and lungs of the premature and very low-birth-weight neonate predispose to obstruction, hypoxia, and ventilation difficulties. Lung compliance is reduced because the alveoli are primarily composed of thick-walled saccular spaces. The very compliant chest wall results in a significant mechanical disadvantage with lower FRC and O_2 reserve, lower-minute ventilation, and early respiratory muscle fatigue. Dead space ventilation as a proportion of tidal volume is increased, which promotes further risk for respiratory failure. Production of surfactant begins between 23 and 24 weeks of gestation, and may be inadequate until 36 weeks of gestation [73]. RDS from surfactant deficiency results in low lung volumes and poor compliance, and increased intrapulmonary shunt and ventilation/perfusion (V/Q) mismatch leading to severe hypoxia. Lung injury associated with inflammatory mediator release related to mechanical ventilation or high concentration of inspired oxygen may contribute to prolonged weaning and chronic lung disease or bronchopulmonary dysplasia (BPD). A recent retrospective multicenter study of premature infants with BPD and CHD evaluated the postoperative course and outcome in these LBWNs after cardiac surgery. The overall 30-day survival postsurgery was 84%, survival to hospital discharge was 68%, and there was a 50% mortality for patients with univentricular hearts and severe BPD. Overall, these patients had increased morbidity and mortality and a prolonged ICU and hospital stay compared with full-term neonates [74].

Persistent cardiac failure or excessive pulmonary flow from certain cardiac defects will increase total lung water and prevent or delay weaning from mechanical ventilation in the LBWN or premature newborn. Although RDS with increased pulmonary vascular resistance will limit pulmonary blood flow initially, as the lung injury resolves and the PVR decreases, pulmonary blood flow will substantially increase. For premature infants without RDS, pulmonary vascular tone is usually very low and pulmonary blood flow may therefore be very high in the circumstance of a cardiac defect with a large left to right shunt, such as truncus arteriosus. Medical management with mechanical ventilation, diuretics, inotropes and va-

sodilators is often ineffective in such cases. A low cardiac output state often persists with significant runoff to the pulmonary circulation. Continuing with medical management while waiting for an appropriate weight gain is frequently ineffective and the only alternative is surgical intervention. Palliation with a PA band to limit pulmonary blood flow is difficult to judge in an LBWN or premature infant because of technical considerations, and subsequent distortion of the pulmonary arteries may severely limit later surgical procedures. Therefore, complete surgical repair early in the course of management may be indicated to provide the optimal conditions for growth and development.

A similar problem arises in LBWN or premature infants who are cyanosed at birth from pulmonary outflow obstruction and ductus-dependent pulmonary blood flow. A longer-term infusion of prostaglandin E_1 may be considered; however, the side effects of apnea and gastric mucosal hyperplasia are limitations. Further, the runoff across a large ductus is difficult to control and systemic hypoperfusion may develop. Palliation with a modified BT shunt is possible, but may be limited by the size of the pulmonary arteries and geometry of the shunt. In addition to distortion of the pulmonary arteries, flow across the shunt could be excessive and result in systemic hypoperfusion and cardiac failure from volume overload. Therefore, the side effects of palliation may not allow for subsequent growth and development, and the best alternative may be early surgical repair. This is the case for some patients with tetralogy of Fallot, with or without pulmonary atresia, and successful repair in LBWN and premature infants has been reported. Nevertheless, the postoperative course of these patients is often prolonged and characterized by restrictive right ventricular physiology; however, if complete repair has been successful without significant residual lesion, this approach with anatomic correction of the circulation provides the best option for longer-term survival and growth.

Premature and LBWN infants with single ventricle physiology or a parallel circulation are difficult to manage, and an adequate balance between the ductus-dependent pulmonary or systemic flow may not be achieved. Prolonged mechanical ventilation using a low inspired O_2 concentration or added CO_2 to the fresh gas flow may be necessary to raise PVR. Systemic hypoperfusion, NEC, renal hypoperfusion, and feed intolerance are common problems. Excessive pulmonary blood flow and cardiac failure means that prolonged mechanical ventilation is necessary. As previously mentioned, a prolonged PGE_1 infusion is also not desirable because of complications including edema, apnea, and gastric outlet obstruction from gastric antral hyperplasia; although low concentrations maybe used (0.01 mcg/kg/min), a clear dose–response relationship between ductal size and PGE_1 dose has not been demonstrated. Size limitations are a considerable problem in newborns who require a Stage I palliation for conditions such as HLHS. It is often very difficult to balance systemic and pulmonary blood flow in an LBWN after a traditional Norwood operation with pulmonary blood flow supplied by a modified BT shunt; the low diastolic pressure from pulmonary runoff may lead to myocardial ischemia, CHF from volume overload to the ventricle, and systemic hypoperfusion. There are alternatives to the Norwood palliation that may be preferable in the LBWN. A modified Stage I operation using a right ventricle to PA shunt to supply pulmonary blood flow (Sano shunt) may allow better postoperative recovery because pulmonary blood flow occurs predominantly during ventricular systole and as such systemic diastolic pressure is higher. A further alternative to Stage I palliation in high-risk neonates (as LBWNs) is to use a hybrid Stage I strategy. This can be performed without needing cardiopulmonary bypass, and thereby obviate the significant risks associated with CPB in these patients related to technical limitations and neurological injury [75, 76]. The hybrid technique is performed in the catheterization laboratory, and via a median sternotomy both pulmonary arteries are banded, and the patents ductus arteriosus is stented via the main PA under fluoroscopic guidance. Although the hybrid approach reduces the initial surgical insult, there is no information on follow-up to date that any of the alternative surgical approaches described above leads to an improvement in longer-term survival and outcomes [76].

The potential for RDS is another important consideration for premature infants undergoing CPB. Lung injury postcardiac surgery is initiated by shear forces and from contact of blood with the nonendothelial surfaces of the extracorporeal circuit resulting in activation of a systemic inflammatory response [77]. However, surfactant depletion may also occur [78], and when combined with endothelial injury may contribute to pulmonary hypertension and altered lung compliance in the immediate postoperative period. However, there is no data to support prophylactic use of surfactant, pre- or post-CPB, and in our experience significant morbidity and lung injury secondary to RDS from surfactant depletion post-CPB is uncommon. Nonetheless, we have tended to use surfactant both intraoperatively and during the early postoperative period in premature infants (<36 weeks gestation) if there is evidence of RDS or altered lung compliance.

Necrotizing enterocolitis

CHD may be an important predisposing factor to developing NEC [79,80]. Using a case-controlled study of neonates admitted to a cardiac ICU over a 4-year period, McEllhaney et al. reported that cardiac defects with the potential for significant runoff from the systemic to pulmonary

circulation, specifically HLHS, aortopulmonary window, truncus arteriosus, and patients who had episodes of poor systemic perfusion, were more likely to develop NEC [81]. This supports the notion that one of the principle underlying mechanism of NEC in patients with CHD may be mesenteric ischemia. Nevertheless, other factors including the stress response induced by cardiac surgery, and CPB-related activation of inflammatory pathways and reperfusion also play a role [79]. Of note, the feeding history or the type of feed, the use of indwelling umbilical catheters, and cardiac catheterization did not correlate with the incidence of NEC.

Although most of the cases of NEC were successfully managed medically without surgical intervention, the duration of hospitalization was significantly prolonged in those with NEC. The incidence of NEC reported by McEllhaney was 3.3%, which was similar to an incidence of 3.5% reported by Cheng et al. [82]. In this study, surgical intervention in neonates with symptomatic congenital disease who develop NEC was retrospectively evaluated. Patients with CHD and diagnosis of NEC had a high mortality of 57%. However, those patients with proven NEC (without perforation) who underwent early cardiac surgery had a higher survival than in those managed medically and had delayed surgery (75% vs 44%).

Clinical signs of NEC include abdominal distention, feed intolerance, temperature and glucose instability, hemepositive or frank blood in the stool, abdominal guarding, and tenderness. Abdominal radiograph may demonstrate distention or an abnormal gas pattern, pneumatosis, portal air or intraperitoneal air consistent with perforation. Thrombocytopenia and leukocytoses are usually evident on blood examination. If NEC results in perforation or severe bowl ischemia, the neonate may develop sepsis syndrome with hypotension, third-space fluid loss, poor perfusion, and edema. On most occasions, patients can be treated medically with fluid restrictions, antibiotics, and vasoactive support; less frequently, laparotomy maybe necessary. The key to management, however, is to improve perfusion and O_2 delivery to the gut. Therefore, once hemodynamically stable without clinical signs of sepsis syndrome, early cardiac surgical intervention to improve splanchnic perfusion is preferable.

Intraventricular hemorrhage

The risk for intraventricular hemorrhage (IVH) decreases with increasing gestational age (risk at 23 weeks varies from 10 to 83%, at 25 weeks the incidence has decreased to 10–22%) [73]. IVH in the newborn infant is determined largely by cerebral immaturity and hemodynamic disturbances, thus even in the term infants with complex CDH there may be an increased incidence of IVH related to fluctuation in perfusion pressure, cerebral "steal" phenomena from excessive diastolic runoff, acidosis, and hypoxia. The diagnosis of IVH before surgery is important, because of the potential for extension of the hemorrhage during CPB related to anticoagulation, increased fibrinolytic activity, and changes in perfusion pressure.

There is no prospective data suggesting an increased risk for IVH in low-birth-weight infants if they undergo early repair and cardiopulmonary bypass [11,83]. As noted previously, there is increasing data from MRI examinations of the newborn brain in the perioperative period that supports the notion that the immature brain is vulnerable to injury related to cardiac surgery and CPB, particular in water-shed vascular distributions. It is unknown whether the premature or LBWN has an even higher risk, and longer-term neurodevelopmental outcomes are also unknown for this group of patients.

As a baseline, we routinely perform a cranial ultrasound in all premature (<35 weeks gestation) neonates prior to cardiac surgery. There are no clear guidelines as to how to manage neonates who have an IVH detected by ultrasound prior to surgery. Delaying surgery as long as possible is prudent to lower the risk for extension and further neurological injury. This may not be possible for some defects; however, in general our practice is to wait approximately 7–10 days before undergoing surgery and CPB.

Outcome

Several studies have evaluated the overall outcome of preterm and very low-birth-weight infants undergoing congenital heart surgery [8,11,72,84–87]. One of the earliest studies addressing patient size and outcome was by Pawade and Karl et al. [88]. They reported a hospital mortality of 16.5% for patients <2.5 kg, with risk factors including univentricular cardiac defects and duration of CPB. Chang et al. [72] reported a 70% survival rate in 100 patients with birth weight ≤2500 g with congenital heart lesions. Patients were divided into three groups: Group 1 ($n = 62$) had early surgical intervention with a survival rate for palliation of 78% and for primary repair of 82%. Group 2 ($n = 26$) had late surgical intervention (at a mean age 4.3 mo) after being managed medically prior to corrective surgery; 23% (6/26) died during medical management, and of the 20/26 undergoing surgery, 90% survived. In Group 3 ($n = 12$), no intervention was undertaken (lethal prognosis) and all died. The conclusion from this paper was that prolonged efforts to achieve medical stability and promote weight gain may not yield superior result compared to early surgical intervention. Rossi et al. [5] reported their experience of 30 patients <2 kg with CHD, citing a hospital survival of 83% and no difference in mortality rates based on age, weight, or type of surgical procedure, although premature infants

tended to have an increased risk for hospital mortality. Reddy et al. [11] reported 102 patients who underwent complete surgical repair for CHD (mean weight of 2100 g and 66 premature <36 weeks). Preoperative morbidity was more common among patients referred late for surgical correction. There were 10 early deaths and the survival at 1 year was 82%. Regression analysis revealed no correlation between weight and gestational age with survival, but the factors that did correlate included longer bypass time, complex anomalies, and diagnosis of truncus arteriosus. No patients suffered postbypass intracerebral hemorrhage.

These initial reports concentrated particularly on neonates <2.5–3 kg. However, the size limits have been decreased even further with recent reports of successful surgery in the very LBWN. Dees et al. [89] reported their retrospective experience of premature low-birth-weight infants undergoing cardiac surgery. The median gestational age of their patients were 33 weeks and mean birth weight 1.85 kg. They noted an increased risk for NEC by factor of 1.7, and an overall mortality twice that of patients in the neonatal ICU of similar age and size who did not have CHD. In our experience at Children's Hospital, Boston, evaluating 116 neonates weighing ≤2000 g at birth with CHD, early age at diagnosis, need for CPR before surgery, presence of multiple congenital anomalies, and more complex cardiac disease characterized the neonates with highest risk for death regardless of gestational age and birth weight. Reddy and Hanley [84] reported the outcomes of 20 infants <1.5 kg who underwent complete repair of congenital heart defects. Modifications of neonatal cardiopulmonary bypass techniques were necessary; however, there were only two early deaths unrelated to the surgical procedure. No patient had evidence of intracranial hemorrhage postbypass and at 14 months follow-up, there was only one late death. Repeat surgical and catheter reinventions were necessary in four patients. There were no neurological sequelae attributable to surgery. Finally, two recent studies in LBWNs once again confirmed that cardiac surgery can be performed in critically ill and LBWNs with acceptable mortality, although at the cost of increased morbidity; early outcome was independent of age, weight, prematurity and type of first intervention, and moreover primary correction appeared to result in an early survival benefit that remained constant over time [7,10].

A conclusion from these studies would seem to support the notion that low birth weight and prematurity do not appear to be limitations to successful repair of complex two-ventricle defects, although long-term follow-up is necessary to determine growth and development patterns. However, these studies are primarily single-center and have relatively small numbers that makes it difficult to draw definite conclusions. Perhaps providing a broader perspective is the recent analysis from the Society of Thoracic Surgeons Congenital Heart Database of the mortality in infants with low birth weight undergoing cardiac surgery [8]. The data collected from 32 centers were analyzed, and included 3022 infants from 0 to 90 days weighing 1–2.5 kg ($n = 517$) and 2505 infants greater than 2.5–4 kg. Infants weighing less than 2.5 kg had a significantly higher mortality following both two-ventricle repairs and single-ventricle palliation, including procedures such as coarctation of the aorta, total anomalous pulmonary venous connection repair, arterial switch operation, systemic to artery shunt, and the stage one palliation. Lower infant weight remained strongly associated with mortality risk after stratifying the population by Risk Adjustment in Congenital Heart Surgery score and Aristotle Basic Complexity levels.

As also demonstrated in this last analysis from Thoracic Surgeons Congenital Heart Database low birth weight and prematurity continue to be reported as significant risk factors for early mortality in patients with complex single-ventricle disease, in particular HLHS. Forbess et al. evaluated anatomic subtypes and preoperative physiologic variables associated with early mortality after Stage I/Norwood procedure and noted that aortic atresia, mitral atresia, a small ascending aorta, metabolic acidosis, and weight <3 kg all increased risk for early mortality [90]. Mahle et al, in a retrospective review of 840 patients who underwent Stage I surgery for HLHS, reported that surgical experience had a significant impact on outcome, with patients operated in the later surgical era having improved survival. In addition, weight <2.5 kg was associated with higher mortality in this study [91]. In a retrospective review by Weinstein et al. of 67 LBWNs with HLHS undergoing Stage I/Norwood palliation (14 patients <2 kg and 2 patients <1.5 kg), early mortality, defined as death within 30 days or before hospital discharge, was 51% (34/67) [92]. Although they were unable to identify patient, procedural, or time-related variables that correlated with increased mortality, the mortality rate in this group of patients remains higher than that reported for patients of larger size who undergo Stage I palliation. A recent single center outcome and risk analysis for the Norwood procedure by Stasik et al. demonstrated a 21% hospital mortality, with weight less than 2.5 kg and extracardiac abnormalities being independent risk factors [93].

Although the advances in surgical and cardiopulmonary bypass techniques and improved outcome as documented above, LBWN remain a challenging population both for surgeons and anesthesiologists. A reasonable conclusion from the above studies would appear that 2.5 kg is an important cut point, with LBWN and premature newborns <2.5 kg having a higher risk for mortality and morbidity regardless of the surgical procedure. In addition to size limitations, end-organ immaturity and co-morbidities are important contributing factors to adverse outcomes. Attention to detail is essential and the optimal management requires the close collaboration of a multidisciplinary perioperative team.

Fetal cardiac intervention and surgery

Advances in fetal echocardiography have improved accuracy in the diagnosis and evaluation of congenital heart lesions and functional pathology, which has in turn led to improved perinatal management and counseling. Studies have shown specifically for HLHS and transposition of the great arteries among other lesions [94,95] that prenatal diagnosis does result in an improved preoperative condition and possibly decreased mortality. However, there are few studies that document the natural history of cardiac growth and physiological changes in individual fetal cardiac malformations or their timing of impact during fetal growth, and we know little about causes for these lesions whether it might be genetic or environmental factors. Unfortunately, there is no specific animal model of cardiac malformations that is similar to the human fetus to provide insights into pathophysiology and effect on development, nor to aid in developing management strategies. However, we know that the normal development of the heart and great vessels in the fetus require normal blood flow patterns. For example, changes in ventricular growth and function can be seen on serial fetal echocardiograms in a fetus with aortic or pulmonary valve stenosis [96] leading to ventricular hypoplasia, fibrosis, and often abnormalities of coronary, systemic arterial, and pulmonary venous morphology [97]. In a worst-case scenario, fetal critical aortic stenosis may progress to HLHS in a proportion of cases, resulting in univentricular circulation. The major reason for intervention in the fetus, therefore, is to improve blood flow patterns to allow for additional in utero development of the heart and improve postnatal outcomes. This "flow theory," at least in part, demonstrates that normal flow across the foramen ovale, atrioventricular, and semilunar valves contributes to normal growth of the ventricles.

The recognition that certain CHD can evolve in utero, and that early intervention may improve outcome has led to the evolution of fetal intervention. To date the main target lesions for fetal intervention are the obstruction of left or right semilunar valves that if not relieved may lead to pulmonary atresia with intact ventricular septum (PA/IVS) [98–100] or severe aortic stenosis, which if not relieved may lead to HLHS [101–104]. The documented transition from normal-sized LV to HLHS in fetuses with aortic stenosis seems to occur in the second or early third semester [105–107], therefore at Children's Hospital, Boston, balloon dilation of the stenotic aortic

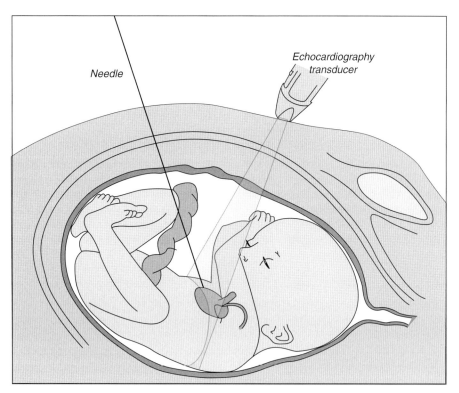

Figure 14.1 Ideal fetal position for fetal intervention. Fetal left chest is anterior and pathway from the maternal abdomen to LV apex is unobstructed (Courtesy of Dr A. Marshall, drawing by E. Flynn)

valve in a fetus is performed between the 21st and the 29th week of the pregnancy. Another fetal intervention involving balloon septostomy of a nearly or completely intact atrial septum in HLHS [98,101,108–110] has been used to lower pulmonary venous pressure and possibly prevent or alter the development of pulmonary hypertension and hydrops fetalis [111–113]. Fetal pacing has been attempted where the fetus is too premature to be delivered and other medical therapies have failed to control heart failure and hydrops [114], but there is yet no successful medium- or long-term outcome in humans.

Fetal cardiac intervention should be considered as innovative therapy. A fetal cardiac intervention program must be multidisciplinary with collaboration between, neonatologists, obstetricians (specialized in prenatal diagnosis and fetal medicine), pediatric cardiologists, and pediatric anesthesiologists (pediatric and obstetric). The procedures are performed in the hospital where the mother is the patient, to provide the best care for the pregnant woman.

A technique used by our fetal intervention team is described. It includes positioning the pregnant mother supine with left lateral displacement and rapid sequence general endothracheal anesthesia is induced with thiopenthal or propofol. General anesthesia is maintained with desflurane in 100% oxygen, intermittent opioids, and

muscle relaxant. Ephedrine is used if needed to maintain maternal blood pressure within 20% of awake baseline level. The mother's abdomen is prepped and draped, and after determining the weight of the fetus and using ultrasound guidance through the uterus, the obstetrician injects intramuscular atropine (20 µg/kg), vecuronium (0.2 mg/kg), and fentanyl (50 µg/kg) into the thigh of the fetus to ensure that the fetus is anesthetized and immobile. The mother is monitored according to ASA guidelines, and the fetus is monitored with ultrasound and heart rate. Under continuous ultrasound guidance, an 18- or a 19-ga cannula and stylet needle is passed through the maternal abdomen, uterine wall, and fetal chest wall into the fetal heart (either LV, RV, or RA, depending on the procedure to be performed) (see Figure 14.1). Balloon positioning for inflation is based on external measurements and ultrasound imaging and inflated when in the correct position [104]. Fetal hemodynamic changes including bradycardia and ventricular dysfunction may occur. From 2000 to 2006, 83 fetuses underwent cardiac intervention at Children's Hospital, Boston, and included ventricular access in 63 patients, atrial access in 17, and both in 3. Fetal hemodynamic instability was evident in 37 patients (45%), 11 of whom had severe hemodynamic instability with bradycardia and ventricular dysfunction lasting more than 10 minutes. Ventricular access was the only independent risk factor for hemodynamic instability. Fetal resuscitation was performed with intramuscular or intracardiac epinephrine and atropine. The heart rate and ventricular function normalized in all fetuses. Overall five fetuses died within 1 day of the cardiac intervention, four of whom had had hemodynamic instability during the procedure. Hemopericardium may be the cause for fetal demise in a subset of patients [115]. All patients are followed postintervention until birth with periodically ultrasound to monitor growth and function of the heart. The longer-term benefits of fetal interventions are still to be determined and there may be significant ethical concerns as two individuals (i.e., the mother and fetus) are now at risk for an adverse event.

Fetal cardiac surgery is not currently a realistic therapeutic option for critical CHD, it is nevertheless a future direction for management. The progress and future potential of in utero cardiac repair may enable salvage of a life-threatening in utero condition and optimize long-term outcome by altering in utero cardiac development.

References

1. Jonas RA (1998) Optimal pH strategy for cardiopulmonary bypass in neonates, infants and children. Perfusion 13:377–387.
2. Newburger JW, Jonas RA, Soul J, et al. (2008) Randomized trial of hematocrit 25% versus 35% during hypothermic cardiopulmonary bypass in infant heart surgery. J Thorac Cardiovasc Surg 135:347–354.
3. Wypij D, Newburger JW, Rappaport LA, et al. (2003) The effect of duration of deep hypothermic circulatory arrest in infant heart surgery on late neurodevelopment: the Boston Circulatory Arrest Trial. J Thorac Cardiovasc Surg 126:1397–1403.
4. Gaynor JW, Wernovsky G, Jarvik GP, et al. (2007) Patient characteristics are important determinants of neurodevelopmental outcome at one year of age after neonatal and infant cardiac surgery. J Thorac Cardiovasc Surg 133:1344–1353.
5. Rossi AF, Seiden HS, Sadeghi AM, et al. (1998) The outcome of cardiac operations in infants weighing two kilograms or less. J Thorac Cardiovasc Surg 116:28–35.
6. Abrishamchian R, Kanhai D, Zwets E, et al. (2006) Low birth weight or diagnosis, which is a higher risk?—A meta-analysis of observational studies. Eur J Cardiothorac Surg 30:700–705.
7. Bove T, Francois K, De Groote K, et al. (2004) Outcome analysis of major cardiac operations in low weight neonates. Ann Thorac Surg 78:181–187.
8. Curzon CL, Milford-Beland S, Li JS, et al. (2008) Cardiac surgery in infants with low birth weight is associated with increased mortality: analysis of the Society of Thoracic Surgeons Congenital Heart Database. J Thorac Cardiovasc Surg 135:546–551.
9. Dimmick S, Walker K, Badawi N, et al. (2007) Outcomes following surgery for CHD in low-birthweight infants. J Paediatr Child Health 43:370–375.
10. Oppido G, Napoleone CP, Formigari R, et al. (2004) Outcome of cardiac surgery in low birth weight and premature infants. Eur J Cardiothorac Surg 26:44–53.
11. Reddy VM, McElhinney DB, Sagrado T, et al. (1999) Results of 102 cases of complete repair of congenital heart defects in patients weighing 700 to 2500 grams. J Thorac Cardiovasc Surg 117:324–331.
12. Anand KJ, Sippell WG, Aynsley-Green A (1987) Randomised trial of fentanyl anaesthesia in preterm babies undergoing surgery: effects on the stress response. Lancet 1 (1):62–66.
13. Friedman WF (1972) The intrinsic physiologic properties of the developing heart. Prog Cardiovasc Dis 15:87–111.
14. Baum VC, Palmisano BW (1997) The immature heart and anesthesia. Anesthesiology 87:1529–1548.
15. Bove AA, Santamore WP (1981) Ventricular interdependence. Prog Cardiovasc Dis 23:365–388.
16. Berman W (1978) The hemodynamics of shunts in CHD. In: Johansen K, Burggren WW (eds) Cardiovascular Shunts: Phylogenetic, Ontogenetic, and Clinical Aspects. Raven Press, New York, pp. 399–410.
17. Keens TG, Bryan AC, Levison H, Ianuzzo CD (1978) Developmental pattern of muscle fiber types in human ventilatory muscles. J Appl Physiol 44:909–913.
18. Mansell A, Bryan C, Levison H (1972) Airway closure in children. J Appl Physiol 33:711–714.
19. Mills AN, Haworth SG (1991) Greater permeability of the neonatal lung. Postnatal changes in surface charge and biochemistry of porcine pulmonary capillary endothelium. J Thorac Cardiovasc Surg 101:909–916.
20. Feltes TF, Hansen TN (1989) Effects of an aorticopulmonary shunt on lung fluid balance in the young lamb. Pediatr Res 1 (26):94–97.
21. Wernovsky G, Rubenstein SD, Spray TL (2001) Cardiac surgery in the low-birth weight neonate. New approaches. Clin Perinatol 28:249–264.
22. Wernovsky G, Wypij D, Jonas RA, et al. (1995) Postoperative course and hemodynamic profile after the arterial switch operation in neonates and infants. A comparison of low-flow cardiopulmonary bypass and circulatory arrest. Circulation 92:2226–2235.
23. Mackie AS, Booth KL, Newburger JW, et al. (2005) A randomized, double-blind, placebo-controlled pilot trial of triiodothyronine in neonatal heart surgery. J Thorac Cardiovasc Surg 130:810–816.
24. de Ferranti S, Gauvreau K, Hickey PR, et al. (2004) Intraoperative hyperglycemia during infant cardiac surgery is not associated with adverse neurodevelopmental outcomes at 1, 4, and 8 years. Anesthesiology 100:1345–1352.
25. Chaturvedi RR, Shore DF, White PA, et al. (1999) Modified ultrafiltration improves global left ventricular systolic function after open-heart surgery in infants and children. Eur J Cardiothorac Surg 15:742–746.
26. Elliott M (1999) Modified ultrafiltration and open heart surgery in children. Paediatr Anaesth 9:1–5.

27. Elliott MJ (1993) Ultrafiltration and modified ultrafiltration in pediatric open heart operations. Ann Thorac Surg 56:1518–1522.

28. Li J, Hoschtitzky A, Allen ML, et al. (2004) An analysis of oxygen consumption and oxygen delivery in euthermic infants after cardiopulmonary bypass with modified ultrafiltration. Ann Thorac Surg 78:1389–1396.

29. Ungerleider RM, Shen I (2003) Optimizing response of the neonate and infant to cardiopulmonary bypass. Semin Thorac Cardiovasc Surg Pediatr Card Surg Annu 6:140–146.

30. Journois D, Israel-Biet D, Pouard P, et al. (1996) High-volume, zero-balanced hemofiltration to reduce delayed inflammatory response to cardiopulmonary bypass in children. Anesthesiology 85:965–976.

31. Rodriguez RA, Ruel M, Broecker L, Cornel G (2005) High flow rates during modified ultrafiltration decrease cerebral blood flow velocity and venous oxygen saturation in infants. Ann Thorac Surg 80:22–28.

32. Keenan HT, Thiagarajan R, Stephens KE, et al. (2000) Pulmonary function after modified venovenous ultrafiltration in infants: a prospective, randomized trial. J Thorac Cardiovasc Surg 119:501–505.

33. Sorof JM, Stromberg D, Brewer ED, et al. (1999) Early initiation of peritoneal dialysis after surgical repair of CHD. Pediatr Nephrol 13:641–645.

34. Dittrich S, Vogel M, Dahnert I, et al. (2000) Acute hemodynamic effects of post cardiotomy peritoneal dialysis in neonates and infants. Intensive Care Med 26:101–104.

35. Bokesch PM, Kapural MB, Mossad EB, et al. (2000) Do peritoneal catheters remove pro-inflammatory cytokines after cardiopulmonary bypass in neonates? Ann Thorac Surg 70:639–643.

36. Hickey PR, Andersen NP (1987) Deep hypothermic circulatory arrest: a review of pathophysiology and clinical experience as a basis for anesthetic management. J Cardiothorac Anesth 1:137–155.

37. Newburger JW, Jonas RA, Wernovsky G, et al. (1993) A comparison of the perioperative neurologic effects of hypothermic circulatory arrest versus low-flow cardiopulmonary bypass in infant heart surgery. N Engl J Med 329:1057–1064.

38. Bellinger DC, Jonas RA, Rappaport LA, et al. (1995) Developmental and neurologic status of children after heart surgery with hypothermic circulatory arrest or low-flow cardiopulmonary bypass. N Engl J Med 332:549–555.

39. du Plessis AJ (1997) Neurologic complications of cardiac disease in the newborn. Clin Perinatol 24:807–826.

40. Greeley WJ, Kern FH, Ungerleider RM, et al. (1991) The effect of hypothermic cardiopulmonary bypass and total circulatory arrest on cerebral metabolism in neonates, infants, and children. J Thorac Cardiovasc Surg 101:783–794.

41. Slogoff S, Girgis KZ, Keats AS (1982) Etiologic factors in neuropsychiatric complications associated with cardiopulmonary bypass. Anesth Analg 61:903–911.

42. Bellinger DC, Wernovsky G, Rappaport LA, et al. (1991) Cognitive development of children following early repair of transposition of the great arteries using deep hypothermic circulatory arrest. Pediatrics 87:701–707.

43. Kern FH, Jonas RA, Mayer JE, Jr., et al. (1992) Temperature monitoring during CPB in infants: does it predict efficient brain cooling? Ann Thorac Surg 54:749–754.

44. Mault JR, Whitaker EG, Heinle JS, et al. (1994) Cerebral metabolic effects of sequential periods of hypothermic circulatory arrest. Ann Thorac Surg 57:96–100.

45. Rogers AT, Prough DS, Roy RC, et al. (1992) Cerebrovascular and cerebral metabolic effects of alterations in perfusion flow rate during hypothermic cardiopulmonary bypass in man. J Thorac Cardiovasc Surg 103:363–368.

46. Shin'oka T, Shum-Tim D, Jonas RA, et al. (1996) Higher hematocrit improves cerebral outcome after deep hypothermic circulatory arrest. J Thorac Cardiovasc Surg 112:1610–1620.

47. Shin'oka T, Shum-Tim D, Laussen PC, et al. (1998) Effects of oncotic pressure and hematocrit on outcome after hypothermic circulatory arrest. Ann Thorac Surg 65:155–164.

48. Wypij D, Jonas RA, Bellinger DC, et al. (2008) The effect of hematocrit during hypothermic cardiopulmonary bypass in infant heart surgery: results from the combined Boston hematocrit trials. J Thorac Cardiovasc Surg 135:355–360.

49. Jonas RA, Wypij D, Roth SJ, et al. (2003) The influence of hemodilution on outcome after hypothermic cardiopulmonary bypass: results of a randomized trial in infants. J Thorac Cardiovasc Surg 126:1765–1774.

50. Fraser CD, Jr., Andropoulos DB (2008) Principles of antegrade cerebral perfusion during arch reconstruction in newborns/infants. Semin Thorac Cardiovasc Surg Pediatr Card Surg Annu 61–68.

51. Nelson DP, Andropoulos DB, Fraser CD, Jr. (2008) Perioperative neuroprotective strategies. Semin Thorac Cardiovasc Surg Pediatr Card Surg Annu 49–56.

52. Petit CJ, Rome JJ, Wernovsky G, et al. (2009) Preoperative brain injury in transposition of the great arteries is associated with oxygenation and time to surgery, not balloon atrial septostomy. Circulation 119:709–716.

53. Johnston MV (2007) CHD and brain injury. N Engl J Med 357:1971–1973.

54. Miller SP, McQuillen PS (2007) Neurology of CHD: insight from brain imaging. Arch Dis Child Fetal Neonatal Ed 92:F435–F437.

55. Miller SP, McQuillen PS, Hamrick S, et al. (2007) Abnormal brain development in newborns with CHD. N Engl J Med 357:1928–1938.

56. Shew SB, Jaksic T (1999) The metabolic needs of critically ill children and neonates. Semin Pediatr Surg 8:131–139.

57. Anand KJ, Sippell WG, Schofield NM, Aynsley-Green A (1988) Does halothane anaesthesia decrease the metabolic and endocrine stress responses of newborn infants undergoing operation? Br Med J 296:668–672.

58. Yaster M (1987) The dose response of fentanyl in neonatal anesthesia. Anesthesiology 66:433–435.

59. Wood M, Shand DG, Wood AJ (1980) The sympathetic response to profound hypothermia and circulatory arrest in infants. Can Anaesth Soc J 27:125–131.

60. Anand KJ, Hansen DD, Hickey PR (1990) Hormonal-metabolic stress responses in neonates undergoing cardiac surgery. Anesthesiology 73:661–670.

61. Anand KJ, Hickey PR (1992) Halothane-morphine compared with high-dose sufentanil for anesthesia and postoperative analgesia in neonatal cardiac surgery. N Engl J Med 326:1–9.

62. Gruber EM, Laussen PC, Casta A, et al. (2001) Stress response in infants undergoing cardiac surgery: a randomized study of fentanyl bolus, fentanyl infusion, and fentanyl-midazolam infusion. Anesth Analg 92:882–890.

63. Kussman BD, Gruber EM, Zurakowski D, et al. (2001) Bispectral index monitoring during infant cardiac surgery: relationship of BIS to the stress response and plasma fentanyl levels. Paediatr Anaesth 11:663–669.

64. Firmin RK, Bouloux P, Allen P, et al. (1985) Sympathoadrenal function during cardiac operations in infants with the technique of surface cooling, limited cardiopulmonary bypass, and circulatory arrest. J Thorac Cardiovasc Surg 90:729–735.

65. Ratcliffe JM, Wyse RK, Hunter S, et al. (1988) The role of the priming fluid in the metabolic response to cardiopulmonary bypass in children of less than 15 kg body weight undergoing open-heart surgery. Thorac Cardiovasc Surg 36:65–74.

66. Pollock EM, Pollock JC, Jamieson MP, et al. (1988) Adrenocortical hormone concentrations in children during cardiopulmonary bypass with and without pulsatile flow. Br J Anaesth 60:536–541.

67. Laussen PC, Murphy JA, Zurakowski D, et al. (2001) Bispectral index monitoring in children undergoing mild hypothermic cardiopulmonary bypass. Paediatr Anaesth 11:567–573.

68. Desborough JP (2000) The stress response to trauma and surgery. Br J Anaesth 85:109–117.

69. Naito Y, Tamai S, Shingu K, et al. (1992) Responses of plasma adrenocorticotropic hormone, cortisol, and cytokines during and after upper abdominal surgery. Anesthesiology 77:426–431.

70. Hansen DD, Hickey PR (1986) Anesthesia for HLHS: use of high-dose fentanyl in 30 neonates. Anesth Analg 65:127–132.

71. Odegard KC, DiNardo JA, Kussman BD, et al. (2007) The frequency of anesthesia-related cardiac arrests in patients with CHD undergoing cardiac surgery. Anesth Analg 105:335–343.

72. Chang AC, Hanley FL, Lock JE, et al. (1994) Management and outcome of low birthweight neonates with congenital heart disease. J Pediatr 124:461–466.

73. Spaeth JP, O'Hara IB, Kurth CD (1998) Anesthesia for the micropremie. Semin Perinatol 22:390–401.

74. McMahon CJ, Penny DJ, Nelson DP, et al. (2005) Preterm infants with CHD and bronchopulmonary dysplasia: postoperative course and outcome after cardiac surgery. Pediatrics 116:423–430.

75. Bacha EA, Daves S, Hardin J, et al. (2006) Single-ventricle palliation for high-risk neonates: the emergence of an alternative hybrid stage I strategy. J Thorac Cardiovasc Surg 131:163–171.

76. Pizarro C, Murdison KA, Derby CD, Radtke W (2008) Stage II reconstruction after hybrid palliation for high-risk patients with a single ventricle. Ann Thorac Surg 85:1382–1388.

77. Griese M (1999) Pulmonary surfactant in health and human lung diseases: state of the art. Eur Respir J 13:1455–1476.

78. McGowan FX, Jr., Ikegami M, del Nido PJ, et al. (1993) Cardiopulmonary bypass significantly reduces surfactant activity in children. J Thorac Cardiovasc Surg 106:968–977.

79. Giannone PJ, Luce WA, Nankervis CA, et al. (2008) Necrotizing enterocolitis in neonates with congenital heart disease. Life Sci 82:341–347.

80. Nankervis CA, Giannone PJ, Reber KM (2008) The neonatal intestinal vasculature: contributing factors to necrotizing enterocolitis. Semin Perinatol 32:83–91.

81. McElhinney DB, Hedrick HL, Bush DM, et al. (2000) Necrotizing enterocolitis in neonates with congenital heart disease: risk factors and outcomes. Pediatrics 106:1080–1087.

82. Cheng W, Leung MP, Tam PK (1999) Surgical intervention in necrotizing enterocolitis in neonates with symptomatic congenital heart disease. Pediatr Surg Int 15:492–495

83. Krull F, Latta K, Hoyer PF, et al. (1994) Cerebral ultrasonography before and after cardiac surgery in infants. Pediatr Cardiol 15:159–162.

84. Reddy VM, Hanley FL (2000) Cardiac surgery in infants with very low birth weight. Semin Pediatr Surg 9:91–95.

85. Bove EL (1998) Current status of staged reconstruction for hypoplastic left heart syndrome. Pediatr Cardiol 19:308–315.

86. Borowski A, Schickendantz S, Mennicken U, Korb H (1997) Open heart interventions in premature low- and very-low-birth-weight neonates: risk profile and ethical considerations. Thorac Cardiovasc Surg 45:238–241.

87. Beyens T, Biarent D, Bouton JM, et al. (1998) Cardiac surgery with extracorporeal circulation in 23 infants weighing 2500 g or less: short and intermediate term outcome. Eur J Cardiothorac Surg 14:165–172.

88. Pawade A, Waterson K, Laussen P, et al. (1993) Cardiopulmonary bypass in neonates weighing less than 2.5 kg: analysis of the risk factors for early and late mortality. J Card Surg 1 (8):1–8.

89. Dees E, Lin H, Cotton RB, et al. (2000) Outcome of preterm infants with congenital heart disease. J Pediatr 137:653–659.

90. Forbess JM, Cook N, Roth SJ, et al. (1995) Ten-year institutional experience with palliative surgery for hypoplastic left heart syndrome. Risk factors related to stage I mortality. Circulation 92:II262–II266

91. Mahle WT, Spray TL, Wernovsky G, et al. (2000) Survival after reconstructive surgery for hypoplastic left heart syndrome: a 15-year experience from a single institution. Circulation 102:III136–III141.

92. Weinstein S, Gaynor JW, Bridges ND, et al. (1999) Early survival of infants weighing 2.5 kilograms or less undergoing first-stage reconstruction for hypoplastic left heart syndrome. Circulation 100:II167–II170.

93. Stasik CN, Gelehrter S, Goldberg CS, et al. (2006) Current outcomes and risk factors for the Norwood procedure. J Thorac Cardiovasc Surg 131:412–417.

94. Kumar RK, Newburger JW, Gauvreau K, et al. (1999) Comparison of outcome when hypoplastic left heart syndrome and transposition of the great arteries are diagnosed prenatally versus when diagnosis of these two conditions is made only postnatally. Am J Cardiol 83:1649–1653.

95. Chang AC, Huhta JC, Yoon GY, et al. (1991) Diagnosis, transport, and outcome in fetuses with left ventricular outflow tract obstruction. J Thorac Cardiovasc Surg 102:841–848.

96. Acharya G, Archer N, Huhta JC (2007) Functional assessment of the evolution of CHD in utero. Curr Opin Pediatr 19:533–537.

97. Gardiner HM (2005) Response of the fetal heart to changes in load: from hyperplasia to heart failure. Heart 91:871–873.

98. Matsui H, Gardiner H (2007) Fetal intervention for cardiac disease: the cutting edge of perinatal care. Semin Fetal Neonatal Med 12:482–489.

99. Galindo A, Gutierrez-Larraya F, Velasco JM, de la Fuente P (2006) Pulmonary balloon valvuloplasty in a fetus with critical pulmonary stenosis/atresia with intact ventricular septum and heart failure. Fetal Diagn Ther 21:100–104.

100. Gardiner HM, Kumar S (2005) Fetal cardiac interventions. Clin Obstet Gynecol 48:956–963.

101. Huhta J, Quintero RA, Suh E, Bader R (2004) Advances in fetal cardiac intervention. Curr Opin Pediatr 16:487–493.

102. Kohl T, Sharland G, Allan LD, et al. (2000) World experience of percutaneous ultrasound-guided balloon valvuloplasty in human fetuses with severe aortic valve obstruction. Am J Cardiol 85:1230–1233.

103. Suh E, Quintessenza J, Huhta J, Quintero R (2006) How to grow a heart: fibreoptic guided fetal aortic valvotomy. Cardiol Young 16 (Suppl 1):43–46.

104. Tworetzky W, Marshall AC (2004) Fetal interventions for cardiac defects. Pediatr Clin North Am 51:1503–1513.

105. Hornberger LK, Barrea C (2001) Diagnosis, natural history, and outcome of fetal heart disease. Semin Thorac Cardiovasc Surg Pediatr Card Surg Annu 4:229–243.

106. Hornberger LK, Sanders SP, Rein AJ, et al. (1995) Left heart obstructive lesions and left ventricular growth in the midtrimester fetus. A longitudinal study. Circulation 92:1531–1538.

107. Simpson JM, Sharland GK (1997) Natural history and outcome of aortic stenosis diagnosed prenatally. Heart 77:205–210.

108. Gardiner HM (2008) In-utero intervention for severe congenital heart disease. Best Pract Res Clin Obstet Gynaecol 22:49–61.

109. Marshall AC, Levine J, Morash D, et al. (2008) Results of in utero atrial septoplasty in fetuses with hypoplastic left heart syndrome. Prenat Diagn 28:1023–1028.

110. Marshall AC, Van Der Velde ME, Tworetzky W, et al. (2004) Creation of an atrial septal defect in utero for fetuses with hypoplastic left heart syndrome and intact or highly restrictive atrial septum. Circulation 110:253–258.

111. Michelfelder E, Gomez C, Border W, et al. (2005) Predictive value of fetal pulmonary venous flow patterns in identifying the need for atrial septoplasty in the newborn with hypoplastic left ventricle. Circulation 112:2974–2979.

112. Taketazu M, Barrea C, Smallhorn JF, et al. (2004) Intrauterine pulmonary venous flow and restrictive foramen ovale in fetal HLHS. J Am Coll Cardiol 43:1902–1907.

113. Vlahos AP, Lock JE, McElhinney DB, Van Der Velde ME (2004) Hypoplastic left heart syndrome with intact or highly restrictive atrial septum: outcome after neonatal transcatheter atrial septostomy. Circulation 109:2326–2330.

114. Assad RS, Zielinsky P, Kalil R, et al. (2003) New lead for in utero pacing for fetal congenital heart block. J Thorac Cardiovasc Surg 126:300–302.

115. Mizrahi-Arnaud A, Tworetzky W, Bulich LA, et al. (2007) Pathophysiology, management, and outcomes of fetal hemodynamic instability during prenatal cardiac intervention. Pediatr Res 62:325–330.

15 Approach to the teenaged and adult patient

Victor C. Baum, M.D. and Duncan G. de Souza, M.D.

University of Virginia, Charlottesville, Virginia, USA

Introduction

Advances in cardiac surgery and perioperative care in the past several decades have meant that over 85% of infants born with congenital heart disease (CHD) are now expected to reach adulthood. There are, though, relatively few conditions for which surgical repair is completely and uniformly totally curative for the entire population [1]. Cure requires that normal cardiovascular function be achieved and maintained, life expectancy is normal, and further medical evaluation for CHD is not required. It is estimated that there are currently over 500,000 adults in the USA with CHD, 55% of whom remain at moderate–high risk, and over 115,000 of whom have truly complex disease [2]. Put another way several years ago, "the number of adults with CHD now equals the number of children

with CHD" [3] and in fact the number of adults with CHD now exceeds the number of children.

These patients bring with them problems related to complex postoperative anatomy and physiology that will not be familiar to physicians used to caring for adults, but also the medical problems that accrue with aging, which will not be familiar to physicians used to caring for children. This problem has resulted in two American College of Cardiology sponsored Bethesda Conferences in the past several years, most recently in 2001 [3]. These panels have recommended the establishment of regionalized adult congenital heart centers that consist of a full coterie of professionals educated and experienced in the care of the adult with CHD. Adult congenital heart fellowships as an additional period of training after adult cardiology fellowships are being offered. A specific recommendation was that noncardiac surgery on CHD patients with moderate–complex disease be performed at an adult CHD center with the consultation of an anesthesiologist experienced with CHD [3, 4]. A recent Practice Guideline published by the American College of Cardiology and American Heart Association is an excellent,

Anesthesia for Congenital Heart Disease 2nd edition. Edited by Dean Andropoulos, Stephen Stayer, Isobel Russell and Emad Mossad.
© 2010 Blackwell Publishing.

comprehensive guide to the management of adults with CHD, including perioperative management [5].

The field of CHD in adults is in actuality two distinct fields, with some overlap. In much of the world, patients live without access to pediatric cardiac or surgical services. These adolescents and adults with CHD may well have had only palliative surgery, and more likely no surgery. These patients have the many potential noncardiac complications of longstanding cyanotic or acyanotic heart disease (described below) superimposed on the natural history of the underlying cardiac disease. In the medically advanced world, where cardiac surgery is available and financially practical for most of the population, practitioners are faced with the sequelae of the unnatural history of surgical repair, and rarely encounter a patient who has been only palliated or remains unrepaired.

This chapter reviews the organ system sequelae of longstanding CHD, both noncardiac and cardiac, and the anatomy, pathophysiology, and surgical approach to the common lesions. Particular attention is given to the patient with single ventricle physiology after the Fontan operation, a large and growing segment of the adolescent and adult congenital heart population. With the routine survival of children with CHD, additional attention is also given to issues of pregnancy and delivery, as anesthesiologists are intimately involved in this care. Finally, perioperative and anesthetic outcomes are reviewed, and specific recommendations made for the anesthetic approach to adults with CHD.

Noncardiac sequelae of longstanding CHD

Pulmonary sequelae

Lesions resulting in increased pulmonary blood flow or in obstruction to free pulmonary venous drainage can cause increased interstitial fluid, with decreased pulmonary compliance [6], and increased work of breathing. Patients with cyanotic disease and chronic hypoxemia have increased minute ventilation with normal $PaCO_2$ [7]. Cyanotic patients appear to have a normal ventilatory response to hypercarbia but a blunted response to hypoxemia [8,9] that resolves after surgical correction [10]. End-tidal PCO_2 underestimates $PaCO_2$ in cyanotic patients with decreased, normal, or increased pulmonary blood flow [11].

Although enlarged, hypertensive pulmonary arteries or an enlarged left atrium can on occasion entrap or obstruct a bronchus causing atelectasis, pneumonia, or focal emphysema in children, this is rare in adults. Hemoptysis is a finding of late stage Eisenmenger physiology, and thrombosis of upper lobe pulmonary arteries can occur in patients with Eisenmenger physiology and erythrocytosis

[12]. Prior thoracic surgery may have resulted in phrenic nerve injury.

The incidence of scoliosis in CHD patients, as high as 19%, is more common in children with cyanotic CHD, and may develop in adolescence, years following surgical correction of cyanosis [13]. The interaction of cyanosis and early lateral thoracotomy in the development of scoliosis remains unclear. Although rare, scoliosis can be severe enough to impact pulmonary function.

The most serious complication of longstanding pulmonary hyperemia is the development of Eisenmenger physiology (see below). The age at which this develops depends on the underlying physiology (earlier at high altitude, for example), and also the level of the shunt. Patients with atrial level shunts may not develop evidence of pulmonary vascular disease until late middle age.

Hematologic sequelae

Hematologic sequelae are predominantly a consequence of longstanding cyanotic CHD and include abnormalities of both red cell regulation and hemostasis. Chronic hypoxemia results in increased renal erythropoietin production. There is a lack of association between oxygen saturation, 2,3-diphosphoglycerate, and red cell mass [14]. The oxygen–hemoglobin dissociation curve is usually normal or minimally right shifted. Most patients establish an equilibrium state. They have a stable hematocrit and are iron replete. Some patients, however, develop excessive hematocrits and are iron deficient, resulting in a hyperviscous state. Symptoms of hyperviscosity are rare at hematocrits <65% if the patient is not iron deficient (Table 15.1). Although it has been taught that iron deficient red cells are less deformable than iron replete red cells and will cause increased viscosity for the same hematocrit, there is conflicting evidence [15]. Iron deficiency can be related to inappropriate, repeated phlebotomies in an attempt to reduce hematocrit and the use of routine or prophylactic phlebotomy to decrease the hematocrit is not indicated [16]. The other indication for phlebotomy is to improve perioperative hemostasis in the face of a high hematocrit [17]. Therapy is recommended for temporary relief of *symptomatic* hyperviscosity only (not due

Table 15.1 Signs and symptoms of hyperviscosity syndrome

Headache
Faintness, dizziness, light headedness
Blurred or double vision
Fatigue
Myalgias, muscle weakness
Paresthesias of fingers, toes, or lips
Depressed mentation, a feeling of dissociation

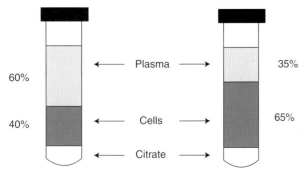

60%

40%

35%

65%

← Plasma →

← Cells →

← Citrate →

Figure 15.1 The effect of a fixed amount of citrate anticoagulant in tubes of blood with normal and increased hematocrit. The fixed anticoagulant volume combined with decreased plasma volume in the erythrocytotic blood results in artifactual elevation of the prothrombin and partial thromboplastin times. Similarly, although the concentrations of platelets are identical in both samples of *plasma*, the platelet count *per milliliter of whole blood* (which is reported by the laboratory) will be lower in erythrocytotic blood (Reproduced and used with permission from Reference [18])

to dehydration). In fact, true, symptomatic hyperviscosity syndrome is quite uncommon [16]. Symptoms usually regress within 24 hours of a partial isovolumic exchange transfusion. It is rare for adult patients to require removal of more than one unit of blood. Phlebotomized blood can be banked for autologous perioperative transfusion if needed. Prolonged preoperative fasting should be specifically avoided in these patients, as rapid increases in hematocrit can accompany dehydration. Each volume of erythrocytotic blood contains less plasma than normal blood (Figure 15.1).

Blood cells will not necessarily be microcytic and hypochromic in the face of erythrocytosis and iron deficiency, possibly due to the concurrent presence of folate or B vitamin deficiencies [19]. Treatment with oral iron should be undertaken with care, as rapid increases in hematocrit can ensue.

A variety of hemostatic abnormalities have been described in cyanotic patients [12]. Bleeding diatheses are uncommon at hematocrits less than 65%, although surgical bleeding can occur. Generally, the degree of the bleeding diathesis mirrors the hematocrit. Platelet counts are typically low normal, and are occasionally low, but bleeding is not related to the thrombocytopenia. When corrected for the decreased plasma volume in each blood sample, total plasma platelet count is closer to normal (Figure 15.1). Abnormalities of platelet function have also been reported [20]. Patients with synthetic vascular anastomoses or low-pressure conduits are often maintained on chronic antiplatelet therapy.

Abnormalities of both the intrinsic and extrinsic coagulation pathways with abnormalities of a variety of specific clotting factors have been inconsistently described in

cyanotic patients. Fibrinolytic pathways are normal [21]. On occasion, patients with both cyanotic and acyanotic CHD have been described with deficiencies of the largest von Willebrand factor multimers that have corrected following corrective cardiac surgery [22].

The decreased plasma volume in erythrocytotic blood may cause spurious results of the prothrombin and partial thromboplastin times. The fixed amount of anticoagulant in the sample tube presumes a normal plasma volume and may be excessive for an erythrocytotic sample (Figure 15.1). If informed about the patient's hematocrit, the clinical laboratory can provide an appropriate tube. Correcting to an idealized hematocrit of 45%, the appropriate amount of citrate can be added to the tube as follows:

$$\text{Millileter citrate} = (0.1 \times \text{blood volume collected}) \times \left[\frac{100 - \text{patient's hematocrit}}{55} \right]$$

Due to the excessive hemoglobin turnover in cyanotic CHD, adult patients with cyanotic CHD have an increased incidence of calcium bilirubinate gallstones, and biliary colic can develop years after cardiac surgery has resolved the cyanosis [12]. Blood glucose can be spuriously low, as the larger than normal numbers of cells in the blood tube can metabolize excessive glucose prior to arrival in the laboratory.

Factors besides intrinsic hemostatic defects can increase the risk of excessive perioperative bleeding in patients with cyanotic CHD, particularly during thoracic surgery. These include increased tissue vascularity, elevated systemic venous pressure, and abnormal aortopulmonary and transpleural collateral vessels. In addition, many patients will have had prior intrathoracic surgery.

Renal sequelae

Abnormal renal histopathology with chronic cyanotic CHD includes hypercellular glomeruli with basement membrane thickening, focal interstitial fibrosis, tubular atrophy, and hyalinization of afferent and efferent arterioles [23]. High plasma uric acid levels can be found in adults with cyanotic CHD. Although one might presume that this is from increased urate production, it is rather due to inappropriately low fractional uric acid excretion [24]. This enhanced urate reabsorption is believed due to renal hypoperfusion with a high filtration fraction. Urate stones and urate nephropathy are, however, rare [25]. Arthralgias are common, but gouty arthritis is less frequent than would be expected from the degree of hyperuricemia [24].

Neurological sequelae

Adults with unmodified or persistent intracardiac shunts remain at risk for paradoxical emboli. Even patients with a predominant left-to-right shunt are at some risk. Although it has been said that unlike children, adults with cyanotic CHD are not at risk for the development of cerebral thrombosis no matter the level of hematocrit [12,26], that conclusion has been challenged [27]. In any event, adults do remain at risk for the development of brain abscesses. A healed childhood brain abscess can serve as a nidus for seizures throughout adulthood.

Prior thoracic surgery can have caused iatrogenic peripheral nerve damage. Surgery at the apices of the lung, such as Blalock–Taussig shunts, patent ductus arteriosus (PDA) ligation, pulmonary arterial band, and coarctation repair in particular, are associated with injury to the recurrent laryngeal nerve, the phrenic nerve, and the sympathetic chain. Resultant injuries can be permanent.

Vascular access considerations

Both congenital abnormalities and alterations due to cardiac catheterization or surgery can affect the suitability of a variety of vessels for cannulation by the anesthesiologist. These are summarized in Table 15.2.

Pregnancy

As more children with CHD grow into adulthood, so will more of them become pregnant. The physiologic changes of pregnancy, labor, and delivery can significantly alter the physiologic status of these patients. Readers are referred to more specialized books for a more complete discussion of the pregnant woman with CHD [28,29]. Pregnancy considerations are included under specific defects listed below.

Heart disease (acquired and congenital) is the second leading cause of maternal death [30,31]. Pregnancy can be carried successfully to term with vaginal delivery for most congenital cardiac lesions. As a generalization, mothers with volume lesions tolerate pregnancy better than mothers with pressure lesions. Pulmonary hypertension, depressed ventricular function, severe left heart obstructive lesions, Marfan syndrome with a dilated aortic root, and cyanosis are predictors of maternal and fetal complications. Patients with Eisenmenger physiology are at particularly high risk. Up to 47% of cyanotic women will develop deterioration of functional capacity during pregnancy [32]. Complications include thrombotic complications, cardiovascular complications, and peripartum endocarditis [33]. Women with cyanotic disease may also have early deliveries due to poor fetal growth. The maternal and fetal course worsens with increasing hypoxemia, as mirrored by increasing hematocrit. Hematocrits greater than 44% are associated with birth weights less than the 50th percentile, and fetal death is about 90% or more with hemoglobin levels greater than18 g/dL or oxygen saturation less than 85%, with most losses in the first trimester. Anticoagulation is recommended for cyanotic women and women with Eisenmenger physiology during the third trimester and the first postpartum month.

The numerous physiologic changes accompanying pregnancy are well known. These may be more or less deleterious based on the cardiac pathophysiology and are summarized in Table 15.3. Women who are marginally compensated prepregnancy may have physiologic deterioration with these changes. Changes in vascular resistance can alter shunting patterns. Increased cardiac output increases the risk of aortic rupture in disorders of the aortic wall such as Marfan syndrome or repaired coarctation. The decrease in systemic vascular resistance that accompanies pregnancy is better tolerated in patients with regurgitant lesions.

Most anesthesiologists will encounter pregnant women near the time of delivery toward the end of term. It should be appreciated that pregnancy itself is somewhat of a stress test, with most hemodynamic changes of pregnancy having occurred by 20–26 weeks. The woman who has successfully carried an infant to term has already

Table 15.2 Vascular access considerations

Vessel	Potential problem
Femoral vein(s)	In older patients may have been ligated if *cardiac catheterization* done by cut down. In younger patients may be thrombosed after use of large therapeutic catheters
Inferior vena cava	Some lesions (particularly *asplenia*) associated with discontinuity of the inferior vena cava. Will not be able to pass a catheter from the groin to the right atrium
Left subclavian and pedal arteries	Blood pressure will be low in the presence of *coarctation* of the aorta or following subclavian flap repair (subclavian artery only), and variably so if postoperative recoarctation
Subclavian artery	Blood pressure low with classic *Blalock–Taussig* shunt on that side, and variably so with modified Blalock–Taussig
Right subclavian artery	Blood pressure artifactually high with *supravalvar aortic stenosis* (Coanda effect)
Superior vena cava	Risk of catheter-related thrombosis with *Glenn operation* or lateral tunnel *Fontan*

Table 15.3 Physiologic changes of pregnancy

50% increase in blood volume
Peripheral vasodilation
Fall in systemic vascular resistance
Fall in pulmonary vascular resistance
50% increase in cardiac output (both heart rate and stroke volume)
Increased oxygen consumption
Activation of the coagulation system with increased thromboembolic risk
Myocardial excitability is increased
Increased minute ventilation and work of breathing
Mild respiratory alkalosis
Anemia
Supine hypotension (aortocaval compression)

demonstrated that she is in a relatively low risk group. In general, there is no reason to favor a spontaneous labor over an induced one. Uterine contractions with a functioning labor epidural are easily tolerated. Active second stage bearing down is a time of significant maternal stress and close observation is necessary. The third stage can be accompanied by an autotransfusion of placental blood or, in the case of uterine atony, significant blood loss with hypovolemia, both of which can affect maternal hemodynamic homeostasis. Oxytocin will decrease systemic vascular resistance and increase heart rate and pulmonary vascular resistance (PVR). Methylergonovine will increase systemic vascular resistance. Patients with fixed cardiac output may have difficulty coping with the rapid changes in loading conditions with labor and delivery and pulmonary edema or heart failure can develop.

Some mothers will be on antiarrhythmic medications. Almost all of these will cross the placenta, and almost all appear to be safe for the fetus. Beta-blockers can interfere with fetal growth and the response of the fetus to the stress of labor, and amiodarone can result in fetal thyroid dysfunction. DC cardioversion appears to be safe for the fetus at all stages, due to the low intensity of the electrical field at the uterus. However, the fetus should be monitored throughout the procedure. Women with implanted internal defibrillators have carried successfully to term [34]. In this series, there was only one fetal death in eight cardioversions, with no maternal deaths.

If cardiac surgery is required during pregnancy, cardiopulmonary bypass carries with it increased risk for the fetus. This is increased with hypothermia.

The recurrence of CHD in infants of mothers with CHD was at one time quoted at approximately 4%, but it has become apparent that the recurrence risk varies with the type of maternal defect and the underlying genetic basis.

Bacterial endocarditis prophylaxis is not recommended for uncomplicated deliveries, although it is probably common clinical practice.

Psychosocial issues

Adolescents often have psychological peculiarities well known to pediatricians, and teenagers with CHD are no different. Issues of denial, sense of immortality, and desire for risk taking can all impact on optimally caring for these adolescents as they transition into adulthood. Body conscious adolescents may struggle with bodies that are scarred due to prior surgery and may have physical limitations. Although most adolescents and adults with CHD function quite well, adults with CHD are less likely to be married or cohabiting, are more likely to be living with their parents [35], and are more likely to have psychological issues [36].

Adult CHD patients may have difficulty in obtaining life and health insurance after they are no longer covered under their parents' policies [37]. Life insurance is somewhat more readily available than in the past, but policies vary widely among insurers [38].

Cardiac sequelae

The hemodynamic effects of an anatomical cardiac defect can be compounded by time and modified by imposed chronic cyanosis or pulmonary vascular disease. Myocardial dysfunction can be inherent to the CHD, but can also be due to surgical injury, including inadequate intraoperative myocardial protection [39,40]. This is particularly true of now middle-aged adults who had surgical repairs several decades ago. Although the basic pathophysiology might be well understood by those caring for children with CHD, the natural history of these lesions may be unexpected. Some patients with dysmorphic syndromes will develop heart disease in adult life. For example, 46% of a young adult Down syndrome population without CHD developed mitral valve prolapse, and a small number developed aortic insufficiency [41]. The large number of cardiac lesions and subtypes, compounded with an array of surgical palliative and corrective procedures, make a complete cataloging of all defects and modifications impossible in this context. This chapter is primarily devoted to the more common and physiologically important defects. Both short- and long-term surgical results from older series may not reflect current results.

Acyanotic lesions

Atrial septal defect and partial anomalous pulmonary venous connection

Both the natural history and the outcome after surgery for partial anomalous pulmonary venous return are similar to that of the physiologically similar secundum atrial septal defect (ASD) [42–44]. Because patients with otherwise uncomplicated ASDs often remain asymptomatic until adulthood, ASDs account for about one-third of CHD discovered in adults. Survival of unrepaired defects into adulthood is routine, but complications developing in adulthood provide the rationale for routine childhood correction. Patients with left-to-right shunts of greater than 1.5:1 are at risk for developing symptoms, but all ASDs carry a lifelong risk of paradoxical emboli. Presenting symptoms are typically dyspnea on exertion or palpitations. There is a mortality of 6% per year over 40 years of age [42–44] and essentially all patients older than 60 years are symptomatic. Patients with large, unrepaired defects often die of right ventricular failure or atrial tachyarrhythmias at age 30–50 [45]. In addition to atrial tachyarrhythmias and paradoxical emboli, left-to-right shunting through the defect can increase with aging. Systemic hypertension and/or ischemic coronary disease can occur with aging, and both decrease left ventricular diastolic compliance, which increases the left-to-right shunt. After the age of 40, patients can develop pulmonary vascular disease, now pressure loading the chronically volume-loaded right ventricle. Mitral insufficiency can develop in adulthood and is significant in about 15% of adult patients [46].

Incomplete resolution of right ventricular dilation has been reported with surgical closure after 5 years of age [47]. Left ventricular dysfunction has been reported by some in patients having surgical closure in adulthood [48] and atrial flutter or fibrillation can arise after late repair. Postoperative survival in patients without pulmonary vascular disease is high if operated on before 24 years of age, but survival is worse if surgery is done between 25 and 41 years of age, and worse yet after 41 years of age [49].

Pregnancy is uncomplicated in the vast majority, but the increased circulating blood volume of pregnancy can cause heart failure in those with larger defects. Acute hypovolemia from intrapartum blood loss can cause right-to-left shunting through the defect. Peripheral venous thrombosis carries with it the risk of paradoxical embolization.

Ventricular septal defect

The long-term natural history of ventricular septal defect (VSD) has been reviewed in detail [50]. More than 75% of small and even moderate-sized VSDs close spontaneously during childhood by a gradual ingrowth of surrounding septum. Over 90% of those defects that will close spontaneously will have closed by 10 years of age. Other mechanisms of natural closure include closure by tricuspid valve tissue, prolapsed aortic valve tissue, and endocarditis. There is an incidence of aortic insufficiency in adults

with VSD from prolapse into the defect [51]. Otherwise, a small VSD in the adult is of no hemodynamic import, other than the continuing risk of endocarditis. A moderately restrictive defect can result in atrial or ventricular failure in adulthood and variable increases in PVR. Pulmonary vascular disease can progress if closure of a large VSD is delayed. VSDs provide a continuing endocarditis risk if unclosed; however, if otherwise uncomplicated, the risk in surgically closed defects does not extend beyond several months of surgery.

Several studies have shown possible ventricular dysfunction years after surgical closure [52–54]. Those patients whose defect was closed via a right ventriculotomy are at greater risk to develop long-term right ventricular dysfunction. However, most of these patients had surgery late by current standards. It appears that the changes of chronic volume overload resolve if surgical correction is undertaken by 5 years of age.

Pregnancy is well tolerated in the absence of pulmonary hypertension (less than three-quarters systemic pressure) or preexisting heart failure. Pregnancy with a spontaneously or surgically closed defect carries no additional risk, in the absence of additional cardiac problems. The acute blood loss accompanying delivery can be associated with shunt reversal in a larger defect.

Patent ductus arteriosus

PDA only rarely closes spontaneously after the neonatal period. In addition to the consequences of chronic left-to-right shunting, in the adult the PDA may become calcified or aneurysmally dilated with the risk of rupture [55,56]. These increase the risk of surgery, which will occasionally require the use of cardiopulmonary bypass [57]. Unrepaired, one-third of patients die of heart failure, pulmonary arterial hypertension, or endocarditis by 40 years of age, and two-thirds by age 60 [58]. Small PDAs are well tolerated (though remain an endocarditis risk) and do not carry a hemodynamic risk for pregnancy. There is no residual endocarditis risk after 6 months following uncomplicated PDA closure.

Coarctation of the aorta

There is a significant morbidity and mortality from unoperated coarctation of the aorta in the adult. There is a 25% mortality by 20 years of age, 50% by age 30, 75% by age 50, and 90% by age 60 [45,59–61]. Causes of death include left ventricular failure, rupture of cerebral aneurysms, and dissection of a postcoarctation aneurysm. Left ventricular failure can develop in unrepaired adults older than 40 years. Half of patients operated on after age 40 have persistent hypertension, and many of the remainder will have abnormal hypertensive responses to exercise. Long-term survival after surgery is worse the older the patient was at the time of surgery, with a 15-year survival of only 50% in patients having surgery at over 40 years of age.

Unless repair is undertaken early in life, there is an incremental risk for the development of premature coronary atherosclerotic disease. Even with operation, coronary artery disease is the leading cause of death 11–25 years after operation [62]. Bicuspid aortic valve is a common coexisting lesion, and often does not become stenotic until middle age or older, although it is always an endocarditis risk. Coarctation can also be associated with functionally significant mitral valve abnormalities.

Although the current approach is by an elongated primary repair, for many years the preferred repair was the Waldhausen, or subclavian flap operation, in which the left subclavian artery was opened and rotated down as a flap to open the area of coarctation. These patients may have poor pulses and an artifactually low blood pressure in the left arm. Patients who have had coarctation repairs in childhood may develop aneurysms or pseudoaneurysms at the site of the repair or restenosis of the repaired area in adolescence or adulthood (Figure 15.2). Reoperation on these sites in adulthood can be complex and

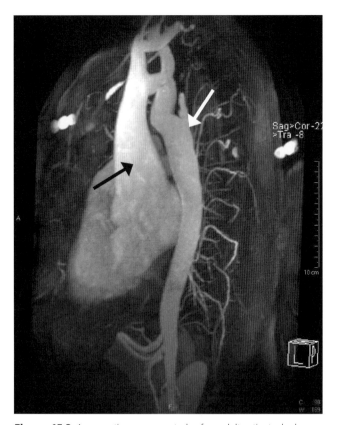

Figure 15.2 A magnetic resonance study of an adult patient who has developed a pseudoaneurysm at the site of an old coarctation repair (*white arrow*). In addition, there is dilation of the ascending aorta, probably related to an associated bicuspid aortic valve (*black arrow*)

involve significant blood loss. Recoarctation or aneurysm formation can be approached endovascularly by balloon angioplasty/stenting [63,64].

Hypertension can be exacerbated during pregnancy in women with unoperated coarctation, with the risks of aortic dissection or rupture, heart failure, angina, and rupture of a circle of Willis aneurysm [65]. Aneurysms with the potential for rupture can also occur at the site of repair. Blood pressure control is of great importance during pregnancy. Most aortic ruptures during pregnancy occur prior to labor and delivery. Epidural analgesia would help minimize hypertension during delivery. Although percutaneous stenting or angioplasty would seem warranted in cases of aortic dissection or severe uncontrolled hypertension, pregnancy predisposes to aortic dissection, so these procedures should be avoided during pregnancy [66]. The incidence of CHD in children of these mothers is about 3%.

Aortic stenosis

Most adult patients with aortic stenosis have a bicuspid aortic valve. Although endocarditis risk is lifelong, symptoms often do not develop until late middle age or later. Once symptoms develop (angina, syncope or near syncope, heart failure), survival is markedly shortened: median survival is 5 years after the development of angina, 3 years after syncope, and 2 years after heart failure [67].

Most mothers with aortic stenosis can have safe pregnancies with vaginal deliveries. Severe aortic stenosis (valve area less than $1.0\ cm^2$) may cause maternal clinical deterioration and significant maternal and fetal mortality. Hemodynamic monitoring during delivery is critical with maintenance of preload and avoidance of vasodilation and hypotension. When required, percutaneous balloon valvuloplasty appears to carry lower risk than open valvotomy during pregnancy.

Pulmonary valve stenosis

Apart from neonates with critical pulmonic stenosis, long-term asymptomatic survival is routine [50]. Mild pulmonic stenosis in the adult does not require surgical correction; there is a 94% survival 20 years after diagnosis [68]. However, with aging right ventricular fibrosis and right ventricular failure can develop, which is the most common cause of death, occurring usually in the fourth decade. Essentially all patients who have relief of stenosis surgically or by balloon valvuloplasty have normal postoperative right ventricular function, but abnormal ventricular function may not completely normalize after late correction. Isolated pulmonary stenosis even of a severe degree is usually well tolerated during pregnancy, despite the volume overload.

Congenitally corrected transposition of the great vessels (l-transposition, ventricular inversion)

Most patients whose anatomic right ventricle is the systemic ventricle as an isolated defect will have normal biventricular function through early adulthood, but often develop right ventricular failure with increasing age [69]. By age 45, two-thirds of those with associated cardiac lesions and 25% of those with isolated l-TGA will have developed heart failure [70]. It has recently been suggested that at least some of these patients would be suitable for cardiac resynchronization therapy to improve function of a failing systemic right ventricle [71]. Second or third degree heart block occurs with an incidence of about 2% per year, and more than 75% of patients have some degree of heart block, although the intrinsic pacemaker remains above the bundle of His with a narrow QRS. L-transposition can be associated with an Ebstein-like deformity of the tricuspid valve (in the systemic ventricle). There is a significant incidence of tricuspid insufficiency (physiologically analogous to mitral insufficiency in the normal heart) even in patients without this Ebstein-like malformation, and the incidence is higher still in patients with this valve deformity [72].

There is the possibility that the systemic right ventricle could fail and tricuspid insufficiency worsen when faced with the stress of pregnancy. This should be monitored during the pregnancy.

Ebstein's anomaly of the tricuspid valve

Following tricuspid valve replacement (the current approach is repair if possible), up to 25% of patients will have high-grade atrioventricular block. There is often associated a right-sided bypass tract resulting in Wolff–Parkinson–White accelerated conduction, allowing rapid ventricular rates and possible development of ventricular fibrillation. This is a particular concern as 25–30% of patients will develop supraventricular tachyarrhythmias in addition to the fraction that will develop atrial fibrillation as a consequence of aging. The atria of these hearts are irritable and there is increased risk of inducing a tachyarrhythmia when introducing central venous catheters. These arrhythmias may need to be aggressively treated as they may be associated with significant hypotension.

In the absence of marked cyanosis or right-sided heart failure, pregnancy and delivery are generally well tolerated, even after valve repair or replacement, although with a somewhat increased risk of fetal loss, prematurity, and low birth weight. In one series although infants of cyanotic mothers were smaller, there was no increased incidence of preterm delivery [73]. The incidence of CHD in offspring is about 6%.

Cyanotic lesions

Tetralogy of Fallot

Tetralogy of Fallot is the most common cyanotic lesion encountered in adults. Unoperated, approximately 25% of patients will survive to adolescence, following which the mortality is 6.6% per year. Only 3% will survive to age 40 [74]. Unlike children, adolescents and adults with tetralogy do not develop hypercyanotic "tet spells." The outcome in patients surgically corrected as adults is worse compared to surgical correction in childhood [75]. Progressive aortic insufficiency can develop in adults with unrepaired tetralogy as the unsupported aortic valve leaflets prolapse into the VSD. It would be very unlikely that adults in medically developed countries will be encountered with unoperated tetralogy of Fallot. However, in medically developed nations patients with complex lesions that were once considered inoperable might be considered operable today. Almost all patients who have had palliation in the USA by means of an aortopulmonary shunt will have gone on to eventual complete repair due to the suboptimal hemodynamics of continued cyanosis.

Long-term survival after surgery has been reported to be as high as 85% at 32–36 years after surgery [76], although symptomatic arrhythmias and diminished exercise tolerance occur in 10–15% at 20 years after the primary repair [76–79]. Although the VSD component is currently approached through the right atrium, adult patients may have had repair via a right ventriculotomy with an obligate right bundle branch pattern on the surface electrocardiogram, although physiologically this reflects only disordered conduction in the region of the ventriculotomy in the right ventricular outflow tract. Right ventricular function in these patients can have an abnormal response to exercise. Repair at an earlier age (less than 12 years old) results in better long-term right ventricular function. In the (now uncommon) unrepaired adult patient, the development of systemic hypertension in adult life will impose an additional load on both ventricles, not just the left ventricle, due to the unrestrictive VSD. The increased systemic resistance can decrease the right-to-left shunt and improve cyanosis, but at the expense of right- or biventricular failure.

Up to 5.5% of patients may have sudden death or require treatment for ventricular tachycardia, often years after surgical correction [80]. Risk factors include older age at repair, left ventricular dysfunction, residual right ventricular hypertension from outflow tract obstruction or pulmonary artery stenosis, severe pulmonary insufficiency, and prolongation of the QRS to greater than 180 msec [81, 82]. This last indicator, though sensitive, has a poor positive prognostic value. The impact of these factors in younger patients, who have not had repairs via a right ventriculotomy, remains unclear. The foci for these arrhythmias are typically in the right ventricular outflow tract and can be ablated. However, premature ventricular contractions and even nonsustained ventricular tachycardia are not uncommon but may not be associated with sudden death [83], making it difficult to know which patients to treat. Additional long-term complications include chronic pulmonary insufficiency and aneurysm formation at a right ventricular outflow tract patch. The development of atrial or ventricular arrhythmias usually reflects the development of hemodynamic deterioration.

Patients with repaired tetralogy may come to reoperation for a variety of reasons [79]. Patients who have required repair using a right ventricle to pulmonary artery conduit will require replacement of the conduit from one to several times. Because these conduits sit close to the sternum, sternotomy may be particularly risky and on occasion sternotomy is done after femoral cannulation for cardiopulmonary bypass. Right ventricle outflow tract patches can also on occasion require surgery for the aneurysmal dilation.

At one time it was taught that a pulmonary valve was not required in the face of a functioning tricuspid valve, and transannular patches, with obligate pulmonary insufficiency, were performed with little concern. However, it has become apparent that many patients with significant pulmonary insufficiency and a chronically overloaded right ventricle will develop right ventricular failure, and we are seeing increasing numbers of these patients, often in their early 20s for placement of a pulmonary valve [84]. The disease process is accelerated if there is further volume stress on the right ventricle. This can occur from a residual VSD or significant tricuspid regurgitation. Although this is typically done as an open procedure utilizing a homograft, there have been recent advances in developing a valve that is delivered transvascularly in the cardiac catheterization laboratory [85]. Placement of a competent pulmonary valve will improve right ventricular function in a significant number of adults, suggesting that this not be delayed when there is evidence if developing right ventricular dysfunction.

Women who have had a good surgical correction without residual defects should tolerate pregnancy and delivery well [86]. However, women who have been left with severe pulmonary insufficiency and a volume-loaded right ventricle are more likely to have complications during pregnancy. In addition, it is thought that pregnancy can have an effect on diminishing right ventricular function that extends beyond pregnancy and delivery, particularly in women with ventricular dysfunction from pulmonary insufficiency. Women with uncorrected tetralogy of Fallot, particularly those with significant cyanosis, have a high incidence of fetal loss (80% with hematocrit greater than 65%). The fall in systemic resistance with pregnancy and delivery can worsen cyanosis, and the physiologic volume load can exaggerate failure of both ventricles. The acute hypovolemia from blood loss during delivery can worsen right-to-left shunting in unrepaired patients. The recurrence risk for CHD in a child of a mother with tetralogy is estimated at 2.5–8%.

Transposition of the great arteries (d-transposition)

With a 1-year mortality of approximately 100%, all adolescents and adults with d-transposition will have had some type of surgical correction. Many adults will have had atrial type repairs, of either the Mustard or Senning type. Teenagers and young adults will be young enough to have had repair by an arterial switch operation. Some will have had repair of d-transposition and VSD with a Rastelli-type repair.

Atrial repairs result in a systemic right ventricle. Patients who have had an atrial type repair have consistently abnormal right ventricular function, with a right ventricular ejection fraction of about 40%. It has been suggested that the earlier the surgery the better the right ventricular function, although it remains abnormal [87]. Right ventricular dysfunction can be progressive [88]. It has recently been suggested that at least some of these patients would be suitable for cardiac resynchronization therapy to improve function of a failing systemic right ventricle [71]. Following atrial repairs, there is also possible late development of tricuspid valve insufficiency. By 20 years, survival after these operations is less than 80%. [89,90] and by 25 years half will have developed right ventricular dysfunction and one-third severe tricuspid insufficiency [90–93]. Selected patients may be candidates for conversion to an arterial switch [94].

There is a significant incidence of late electrophysiologic sequelae after atrial repair, including sinus node dysfunction (bradycardia), junctional escape rhythms, atrioventricular block, and supraventricular tachyarrhythmias. These atrial arrhythmias can result in sudden death, presumably from 1:1 conduction causing ventricular fibrillation [95]. The frequency of tachyarrhythmias increases after the 10th postoperative year and about 20% of patients will have developed them by age 20.

It is still too premature to know the very long-term outcome after the arterial switch operation. Many of these children have abnormal resting myocardial perfusion, and the implication for the development of coronary artery disease in adulthood remains unknown.

Since the arterial switch operation was introduced in the early 1980s, most parturients now will have had this rather than an atrial repair. Pregnancy and delivery are generally well tolerated after an atrial or Rastelli repair if baseline right ventricular function is good; however, right

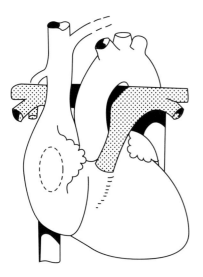
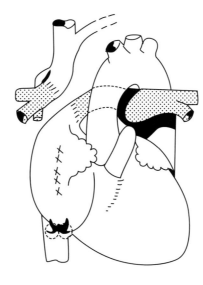

Figure 15.3 The Fontan operation as originally proposed. There is a classic Glenn shunt to the right pulmonary artery, and homograft valves at the origin of the inferior vena cava to the right atrium and connecting the right atrium to the left pulmonary artery (Reproduced and used with permission from Reference [98])

ventricular failure and worsening functional capacity can occur [96]. There is an increased incidence of prematurity and small infants in the offspring of these women. Women who have had an uncomplicated course after an arterial switch repair should not be at increased risk.

Single ventricle anatomy/Fontan physiology

This large rubric includes such lesions as tricuspid atresia and more complex anatomy with a single ventricle, and thus long-term survival depends to some degree on the type and degree of coexisting cardiac malformations. Both pulmonary stenosis (protecting the pulmonary vasculature from excessive flow) and a competent atrioventricular valve improve long-term survival. A single ventricle of left ventricular morphology allows for better ventricular function than does one of the right ventricular type [97]. In the absence of a fortuitous degree of pulmonary stenosis protecting the lungs without excessive cyanosis, survival to adulthood is uncommon without palliation. Palliation with an aortopulmonary shunt is associated with volume loading of the single ventricle and decreasing function with age. In this era, almost all patients will have had some type of Fontan surgery.

The Fontan operation was revolutionary (Figure 15.3) [98]. Kreutzer's modification of the original operation became known as the atriopulmonary Fontan or modified Fontan (Figure 15.4) [99]. The driving force after this operation is central venous pressure as the right atrium soon loses its contractile function, necessitating the strict selection criteria that are still relevant today [100]. Success of Fontan circulation is based on an unobstructed pathway from systemic veins to pulmonary artery, a pulmonary vasculature that is free from anatomic distortion, low PVR and good systemic ventricular function without significant atrioventricular valve insufficiency.

The presence of the right atrium as a large, dilated chamber played a direct role in the three major long-term complications. The poor flow dynamics of the atriopulmonary connection lead to the conception of a lateral tunnel Fontan combined with a bidirectional Glenn shunt [101] (Figure 15.5a). Benefits for this total cavopulmonary connection were:
1 Improved pulmonary blood flow
2 Decreased atrial arrhythmia because less of the atrium would be subjected to long-term central venous hypertension
3 Reduced incidence of thrombosis with the exclusion of the atrium as a large venous reservoir

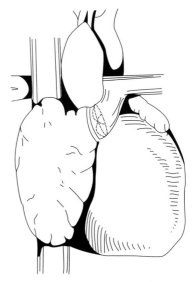

Figure 15.4 The atriopulmonary modification of the Fontan operation as proposed by Kreutzer et al. The right atrium is anastomosed directly to the pulmonary artery without an interposed homograft (Reproduced and used with permission from Reference [99])

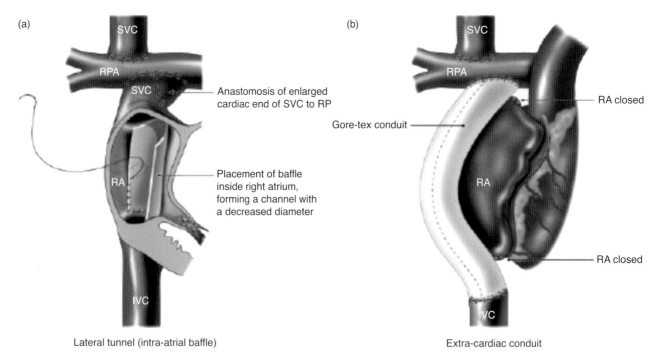

(a)

SVC

RPA

SVC

—— Anastomosis of enlarged
cardiac end of SVC to RP

RA

—— Placement of baffle
inside right atrium,
forming a channel with
a decreased diameter

IVC

Lateral tunnel (intra-atrial baffle)

(b)

SVC

RPA

RA closed ——

Gore-tex conduit ——

RA

RA closed ——

IVC

Extra-cardiac conduit

Figure 15.5 The modern Fontan operation, showing both the lateral tunnel (left) and extracardiac (right) modifications (Reproduced and used with permission from Reference [102])

A further modification is the extracardiac Fontan. The Fontan pathway is entirely "extracardiac" with a prosthetic tube used to connect the inferior vena cava to the right pulmonary artery. The extracardiac Fontan greatly reduces the number of atrial incisions and hopefully the long-term development of atrial arrhythmias (Figure 15.5b). A large retrospective single-center review found a reduced incidence of atrial arrhythmias and improved long-term survival with the extracardiac Fontan [102]. Results, however, are limited by the shorter duration of follow-up.

Thrombosis

The dilated right atrium became a large reservoir of slowly swirling blood and ready substrate for thrombosis. Thrombus in the Fontan pathway causes raised central venous pressures. Embolization to the pulmonary circulation raises PVR and causes hemodynamic compromise. Clot can also embolize to the systemic circulation through fenestrations or residual right-to-left shunts. Thrombus can also form in the pulmonary veins, systemic atrium, or single ventricle. Embolism of clot from these locations leads most often to stroke or myocardial infarction. The presence of clot forming outside the Fontan pathway challenges the simple explanation of stagnant blood in the dilated atrium being the sole cause.

Good prospective studies leading to evidence-based recommendations are rare. Monagle's review found a venous thrombosis incidence of 3–16% and an arterial thrombosis incidence of 3–19%, and no consensus on ideal prophylaxis could be derived [103]. Coon et al. found an incidence of 8.8% with no difference between atriopulmonary and lateral tunnel connections [104]. Varma et al. found an incidence of 17% of subclinical pulmonary emboli [105]. There is also evidence that Fontan patients exist in a hypercoagulable state. Alterations in procoagulant and anticoagulant factors have been documented with the overall balance tipped in favor of thrombosis due to reductions in antithrombin III and protein C and an increase in factor VIII [106,107]. Thromboprophylaxis is a dilemma. Jacobs' group found success with low-dose aspirin [108]. Given the morbidity of thromboembolism, it seems reasonable to put all Fontan patients on aspirin. Those who display further potential for thrombosis such as low cardiac output state, atrial arrhythmia with significant atrial dilation, or marked venous hypertension may benefit from coumadin.

Atrial arrhythmia

Long-term follow-up of Fontan patients shows a steady increase in atrial tachyarrhythmias with an incidence of over 50% at 20 years [109]. Multivariate risk models have identified older age at time of Fontan surgery, early postoperative arrhythmias, sinus node dysfunction, and double inlet left ventricle as risk factors. It was hoped that the lateral tunnel Fontan would decrease the rate of atrial arrhythmias. While initial results were promising [110], much of this benefit is lost with longer-term follow-up [111].

Atrial tachyarrhythmias cause hemodynamic deterioration, both short and long term. Patients with Fontan physiology tolerate tachycardia poorly. Filling pressures rise in the systemic atrium and subsequently throughout the Fontan pathway. Decreased ventricular filling further reduces cardiac output leading to a dangerous combination of a low output state with elevated Fontan pressures. Medical therapy to rapidly control the ventricular rate is urgently required. A frequent dilemma is the possibility of atrial thrombus if the arrhythmia has persisted for more than 24 hours. Transesophageal echocardiography (TEE) is the gold standard for excluding clot in the left atrial appendage of two-ventricle patients with atrial fibrillation. The sensitivity and specificity of TEE is, however, reduced in patients with large, dilated atria [112]. Weighing the risks of stroke with the benefits of restoration of sinus rhythm will determine if the patient requires cardioversion (pharmacological or electrical) or simply control of ventricular rate.

Late onset atrial tachyarrhythmias usually occur between 6 and 10 years [113]. The most common tachyarrhythmia is right intra-atrial reentrant tachycardia. Over time, episodic attacks of tachycardia become more frequent. The natural history is that once tachycardia develops, it becomes increasingly hard to control and many patients end up in atrial fibrillation. Sinus rhythm is critical in maintaining preload. The onset of atrial tachyarrhythmias mandates an evaluation of the Fontan pathway with attention turned to treating any significant obstructions, percutaneously or surgically. With passive pulmonary blood flow, even small gradients can be very hemodynamically significant [114]. Therapy for chronic atrial arrhythmias consists of medication, catheter ablation, or surgery. The atrial dilation along with scar from previous suture lines makes arrhythmias often refractory to medical treatment. Catheter ablation typically has good initial success but a high recurrence [115].

Bradyarrhythmias constitute the other major cardiac rhythm problem. Driscoll found the incidence of bradyarrhythmias requiring pacemakers to be 13% [115]. The incidence of sinus node dysfunction is less in the modern Fontan operation [116]. A clear benefit from an extracardiac connection when compared to the lateral tunnel approach has been difficult to prove [117,118].

Bradyarrhythmias are believed to be caused by surgical dissection near the sinus node. The rising incidence with time suggests progressive fibrosis and scar around the sinus node leads to ischemia. Sinus bradycardia causes a decrease in cardiac output that may be asymptomatic at rest but clinically significant with exercise. Junctional escape rhythms with loss of atrioventricular synchrony decrease ventricular filling while raising atrial pressure. Premature atrial beats that occur more often with slow heart rates may precipitate an intra-atrial reentry tachycardia. Thus, sinus node dysfunction serves as a risk factor for the development of atrial tachyarrhythmias. Pacemakers pose special problems in the Fontan patient because of the altered venous anatomy. Fontan patients require epicardial leads placed via repeat sternotomy. The generator battery is placed in an abdominal subcutaneous pocket and can be replaced easily but lead malfunction requiring replacement necessitates another sternotomy. Although atrioventricular synchrony can be achieved with pacing, it remains inferior to sinus rhythm.

Protein losing enteropathy

Protein losing enteropathy (PLE) is confounding and serious. The quoted incidence is 10–15% but a large international multicenter study found a rate of 3.7% [119]. The patient is edematous with ascites and pleural–pericardial effusions. Serum albumin is low and the diagnosis is confirmed by finding enteric protein loss with elevated levels of stool alpha-1 antitrypsin. Most ominously, PLE is accompanied by a 50% 5-year mortality.

It was believed that PLE constituted a straightforward situation of elevated portal pressures in the setting of central venous hypertension. However, there is not a good correlation between central venous pressures and PLE, leading to a broader understanding of PLE as a multifactorial phenomenon [119]. Firstly, patients with Fontan circulation exhibit a low cardiac output state. It is postulated that blood is shunted away from the mesenteric vasculature in a manner similar to that of hemorrhagic shock. Secondly, a low cardiac output state may induce an inflammatory response. Lastly, patients with congenital disorders of glycosylation have decreased levels of enterocyte heparan sulfate and episodic PLE. Anecdotal success has been reported with both corticosteroids and heparin therapy in Fontan PLE [120, 121]. Weaving these diverse theories into unified whole is difficult. Ostrow noted a reduced mesenteric to celiac artery flow ratio correlated with PLE. All other markers of inflammation, coagulation, and liver function were not predictive of PLE [122].

Pathophysiologic factors other than raised central venous pressures are at work in the development of PLE. Patients who present with PLE should have a complete hemodynamic evaluation because interventions that improve cardiac output have proven success. Cardiac output should be optimized with medical therapy, fenestration, or pacing. In the absence of correctable obstructions, PLE is poorly prognostic. Symptomatic relief can be obtained with intermittent infusion of albumin but this does not address the underlying problem. Although there are case reports of successful cardiac transplantation or Fontan conversion, these major surgeries are high risk and even if the patient survives, PLE has been known to recur.

Preoperative assessment for noncardiac surgery

Patients with Fontan circulation can have a low cardiac output state despite the presence of good ventricular function, minimal AV valve regurgitation, and low PVR [123]. Complicating the issue is that 90% of these patients described themselves as having good functional status. Others have noted this large discrepancy between patients' subjective assessment of their function and performance on objective testing. This places the anesthesiologist in a dilemma when faced with a Fontan patient rating their functional status as "good." We believe that transthoracic echocardiography should be the initial preoperative investigation and is mandatory except in cases of very minor surgery. Good functional status stratifies the patient as "low risk" only within the context of patients with Fontan circulation.

Patients who manifest refractory arrhythmias, cirrhosis, PLE, hypoxemia, ventricular dysfunction, or significantly elevated PVR are described as having failing Fontan physiology. A search is required for correctable lesions [124], as discussed above. In addition, some patients develop collateral vessels. Aortopulmonary collaterals result in a progressive volume load on the single ventricle. Collaterals from the venous system to the systemic atrium or ventricle cause hypoxemia. In both cases, large collaterals should be coil occluded in the catheterization laboratory. Another option is the creation of a fenestration, which can improve cardiac output and lower central venous pressures, but at the expense of a right-to-left shunt. Unfortunately, not all of these therapeutic options are indicated or successful in every patient. At this point if no realistic hope of further improvement exists, the patient should be listed for cardiac transplantation.

The functional state of Fontan patients exists across a spectrum but generally falls into two groups. The largest group is those who report NYHA I–II level of function but have been shown to possess much less cardiorespiratory reserve than age matched two-ventricle controls. These patients will tolerate most surgical procedures with an acceptably low risk. The second group is smaller but consists of those patients who have manifested one or more of the failing Fontan criteria. Surgery in these patients carries much greater risk and should only be undertaken after careful consultation with physicians experienced in adult CHD.

When it comes to a discussion of anesthetic management, the knowledge one has is far more important than the drugs one uses. There is no "right" drug for these patients, nor is there a single "best" anesthetic technique. The critical issue is to have clear understanding of the patient's pathophysiology. Certain principles for patients with Fontan physiology are important and need to be stressed. Our recommendations for anesthesia in the Fontan patient are:

1 Maintenance of preload is essential. Intravenous hydration is required during the NPO period.
2 Regional and neuraxial techniques are attractive options. Neuraxial techniques demand careful attention to volume status because of the resulting sympathectomy. A neuraxial anesthetic is a poor choice if a high level of block is required. A slowly titrated epidural is preferable to a rapid acting spinal anesthetic. The patient's anticoagulation regimen must be carefully managed when neuraxial techniques are being considered.
3 Airway management must be skilled to avoid hypercarbia and elevations in PVR.
4 Adequate levels of anesthesia must be established before stimulating events such as laryngoscopy are undertaken. A surge of catecholamines may precipitate dangerous tachycardia.
5 Spontaneous ventilation that augments pulmonary blood flow is desirable but must not be pursued at all costs. Spontaneous ventilation under deep levels of anesthesia will result in significant hypercarbia. The benefit of spontaneous ventilation maybe completely overwhelmed by the rise in PVR secondary to hypercarbia.
6 A plan must be in place to treat tachyarrhythmias.
7 Patients with pacemakers must have the device interrogated prior to surgery. The degree of pacemaker dependence and the response to a magnet needs to be noted. A plan is required to deal with pacemaker interference from electrocautery.
8 If large volume shifts are anticipated, invasive monitoring with central lines and TEE is recommended. Small central venous catheters are appropriate for delivering inotropic drugs and monitoring, but some centers will prefer to avoid right jugular catheters for fear of thrombosing the Glenn/Fontan pathway.
9 An appropriate plan for postoperative pain management should be established. The need for anticoagulation in many Fontan patients may preclude the use of epidural analgesia.
10 A cardiologist experienced in caring for patients with CHD should be involved in pre- and postoperative care.

Fontan conversion surgery

The first 20 years of the Fontan era consisted of the atriopulmonary connection. Thus, there is a large cohort of patients who may be candidates for conversion to the modern Fontan. The need for this procedure is predicted to substantially increase. Fontan conversion surgery is the most commonly performed high-risk operation in the adult CHD population.

The profile of the early patients undergoing Fontan conversion surgery was one of refractory atrial arrhythmias and poor functional state. Sheikh et al. reported their experience with 15 Fontan conversions [125]. Two general tends were evident. First, in this very high-risk group of patients, there were no perioperative deaths. Second, arrhythmia control was much better in the group that underwent extracardiac connection with arrhythmia surgery. Those patients who underwent Fontan conversion without a procedure to treat their arrhythmia had disappointing results. The large case series of Mavroudis confirms these trends [126]. Their preferred technique is conversion to an extracardiac Fontan connection without fenestration. Intraoperative electrophysiologic mapping was done in all patients. Over time they modified their practice to include more extensive arrhythmia ablation techniques. This decreased their arrhythmia recurrence rate from 13.5 to 7.8%. The risk factors for death or transplantation were right or ambiguous ventricular morphology, PLE, moderate or worse atrioventricular valve insufficiency, and long cardiopulmonary bypass duration.

The success of the conversion operation suggests that patients should not have multiple failed attempts at arrhythmia ablation in the catheterization laboratory because of a fear that surgery is associated with an unacceptably high mortality. Proper selection criteria include patients with pathway obstruction, refractory arrhythmia, and poor functional status despite adequate ventricular function. The higher-risk groups of patients are those with significant ventricular dysfunction or atrioventricular valve insufficiency and those with PLE. Among this higher-risk group consideration should be given to cardiac transplantation, especially in those with PLE, and even this remains a high-risk option.

Principles of anesthesia management are listed earlier in this section, but a few added points deserve mention for Fontan conversion surgery. Since the most common indication for surgery is atrial arrhythmia, these patients have the ability to become tachycardic very easily with prompt hemodynamic deterioration. Underlying ventricular function may be poor with prolonged intravenous induction as blood moves sluggishly through the huge atrium. Repeat sternotomy in Fontan patients can incur especially large blood loss because of the raised central venous pressure. Maintenance of preload and the ability for large volume transfusion is required. Extensive electrocautery is used in the repeat sternotomy, which can interrupt pacemaker function. If pacemaker dependent, consider reprogramming the device to an asynchronous mode. The ability to pace or cardiovert using transcuta-

neous patches is necessary. Prior to separation from bypass, ventilation should be optimized to keep PVR low. Long bypass times can precipitate a potent inflammatory response raising PVR. Milrinone's pulmonary vasodilating properties make it an attractive choice. Despite long bypass duration, aortic cross-clamp time usually is short. Ventricular function after bypass is generally good but must be supported as necessary. Lastly, aggressive management of coagulation is required and in this regard there is no substitute for point of care testing to guide transfusion.

Pregnancy in the Fontan patient

Since pregnancy is a "stress test," who will pass this test and who will fail? Drenthen et al. identified 38 patients from a large registry of Fontan patients [127]. Ten pregnancies from six women resulted in four live births, five miscarriages, and one ectopic pregnancy. The live birth pregnancies were complicated by functional deterioration, atrial arrhythmias, prematurity, and intrauterine growth retardation. They end with the controversial statement that "pregnancy is not advisable." Ten years earlier, however, Canobbio came to a different conclusion [128]. In the largest review to date, they described 33 pregnancies from 21 women. The outcomes were 15 live births, 13 miscarriages, and 5 elective abortions. Functional status remained good throughout the pregnancies in all but one case. There was no significant risk of prematurity and no increased risk of CHD in the infants. The authors conclude that "the tendency to routinely discourage pregnancy may need to be reconsidered."

Despite the problems of retrospective review and self-reporting, these case series provide reassurance. Firstly, pregnancy is usually undertaken only in those patients with relatively good functional status, thereby removing the highest risk patients. Undoubtedly, most adult congenital cardiologists would counsel against pregnancy in any patient with evidence of failing Fontan circulation. In addition, by the time of parturition, the stresses of the hemodynamic alterations of pregnancy have already been successfully faced. In patients with good functional status, pregnancy can successfully be carried to term, albeit with increased risk of miscarriage and premature delivery. A review of the case reports in the anesthetic literature shows that epidural analgesia is well tolerated and indeed recommended for the first stage of labor. The caesarian section rate approaches 50% [127]. Neuraxial anesthesia for caesarian section, in addition to its usual benefits, preserves spontaneous ventilation, which is desirable in Fontan patients. However, no increased risk from general anesthesia was identified. Perioperative complications are low, and peripartum cardiac decompensation is rare.

Truncus arteriosus

Essentially all patients who survive to adolescence will have had surgical repair. Although conduits placed in early childhood will be outgrown, valved conduits placed in late childhood should suffice for adult size. There can be ongoing problems with incompetence or stenosis of both the truncal valve, now analogous to the aortic valve, and the valved right ventricle to pulmonary artery conduit. Truncal (aortic) valve insufficiency or stenosis, in addition to obligate conduit replacement, can require surgery later in life. Because the conduit often lies immediately behind and in close proximity to the sternum, it can be at very high risk of accidental incision during later sternotomy. Mothers with otherwise good cardiac function should not be at increased risk for pregnancy or delivery.

Eisenmenger syndrome

Eisenmenger syndrome refers to fixed, irreversible pulmonary hypertension from unrepaired or incompletely repaired intracardiac lesions such as complete atrioventricular canal or VSD. This syndrome is often present in patients with Trisomy 21, who were not regularly offered cardiac surgery in earlier eras. This fixed pulmonary hypertension results in extensive muscularization of the pulmonary vasculature, leading to permanent right-to-left shunting, increased cyanosis, erythrocytosis, and a number of additional sequelae listed in Table 15.4 [129]. Eisenmenger physiology is compatible with survival into adulthood [130–132]. Survival is 80% 10 years after diagnosis and 42% at 25 years [133]. Worse prognosis is associated with syncope, elevated right atrial pressure, and systemic oxygen saturation less than 85% [130]. The most common cause of death is sudden cardiac death, but others are heart failure, hemoptysis, brain abscess, thromboembolism, and the complications of pregnancy and noncardiac surgery [134]. Supraventricular arrhythmias are common [134]. Although alarming, hemoptysis does not seem to be a predictor of impending death. The onset of irreversible pulmonary vascular disease depends on the degree of shear rate, and for atrial level shunts such as ASDs it may not develop until midlife. Patients with pulmonary vascular disease face significant potential perioperative risks and can constitute a major proportion of adults referred for anesthetic evaluation prior to noncardiac surgery.

These patients are at risk for both bleeding (although usually minor and mucosal) and thrombosis as well as the other problems due to chronic hypoxemia and erythrocytosis (see above). Approximately one-third of adults with Eisenmenger syndrome will develop intrapulmonary thromboses [135].

Over the past several years, oral therapies for pulmonary hypertension have been developed. Patients may be on chronic therapy with sildenafil (Viagra®), a phosphopdiesterase-5 inhibitor, or more likely bosentan (Tracleer®), an antagonist at both the endothelin-1 and -2 receptors, or similar drugs.

Fixed PVR precludes rapid adaptation to perioperative hemodynamic changes. Changes in systemic vascular resistance are mirrored by changes in the degree of right-to-left shunting. Systemic vasodilators, including regional anesthesia, must be used with caution, and close assessment of intravascular volume is important. Extended preoperative fasting should be avoided. Epidural anesthesia has been used successfully in these patients, but the local anesthetic should be delivered in small increments [136].

Table 15.4 Signs, symptoms, and findings with Eisenmenger syndrome

Physical examination: Right ventricular heave, loud pulmonic component of the second heart sound, single or narrowly split second heart sound, Graham–Steell murmur of pulmonary insufficiency, pulmonic ejection sound ("click"), clubbing, peripheral edema. Prior left-to-right shunt murmurs will have receded

Chest radiography: Decreased peripheral pulmonary arterial markings with prominent central pulmonary vessels ("pruning") are possible but not as frequent as in primary pulmonary hypertension. Possible calcification of the pulmonary arteries. Right atrial and right ventricular enlargement

Chest CT: Can show pulmonary artery thromboses

Electrocardiogram: Right ventricular hypertrophy

Symptoms

Impaired exercise tolerance

Exertional dyspnea

Palpitations (often due to atrial fibrillation or flutter)

Complications from erythrocytosis/hyperviscosity (see text)

Hemoptysis from pulmonary thrombosis/infarction or rupture of pulmonary vessels or aortopulmonary collateral vessels

Complications from paradoxical embolization

Syncope from inadequate cardiac output or arrhythmias

Heart failure (usually end-stage)

Postoperative postural hypotension can increase the degree of right-to-left shunting, and these patients should be cautioned to change position slowly.

Placement of pulmonary artery catheters is problematic and not without potential complication in patients with pulmonary vascular disease and who can also have hemostatic defects associated with erythrocytosis [137]. Pulmonary hypertension is a risk factor for pulmonary artery rupture. Right-to-left intracardiac shunting and abnormal cardiac anatomy may make passage to the pulmonary artery difficult without fluoroscopy. Given that the relative resistances of the systemic and pulmonary beds will be reflected in systemic oxygen saturation, which is readily measured by pulse oximetry, and measurements of thermodilution output will not accurately reflect systemic output, the value of a pulmonary artery catheter in these patients is minimal at best and they are essentially never indicated. One possible exception is the patient with pulmonary vascular disease and an ASD who is at risk to develop right ventricular failure if suprasystemic right ventricular pressures develop [138].

Fixed PVR is by definition unresponsive to pharmacologic manipulation. Nevertheless it would seem prudent to avoid those factors known to exacerbate pulmonary resistance including hypothermia, hypercarbia, acidosis, hypoxia, and α-adrenergic agonists. Although the last of those is commonly listed, in the context of pulmonary vascular disease due to a shunt lesion systemic vasoconstrictive effects predominates and systemic oxygen saturation will increase.

Appropriate nerve blocks offer an attractive alternative to general anesthesia. If patients undergo general anesthesia, consideration should be given to returning them to an intensive care unit for gradual emergence and close observation. Because of the increased perioperative risk, patients should be observed at least overnight in an intensive care type of unit, particularly if they have not had any recent surgery or anesthesia and their response will be unknown. Ambulatory surgery is possible, however, for patients having uncomplicated minor surgical procedures with sedation or nerve block.

Pregnancy carries with it a very high mortality risk—30% of all pregnancies end in maternal death, and a successful first pregnancy does not preclude maternal death during a subsequent pregnancy [139]. Maternal deaths are most frequently due to thromboembolism, but other common causes are hypovolemia, preeclampsia, worsening heart failure, and worsening hypoxemia. The changes in hemodynamics of both pregnancy and delivery increase maternal risk. Pulmonary embolism (macro and micro) has caused peripartum deaths, and death can occur days after delivery. Although there is no consensus, subcutaneous low-molecular-weight heparin appears to be effective, and may need to be continued through the puerperium, the time of greatest thrombotic risk. Continuous nasal cannula oxygen can raise maternal oxygen saturation by several percent, and there is a suggestion that this will improve fetal growth. The elevated PVR limits pulmonary blood flow while the drop in systemic vascular resistance favors increasing right-to-left shunting. Excessive acute blood loss with delivery will be poorly tolerated. Even with a successful delivery, mothers can die in the next several days from worsening hemodynamics or pulmonary embolism. Many of these case series are several decades old, and it is suggested that current obstetric and anesthetic management (as of 1998) have significantly improved outcomes [140]. Women should be carefully monitored, with arterial catheters, during delivery. Epidural analgesia, delivered slowly and carefully, can mitigate many of the deleterious hemodynamic changes of active labor. Single-shot spinal anesthesia is not indicated due to the rapid, deleterious hemodynamic effects. General anesthesia has been used successfully for operative delivery. Whether scheduled cesarean section or vaginal birth is to be preferred remains unclear [141]. It seems that the mortality rates for both are similar, and higher than the mortality rate for spontaneous abortion. There is a high incidence of premature deliveries. Pulmonary hypertension and pregnancy has been reviewed in detail [140,142].

Perioperative and anesthetic outcome

Given the wide spectrum of both longstanding cyanotic and acyanotic heart disease and the various medical issues that accrue with aging, it is difficult to adequately derive specific anesthetic outcome data for each of the many clinical permutations. In a retrospective review from Texas Children's Hospital [143] the anesthetic management and immediate outcome of 85 adult and teenaged patients undergoing surgery for CHD were compared to lesion matched control patients younger than 6 years. The primary outcome variable was death within 30 days of surgery, and secondary outcomes were major neurological morbidity, mechanical ventilation beyond 24 hours postoperatively, and length of ICU and hospital stay.

All patients who experienced major neurological morbidity or perioperative mortality were in the older patient group, and all of those were undergoing repeat operations. Four patients died within 30 days of surgery, none in the operating room. No deaths or other major intraoperative events occurred in any patient undergoing a first-time operation, whether in the younger or older patient group.

The anesthetic agents used for both younger and older patients were very similar. Also there was no difference between groups regarding the use of single or multiple inotropic agents.

Fifty-nine percent of the older patients versus 15% of younger patients required antiarrhythmic treatment, and greater numbers of older patients received lidocaine, amiodarone, and magnesium sulfate. Temporary cardiac pacing was used, and defibrillation performed more frequently in the older patients. Of the arrhythmias requiring treatment, 58% were ventricular in the adults compared to 24% in the control patients.

Another published study regarding perioperative outcome of adults with CHD is from the Royal Brompton Hospital [144]. These authors report a slightly greater overall mortality, 6.8% compared to 4.7% in the Texas study. They also found reoperation to be a significant risk factor for early postoperative mortality, and that the number of previous operations correlated with increased mortality. Cyanosis and increasing age were also correlated with increased mortality. Compared to the Texas study, patients in the Brompton study were significantly older, mean age 31 years, and one-third of the nonsurvivors in that study were greater 50 years.

From these retrospective reviews, there appears to be an increased incidence of perioperative morbidity among older patients with CHD undergoing cardiac surgery, and certain groups of patients have the greatest risk, particularly the single-ventricle patient.

Another group of patients with greater risk of mortality or major morbidity are those with cyanosis, especially those requiring repeat sternotomy. These two factors were the best predictors of early mortality in the Brompton study, and all deaths and major complications occurred among these patients in the Texas study. There are several reasons for this observation. First, longstanding cyanosis leads to increased risk for coagulopathy and organ dysfunction. Second, most of these patients had ventricular dysfunction, which renders the myocardium more vulnerable to the ischemic insult from cardiopulmonary bypass and aortic cross-clamping, thereby increasing the possibility of postoperative ventricular failure and arrhythmias.

Anesthetic management

Based on the above data and our experience, we recommend the following management for adult patients undergoing repeat sternotomy for congenital heart surgery:

Preoperative preparations:
1 Patient data should be presented to a multidisciplinary group consisting of cardiologists, surgeons, and anesthesiologists. Data analysis includes laboratory results, cardiac catheterization, echocardiography, Holter monitor results, chest radiograph, and magnetic resonance imaging. Among this group of specialists, a consensus can be developed regarding the timing of surgery and surgical options.
2 The patient's cardiac rhythm should be assessed, particularly the functioning of pacemakers and underlying cardiac rhythm in case of pacemaker failure.
3 An anesthetic plan with the patient's unique pathophysiology and anticipated response to anesthetic interventions should be developed. This is particularly important for the single-ventricle patient with poor ventricular function, who may be intolerant to myocardial depressants, positive pressure ventilation, or loss of sinus rhythm.

General operating room care:
1 Establish large bore intravenous access and provisions for rapid infusion of volume. A pressurized rapid infusion system capable of delivering at least 500 mL/min of warmed fluid or blood is recommended. In the case of massive bleeding, rapid infusion can be established utilizing the bypass machine. Tubing from the venous reservoir is passed through a roller pump head and connected to large bore venous access. The patient is heparinized, and large volumes can be transfused while preparations are made to rapidly institute bypass via the femoral route.
2 Multifunction external pacing, defibrillating, and cardioversion pads should be applied and antiarrhythmic drugs immediately available.
3 Preparations should be made to treat postoperative hemorrhage. Tranexamic acid and ε-aminocaproic acid are effective in reducing bleeding in these patients [7]. Aprotinin is no longer available to prevent hemorrhage, but recombinant factor VIIa has gained increasing use to reduce established postcardiotomy hemorrhage and should be considered in these patients [145]. Adequate blood products, including platelets, fresh frozen plasma, and cryoprecipitate should be available. Cell salvage, with reinfusion of washed autologous red blood cells, is appropriate [146]. Thromboelastography [147] during bypass, with heparinase added to neutralize heparin, may be particularly useful to predict the need for blood products postbypass, particularly in patients with baseline coagulopathy of cyanosis.
4 TEE is indicated for congenital heart surgery in infants and children; these guidelines are also applicable to adult congenital heart surgery [148–150].
5 Neurological monitoring with transcranial Doppler ultrasound (to assist in detecting and limiting cerebral emboli), bispectral index, and near infrared spectroscopy may be helpful in minimizing neurological complications [151].

Noncardiac surgery in the adult with CHD

As increasing numbers of adults with CHD survive well into adulthood, they will also require noncardiac surgical procedures of all types [152]. These will include vaginal and operative deliveries as discussed earlier in this chapter, as well as common gynecological, general surgery, orthopedic, dental, and urologic surgeries. With simple repaired CHD, and peripheral surgery, standard preoperative evaluation and attention to infective endocarditis prophylaxis, along with standard anesthetic care, are usually all that is necessary. With complex or palliated CHD with significant residua, or in extensive or more invasive surgery, careful evaluation of the patient in consultation with their cardiologist, as well as communication with the surgeon about the necessity and the goals of the procedure, as well as the techniques planned, is essential. Common surgeries normally well tolerated by patients with normal hearts, but that may introduce significant physiologic tresspass in the patient with CHD, include laparoscopic surgery, and spinal fusion surgery. Both insufflation of the periotoneal cavity with carbon dioxide for laparoscopy, or the significant blood loss and prone position with extensive spinal fusion surgery, may not be well tolerated by patients with limited cardiac reserve, especially single ventricle patients with Fontan physiology. Invasive monitoring and recovery in an intensive care unit in a setting with experience in caring for adults with CHD may be necessary to maximize perioperative outcomes. General recommendations for perioperative care of these patients are listed in Table 15.5 [5].

Conclusions

As the number of operations for adult CHD increases, these surgeries will be performed in a variety of institutions and systems. The optimal environment for performing congenital heart surgery on adult patients may be lacking in many situations. In our opinion, this type of surgery is best accomplished in a system designed for adults with CHD. Optimal care for these patients is provided by cardiologists trained and experienced in both pediatric and adult cardiology, by surgeons with training and experience with CHD, and by anesthesiologists with interest and experience in caring for the adult with CHD. Whatever the setting, the cardiac anesthesiologists performing these cases must be thoroughly aware of the anesthetic implications for the unique pathophysiology of each patient, and must not rely on their "usual" expectations of either true pediatric CHD or acquired adult heart disease.

Table 15.5 Recommendations for noncardiac surgery in adults with congenital heart disease

Class I

1. Basic preoperative assessment for ACHD patients should include systemic arterial oximetry, an ECG, chest x-ray, TTE, and blood tests for full blood count and coagulation screen (*Level of evidence: C*)
2. It is recommended that when possible, the preoperative evaluation and surgery for ACHD patients be performed in a regional center specializing in congenital cardiology, with experienced surgeons and cardiac anesthesiologists (*Level of evidence: C*)
3. Certain high-risk patient populations should be managed at centers for the care of ACHD patients under all circumstances, unless the operative intervention is an absolute emergency. High-risk categories include patients with the following:
   a. Prior Fontan procedure (*Level of evidence: C*)
   b. Severe pulmonary arterial hypertension (PAH) (*Level of evidence: C*)
   c. Cyanotic CHD (*Level of evidence: C*)
   d. Complex CHD with residua such as heart failure, valve disease, or the need for anticoagulation (*Level of evidence: C*)
   e. Patients with CHD and malignant arrhythmias (*Level of evidence: C*)
4. Consultation with ACHD experts regarding the assessment of risk is recommended for patients with CHD who will undergo noncardiac surgery (*Level of evidence: C*)
5. Consultation with a cardiac anesthesiologist is recommended for moderate- and high-risk patients (*Level of evidence: C*)

Class I evidence: benefits significantly outweigh risk, and procedures *should* be performed. Level C evidence: very limited populations evaluated; only consensus opinion of experts, case studies, or standard of care. A recommendation with Level C evidence does not imply that it is weak; recommendations for perioperative care of adults with CHD for noncardiac surgery do not lend themselves to clinical trials.
Source: Reproduced and used with permission from Reference [5].

Summary of anesthetic issues for congenital heart lesions most commonly encountered in adults

ASD
- Primarily left-to-right shunt, but may have paradoxical emboli
- Many patients with hemodynamically insignificant ASDs present after embolic stroke
- Pulmonary vascular disease usually does not develop until age 40 or later

VSD
- Left-to-right shunt
- Delayed closure may leave longstanding ventricular dysfunction or irreversible pulmonary hypertension
- Increased incidence of aortic insufficiency

PDA
- Longstanding left-to-right shunt
- May develop end-stage pulmonary hypertension

- Ductus may be calcified or aneurismal when repaired in adulthood

Coarctation of the aorta
- Arterial monitoring in right arm
- Primary repair in adulthood is associated with poor outcome
- Revision of childhood repair common, either surgically or via cardiac catheterization
- Open repair of recoarctation may have excessive blood loss

Transposition of the great arteries (dTGA)
- Atrial arrhythmias and/or sick sinus syndrome after Mustard or Senning procedure
- Progressive RV failure or tricuspid insufficiency may develop after Mustard or Senning procedure
  - Tricuspid valve repair or replacement
  - Conversion to the arterial switch procedure may be indicated, usually preceded by pulmonary artery banding

Congenitally corrected transposition of the great arteries
- Heart block is common
- Right (systemic) ventricular failure develops with increasing age
- Double switch procedure places the left ventricle as the systemic pump

Ebstein's anomaly
- Adults may show congestive heart failure or cyanosis depending on right ventricular output
- Atrial arrhythmias are common, and AV block is common after tricuspid replacement

Tetralogy of Fallot
- Primary repair can be performed in adults with good outcome
- Reoperation most commonly needed for pulmonary insufficiency or conduit failure
- Ventricular arrhythmias are common years after repair

Atrioventricular canal
- Most frequently associated with Down syndrome
- Residual or progressive mitral regurgitation may necessitate surgery later in life

Truncus arteriosus
- Essentially all patients require repeat operations for RV to PA conduit revision
- Some patients will require truncal (neo-aortic) valve repair or replacement

Single ventricle
- Variable anatomy (usually atresia of AV valve or semilunar valve) with mixing of systemic and pulmonary venous blood
- Fontan procedure performed as staged surgical repair
  - CVP is the driving force for pulmonary blood flow
  - Positive pressure ventilation will increase intrathoracic pressure, decrease pulmonary blood flow, thereby decreasing cardiac output
- Conversion of atriopulmonary Fontan to extracardiac Fontan has been performed in adults with improvement in cardiac function

References

1. Mahoney LT, Skorton DJ (1991) Insurability and employability. J Am Coll Cardiol 18:334–336.
2. Warnes CA, Liberthson R, Danielson GK, et al. (2001) Task force 1: the changing profile of congenital heart disease in adult life. J Am Coll Cardiol 37:1170–1175.
3. Webb GD, Williams RG (2001) Care of the adult with congenital heart disease: introduction. J Am Coll Cardiol 37:1166.
4. Landzberg MJ, Murphy DJ, Jr, Davidson WR, Jr, et al. (2001) Task force 4: organization of delivery systems for adults with congenital heart disease. J Am Coll Cardiol 37: 1187–1193.
5. Warnes CA, Williams RG, Bashore TM, et al. (2008) ACC/AHA 2008 guidelines for the management of adults with congenital heart disease. J Am Coll Cardiol 52:e1–e121.
6. Bancalari E, Jesse MJ, Gelband H, et al. (1977) Lung mechanics in congenital heart disease with increased and decreased pulmonary blood flow. J Pediatr 90:192–195.
7. Sietsema KE, Perloff JK (1991) Cyanotic congenital heart disease: dynamics of oxygen uptake and control of ventilation during exercise. In: Perloff JK, Child JS (eds) Congenital Heart Disease in Adults. WB Saunders, Philadelphia, pp. 104–110.
8. Sorensen SC, Severinghaus JW (1968) Respiratory insensitivity to acute hypoxia persisting after correction of tetralogy of Fallot. J Appl Physiol 25:221–223.
9. Edelmann NH, Lahiri S, Braudo L, et al. (1970) The ventilatory response to hypoxia in cyanotic congenital heart disease. N Engl J Med 282:405–411.
10. Blesa MI, Lahiri S, Rashkind WJ, et al. (1977) Normalization of the blunted ventilatory response to acute hypoxia in congenital cyanotic heart disease. N Engl J Med 296:237–241.
11. Burrows FA (1989) Physiologic dead space, venous admixture, and the arterial to end-tidal carbon dioxide difference in infants and children undergoing cardiac surgery. Anesthesiology 70:219–225.
12. Perloff JK, Rosove MH, Child JS, et al. (1988) Adults with cyanotic congenital heart disease: hematologic management. Ann Intern Med 109:406–413.

13. Kawakami N, Mimatsu K, Deguchi M, et al. (1995) Scoliosis and congenital heart disease. Spine 20:1252–1255.

14. Berman WJ, Wood SC, Yabek SM, et al. (1987) Systemic oxygen transport in patients with congenital heart disease. Circulation 75:360–368.

15. Broberg CS, Bax BE, Okonko DO, et al. (2006) Blood viscosity and its relationship to iron deficiency, symptoms, and exercise capacity in adults with cyanotic congenital heart disease. J Am Coll Cardiol 48:356–365.

16. Spence MS, Balaratnam MS, Gatzoulis MA (2007) Clinical update: cyanotic congenital heart disease. Lancet 370:1530–1532.

17. Thorne SA (1988) Management of polycythaemia in adults with cyanotic congenital heart disease. Heart 79:315–316.

18. Baum VC (1996) The adult with congenital heart disease. J Cardiothorac Vasc Anesth 10:261–282.

19. Kaemmerer H, Fratz S, Braun SL, et al. (2004) Erythrocyte indexes, iron metabolism, and hyperhomocysteinemia in adults with cyanotic congenital cardiac disease. Am J Cardiol 94:825–828.

20. Ware JA, Reaves WH, Horak JK, et al. (1983) Defective platelet aggregation in patients undergoing surgical repair of cyanotic congenital heart disease. Ann Thorac Surg 36:289–294.

21. Rosove MH, Hocking WG, Harwig SS, et al. (1983) Studies of beta-thromboglobulin, platelet factor 4, and fibrinopeptide A in erythrocytosis due to cyanotic congenital heart disease. Thromb Res 29:225–235.

22. Weinstein M, Ware JA, Troll J, et al. (1988) Changes in von Willebrand factor during cardiac surgery: effect of desmopressin acetate. Blood 71:1648–1655.

23. Spear GS (1977) The glomerular lesion of cyanotic congenital heart disease. Johns Hopkins Med J 140:185–188.

24. Ross EA, Perloff JK, Danovitch GM, et al. (1986) Renal function and urate metabolism in late survivors with cyanotic congenital heart disease. Circulation 73:396–400.

25. Young D (1980) Hyperuricemia in cyanotic congenital heart disease. Am J Dis Child 134:902–903.

26. Perloff JK, Marelli AJ, Miner PD (1993) Risk of stroke in adults with cyanotic congenital heart disease. Circulation 87:1954–1959.

27. Ammash N, Warnes CA (1996) Cerebrovascular events in adult patients with cyanotic congenital heart disease. J Am Coll Cardiol 28:768–772.

28. Oakley C, Warnes CA (2007) Heart Disease in Pregnancy, 2 edn. Blackwell, Oxford.

29. Warnes CA, Elkayam U (1998) Congenital heart disease and pregnancy. In: Elkayam U, Gleicher N (eds) Cardiac Problems in Pregnancy, 3 edn. Wiley-Liss, New York, pp. 39–53.

30. Lewis G, Drife J (2004) Why Mothers Die 2000–2002. Confidential Enquiry into Maternal and Child Health. RCOG Press, London.

31. Malhotra S, Yentis SM (2006) Reports on confidential enquiries into maternal deaths: management strategies based on trends in maternal cardiac deaths over 30 years. Int J Obstet Anesth 15:223–226.

32. Shime J, Mocarski EJ, Hastings D, et al. (1987) Congenital heart disease in pregnancy: short- and long-term implications. Am J Obstet Gynecol 156:313–322.

33. Presbitero P, Somerville J, Stone S, et al. (1994) Pregnancy in cyanotic congenital heart disease. Outcome of mother and fetus. Circulation 89:2673–2676.

34. Natale A, Davidson T, Geiger MJ, et al. (1997) Implantable cardioverter-defibrillators and pregnancy: a safe combination? Circulation 96:2808–2812.

35. Foster E, Graham TP, Jr, Driscoll DJ, et al. (2001) Task force 2: special health care needs of adults with congenital heart disease. J Am Coll Cardiol 37:1176–1183.

36. van Rijen EH, Utens E, Roos-Hesselink JW, et al. (2005) Longitudinal development of psychopathology in an adult congenital heart disease cohort. Int J Cardiol 99:315–323.

37. Skorton DJ, Garson A, Jr, Allen HD, et al. (2001) Task force 5: adults with congenital heart disease: access to care. J Am Coll Cardiol 37:1193–1198.

38. Truesdell SC, Clark EB (1991) Health insurance status in a cohort of children and young adults with congenital cardiac diagnoses. Circulation 84 (Suppl 2):II-386.

39. Humes RA, Mair DD, Porter CB, et al. (1988) Results of the modified Fontan operation in adults. Am J Cardiol 61:602–604.

40. Graham TP, Jr, Cordell GD, Bender HW (1995) Ventricular function following surgery. In: Kidd BS, Rowe RD (eds) The Child With Congenital Heart Disease After Surgery. Futura Publishing Co, Mt. Kisco

41. Geggel RL, O'Brien JE, Feingold M (1993) Development of valve dysfunction in adolescents and young adults with Down syndrome and no known congenital heart disease. J Pediatr 122:821–823.

42. Markman P, Howitt G, Wade EG (1965) Atrial septal defect in the middle-aged and elderly. Q J Med 34:409–426.

43. Craig RJ, Selzer A (1968) Natural history and prognosis of atrial septal defect. Circulation 37:805–815.

44. Mattila S, Merikallio E, Tala P (1979) ASD in patients over 40 years of age. Scand J Thorac Cardiovasc Surg 13:21–24.

45. Campbell M (1970) Natural history of coarctation of the aorta. Br Heart J 32:633–640.

46. Boucher CA, Liberthson RR, Buckley MJ (1979) Secundum atrial septal defect and significant mitral regurgitation: incidence, management and morphologic basis. Chest 75:697–702.

47. Liberthson RR, Boucher CA, Strauss HW, et al. (1981) Right ventricular function in adult atrial septal defect. Preoperative and postoperative assessment and clinical implications. Am J Cardiol 47:56–60.

48. Davies H, Oliver GC, Rappoport WJ, et al. (1970) Abnormal left heart function after operation for atrial septal defect. Br Heart J 32:747–753.

49. Murphy JG, Gersh BJ, McGoon MD, et al. (1990) Long-term outcome after surgical repair of isolated atrial septal defect. Follow-up at 27 to 32 years. N Engl J Med 323:1645–1650.

50. O'Fallon WM, Weidman WH (1993) Long-term follow-up of congenital aortic stenosis, pulmonary stenosis and ventricular septal defect. Circulation 87 (Suppl I):I1–I126.

51. Wilson NJ, Neutze JM (1993) Adult congenital heart disease: principles and management guidelines: part II. Aust N Z J Med 23:697–705.

52. Jarmakani JM, Graham TP, Jr, Canent RV, Jr, et al. (1971) The effect of corrective surgery on left heart volume and mass in children with ventricular septal defect. Am J Cardiol 27:254–258.

53. Jarmakani JM, Graham TPJ, Canent RVJ (1972) Left ventricular contractile state in children with successfully corrected ventricular septal defect. Circulation 45 (Suppl 1): 102–110.

54. Maron BJ, Redwood DR, Hirshfeld JWJ, et al. (1973) Postoperative assessment of patients with ventricular septal defect and pulmonary hypertension. Response to intense upright exercise. Circulation 48:864–874.

55. Hankins G, Brekken A, Davis L (1985) Maternal death secondary to a dissecting aneurysm of the pulmonary artery. Obstet Gynecol 65:45–48.

56. Guthrie W, McLean H (1972) Dissecting aneurysms of arteries other than the aorta. J Pathol 108:210–235.

57. Fisher RG, Moodie DS, Sterba R, et al. (1986) Patent ductus arteriosus in adults—long-term follow-up: nonsurgical versus surgical treatment. J Am Coll Cardiol 8:280–284.

58. Campbell M (1968) Natural history of patent ductus arteriosus. Br Heart J 30:4–13.

59. Mitchell SC, Korones SB, Berendes HW (1971) Congenital heart disease in 56,109 births. Incidence and natural history. Circulation 43:323–332.

60. Abbott ME (1928) Coarctation of the aorta of adult type: II. A statistical study and historical retrospect of 200 recorded cases with autopsy, of stenosis or obliteration of the descending arch in subjects above the age of two years. Am Heart J 3:392–421.

61. Reifenstein GH, Levine SA, Gross RE (1947) Coarctation of the aorta: a review of 104 autopsied cases of the "adult type", 2 years of age or older. Am Heart J 33:146–168.

62. Maron BJ, Humphries JO, Rowe RD, et al. (1973) Prognosis of surgically corrected coarctation of the aorta. A 20- year postoperative appraisal. Circulation 47:119–126.

63. Golden AB, Hellenbrand W (2007) Coarctation of the aorta: stenting in children and adults. Catheter Cardiovasc Interv 69:289–299.

64. Kutty S, Greenberg RK, Fletcher S, et al. (2008) Endovascular stent grafts for large thoracic aneurysms after coarctation repair. Ann Thorac Surg 85:1332–1338.

65. Beauchesne L, Connolly H, Ammash N, et al. (2001) Coarctation of the aorta. Outcome of pregnancy. J Am Coll Cardiol 38:1728–1733.

66. Oakley C, Connolly HM (2007) Acyanotic congenital heart disease. In: Oakley C, Warnes CA (eds) Heart Disease in Pregnancy. Blackwell, Oxford, pp. 29–42.

67. Carabello BA, Carawford FAJ (1997) Valvular heart disease. N Engl J Med 337:32–41.

68. Hayes CJ, Gersony WM, Driscoll DJ, et al. (1993) Second natural history study of congenital heart defects. Results of treatment of patients with pulmonary valvar stenosis. Circulation 87:I28–I37.

69. Graham TP, Jr, Parrish MD, Boucek RJJ, et al. (1983) Assessment of ventricular size and function in congenitally corrected transposition of the great arteries. Am J Cardiol 51:244–251.

70. Graham TP, Jr, Bernard YD, Mellen BG, et al. (2000) Long-term outcome in congenitally corrected transposition of the great arteries: a multi-institutional study. J Am Coll Cardiol 36:255–261.

71. Diller GP, Okinko D, Uebing A, et al. (2006) Cardiac resynchronization therapy for adult congenital heart disease patients with a systemic right ventricle: analysis of feasibility and review of early experience. Eurospace 8:267–272.

72. Connelly MS, Robertson P, Liu P, et al. (1994) Congenitally corrected transposition of the great arteries in adults: natural history. Circulation 90:I51.

73. Connolly HM, Warnes CA (1994) Ebstein's anomaly: outcome of pregnancy. J Am Coll Cardiol 1194–1198.

74. Bertranou EG, Blackstone EH, Hazelrig JB, et al. (1978) Life expectancy without surgery in tetralogy of Fallot. Am J Cardiol 42:458–466.

75. Rammohan M, Airan B, Bhan A, et al. (1998) Total correction of tetralogy of Fallot in adults—surgical experience. Int J Cardiol 63:121–128.

76. Nollert G, Fischlein T, Bouterwek S, et al. (1997) Long-term survival in patients with repair of tetralogy of Fallot: 36-year follow-up of 490 survivors of the first year after surgical repair. J Am Coll Cardiol 30:1374–1383.

77. Murphy JG, Gersh BJ, Mair DD, et al. (1993) Long-term outcome in patients undergoing surgical repair of tetralogy of Fallot. N Engl J Med 329:593–599.

78. Harrison DA, Harris L, Siu SC, et al. (1997) Sustained ventricular tachycardia in adult patients late after repair of tetralogy of Fallot. J Am Coll Cardiol 30: 1368–1373.

79. Oechslin EN, Harrison DA, Harris L, et al. (1999) Reoperation in adults with repair of tetralogy of Fallot: indications and outcomes. J Thorac Cardiovasc Surg 118:245–251.

80. Kavey RE, Blackman MS, Sondheimer HM (1982) Incidence and severity of chronic ventricular dysrhythmias after repair of tetralogy of Fallot. Am Heart J 103:342–350.

81. Gatzoulis MA, Balaji S, Webber SA, et al. (2000) Risk factors for arrhythmia and sudden cardiac death late after repair of tetralogy of Fallot: a multicentre study. Lancet 356: 975–981.

82. Abd El Rahman MY, Abdul-Khaliq H, Vogel M, et al. (2000) Relation between right ventricular enlargement, QRS duration, and right ventricular function in patients with tetralogy of Fallot and pulmonary regurgitation after surgical repair. Heart 84:416–420.

83. Cullen S, Celermajer DS, Franklin RC, et al. (1994) Prognostic significance of ventricular arrhythmia after repair of tetralogy of Fallot: a 12-year prospective study. J Am Coll Cardiol 23:1151–1155.

84. Discigil B, Dearani JA, Puga FJ, et al. (2001) Late pulmonary valve replacement after repair of tetralogy of Fallot. J Thorac Cardiovasc Surg 121:344–351.

85. Lurz P, Coats L, Khambadkone S, et al. (2008) Percutaneous pulmonary valve implantation: impact of evolving technology and learning curve on clinical outcome. Circulation 117:1964–1972.

86. Singh H, Bolton PJ, Oakley CM (1982) Pregnancy after surgical correction of tetralogy of Fallot. BMJ 285:168–170.

87. Graham TP, Jr, Burger J, Bender HW, et al. (1985) Improved right ventricular function after intra-atrial repair of transposition of the great arteries. Circulation 72:II45–II51.

88. Graham TP (1991) Ventricular performance in congenital heart disease. Circulation 84:2259–2274.

89. Gelatt M, Hamilton RM, McCrindle BW, et al. (1997) Arrhythmia and mortality after the Mustard procedure: a 30-year single-center experience. J Am Coll Cardiol 29:194–201.

90. Wilson NJ, Clarkson PM, Barratt-Boyes BG, et al. (1998) Long-term outcome after the Mustard repair for simple transposition of the great arteries. 28-year follow-up. J Am Coll Cardiol 32:758–765.

91. Warnes CA, Somerville J (1987) Transposition of the great arteries: late results in adolescents and adults after the Mustard procedure. Br Heart J 58:148–155.

92. Myridakis DJ, Ehlers KH, Engle MA (1994) Late follow-up after venous switch operation (Mustard procedure) for simple and complex transposition of the great arteries. Am J Cardiol 74:1030–1036.

93. Puley G, Siu S, Connelly M, et al. (1999) Arrhythmia and survival in patients >18 years of age after the mustard procedure for complete transposition of the great arteries. Am J Cardiol 83:1080–1084.

94. Mavroudis C, Backer CL (2000) Arterial switch after failed atrial baffle procedures for transposition of the great arteries. Ann Thorac Surg 69:851–857.

95. Garson AJ (1990) The emerging adult with arrhythmias after congenital heart disease: management and financial health care policy. Pacing Clin Electrophysiol 13:951–954.

96. Clarkson PM, Wilson NJ, Neutze JM, et al. (1994) Outcome of pregnancy after the Mustard operation for transposition of the great arteries with intact ventricular septum. J Am Coll Cardiol 24:190–193.

97. Sano T, Ogawa M, Taniguchi K, et al. (1989) Assessment of ventricular contractile state and function in patients with univentricular heart. Circulation 79:1247–1256.

98. Fontan F, Baudet E (1971) Surgical repair of tricuspid atresia. Thorax 26:240–248.

99. Kreutzer G, Galindez E, Bono H, et al. (1973) An operation for the correction of tricuspid atresia. J Thorac Cardiovasc Surg 66:613–621.

100. Choussat A, Fontan F, Besse P (1978) Selection criteria for Fontan's procedure. In: Anderson RH, Shinebourne EA (eds) Pediatric Cardiology. Churchill Livingstone, Edinburgh, pp. 559–566.

101. de Leval MR, Kilner P, Gewillig M, et al. (1988) Total cavopulmonary connection: a logical alternative to atriopulmonary connection for complex Fontan operations. Experimental studies and early clinical experience. J Thorac Cardiovasc Surg 96:682–695.

102. d'Udekem Y, Iyengar AJ, Cochrane AD, et al. (2007) The Fontan procedure: contemporary techniques have improved long-term outcomes. Circulation 116:I157–I164.

103. Monagle P, Karl TR (2002) Thromboembolic problems after the Fontan operation. Pediatr Card Surg Annu Semin Thorac Cardiovasc Surg 5:36–47.

104. Coon PD, Rychik J, Novello RT, et al. (2001) Thrombus formation after the Fontan operation. Ann Thorac Surg 71:1990–1994.

105. Varma C, Warr MR, Hendler AL, et al. (2003) Prevalence of "silent" pulmonary emboli in adults after the Fontan operation. J Am Coll Cardiol 41:2252–2258.

106. Cromme-Dijkhuis AH, Henkens CM, Bijleveld CM, et al. (1990) Coagulation factor abnormalities as possible thrombotic risk factors after Fontan operations. Lancet 336:1087–1090.

107. Odegard K, McGowan FXJ, Zurakowski D, et al. (2003) Procoagulant and anticoagulant factor abnormalities following the Fontan procedure: increased factor VIII may predispose to thrombosis. J Thorac Cardiovasc Surg 125:1260–1267.

108. Jacobs ML, Pourmoghadam KK, Geary EM, et al. (2002) Fontan's operation: is aspirin enough? Is coumadin too much? Ann Thorac Surg 73:64–68.

109. Weipert J, Noebauer C, Schreiber C, et al. (2004) Occurrence and management of atrial arrhythmia after long-term Fontan circulation. J Thorac Cardiovasc Surg 127:457–464.

110. Gelatt M, Hamilton RM, McCrindle BW, et al. (1994) Risk factors for atrial tachyarrhythmias after the Fontan operation. J Am Coll Cardiol 24:1735–1741.

111. Durongpisitkul K, Porter CJ, Cetta F, et al. (1998) Predictors of early- and late-onset supraventricular tachyarrhythmias after Fontan operation. Circulation 98:1099–1107.

112. Kim PJ, Franklin WH, Duffy E, et al. (2003) Accuracy of transesophageal echocardiography in detecting right atrial thrombus in patients after the Fontan operation [abstract]. Circulation 108:IV667.

113. Kirsh JA, Walsh EP, Triedman JK (2002) Prevalence of and risk factors for atrial fibrillation and intra-atrial reentrant tachycardia among patients with congenital heart disease. Am J Cardiol 90:338–340.

114. Deal BJ, Mavroudis C, Backer CL (2007) Arrhythmia management in the Fontan patient. Pediatr Cardiol 28:448–456.

115. Driscoll DJ, Offord KP, Feldt RH, et al. (1992) Five- to fifteen-year follow-up after Fontan operation. Circulation 85:469–496.

116. Balaji S, Gewillig M, Bull C, et al. (1991) Arrhythmias after the Fontan procedure. Comparison of total cavopulmonary connection and atriopulmonary connection. Circulation 84:III162–III167.

117. Cohen MI, Bridges ND, Gaynor JW, et al. (2000) Modifications to the cavopulmonary anastomosis do not eliminate early sinus node dysfunction. J Thorac Cardiovasc Surg 120:891–900.

118. Giannico S, Hammad F, Amodeo A, et al. (2006) Clinical outcome of 193 extracardiac Fontan patients: the first 15 years. J Am Coll Cardiol 47:2065–2073.

119. Mertens L, Hagler DJ, Sauer U, et al. (1998) Protein-losing enteropathy after the Fontan operation: an international multicenter study. PLE study group. J Thorac Cardiovasc Surg 115:1063–1073.

120. Rychik J, Piccoli DA, Barber G (1991) Usefulness of corticosteroid therapy for protein-losing enteropathy after the Fontan procedure. Am J Cardiol 68:819–821.

121. Donnelly JP, Rosenthal A, Castle VP, et al. (1997) Reversal of protein-losing enteropathy with heparin therapy in three patients with univentricular hearts and Fontan palliation. J Pediatr 130:474–478.

122. Ostrow A, Freeze H, Rychik J (2006) Protein-losing enteropathy after Fontan operation: investigations into possible pathophysiologic mechanisms. Ann Thorac Surg 82:695–701.

123. Harrison DA, Liu P, Walters JE, et al. (1995) Cardiopulmonary function in adult patients late after Fontan repair. J Am Coll Cardiol 26:1016–1021.

124. Ghanayem NS, Berger S, Tweddell JS (2007) Medical management of the failing Fontan. Pediatr Cardiol 28:465–471.

125. Sheikh AM, Tang AT, Roman K, et al. (2004) The failing Fontan circulation: successful conversion of atriopulmonary connections. J Thorac Cardiovasc Surg 128:60–66.

126. Mavroudis C, Deal BJ, Backer CL, et al. (2007) J. Maxwell Chamberlain Memorial Paper for congenital heart surgery. 111 Fontan conversions with arrhythmia surgery: surgical lessons and outcomes. Ann Thorac Surg 84:1457–1465.

127. Drenthen W, Pieper PG, Roos-Hesselink JW, et al. (2006) Pregnancy and delivery in women after Fontan palliation. Heart 92:1290–1294.

128. Canobbio MM, Mair DD, Van Der Velde M, et al. (1996) Pregnancy outcomes after the Fontan repair. J Am Coll Cardiol 28:763–767.

129. Diller GP, Gatzoulis MA (2007) Pulmonary vascular disease in adults with congenital heart disease. Circulation 115:1039–1050.

130. Vongpatanasin W, Brickner ME, Hillis LD, et al. (1998) The Eisenmenger syndrome in adults. Ann Intern Med 128:745–755.

131. Cantor WJ, Harrison DA, Moussadji JS, et al. (1999) Determinants of survival and length of survival in adults with Eisenmenger syndrome. Am J Cardiol 84:677–681.

132. Diller GP, Dimopoulos K, Broberg CS, et al. (2006) Presentation, survival prospects, and predictors of death in Eisenmenger syndrome: a combined retrospective and case-control study. Eur Heart J 27:1737–1742.

133. Saha A, Balakrishnan KG, Jaiswal PK, et al. (1994) Prognosis for patients with Eisenmenger syndrome of various aetiology. Int J Cardiol 45:199–207.

134. Daliento L, Somerville J, Presbitero P, et al. (1998) Eisenmenger syndrome. Factors relating to deterioration and death. Eur Heart J 19:1845–1855.

135. Silversides CK, Granton JT, Konen E, et al. (2003) Pulmonary thrombosis in adults with Eisenmenger syndrome. J Am Coll Cardiol 42:1982–1987.

136. Holzman RS, Nargozian CD, Marnach R, et al. (1992) Epidural anesthesia in patients with palliated cyanotic congenital heart disease. J Cardiothorac Vasc Anesth 6:340–343.

137. Devitt JH, Noble WH, Byrick RJ (1982) A Swan-Ganz catheter related complication in a patient with Eisenmenger's syndrome. Anesthesiology 57:335–337.

138. Perloff JK (1987) The Clinical Recognition of Congenital Heart Disease, 3rd edn. WB Saunders, Philadelphia.

139. Gleicher N, Midwall J, Hochberger D, et al. (1979) Eisenmenger's syndrome and pregnancy. Obstet Gynecol Surv 34:721–741.

140. Weiss BM, Zemp L, Seifert B, et al. (1998) Outcome of pulmonary vascular disease in pregnancy: a systematic overview from 1978 through 1996. J Am Coll Cardiol 31:1650–1657.

141. Bonnin M, Mercier FJ, Sitbon O, et al. (2005) Severe pulmonary hypertension during pregnancy: mode of delivery and anesthetic management of 15 consecutive cases. Anesthesiology 102:1133–1137.

142. Weiss BM, Hess OM (2000) Pulmonary vascular disease and pregnancy: current controversies, management strategies, and perspectives. Eur Heart J 21:104–115.

143. Andropoulos DB, Stayer SA, Skjonsby BS, et al. (2002) Anesthetic and perioperative outcome of teenagers and adults with congenital heart disease. J Cardiothorac Vasc Anes 16:731–736.

144. Dore A, Glancy DL, Stone S, et al. (1997) Cardiac surgery for grown-up congenital heart patients: survey of 307 consecutive operations from 1991 to 1994. Am J Cardiol 80:906–913.

145. Masud F, Bostan F, Chi E, et al. (2009) Recombinant factor VIIa treatment of severe bleeding in cardiac surgery patients: a retrospective analysis of dosing, efficacy, and safety outcomes. J Cardiothorac Vasc Anesth 23:28–33.

146. McGill N, O'Shaughnessy D, Pickering R, et al. (2002) Mechanical methods of reducing blood transfusion in cardiac surgery: randomised controlled trial. BMJ 324:1299.

147. Royston D, von Kier S (2001) Reduced haemostatic factor transfusion using heparinase-modified thrombelastography during cardiopulmonary bypass. Br J Anaes 86:575–578.

148. Fyfe DA, Ritter SB, Snider AR, et al. (1992) Guidelines for transesophageal echocardiography in children. J Am Soc Echocardiogr 5:640–644.

149. Cheitlin MD, Alpert JS, Armstrong WF, et al. (1997) ACC/AHA Guidelines for the Clinical Application of Echocardiography. A report of the American College of Cardiology/American Heart Association Task Force on Practice Guidelines (Committee on Clinical Application of Echocardiography). Developed in collaboration with the American Society of Echocardiography. Circulation 95:1686–1744.

150. American Society of Anesthesiologists (1996) Practice guidelines for perioperative transesophageal echocardiography. A report by the American Society of Anesthesiologists and the Society of Cardiovascular Anestheisologists Task Force on Transesophageal Echocardiography. Anesthesiology 84:986–1006.

151. Edmonds HL, Jr, Rodriguez RA, Audenaert SM, et al. (1996) The role of neuromonitoring in cardiovascular surgery. J Cardiothorac Vasc Anesth 10:15–23.

152. Galli KK, Myers LB, Nicolson SC (2001) Anesthesia for adult patients with congenital heart disease undergoing noncardiac surgery. Int Anesthesiol Clin 39:43–71.

4 Management

16 Hemodynamic management*

Dean B. Andropoulos, M.D.

Texas Children's Hospital, Baylor College of Medicine, Houston, Texas, USA

Introduction

Congenital heart disease (CHD) encompasses a diverse group of diseases with dramatic differences between patients, even with same or similar diagnoses. Because of these dramatic differences, it is fair to say that each patient is unique and requires an individually tailored approach for optimal hemodynamic management. Before deciding on the medications or the interventions that one will employ to improve the hemodynamic status of these patients, one has to understand the anatomy and physiology of the congenital heart lesion as well as the comorbid conditions that may influence the choice of inotrope and vasoactive drugs that one will use. Hemodynamic management of patients is also impacted by long-term hemodynamic perturbations that arise as a result of disease itself or compensatory changes due to uncorrected lesions and the sequelae after surgical palliation or correction (Table 16.1).

Pathophysiology of congenital cardiac lesions

CHD includes a wide spectrum of lesions; however, all CHDs include in part or in their entirety one or more of the following four lesions:
1 Obstructive lesions
2 Regurgitant lesions
3 Shunt lesions
4 Mixing lesions
It is important for the anesthesiologists to understand how the presence of one or a combination of these lesions impacts the hemodynamic management of a patient with CHD.

Obstructive lesions

Obstructive lesions, whether they are on the right or left side, impose a pressure load on the chamber proximal to the obstruction, which over a period of time leads to chamber hypertrophy and/or enlargement. Increases in oxygen demands by the hypertrophied myocardium may eventually outstrip the coronary blood supply and cause myocardial ischemia. The primary derangement seen in right-sided obstructive lesions is reduction of pulmonary blood flow and possible hypoxemia. Left-sided obstructive lesions (coarctation of aorta, hypoplastic left heart syndrome) mainly present as decreased cardiac output

---

*Portions of this chapter were published as Chapter 14: Hemodynamic Management, by Aman Mahajan, M.D., and Jure Marijic, M.D., in *Anesthesia for Congenital Heart Disease*, 1st edn.

Anesthesia for Congenital Heart Disease 2nd edition. Edited by
Dean Andropoulos, Stephen Stayer, Isobel Russell and Emad Mossad.
© 2010 Blackwell Publishing.

Table 16.1 Hemodynamic stigmata in congenital heart disease

Pulmonary hypertension and pulmonary vascular disease
Valvular regurgitation or stenosis
Ventricular enlargement
Ventricular hypertrophy
Impaired diastolic and systolic ventricular function
Outflow tract obstruction
Polycythemia and Hyperviscosity
Autonomic denervation in the transplanted heart

and systemic perfusion. Hemodynamic management (Figure 16.1) in patients with obstructive lesions requires the knowledge of the degree of stenosis or obstruction in the vascular tree and the ability to keep the proximal pressure higher in order to overcome the resistance and maintain antegrade flow in the circulation. It is very important to distinguish between fixed and dynamic obstruction since the management of the obstruction caused by these two mechanisms is very different. The degree of dynamic obstruction (e.g., right ventricular outflow tract obstruction or hypertrophic cardiomyopathy) is dependent upon end-diastolic volume; and increased

preload, decreased heart rate, and decreased contractility decrease obstruction and gradient, increasing forward flow as well as decreasing myocardial work and oxygen consumption. Obstructive lesions frequently coexist with shunting or mixing lesions. Under these conditions, the degree of obstruction will dramatically alter the shunt fraction and in some cases may even change the direction of the shunt. Changes in systemic (SVR) and pulmonary (PVR) vascular resistances will also effect pulmonary-to-systemic blood flow ratio (Qp:Qs) in such combined lesions.

Regurgitant lesions

Valvular regurgitation can be seen as a primary congenital anomaly in certain congenital cardiac lesions (Ebstein's anomaly, atrioventricular canal defect, cleft mitral valve), but more commonly develops as a long-term sequelae of anatomical and physiological changes induced by pressure or volume loads that have been imposed by other associated lesions. The regurgitant fraction (portion of the total stroke volume) is dependent upon preload (may change geometry of the ventricle and mitral valve), afterload (changes impedance to forward flow), and heart rate

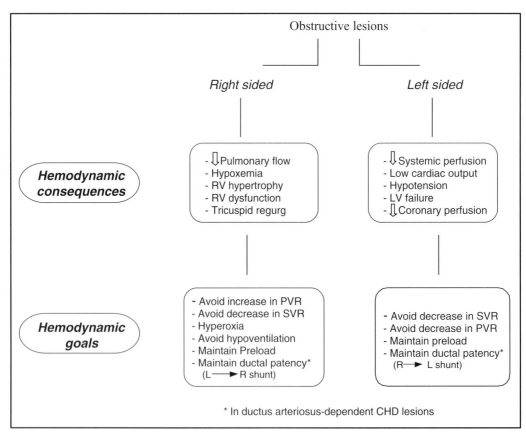

Figure 16.1 Hemodynamic consequences and goals for obstructive lesions. RV, right ventricle; LV, left ventricle; PVR, pulmonary vascular resistance; SVR, systemic vascular resistance; R, right; L, left; CHD, congenital heart disease

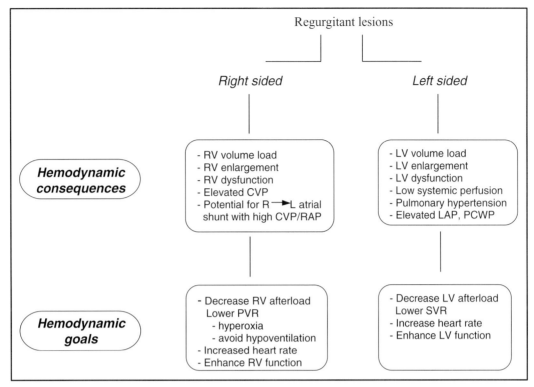

Figure 16.2 Hemodynamic consequences and goals for regurgitant lesions. RV, right ventricle; CVP, central venous pressure; RAP, right atrial pressure; LV, left ventricle; LAP, left atrial pressure; PCWP, pulmonary capillary wedge pressure; PVR, pulmonary vascular resistance; SVR, systemic vascular resistance; R, right; L, left

(through changes in ventricular end-diastolic volume, systolic and diastolic time). Appropriate management of the heart rate, preload, and afterload helps minimize the negative hemodynamic effect of valvular regurgitation (Figure 16.2). Poor ventricular function results from volume loading associated with significant valvular regurgitation and alters the severity of regurgitation. This is especially true for atrioventricular valves since the ventricle is an integral part of valvular apparatus.

Shunt lesions

Shunts can be intracardiac (ASD/VSD) or extracardiac (PDA or surgically created, e.g., systemic to pulmonary artery shunt). Flow in a shunt is dependent upon the pressure gradient and relative vascular resistance in the vascular bed distal to the shunt. The degree to which each of these factors affects the amount and direction of shunting depends upon the size of the anatomical defect. In general, if the shunt size is large (nonrestrictive), the pressure gradient across the defect will be small and flow across the shunt will be affected more by the vascular resistance in the respective vascular beds and less dependent upon the pressure gradient. The converse is also true

when the anatomical size of the shunt is small (restrictive flow).

In the case of a left-to-right shunt, increasing the SVR (systemic arterial pressures) or decreasing the PVR increases the amount of shunting leading to an excess of pulmonary blood flow (Qp) relative to systemic blood flow (Qs). This increased Qp:Qs ratio predisposes to pulmonary edema and development of pulmonary vascular disease. At the same time, systemic blood flow and oxygen supply delivery decrease. Hemodynamic management (Figure 16.3) of patients with left-to-right shunting includes lowering of SVR and avoiding maneuvers that decrease PVR (hyperoxia, hypocarbia). In extreme cases, one may need to increase the PVR above normal by providing either hypoxic inspired gas mixtures or hypercapneic ventilation. Inotropes and vasodilators should be selected and used with these goals in mind. On the other hand, right-to-left shunts are optimally managed by lowering the PVR as well as avoiding decreases in SVR. Hyperventilation and higher concentrations of inspired oxygen have been used to lower PVR in patients with CHD to test the reactivity of PVR as well as for therapy. Other options include the use of selective pulmonary vasodilators such as inhaled nitric oxide (iNO), prostacyclin, calcium channel blockers, and sildenafil.

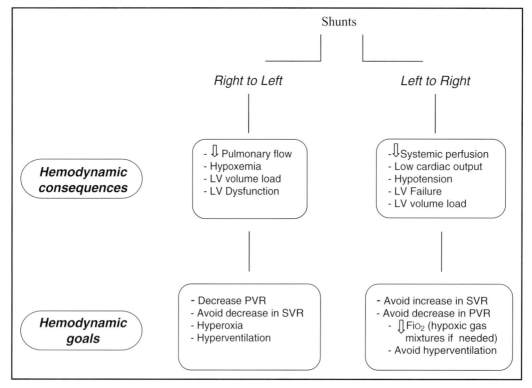

Figure 16.3 Hemodynamic consequences and goals for intracardiac and extracardiac shunting Lesions. LV, left ventricle; LAP, left atrial pressure; PCWP, pulmonary capillary wedge pressure; PVR, pulmonary vascular resistance; SVR, systemic vascular resistance; FiO₂, fraction of inspired oxygen

Mixing lesions

Congenital heart defects in which there is a complete mixing of oxygenated and deoxygenated blood in the cardiac chambers or the great vessels are termed mixing lesions (tricuspid atresia, univentricular hearts, truncus arteriosus, anomalies of pulmonary venous return). This complete mixing is due to the unrestricted flow of blood from right-sided structures to left and vice versa across a large communication between the two sides, leading to arterial hypoxemia of varying degrees. As in the case of large shunts, the flow of blood is significantly affected by the vascular resistance of pulmonary and systemic circulation (Figure 16.4).

Complete mixing (as well as right-to-left intracardiac shunting) results in partially desaturated blood in systemic circulation and over a period of time, to compensatory changes in the oxygen carrying capacity of the blood (increased hemoglobin and red cell mass) and oxygen delivery to the tissues (increased 2,3 DPG and fall in oxygen consumption). Potentially large increases in blood viscosity occurring as a result of elevation in serum hematocrit to 65–70% may compromise blood flow to vital organs and decrease oxygen delivery to the tissues rather than increase it.

Determinants of cardiac output and oxygen delivery

Besides the unique factors discussed earlier, that alter the hemodynamic management in patients with CHD, it is important to recognize that alterations of preload, afterload, contractility, and heart rate are four cornerstones that affect cardiac output, before and after surgical correction of congenital cardiac disease (Figure 16.5). The oxygen-carrying capacity of blood is improved by increasing the hemoglobin concentration. Each of these factors should be adjusted for the specific congenital cardiac lesion and the cardiovascular physiology that is associated with the lesion.

Pharmacologic therapy for CHD

The goal of drug therapy in an acute setting should be to optimize cardiac output; improve perfusion pressure to vital organs such as brain, heart, and kidneys; and maintain an optimal balance between systemic and pulmonary blood flows with an appropriate level of oxygenation.

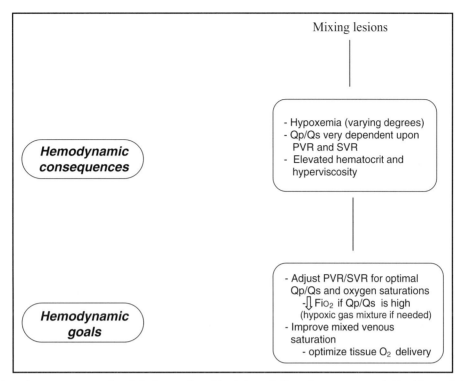

Figure 16.4 Hemodynamic consequences and goals for intracardiac mixing lesions. Qp/Qs, pulmonary to systemic blood flow ratio; PVR, pulmonary vascular resistance; SVR, systemic vascular resistance; FiO$_2$, fraction of inspired oxygen

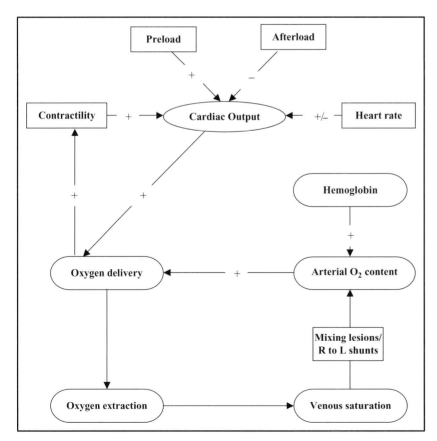

Figure 16.5 Determinants of cardiac output and oxygen delivery. R, right; L, left

Table 16.2 Cardioactive and vasoactive drugs

Drug	Dose	Receptors	Inotropy	HR	SVR	PVR	Renal vascular resistance
Epinephrine	0.02–0.2 µg/kg/min						
	Lower dose	β_1, $\beta_2 > \alpha_1$	↑	↑	↔, ↓	↔, ↓	↓
	Higher dose	$\alpha_1 > \beta_1$, β_2	↑	↑	↑	↑	↑
Norepinephrine	0.02–0.2 µg/kg/min	$\alpha_1 > \beta_1$, β_2	↑	↑	↑	↑	↓
Dopamine	2–5 µg/kg/min	DA_1, DA_2	↔	↔	↔	↔	↓
	5–10 µg/kg/min	β_1, $\beta_2 > \alpha_1$	↑	↑	↔, ↓	↔	↑
	>10 µg/kg/min	$\alpha_1 > \beta_1$, β_2	↑	↑	↑	↑	
Dobutamine	2–20 µg/kg/min	$\beta_1 > \beta_2$, α_1	↑	↑	↓	↓	↔
Isoproterenol	0.01–0.2 µg/kg/min	β_1, β_2	↑	↑	↓	↓	↓
Milrinone	Loading 25–100 µg/kg	Phosphodiesterase III inhibitor/↑ cAMP	↑	↑	↓	↓	↓
	Infusion 0.25–0.75 µg/kg/min						
Calcium chloride	5–10 mg/kg IV bolus; 10 mg/kg/hr infusion	Contractile proteins	↑	↔, ↓	↑	↔, ↑	↔

HR, heart rate; SVR, systemic vascular resistance; PVR, pulmonary vascular resistance; DA, dopamine.

The drugs that may be used in the acute hemodynamic management of patients can be categorized as being belonging to one or more of these functional classes:

1 Inotropes (epinephrine, dopamine, dobutamine, milrinone, amrinone, calcium, digoxin)
2 Chronotropes (isoproterenol)
3 Vasoconstrictors (norepinephrine, phenylephrine, vasopressin)
4 Vasodilators (nitroglycerin, nitroprusside, prostaglandins, nitric oxide (NO), hydralazine, phentolamine, phenoxybenzamine)
5 Beta-adrenergic antagonists;
6 Newer cardiotonic and vasoactive agents

These drugs will now be reviewed, and the pediatric cardiovascular anesthesiologist must keep in mind that the indications for and doses of these drugs in an individual patient are highly variable. Tables 16.2 and 16.3 summarize the effects and recommended dosages for these drugs.

Affects such as age, disease state, and adrenergic receptor up- or downregulation necessitate frequent titration of drugs to effect.

Inotropes

Epinephrine

Epinephrine is an endogenous catecholamine that is secreted primarily by the adrenal glands and has strong alpha- and beta-adrenergic receptor activation. This action on both types of adrenergic receptors leads to the complexity of response in different organs and tissue beds. The response of exogenously administered epinephrine is to a large part dependent upon the ratio of alpha- to beta-receptors in the individual tissue beds as well as to the dose of epinephrine given (Figure 16.6). At lower doses (<0.05 mcg/kg/min), epinephrine causes a moderate

Table 16.3 Vasoactive drugs

Drug	Dose	Receptors	Inotropy	HR	SVR	PVR	Renal vascular resistance
Vasopressin	0.01–0.05 Units/kg/h	V_1, V_2	↔	↔, ↓	↑	↑	↑
Phenylephrine	0.02–0.3 mcg/kg/min	α_1 (agonist)	↔	↓	↑	↑	↑
Nitroglycerin	0.2–10 µg/kg/min	Vascular myocyte/guanylyl cyclase, cGMP ↑	↔	↔, ↑	↓	↓	↓
Nitroprusside	0.2–5 µg/kg/min	Vascular myocyte/Guanylyl Cyclase, cGMP ↑	↔	↔, ↑	↓	↓	↓
Phentolamine	0.2–2 µg/kg/min	α_1 (antagonist)	↔	↔, ↑	↓	↓	↓
Inhaled nitric oxide	10–40 ppm	Vascular myocyte/cGMP ↑	↔	↔	↔	↓	↔
Prostaglandin E_1	0.01–0.2 µg/kg/min	Vascular myocyte/cAMP ↑	↔	↔, ↑	↓	↓	↓

V, vasopressin; HR, heart rate; SVR, systemic vascular resistance; PVR, pulmonary vascular resistance.

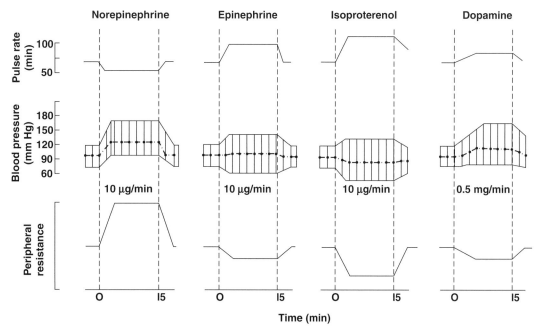

Figure 16.6 Effects of infusions of norepinephrine, epinephrine, isoproterenol, and dopamine in dogs (Reproduced and used with permission from Reference [1])

increase in systolic blood pressure that is mainly due to the increased ventricular contraction [1]. Activation of the beta-2 receptors in the vascular smooth muscles of the skeletal muscles usually leads to a decrease in the SVR and slight decrease in the diastolic pressure. As the dose is progressively increased, more prominent peripheral vasoconstriction is seen due to the activation of the alpha-receptors in other vascular beds [2]. Renal blood flow is consistently decreased as vascular resistance in all segments of the renal vasculature increases [3]. Epinephrine has been used as a strong inotrope in the supporting the function of a failing myocardium. Epinephrine's action on the predominant beta-1 receptors in the heart leads to an increase in contractility and an increase in the heart rate. Higher doses will lead to a decrease in the refractory period of the atrioventricular node and an increase in the automaticity of the myocardium, which may predispose to the development of atrial or ventricular arrhythmias.

During cardiopulmonary resuscitation, epinephrine is the vasopressor of choice since it has profound alpha-adrenergic stimulation that aid in maintaining the cerebral and coronary perfusion pressure in the face of cardiovascular collapse [4]. Current American Heart Association (AHA) recommendations for cardiopulmonary resuscitation dosing of epinephrine in adults is 0.5–1 mg IV, repeated as necessary every 3–5 minutes.

The AHA-recommended dose of epinephrine in children for bradycardia, asystolic, or pulseless arrest is 0.01

mg/kg intravenously, repeated at 3–5-minute intervals. Higher doses of epinephrine are no longer recommended [5,6]. Prolonged exposure of epinephrine and other catecholamine compounds to alkaline solutions (e.g., sodium bicarbonate) leads to the auto-oxidation and loss of their activity. Epinephrine should not be mixed with infusion bags or bottles that have alkaline solutions.

Epinephrine is used as an infusion primarily in the dose range from 0.02 to 0.2 mcg/kg/min, although doses up to 0.5 mcg/kg/min or higher are occasionally required in the short term for acute severe low cardiac output in situations such as weaning from bypass, or during extracorporeal membrane oxygenation cannulation or emergency institution of bypass. Prolonged exposure to high doses of epinephrine, i.e., 0.2 mcg/kg/min or higher for more than several hours, may cause myocardial necrosis in infants, and consideration should be given for mechanical circulatory support in this instance [7].

Dopamine

Dopamine is another naturally occurring catecholamine that is an immediate precursor of norepinephrine. Most of the functions of endogenously excreted dopamine are as a central neurotransmitter, though it has been found in the peripheral circulation as well. The cardiovascular effects of exogenously administered dopamine are due to the activation of a variety of receptors that have different affinity for the drug [8]. At a lower dose (<5 μg/kg/min), the primary receptors that are activated are the dopaminergic-1 (DA-1) receptors present in the renal, mesenteric, and coronary vascular beds. Infusion of low-dose dopamine can lead to an increase in renal blood flow and an increase in glomerular filtration rate [9]. Even though there is promising data in animals as well as some uncontrolled human studies [10], no prospective randomized controlled trial has evaluated the role of dopamine in improving acute renal failure, either alone or in combination with diuretics. It is therefore unclear, if renal dose dopamine has direct beneficial effects in improving renal function. As the dose of the drug is increased, stimulation of the beta-1 receptors in the myocardium leads to an increase in inotropy and chronotropy of the heart [11]. At these doses, dopamine causes an increase in cardiac output, decrease in pulmonary capillary wedge pressure, and there is usually a decrease in SVR with only slight changes in blood pressure. The increase in heart rate is much less as compared to isoproterenol. Total peripheral resistance is usually unchanged with low or intermediate doses of dopamine, due to vasodilatory action of dopamine on regional vascular beds. At higher doses (>10 μg/kg/min), more alpha-1 receptors are activated leading to a more intense peripheral vasoconstriction and an increase in vascular resistance. Dopamine causes release of norepinephrine from nerve endings; this also adds to its pharmacologic effect of adrenergic stimulation.

In a study of dopamine pharmacokinetics in infants and children who were recovering from cardiac surgery or sepsis and had stable hemodynamics, the drug was reported to have a distribution half-life of 1.8 ± 1.1 minutes [12]. The volume of distribution (2952 ± 2332 mL/kg) and the clearance (454 ± 900 mL/kg/min) were found to be highly variable, underscoring the principle of titrating this drug to effect in the individual patient. Dopamine in the dose range 5–15 μg/kg/min is commonly used as an inotropic support to assist in the weaning of the heart from cardiopulmonary bypass (CPB). In recent years, some practitioners have avoided dopamine because of its role as a neurotransmitter, which can cross the blood–brain barrier and is known to suppress pituitary function, particularly thyroid releasing hormone, in infants and children [13].

This potential adverse effect is not seen with other natural or synthetic catecholamines [14].

Dobutamine

A synthetic congener of dopamine, dobutamine's pharmacological actions are due to its activation of alpha- and beta-adrenergic receptors. Dobutamine has not been shown to have any effect on the dopaminergic receptors or lead to the release of norepinephrine from nerve endings. The primary action of dobutamine is on the beta-1 receptors with only a small action on the beta-2 or alpha-1 receptors. This action manifests as an increase in inotropy and chronotropy. Cardiac output is markedly enhanced and the left-sided filing pressures are decreased. Total peripheral resistance is unchanged or may be decreased with the use of dobutamine. This effect may be especially beneficial in treating patients with ventricular dysfunction.

There is little direct increase in renal blood flow as is seen with dopamine. Dobutamine has been shown to be effective in improving depressed cardiac index after CPB in children with CHD in doses ranging from 5 to 15 mcg/kg/min [15]. Comparison with newer inotropic drugs such as milrinone demonstrates similar improvements in stroke volume but a more profound decrease in left ventricular filling pressures and vascular resistance with the phosphodiesterase inhibitors [16]. Increased heart rate is more prominent with dobutamine than with milrinone. At equivalent inotropic doses, dobutamine enhances the automaticity of the sinoatrial node to a much less extent than isoproterenol [17]. Higher doses of dobutamine (>15 mcg/kg/min) can predispose to the development of atrial or ventricular arrhythmias.

The dose range of a dobutamine infusion ranges from 3 to 20 mcg/kg/min. Steady state levels were achieved in 10 minutes and the half-life was 2.37 minutes in a pharmacokinetic study in adult patients with heart failure [18]. Since almost all tissues metabolize dobutamine, dosage adjustment need not be performed even in patients with renal, hepatic, or any other organ dysfunction. Tolerance to long-term infusions (>72 h) may develop due to downregulation of beta-receptors [19]. Despite the fact that dobutamine will increase cardiac output in neonates by increasing stroke volume, heart rate, and cardiac output, it is frequently used to stress the myocardium, and will increase myocardial oxygen consumption, and produce diastolic dysfunction in some patients with repaired CHD [20,21].

Milrinone

Milrinone is a bipyridine derivative that induces vasodilatation and exerts a positive inotropic effect by blocking the phosphodiesterase III enzyme. The inhibition of phosphodiesterase leads to the accumulation of cyclic adenosine monophosphate (cAMP), independent of adrenergic receptor stimulation [22]. The increase in cAMP in cardiac myocytes improves systolic and diastolic function by altering calcium influx [23], and by altering uptake and binding of calcium to myofilaments. Whereas in vascular smooth muscle, accumulation of cAMP predominantly effects the removal of calcium across sarcolemma and therefore vasodilatation. The decrease in SVR allows phosphodiesterase inhibitors to increase cardiac output and oxygen delivery without increasing myocardial work and oxygen demand. Because of the dual effects on the inotropic state of the heart and the vascular resistance, milrinone has been used extensively in the treatment of congestive heart failure, pulmonary hypertension, and postoperative low cardiac output.

Milrinone has been shown to be an effective inotrope in adults as well as children with CHD [24,25]. Peripheral vasodilation also ensues as a result of vascular smooth muscle relaxation. Chang et al. reported that milrinone (loading 50 μg/kg followed by an infusion of 0.5 μg/kg/min), when administered to neonates with low cardiac output after cardiac surgery, was able to lower filling pressures, SVR, and PVR (>25%), and improve cardiac index (from 2.1 to 3.1) [26]. Similarly, Bailey et al. found a mean increase in cardiac output of 18% after milrinone therapy in 20 children undergoing corrective surgery for congenital cardiac defects [27]. Milrinone also improves diastolic function. In adult patients undergoing CPB, administration of 0.5 μg/kg/min milrinone decreased endotoxemia and other markers of inflammation, likely because of improved splanchnic perfusion. In the pediatric population, where hemodilution and activation of the inflammatory response during CPB is an even greater problem, the administration of phosphodiesterase inhibitors could potentially be of greater benefit. Hypotension and reflex tachycardia may result as a side effect of milrinone therapy. Mehra et al. reported a 4% incidence of thrombocytopenia in 71 patients who received long-term intravenous milrinone therapy (>3 days) [28]. Milrinone is primarily renally excreted and higher bolus doses (50–75 μg/kg) may show prolonged hemodynamic effects in patients with impaired renal function. Serum half-life was found to be 0.8 hours in patients with congestive heart failure [29]. Milrinone has also been suggested to have a higher volume of distribution and a faster clearance in infants and children as compared to adults [29]. The dose recommended for milrinone therapy in patients with normal renal function is a bolus of 50 μg/kg followed by an infusion of 0.25–0.75 μg/kg/min. Hypotension seen with a loading dose may be avoided by reducing or eliminating the loading dose and simply beginning the infusion, recognizing that therapeutic plasma levels will not be achieved for several hours.

In recent years, milrinone has gained widespread use in congenital cardiac anesthesia, and is one of the few regimens that have been subjected to prospective, randomized, double blind, controlled study. In 227 infants and children undergoing cardiac surgery with bypass, high-dose milrinone (75 mcg/kg loading dose after bypass, followed by 0.75 mcg/kg/min infusion) reduced the incidence of low cardiac output syndrome by 55% compared to placebo or low-dose milrinone (25 mcg/kg load and 0.25 mcg/kg/min) [30]. In a pharmacokinetic study of 16 neonates undergoing Norwood Stage I palliation, a loading dose of 100 mcg/kg into the bypass circuit at the

start of rewarming provided therapeutic plasma concentrations, but an infusion of 0.5 mcg/kg/min caused a significant increase in plasma milrinone concentration over the first 12 hours; impaired renal function was thought to be the cause, and neonates may require lower doses of 0.2 mcg/kg/min [31].

Calcium

The calcium ion is an integral part of the excitation–contraction coupling and impulse generation in myocardial cells and is a major determinant of vascular smooth muscle tone. Administration of calcium in the form of calcium chloride or calcium gluconate helps improve the inotropic function of the heart in the presence of hypocalcemia [32] (decreased serum ionized calcium levels). Calcium functions primarily as a vasoconstrictor when the serum ionized calcium levels are normal. Routine administration of calcium salts upon termination of CPB is a subject of debate. The incidence of hypocalcemia during CPB is relatively high, but the ionized calcium levels usually are corrected to normal levels as weaning from CPB is attempted [33], and therefore calcium administration may not be required for most patients. Moreover, increasing evidence suggests that elevated intracellular calcium levels are associated with cell death and injury during ischemia and reperfusion injury [34]. A recent study also suggests that no significant improvement in cardiac index was observed in adult patients with good ventricular function upon administration of calcium chloride at the termination of CPB [35]. Murdoch et al. reported an increase in the systemic vascular resistance index (885–1070 dyne s/cm^5/m^2) and a decrease in CI (4.44–3.85 L/min/m^2) after administration of 10 mg/kg of CaCl$_2$ in 12 children following cardiac surgery [36]. Rapid administration of calcium can slow the heart rate transiently and it should be used cautiously in patients who are taking digoxin as it may precipitate digoxin toxicity.

Calcium administration is not recommended in bradyasystoles unless severe hypocalcemia or hyperkalemia coexists or if the arrest is secondary to calcium channel antagonist drugs [5,6].

A higher and more predictable amount of elemental calcium is available from the intravenous administration of calcium chloride than calcium gluconate or gluceptate [37].

Because the neonatal myocardial sarcoplasmic reticulum is not well organized, and release and reuptake of Ca^{++} is not efficient, some anesthesiologists administer a CaCl$_2$ infusion of 10 mg/kg/h to neonates after CPB, especially when they require citrated blood products for postcardiotomy bleeding. However, a recent retrospective review of infants younger than 1 year demonstrated that mortality after cardiac surgery with bypass was correlated with higher Ca^{++} supplementation, suggesting that this agent should be used only with documented hypocalcemia with associated myocardial dysfunction, or in neonates receiving significant amounts of citrated blood products, and discontinued as soon as possible [38].

Chronotropes

Isoproterenol

Isoproterenol is a potent nonselective beta-adrenergic agonist with only very minimal actions on alpha-receptors. Due to its vasodilatory beta-2 stimulatory actions as well as lack of alpha-receptor stimulation, isoproterenol leads to lowering of peripheral vascular resistance [1,39] (Figure 16.6). Its vasodilatory actions may be seen in renal, mesenteric, and pulmonary vascular beds. Cardiac output is increased in patients with heart failure as a result of the increased inotropy and chronotropy in the face of diminished SVR [17]. An intravenous infusion of isoproterenol has more chronotropic than inotropic as opposed to dopamine or dobutamine. Myocardial oxygen demands are greatly exacerbated by isoproterenol and this may exacerbate or induce ischemia [40]. Higher doses of isoproterenol can be arrhythmogenic and may induce ventricular tachycardia or fibrillation.

Isoproterenol has been shown to cause less hyperglycemia as compared to epinephrine, since insulin secretion is stimulated by the strong beta-adrenergic stimulation. The drug has been shown to be effective in increasing the heart rate in patients with severe bradycardia or a heart block [5,6]. This chronotropic effect of isoproterenol remains the principal use of the drug, and it is often used in electrophysiologic studies to increase heart rate and incite atrial and ventricular arrhythmias, and principal use in cardiac anesthesia is in the denervated heart immediately after heart transplant, or in cases of complete atrioventricular block. Isoproterenol is generally not used as a first line drug in the management of myocardial dysfunction or in the treatment of heart failure. The dose for isoproterenol infusion ranges from 0.01 to 0.2 µg/kg/min.

Vasoconstrictors

Norepinephrine

Norepinephrine is an endogenous catecholamine that is primarily released by the postganglionic adrenergic nerve endings. Besides being a major source of epinephrine, the adrenal medulla also contains norepinephrine in a smaller fraction (10–20%).

The actions of norepinephrine are very similar to epinephrine on the heart with strong stimulation of the beta-1 receptors and increase in myocardial contractility

[3]. There is a substantial difference in the peripheral action of the two drugs [1] and these differences account for the difference in the clinical use of these two drugs. Norepinephrine is a potent alpha-1 agonist at all doses with minimal effects on the vasodilatory beta-2 receptors [1]. As a result, even low doses of norepinephrine lead to an increase in the systolic and diastolic blood pressure. SVR is increased as a result of the vasoconstriction of most peripheral vascular beds. Cardiac output is usually decreased or unchanged, depending upon the increase in total peripheral resistance. Heart rate may be slowed as a result of reflex increase in vagal tone, or may increase if the beta-1 effects predominate in an individual patient. Both of the endogenous catecholamines, epinephrine, and norepinephrine can lead to hyperglycemia with prolonged infusions [41]. Norepinephrine usually causes these effects at much higher doses than epinephrine.

Norepinephrine functions as a strong vasoconstrictor and is useful in the clinical situation of decreased SVR; however, it is used infrequently in infants and children. Dose range of norepinephrine infusion varies from 0.02 to 0.2 µg/kg/min. It is effective in raising SVR in cases of profound vasodilatory shock unresponsive to high doses of dopamine or dobutamine, such as from sepsis in neonates [42].

Phenylephrine

Phenylephrine is a pure peripheral alpha-1 receptor agonist used as a bolus or infusion where low systemic blood pressure or SVR must be treated acutely. The pure α effects often result in reflex slowing of the heart rate, although this is not as pronounced in young infants. Its principle use in CHD is to acutely raise SVR when either ventricle is compromised by outflow obstruction, e.g., tetralogy of Fallot (TOF) with low SVR leading to increased right-to-left intracardiac shunting and cyanosis during a "Tet Spell" [43], and hypertrophic cardiomyopathy [44] or other left-sided lesions where the gradient across the obstruction is increased by low SVR. On CPB, small phenylephrine boluses can be used to increase perfusion pressure when other measures such as increasing bypass flow are ineffective, until SVR on bypass equilibrates with cooling, and viscosity changes from redistribution of red cells in the patient-bypass circuit. Infusions can be used when frequent boluses are necessary, such as in the TOF patient with continuous spelling before bypass. Phenylephrine is very effective at increasing the blood pressure, but its principle adverse effect is vasoconstriction of peripheral tissue beds, including skeletal muscle, skin, renal, and mesenteric. This vasoconstriction may be intense, and theoretically may compromise end organ blood flow and function, leading many practitioners to limit its use to extreme situations. Extravasation of phenylephrine into the skin and subcutaneous tissues may lead to ischemia, necrosis, and tissue loss.

Bolus dosing of phenylephrine is 0.5–5 mcg/kg, and infusion dosing ranges from 0.02 to 0.3 mcg/kg/min, through a central venous catheter if possible.

Vasopressin

Vasopressin is a neurogenic polypeptide produced by the paraventricular nucleus of the midbrain in response to low blood pressure and is secreted by the posterior lobe of the pituitary. Vasopressin produces intense vasoconstriction and an antidiuretic effect. Vasopressin exerts these effects via V1 (vasoconstriction) and V2 receptors (antidiuresis). In the past, the most common use of vasopressin was to treat gastrointestinal bleeding. More recently, vasopressin has been used as an alternative to epinephrine in the acute resuscitation; however, the superiority of vasopressin over epinephrine for this indication is not clear. A theoretical advantage of vasopressin is that vasopressin does not rely on adrenergic receptors, which may be downregulated in chronically elevated catecholamine states. In conditions of metabolic acidosis signal transmission via adrenergic receptors is also ineffective. Some conditions producing low blood pressure (i.e., septic shock) were associated with low plasma vasopressin concentration, suggesting inappropriately low vasopressin secretion. In some of these patients, hypersensitivity to the administration of vasopressin has been described, possibly due to upregulation of vasopressin receptors, and is in agreement with studies showing rapid desensitization to vasopressin [45].

There is a paucity of information about vasopressin use in the pediatric population. Rosenzweig et al. reported their experience with use of vasopressin in moribund pediatric patients after postcardiac surgery [46]. These patients were classified as unresponsive to standard vasopressors, although in some of these patients a trial of epinephrine or dopamine was not attempted, and some of these 11 patients were clearly on extremely high doses of adrenergic stimulators. The dosage of vasopressin they used varied from 0.0003 to 0.002 U/kg/min. These doses of vasopressin produced an average increase in systolic blood pressure of 22 mm Hg (65–87 mm Hg). The authors measured plasma vasopressin levels in three patients before treatment and all had low levels of vasopressin. Patients who had low blood pressure and poor cardiac function before the initiation of vasopressin therapy died. Vasoconstrictor use is ill advised in the presence of a low cardiac output state; therefore, we suggest one ensure good cardiac output either by a clinical exam or a direct measurement before resorting to vasoconstrictors. Vasopressin is particularly useful in cases of low SVR induced by excessive alpha-adrenergic blockade, such as with phenoxybenzamine or phentolamine [47]. Doses are most commonly calculated in units/kg/h, and range from 0.01 to a maximum of 0.05 units/kg/h, and should be weaned and discontinued as soon as possible.

Vasodilators

Nitroglycerin

Nitroglycerin, like all other nitrates produces vasodilatation by releasing NO. The release of NO from nitroglycerin, unlike that of some other NO donors is enzymatically mediated. Nitroglycerin is frequently referred to as a venodilator, while sodium nitroprusside (SNP) is thought of as a preferential dilator of arteries, although these differences are difficult to demonstrate. The major indications for the use of nitroglycerin are myocardial ischemia, systemic hypertension, pulmonary hypertension, volume overload, congestive heart failure, and pulmonary edema. Venodilation associated with nitroglycerin therapy leads to a decrease in venous return. The decrease in preload leads to a lowering of the left ventricular end-diastolic volume and pressure, and therefore diminished of wall stress. The net effect is usually an improvement in the ratio of myocardial oxygen demand to delivery. Nitroglycerin also dilates both diseased and normal coronary arteries [48]. Hypotension and reflex tachycardia are the potentially undesirable side effects. Nitroglycerin is used in the cardiac surgical patients for the treatment of systemic or pulmonary hypertension as well as to decrease filling pressure and improve cardiac index. In a study including 20 pediatric patients with CHD, of whom 14 had preoperative pulmonary hypertension, nitroglycerin (>2 mcg/kg/min) reduced both SVR and PVR [49]. Improved cardiac index was seen only with higher doses. The authors suggest that the effect of the drug on the systemic and pulmonary arteries and on capacitance vessels is dose related. In lower doses (<2 mcg/kg/min), nitroglycerin mainly produced venodilation, as evidenced by an increased requirement of volume to maintain a constant right and left atrial pressure.

Tolerance to the drug is known to occur after more than 24 hours of intravenous therapy. In patients who have been on a prolonged therapy, the drug infusion should be tapered slowly to avoid rebound hypertension. Methemoglobinemia and cyanide toxicity from the release of nitrite ions upon metabolism is an extremely rare side effect [50].

The usual doses of intravenous nitroglycerin infusion are 0.5–5 mcg/kg/min.

Sodium nitroprusside

The hypotensive properties of SNP were described in the late 1800s; however, the drug was not approved for clinical use until 1974. Frequently, nitroprusside is incorrectly referred to as a direct, preferential arterial vasodilator. Nitroprusside dilates both arteries and veins by releasing NO in an interaction with tissue compounds containing sulfhydryl groups. The released NO activates soluble guanyl cyclase that increases cGMP. Nitroprusside is most commonly used to control blood pressure in hypertensive patients, and decrease SVR, thereby improving forward flow in patients with poor LV function or regurgitant lesions (mitral or aortic regurgitation). Because of its short half-life, SNP allows precise control of blood pressure and SVR. In patients with diminished myocardial function, cardiac output is increased from an increased stroke volume as a result of decreased aortic impedance. Despite significant reductions in SVR, the blood pressure drop is usually modest since an increase in cardiac output compensates for the decrease in SVR. The drop in blood pressure is more dramatic in patients with preexisting hypovolemia or obstructive cardiac lesions. In patients with hypertrophic cardiomyopathy, SNP may increase outflow obstruction, and patients with aortic or mitral stenosis may not be able to compensate with an increase in cardiac output, resulting in profound hypotension. Because of dilatation of both pulmonary and systemic vasculature, SNP is of little value in patients with shunts and mixing lesions. Although frequently used in the pediatric population, the reported experience of use of SNP in neonates is limited. In one of those reports, Benitz et al. administered SNP (0.2–6 μg/kg/min) to 58 neonates with various diagnoses including shock, respiratory distress syndrome (RDS), and persistent pulmonary hypertension [51]. Patients with RDS had an increased PaO_2, decreased $PaCO_2$ and peak inspiratory pressures and 82% survived. Patients in shock showed signs of improved perfusion, increased urine output, and decreased acidosis. Response to SNP was suggested to be good predictor of survival. Adverse effects were uncommon and there was no evidence of toxicity. The authors concluded that SNP is safe and effective in controlling these circulatory disorders in the neonates.

One of the dangers associated with the use of nitroprusside use is toxicity from the formation of cyanide. Cyanide, a byproduct of SNP metabolism, is taken up by red cells and inactivated predominantly in the liver by reacting with thiosulfate. This reaction is catalyzed by the enzyme rhodanase and patients with liver failure are more susceptible to cyanide toxicity. If cyanide toxicity occurs, SNP should be stopped immediately, and after confirmation of diagnosis, the patient should be treated with 3% sodium nitrate followed by the administration of sodium thiosulfate. SNP should be used cautiously in patients with renal failure since they may have difficulty metabolizing the thiocyanate produced during breakdown of SNP. In a retrospective review of 63 children after cardiac surgery to control blood pressure, or lower SVR for hemodynamic purposes, 11% of patients experienced an elevated cyanide concentration. Mean SNP dose was 2.8 mcg/kg/min in those patients with elevated cyanide levels, and 1.1 mcg/kg/min for those without elevated levels; with an increased risk of elevated cyanide levels starting at 1.8 mcg/kg/min [52].

The starting dose of SNP is 0.5–1 mcg/kg/min and the dose can be titrated up to 5 mcg/kg/min. The high doses pose greater risk for toxicity, so doses exceeding 3 mcg/kg/min should not be administered for longer than several hours. Sodium thiosulfate can be added to the infusion to eliminate cyanide; but alternative methods of hypertension treatment should be instituted. In a multicenter study of 118 infants and children receiving esmolol for blood pressure control on admission to the ICU after coarctation repair via thoracotomy, only 15–20% of neonates required SNP, 50% of patients aged 1–24 months, and 80% of patients aged 2–6 years required SNP for blood pressure control. The median maximal SNP dose was 3 mcg/kg/min, and there was no mortality, neurological complication, or significant acidosis [53].

Prostaglandins

Prostaglandins such as PGE_1 and PGI_2 are the main metabolites of the arachidonic acid pathway. In the vascular tissues, they are predominantly generated and subsequently released by the endothelium to bind to specific receptors on the underlying smooth muscle cells. This leads to the activation of adenylate cyclase and an increase in cAMP levels, which lowers intracellular Ca^{++} and produces vascular smooth muscle relaxation.

PGE_1 is used to relax the smooth muscle and maintain the patency of the ductus arteriosus in neonates whose systemic or pulmonary circulation is dependent on ductal patency. PGE_1 when administered to 27 neonates in whom pulmonary or systemic blood flow was entirely or significantly dependent upon ductal patency, led to an improvement in hypoxemia and acidemia, as well as ductus dilatation [54]. It has been demonstrated to maintain ductal patency for as long as 2 months [55] and to reopen a recently closed ductus. Preoperative drug therapy with PGE_1 has lowered the mortality and allowed planned surgeries, rather than desperate attempts at emergency palliation, which was frequently the case in the past. Side effects of PGE_1 therapy occur in (20–40%) of patients at higher doses (0.05–0.1 mcg/kg/min) but they are usually reversible upon lowering the dose or discontinuation of the drug. Hypotension, apnea, hyperpyrexia, and jitteriness are some of the adverse effects.

Besides management of neonatal CHD, PGE_1 has been used to treat pulmonary hypertension secondary to mitral valve disease [56], after congenital cardiac surgery [57] and after heart transplantation [58]. There has been only limited research conducted in the use of inhaled PGE$_1$.

PGI$_2$ or prostacyclin (epoprostenol) is a relatively recent addition to the drug therapy for the management of pulmonary vascular disease. Even though PGI$_2$ is probably the most selective pulmonary vasodilator of all the currently available intravenous drugs, administration of PGI$_2$ via this route will lower systemic arterial pressure. PGI$_2$ is spontaneously hydrolyzed to 6-keto-prostaglandin F$_{1\alpha}$ with a half-life of 1–3 minutes. The relatively selective effect on lowering PVR is due to rapid inactivation in the pulmonary vasculature bed during a single circulation time. Intravenous infusions of PGI$_2$ (epoprostenol) have been shown to be useful in decreasing the PVR in patients with primary pulmonary hypertension, and after cardiac surgery in neonates [59]. Due to its short half-life, aerosolized PGI$_2$, like NO, can selectively dilate pulmonary vessels with minimal affects on the systemic arterial pressure. Several anecdotal reports and a few small clinical studies suggest that inhaled PGI$_2$ can reduce elevated pulmonary artery pressures (PAPs) and PVR. Schulze-Neick et al. reported inhaled PGI$_2$ and NO to have similar advantageous effects on reducing PVR in patients with CHD after cardiac surgery [60]. Another study demonstrated reduction of PAPs and improvement in the right ventricular function following inhaled PGI$_2$ therapy with bolus dosing (2.5, 5, 10 µg) in nine patients undergoing cardiac surgery including heart transplantation [61]. The optimal dosing of epoprostenol remains undefined and dosing of inhaled PGI$_2$ ranging from 1 to 50 ng/kg/min has been shown to efficacious [62]. This agent has also been demonstrated to lower elevated PAP and PVR in infants after congenital heart surgery with bypass [63].

Sildenafil

Sildenafil is a phosphodiesterase-5 inhibitor, which in its intravenous form, appears to be a selective and highly effective pulmonary vasodilator in a piglet model of meconium aspiration with severe pulmonary hypertension [64]. Sildenafil has been shown in case reports to ameliorate the effects of NO withdrawal in a patient after cardiac surgery with persistent pulmonary hypertension [65]. In doses of 0.5–2.0 mg/kg given via nasogastric tube, sildenafil was effective at lowering mean PAP in infants after atrioventricular septal defect repairs [66].

Inhaled nitric oxide

A ubiquitous compound in the human body, NO, is produced as a result of the conversion of the amino acid arginine to citrulline, a reaction that is facilitated by the enzyme nitric oxide synthase (NOS). NO, being a very small and lipophilic molecule, diffuses into the underlying smooth muscle cells producing an increase in intracellular cGMP levels and subsequent vasodilation [67]. NO, when delivered via the inhaled route, readily crosses the alveolar–capillary membrane leading to pulmonary vasodilation and a decrease in PVR. High affinity binding and immediate inactivation of iNO activity by hemoglobin limits the action of the drug to the pulmonary circulation. iNO therapy has been shown to be useful in the treatment of pulmonary hypertension, which is frequently seen in CHD [67, 68]. Pulmonary hypertension in patients with CHD is multifactorial, due to chronic hypoxemia or due to chronic elevation of pulmonary blood flow and/or pulmonary venous pressures. PVR is also increased immediately after CPB due to the endothelial dysfunction. iNO is ideally suited in selectively reducing PVR in this critical period. Miller et al. reported a lowering of PVR (37%), while increasing CO by 14% using low doses of iNO, in CHD patients who had high PVR (PAP/SAP > 0.5, mean PAP > 37 mm Hg) shortly after their surgery. LAP, SVR, and SAP remained unaffected. Patients with low postoperative PVR did not show any hemodynamic effect in response to iNO [68]. The pulmonary vascular selectivity of iNO may be especially useful in reducing the right ventricular afterload in patients undergoing heart transplant, where the donor hearts may not be accustomed to high PVR of that is usually seen in these patients [69]. Several investigators have reported the use of iNO in the preoperative period as a test of reversibility of PVR and in predicting post-CPB pulmonary hypertension, as well as using the preoperative evaluation to predict the use of the drug in the immediate post-CPB period [67,70–72]. In a study of 20 patients with VSDs and/or ASDs, Winberg et al. reported the lowering of PAP (from 50 to 38 mm Hg) and a decrease in PVR by 34%, after administration of 40 ppm iNO in patients with elevated PVR at the time of preoperative cardiac catheterization. Systemic pressures remained unchanged [72].

Others have reported the benefit of iNO in improving oxygenation, likely by improving pulmonary blood flow and ventilation–perfusion balance in congenital cardiac surgery patients [73]. Even though iNO has been shown to be effective in a variety of congenital heart lesions, it may not be helpful in reducing PVR in all patients. In a double-blind study, the combination of milrinone 0.5 mcg/kg/min and NO 30 PPM was more effective at lowering PAP than either agent alone [74]. The nonresponders are usually those who have long-standing pulmonary hypertension and extensive remodeling of the pulmonary vasculature. NO also has not been shown to improve postoperative outcome, the cost is prohibitive at several thousand dollars per day of use, the delivery system setup is complex, as is transport with NO, and there are toxicity issues (see below). All of these issues suggest that

NO should only be used as a last resort in a patient with known or suspected severe pulmonary hypertension resulting in low cardiac output (in two-ventricle patients), or severe desaturation in single ventricle patients after systemic arterial or venous to pulmonary artery shunts.

NO can be administered using a face mask in a spontaneously ventilating patient, or added to the inspiratory limb of the breathing circuit in a mechanically ventilated patient. The most commonly used dose range is 20–40 ppm, though a decrease in PVR has been demonstrated with doses as low as 2–5 ppm. Side effects of iNO at these doses are minimal, even with prolonged therapy.

A novel approach is to administer IV L-citrulline, an amino acid precursor of NO, as a potential therapy to increase NO concentrations and prevent pulmonary hypertensive crises in susceptible patients. Initial phase I and phase II trials have demonstrated predictable pharmacokinetics and no safety issues so far with this approach [75].

Abrupt withdrawal of NO or rapid reductions in drug dosage may lead to rebound pulmonary hypertension [76]. The binding of NO to hemoglobin gives rise to methemoglobin [77], and methemoglobin levels should be routinely monitored especially with prolonged therapy.

Nitrogen dioxide is also formed as a byproduct of NO administration, and its levels should be maintained below 5 ppm. Nitrogen dioxide in high concentrations can lead to injury of the lungs [67].

Phentolamine

Phentolamine binds reversibly to and blocks the alpha-receptors, and several groups have demonstrated the beneficial effects of phentolamine on reducing SVR as a result of its strong vasodilating properties. In one study of patients undergoing cardiac surgery, administration of 0.2 mg/kg of phentolamine during cooling and rewarming periods reduced plasma lactate levels, indicating better tissue perfusion. In addition, the nasopharyngeal–rectal temperature difference was fourfold higher in the control group, while systemic oxygen consumption was higher and blood pressure was lower in the phentolamine group (59 ± 6 vs 63 ± 7 mm Hg) [78]. The superiority of one vasodilator over another has not been demonstrated in cardiac surgery, but because one of the most important reasons for the increase in SVR during and after CPB is an elevation in plasma catecholamines, administration of an alpha-adrenergic blocker seems logical.

Another potential use of phentolamine is in the treatment of extravasation of vasoconstrictors like phenylephrine, norepinephrine, or epinephrine. Local infiltration of 0.5–1% phentolamine is recommended for this use.

Phenoxybenzamine

Phenoxybenzamine is an irreversible alpha-1 receptor blocker that is advocated by some groups for routine perioperative management in infants undergoing cardiac surgery with the use of hypothermic CPB. The advantage of phenoxybenzamine over other vasodilators is its irreversibility and unparalleled potency to dilate peripheral vasculature and shift blood from pulmonary to systemic circulation (decreased Qp:Qs ratio) leading to an increase in cardiac output and oxygen delivery. Phenoxybenzamine was prospectively studied by Tweddell et al. [79] for patients undergoing the Norwood operation. They administered 0.25 mg/kg phenoxybenzamine at the start of CPB. In patients that did not reach target O_2 delivery ($SvO_2 > 50\%$) and target Qp:Qs (0.8–1.2) infusion of 0.25 mg/kg/24 h phenoxybenzamine was administered for up to 48 hours. They concluded that phenoxybenzamine improves systemic oxygen delivery in early postoperative period when compared to standard hemodynamic management [79]. In a follow-up study from the same group, postoperative single ventricle neonatal patients receiving phenoxybenzamine had a higher SvO_2 and better systemic oxygen delivery at a higher systemic oxygen saturation than those who did not [80].

Beta-adrenergic antagonists

Beta-blockers, like digoxin and ACE inhibitors, are more beneficial in the management of chronic heart failure where they have been shown to improve the functional status in both pediatric and adult CHD [81, 82]. This effect is due to the modulation of the endogenous neurohumoral system. Several studies have demonstrated down-regulation of beta-adrenoceptors in chronic heart failure as a result of elevated sympathetic tone [83, 84]. Therapy with beta-blockers such as propranolol, metoprolol, and carvedilol increase the number of myocardial beta-adrenoceptors and improve myocardial function in heart failure secondary to CHD [85, 86]. Responsiveness to catecholamines may be preserved in these patients during the perioperative period as a result of beta-blocker therapy. Besides their use in the management of chronic heart failure, these medications have several uses in the acute hemodynamic management of patients with CHD. By reducing the effects of increased sympathetic tone on the right ventricular infundibulum in TOF, beta-blockers are effective in the treatment of cyanotic spells [87]. Also, a decrease in heart rate allows for a longer diastolic filling time and improved preload. The use of esmolol, a short-acting beta-1 selective antagonist, is well suited for the hemodynamic management of TOF in the perioperative setting [88]. Esmolol in doses of 100–700 mcg/kg/min has also been successfully used to control postoperative hypertension after repair of aortic coarctation in children [53,89].

Newer cardiotonic and vasoactive agents

Currently, there exists limited scientific literature regarding the use of some new vasoactive drugs in patients with CHD, though a few of them have been well researched in other patient groups. A brief description of some of these newer agents is as follows.

Levosimendan

Levosimendan is a positive inotrope and vasodilator. Most other positive inotropes work through stimulation of adrenergic receptors and increase intracellular calcium that may be already elevated in the failing heart. Unlike these drugs, levosimendan works by causing conformational changes in the myofilaments making them more sensitive to intracellular calcium. The vasodilatation produced is mediated by opening of potassium channels. Although drug is not approved for routine clinical use in the USA, there are extensive clinical studies involving large number of patients with end-stage cardiac failure demonstrating that levosimendan is both safe and effective in providing symptomatic relief. Levosimendan was also more effective in decreasing pulmonary artery wedge pressure and increasing cardiac output [90]. Experience with the use of levosimendan in the perioperative period is limited. In a prospective randomized placebo-controlled trial in patients undergoing cardiac surgery, levosimendan given before separation from CPB enhanced cardiac performance, decreased SVR, increased myocardial oxygen consumption, and significantly decreased blood pressure, occasionally leading to hypotension [91]. The hypotension was responsive to volume administration and did not require vasoconstrictors. In 15 children with acute heart failure, levosimendan improved ejection fraction in all while allowing a reduction in the dobutamine dose, in levosimendan doses of 6–12 mcg/kg load and 0.05–0.1 mcg/kg/min, with other hemodynamics unchanged [92]. Despite exhibiting the expected hemodynamic effects, the drug has shown little or no effect on survival in adult patients with heart failure, and thus the drug has not been further developed for use in the USA.

Nesiritide (B-natriuretic peptide)

Nesiritide is a human recombinant form of B-type natriuretic peptide (BNP) that is identical to and has actions that are similar to the endogenous BNP. Human BNP stimulates increases in intracellular cGMP in the vascular endothelial cells and smooth muscles. Elevated cGMP levels with nesiritide therapy lead to venodilation and arteriodilation. Nesiritide has natriuretic, diuretic, and vasodilatory properties. Currently, the primary use of nesiritide is in the treatment of acute decompensated heart failure. It produces dose-dependent reductions in the pulmonary capillary wedge pressure (PCWP) and systemic arterial pressure in patients with heart failure. In addition, vasodilation occurs without a change in heart rate and is associated with increases in stroke volume and cardiac output. In a randomized controlled trial involving 489 subjects, nesiritide, when given as a bolus dose of 2 μg/kg and followed by an infusion at 0.01–0.03 μg/kg/min, was more effective in lowering the PCWP as compared to nitroglycerin [93]. In another randomized controlled trial that included 103 patients with heart failure and systolic dysfunction, nesiritide was reported to decrease the PCWP by up to 39% as well as lower the right atrial pressure and SVR, along with a significant improvement in the cardiac index [94]. Colucci et al. reported that nesiritide was effective as the standard drug therapy (dobutamine, milrinone, dopamine, or nitroglycerin) in treating heart failure [95]. The renal hemodynamic effects of nesiritide (BNP) appear to be that of arteriolar vasoconstriction, which would likely augment glomerular filtration rate and filtration fraction in the setting of compromised renal perfusion. Additionally, BNP leads to an increase in both urinary sodium excretion as well as fractional excretion of sodium (FENA) [96]. Mild diuretic effect of nesiritide therapy has been reported in a few clinical trials [96, 97]. In a limited pediatric experience of 17 patients after cardiac surgery, a loading dose of 1 mcg/kg was administered on bypass, and then an infusion of 0.1 and then 0.2 mcg/kg/min was continued. There was a 7% decrease in mean arterial pressure, with no adverse effects [98]. Use of this agent has been limited in the pediatric population, likely because multiple controlled adult trials have not demonstrated any survival benefit with this agent.

Fenoldopam

Fenoldopam is a selective dopamine-1 receptor agonist with moderate affinity for alpha-2 receptors. Despite its binding to alpha-2 receptors, fenoldopam has no significant sedative effect. Fenoldopam can be given intravenously as an infusion or administered parenterally. Fenoldopam administration produces dramatic vasodilatation of the peripheral vasculature including renal, mesenteric coronary, and skeletal muscle. The main indication for the use of fenoldopam is in the treatment of hypertensive emergencies and postoperative hypertension [99, 100]. The theoretical advantage of use of fenoldopam is that it maintains renal perfusion while decreasing blood pressure. This is especially important in patients with decreased renal function, since in these patients rapid drop in blood pressure may lead to decreased renal blood flow, glomerular filtration rate, and even acute renal insufficiency. In one retrospective case series Tobias reports use of fenoldopam for controlled hypotension during posterior spinal fusion in children and adolescence (8–14 years old) [101]. Target MAP of 50–65 mm Hg was reached in an average of 7 minutes. The starting infusion rate in this report was 0.3–0.5 µg/kg/min and target blood pressure was achieved with infusion of 0.2–2.5 µg/kg/min (mean 1.0 ± 0.3 µg/kg/min). The infusion of fenoldopam was associated with significant increase in heart rate (87–114 bpm), most likely due to reflex response to hypotension along with a small but significant decrease in PO_2 suggestive of increased shunting due to pulmonary vasodilatation. During prolonged infusion of fenoldopam, there is development of tolerance with a half-life (predicted loss of 50% effectiveness of the drug) of 60 hours, without a prolonged pharmacodynamic effect or rebound hypertension upon discontinuation of fenoldopam. Infusion of fenoldopam in healthy, normotensive awake individuals produced decrease in global and regional blood flow. The decrease in cerebral blood flow was not due to decrease in cerebral blood pressure since normalization of blood pressure with concurrent infusion of phenylephrine failed to restore blood flow. The authors postulated that the decrease in cerebral blood flow was mediated by fenoldopam's alpha-2 agonist activity. It remains unclear if the reduction of cerebral blood flow may have negative consequences in patients during intraoperative controlled hypotension or in treatment of hypertensive emergencies where brain ischemia is a real concern. In a retrospective study of 25 postoperative cardiac neonates with inadequate urine output despite conventional diuretic therapy, fenoldopam increased urine output by 50% and had minimal effect on hemodynamics [102].

Assessment of systemic oxygen delivery and cardiac output

Somatic near-infrared oximetry

In the operating room during congenital cardiac surgery conventional physical examination measures of cardiac output and systemic oxygen delivery, such as peripheral perfusion assessed by examination of pulses and capillary refill are not accessible. In the intensive care unit, these signs may be obscured by vasoactive agents used to achieve hemodynamic goals. Invasive hemodynamic monitoring is used, and this topic is covered in Chapter 9. It is becoming increasingly clear that a single physiologic variable, i.e., blood pressure, heart rate, oxygen saturation that is in a desired range does not necessar-

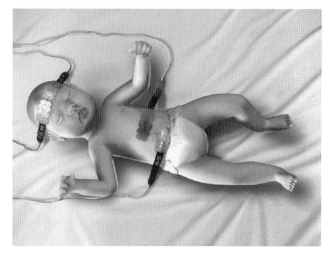

Figure 16.7 Cerebral and somatic near-infrared spectroscopy probes. Somatic probes can be placed on flank at T10–11 level for muscle and renal rSO_2 measurement, infraumbilical for mesenteric rSO_2, or on quadriceps for muscle rSO_2 (Courtesy of Somanetics Corp.)

ily mean that cardiac output and oxygen delivery to organs and tissues is adequate [103]. Noninvasive technologies for measuring oxygen delivery and among them somatic near-infrared spectroscopy (NIRS) to measure regional oxygen saturation (rSO_2) in flank muscle, kidney, intestine, and extremity muscles (Figures 16.7 and 16.8) have all been studied as a continuous method for assessing cardiac output. The principles of NIRS are discussed in Chapter 10; briefly, near infrared light at 700–900 nm at 2–4 different wavelengths is shone into tissues containing hemoglobin, and the distinctive light absorption spectra of oxy- and deoxy hemoglobin are used to estimate or measure directly the oxyhemoglobin saturation in the tissue in the path of the light. The most common use of NIRS is for cerebral oximetry, but this technique is now US FDA approved for measurement of somatic tissue oxygenation. At rest and with normal physiology including cardiac output and oxygen delivery, somatic rSO_2 in muscles is high, i.e., 70–80%. With either decreased oxygen delivery from low cardiac output from shock or anemia, or increased consumption with vigorous exercise [104], somatic rSO_2 decreases rapidly in real time, making this technology a potentially sensitive indicator of somatic oxygen delivery if oxygen consumption is steady state [105]. Somatic NIRS has been demonstrated to decline rapidly and consistently with aortic cross-clamping for coarctation repair during thoracotomy [106], with dehydration and hypovolemia from acute gastroenteritis [107], and with low cardiac output states in postoperative single ventricle neonates after Norwood stage I palliation [103]. Somatic rSO_2 in the muscle and kidney is normally at least 10–15% higher than cerebral rSO_2; a decrease in somatic rSO_2 to less than 10% above cerebral rSO_2 increases

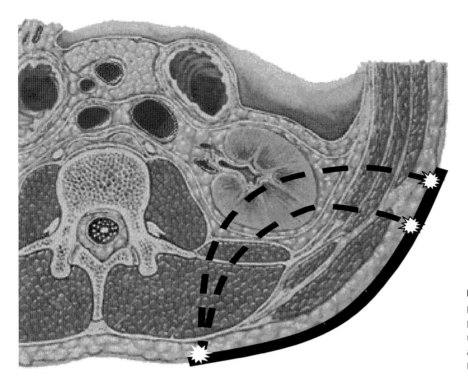

Figure 16.8 Cross-sectional view of light path of somatic near-infrared spectroscopy probe placed on flank at T10–11 level in a neonate. rSO_2 of psoas and intercostal muscles, and kidney is measured (Courtesy George M. Hoffman, M.D.)

likelihood of circulatory shock, inadequate oxygen delivery, and anaerobic metabolism; if the somatic rSO_2 is equal to or below the cerebral rSO_2, probability of anaerobic conditions is greater than 50% [103] (Figure 16.9). This technology can thus be used as an early warning system and has potential to improve outcomes in critically ill infants after congenital heart surgery. Splanchnic oximetry using NIRS probes placed on the abdominal wall is a sensitive indicator of intestinal ischemia, correlating with gastric pH measured by tonometry as well as serum lactate levels [108].

Serum lactate levels

Inadequate tissue oxygen delivery may manifest as anaerobic metabolism with metabolic acidosis and elevated lactate levels in the plasma. However, there are other reasons for elevated lactate in the cardiac surgery patient, such as elevated lactate levels in banked blood used to prime the bypass circuit, or periods of low-flow CPB of circulatory arrest. Therefore, lactate levels immediately after bypass or on admission to the ICU have not shown a strong correlation with low cardiac output, adverse outcomes, and

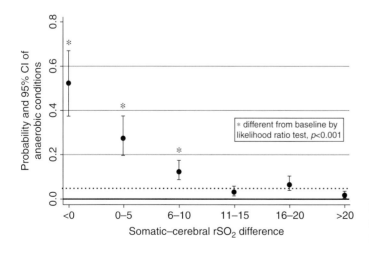

Figure 16.9 Probability of anaerobic conditions with somatic–cerebral rSO_2 difference in neonates after Norwood Stage I palliation (Reproduced and used with permission from Reference [103]

death. Other lactate measures such as the total time of lactate >2 mMol/L, persistent lactate levels >8 mMol/L, and rate of increase of decrease of serum lactate over time did have a stronger predictive value [109, 110]. Therefore, a single spot lactate level is of limited value; rather the trend over time and persistence of elevated lactate levels are important indicators of low cardiac output and inadequate oxygen delivery. And, serum lactate levels are a single data point in the assessment of cardiac output and oxygen delivery; and values must be used in the context of the array of other data in the patient undergoing congenital heart surgery.

Conclusions

The choice of a therapeutic drug in patients with CHD should be made after careful consideration of the alteration in hemodynamics that may occur as a result of the drugs' pharmacological effects. This requires an understanding of the anatomy and associated physiology of the various congenital heart lesions. The anesthesiologist must also consider the adequacy of each of the determinants of cardiac output, including heart rate, preload, afterload, and contractility. Clinical management should be based upon the risks and benefits of the various therapies.

References

1. Allwood M, Cobbold A, Ginsburg J (1963) Peripheral vascular effects of noradrenaline, isopropylnoradrenaline and dopamine. Br Med Bull 19:132–136.
2. Zaritsky A, Chernow B (1981) Catecholamines in critical care medicine. Crit Care Med 9:39–47.
3. Gambos E, Hulet W, Bopp P, et al. (1962) Reactivity of renal systemic circulation to vasoconstrictor agents in normotensive and hypertensive subjects. J Clin Invest 41:203–217.
4. Michael J, Guerci A, Koehler R, et al. (1984) Mechanism by which epinephrine augments cerebral and myocardial perfusion during cardiopulmonary resuscitation in dogs. Circulation 69:822–835.
5. International Liaison Committee on Resuscitation (2005) 2005 International consensus on cardiopulmonary resuscitation and emergency cardiovascular care science with treatment recommendation. Circulation 112:III-1–III-136.
6. American Heart Association (2006) 2005 American Heart Association (AHA) guidelines for cardiopulmonary resuscitation (CPR) and emergency cardiovascular care (ECC) of pediatric and neonatal patients: pediatric advanced life support. Pediatrics 117:e1005–e1028.
7. Booker PD (2002) Pharmacological support for children with myocardial dysfunction. Paediatr Anaesth 12:5–25.
8. Goldberg L, Rajfer E (1985) Dopamine receptors: applications in clinical cardiology. Circulation 72:245–248.
9. Parker S, Carlon G, Isaacs M, et al. (1981) Dopamine administration in oliguria and oliguric renal failure. Crit Care Med 9:630–632.
10. Henderson I, Beattie T, Kennedy A (1980) Dopamine hydrochloride in oliguric renal states. Lancet 2:827–828.
11. Goldberg L (1974) Dopamine. Clinical uses of endogenous catecholamine. N Engl J Med 291:707–710.
12. Eldadah M, Schwartz P, Harrison R (1991) Pharmacokinetics of dopamine in infants and children. Crit Care Med 19:1008–1011.
13. Van Den Berghe G, de Zegher F, Lauwers P (1994) Dopamine suppresses pituitary function in infants and children. Crit Care Med 22:1747–1753.
14. Filippi L, Pezzati M, Poggi C, et al. (2007) Dopamine versus dobutamine in very low birthweight infants: endocrine effects. Arch Dis Child Fetal Neonatal Ed 92:F367–F371.
15. Bohn D, Poirier C, Edmonds J, et al. (1980) Hemodynamic effects of dobutamine after cardiopulmonary bypass in children. Crit Care Med 367–371.
16. Gross R, Strain J, Greenberg M, et al. (1986) Systemic and coronary effects of intravenous milrinone and dobutamine in congestive heart failure. J Am Cardiol 7:1107–1113.
17. Loeb H, Khan M, Saudaye A, et al. (1976) Acute hemodynamic effects of dobutamine and isoproterenol in patients with low output cardiac failure. Circ Shock 3:55–59.
18. Kates R, Leier C (1978) Dobutamine pharmacokinetics in severe heart failure. Clin Pharmacol Ther 24:537–541.
19. Unverferth D, Blanford M, Kates R, et al. (1980) Tolerance to dobutamine after a 72 hour continuous infusion. Am J Med 69:262–266.
20. Robel-Tillig E, Knüpfer M, Pulzer F, Vogtmann C (2007) Cardiovascular impact of dobutamine in neonates with myocardial dysfunction. Early Hum Dev 83:307–312.
21. Van Den Berg J, Wielopolski PA, Meijboom FJ, et al. (2007) Diastolic function in repaired tetralogy of Fallot at rest and during stress: assessment with MR imaging. Radiology 243:212–219.
22. Kariya T, Willie L, Dage R (1982) Biochemical studies on the mechanism of cardiotonic activity of MDL 17043. J Cardiovasc Pharmacol 4:509–514.
23. Benotti J, Grossman W, Braunwald E (1978) Hemodynamic assessment of amrinone: a new inotropic agent. N Engl J Med 199:1373–1377.
24. Wright E, Skoyles J, Sherry M (1992) Milrinone in the treatment of low cardiac output states following cardiac surgery. Eur J Anesthesiol 5 (Suppl):21–26.
25. Ramamoorthy C, Anderson G, Williams G, et al. (1998) Pharmacokinetics and side effects of Milrinone in infants and children after open heart surgery. Anesth Analg 86:283–289.
26. Chang A, Atz A, Wernovsky G, et al. (1995) Milrinone: systemic and pulmonary hemodynamic effects in neonates after cardiac surgery. Crit Care Med 23:1907–1914.
27. Bailey JM, Miller BE, Lu W, et al. (1999) The pharmacokinetics of milrinone in pediatric patients after cardiac surgery. Anesthesiology 90:1012–1018.

28. Mehra M, Ventura H, Kapoor C, et al. (1997) Safety and clinical utility of long term intravenous milrinone in advanced heart failure. Am J Cardiol 80:61–64.

29. Edelson J (1986) Pharmocokinetics of bipyridines amrinone and milrinone. Circulation 73:145–155.

30. Hoffman TM, Wernovsky G, Atz AM, et al. (2003) Efficacy and safety of milrinone in preventing low cardiac output syndrome in infants and children after corrective surgery for congenital heart disease. Circulation 107:996–1002.

31. Zuppa AF, Nicolson SC, Adamson PC, et al. (2006) Population pharmacokinetics of milrinone in neonates with hypoplastic left heart syndrome undergoing stage I reconstruction. Anesth Analg 102:1062–1069.

32. Drop L, Geffin G, O'Keefe D, et al. (1981) Relation between ionized calcium concentration and ventricular pump performance in the dog under hemodynamically controlled conditions. Am J Cardiol 47:1041–1051.

33. Robertie P, Butterworth J, Royster R, et al. (1991) Normal parathyroid hormone responses to hypocalcemia during cardiopulmonary bypass. Anesthesiology 75:43–48.

34. Elz J, Panagiotopoulos S, Nayker W, et al. (1989) Reperfusion induced calcium gain after ischemia. Am J Cardiol 63:7E–13E.

35. Royster R, Butterworth J, Prielipp R, et al. (1992) A randomized blinded, placebo-controlled evaluation of calcium chloride and epinephrine for inotropic support after emergence from cardiopulmonary bypass. Anesth Analg 74:3–13.

36. Murdoch I, Qureshi S, Huggon I (1983) Perioperative hemodynamic effects of an intravenous infusion of calcium chloride in children following cardiac surgery. Acta Paediatr 83:658–661.

37. Broner CW, Stidham GL, Westenkirchner DF, Watson DC (1990) A prospective, randomized, double-blind comparison of calcium chloride and calcium gluconate therapies for hypocalcemia in critically ill children. J Pediatr 117:986–989.

38. Dyke PC, Yates AR, Cua CL, et al. (2007) Increased calcium supplementation is associated with morbidity and mortality in the infant postoperative cardiac patient. Pediatr Crit Care Med 8:254–257.

39. Walters P, Cooper T, Denison A, et al. (1955) Dilator responses to isoproterenol in cutaneous and skeletal muscle vascular beds of adrenergic blocking drugs. J Pharmacol Exp Ther 115:323–327.

40. Vatner S, Baig H (1978) Comparison of the effects of ouabain and isoproterenol on ischemic myocardium of conscious dogs. Circulation 58:654–662.

41. Clutter W, Bier D, Shah S, et al. (1980) Epinephrine plasma metabolic clearance rates and physiologic thresholds for metabolic and hemodynamic actions in man. J Clin Invest 66:94–101.

42. Tourneux P, Rakza T, Abazine A, et al. (2008) Noradrenaline for management of septic shock refractory to fluid loading and dopamine or dobutamine in full-term newborn infants. Acta Paediatr 97:177–180.

43. Oshita S, Uchimoto R, Oka H, et al. (1989) Correlation between arterial blood pressure and oxygenation in Tetralogy of Fallot. J Cardiothorac Anesth 3:597–600.

44. Stewart WJ, Schiavone WA, Salcedo EE, et al. (1987) Interperative Doppler echocardiography in hypertrphic cardiomyopathy: correlations with the obstructive gradient. J Am Coll Cardiol 10:327–335.

45. Holmes CL, Patel BM, Russell JA, et al. (2001) Physiology of vasopressin relevant to management of septic shock. Chest 120:989–1002.

46. Rosenzweig E, Starc T, Chen J, et al. (1999) Intravenous arginine-vasopressin in children with vasodilatory shock after cardiac surgery. Circulation 9 (100):182–186.

47. O'Blenes SB, Roy N, Konstantinov I, et al. (2002) Vasopressin reversal of phenoxybenzamine-induced hypotension after the Norwood procedure. J Thorac Cardiovasc Surg 123:1012–1013.

48. Strauer B, Scherpe A (1978) Ventricular function and coronary hemodynamics after intravenous nitroglycerin in coronary artery disease. Am Heart J 95:210–219.

49. Ilbawi M, Farouk I, Serafin D, et al. (1985) Hemodynamic effects of intravenous nitroglycerin in pediatric patients after heart surgery. Circulation 72 (II):101–107.

50. Gibson G, Hunter J, Rabe D, et al. (1982) Methemoglobinemia produced by high dose nitroglycerin. Ann Intern Med 96:615–616.

51. Benitz WE, Malachowski N, Cohen RS, et al. (1985) Use of sodium nitroprusside in neonates: efficacy and safety. J Pediatr 106:102–110.

52. Moffett BS, Price JF (2008) Evaluation of sodium nitroprusside toxicity in pediatric cardiac surgical patients. Ann Pharmacother 42:1600–1604.

53. Tabbutt S, Nicolson SC, Adamson PC, et al. (2008) The safety, efficacy, and pharmacokinetics of esmolol for blood pressure control immediately after repair of coarctation of the aorta in infants and children: a multicenter, double-blind, randomized trial. J Thorac Cardiovasc Surg 136:321–328.

54. Ohara T, Ogata H, Fujiyama J, et al. (1985) Effects of prostaglandin E1 infusion in the pre-operative management of critical congenital heart disease. Tohoku J Exp Med 146 (2):237–249.

55. Freed M, Heyman M, Rudolph A, et al. (1981) Prostaglandin E1 in ductus arteriosus dependent congenital heart disease. Circulation 64:889–905.

56. D'Ambra M, LaRaia P, Philbin D, et al. (1985) Prostaglandin E1: a new therapy for refractory right heart failure and pulmonary hypertension after mitral valve replacement. J Thorac Cardiovasc Surg 89:567–572.

57. Rubis L, Stephenson L, Johnston M, et al. (1981) Comparison of effects of prostaglandin E1 and nitroprusside on pulmonary vascular resistance in children after open-heart surgery. Ann Thorac Surg 32 (6):563–570.

58. Armitage J, Hardesty R, Griffith B, et al. (1987) Prostaglandin E1: an effective treatment of right heart failure after orthotopic heart transplantation. J Heart Transplant 6:348–351.

59. Kermode J, Butt W, Shann F (1991) Comparison between prostaglandin E1 and epoprostenol in infants after heart surgery. Br Heart J 66:175–178.

60. Schulze-Neick I, Uhlemann F, Nurnberg J, et al. (1997) Aerosolized prostacyclin for preoperative evaluation and post-cardiosurgical treatment of patients with pulmonary hypertension. Z Kardiol 86:71–80.

61. Haraldsson A, Kieler J, Ricksten S (1996) Inhaled prostacyclin for the treatment of pulmonary hypertension after

cardiac surgery or heart transplantation: a pharmacodynamic study. J Cardiothorac Vasc Anesth 10:864–868.

62. Zwissler B, Kemming G, Habler O, et al. (1996) Inhaled prostacyclin (PGI2) versus inhaled nitric oxide in adult respiratory distress syndrome. Am J Respir Crit Care Med 154:1671–1677.

63. Müller M, Scholz S, Kwapisz M, et al. (2003) Use of inhaled iloprost in a case of pulmonary hypertension during pediatric congenital heart surgery. Anesthesiology 99:743–744.

64. Shekerdemian LS, Ravn HB, Penny DJ (2002) Intravenous sildenafil lowers pulmonary vascular resistance in a model of neonatal pulmonary hypertension. Am J Respir Crit Care Med 165:1098–1102.

65. Atz AM, Wessel DL (1999) Sildenafil ameliorates effects of inhaled nitric oxide withdrawal. Anesthesiology 91:307–310.

66. Raja SG, Danton MD, MacArthur KJ, Pollock JC (2007) Effects of escalating doses of sildenafil on hemodynamics and gas exchange in children with pulmonary hypertension and congenital cardiac defects. J Cardiothorac Vasc Anesth 21:203–207.

67. Roberts J, Lang P, Bigatello L, et al. (1993) Inhaled nitric oxide in congenital heart disease. Circulation 87:447–453.

68. Miller O, Celermyer D, Deanfield J, et al. (1994) Very low dose inhaled nitric oxide: a selective pulmonary vasodilator after operations for congenital heart disease. J Thorac Cardiovasc Surg 108:487–494.

69. Kieler-Jensen N, Lundin S, Ricksten S (1995) Vasodilator therapy after heart transplantation: effects of inhaled nitric oxide and intravenous prostacyclin, prostaglansin E1 sodium nitroprusside. J Heart Lung Transplant 14:436–443.

70. Turanlahti M, Laitinen P, Pesonen E (2000) Preoperative and postoperative response to inhaled nitric oxide. Scand Cardiovasc J 34:46–52.

71. Kadosaki M, Kawamura T, Oyama K, et al. (2002) Usefulness of nitric oxide treatment for pulmonary hypertensive infants during cardiac anesthesia. Anesthesiology 96:835–840.

72. Winberg P. Lundell B, Gustafsson L (1994) Effects of inhaled nitric oxide on raised pulmonary vascular resistance in children with congenital heart disease. Br Heart J 71:282–286.

73. Sadao K, Masahiro S, Toshihiko M, et al. (1997) Effect of nitric oxide on oxygenation and hemodynamics in infants after cardiac surgery. Artif Organs 21 (1):14–16.

74. Khazin V, Kaufman Y, Zabeeda D, et al. (2004) Milrinone and nitric oxide: combined effect on pulmonary artery pressures after cardiopulmonary bypass in children. J Cardiothorac Vasc Anesth 18:156–159.

75. Barr FE, Tirona RG, Taylor MB, et al. (2007) Pharmacokinetics and safety of intravenously administered citrulline in children undergoing congenital heart surgery: potential therapy for postoperative pulmonary hypertension. J Thorac Cardiovasc Surg 134:319–326.

76. Miller O, Tang S, Keech A, et al. (1995) Rebound pulmonary hypertension on withdrawal from inhaled nitric oxide. Lancet 346:51–52.

77. Chiodi H, Mohler J (1985) Effects of exposure of blood hemoglobin to nitric oxide. Environ Res 37:355–363.

78. Koner O, Tekin S, Koner A, et al. (1999) Effects of phentolamine on tissue perfusion in pediatric cardiac surgery. J Cardiothorac Vasc Anesth 13 (2):191–197.

79. Tweddell J, Hoffman G, Fedderly R, et al. (1999) Phenoxybenzamine improves systemic oxygen delivery after the Norwood procedure. Ann Thorac Surg 67:161–167.

80. Hoffman GM, Tweddell JS, Ghanayem NS, et al. (2004) Alteration of the critical arteriovenous oxygen saturation relationship by sustained afterload reduction after the Norwood procedure. J Thorac Cardiovasc Surg 127:738–745.

81. Buchhorn R, Bartmus D, Siekmeyer D, et al. (1998) Beta-blocker therapy of severe congestive heart failure in infants with left to right shunts. Am J Cardiol 81:1366–1368.

82. Consensus recommendation (1999) Consensus recommendation for the management of chronic heart failure. On behalf of the membership of the advisory council to improve outcomes nationwide in heart failure. Am J Cardiol 83:1A.

83. Bristow M, Ginsberg R, Minobe W, et al. (1981) Decreased catecholamine sensitivity and beta receptor density in failing human hearts. N Engl J Med 307:205–211.

84. Buchhorn R, Hulpke-Wette M, Russchewki W, et al. (2002) Beta-receptor downregulation in congenital heart disease: a risk factor for complications after surgical repair? Ann Thorac Surg 73:610–613.

85. Bruns L, Chrisant M, Lamour J, et al. (2001) Carvedilol as therapy in pediatric heart failure: an initial multicenter experience. J Pediatr 138:505–511.

86. Buchhorn R, Hulpke-Wette M, Hilgers R, et al. (2001) Propranolol treatment of congestive heart failure in infants with congenital heart disease: the CHF-PRO-INFANT Trial. Int J Cardiol 79:167–173.

87. Garson A, Gillette P, McNamara P (1981) Propranolol: the preferred palliation for tetralogy of Fallot. Am J Cardiol 47:1098–1104.

88. Nussbaum J, Zane E, Thys D (1989) Esmolol infor the treatment of hypercyanotic spells in infants with tetralogy of Fallot. J Cardiothrac Anesth 3:200–202.

89. Wiest D, Garner S, Uber W, et al. (1997) Esmolol for the management of pediatric hypertension after cardiac operations. J Thorac Cardiovasc Surg 115:890–897.

90. Follath F, Cleland J, Just H, et al. (2002) Efficacy and safety of intravenous levosimendan compared with dobutamine in severe low-output heart failure (the LIDO study): a randomised double-blind trial. Lancet 360:196–202.

91. Nijhawan N, Nicolosi A, Montgomery M, et al. (1999) Levosimendan enhances cardiac performance after cardiopulmonary bypass: a prospective, randomized placebo-controlled trial. J Cardiovasc Pharmacol 34:219–228.

92. Namachivayam P, Crossland DS, Butt WW, Shekerdemian LS (2006) Early experience with Levosimendan in children with ventricular dysfunction. Pediatr Crit Care Med 7:445–448.

93. Young J, Abraham W, Stevenson L, et al. (2000) Results of the VMAC trial: vasodilation in the management of acute congestive heart failure. Circulation 102:2794.

94. Mills R, LeJemtel T, Horton D, et al. (1999) Sustained hemodynamic effects of nesiritide in heart failure: a randomized,

double blind, placebo controlled clinical trials. Natrecor study group. J Am Coll Cardiol 34 (1):155–162.

95. Colucci W, Elkayam U, Horton D, et al. (2000) Intravenous nesiritide, a natriuretic peptide, in the treatment of decompensated congestive heart failure. N Eng J Med 343:246–253.

96. Jensen K, Eiskjaer H, Carstens J (1999) Renal effects of brain natriuretic peptide in patients with congestive heart failure. Clin Sci 96:5–15.

97. Marcus L, Hart D, Packer M, et al. (1996) Hemodynamic and renal excretory effects of human brain natriuretic peptide infusions in patients with congestive heart failure: a double blind, placebo controlled, randomized crossover trial. Circulation 94:3184–3189.

98. Simsic JM, Scheurer M, Tobias JD, et al. (2006) Perioperative effects and safety of nesiritide following cardiac surgery in children. J Intensive Care Med 21:22–26.

99. Panacek E, Bednarczyk E, Dunbar L, et al. (1995) Randomized, prospective trial of fenoldopam vs sodium nitroprusside in the treatment of acute severe hypertension. Fenoldopam Study Group. Acad Emerg Med 2:959–965.

100. Goldberg ME, Cantillo J, Nemiroff MS, et al. (1993) Fenoldopam infusion for the treatment of post-operative hypertension. J Clin Anesth 5:386–391.

101. Tobias J (2001) Fenoldopam for controlled hypotension during spinal fusion in children and adolescents. Paediatr Anaesth 10:261–266.

102. Costello JM, Thiagarajan RR, Dionne RE, et al. (2006) Initial experience with fenoldopam after cardiac surgery in neonates with an insufficient response to conventional diuretics. Pediatr Crit Care Med 7:28–33.

103. Hoffman GM, Ghanayem NS, Mussatto KA, et al. (2005) Perioperative perfusion assessed by somatic NIRS predicts postoperative renal dysfunction. Anesthesiology 103:A1327.

104. Rao RP, Danduran MJ, Frommelt PC, et al. (2009) Measurement of regional tissue bed venous weighted oximetric trends during exercise by near infrared spectroscopy. Pediatr Cardiol 30 (4):465–471.

105. Hoffman GM, Ghanayem NS, Tweddell JS (2005) Noninvasive assessment of cardiac output. Semin Thorac Cardiovasc Surg Pediatr Card Surg Annu 12–21.

106. Berens RJ, Stuth EA, Robertson FA, et al. (2006) Near infrared spectroscopy monitoring during pediatric aortic coarctation repair. Paediatr Anaesth 16:777–781.

107. Hanson SJ, Berens RJ, Havens PL, et al. (2009) Effect of volume resuscitation on regional perfusion in dehydrated pediatric patients as measured by two-site near-infrared spectroscopy. Pediatr Emerg Care 25 (3):150–153.

108. Kaufman J, Almodovar MC, Zuk J, Friesen RH (2008) Correlation of abdominal site near-infrared spectroscopy with gastric tonometry in infants following surgery for congenital heart disease. Pediatr Crit Care Med 9:62–68.

109. Kalyanaraman M, DeCampli WM, Campbell AI, et al. (2008) Serial blood lactate levels as a predictor of mortality in children after cardiopulmonary bypass surgery. Pediatr Crit Care Med 9:285–288.

110. Seear MD, Scarfe JC, LeBlanc JG (2008) Predicting major adverse events after cardiac surgery in children. Pediatr Crit Care Med 9:606–611.

17 Arrhythmias: diagnosis and management

Jeffrey J. Kim, M.D.
Texas Children's Hospital, Baylor College of Medicine, Houston, Texas, USA

Kathryn K. Collins, M.D.
The Children's Hospital, Aurora, and University of Colorado at Denver Health Sciences Center, Denver, Colorado, USA

Wanda C. Miller-Hance, M.D.
Texas Children's Hospital, Baylor College of Medicine, Houston, Texas, USA

Introduction

The practice of pediatric cardiovascular anesthesiology has evolved significantly over the years, expanding beyond the operative setting to many nonsurgical environments. Anesthetic care for infants and children known to have or who may develop cardiac rhythm disturbances is now provided at various locations, including operating rooms, intensive care units, emergency facilities, treatment rooms, cardiac catheterization/electrophysiology laboratories, and other sites. General knowledge of arrhythmia diagnosis and management is essential when caring for patients at any of these settings, although in some cases, guidance and input from a specialist may be necessary.

This chapter provides a practical approach to pediatric cardiac arrhythmias with discussions focused on diagnosis, mechanisms, and acute management strategies. A brief review of antiarrhythmic drug therapy and basic

Anesthesia for Congenital Heart Disease 2nd edition. Edited by Dean Andropoulos, Stephen Stayer, Isobel Russell and Emad Mossad. © 2010 Blackwell Publishing.

principles of cardiac pacing in children, as applicable to the practice of anesthesia, are presented as well.

Cardiac rhythm disturbances

Sinus bradycardia

Slow heart rates can be observed during sleep or at times of high vagal tone. When there is significant sinus bradycardia, atrial, junctional, or ventricular escape rhythms may ensue. In otherwise healthy children, this is usually a benign finding, particularly if hemodynamic stability is maintained. Certain forms of congenital heart disease (CHD), however, may be more prone to slow heart rhythms that may indeed be clinically significant. Patients with heterotaxy syndromes may be included in this category due to absence, displacement, or hypoplasia of the true sinus node [1].

In the intraoperative setting, particularly upon induction of anesthesia, with laryngoscopy, endotracheal intubation, or tracheal suctioning, sinus bradycardia may occur due to vagal stimulation. Sinus bradycardia may also be related to drug administration (i.e., opioids) or other mechanisms of increased parasympathetic activity. This type of sinus bradycardia rarely results in significant hemodynamic compromise, and, if present, can usually be treated with removal of the stimulus or the administration of chronotropic agents such as atropine or epinephrine (Table 17.1). Slow sinus rates may be seen following interventions such as closure of atrial septal defects and cardiac transplantation.

Sinus bradycardia can also be secondary to hypoxemia, hypothermia, drugs, acidosis, electrolyte abnormalities, or increased intracranial pressure. Bradycardia related to hypoxemia should be treated promptly with supplemental oxygen and appropriate airway management. The approach to other forms of secondary sinus bradycardia should focus on addressing the underlying cause. For worrisome low heart rates, particularly in small infants, or if there is clinical evidence of a low cardiac output state, pharmacologic therapy (isoproterenol, atropine) or temporary pacing should be considered.

Sinus node dysfunction

Sinus node dysfunction, often termed sick sinus syndrome, encompasses a spectrum of disorders characterized by slow or irregular heart rates with a variety of escape rhythms frequently alternating with periods of tachycardia. The respondent tachycardia may be atrial tachycardia, atrial flutter, or atrial fibrillation. The term tachycardia–bradycardia syndrome is frequently used to characterize this association. Surgical interventions most likely to be associated with sinus node dysfunction include extensive atrial baffling procedures, such as Mustard or Senning operations, and the Fontan procedure. Management of symptomatic patients may include pacemaker implantation, pharmacological therapy for tachyarrhythmias, atrial antitachycardia pacing, and in some cases, transcatheter or surgical ablation.

Sinus tachycardia

Sinus tachycardia is more commonly seen in the perioperative period than sinus bradycardia. It is often the result of stress or painful stimuli, hypovolemia, anemia, fever, medications (i.e., inotropic agents), a high catecholamine state, surgical manipulation, or the presence of effusions. Sinus tachycardia can often times be differentiated from pathologic supraventricular arrhythmias by its variability in rate and its normal P wave axis. Treatment is directed at the underlying cause. Prolonged periods of sinus tachycardia may impair diastolic filling time, limit ventricular preload, and compromise systemic cardiac output (decreased urine output, poor peripheral perfusion, metabolic acidosis). Patient groups at higher risk of

Table 17.1 Acute therapy of bradycardia

Treat primary causes	
Hypoxemia, hypothermia, acidosis, hypotension, anemia, hypoglycemia, hypothyroidism	
Consider causative drugs	
Opioids, beta-blockers, digoxin	
Drug therapy	
Drug	Dosage
Atropine	0.02–0.04 mg/kg IV (minimum dose 0.1 mg; maximum dose child 0.5 mg, adolescent 1.0 mg)
Epinephrine	1 μg/kg IV bolus (lower dose may also be effective)
	Infusion: start at 0.02 μg/kg/min, may increase to 2.0 μg/kg/min
Isoproterenol	Infusion: 0.01–2.0 μg/kg/min
Temporary atrial pacing	
Transcutaneous, esophageal, intracardiac, epicardial	

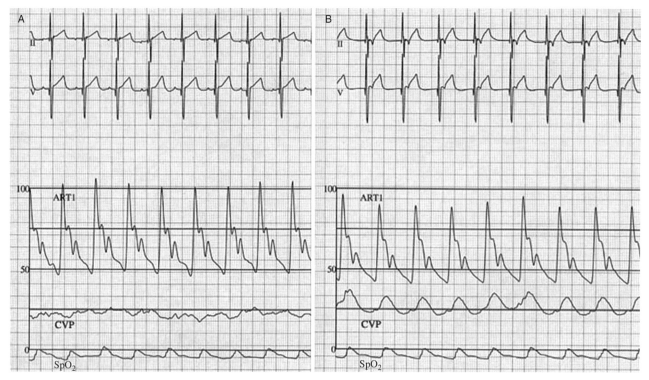

Figure 17.1 (a) Normal sinus rhythm. The normal atrioventricular activation sequence is shown in this intraoperative recording (P wave precedes each QRS complex). Baseline hemodynamic and oxygen saturation tracings are shown. ART1, systemic arterial blood pressure (scale 0–100 mm Hg); CVP, central venous pressure (scale 0–60 mm Hg); SpO₂, oxygen saturation by pulse oximetry. (b) Junctional rhythm. The electrocardiographic features of junctional rhythm are demonstrated in the same patient during the prebypass period. Retrograde P waves are seen following the QRS complexes. Associated hemodynamic changes include a reduction in the systemic arterial blood pressure and prominent *v* waves on the CVP tracing related to the loss of atrioventricular synchrony

hemodynamic compromise are those with significant degrees of ventricular hypertrophy or noncompliant ("stiff") ventricles with associated diastolic dysfunction, such as in certain types of cardiomyopathies or chronic obstructive outflow lesions.

Junctional rhythm

Junctional rhythm is characterized by QRS complexes of morphology identical to that of sinus rhythm without preceding P waves and is thought to originate in the bundle of His. It often occurs in the context of sinus bradycardia or sinus node dysfunction. In this rhythm, there is normal atrioventricular (AV) nodal conduction, but it is sometimes difficult to determine this as the junctional beats are slightly faster than the atrial beats or there is 1:1 ventriculoatrial (V:A) conduction retrograde through the AV node. In the intraoperative setting, this is a fairly common rhythm resulting from cardiac manipulation and dissection around the right atrium. In addition to the electrocardiographic findings described above, the invasive pressure tracings may display waveform changes. The central venous pressure contour may demonstrate prominent *v*

waves (right atrial pressure wave at the end of systole) due to the loss of AV synchrony (Figure 17.1). An associated decrease in cardiac output may manifest as a reduction in systemic arterial blood pressure as a result of the lack of normal atrial systolic contribution to ventricular filling. Temporary atrial pacing at 10–20 beats per minute (bpm) above the junctional rate would document normal AV nodal conduction and restore AV synchrony.

Conduction disorders

Bundle branch block

In the unoperated patient, bundle branch block is an uncommon finding on the electrocardiogram (ECG), although incomplete right bundle branch or intraventricular conduction delays may be seen in patients with right ventricular volume overload (atrial septal defects, anomalous pulmonary venous return, etc.). On rare cases, a right bundle branch block (RBBB) can also be congenital and idiopathic. In the postoperative patient, an RBBB pattern is a frequent finding after interventions for various congenital heart defects including tetralogy of Fallot, right ventricular outflow tract reconstructions, ventricular septal defects, and AV septal defects (also referred as AV canal or endocardial cushion defects). The bundle branch block pattern may be related to a ventriculotomy incision, damage to the moderator band, ventricular septal defect repair, or resection of infundibular muscle. Left bundle branch block (LBBB) patterns are uncommon in children but can be seen in some patients following surgery involving the left ventricular outflow tract.

Atrioventricular block

First-degree atrioventricular block

First-degree AV block is characterized by prolongation of the PR interval beyond the normal for age. Each P wave is followed by a conducted QRS complex. This can be a normal variant in healthy individuals but can also been seen in various disease states (i.e., rheumatic fever, structural heart lesions associated with stretching of the atria). In general, first-degree AV block in an otherwise healthy child is a benign condition and requires no specific treatment.

Second-degree atrioventricular block

Second-degree AV block has two predominant forms: Mobitz type I (Wenckebach) and Mobitz type II. Both forms show a periodic failure to conduct atrial impulses to the ventricle. In type I second-degree AV block, there is a progressive lengthening of the PR interval with eventual failure to conduct the next atrial impulse to the ventricle (P waves without associated QRS complexes) (Figure 17.2). The RR intervals concomitantly shorten. This condition can occur during periods of high vagal tone and is generally considered a benign phenomenon that needs no therapy. In the less frequent type II second-degree AV block, there is a constant PR interval prior to an atrial impulse that suddenly fails to conduct. This type of AV block is considered more worrisome due to its potential for progression. It can be seen in patients following surgery for CHD and is thought to be secondary to damage to the His bundle or distal conduction system. The degree of

conduction deficit in second-degree AV block can be expressed as the ratio of P waves per QRS complexes (i.e., 2:1, 3:2). High-grade AV block is defined as two or more nonconducted P waves in succession that would normally be expected to conduct. Temporary pacing and close patient observation may be warranted as hemodynamically significant bradycardia or continued progression of conduction deficit may ensue.

Third-degree (complete) atrioventricular block

Third-degree AV block is characterized by total failure of atrial impulses to be conducted to the ventricle. There is complete dissociation between the atria and ventricles and the ventricular rate is usually slow and regular. In AV dissociation, the ventricular escape rate may be narrow (if originating from the perinodal region) or it may be wide (if originating from within the ventricle). The diagnostic feature on the ECG is that all atrial impulses that should be propagated to the ventricle fail to do so (Figure 17.3). Complete AV may be either congenital or acquired. Congenital complete AV block in infants with otherwise structurally normal hearts may be due to intrauterine exposure to maternal antibodies associated with collagen vascular diseases. Anatomic substrates at high risk of complete AV block include patients with *l*-transposition of the great arteries with ventricular inversion (congenitally corrected transposition) and those with polysplenia/left atrial isomerism [1]. Acquired postoperative AV block is thought to occur from damage to the compact AV node or bundle of His and may be of a transient or permanent nature. The surgical procedures most commonly associated with complete AV block include repair of AV septal defects, ventricular septal defects, resection of subaortic obstruction, and interventions in patients with *l*-transposition of the great arteries [2]. The incidence of surgical AV block has been reported as high as in 2–4% of pediatric patients. Eventual recovery of normal conduction occurs in over 60% of subjects and usually does so within the first 10 postoperative days with a smaller percentage showing later recovery [3,4]. Acute treatment includes temporary pacing (either AV sequential or ventricular pacing only). If the junctional escape rhythm is of adequate rate to support stable hemodynamics, then temporary pacing may be set as a back up

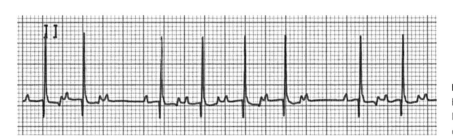

Figure 17.2 Mobitz type I second-degree AV block (Wenckebach) is shown with progressive lengthening of the PR interval and eventual failure of an atrial impulse to conduct

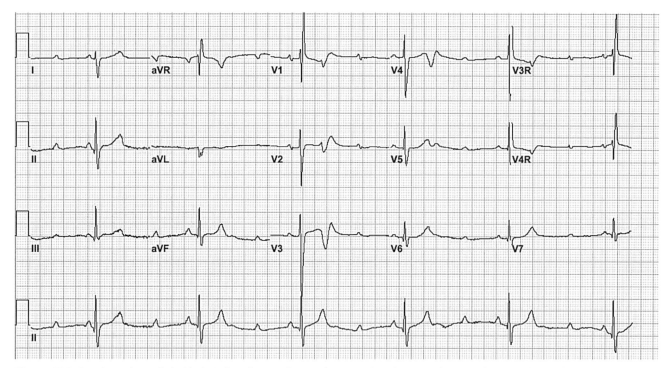

Figure 17.3 Complete atrioventricular block. Surface electrocardiogram shows complete dissociation between the atria and ventricles related to inability of the atrial impulses to be propagated to the ventricular myocardium. The ventricular rate is fairly regular

and the patient monitored closely. Postoperative surveillance in the patient with surgical AV block includes close observation for return of AV conduction and daily evaluation of thresholds of the temporary pacing wires. The ventricular output of the temporary pacemaker should be set well above the capture threshold for an increased margin of safety. Permanent cardiac pacing is generally indicated in patients who have not recovered from complete AV block within 10–14 days after surgical intervention.

When providing anesthetic care to a patient in the setting of complete AV block and no pacemaker, the following should be considered: placement of transcutaneous pacing pads, access to temporary transvenous pacing, availability of isoproterenol, emergency drugs, and resuscitation equipment. Although insertion of a temporary pacemaker has been suggested prior to general anesthesia in children with complete AV block, a retrospective 10-year chart review that examined this issue concluded that there was no benefit to the routine use of this approach [5].

Supraventricular arrhythmias

Premature atrial contractions

Isolated premature atrial contractions (PACs) are relatively common in the younger age group (infants and small children). The early P waves on the ECG frequently have an axis and morphology differing from those in normal sinus rhythm and are typically followed by a normal appearing QRS. On occasion, the PACs may block at the AV node or conduct aberrantly (abnormal wider QRS). Blocked PACs may mimic bradycardia and aberrantly conducted PACs may mimic ventricular ectopy. PACs are usually benign requiring no therapy. Investigation may be warranted in cases of symptomatic, frequent, or complex (multifocal) PACs. If a central venous catheter or other type of intracardiac line is present, radiographic or echocardiographic assessment of the tip position should be considered, as appropriate adjustments can eliminate direct atrial irritability as a potential etiology.

Supraventricular tachycardia

Supraventricular tachycardia (SVT) is the most common clinically significant arrhythmia in infants and children. This rhythm disturbance is characterized by a narrow or "usual" complex QRS morphology and can occur in structurally normal hearts as well as in various forms of CHD. "Usual" complex implies that the QRS morphology in tachycardia is similar to that in normal sinus rhythm. This differentiation is made because patients with CHD often have abnormalities on their baseline ECG including a bundle branch block. On occasion, widening of the QRS in SVT may also be secondary to aberrancy in the right or left bundle branches or because of the tachycardia mechanism

Table 17.2 Characteristics of supraventricular tachycardia mechanisms

	Automatic	Reentrant
Onset and termination	"Warm-up" at initiation "Cool-down" at termination	Abrupt
Mode of initiation	Spontaneous	Premature beats
Ability to initiate/terminate with timed premature beats	No	Yes
Variation in tachycardia rate	Wide	Narrow
Response to catecholamines	Increased rate	None or slight rate increase
Response to adenosine	None	Termination
Response to drugs that increase refractoriness	Variable	Slowing or termination
Response to overdrive pacing	Transient suppression, quick resumption	Termination
Response to cardioversion	None	Termination

itself. When the QRS complex is wide, the distinction between supraventricular and ventricular tachycardia may be difficult.

There are two general types of SVT: automatic and reentrant. These can be differentiated by evaluating characteristics of the tachycardia, as listed in Table 17.2. The most common mechanisms of SVT and their electrographic features are noted in Table 17.3. Evaluation of a tachyarrhythmia typically includes a surface 12-lead ECG and a continuous rhythm strip to document onset, termination, response to medications (i.e., adenosine), or pacing maneuvers. Bedside or transport monitor strips are helpful to determine tachycardia rate, but are usually not sufficient for diagnosis or to differentiate among tachycardia mechanisms.

In the postoperative patient, an atrial electrogram can be useful in both diagnosis and management. The ECG recording is obtained from temporary wires typically placed on the atrial myocardium at the conclusion of surgery. Although both, a standard 12-lead ECG and an atrial electrogram, record the same cardiac electrical activity, these electrical sequences display distinct configurations in different leads. The P waves on an atrial electrogram are amplified, appearing much larger. Thus, if

Table 17.3 Mechanisms of supraventricular tachycardia and electrographic features

Diagnosis	Electrocardiographic features
Automatic tachycardias	
Ectopic atrial tachycardia	Atrial rates of 90–330 bpm Incessant rhythm From atrial focus distinct from sinus node Abnormal P wave morphology and/or axis Distinct P waves preceding QRS complexes No influence of AV block on tachycardia
Junctional ectopic tachycardia	Narrow QRS tachycardia Incessant rhythm AV dissociation frequent feature Atrial rate slower than ventricular rate Capture beats frequently seen (QRS complexes slightly earlier than expected from antegrade conduction of normal sinus impulses)
Reentrant tachycardias	
Atrial flutter	Sawtooth pattern or more discrete undulating P waves (leads II, II, AVF) Variable rates of AV conduction seen (1:1, 2:1, 3:1, or 4:1)
Atrioventricular reentrant tachycardia (accessory pathway mediated)	P waves immediately following the QRS complex, on ST segment or T wave
Concealed bypass tract Wolff-Parkinson-White Syndrome	AV block results in termination of tachycardia
Atrioventricular nodal reentry tachycardia	P waves buried within QRS and not discernible AV block results in termination of tachycardia

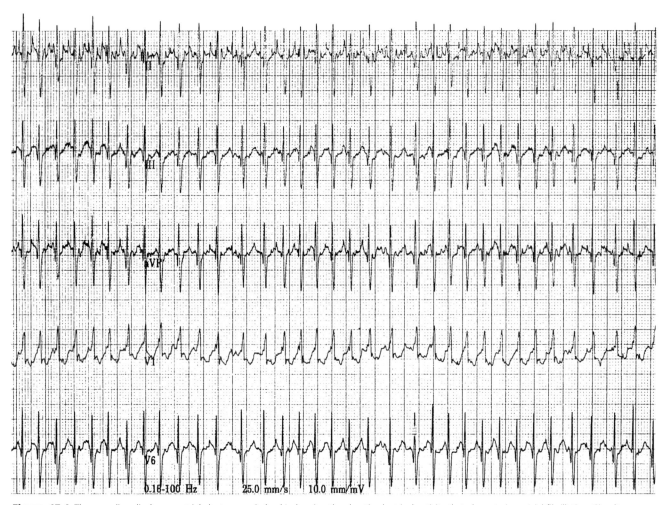

Figure 17.4 The recording displays an atrial electrogram in lead I, showing the chaotic electrical activity that characterizes atrial fibrillation. Simultaneous chest lead tracings (V1 and V6) demonstrate an irregular heart rate due to variable atrioventricular conduction (varying RR intervals)

it is difficult to discern P waves on the surface ECG, an atrial electrogram may assist to clearly define atrial activity and the relationship between atrial and ventricular depolarization (Figure 17.4). This may be of benefit in the differentiation of atrial and junctional arrhythmias, and defining the nature of an AV block if present.

Atrial electrograms can be recorded by using a bedside monitor or a standard 12-lead ECG machine; however, in most cases the latter is used. When using a bedside monitor, a rhythm strip with two or more channels should be used in order to display the atrial electrogram along with ECG recording(s) from surface lead(s). There are various ways to obtain an atrial electrogram along with a standard tracing depending on the recorder, epicardial wires, and lead configuration.

The following is one such arrangement using a standard 12-lead ECG machine:
1 If two atrial wires are present, each lead is attached to the connectors that usually go to the right and left arm leads. An alligator clip may be used if necessary. This allows for a bipolar atrial electrogram to be recorded in lead I (large deflection of atrial depolarization with trivial or no signal representative of ventricular activity). The chest leads will provide standard tracings. By evaluating the atrial activity as displayed by the atrial electrogram (lead I) and the ventricular impulses represented by the QRS complex on the chest leads (V1–V6), an assessment of the electrical sequence of cardiac events can be made. If only a single atrial lead is available, this can be attached to one of the chest leads to obtain a corresponding atrial electrogram. In this case, the limb leads can be used to provide a reference for the ventricular activity. An alternate lead configuration may utilize a single atrial lead and skin lead as a substitute for the arm leads to obtain an atrial tracing in lead I and other leads serve as a reference. Typically, atrial wires emerge on the right side of the chest and ventricular wires on the left, although this may vary.
2 A rhythm strip should be printed out in order to examine the recordings.

While maximizing atrial waveforms, the atrial electrogram should facilitate arrhythmia diagnosis and the institution of appropriate treatment. In addition, these temporary wires may be used for rapid atrial pacing in attempts to terminate SVT due to reentrant mechanisms or to overdrive suppress an automatic focus.

Management of SVT depends on the clinical status of the patient, type of tachycardia and precise electrophysiologic mechanism (Table 17.4). If the tachyarrhythmia is associated with significant hemodynamic compromise, emergent therapy is indicated. Synchronized direct current cardioversion should be considered for any acute tachyarrhythmia associated with low cardiac output, recognizing that this approach may not always result in restoration of normal sinus rhythm.

Atrial tachycardias

Automaticity of atrial tissue accounts for the majority of supraventricular arrhythmias in this group [6]. In general, these rhythm disorders are more difficult to treat than reentrant types.

Focal atrial tachycardia

Focal atrial tachycardia (AT) is a rhythm disturbance originating from a single focus in the atrium outside of the sinus node. In the past, focal AT was thought to solely be due to enhanced automaticity. Thus, it was often referred to as an automatic or ectopic atrial tachycardia (EAT). It has recently become apparent that in some rare cases focal AT is triggered or microreentrant in etiology, and is not due to a true ectopic focus. These forms of AT can not be easily distinguished on the basis of the surface ECG alone. The clinical characteristics of EAT follow those outlined in Table 17.2 for automatic tachycardias. EAT may be incessant or episodic. The diagnosis is made by evaluation of the surface ECG or rhythm strips, demonstrating an abnormal P wave morphology and/or axis (Figure 17.5). The PR interval may also differ from that in sinus rhythm. Atrial rates in EAT are faster than usual sinus rates for age and physiologic state of the patient. If the atrial rates are very rapid, some of the atrial impulses may not be conducted to the ventricles due to AV node refractoriness.

EAT is relatively rare and is generally found in two different clinical scenarios [7,8]. A patient with a structurally normal heart can develop EAT as a primary phenomenon. In older children, EAT can be incessant and, on rare occasion, lead to the development of myocardial dysfunction or dilated cardiomyopathy because of the chronicity of the tachycardia. In neonates and infants, EAT often follows a more benign course and frequently resolves spontaneously early in life. A patient with CHD can also develop EAT in the postoperative period related to car-

diac surgery. In this setting, EAT tends to be episodic and transient, usually resolving within days. In a recent report, postoperative patients who developed EAT tended to have lower preoperative oxygen saturations, increased inotropic support both pre- and postoperatively, and had undergone an atrial septostomy prior to surgical intervention [9]. No specific cardiac repair was associated with the development of EAT.

The management of postoperative EAT includes the treatment of fever if present, adequate sedation, correction of electrolyte abnormalities, and the withdrawal of medications associated with sympathetic stimulation (i.e., inotropic agents) or with vagolytic properties (i.e., pancuronium). The institution of antiarrhythmic medications is based on overall heart rates and the hemodynamic status of the patient. The choice of therapy is based on clinical judgment and ventricular function. There are no large clinical series investigating antiarrhythmic drug efficacy in postoperative EAT. Intravenous medications such as esmolol, procainamide, and amiodarone can be effective in slowing the tachycardia rate [10]. Oral agents (class I and class III drugs) may also be of benefit. Digoxin has minimal effect on the atrial focus, but can slow the overall heart rates by slowing AV conduction [11]. In very rare cases in the postoperative patient, EAT may be incessant and life threatening and consideration should be given to transcatheter ablation of the atrial focus [12]. Atrial pacing and cardioversion are not likely to be effective.

Multifocal atrial tachycardia

Multifocal atrial tachycardia (MAT), also known as chaotic atrial rhythm, is an uncommon atrial arrhythmia characterized by multiple (at least three) P wave morphologies [13]. These different morphologies correspond to multiple foci of automatic atrial activity. Characteristic ECG features include variable PP, RR, and PR intervals, and typical atrial rates exceed 100 bpm. MAT may be seen in young infants without structural heart disease, in patients with cardiac defects after surgical intervention, and in children with noncardiac medical conditions [14,15]. Treatment focuses on ventricular rate control and/or decreasing automaticity. Drugs such as digoxin, procainamide, flecainide, amiodarone, and propafenone have been found to be successful in converting MAT to sinus rhythm in children [16]. Adenosine, pacing, and direct current cardioversion are usually ineffective.

Junctional tachycardias

Automaticity of junctional tissue accounts for the majority of supraventricular arrhythmias in this group [6]. These rhythm disorders also tend to be somewhat resistant to standard pharmacological therapy.

Table 17.4 Acute therapy of perioperative arrhythmias without evidence of hemodynamic compromise

Rhythm disturbance	Treatment considerations
Sinus bradycardia	See Table 17.1
Sinus tachycardia	Correct underlying cause
Premature atrial contractions	Evaluate position of central venous line or intracardiac catheter
	Assess/correct electrolyte disturbances (i.e., hypokalemia)
Focal atrial tachycardia (ectopic atrial tachycardia)	Correct fever, electrolyte abnormalities
	Adequate sedation
	Consider possible role or inotropes/vagolytics
	Digoxin, usually first drug but rarely effective as single agent
	Beta-blockers, use with caution if depressed cardiac function
	Procainamide
	Amiodarone, Sotalol
	Flecainide, Propafenone
Multifocal atrial tachycardia (chaotic atrial tachycardia)	As in ectopic atrial tachycardia
	Goals are rate control and decreased automaticity
Accelerated junctional rhythm	Correct fever
	Consider possible role or inotropic agents
	Temporary atrial pacing
Junctional ectopic tachycardia	Correct fever, electrolyte abnormalities
	Consider possible role or inotropes/vagolytics
	Surface cooling to 34–35°C
	Temporary atrial pacing (for JET rates below 180 bpm)
	Amiodarone
	Hypothermia plus procainamide
Atrial flutter	Adenosine to confirm diagnosis
	Atrial overdrive pacing
	Digoxin
	Procainamide
	Amiodarone, Sotalol
	Propafenone
Atrial fibrillation	Digoxin (except in WPW)
	Beta-blockers
	Procainamide, Quinidine
	Amiodarone, Sotalol
Atrioventricular reentrant tachycardia or atrioventricular nodal reentry tachycardia	Consider vagal maneuvers
	Adenosine
	Atrial overdrive pacing
	Procainamide
	Amiodarone
Premature ventricular contractions	Consider and treat underlying cause
	Lidocaine
Ventricular tachycardia	Lidocaine
	Amiodarone
	Procainamide
	Magnesium (for torsade de pointes)
	Beta-blockers
	Phenytoin (for digitalis toxicity)
Ventricular fibrillation	Check for loose ECG electrode mimicking VF
	Lidocaine
	Amiodarone (to prevent recurrence)

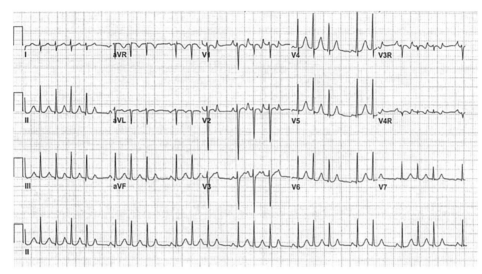

Figure 17.5 Fifteen-lead electrocardiogram in a 6-year-old child with ectopic atrial tachycardia. The characteristic features of the tachycardia are shown including a faster than expected heart rate for age, an abnormal P wave axis (left atrial focus), and maintenance of the arrhythmia in the presence of atrioventricular block

Accelerated junctional rhythm

Accelerated junctional rhythm is an automatic rhythm that arises from the AV junction. Characteristics of this arrhythmia include a narrow or "usual" QRS pattern with no preceding P wave. There is either VA dissociation with ventricular rates faster than atrial rates or the presence of 1:1 VA conduction retrograde via the AV node. Temporary atrial pacing at a rate 10–20 bpm faster than the junctional rate often reestablishes AV synchrony and effectively suppresses the automatic junctional rhythm. Changes in the patient's physiologic state including fever, chronotropic agents, and endogenous catecholamines may act to stimulate the automatic junctional focus and increases in junctional rates may be seen. This rhythm is usually well tolerated and easily managed with temporary pacing and control of the patient's underlying physiologic state.

Junctional ectopic tachycardia

Junctional ectopic tachycardia (JET) is also an automatic rhythm that arises from the AV junction and is a narrow or "usual" complex tachycardia without preceding P waves. It is differentiated from accelerated junctional rhythm by the heart rate and hemodynamic status of the patient. This tachyarrhythmia has been classically defined by heart rates above 160 or 170 bpm with resultant hemodynamic compromise [17]. In the recent past, however, JET has also been considered if the junctional rate exceeded >95% of heart rate for age [18]. There is either VA dissociation with ventricular rates faster than atrial rates or the presence of 1:1 VA conduction (Figure 17.6). If 1:1 VA con-

duction is noted, then a trial of adenosine or rapid atrial pacing may be beneficial to differentiate JET from other reentrant forms of SVT on an atrial electrogram.

This type of tachycardia typically occurs in the immediate postoperative period and usually results in hemodynamic instability and significant morbidity and may contribute to mortality [19–21]. It occurs most commonly following surgical intervention for tetralogy of Fallot, repair of ventricular septal defects, AV septal defects, transposition of the great arteries, and total anomalous pulmonary venous connections [22].

Numerous therapies have been advocated for JET [20–24]. In the acute setting strategies include:

1 Control of fever to at least normothermia. Core temperature cooling (to 34 or 35°C) in the younger patient by the use of cooling blankets, fans, or cold compresses has been shown to be of benefit in reducing the tachycardia rate [25–27]. Shivering, if significant, should be avoided by the use of muscle relaxants in view of potential detrimental increases in oxygen consumption.

2 Decreasing or withdrawing medications associated with catecholamine stimulation or vagolytic agents.

3 Correction of electrolyte abnormalities, especially potassium and calcium.

4 Temporary atrial pacing at heart rates 10–20 bpm above the JET rate. This establishes AV synchrony and often benefits the hemodynamic status of the patient. However, if the JET rates are faster than 180 or 190 bpm, there is often little benefit with overdrive atrial pacing.

5 Initiation of antiarrhythmic medications. The two most widely used drugs for JET are amiodarone and procainamide [23,24,28–30]. Amiodarone has a longer

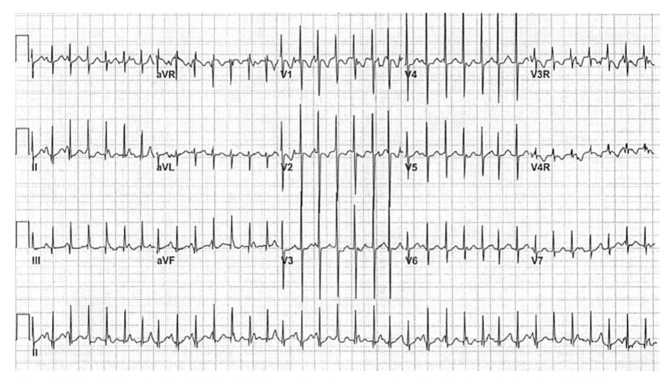

Figure 17.6 Junctional ectopic tachycardia. Fifteen-lead electrocardiogram in a postoperative patient following repair of tetralogy of Fallot. The tachycardia is characterized by a narrow QRS complex and atrioventricular dissociation

onset of action and a longer half-life as compared to procainamide. It has been shown to reduce the heart rate in JET during the initial bolus infusion [28,29]. Core cooling is often continued but is not generally needed for efficacy. This may avoid the challenge of having to evaluate clinical signs reflecting the adequacy of cardiac output (distal peripheral perfusion, skin temperature) in a hypothermic tachycardic patient. Amiodarone does not influence ventricular function and generally causes less blood pressure change during the initial bolus infusion, as compared to procainamide. The benefits of procainamide are that it has a faster onset of action and a shorter half-life. The concerns are that it appears to be efficacious predominantly with the use of core cooling. It may also cause a decrease in peripheral vascular resistance and hypotension, especially during bolus infusions. Procainamide may also have negative inotropic properties. Usually, a normal saline bolus or other volume expander should be administered prior to or during procainamide therapy to maintain adequate hemodynamics. Both drugs have been shown to be effective in the treatment of JET in published retrospective studies; however, drug choice may be influenced by physician/center preference. Because amiodarone and procainamide can each result in QT prolongation and

proarrhythmic side effects, concomitant drug administration should be avoided. Anecdotally, digoxin loading may slow the JET rate, but this has not well documented in the literature. Beta-blockers and calcium-channel blockers can depress myocardial contractility, a feature that limits their application in the immediate postoperative period. The use of intravenous class IC agents such as propafenone and flecainide has been reported, but these agents have not been studied extensively for JET [31–33].

6 Overdrive pacing and cardioversion are generally considered ineffective to terminate JET.

The natural history of perioperative JET is that it resolves within 2–5 days from the surgical intervention. Long-term antiarrhythmic therapy is usually not necessary. In extreme cases where JET cannot be controlled medically, transcatheter ablation can be considered [34,35].

Reentrant supraventricular tachycardias

Reentry, also known as "circus" movement or reciprocation, implies that a single stimulus or excitation wave front returns and reactivates the same site or tissue where it came from. Reentrant forms of SVT may or may not involve accessory pathways.

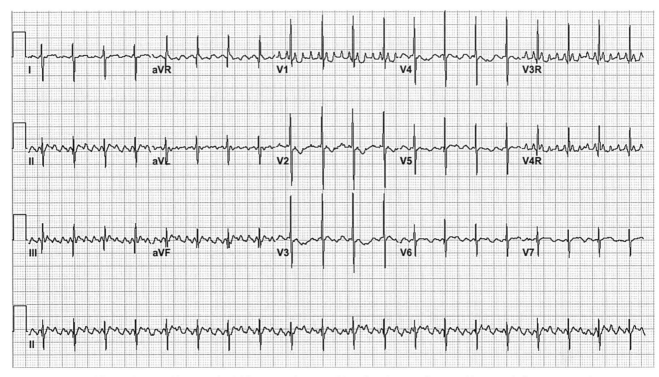

Figure 17.7 Atrial flutter. The typical features of atrial flutter are shown on this surface electrocardiogram with sawtooth flutter waves and 4:1 atrioventricular conduction

Atrial flutter

Atrial flutter is an arrhythmia confined to the atrial myocardium. The electrophysiologic basis for this rhythm disturbance involves reentry within the atrium itself. The typical or classic form of atrial flutter is characterized by a negative sawtooth P wave pattern and atrial rates greater than 300 bpm (Figure 17.7). This form of atrial flutter may occasionally be seen in an otherwise healthy neonate but is relatively uncommon in children. In patients with CHD, slower atrial rates and varying P wave morphologies are more frequently seen, likely due to anatomic abnormalities related to suture lines, scars, or fibrosis from previous surgical interventions in atrial tissue. This form of "scar flutter" is commonly termed intra-atrial reentrant tachycardia (IART) [36]. This is one of the most common arrhythmias in the postoperative patient with structural heart disease and considered the cause of significant morbidity following certain types of surgical interventions [37]. Procedures that involve extensive atrial manipulations, such as atrial redirection procedures (Senning or Mustard operations) and those associated with atrial dilation (Fontan surgery), are particularly at high risk. The diagnosis of atrial flutter is suggested by abrupt onset of a rapid atrial rhythm that remains relatively regular over time. AV nodal conduction accounts for the ventricular response rate that may be variable. Rapid clinical deterioration is likely with fast ventricular rates and prompt intervention is frequently necessary.

Management approaches for atrial flutter include:

1 Although adenosine will not terminate atrial flutter, it may assist in confirmation of the diagnosis by enhancing AV block and uncovering flutter waves.
2 Atrial overdrive pacing (via esophagus, intracardiac pacing catheter, or epicardial wires) has been shown to be safe and effective in the acute termination of atrial flutter [38]. After determination of the atrial cycle length, rapid atrial stimulation is performed in short bursts to attempt interruption of the reentry circuit.
3 Synchronized cardioversion is the treatment of choice for any patient with unstable hemodynamics associated with atrial flutter.
4 Pharmacologic agents such as digoxin, procainamide, and amiodarone may be used in acute situations. Drug therapy for controlling the ventricular response in atrial flutter may include in some cases beta-blockers or calcium-channel blockers. Important considerations regarding drug selection are patient age, underlying ventricular function and presence of sinus node dysfunction (a concomitant problem in patients with recurrent atrial flutter). Ibutilide, a class III agent, is available for acute termination of atrial flutter and has been used in the postoperative adult with CHD.

5 Chronic drug therapy is frequently required in patients with CHD because of the potential for recurrence and associated rapid AV conduction.

6 Pacemaker therapy, atrial antitachycardia pacing, and radiofrequency ablation are additional modalities more applicable to long-term management.

Atrial fibrillation

Atrial fibrillation is a complex arrhythmia that is thought to be due to multiple reentrant circuits versus originating from focal points within the pulmonary veins. In most cases, atrial fibrillation originates in the left atrium, while atrial flutter is generally considered a right atrial disease. In the pediatric age group, this tachyarrhythmia is less frequent than atrial flutter. The atrial rates are rapid and irregular ranging from 400 to 700 bpm. Ventricular response rates are variable but generally range between 80 and 150 bpm. Patients at potential risk for atrial fibrillation include those with an enlarged left atrium (i.e., rheumatic heart disease, severe AV valve regurgitation), preexcitation syndromes, structural heart disease (Ebstein's anomaly, tricuspid atresia, atrial septal defects), and cardiomyopathies.

Management principles in atrial fibrillation are similar to those for atrial flutter except that atrial overdrive pacing is not effective in terminating the arrhythmia. Cardioversion is more likely to be required and higher amounts of energy may be needed. An orientation of the cardioversion pads over the front and back of the heart may be necessary to provide a shock vector through the entire atrium. Anticoagulation and consideration of transesophageal echocardiography for evaluation of intracardiac thrombi is recommended prior to cardioversion if atrial fibrillation has been present more than a few days [39, 40].

Atrioventricular reentrant tachycardia and atrioventricular nodal reentrant tachycardia

Atrioventricular reentrant tachycardia (AVRT) mediated by an accessory pathway between the atrium and ventricle is the most common form of SVT in infancy and childhood. Typically, the tachycardia circuit consists of conduction from the atrium, down the AV node, through the His bundle and ventricles, up the accessory pathway, and back to the atrium. This form of SVT is called "orthodromic" SVT and occurs in patients with Wolff-Parkinson-White syndrome (WPW), concealed accessory pathways, and permanent junctional reciprocating tachycardia (PJRT). In contrast, in "antidromic" SVT, conduction travels from the atrium, down the accessory pathway, through the ventricles, up the AV node, and back to the atrium. The QRS complex in this form of SVT is obligatorily wide. Antidromic tachycardia can occur in patients with WPW and other preexcitation variants (Mahaim tachycardia).

Atrioventricular nodal reentrant tachycardia (AVNRT), or reentry within the AV node, is more likely in the adolescent or young adult. In AVNRT there are two physiologically distinct components of the AV node designated as "slow" and "fast" AV nodal pathways. The typical form of AVNRT consists of antegrade conduction (from the atrium to the ventricle) via the slow pathway followed by retrograde conduction (back to the atrium) via the fast pathway.

Both AVRT (Figure 17.8) and AVNRT (Figure 17.9) have clinical characteristics of reentrant tachycardia mechanisms listed in Table 17.2. The two can often be distinguished by close evaluation of the surface ECG in tachycardia and at baseline. In AVRT (of the orthodromic form), the P wave can be seen immediately following the QRS complex or in the ST segment or T wave. The reason for this P wave location is that a set time period is necessary for conduction to proceed from the ventricles through the accessory pathway back to the atrium. In contrast, in AVNRT, the P wave is buried in the QRS complex and is often not discernible. This is because the tachycardia circuit is within the AV node and the atria and the ventricles are activated almost simultaneously. Patients with structurally normal hearts as well as those with CHD can have either AVRT or AVNRT. Ebstein's anomaly of the tricuspid valve is frequently associated with AVRT secondary to one or multiple accessory pathways [41]. The accessory pathway(s) in this condition is (are) usually right-sided. L-transposition of the great arteries can be associated with Ebstein's-like features of the left-sided AV valve and left-sided accessory pathways can be identified in a subset of these patients.

Management principles of AVRT or AVNRT include the following:

1 If the patient is hemodynamically unstable, emergent direct current cardioversion (0.5–1.0 joule/kg) should be carried out. A lower energy setting is adequate for epicardial paddles. This should also be considered in the stable patient when potential rapid clinical deterioration is anticipated or after unsuccessful conventional therapy.

2 In the stable patient, various modalities can be utilized to acutely terminate the tachycardia. Vagal maneuvers (Valsalva maneuver, coughing, gag reflex stimulation, Trendelenburg position) enhance parasympathetic influences and may acutely terminate the tachycardia [42]. Adenosine has become the first line pharmacologic therapy for SVT [43–45]. Other agents (digoxin, edrophonium, beta-blockers, calcium-channel blockers, phenylephrine) have been used in the acute setting with variable results; however, serious adverse effects may be seen. Continuous ECG monitoring is recommended

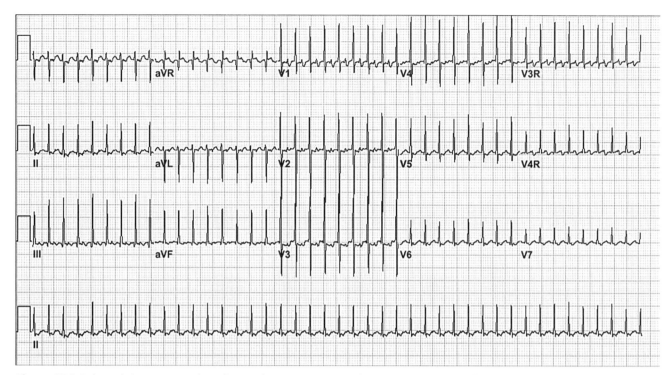

Figure 17.8 Atrioventricular reentrant tachycardia secondary to an accessory pathway in a patient with Wolff-Parkinson-White syndrome. This electrocardiogram shows a narrow complex tachycardia with a very regular rate and a distinct retrograde P wave approximately 80 msec after the QRS complex

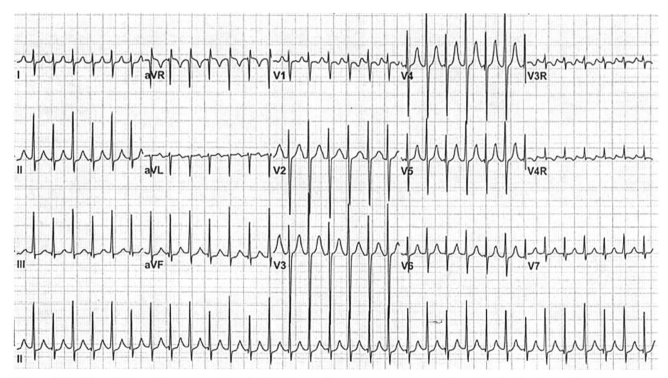

Figure 17.9 Atrioventricular nodal reentrant tachycardia. This electrocardiogram shows a narrow complex tachycardia. There is no evidence of a retrograde P wave as it is obscured by the QRS complex, secondary to simultaneous atrial and ventricular depolarization

as well as the availability of atropine as transient brady-cardia following tachycardia termination may be seen.

3 Rapid atrial pacing may be conducted via a trans-esophageal electrode catheter or via temporary atrial pacing wires. One should first establish that at the pacing outputs utilized, the electrode catheter or the temporary wires do not capture the ventricle and cause ventricular contraction. Then, rapid atrial pacing is performed by pacing the atrium at 10–20% faster than the SVT rate for a period of up to 15 seconds, which typically terminates the arrhythmia. In patients with high catecholamine states, termination of SVT can be successful but rapid recurrence may be seen. In this instance, it is helpful to sedate the patient and limit catecholamine stimulation if possible.

4 Once the tachycardia has terminated or if it terminates and then reinitiates, antiarrhythmic medication can be instituted. For perioperative patients unable to take oral medications, parenteral therapy may include procainamide or amiodarone. Beta-blockers and calcium-channel blockers may be less desirable in the immediate perioperative period due to their negative effects on myocardial contractility. A short-acting agent, such as esmolol, may offer a larger margin of safety in this case.

5 If the patient has incessant tachycardia and cannot be controlled with medications, transcatheter ablation may be warranted.

Ventricular arrhythmias

Ventricular arrhythmias are disorders that arise distal to the bifurcation of the common His bundle. These are relatively rare in young children and more commonly seen in the adolescent or young adult with a history of operated CHD. Patients with ventricular rhythm abnormalities may have minimal to no symptomatology or be gravely ill. Evaluation of ventricular arrhythmias should include a review of the medical history for the presence of associated cardiovascular pathology or potential cause, analysis of the ECG, and most importantly, assessment of the hemodynamic state of the patient.

Premature ventricular contractions

Premature ventricular contractions (PVCs) are premature beats that originate in the ventricular myocardium. These are characterized by (1) prematurity of the QRS complex not preceded by premature atrial activity, (2) a QRS morphology that differs from that in sinus rhythm, (3) prolongation of the QRS duration for age (this is a frequent finding but may not always be the case), and (4) abnormalities of repolarization. In patients with structurally normal hearts, PVCs of a single QRS morphology (uniform) with-

out associated symptoms are generally considered benign. Patients that merit further investigation include those with PVCs of multiple morphologies (multiform) on ECG and those that occur with moderate frequency and are associated with symptoms or present in the context of an abnormal heart.

Ventricular ectopy in the perioperative period may be secondary to myocardial irritation from intracardiac catheters or direct surgical stimulation. Additional etiologies include respiratory (hypoxemia), electrolyte (hypokalemia), or metabolic (acidosis) derangements. Isolated PVCs may also be due to pharmacological agents (including recreational drugs), myocardial injury, poor hemodynamics, and prior complex surgical intervention.

Ventricular tachycardia

Ventricular tachycardia (VT) is defined as three or more consecutive ventricular beats occurring at a rate greater than 120 bpm in adults or more than 20% greater than the preceding sinus rate in children. The QRS morphology in VT is different than that in sinus rhythm and is usually wide for the patient's age, although not necessarily. Electrocardiographic features that favor this diagnosis include (1) AV dissociation, (2) intermittent fusion (QRS complex of intermediate morphology between two other distinct QRS morphologies), (3) QRS morphology of VT similar to that of isolated PVCs, and (4) tachycardia rate in children usually below 250 bpm. An RBBB QRS morphology is most common in infants with VT, whereas in older children an LBBB pattern is more frequent with wider QRS morphologies.

Various qualifiers have been proposed to further characterize VT. The classification as monomorphic (one QRS morphology) or polymorphic (multiple QRS morphologies) is based on the evaluation of the QRS pattern in multiple ECG leads. Ventricular tachycardia is considered to be sustained or nonsustained if it lasts more or less than 10 seconds respectively.

Acute onset of VT in pediatric patients may be due to hypoxia, acidosis, electrolyte imbalance, or metabolic problems. In the perioperative or immediate postoperative setting, the presence of VT may suggest coronary artery injury and/or myocardial ischemia. This arrhythmia may also occur in the context of depressed myocardial function, poor hemodynamics, prior surgical interventions, myocardial tumors, cardiomyopathies (hypertrophic, dilated, left ventricular noncompaction, arrhythmogenic right ventricular cardiomyopathy), myocarditis, acute injury (trauma), and primary channelopathies (long QT syndrome, Brugada syndrome). Among patients with CHD and ventricular arrhythmias, those at higher risk include older patients following tetralogy of Fallot repair or those with significant residual hemodynamic abnormalities.

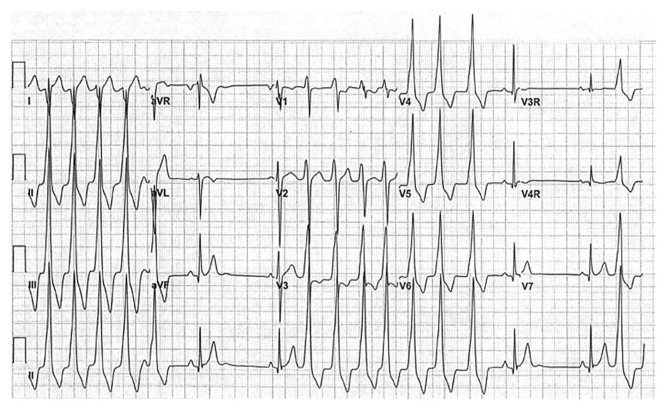

Figure 17.10 Ventricular tachycardia. Runs of a uniform, wide complex rhythm are seen, separated by a few beats of normal sinus rhythm

The following potential causes of ventricular ectopy in patients with structural heart disease have been proposed: inadequate myocardial protection during the surgical procedure, chronic pressure or volume loads, residual or recurrent pathology, and scar formation at the ventriculotomy site.

Monomorphic ventricular tachycardia

Although occasionally seen in patients with otherwise normal hearts, monomorphic VT is a more common phenomenon in patients with underlying cardiac abnormalities. In the abnormal heart, the tachycardia is thought to originate from a reentrant focus in scarred or damaged myocardial tissue. The electrocardiographic findings are those of a wide regular QRS rhythm of uniform morphology (Figure 17.10).

Polymorphic ventricular tachycardia

Torsade de pointes

Torsade de pointes ("twisting of the peaks") refers to a form of polymorphic VT. The characteristic electrocardiographic feature of this arrhythmia is that of a varying QRS morphology manifested as positive and negative oscilla-

tions of the QRS direction that twists around an isoelectric baseline (Figure 17.11). Polymorphic VT may occur in long QT syndromes, can be secondary to drug therapy or neurologic pathology, or be the result of myocardial ischemia. Torsade may terminate spontaneously or degenerate into ventricular fibrillation (VF).

Long QT syndromes

The long QT syndromes can occur in the congenital (inherited) or acquired forms. This distinction is relevant to management strategies. The congenital varieties are predominantly the result of genetic defects in the sodium or potassium channels responsible for maintaining electrical homeostasis in the heart. Genetic testing is commercially available for long QT defects. Although the eventual direction is toward gene-specific therapies, at the present, all patients with prolong QT syndrome are treated similarly. Clinical diagnostic criteria have been suggested for long QT syndrome on the basis of ECG findings, clinical history, and family history [46]. The hallmark of the disease is prolongation of the corrected QT interval (QTc) on the resting ECG (Figure 17.12). The QTc is derived as follows:

$$\text{Corrected QT} = \frac{\text{Measured QT interval}}{\text{Square root of preceding RR interval}}$$

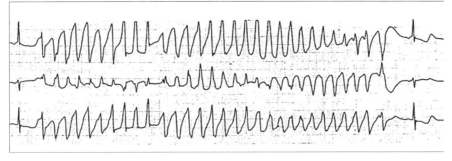

Figure 17.11 Torsade de pointes. The typical positive and negative oscillations of the QRS complexes in torsade are shown

A QTc greater than 0.46 seconds is considered abnormal regardless of age. In addition to torsade de pointes, potential arrhythmias in patients with long QT syndrome include VF and bradyarrhythmias. An important consideration in the care of these patients is ensuring adequate beta-adrenergic blockade preoperatively and minimizing adrenergic stimulation as this may trigger tachyarrhythmias. Conditions and drugs associated with QT interval prolongation should also be avoided. Intraoperative tachyarrhythmias can be treated with additional doses of beta-blockers. Others drugs to be considered include phenytoin and lidocaine. Despite the fact that several anesthetics (intravenous medications and volatile agents)

increase the QT interval, in most cases these drugs are used without untoward effects. A comprehensive list of drugs that prolong the QT interval and/or may induce torsade de pointes is included in The Arizona Center for Education and Research on Therapeutics frequently updated website (http://www.azcert.org/medical-pros/drug-lists/drug-lists.cfm).

Acquired forms of long QT may result from electrolyte disturbances (hypokalemia, hypocalcemia, hypomagnesemia), drug therapy (antiarrhythmic agents, antipsychotic drugs), and neurologic or endocrine abnormalities. Therapy in this setting should focus on correction of the underlying cause.

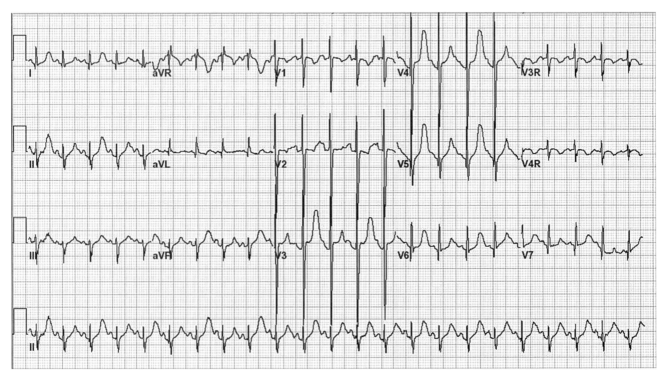

Figure 17.12 Electrocardiogram of a child with long QT syndrome. The corrected QT interval measure 500 msec. Note the T wave alternans (alternating T wave morphologies), a classic but not common finding in patients with long QT syndrome

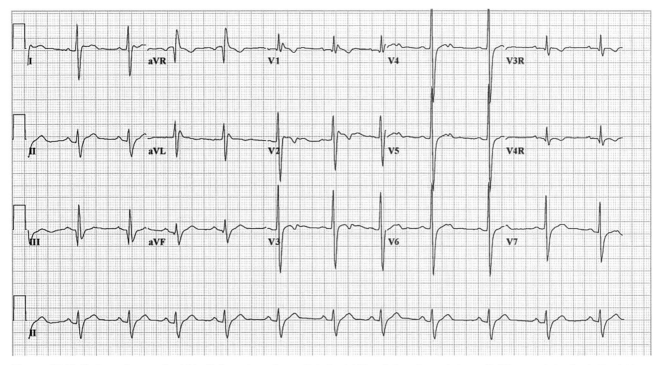

Figure 17.13 Electrocardiogram of a child with Brugada syndrome. Note the right bundle branch morphology with ST segment elevation in the right precordial leads

General considerations in the management of VT are as follows:

1 A wide QRS tachycardia should always be considered of ventricular origin until proven otherwise, although some atypical forms of supraventricular arrhythmias may mimic VT.

2 The primary approach in caring for a patient with an acute ventricular arrhythmia is prompt evaluation of hemodynamics. In general, sustained ventricular arrhythmias are poorly tolerated and require immediate attention. Cardiopulmonary resuscitation should be instituted in the unstable patient and electrical cardioversion should be performed.

3 Pharmacological therapy may be indicated in the stable patient with VT or for the prevention of recurrence. Recommended agents include amiodarone, lidocaine, procainamide, or beta-blockers. The choice of agent is dependent on the associated clinical scenario.

4 Electrical cardioversion in torsade de pointes should be performed only if the arrhythmia is sustained. In patients with frequent but nonsustained runs of torsade de pointes, cardioversion is of no benefit and may be detrimental. Magnesium sulfate is considered the first line drug and lidocaine may also have a role in therapy. Procainamide and amiodarone are relatively contraindicated due to QT prolongation.

5 For polymorphic VT associated with acquired QT prolongation such as that related to the proarrhythmic ef-

fects of certain drugs, pacing and isoproterenol may also be considered, particularly in the setting of long pauses in the cardiac cycle.

Brugada syndrome

Brugada syndrome is a genetically determined disease characterized by a distinct ECG pattern (RBBB with coved or saddle-shaped ST elevation in leads V1–V3) (Figure 17.13) [47,48]. Various genetic defects leading to abnormalities in sodium and calcium currents have been identified in affected patients [49]. The inheritance pattern is usually autosomal dominant, although there is a vast array of genetic heterogeneity. Fortunately, this syndrome has been reported rarely in children [50].

Clinically, the importance of Brugada syndrome is related to its strong propensity for ventricular arrhythmias. By current estimates, it is responsible for between 5 and 20% of all sudden deaths in structurally normal hearts. It is likely underdiagnosed with a national incidence of approximately 5 per 10,000 individuals. The ECG findings are often concealed or transient. In cases of suspected Brugada syndrome with a normal ECG pattern, administration of a sodium-channel blocker can be used to unmask the classic pattern. Antiarrhythmic medications appear to have limited efficacy in preventing recurrences of ventricular arrhythmias and prolonging survival in Brugada syndrome. Only patients with implantable defibrillators appear to be protected from sudden death. From a standpoint of anesthetic care, it is important to note that many events in patients with Brugada syndrome occur during rest or sleep. Theoretically, this may implicate sedation and anesthesia as a time of risk, therefore close monitoring is warranted.

Ventricular fibrillation

VF is an uncommon arrhythmia in children characterized by chaotic, asynchronous ventricular depolarizations failing to generate an effective cardiac output. The ECG morphology in VF demonstrates low amplitude irregular deflections without identifiable QRS complexes. A loose ECG electrode may mimic these surface ECG features; therefore, immediate clinical assessment of cardiac output (checking for a pulse) and adequate pad contact should be performed when VF is suspected.

Considerations in the management of VF are as follows:
1 This is a lethal arrhythmia if untreated; therefore, immediate defibrillation (initial dose 2 joules/kg for the transthoracic approach) is the definitive therapy. If this is unsuccessful, the energy dose should be doubled (4 joules/kg) and repeated. Infant paddles are generally recommended for those weighing less than 10 kg. Adult paddles are suggested for children weighing over 10 kg in order to reduce impedance and maximize current flow.
2 Adequate airway control (oxygenation, ventilation) and chest compressions should be rapidly instituted while preparing for defibrillation or between shocks if several defibrillation attempts are needed.
3 Adjunctive pharmacologic agents for VF include lidocaine and amiodarone. The intravenous preparation of sotalol may be an option in countries where available. Bretylium use in children with VF is not well documented and it is no longer considered an appropriate agent.
4 Additional therapies such as mechanical circulatory support may be an option in selected cases.

The most generally accepted management strategies for acute therapy of perioperative rhythm disturbances without associated hemodynamic compromise are summarized in Table 17.4.

Pharmacologic therapy of cardiac arrhythmias

Antiarrhythmic drugs exert their effects primarily by blocking sodium, potassium, or calcium- channels, or by altering adrenergic tone. These pharmacologic agents are generally classified according to their presumed mechanism of action and electrophysiologic properties. The drug classification scheme described by Vaughan Williams in the 1960s (Table 17.5) and modified over the years is one frequently used. Although an oversimplification, this classification may be helpful in predicting response to therapy. Appropriate selection of a pharmacologic agent requires an understanding of the mechanism of the arrhythmia and the proposed effects of the drug. This section discusses antiarrhythmic drug therapy focusing on agents most frequently used for acute management in the pediatric age group (Table 17.6) [51]. It should be emphasized that perioperative consultation with a cardiologist should be considered during the care of patients with rhythm disturbances or in those receiving chronic antiarrhythmic therapy.

Class I agents

The largest group of antiarrhythmic drugs is the sodium-channel blockers. The relatively large size of this class has led to subclassification of these agents into IA, IB, and IC groups on the basis of their cellular actions. Group IC is for oral therapy only and is not discussed in this chapter.

Class IA agents

The class IA drugs include procainamide, quinidine, and disopyramide. The predominant electrophysiologic effects of these agents are prolongation of myocardial repolarization (QT interval) and duration of the action potential. Their mechanism of action is primarily related to inhibition of the fast sodium channels. The anticholinergic (vagolytic) properties of these drugs account for their more pronounced effects at fast heart rates.

Procainamide

Procainamide is a potent sodium-channel blocker, and to a lesser extent, a potassium-channel blocker. This agent slows atrial conduction (prolongs PR interval) and lengthens the QRS duration and QT interval. Procainamide is useful in the management of both atrial and ventricular arrhythmias [23,30,52,53]. The suppression of abnormal automaticity accounts for the role of this agent in the treatment of EAT, JET, and VT. This drug is generally more effective than lidocaine in acutely terminating sustained VT.

Procainamide may be administered via the oral, intravenous, or intramuscular routes. For the treatment of acute arrhythmias, intravenous loading (doses of 10–15 mg/kg) is usually required. This is administered over a period of 30–45 minutes. The lower end of the loading dose spectrum is recommended for younger patients. Continuous ECG monitoring and frequent blood pressure assessments are recommended during the loading phase. The drug is

Table 17.5 Classification of antiarrythmic agents

Class and action	Drugs
Class I: sodium-channel blockers. Drugs may be subclassified into IA, IB, and IC categories. **IA agents:** moderately depress phase zero upstroke of the action potential, slow conduction and prolong repolarization. Effectively slow conduction in atria, ventricles, and accessory connections.	Procainamide Quinidine Disopyramide
IB agents: shorten action potential duration and result in minimal alteration of conduction. These agents are usually not effective in the treatment of supraventricular tachycardia.	Lidocaine Mexiletine Phenytoin
IC agents: significantly depress phase zero upstroke, with marked slowing of conduction but impart little change in refractoriness.	Flecainide Propafenone
Class II: beta-adrenergic receptor blockers. Antiarrhythmic effects result from conduction and decreasing automaticity, particularly in the sinoatrial and atrioventricular nodes.	Esmolol Atenolol Metoprolol Propranolol
Class III: potassium-channel blockers. Primarily prolong action potential duration with resultant prolongation of refractoriness.	Amiodarone Sotalol Bretylium Ibutilide
Class IV: calcium-channel blockers with predominant sites of action in the sinoatrial and atrioventricular nodes.	Verapamil Diltiazem
Others	Atropine Digoxin Adenosine Magnesium sulfate

rapidly distributed following intravenous injection. An infusion is frequently initiated at 30–50 μg/kg/min. Monitoring of plasma levels is advisable during maintenance infusion. The infusion rate is adjusted accordingly to maintain therapeutic levels between 4 and 8 μg/mL. The drug is eliminated by the kidneys (50–60%) and via hepatic metabolism (10–30%). Hepatic acetylation accounts for the generation of *N*-acetylprocainamide (NAPA), a metabolite with antiarrhythmic (class III) properties.

Potential side effects include hypotension due to blocking of alpha-adrenergic receptors and decreased peripheral vascular resistance during rapid intravenous administration. Significant QT prolongation and proarrhythmia is also well described. Additional nontherapeutic effects include negative inotropy and AV block. Gastrointestinal symptoms, a lupus-like syndrome and blood dyscrasias may also occur.

Class IB agents

Class IB drugs include lidocaine, mexiletine, phenytoin, and tocainide. These inhibit fast sodium channels and shorten the action potential duration and refractory period.

Lidocaine

Lidocaine is a short-acting antiarrhythmic agent with primary effects on ventricular myocardium. It shortens action potential duration and refractory period. Lidocaine is one of the antiarrhythmic drugs more commonly employed in operating rooms and intensive care environments. It is proven to be effective for suppression of frequent ventricular ectopy, warning arrhythmias, and for prevention of recurrence of VT/VF [54–57].

Table 17.6 Intravenous antiarrhythmic agents

Agent	Dosing
Adenosine	100 μg/kg rapid bolus, increase by 50 μg/kg every 2 min, up to 300 μg/kg maximum
Amiodarone	*Load*: 5 mg/kg over 30–60 min *Infusion*: 5–10 μg/kg/min
Digoxin	*Load*: 20–30 μg/kg (divide as $\frac{1}{2}$ dose, $\frac{1}{4}$ dose, $\frac{1}{3}$ dose every 8 h), dose is age dependent *Maintenance*: 7–10 μg/kg/day divided every 12 h orally
Diltiazem	*Load*: 0.25 mg/kg up to 20 mg bolus over 2 min *Infusion*: 0.1–0.3 mg/kg/h, may increase up to 15 mg/h
Esmolol	*Load*: 500 μg/kg over 1–2 min *Infusion*: 50 μg/kg/min starting dose, may increase gradually to 400 μg/kg/min
Flecainide	1–2 mg/kg over 5–10 min (not available in the USA)
Magnesium sulfate	25–50 mg/kg (up to 2 g) over 20–30 min
Lidocaine	*Load*: 1 mg/kg every 5 min up to three times *Infusion*: 20–50 μg/kg/min
Phenytoin	1–3 mg/kg over 10–15 min
Procainamide	*Load*: 10–15 mg/kg over 30–45 min *Infusion*: 40–50 μg/kg/min
Propafenone	*Load*: 1 mg/kg over 10 min (not available in the USA) *Infusion*: 4–7 μg/kg/min
Propanolol	0.05–0.15 mg/kg over 5 min
Sotalol	*Load*: 0.2–1.5 mg/kg (not available in the USA)
Verapamil	0.05–0.30 mg/kg over 3–5 min, maximum 10 mg, not under 12 mo of age

The recommended dosage includes an initial bolus of 1 mg/kg intravenously, and if ineffective, may be repeated after several minutes. The maintenance infusion rate ranges between 20 and 50 μg/kg/min. Lidocaine is rapidly metabolized in the liver by microsomal enzymes. Therefore, drugs associated with altered microsomal enzyme activity or conditions with potential reductions in hepatic blood flow (i.e., severe congestive heart failure) may result in decreased drug metabolism. Monitoring of drug levels is advisable during continuous infusion.

Lidocaine toxicity from excessive plasma concentrations may result from poor cardiac output or hepatic or renal failure. Elevated plasma levels beyond the therapeutic range may cause gastrointestinal symptoms (nausea and vomiting), central nervous system pathology (paresthesias, tremor, confusion, seizures), and in rare instances hemodynamic perturbations.

Class II agents

The class II drugs (esmolol, atenolol, metoprolol, and propranolol) block beta-adrenergic receptors to variable extents (receptor selectivity and intrinsic sympathomimetic activity) depending on the specific agent. Antiarrhythmic effects result from slowing conduction and decreasing automaticity, particularly in the sinoatrial and AV nodes. These agents universally decrease sympathetic activity thorough beta-receptor blockade.

Esmolol

Esmolol is a predominant beta-1-selective (cardioselective) adrenergic receptor-blocking agent with a rapid onset and very short duration of action. The primary electrophysiologic drug property is inhibition of sinoatrial and AV conduction. The brief elimination half-life of this drug after intravenous injection (approximately 9 minutes) is a feature that has made it desirable in the perioperative and intensive care settings. Esmolol is commonly used for heart rate and blood pressure control and management of a wide number of tachyarrhythmias (supraventricular and ventricular) [58,59].

An intravenous loading dose of 100–500 μg/kg (over 1–2 minutes) can be administered. This is followed by a continuous infusion starting at 50–100 μg/kg/min and titrated to effect. Because of its short half-life, blood levels of esmolol can be rapidly altered by increasing or decreasing the infusion rate and rapidly eliminated by discontinuing the infusion.

Most adverse effects related to esmolol therapy have been mild and transient. Reported cardiovascular side effects include bradycardia, sinus pauses, AV block, hypotension, and negative inotropy. These are more likely to be seen during bolus therapy.

Class III agents

The class III drugs (amiodarone, sotalol, bretylium, ibutilide) block potassium channels and increase action potential duration and refractoriness in atrial and ventricular muscle and in Purkinje fibers.

Amiodarone

Amiodarone has a wide spectrum of actions with multiple and complex electrophysiologic effects that encompass all four antiarrhythmic drug classes. Class I actions include inhibition of fast sodium channels. Class II and IV effects result in depression of sinus node automaticity and function, and slowing of AV and His–Purkinje system conduction. As a class III agent, amiodarone delays repolarization and increases action potential duration resulting in prolongation of refractoriness in all cardiac tissues and accessory connections if present. In addition to blocking potassium channels, amiodarone exhibits vagolytic properties, weakly blocks calcium channels and noncompetitively blocks alpha- and beta-adrenergic receptors. The efficacy of this agent has been documented against many supraventricular (EAT, atrial flutter and fibrillation, reentrant arrhythmias involving accessory pathways, JET) and ventricular arrhythmias (VT and VF) [29,60–62]. The usefulness of this drug in the treatment of life-threatening tachyarrhythmias accounts for its increasing role in emergency cardiovascular management.

Intravenous therapy requires a loading dose because of its rapid plasma disappearance during the distribution phase. In children the suggested dose is 5 mg/kg over 1 hour. The same dose is then infused over 12 hours, and repeated if necessary. Amiodarone binds extensively to most tissues, accounting for its extremely prolonged elimination. The slow elimination rate of amiodarone leads to an unusually long half-life (25–110 days).

Amiodarone administration may result in sinus bradycardia and AV block. Hypotension is another potential complication of intravenous therapy, likely due to calcium chelation. Electrocardiographic effects include PR, QRS, and QTc prolongation. There are significant drug interactions with amiodarone that merit attention. Coadministration with other antiarrhythmic agents (digoxin, procainamide, flecainide, quinidine, phenytoin) may result in increased levels of these drugs. The concomitant use of amiodarone with beta-blockers or calcium-channel antagonists should raise concerns of potential synergistic effects on conduction tissue. A number of adverse effects have been reported with long-term oral therapy in children. These include skin discoloration, corneal microdeposits, alterations in hepatic and thyroid function, pulmonary fibrosis, and neurologic disturbances.

Bretylium

Clinical experience with bretylium is limited in the pediatric age group [55,63]. Indications in the past included VT or VF unresponsive to standard therapy. Bretylium is no longer listed in the American Heart Association guidelines for pediatric resuscitation because of the risk of hypotension, the lack of demonstrable effectiveness in VT, and the absence of published studies of its use in children [64].

Ibutilide

Ibutilide is an intravenous class III agent approved in the adult population for the acute conversion of atrial flutter and fibrillation of recent onset (<90 days) to sinus rhythm [65–67]. Like other drugs that prolong ventricular repolarization, this agent may be associated with excessive QT prolongation and polymorphic VT requiring careful patient selection and monitoring during drug administration. The clinical experience with ibutilide in the pediatric age group is extremely limited [68].

Class IV agents

The class IV drugs, also known as calcium-channel blockers (verapamil, diltiazem, nifedipine), inhibit the slow inward calcium current.

Verapamil

The actions of this drug are mediated through prolongation of conduction time and refractory period in nodal tissue. Verapamil has been shown to be efficacious in the management of SVT and certain types of VT [69–71].

Verapamil should not be used in young children (<1 year of age) in view of the potential for severe hemodynamic compromise (refractory hypotension, myocardial depression, asystole and cardiovascular collapse) following its administration [72,73]. The detrimental effects are related to calcium-channel blockade and uncoupling of excitation–contraction in myocardial cells. In older children (>1 year of age), verapamil is infused in a dose of 0.1 mg/kg. The concomitant use of verapamil and beta-blocking agents may result in serious cardiovascular side effects and is therefore not recommended. In the setting of WPW syndrome, verapamil may enhance the ventricular response rate of atrial fibrillation leading to hemodynamic compromise.

Other agents

Atropine

Atropine sulfate, an antimuscarinic, parasympatholytic drug, accelerates sinus or atrial pacemakers and enhances AV conduction. Atropine is recommended in the treatment of symptomatic bradycardia caused by increased vagal activity or AV block, such as vagally mediated bradycardia during intubation. Atropine may be used to treat bradycardia accompanied by poor perfusion or hypotension; however, epinephrine may be a more effective therapy in this setting. Efforts to ensure adequate oxygenation and ventilation and exclude hypothermia should precede pharmacologic therapy of bradycardia.

The recommended dose is 0.02 mg/kg with a minimum single dose of 0.1 mg and a maximum single dose of 0.5 mg in a child, and 1.0 mg in an adolescent or young adult. The dose may be repeated in 5 minutes, to a maximum total dose of 1.0 mg in a child and 2.0 mg in an adolescent. In the absence of intravenous access, atropine (0.02 mg/kg) may be administered tracheally or intramuscularly, although with less reliable absorption than through the intravenous route. Small doses of atropine may be associated with transient heart rate slowing. Atropine may also rarely cause cardiac arrhythmias.

Digoxin

Digitalis glycosides have been used for many years as pharmacologic agents in the management of certain arrhythmias. The electrophysiologic properties of digoxin are the result of direct effects on cardiac tissues (through inhibition of the sarcolemmal sodium pump) and indirect effects via the autonomic (parasympathetic) nervous system. Digoxin is known to increase the refractory period and decrease the conduction velocity of the specialized cardiac conduction system, slow the sinus rate (primarily by enhancing vagal discharge), and shorten the refractory period in atrial and ventricular muscle.

Digoxin can be effective in the treatment of a wide spectrum of supraventricular arrhythmias such as SVT, atrial flutter, atrial fibrillation, and chaotic AT. In patients with WPW, digoxin is not recommended because it may alter the conduction properties of the accessory pathway and lead to malignant arrhythmias (VT and VF) during atrial flutter or fibrillation.

Digoxin can be administered orally or parenterally. In view of the fact that the onset of its effect may be delayed (up to 5 h), this drug is less than ideal in the treatment of acute symptomatic tachycardias. Despite this limitation, digitalis glycosides remain useful in controlling the ventricular response in atrial tachyarrhythmias, particularly during atrial flutter or fibrillation. A common loading algorithm utilizes a total digitalizing dose of 30–50 μg/kg. Half of this amount is given initially, followed by two doses at 6-hour intervals of 25% of the total dose. For intravenous use, the total digitalizing dose is reduced to 75% of the total oral dose given following a similar scheme. Maintenance doses of digoxin are 7–10 μg/kg/day. Digoxin is tightly bound to peripheral tissue proteins. Drug excretion is via the kidneys. Doses adjustments are indicated in cases of renal impairment or congestive heart failure.

The coadministration of digoxin with other antiarrhythmic agents (amiodarone, quinidine, verapamil) requires an adjustment (reduction) in the digoxin dose and monitoring of plasma levels. Toxic manifestations of digitalis therapy may be classified as cardiac and noncardiac. Digoxin toxicity can cause virtually any type of cardiac rhythm disturbance. Noncardiac manifestations of digitalis toxicity include gastrointestinal (nausea, vomiting, anorexia) and neurologic symptoms (headache, lethargy, weakness, confusion, seizures), and visual disturbances. Although nonspecific, noncardiac symptoms are the earliest manifestations of digitalis toxicity.

Adenosine

Adenosine is a purine agonist, with effects mediated via the activation of the A_1 adenosine receptor (leading to activation of adenylate cyclase and intracellular cyclic-AMP production). The electrophysiologic effects are secondary to an increase in potassium conductance and depression of the slow inward calcium current resulting in transient sinus slowing or AV nodal block. This accounts for its therapeutic value in terminating arrhythmias that involve the AV node. Adenosine is the drug of choice for acute treatment of SVT [43,44,64,74–76]. Adenosine can also provide aid in the diagnosis of atrial tachyarrhythmias and may also be useful in the differentiation of wide QRS tachycardias [76].

To terminate SVT, a bolus of adenosine is rapidly injected intravenously, preferably into a central vein, at initial doses of 100–150 μg/kg/min, followed by a rapid normal saline flush. The dose can be doubled up to a maximum of 300 μg/kg (or adult dose of 6–12 mg). The effects of the drug are seen within a period of 10–20 seconds. It is extremely useful to obtain an ECG recording during its administration as the response to adenosine may provide insight into the mechanism of the tachycardia. Adenosine is rapidly metabolized by erythrocytes and endothelial cells, accounting for its extremely short half-life (<10 s).

Cardiac side effects include sinus pauses, sinus bradycardia, AV block, and reflex sinus tachycardia. These effects are generally transient and may only require supportive care. However, some suggest availability of temporary pacing. Adenosine should be used with caution in patients following cardiac transplantation in view of increased duration of the electrophysiologic effect of this agent in the denervated heart. Other unwanted effects are transient and generally well tolerated. These include flushing, shortness of breath, bronchospasm, and chest pressure. On very rare occasions hypotension may occur.

Magnesium sulfate

Magnesium is a major intracellular cation, cofactor in multiple enzymatic reactions, and important regulator of numerous cardiovascular processes. Magnesium sulfate therapy is indicated as adjunct management for arrhythmias in patients with documented hypomagnesemia or torsade de pointes [59]. Magnesium deficiency is frequently seen in the context of other electrolyte abnormalities (hypokalemia and hypocalcemia). Rhythm disturbances associated with hypomagnesemia resemble those with hypokalemia or digitalis toxicity.

In the setting of torsade de pointes, intravenous infusion (over several minutes) of 25–50 mg/kg (up to 2 g) is recommended. Approximately 70% of plasma Mg^{2+} is ultrafiltered by the kidney and the remainder is bound to protein. Side effects associated with magnesium administration include flushing, diaphoresis, muscle weakness, and central nervous system depression. Magnesium levels well above the therapeutic range can lead to serious morbidity such as cardiac conduction defects, respiratory depression, and circulatory collapse.

Pacemaker therapy in children

Pacemaker nomenclature

Pacemaker nomenclature as established by the North American Society of Pacing and Electrophysiology and the British Pacing and Electrophysiology Group is detailed in Table 17.7 [77]. The generic pacemaker (NBG) code has five positions. The first position or letter of the code refers to the chamber(s) paced, the second to the chamber(s)

sensed, the third to the pacemaker's response to sensing, and the fourth to programmability and rate modulation. The fifth position is restricted to antitachycardia function and is used infrequently.

Permanent cardiac pacing

Advances in pacemaker technology, enhancements in programmability, and miniaturization of units have resulted in the increasing use of these devices in the pediatric age group [78]. The American Heart Association, American College of Cardiology, and Heart Rhythm Society recently updated their guidelines for permanent pacing in children and adolescents in 2008 [79]. Table 17.8 lists indications for which there is general agreement that the device should be implanted (Class I) and for which pacemakers are used frequently but diverging opinions exist regarding benefits (Class II).

In general terms, potential indications can be summarized as follows:
1 Symptomatic sinus bradycardia
2 Recurrent bradycardia–tachycardia syndromes
3 Congenital complete AV block
4 Advanced second- or third-degree AV block

An important consideration in the setting of CHD is correlation of symptoms with recommended criteria for pacemaker placement in view of the physiologic alterations associated with structural heart disease or following surgical intervention. The use of these devices in young patients and those with CHD presents unique challenges and considerations, some of which are highlighted in the following sections [80,81].

Implantation techniques

Permanent pacemaker implantation is accomplished via the transvenous or epicardial approach. These procedures are typically performed under sterile conditions in the cardiac catheterization laboratory, electrophysiology suite, or operating room. Local anesthesia with supplemental

Table 17.7 Generic pacemaker code

Position I, chamber(s) paced	Position II, chamber(s) sensed	Position III, response to sensing	Position IV, programmability, rate modulation	Position V, antitachyarrhythmic function(s)
O, none	O, none	O, none	O, none	O, none
A, atrium	A, atrium	I, inhibited	P, simple programmable	P, pacing
V, ventricle	V, ventricle	T, triggered	M, multiprogramable	S, shock
D, dual (A + V)	D, dual (A + V)	D, dual (I + T)	C, communicating	D, dual (P + S)
			R, rate modulation	

Source: Reproduced with permission from Reference [77].

Table 17.8 Recommendations for permanent pacing in children, adolescents, and patients with congenital heart disease

---

Class I (Benefit >>> Risk)

Advanced second- or third-degree AV block associated with symptomatic bradycardia, ventricular dysfunction, or low cardiac output.

Sinus node dysfunction with correlation of symptoms during age-inappropriate bradycardia. The definition of bradycardia varies with the patient's age and expected heart rate.

Postoperative advanced second- or third-degree AV block that is not expected to resolve or persists at least 7 days after cardiac surgery.

Congenital third-degree AV block with a wide QRS escape rhythm, complex ventricular ectopy, or ventricular dysfunction.

Congenital third-degree AV block in the infant with a ventricular rate <55 bpm or with congenital heart disease and a ventricular rate <70 bpm.

Class IIa (Benefit >> Risk)

Patients with CHD and sinus bradycardia for the prevention of recurrent episodes of IART; sinus node dysfunction may be intrinsic or secondary to antiarrhythmic therapy.

Congenital third-degree AV block beyond the first year of life with an average heart rate <50 bpm, abrupt pauses in ventricular rate that are two or three times the basic cycle length, or associated with symptoms due to chronotropic incompetence.

Sinus bradycardia with complex CHD with a resting heart rate <40 bpm or pauses in ventricular rate >3 s.

Patients with CHD and impaired hemodynamics due to sinus bradycardia or loss of AV synchrony.

Unexplained syncope in patient with prior congenital heart surgery complicated by transient complete heart block with residual fascicular block after careful evaluation to exclude other causes of syncope.

Class IIb (Benefit ≥ Risk)

Transient postoperative third-degree AV block that reverts to sinus rhythm with residual bifascicular block.

Congenital third-degree AV block in the asymptomatic children or adolescents with an acceptable rate, narrow QRS complex, and normal ventricular function.

Asymptomatic sinus bradycardia after biventricular repair of CHD with a resting heart rate <40 bpm or pauses in ventricular rate >3s.

Source: Reproduced with permission from Reference [79].

intravenous sedation may be used in the older age group; however, most infants and small children require a general anesthetic.

The transvenous technique uses the subclavian, cephalic, and axillary vein for access [82]. Under fluoroscopic guidance, pacing leads are advanced into the right atrium and/or ventricle and fixed to the endocardium. After adequate sensing, capture thresholds, and lead impedances are documented, the leads are attached to a generator typically positioned in the pectoral region. The following are considered contraindications to transvenous pacing: intracardiac communication with the potential for right-to-left shunting, prosthetic tricuspid valve, anatomy not suitable for transvenous access to cardiac chambers, and small patient size (<10 kg). Advantages of the transvenous route include longer generator longevity because of lower pacing thresholds and lower incidences of lead fractures [83]. Disadvantages are potential narrowing or thrombosis of venous pathways, lead dislocation, risk of systemic embolization in the presence of an intracardiac shunt, and possible endocarditis.

For epicardial implantation, the leads are attached to the epimyocardial surface of the heart and after appropriate testing, these are tunneled to the generator pocket [84]. This approach requires a subcostal, subxiphoid, thoracotomy, or sternotomy incision. Advantages of epicardial implantation include ability for placement independent of intracardiac pathology and avoidance of considerations regarding venous thrombosis. Disadvantages include the invasiveness of the approach, higher incidence of lead failure, and early generator battery depletion.

Hardware selection and programming of devices

A variety of hardware options are available for cardiac pacing in infants and children. The selection of the particular generator system, mode for pacing, and pacing leads are dependent on a number of factors. In general terms, considerations include patient size, indications for pacing, requirement for specific programmability options, underlying cardiac pathology, and anticipated need for generator longevity.

Both single- and dual-chamber units are commercially available for permanent pacing in the pediatric age group. Dual-chamber devices provide the benefit of AV synchrony. Biventricular pacing systems have also been utilized in children to a limited degree [85]. These devices provide for optimization of hemodynamics in the presence of heart failure. Primary indications have included ventricular dyssynchrony related to a variety of cardiac diagnoses [86,87].

Under specific circumstances such as during surgical interventions, it may be necessary to reprogram a pacemaker to an asynchronous (nonsensing) mode (AOO, VOO, or DOO) in order to prevent erratic pacemaker behavior. If active, the rate-responsiveness feature of the unit should also be disabled prior to anesthetic induction.

Pacemaker malfunction

Problems most frequently accounting for pacemaker malfunction include complications related to lead placement and integrity, failure to pace, failure to capture, under- or oversensing, phrenic nerve stimulation, and pacemaker-mediated tachycardia [88]. Pacemaker troubleshooting may require a combination of chest radiograph, 12-lead ECG, rhythm strip, and device interrogation to determine pacing and sensing thresholds, lead impedances, battery status, and magnet rate.

Children are considered to be at higher risk for lead failure and fracture than their adult counterparts. These problems result in inappropriate pacemaker sensing or capture (under- or overpacing) and potential need for pacemaker revision. Adjustments in pacemaker settings may temporarily remedy these potential issues.

Perioperative considerations

The preoperative assessment of the patient with a pacemaker should include a complete history, emphasizing indications for initial pacemaker implantation, coexistent cardiovascular pathology (structural or acquired), functional status of the patient, and the presence of symptomatology. In addition, a focused physical examination should be performed that includes planned or existent pocket generator location. Preoperative testing should be performed as indicated, including a chest radiograph that allows for identification of the number, position, and integrity of the pacing leads. In some cases, when the pacemaker details are not available, a chest radiograph may display a code that can be used to identify the unit's manufacturer/model.

Device interrogation should be part of a complete preoperative evaluation in all patients with implanted pacemakers scheduled for surgical interventions (cardiac or noncardiac) [89–91]. Consultation with a pediatric cardiologist/electrophysiologist to obtain details of unit type, settings, date of and indications for implantation, and underlying rhythm is highly recommended. The patient's pacemaker card, if available, may also provide relevant information. Results of a recent 12-lead ECG should also be reviewed. Reprogramming may be required prior to the planned procedure to avoid potential problems with pacemaker malfunction related to electromagnetic interference (electrocautery). The rate-responsive mode, if turned on, should be deactivated as well as antitachycardia modes.

Regarding intraoperative management, it should be considered that unipolar electrocautery may interfere with pacemaker function, thus bipolar electrocautery is preferred. In addition to routine perioperative monitoring that includes electrocardiography and pulse oximetry, other modalities that confirm pulse generation during pacing such as manual pulse palpation, auscultation (via precordial or esophageal stethoscope), and/or invasive arterial blood pressure monitoring should be considered. Chronotropic agents and alternate pacing modalities (transcutaneous, transvenous transesophageal, epicardial) should be readily available as appropriate in the event of pacemaker malfunction and inadequate underlying heart rate. If defibrillation is required, the current should not be applied to or passed directly through the pulse generator as this may damage the device circuitry.

A magnet should be accessible to allow for transient asynchronous pacing if required. Most generators respond to magnet application by pacing at a fixed rate asynchronously (AOO, VOO, or DOO). It should be emphasized, however, that the nature of the asynchronous programmed stimuli for magnet mode varies among pacemaker units. Furthermore, at generator end of life, the pacing rate upon magnet application may differ (slower) than the prespecified magnet rate. In some cases, the application of a magnet over a programmable pacemaker during electromagnetic interference (i.e., cautery) may result in generator reprogramming [92]. Therefore, it is emphasized that the use of a magnet should not be considered a substitute for preoperative pacemaker interrogation/programming, nor should it be used routinely over a pacemaker generator during surgery or to offset potential electromagnetic interference. After completion of the procedure, the device should be retested and programmed to baseline settings as appropriate.

Temporary cardiac pacing

The transvenous and epicardial routes are commonly used for temporary pacing, although the transthoracic (transcutaneous) and transesophageal approaches are also suitable in some circumstances. Indications for temporary cardiac pacing are not as clearly defined as in the case of permanent pacing [93]. However, temporary pacing is utilized as an option during some cardiothoracic procedures by placement of pacing wires in the atrial and/or ventricular epimyocardium near the completion of the intervention. Basic programmable settings in the external temporary pulse generator (single or dual chamber device) include (1) pacing rate, (2) atrial and/or ventricular output amplitude (mA), (3) atrial and/or ventricular sensitivity (mV) or asynchronous mode, and (4) A–V interval (ms).

Temporary pacing may be necessary for maintenance of adequate cardiac output in the context of bradyarrhythmias, abnormal AV conduction, AV asynchrony, and heart rates inadequate for physiologic state [94]. Temporary pacing may also be helpful in individuals at risk of high degree AV block and can be used to suppress, overdrive, or terminate tachyarrhythmias. As mentioned earlier in this chapter, atrial recordings obtained through temporary pacing wires may also provide diagnostic information in certain types of rhythm disorders. In the care of patients who depend on temporary pacing for maintenance of adequate hemodynamics, it is extremely important to be attentive to pacemaker settings and capture thresholds, which should be interrogated on a daily basis [95]. Alternate means of pacing should be available in the event of lead/pacemaker failure or malfunction. Temporary pacing can be discontinued with resolution of the indication for pacing or transition to a permanent pacing system must be considered.

External transcutaneous pacing

In the early 1980s, a transcutaneous external pacing unit with features superior to earlier systems was patented and introduced by Dr Paul Zoll. This led to renewed interest in the field and further enhancements of the technology. Most devices currently available for commercial use combine defibrillation/cardioversion capabilities and external pacing features. In pediatric patients, emergency transthoracic pacing may be considered as a temporizing measure in those with symptomatic bradycardia (secondary to abnormal sinus node function or to complete AV block) [96]. It is important to understand that transcutaneous pacing results in simultaneous atrial and ventricular activation, thus optimal hemodynamics may not be feasible. This pacing approach has not been found to be effective in the treatment of asystole in children.

The pacing electrodes should be selected according to size of the patient size (patients under 15 kg require smaller adhesive pads). Device settings typically include heart rate and current output (mA). Most current models provide the option for fixed rate (asynchronous) and demand (synchronous) pacing. After selection of a desired heart rate and pacing modality, the current is increased as tolerated until capture is achieved. If the patient is not anesthetized, sedation may be necessary to improve tolerance to pacing. Prolonged periods of transcutaneous pacing may result in serious burns or skin trauma in infants and young children. In addition to monitoring for pace-

maker capture by an ECG, ongoing clinical assessment of the adequacy of cardiac output should be undertaken.

Esophageal overdrive pacing

An esophageal catheter may be used for atrial sensing allowing for diagnostic information and discrimination of supraventricular tachyarrhythmias. The esophageal route also allows for overdrive pacing of a variety of supraventricular rhythm disorders (atrial flutter, SVT). For this purpose, an electrode catheter is placed into the esophagus, advanced to a location that corresponds roughly to the region behind the atrial mass, and an atrial electrogram is obtained to refine the catheter position. Local anesthesia to the nasopharynx or oropharynx and/or sedation is generally required in order to introduce the catheter and to prevent discomfort during atrial pacing. Standard cardiorespiratory monitoring should be undertaken during the procedure, in addition to airway support as necessary. Emergency drugs and cardioversion/defibrillation equipment should be readily available.

Implantable cardioverter-defibrillators

The primary goal of the internal cardioverter-defibrillator (ICD) is the reduction of sudden death in patients at high risk. Although sudden cardiac death is an uncommon occurrence in pediatrics, certain patient groups may have a definitive risk, deriving potential benefits from these devices. Individuals with arrhythmogenic right ventricular cardiomyopathy, long QT syndrome, Brugada syndrome, hypertrophic cardiomyopathy, and those with a history of near sudden death events may be considered suitable candidates for ICD implantation [97,98]. Additional patients are those with operated CHD and a history of malignant arrhythmias. At the present, experience in the pediatric age group with these devices has been limited and reported mostly in retrospective fashion [99–102]. Prospective trials are required to establish guidelines for use, address safety concerns, and evaluate long-term issues specific to children.

Anesthetic considerations in patients with ICDs relate primarily to potential surgical electromagnetic interference (electrocautery) and the need for an available external cardioverting/defibrillating device. Perioperative consultation with a cardiologist/electrophysiologist is therefore essential in the care of these patients. In many cases, the devices may need to be adjusted or deactivated prior to surgery. In most, but not all devices, application of a magnet temporarily deactivates therapies; however, this is not a substitute to reprogramming and should only be considered in emergencies. Careful evaluation and device programming is advisable at the conclusion of the surgical intervention to ensure patient safety.

References

1. Wu MH, Wang JK, Lin JL, et al. (2001) Cardiac rhythm disturbances in patients with left atrial isomerism. Pacing Clin Electrophysiol 24:1631–1638.
2. Fryda RJ, Kaplan S, Helmsworth JA (1971) Postoperative complete heart block in children. Br Heart J 33:456–462.
3. Weindling SN, Saul JP, Gamble WJ, et al. (1998) Duration of complete atrioventricular block after congenital heart disease surgery. Am J Cardiol 82:525–527.
4. Bruckheimer E, Berul CI, Kopf GS, et al. (2002) Late recovery of surgically-induced atrioventricular block in patients with congenital heart disease. J Interv Card Electrophysiol 6:191–195.
5. Bennie RE, Dierdorf SF, Hubbard JE (1997) Perioperative management of children with third degree heart block undergoing pacemaker placement: a ten year review. Paediatr Anaesth 7:301–304.
6. Ko JK, Deal BJ, Strasburger JF, et al. (1992) Supraventricular tachycardia mechanisms and their age distribution in pediatric patients. Am J Cardiol 69:1028–1032.
7. Koike K, Hesslein PS, Finlay CD, et al. (1988) Atrial automatic tachycardia in children. Am J Cardiol 61:1127–1130.
8. Naheed ZJ, Strasburger JF, Benson DW, Jr, et al. (1995) Natural history and management strategies of automatic atrial tachycardia in children. Am J Cardiol 75:405–407.
9. Rosales AM, Walsh EP, Wessel DL, et al. (2001) Postoperative ectopic atrial tachycardia in children with congenital heart disease. Am J Cardiol 88:1169–1172.
10. Mehta AV, Sanchez GR, Sacks EJ, et al. (1988) Ectopic automatic atrial tachycardia in children: clinical characteristics, management and follow-up. J Am Coll Cardiol 11:379–385.
11. Case CL, Gillette PC (1993) Automatic atrial and junctional tachycardias in the pediatric patient: strategies for diagnosis and management. Pacing Clin Electrophysiol 16:1323–1335.
12. Dhala AA, Case CL, Gillette PC (1994) Evolving treatment strategies for managing atrial ectopic tachycardia in children. Am J Cardiol 74:283–286.
13. Bradley DJ, Fischbach PS, Law IH, et al. (2001) The clinical course of multifocal atrial tachycardia in infants and children. J Am Coll Cardiol 38:401–408.
14. Liberthson RR, Colan SD (1982) Multifocal or chaotic atrial rhythm: report of nine infants, delineation of clinical course and management, and review of the literature. Pediatr Cardiol 2:179–184.
15. Salim MA, Case CL, Gillette PC (1995) Chaotic atrial tachycardia in children. Am Heart J 129:831–833.
16. Dodo H, Gow RM, Hamilton RM, et al. (1995) Chaotic atrial rhythm in children. Am Heart J 129:990–995.
17. Garson AJ, Gillette PC (1979) Junctional ectopic tachycardia in children: electrocardiography, electrophysiology and pharmacologic response. Am J Cardiol 44:298–302.
18. Saul JP, Scott WA, Brown S, et al. (2005) Intravenous amiodarone for incessant tachyarrhythmias in children: a randomized, double-blind, antiarrhythmic drug trial. Circulation 112:3470–3477.
19. Grant JW, Serwer GA, Armstrong BE, et al. (1987) Junctional tachycardia in infants and children after open heart surgery for congenital heart disease. Am J Cardiol 59:1216–1218.
20. Gillette PC (1989) Diagnosis and management of postoperative junctional ectopic tachycardia. Am Heart J 118:192–194.
21. Azzam FJ, Fiore AC (1998) Postoperative junctional ectopic tachycardia. Can J Anaesth 45:898–902.
22. Dodge-Khatami A, Miller OI, Anderson RH, et al. (2002) Surgical substrates of postoperative junctional ectopic tachycardia in congenital heart defects. J Thorac Cardiovasc Surg 123:624–630.
23. Walsh EP, Saul JP, Sholler GF, et al. (1997) Evaluation of a staged treatment protocol for rapid automatic junctional tachycardia after operation for congenital heart disease. J Am Coll Cardiol 29:1046–1053.
24. Laird WP, Snyder CS, Kertesz NJ, et al. (2003) Use of intravenous amiodarone for postoperative junctional ectopic tachycardia in children. Pediatr Cardiol 24:133–137.
25. Bash SE, Shah JJ, Albers WH, et al. (1987) Hypothermia for the treatment of postsurgical greatly accelerated junctional ectopic tachycardia. J Am Coll Cardiol 10:1095–1099.
26. Balaji S, Sullivan I, Deanfield J, et al. (1991) Moderate hypothermia in the management of resistant automatic tachycardias in children. Br Heart J 66:221–224.
27. Pfammatter JP, Paul T, Ziemer G, et al. (1995) Successful management of junctional tachycardia by hypothermia after cardiac operations in infants. Ann Thorac Surg 60:556–560.
28. Raja P, Hawker RE, Chaikitpinyo A, et al. (1994) Amiodarone management of junctional ectopic tachycardia after cardiac surgery in children. Br Heart J 72:261–265.
29. Perry JC, Fenrich AL, Hulse JE, et al. (1996) Pediatric use of intravenous amiodarone: efficacy and safety in critically ill patients from a multicenter protocol. J Am Coll Cardiol 27:1246–1250.
30. Mandapati R, Byrum CJ, Kavey RE, et al. (2000) Procainamide for rate control of postsurgical junctional tachycardia. Pediatr Cardiol 21:123–128.
31. Garson AJ, Moak JP, Smith RTJ, et al. (1987) Usefulness of intravenous propafenone for control of postoperative junctional ectopic tachycardia. Am J Cardiol 59:1422–1424.
32. Wren C, Campbell RW (1987) The response of paediatric arrhythmias to intravenous and oral flecainide. Br Heart J 57:171–175.
33. Paul T, Reimer A, Janousek J, et al. (1992) Efficacy and safety of propafenone in congenital junctional ectopic tachycardia. J Am Coll Cardiol 20:911–914.
34. Gillette PC, Garson A, Jr, Porter CJ, et al. (1983) Junctional automatic ectopic tachycardia: new proposed treatment by transcatheter His bundle ablation. Am Heart J 106:619–623.
35. Braunstein PW, Jr, Sade RM, Gillette PC (1992) Life-threatening postoperative junctional ectopic tachycardia. Ann Thorac Surg 53:726–728.
36. Van Hare GF (2001) Intra-atrial reentry tachycardia in pediatric patients. Prog Pediatr Cardiol 13:41–52.
37. Garson AJ, Bink-Boelkens M, Hesslein PS, et al. (1985) Atrial flutter in the young: a collaborative study of 380 cases. J Am Coll Cardiol 6:871–878.

38. Rhodes LA, Walsh EP, Saul JP (1995) Conversion of atrial flutter in pediatric patients by transesophageal atrial pacing: a safe, effective, minimally invasive procedure. Am Heart J 130:323–327.

39. Klein AL, Grimm RA, Murray RD, et al. (2001) Use of transesophageal echocardiography to guide cardioversion in patients with atrial fibrillation. N Engl J Med 344:1411–1420.

40. Seidl K, Rameken M, Drogemuller A, et al. (2002) Embolic events in patients with atrial fibrillation and effective anticoagulation: value of transesophageal echocardiography to guide direct-current cardioversion. Final results of the Ludwigshafen Observational Cardioversion Study. J Am Coll Cardiol 39:1436–1442.

41. Smith WM, Gallagher JJ, Kerr CR, et al. (1982) The electrophysiologic basis and management of symptomatic recurrent tachycardia in patients with Ebstein's anomaly of the tricuspid valve. Am J Cardiol 49:1223–1234.

42. Muller G, Deal BJ, Benson DW, Jr (1994) "Vagal maneuvers" and adenosine for termination of atrioventricular reentrant tachycardia. Am J Cardiol 74:500–503.

43. Stemp LI, Roy WL (1992) Adenosine for the cardioversion of supraventricular tachycardia during general anesthesia and open heart surgery. Anesthesiology 76:849–852.

44. Paul T, Pfammatter JP (1997) Adenosine: an effective and safe antiarrhythmic drug in pediatrics. Pediatr Cardiol 18:118–126.

45. Wilbur SL, Marchlinski FE (1997) Adenosine as an antiarrhythmic agent. Am J Cardiol 79:30–37.

46. Schwartz PJ, Moss AJ, Vincent GM, et al. (1993) Diagnostic criteria for the long QT syndrome. An update. Circulation 88:782–784.

47. Brugada P, Brugada J (1992) Right bundle branch block, persistent ST segment elevation and sudden cardiac death: a distinct clinical and electrocardiographic syndrome. A multicenter report. J Am Coll Cardiol 20:1391–1396.

48. Wilde AA, Antzelevitch C, Borggrefe M, et al. (2002) Proposed diagnostic criteria for the Brugada syndrome: consensus report. Circulation 106:2514–2519.

49. Chen PS, Priori SG (2008) The Brugada syndrome. J Am Coll Cardiol 51:1176–1180.

50. Probst V, Denjoy I, Meregalli PG, et al. (2007) Clinical aspects and prognosis of Brugada syndrome in children. Circulation 115:2042–2048.

51. Bink-Boelkens MT (2000) Pharmacologic management of arrhythmias. Pediatr Cardiol 21:508–515.

52. Luedtke SA, Kuhn RJ, McCaffrey FM (1997) Pharmacologic management of supraventricular tachycardias in children. Part 1: Wolff-Parkinson-White and atrioventricular nodal reentry. Ann Pharmacother 31:1227–1243.

53. Luedtke SA, Kuhn RJ, McCaffrey FM (1997) Pharmacologic management of supraventricular tachycardias in children. Part 2: Atrial flutter, atrial fibrillation, and junctional and atrial ectopic tachycardia. Ann Pharmacother 31:1347–1359.

54. Nolan PE, Jr (1997) Pharmacokinetics and pharmacodynamics of intravenous agents for ventricular arrhythmias. Pharmacotherapy 17:65S–75S, discussion 89S–91S.

55. Ushay HM, Notterman DA (1997) Pharmacology of pediatric resuscitation. Pediatr Clin North Am 44:207–233.

56. Kudenchuk PJ (1999) Intravenous antiarrhythmic drug therapy in the resuscitation from refractory ventricular arrhythmias. Am J Cardiol 84:52R–55R.

57. Kudenchuk PJ (2002) Advanced cardiac life support antiarrhythmic drugs. Cardiol Clin 20:79–87.

58. Group TER (1986) Intravenous esmolol for the treatment of supraventricular tachyarrhythmia: results of a multicenter, baseline-controlled safety and efficacy study in 160 patients. Am Heart J 112:498–505.

59. Trippel DL, Wiest DB, Gillette PC (1991) Cardiovascular and antiarrhythmic effects of esmolol in children. J Pediatr 119:142–147.

60. Garson AJ, Gillette PC, McVey P, et al. (1984) Amiodarone treatment of critical arrhythmias in children and young adults. J Am Coll Cardiol 4:749–755.

61. Perry JC, Knilans TK, Marlow D, et al. (1993) Intravenous amiodarone for life-threatening tachyarrhythmias in children and young adults. J Am Coll Cardiol 22:95–98.

62. Figa FH, Gow RM, Hamilton RM, et al. (1994) Clinical efficacy and safety of intravenous Amiodarone in infants and children. Am J Cardiol 74:573–577.

63. Mongkolsmai C, Dove JT, Kyrouac JT (1984) Bretylium tosylate for ventricular fibrillation in a child. Clin Pediatr (Phila) 23:696–698.

64. American Heart Association (2006) 2005 American Heart Association (AHA) guidelines for cardiopulmonary resuscitation (CPR) and emergency cardiovascular care (ECC) of pediatric and neonatal patients: pediatric basic life support. Pediatrics 117:e989–e1004.

65. Ellenbogen KA, Clemo HF, Stambler BS, et al. (1996) Efficacy of ibutilide for termination of atrial fibrillation and flutter. Am J Cardiol 78:42–45.

66. Ellenbogen KA, Stambler BS, Wood MA, et al. (1996) Efficacy of intravenous ibutilide for rapid termination of atrial fibrillation and atrial flutter: a dose-response study. J Am Coll Cardiol 28:130–136.

67. Howard PA (1999) Ibutilide: an antiarrhythmic agent for the treatment of atrial fibrillation or flutter. Ann Pharmacother 33:38–47.

68. Hoyer AW, Balaji S (2007) The safety and efficacy of ibutilide in children and in patients with congenital heart disease. Pacing Clin Electrophysiol 30:1003–1008.

69. Bolens M, Friedli B, Deom A (1987) Electrophysiologic effects of intravenous verapamil in children after operations for congenital heart disease. Am J Cardiol 60:692–696.

70. Porter CJ, Gillette PC, Garson A, Jr, et al. (1981) Effects of verapamil on supraventricular tachycardia in children. Am J Cardiol 48:487–491.

71. Porter CJ, Garson A, Jr., Gillette PC (1983) Verapamil: an effective calcium blocking agent for pediatric patients. Pediatrics 71:748–755.

72. Epstein ML, Kiel EA, Victorica BE (1985) Cardiac decompensation following verapamil therapy in infants with supraventricular tachycardia. Pediatrics 75:737–740.

73. Garland JS, Berens RJ, Losek JD, et al. (1985) An infant fatality following verapamil therapy for supraventricular tachycardia: cardiovascular collapse following intravenous verapamil. Pediatr Emerg Care 1:198–200.

74. Till J, Shinebourne EA, Rigby ML, et al. (1989) Efficacy and safety of adenosine in the treatment of supraventricular tachycardia in infants and children. Br Heart J 62:204–211.

75. Rossi AF, Steinberg LG, Kipel G, et al. (1992) Use of adenosine in the management of perioperative arrhythmias in the pediatric cardiac intensive care unit. Crit Care Med 20:1107–1111.

76. Ralston MA, Knilans TK, Hannon DW, et al. (1994) Use of adenosine for diagnosis and treatment of tachyarrhythmias in pediatric patients. J Pediatr 124:139–143.

77. Bernstein AD, Camm AJ, Fletcher RD, et al. (1987) The NASPE/BPEG generic pacemaker code for antibradyarrhythmia and adaptive-rate pacing and antitachyarrhythmia devices. Pacing Clin Electrophysiol 10:794–799.

78. Bevilacqua L, Hordof A (1998) Cardiac pacing in children. Curr Opin Cardiol 13:48–55.

79. Epstein AE, DiMarco JP, Ellenbogen KA, et al. (2008) ACC/AHA/HRS 2008 Guidelines for Device-Based Therapy of Cardiac Rhythm Abnormalities: a report of the American College of Cardiology/American Heart Association Task Force on Practice Guidelines (Writing Committee to Revise the ACC/AHA/NASPE 2002 Guideline Update for Implantation of Cardiac Pacemakers and Antiarrhythmia Devices) developed in collaboration with the American Association for Thoracic Surgery and Society of Thoracic Surgeons. J Am Coll Cardiol 51:e1–e62.

80. Silka MJ, Bar-Cohen Y (2006) Pacemakers and implantable cardioverter-defibrillators in pediatric patients. Heart Rhythm 3:1360–1366.

81. Stephenson EA, Kaltman JR (2006) Current state of the art for use of pacemakers and defibrillators in patients with congenital cardiac malformations. Cardiol Young 16 (Suppl 3):151–156.

82. Molina JE, Dunnigan AC, Crosson JE (1995) Implantation of transvenous pacemakers in infants and small children. Ann Thorac Surg 59:689–694.

83. Gillette PC, Shannon C, Blair H, et al. (1983) Transvenous pacing in pediatric patients. Am Heart J 105:843–847.

84. Villain E, Martelli H, Bonnet D, et al. (2000) Characteristics and results of epicardial pacing in neonates and infants. Pacing Clin Electrophysiol 23:2052–2056.

85. Dubin AM, Janousek J, Rhee E, et al. (2005) Resynchronization therapy in pediatric and congenital heart disease patients: an international multicenter study. J Am Coll Cardiol 46:2277–2283.

86. Cecchin F, Frangini PA, Brown DW, et al. (2009) Cardiac resynchronization therapy (and multisite pacing) in pediatrics and congenital heart disease: five years experience in a single institution. J Cardiovasc Electrophysiol 20:58–65.

87. Blom NA (2009) The role of cardiac resynchronization therapy in the young. J Cardiovasc Electrophysiol 20:66–68.

88. Atlee JL, Bernstein AD (2001) Cardiac rhythm management devices (part II): perioperative management. Anesthesiology 95:1492–1506.

89. Senthuran S, Toff WD, Vuylsteke A, et al. (2002) Implanted cardiac pacemakers and defibrillators in anaesthetic practice. Br J Anaesth 88:627–631.

90. American Society of Anesthesiologists Task Force (2005) Practice advisory for the perioperative management of patients with cardiac rhythm management devices: pacemakers and implantable cardioverter-defibrillators: a report by the American Society of Anesthesiologists Task Force on Perioperative Management of Patients with Cardiac Rhythm Management Devices. Anesthesiology 103:186–198.

91. Rozner MA (2007) The patient with a cardiac pacemaker or implanted defibrillator and management during anaesthesia. Curr Opin Anaesthesiol 20:261–268.

92. Bourke ME (1996) The patient with a pacemaker or related device. Can J Anaesth 43:R24–R41.

93. Reade MC (2007) Temporary epicardial pacing after cardiac surgery: a practical review. Part 1: general considerations in the management of epicardial pacing. Anaesthesia 62:264–271.

94. Janousek J, Vojtovic P, Chaloupecky V, et al. (2000) Hemodynamically optimized temporary cardiac pacing after surgery for congenital heart defects. Pacing Clin Electrophysiol 23:1250–1259.

95. Reade MC (2007) Temporary epicardial pacing after cardiac surgery: a practical review. Part 2: selection of epicardial pacing modes and troubleshooting. Anaesthesia 62:364–373.

96. Beland MJ, Hesslein PS, Finlay CD, et al. (1987) Noninvasive transcutaneous cardiac pacing in children. Pacing Clin Electrophysiol 10:1262–1270.

97. Gradaus R, Wollmann C, Kobe J, et al. (2004) Potential benefit from implantable cardioverter-defibrillator therapy in children and young adolescents [letter]. Heart 90 (3):328–329.

98. Berul CI (2008) Defibrillator indications and implantation in young children. Heart Rhythm 5:1755–1757.

99. Silka MJ (1996) Implantable cardioverter-defibrillators in children. A perspective on current and future uses. J Electrocardiol 29:223–225.

100. Friedman RA, Garson AJ (2001) Implantable defibrillators in children: from whence to shock. J Cardiovasc Electrophysiol 12:361–362.

101. Shannon KM (2002) Use of implantable cardioverter-defibrillators in pediatric patients. Curr Opin Cardiol 17:280–282.

102. Berul CI, Van Hare GF, Kertesz NJ, et al. (2008) Results of a multicenter retrospective implantable cardioverter-defibrillator registry of pediatric and congenital heart disease patients. J Am Coll Cardiol 51:1685–1691.

18 Airway and ventilatory management

Stephen A. Stayer, M.D.
Texas Children's Hospital, Baylor College of Medicine, Houston, Texas, USA

Gregory B. Hammer, M.D.
Lucile Packard Children's Hospital, Stanford University School of Medicine, Stanford, CA, USA

Introduction

Airway and ventilatory management of infants and children with congenital heart disease (CHD) during diagnostic and surgical procedures present unique challenges to the anesthesiologist owing to a range of congenital airway abnormalities, cardiopulmonary interactions, and adverse effects of surgery and cardiopulmonary bypass (CPB). Few other clinical situations will tax the skills of an anesthesiologist as the management of a child with CHD and a difficult airway. Children with cardiovascular disease may be intolerant of the myocardial depressant effects of many anesthetics, limiting the options available in managing their airway during induction of anesthesia. Children with cyanotic CHD experience rapid oxygen desaturation during periods of apnea associated with tracheal intubation. Developing a plan that allows safe airway and ven-

Anesthesia for Congenital Heart Disease 2nd edition. Edited by Dean Andropoulos, Stephen Stayer, Isobel Russell and Emad Mossad.
© 2010 Blackwell Publishing.

tilatory management without hemodynamic compromise requires preparation, skill, and familiarity with a range of techniques of tracheal intubation.

Choosing the appropriate endotracheal tube

The narrowest portion of the of a child's larynx is at the level of the cricoid cartilage, as opposed to adult patients whose limiting airway diameter is at the level of the vocal cords (rima glottidis). Uncuffed endotracheal Tubes (ETTs) are commonly used in children because a seal is created between the tracheal mucosa and the tube at the level of the cricoid cartilage [1]. The adequacy of this seal is usually assessed by performing a leak test in which a gradual increase in positive pressure is delivered through the breathing circuit while the practitioner listens over the mouth or neck for the sound of escaping gas. The circuit pressure at which a leak is auscultated is then documented. The leak test provides the best assessment of tube fit; however, significant interobserver variability has been demonstrated [2]. While the appropriate ETT size may be predicted by the patient's age (Table 18.1), a tube smaller or larger than predicted should be inserted to achieve the most appropriate tracheal fit.

A tight fitting ETT (e.g., no gas leak up to 30–35 cmH_2O) may cause ischemic injury to the tracheal mucosa and submucosa at the level of the cricoid cartilage. Mild ischemia and subsequent swelling may be manifest as postextubation stridor, whereas subglottic stenosis may result from more severe injury [3]. On the other hand, placement of an ETT with a gas leak at low inflating pressures (e.g., <15 cmH_2O) results in excessive leak around the endotracheal tube. This is particularly important for thoracic or cardiovascular surgery because lung compliance may be reduced as a result of surgical traction or pulmonary edema, resulting in the delivery of greater inflating pressures to provide physiologic tidal volumes (VTs). With a loose-fitting ETT in place, the volume of gas leak around the ETT increases as the peak inflating pressure is increased, while alveolar ventilation decreases. Gas leakage representing more than 50% of VT has been demonstrated in the setting of decreasing lung compliance [4]. Associated decreases in minute ventilation may lead to dangerous elevations in $PaCO_2$.

In addition to the risk of inadequate alveolar ventilation, there are other hazards associated with placement of a loose-fitting ETT. Lung function measurements are commonly used to guide mechanical ventilation in the postoperative period. A variable leak around the ETT results in inaccurate measurements of exhaled VTs, lung compliance, and airway resistance. Eliminating or minimizing the gas leak around the ETT will decrease the environmental pollution from either inhaled anesthetic agents or nitric oxide (NO) [5]. Lastly, an adequate seal around the ETT may decrease the risk of pulmonary aspiration should gastric contents be regurgitated following tracheal intubation.

Traditional teaching has recommended the use of uncuffed ETTs in children younger than 8 years. However, there is limited scientific evidence to support this practice. Cuffed endotracheal tubes have been used in more than 15,000 children, none of whom developed clinically significant airway complications [6], and the use of cuffed ETTs for short cases in the operating room reduces the need for repeated laryngoscopy, allows use of lower fresh gas flows, and limits environmental contamination with anesthetic gases [5]. There is no difference in the incidence of airway complications among pediatric intensive care patients intubated with cuffed versus uncuffed endotracheal tubes [7]. Alterations in mucosal edema and lung compliance from the effects of CPB or altering pulmonary blood flow (PBF) may increase the leak around the endotracheal tube in children after heart surgery, and a cuffed ETT may be inflated to compensate for such changes. In a retrospective review of 809 children younger than 2 years

Table 18.1 Endotracheal tube sizes used in pediatric patients

Age	Size (mm ID)
Preterm	
<1000 g	2.5
1000–2500 g	3.0
Term neonate to 6 mo	3.5
6 mo to 1 yr	4.0
1–2 yr	4.0–5.0
Beyond 2 yr	$\dfrac{\text{Age (yr)} + 16}{4}$

ID, internal diameter.

undergoing cardiac surgery over a 4-year period, the incidence of subglottic stenosis (17/809 or 1.08%) was not affected by the common use of cuffed ETT in the series. The most important risk factors were younger age and prolonged (>96 h) postoperative ventilation [8].

A disadvantage of using cuffed ETTs is that their outer diameter is approximately 0.3–0.5 mm larger than uncuffed ETTs with the same inner diameter. As a result, a tube with an inner diameter one size (i.e., 0.5 mm) smaller must be used when a cuffed ETT is placed. This results in greater resistance to gas flow and an increased risk of occlusion of the ETT with blood and tracheal secretions. While a reduction of the tracheal tube diameter by only 0.5 mm might not be expected to effect a clinical change, gas flow resistance increases exponentially at smaller tube diameters. While a reduction in tracheal tube size from 8.0 mm internal diameter (ID) to 7.5 mm ID increases airway resistance by 29%, a change from a size 4.0-mm ID to a 3.5-mm ID tube results in an increase of 71%, and a change from a 3.5-mm ID tube to a 3.0-mm ID tube increases resistance by 85%. The increase in resistance is even more profound if turbulent airflow occurs in smaller tracheal tubes.

A new microcuff endotracheal tube (Kimberly Clark; Roswell, GA, USA) has been developed for pediatric patients that provides a true high-volume low-pressure cuff, eliminates the Murphy eye in order to optimize cuff position at the tip of the endotracheal tube, and an ultrathin cuff that provides an outer diameter to inner diameter ratio similar to uncuffed endotracheal tubes. Two studies including 575 patients aged 0–5 years have found a low incidence of postextubation stridor, and a tracheal tube exchange rate of <3% [9,10].

Orotracheal versus nasotracheal intubation

While orotracheal intubation is performed more commonly than nasotracheal intubation for routine surgery in children, there may be advantages to the use of nasal tubes in children undergoing cardiac surgery. Transesophageal echocardiography (TEE), which is performed in many centers, may cause compression or dislodgement of an orotracheal tube in the oropharynx. However, Stevenson found a low incidence of airway complications during pediatric TEE among children who were orally intubated [11]. Of the 1650 patients he studied, 3 (0.2%) developed a right mainstem advancement of the endotracheal tube, and 8 (0.5%) were inadvertently extubated. Nasal ETTs are more readily secured to the face, and movement of the ETT is less likely during manipulation of the TEE probe. At Texas Children's Hospital, over 4000 TEE studies have been performed in children who were nasally intubated with one inadvertent extubation in the past 10 years. There is a greater risk of damage to nasal alae and, in older children, of sinusitis from long-term nasotracheal intubation [12–14]. The risk of bleeding from adenoidal trauma is especially problematic in the fully anticoagulated patient. This risk is minimized by the routine use of topical vasoconstrictor drugs (e.g., oxymetazoline) and adequate lubrication of the ETT. Excessive pressure should not be used during advancement of the tube through the nose and nasopharynx. Prior to advancing the ETT into the nasopharynx, a soft, lubricated suction catheter can be passed through the ETT through the nasopharynx into the oral cavity. This will act as a guide permitting easier passage of the nasal ETT [15]. Because ETTs can be placed more easily and rapidly via the oral route, oral intubation is preferred for rapid sequence intubation or when intubating cyanotic infants. Once adequate ventilation and oxygenation have been provided and the stomach is suctioned, the ETT may be exchanged for a nasal tube under direct visualization. Because it is important to properly determine the appropriate size of the ETT, we intubate most children orally, perform a leak test, and alter the size of the tube or use a cuffed ETT if necessary via the nasal route. In general, the nasal passages of children will accommodate the same size ETT as would be used for oral intubation.

The difficult airway

The incidence of congenital airway anomalies is believed to be greater among children with CHD than in the general population. Genetic syndromes associated with both airway anomalies and CHDs are frequent, and patients with syndromes such as the CHARGE association and velocardiofacial syndrome must have a complete airway examination. A thorough history should be taken on all patients receiving sedation or anesthesia with attention to the recent presence of an upper respiratory tract infection (URI), snoring or noisy breathing during sleep, inspiratory stridor, and previous problems associated with tracheal

Table 18.2 Suggested contents of difficult airway management cart

Rigid laryngoscope blades of alternate design and size from those routinely used

Endotracheal tubes of assorted size. Nasal and oral airways of assorted sizes

Endotracheal tube guides and tube exchangers. Examples include (but are not limited to) semirigid stylets with or without a hollow core for jet ventilation and light wands

Jet ventilation equipment

Fiberoptic intubation equipment

Laryngeal mask airways of assorted size

Equipment suitable for emergency surgical airway access (e.g., percutaneous cricothyrotomy). Size 3.5, 4.0, 6.0

An exhaled CO_2 detector

intubation or following extubation. In older, cooperative patients, the airway should be examined as with adult patients including mouth opening, dentition, mandibular size (hyomental distance), and neck mobility. Studies in adults have shown that examination of the airway can help predict difficulty of intubation and mask ventilation [16]. No such studies have been performed in infants and children, and it is not known whether assessing mouth opening using a tongue depressor in a nonverbal child is predictive of difficulty with intubation. Assessment of an infant's airway should include an assessment of neck mobility and the appearance of the mandibular size when viewed in profile. Children with micro- or retrognathia are more likely to manifest difficult mask ventilation and/or difficult intubation.

Intubation of the patient with a difficult airway

A modification of the American Society of Anesthesiologists algorithm for the management of the patient with a difficult airway can be applied to children [17]. (Figure 18.1). Specialized airway equipment should be prepared, checked, and available in the operating room. Table 18.2 lists recommendations for equipping a difficult airway cart. In addition to equipment, additional personnel skilled in airway management should be immediately available for assistance.

When the difficult airway is recognized prior to the induction of anesthesia, control of the airway can be performed with the patient awake, following sedation, or after the induction of anesthesia with inhalation agents. Awake, nonsedated, direct laryngoscopy can be accomplished in neonates but may be difficult, traumatic, and have significant adverse hemodynamic consequences. Placement of a laryngeal mask airway (LMA) after application of topical anesthesia to the airway in an awake infant has been described as an alternative to awake direct laryngoscopy [18]. Fiberoptic-guided intubation

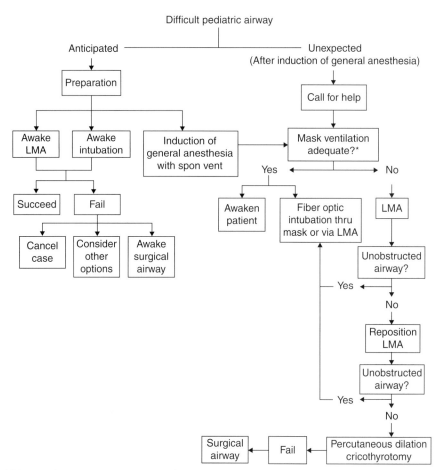

Figure 18.1 Management of the difficult pediatric airway. LMA, laryngeal mask airway (From reference [17])

* May need two person technique and/or oral airway

of the older, cooperative patient using topical anesthesia and intravenous sedation is a safe and effective alternative.

Inhalation induction of anesthesia using sevoflurane with maintenance of spontaneous ventilation is commonly performed in infants and children with a difficult airway. Intravenous access is established prior to mask induction. If the patient develops airway obstruction during the induction of anesthesia, immediate attempts are made to relieve the obstruction by jaw thrust, head extension, use of continuous positive airway pressure (CPAP), and insertion of an oropharyngeal or nasopharyngeal airway. If mask ventilation is inadequate and not improved with the above maneuvers, insertion of an LMA should be attempted. If positive pressure ventilation can be delivered via the LMA, the LMA can be used as a guide for insertion of an ETT or can be exchanged for an ETT with the use of a fiberoptic bronchoscope (FOB). If an LMA fails to provide a patent airway, preparations should be made for an emergency cricothyrotomy (see below). If mask ventilation is possible with either a face mask or LMA, neuromuscular relaxation can be used in order to optimize laryngoscopy.

If mask ventilation is possible, but tracheal intubation is not readily achieved, one should optimize head and neck positioning and consider use of an alternate laryngoscope blade to better visualize the larynx. Repeated attempts at direct laryngoscopy may lead to swelling and/or bleeding in the airway and the inability to perform adequate mask ventilation. After three failed attempts at direct laryngoscopy, use of an LMA should be considered. For the majority of pediatric patients, insertion of an LMA provides a patent airway and a method of delivering positive pressure ventilation, and facilitates fiberoptic intubation.

Fiberoptic-guided tracheal intubation

The development of FOBs with small diameters has facilitated the use of fiberoptic-guided intubation in infants and young children. A pediatric FOB with a 2.2-mm outer diameter that will fit through a 2.5-mm (ID) ETT tube is available (Olympus LF-P, Olympus America Inc., Melville, NY, USA). An FOB with an outer diameter of

2.4 mm that passes through a 3.0-mm (ID) ETT is also manufactured (Pentax Intubation FI-7P, Pentax Precision Instrument Corporation, Orangeburg, NY, USA). Neither of these FOBs has a suction channel. Currently, the smallest FOB that has a suction channel is 2.8 mm in diameter (available from Karl Storz, Tuttlingen, Germany and Oympus America Inc., Melville, NY, USA). Fiberoptic-guided tracheal intubation can be performed via the nose, mouth, or LMA, under sedation and topical anesthesia or under general anesthesia. The nasal route may be preferred because it tends to maintain the scope in the midline, facilitating visualization of the larynx. Repeated practice in children with normal airways is recommended in order to acquire and maintain the skills essential to be proficient with the use of this equipment.

Fiberoptic guided tracheal intubation can also be performed through an LMA. Once the LMA is appropriately positioned, the FOB is passed through the opening of the LMA into the trachea. An ETT is passed into the trachea over the FOB, which is then used to confirm appropriate positioning. When a standard ETT is used, only a short length of the ETT remains outside the LMA, making maintenance of ETT position and removal of the LMA difficult. A variety of techniques have been described to facilitate safe removal of the LMA while maintaining the ETT in place. First, a specially designed, long ETT can be placed over the FOB. Second, a tracheal tube exchange catheter (Cook Critical Care, Inc., Bloomington, IN, USA) can be passed through the ETT into the trachea after which both the ETT and LMA are removed. An ETT is passed over the exchange catheter into the trachea. Third, the ETT can be made temporarily longer by wedging a half size smaller ETT into the proximal end, or by cutting the 15-mm adapter and using it to connect two ETTs of the same size together. After placement of the combined ETTs through the LMA, the LMA and proximal ETT are removed and the 15-mm adapter is replaced. An alternative to fiberoptic intubation through the LMA is "blind" passage of the ETT through the LMA into the trachea. An intubating LMA has been developed for this purpose and is available as small as size #3. In younger children, the epiglottis frequently folds inside the LMA [19]. While this may not cause airway obstruction, traumatic injury to the epiglottis may occur from blind passage of an ETT.

Several other methods for controlling the airway of patients with a difficult airway have been described. These include the use of a lighted stylet, combitube, retrograde transtracheal intubation, blind nasal intubation, use of other specialized laryngoscopes with or without video capability, and digital (tactile) techniques [1,20,21]. The reader is referred to a textbook of general pediatric anesthesiology for more detailed descriptions of these alternative techniques for intubation.

Emergency cricothyrotomy

In the rare instance in which mask ventilation and placement of an LMA do not provide adequate oxygenation and ventilation and tracheal intubation cannot be performed, percutaneous cricothyrotomy may be life saving. Percutaneous tracheotomy kits are available (Cook Critical Care, Inc., Bloomington, IN, USA) that are designed to facilitate pediatric tracheotomy tube placement through the cricoid membrane using the Seldinger technique [22].

The difficult extubation

Tracheal extubation of patients with risk factors for difficult reintubation presents a challenge to the anesthesiologist and intensive care physician. Infants and children with CHD are at high risk for adverse consequences associated with oxygen desaturation, hypercapnia, and hemodynamic instability prior to or during attempted reintubation. Respiratory distress signaling the need for reintubation may develop at a time when a physician with the greatest expertise in airway management is not immediately available. This can occur in the recovery room or intensive care unit, where equipment and other conditions may be less optimal than those encountered in the operating room. In addition, reintubation may be technically more difficult than the initial intubation due to airway edema, bleeding, secretions, and poor patient cooperation. Fiberoptic intubation or other alternative techniques may be extremely difficult or impossible under these circumstances.

Practice guidelines set forth by the American Society of Anesthesiologists Task Force for the Management of the Difficult Airway re commend that anesthesiologists have a preformulated strategy for extubating patients with a difficult airway [17]. This may include placement of a device through the indwelling ETT that serves as a stent over which the ETT can be replaced if the patient fails extubation. Accordingly, tracheal extubation of patients with a difficult airway has been performed over a FOB, gum-elastic bougie, and a jet stylet [23–25]. The "endotracheal ventilation catheter" (ETVC) is a modification of the jet stylet. This device includes a Luer-lock connector in place of the removable 15-mm adaptor, allowing attachment to a high-pressure circuit for jet ventilation, capnography, or oxygen insufflation. The ETVC was used by Cooper in 202 patients over a 3-year period to maintain airway access in patients with difficult airways [26]. Oxygen insufflation and capnography were continued for up to 72 hours following tracheal extubation, during which time the catheter was well tolerated in most patients. Tracheal tube exchange and reintubation were successful in 20 of 22 attempts, with failure in two patients attributed to excessive pliability of a prototype catheter in one patient and operator inexperience in the other.

The Cook Airway Exchange Catheter (CAEC, Cook Critical Care, Bloomington, IN, USA) has been used to maintain airway access in adult patients who were at risk for difficult reintubation [27]. Like the ETVC, this polyurethane catheter has multiple side ports proximal to its blunt tip. It is packaged with both 15-mm and Luer-locking connectors. The catheter was placed prior to tracheal extubation, after which humidified oxygen was insufflated through the lumen for a mean duration of 9.4 hours until it was deemed unlikely that tracheal reintubation would be necessary. In this study, four reintubations were performed over the CAEC on the first attempt and no complications were observed.

Because of their relatively large outer diameter, airway exchange catheters are not suitable for use in infants or small children for maintenance of airway access following tracheal extubation. The smallest available CAEC, e.g., has a 3.0-mm outer diameter. In infants, this may severely limit gas flow around the catheter during spontaneous breathing. For young children, the use of a 0.018-in. guidewire for maintenance of airway access following tracheal extubation has been reported [28]. The guidewire used was Teflon coated and had a floppy, curved tip designed to minimize tissue trauma during placement. This guidewire facilitates placement of the smallest CAEC over which a 3.5-mm ID ETT may be advanced, a method similar to previously described reports [29, 30].

Airway and ventilatory management for thoracic surgery

Ventilation/perfusion in the lateral decubitus position

Several pediatric cardiovascular surgical procedures are performed in the lateral decubitus position, including patent ductus arteriosus (PDA) ligation, insertion of a systemic to pulmonary shunt, repair of coarctation of the aorta, and unifocalization of the pulmonary arteries. Ventilation is normally distributed preferentially to dependent regions of the lung so that there is a gradient of increasing ventilation from the most nondependent to the most dependent lung segments. Because of gravitational effects, perfusion normally follows a similar distribution, with increased blood flow to dependent lung segments. Therefore, ventilation and perfusion are normally well matched. During thoracic surgery, several factors act to adversely affect ventilation/perfusion (V/Q) matching. First, general anesthesia, neuromuscular blockade, and mechanical ventilation cause a decrease in functional residual capacity (FRC) of both lungs. Second,

compression of the dependent lung in the lateral decubitus position may cause atelectasis. Third, surgical retraction and/or single-lung ventilation (SLV) result in collapse of the operative lung. Lastly, hypoxic pulmonary vasoconstriction (HPV), which acts to divert blood flow away from under-ventilated lung, thereby minimizing V/Q mismatch, may be diminished by inhalational anesthetic agents and other vasodilating drugs. These factors apply equally to infants, children, and adults.

The overall effect of the lateral decubitus position on V/Q mismatch, however, is unique in infants. In adults with unilateral lung disease, oxygenation is optimal when the patient is placed in the lateral decubitus position with the healthy lung dependent "down" and the diseased lung nondependent "up" [31]. Presumably, this is related to an increase in blood flow to the dependent, healthy lung and a decrease in blood flow to the nondependent, diseased lung due to the hydrostatic pressure (or gravitational) gradient between the two lungs. This phenomenon optimizes V/Q matching in the adult patient undergoing thoracic surgery in the lateral decubitus position.

In infants with unilateral lung disease, however, oxygenation is improved with the healthy lung "up" [32]. Several factors account for this discrepancy between adults and infants. Infants have a soft, easily compressible rib cage that cannot fully support the underlying lung. Therefore, FRC is closer to residual volume, making airway closure likely to occur in the dependent lung even during tidal breathing [33]. When the adult is placed in the lateral decubitus position, the dependent diaphragm has a mechanical advantage, since it is "loaded" from abdominal pressure. This pressure is reduced in infants, thereby reducing the functional advantage of the dependent diaphragm. The infant's small size also results in a reduced hydrostatic pressure gradient between the nondependent and dependent lungs. Consequently, the favorable increase in perfusion to the dependent, ventilated lung is reduced in infants. This may be especially true for infants with systemic-to-pulmonary artery shunts, e.g., modified Blalock–Taussig (BT), PDA, or multiple aortopulmonary collateral arteries (MAPCAs), in whom systemic pressure may be maintained in the pulmonary arterial circulation.

Finally, all infants have increased oxygen consumption that predisposes them to hypoxemia. Infants normally consume 6–8 mL of oxygen per kg per minute compared with adult's 2–3 mL/kg/min [34]. The FRC of the lung functions as an oxygen reservoir when ventilation ceases. An infant will more rapidly consume oxygen from the diminished oxygen reservoir that is produced during surgery in the lateral decubitus position. Infants with cyanotic CHD are at increased risk of life-threatening oxygen desaturation during thoracic surgery.

Single-lung ventilation

Prior to 1995, nearly all thoracic surgery in children was performed by thoracotomy. In the majority of cases, anesthesiologists ventilated both lungs with a conventional tracheal tube and the surgeons retracted the operative lung in order to gain exposure to the surgical field. During the past decade, the use of video-assisted thoracoscopic surgery (VATS) has dramatically increased in both adults and children. Reported advantages of thoracoscopy include smaller chest incisions, reduced postoperative pain, and more rapid postoperative recovery compared with thoracotomy [35–37]. Recent advances in surgical technique and technology, including high-resolution microchip cameras and smaller endoscopic instruments, have facilitated the application of VATS in smaller patients. VATS is now being utilized for PDA occlusion in many centers. Open thoracotomy is generally performed for more complex procedures, including repair of coarctation of the aorta and pulmonary artery unifocalization.

SLV is desirable during VATS as well as open thoracotomy because lung deflation improves visualization of thoracic contents and may reduce lung injury caused by the use of retractors. There are several different techniques that can be used for SLV in children.

Single-lumen endotracheal tube

The simplest means of providing SLV is to intentionally intubate the ipsilateral mainstem bronchus with a conventional single-lumen ETT. When the left bronchus is to be intubated, the bevel of the ETT is rotated 180° and the head turned to the right [38]. The ETT is advanced into the bronchus until breath sounds on the operative side disappear. An FOB may be passed through or alongside the ETT to confirm or guide placement. When a cuffed ETT is used, the distance from the tip of the tube to the proximal cuff must be shorter than the length of the bronchus so that the cuff is entirely in the bronchus [39]. This technique is simple and requires no special equipment other than an FOB, and may be the preferred technique of SLV in emergency situations such as airway hemorrhage or contralateral tension pneumothorax.

Problems can occur when using a single-lumen ETT for SLV. If a smaller, uncuffed ETT is used, it may be difficult to provide an adequate seal of the intended bronchus. This may prevent the operative lung from collapsing adequately, or fail to protect the healthy, ventilated lung from contamination by purulent material from the contralateral lung. It is not possible to suction the operative lung using this technique. Hypoxemia may occur due to obstruction of the upper lobe bronchus, especially when the short right mainstem bronchus is intubated. Newly available microcuff endotracheal tubes (Kimberly Clark, Roswell, GA, USA) have a thinner walled cuff positioned at the tip of the endotracheal tube and therefore may be advantageous for use in SLV.

Variations of this technique have been described, including intubation of both bronchi independently with small ETTs [40–43]. One mainstem bronchus is initially intubated with an ETT, after which another ETT is advanced over an FOB into the opposite bronchus.

Balloon-tipped bronchial blockers

A Fogarty embolectomy catheter or an end-hole, balloon wedge catheter may be used for bronchial blockade to provide SLV [44–47]. Placement of a Fogarty catheter is facilitated by bending the tip of its stylet toward the bronchus on the operative side. An FOB may be used to reposition the catheter and confirm appropriate placement. When an end-hole catheter is placed outside the ETT, the bronchus on the operative side is initially intubated with an ETT. A guidewire is then advanced into that bronchus through the ETT. The ETT is removed and the blocker is advanced over the guidewire into the bronchus. An ETT is then reinserted into the trachea alongside the blocker catheter. The catheter balloon is positioned in the proximal mainstem bronchus under fiberoptic visual guidance. With an inflated blocker balloon, the airway is completely sealed, providing more predictable lung collapse and better operating conditions than with an ETT in the bronchus.

A potential problem with this technique is dislodgement of the blocker balloon into the trachea. The inflated balloon will then block ventilation to both lungs and/or prevents collapse of the operated lung. The balloons of most catheters currently used for bronchial blockade have low-volume, high-pressure properties and overdistension can damage or even rupture the airway [48]. Guyton et al., however, reported that bronchial blocker cuffs produced lower "cuff to tracheal" pressures than double-lumen tubes [49]. When closed tip bronchial blockers are used, the operative lung cannot be suctioned and CPAP cannot be provided to the operative lung if needed.

Adapters are available that facilitate ventilation during placement of a bronchial blocker through an indwelling ETT [50, 51]. A 5-Fr endobronchial blocker that is suitable for use in children with a multiport adapter and FOB is commercially available (Cook Critical Care, Inc., Bloomington, IN, USA) [52]. The risk of hypoxemia during blocker placement is diminished, and repositioning of the blocker may be performed with fiberoptic guidance during surgery. Even with use of an FOB with a diameter of 2.2 mm, however, the indwelling ETT must be at least 4.5-mm ID to allow passage of the catheter and FOB. The use of this technique, therefore, is generally limited to children older than 18 months.

Univent tube

The Univent tube (Fuji Systems Corporation, Tokyo, Japan) is a conventional ETT with a second lumen containing a small tube that can be advanced into a bronchus [53–55]. A balloon located at the distal end of this small tube serves as a blocker. Univent tubes require FOB for successful placement. Univent tubes are available in sizes as small as a 3.5- and 4.5-mm ID for use in children older than 6 years[56]. Because the blocker tube is firmly attached to the main ETT, displacement of the Univent blocker balloon is less likely than when other blocker techniques are used. The blocker tube has a small lumen that allows egress of gas and can be used to insufflate oxygen or suction the operated lung, but this feature is only present in size 6.0 and larger Univent tubes.

A disadvantage of the Univent tube is the large amount of cross-sectional area occupied by the blocker channel, especially in the smaller size tubes which have a disproportionately high resistance to gas flow [57]. The Univent tube's blocker balloon has low-volume, high-pressure characteristics so mucosal injury can occur during normal inflation [58,59].

Double-lumen tubes

All double-lumen tubes (DLTs) are essentially two tubes of unequal length molded together. The shorter tube ends in the trachea and the longer tube in the bronchus. DLTs for older children and adults have cuffs located on the tracheal and bronchial lumens. The tracheal cuff, when inflated, allows positive pressure ventilation. The inflated bronchial cuff allows ventilation to be diverted to either or both lungs, and protects each lung from contamination from the contralateral side.

Conventional plastic DLTs, once only available in adult sizes (35, 37, 39, and 41 Fr), are now available in smaller sizes. The smallest cuffed DLT is 26 Fr (Rusch, Duluth, GA, USA) that may be used in children as young as 8 years old. DLTs are also available in sizes 28 and 32 Fr (Mallinckrodt Medical, Inc., St. Louis, MO, USA) suitable for children 10 years and older.

DLTs are inserted in children using the same technique as in adults [60]. The tip of the tube is inserted just past the vocal cords and the stylet is withdrawn. The DLT is rotated 90° to the appropriate side and then advanced into the bronchus. In the adult population, the depth of insertion is directly related to the height of the patient [61]. No equivalent measurements are yet available in children. If fiberoptic bronchoscopy is to be used to confirm tube placement, a scope with a small diameter and sufficient length must be available [62].

A DLT offers the advantage of ease of insertion as well as the ability to suction and oxygenate the operative lung

Table 18.3 Tube selection for single lung ventilation in children

Age (yr)	ETT (ID)*	BB[†] (Fr)	Univent®[‡]	DLT (Fr)[§]
0.5–1	3.5–4.0	5		
1–2	4.0–4.5	5		
2–4	4.5–5.0	5		
4–6	5.0–5.5	5		
6–8	5.5–6	6	3.5	
8–10	6.0 cuffed	6	3.5	26
10–12	6.5 cuffed	6	4.5	26–28
12–14	6.5–7.0 cuffed	6	4.5	32
14–16	7.0 cuffed	7	6.0	35
16–18	7.0–8.0 cuffed	7	7.0	35

* Sheridan® Tracheal Tubes, Kendall Healthcare, Mansfield, MA, USA.
† Arrow International Corp., Redding, PA, USA.
‡ Fuji Systems Corporation, Tokyo, Japan.
§ 26 Fr: Rusch, Duluth, GA, USA; 28–35 Fr: Mallinckrodt Medical, Inc., St. Louis, MO, USA.

ETT, endotracheal tube; ID, internal diameter; Fr, French size; DLT, double-lumen tube.

with CPAP. Left DLTs are preferred to right DLTs because of the shorter length of the right main bronchus [63]. Right DLTs are more difficult to position accurately because of the greater risk of right upper lobe obstruction.

DLTs are safe and easy to use. There are very few reports of airway damage from DLTs in adults, and none in children. Their high-volume, low-pressure cuffs should not damage the airway if they are not overinflated with air or distended with nitrous oxide while in place.

Guidelines for selecting appropriate tubes (or catheters) for SLV in children are shown in Table 18.3. There is significant variability in overall size and airway dimensions in children, particularly in teenagers. The recommendations shown in Table 18.3 are based on average values for airway dimensions. Larger DLTs may be safely used in large teenagers.

Ventilatory management during thoracic surgery

During two-lung ventilation, VTs of 10–12 mL/kg are typically used at a respiratory rate that provides normocapnia. When one lung is ventilated, the delivered VT should be reduced to 6–8 mL/kg and the respiratory rate increased by 20% in order to avoid excess inspiratory pressure and volume to the ventilated lung. Pulse oximetry and capnography are useful to reflect trends in the changes in oxygenation and ventilation, but monitoring of arterial blood gas tensions is important to accurately determine PaO_2 and $PaCO_2$ during SLV in infants and children with congenital cardiac disease.

Hypoxemia is commonly encountered during thoracic surgical procedures, especially in children with CHD and preexisting hypoxemia, pulmonary hypertension, or impaired myocardial function. Hypoxemia develops from one or more possible mechanisms. The conducting passages of the operative lung are intentionally obstructed during SLV and/or from surgical retraction and compression of the operative lung. Secretions in the airways, surgical and hydrostatic compression may also compromise gas flow through the conducting passages of the dependent lung. The reduction in ventilation to the operative lung produces regional hypoxemia, inducing HPV, which will reduce V/Q mismatch. However, HPV may be impaired and will not improve V/Q matching in children with CHD. In a dog model, it has been shown that HPV is impaired by elevated pulmonary arterial pressure and by low mixed venous oxygen tension, both of which are commonly encountered among children with CHD [64,65]. Lastly, retraction of the operative lung may compress the mediastinum impairing cardiac filling and reducing cardiac output, which decreases mixed venous oxygen concentration thereby worsening hypoxemia from either intracardiac or intrapulmonary shunting.

Hypoxemia should be treated immediately by increasing the FiO_2 to 1.0 and by confirming patency of the ETT. A suction catheter should be passed through the ETT to clear secretions and/or blood from the lumen. Irrigation with sterile saline may be performed. If the ETT remains occluded, an FOB may be used to determine the site of obstruction and to reestablish patency of the ETT. The surgeon should be informed, and compression of the lung and/or mediastinum should be minimized. Administration of intravenous fluids may improve cardiac output and improve V/Q matching by increasing perfusion pressure to the lungs. Application of CPAP to the nondependent lung will reduce shunt through this lung and improve oxygenation during SLV. If hypoxemia persists despite these maneuvers, the operative lung should be reinflated with 100% oxygen. Although NO might be expected to increase PBF to the ventilated lung and improve oxygenation, two studies in adults failed to show benefit from NO during SLV [66,67].

Changes in lung function in children with CHD

Ventilation may be impaired in children with increased PBF due to left-to-right shunts. Both decreased lung compliance and increased airway resistance have been demonstrated in these children. Two studies in infants and young children with CHD found strong correlation between echocardiographic evidence of pulmonary artery

engorgement and decreased lung compliance [68,69]. A study of neonatal patients undergoing thoracotomy for BT shunts or repair of coarctation of the aorta [70] determined that lung compliance decreased and airway resistance was significantly increased after surgery. However, the return to baseline pulmonary function was prolonged after BT shunt placement when compared to coarctation repair, suggesting that increases in PBF worsens pulmonary mechanics [70]. Some infants develop substantial increases in total lung resistance following heart surgery, the severity of which can be predictive of postoperative respiratory failure [71]. Acute increases in pulmonary artery pressure also produce significant changes in lung mechanics. Airway resistance increases 43% and compliance decreases 11% during periods of acute pulmonary hypertension [72]. In this study, lung biopsy specimens from patients with the greatest increase in pulmonary artery pressure had increased bronchial smooth muscle mass, suggesting that the same local mediators that affect increases in pulmonary arterial pressure produce bronchospasm. Changes in lung mechanics correlate better with the magnitude of pulmonary vascular engorgement than with pulmonary artery hypertension. During cardiac catheterization, the degree of increased PBF is proportionate with increases in respiratory resistance among infants who are mechanically ventilated [73]. Infants with CHD and pulmonary overcirculation have reduced dynamic compliance and increased respiratory resistance that improves following surgery [74].

Extrinsic compression of larger airways by the heart and vascular structures can also affect lung function in children with CHD. Both left and right mainstem bronchial compression have been described from enlarged pulmonary arteries. An enlarged left atrium can compress the left mainstem bronchus, and bronchial compression can occur from extrinsic compression by a right ventricle-to-pulmonary artery conduit [75].

Changes in lung function from CPB

Pulmonary dysfunction is common after cardiac surgery [76]. Children with increased PBF may develop up to a threefold increase in lung water in the immediate postoperative period, the degree of which appears to be related to the presence of pulmonary hypertension [77,78]. In addition, both quantitative and qualitative differences in surfactant have been described in children after CPB [79]. Others have found the most common adverse pulmonary effect is the development of atelectasis, reported to be as high as 82% among children undergoing CPB [80]. Both noncardiogenic pulmonary edema and acute bronchospasm have also been reported following CPB in children and adults [81,82], although the incidence of these complications in children is unknown. Some authors found correlation between the duration of CPB and the severity of lung injury, while others found only minor changes in pulmonary mechanics related to CPB [80,83–85]. These differences may be related to improvements in CPB management over the past decade. In a study of over 100 infants undergoing heart surgery at Texas Children's Hospital, we found no correlation between the duration of CPB, the duration of aortic cross clamp, the use of deep hypothermic circulatory arrest, and pulmonary outcomes [86].

Cardiopulmonary interactions

Positive intrathoracic pressure typically has adverse hemodynamic effects on the right ventricle and variable hemodynamic effects on the left ventricle in patients with normal cardiac anatomy and function. Intrathoracic pressure is transmitted to the thin-walled, compressible superior and inferior vena cava, reducing venous blood return to the right atrium and leading to a decrease in right ventricular filling [87]. In addition, right ventricular output will decrease if pulmonary vascular resistance (PVR) increases from hyperinflation of the lungs. With acute rises in PVR, the right ventricle may become dilated, resulting in decreased left ventricular filling as the intraventricular septum is displaced to the left [88].

PVR is affected by mechanical factors, chemical factors, and local humoral factors. PVR is optimal when the resting lung volume is at FRC and becomes elevated when lung volumes are above or below FRC. As lung volume decreases below FRC, extra-alveolar (large) blood vessels are compressed. In addition, atelectasis develops when lung volume decreases, leading to HPV with associated elevation in PVR. When lung volumes exceed FRC, alveolar distension causes compression of smaller arterioles and capillaries, also resulting in an increase in PVR [89] (Figure 18.2). Both oxygen tension and pH have significant effects on PVR [90], with alveolar hypoxemia and acidemia causing an increase in PVR, and alkalemia reducing PVR. Local pH has the greatest affect on pulmonary vascular tone, and PVR is reduced by producing either respiratory or metabolic alkalemia. Finally, lung expansion from positive pressure ventilation causes a local release of prostaglandins, leading to pulmonary vasodilation. This may explain the decrease in PVR associated with the onset of hyperventilation that occurs before CO_2 is reduced [90].

Changes in pleural pressure also affect left ventricular function. Ventricular output is affected by changes in afterload of the ventricle from transmitted intrathoracic pressure to the ventricular wall. The left ventricle lies within the thoracic cavity, whereas most of the systemic arterial tree lies outside the thoracic cavity. Therefore, changes in pleural pressure affect the left ventricle and not the systemic vasculature. Afterload is affected by the ventricu-

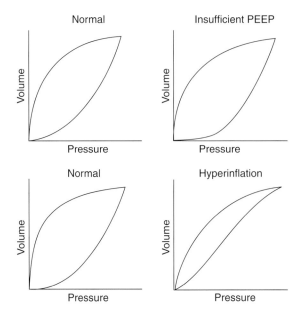

Figure 18.2 Effect of positive end-expiratory pressure (PEEP) on pressure–volume relationship in the lung

lar transmural pressure, i.e., the intracavitary pressure minus the pleural pressure. During spontaneous ventilation, negative intrapleural pressure is transmitted to the ventricular wall. During systole, the ventricle must overcome systemic vascular resistance and pleural pressure, therefore afterload is increased when negative pleural pressure develops as occurs during spontaneous ventilation. With positive pressure ventilation, systemic vascular resistance is unchanged, but afterload to the ventricle is reduced because positive intrapleural pressure will reduce ventricular transmural pressure [91–93] (Figure 18.3).

Mechanical ventilation for children with CHD

Changes in pleural pressure during inspiration have different hemodynamic effects on patients with cardiac and/or pulmonary disease. In healthy individuals, spontaneous inspiration augments venous return and increases right ventricular output, while increasing left ventricular afterload and decreasing left ventricular output. The net effect on total cardiac output is minor, and the conversion to positive pressure ventilation will have minimal effects on cardiac output. However, in hypovolemic patients, total cardiac output decreases from positive pressure ventilation because the decrease in right ventricular preload becomes the predominate hemodynamic effect.

In patients with right heart failure, mechanical ventilation parameters should be selected that will minimize intrathoracic pressure, maintain lung volume at FRC,

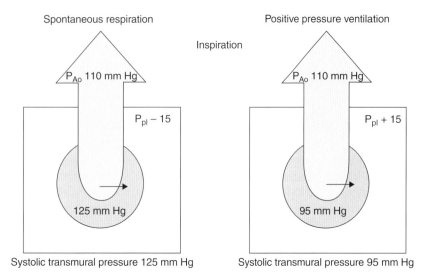

Spontaneous respiration

Positive pressure ventilation

Inspiration

P_{Ao} 110 mm Hg

P_{pl} – 15

125 mm Hg

Systolic transmural pressure 125 mm Hg

P_{Ao} 110 mm Hg

P_{pl} + 15

95 mm Hg

Systolic transmural pressure 95 mm Hg

Figure 18.3 The effect of positive pressure ventilation on systemic ventricular transmural pressure

avoid hypoxemia, and optimize pH in order to minimize PVR. Intrathoracic pressure should be minimized by avoiding excess positive end-expiratory pressure (PEEP) and excessively large VTs. However, inadequate PEEP will cause lung volumes to decrease below FRC, thereby increasing PVR. Pressure volume loops can be used to optimize pulmonary mechanics. (Figure 18.4). Hyperventilation is the traditional maneuver performed to reduce PVR because the associated hypocarbia produces alkalemia. However, both metabolic and respiratory alkalosis reduce PVR [90,94]. Local tissue pH is the most significant factor affecting tone in pulmonary vessels. Because hyperventilation requires an increase in minute ventilation, greater intrathoracic pressure must be used that may reduce right ventricular preload. Creating a metabolic alkalosis through the administration of sodium bicarbonate will produce the same beneficial effect on reducing PVR without interfering with right ventricular filling. Inhaled NO may further reduce PVR in patients with pulmonary hypertension and will improve right heart output.

Positive pressure ventilation will often improve cardiac output among patients with left ventricular failure [95, 96]. As the left ventricle fails, left atrial pressure is increased, leading to pulmonary venous congestion and decreased lung compliance. Work of breathing is increased and greater negative pressure is generated during spontaneous ventilation, which, in turn, increases left ventricular afterload. Positive pressure ventilation will decrease the work of breathing and thereby decrease oxygen consumption. In addition, positive intrathoracic pressure will reduce ventricular afterload enhancing cardiac output.

Patients with nonpulsatile PBF (e.g., following the bidirectional cavopulmonary shunt and Fontan procedures) show the most dramatic interactions between alterations in intrathoracic pressure, PBF, and cardiac output. Because they lack pulsatile flow in their pulmonary arteries, positive intrathoracic pressure interferes with PBF. Likewise, elevations in PVR will reduce PBF. Reductions of PBF impair ventricular filling and reduce cardiac output. The goals of lowering $PaCO_2$ in order to reduce PVR while diminishing intrathoracic pressure are diametrically opposed. A pattern of ventilation providing large VTs, e.g., 10–15 mL/kg, with lower respiratory rates is believed to optimize carbon dioxide elimination and PBF. PEEP is generally avoided in order to diminish intrathoracic pressure. However, atelectasis and lung volumes below FRC will increase PVR and these problems can be minimized through the use of PEEP. High-frequency jet ventilation effectively reduces $PaCO_2$ at a lower mean airway pressure than conventional mechanical ventilation and has been shown to improve cardiac output when

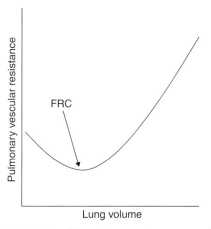

FRC

Pulmonary vescular resistance

Lung volume

Figure 18.4 Relationship of lung volume to pulmonary vascular resistance (PVR). FRC, functional residual capacity

compared to conventional ventilation in postoperative Fontan patients [97].

In patients with lung diseases associated with collapsed or fluid-filled alveoli (atelectasis, pulmonary edema, pneumonia, adult respiratory distress syndrome), gas exchange will improve when FRC is reestablished through the use of PEEP. In this setting, the application of positive pressure and PEEP will have variable cardiovascular effects depending on lung compliance. Even high levels of PEEP have limited effect on cardiac output when lung compliance is reduced, because the higher airway pressures are not transmitted to the heart and pulmonary vasculature [98]. Some congenital heart defects such as tetralogy of Fallot with absent pulmonary valve are associated with small and large airway compression from engorged pulmonary arteries. These patients develop airway collapse during exhalation and typically manifest hyperinflation of some lung segments and/or atelectasis in other areas [99]. Such children benefit from a ventilatory strategy that increases exhalation time, i.e., a slower ventilatory rate allowing prolonged exhalation. The optimal level of PEEP can be determined through the use of pressure–volume and flow–volume loops (Figure 18.4).

Lung management during CPB

Studies performed in animal models and adult patients have compared use of continuous mechanical ventilation, intermittent sigh breaths, and CPAP during CPB. Most studies show improvement in postoperative gas exchange with CPAP; however, this difference appears to be short lived [100, 101]. No such studies have been performed in children. Because closing capacity is higher in infancy, maintaining airway patency through the application of CPAP would theoretically be beneficial. Lung inflation from CPAP, however, may interfere with adequate surgical access to the heart and complete lung collapse is usually required. An F_{IO_2} of 0.21 versus 1.0 has the theoretical benefit of diminishing absorption atelectasis during CPB, although this also has not been studied in children. Before weaning from CPB and after confirmation of the absence of air in the left atrium and ventricle, several vital capacity breaths should be administered in order to reestablish patency of collapsed airways, reinflate atelectatic areas of the lung [102], and to mobilize secretions into the larger airways. The tracheal tube should be suctioned prior to weaning from CPB to assure patency of the tracheal tube and large airways, but care must be taken in order to avoid tracheal mucosal injury producing hemorrhage in a fully anticoagulated patient. Inhaled beta-2 agonists are commonly administered before weaning from CPB in order to decrease airway re-

activity; however, the efficacy of this practice has not been proven.

Volume control versus pressure control ventilation

Volume-limited ventilation delivers a relatively constant VT despite changes in the patient's total pulmonary compliance. During volume controlled ventilation, the peak inspiratory pressure varies and is dependent on the set VT, PEEP, gas flow rate, gas flow resistance, and respiratory system compliance. The presence of high inflation pressures signals decreased pulmonary compliance or conductance (e.g., offset of neuromuscular blockade, bronchospasm) or obstruction of the breathing circuit (e.g., occluded ETT). Disadvantages of volume-limited ventilation include the potential to produce very high inflating pressures and increase the risk of barotrauma. With proper monitoring of inspiratory pressure, including the use of appropriate limits and alarms, changes in the patient's pulmonary mechanics can be observed and the risk of barotrauma minimized. Because of technical difficulties in accurately delivering very small VTs (e.g., <100 cc), volume-limited ventilators have been primarily used in patients over 10 kg body weight. More recently, however, ventilators have been introduced that may be used in a volume-limited mode for smaller patients [103, 104].

In the neonate and infant, ventilators that are pressure-limited and time-cycled are commonly used. These ventilators offer the advantages of avoiding excessive inflating pressures and barotrauma. However, a decrease in the compliance or conductance of the patient's respiratory system, ventilator circuit, or tracheal tube will cause a reduction in delivered VT. An increase in compliance, conversely, will result in an increased VT and the risk of "volutrauma." Pressure limited or pressure control ventilation (PCV) is frequently applied to infants and children receiving mechanical ventilatory support in which severe pulmonary pathology dictates the need for rapid respiratory rates or high inflating pressures. Advantages of this mode of ventilation include limiting the peak inflating pressure delivered by the ventilator, thereby limiting the transalveolar pressure and ventilator-induced lung injury [105]. The decelerating flow used to produce PCV is thought to improve the distribution of gas flow to the lungs [106]. When compared to volume control ventilation, there is a more rapid improvement in lung compliance and oxygenation with PCV [107]. Some anesthesia ventilators may not deliver small VTs accurately because of the proportionately large compression volume loss in the ventilator and circuit [108]. Therefore, setting an anesthesia ventilator in pressure control mode will deliver more consistent ventilation to infants when the anesthesia machine cannot compensate for compression volume loss in the entire circuit [104].

Monitoring ventilation

Ventilation is the tidal exchange of gas between lungs and the atmosphere, and is measured by the concentration of CO_2 in arterial blood ($PaCO_2$). In the operating room, the most common noninvasive method of measuring CO_2 is capnography, which closely reflects changes in $PaCO_2$ among patients without lung or heart disease. Capnography is less accurate in infants when there is a leak around the ETT and when CO_2 is measured at the Y piece due to fresh gas washout of the small volume of CO_2 sampled [109]. Another measurement of alveolar ventilation is the measurement of exhaled VTs. Exhaled VT is usually measured by a spirometer located at the end of the expiratory limb. This measurement tends to be an overestimate because it reflects the patient's exhaled VT and the compression volume in the breathing circuit. As a result, the measured exhaled VT may be grossly inaccurate in infants. If there is a leak around the ETT, the spirometer will underestimate the exhaled gas volume. Without reliable $ETCO_2$ monitoring or exhaled VT measurements, the pediatric cardiovascular anesthesiologist must rely on chest expansion and peak inspiratory measurement (PIP) to make ventilator adjustments. Because adult anesthesia ventilators have large compression volumes, only profound changes in lung compliance are reflected in changes in PIP. For these reasons, blood gases should be measured frequently in order to assure adequate ventilation and to recognize changes in acid–base status. Newer monitoring systems allow for measurement of flow and pressure at the ETT, assisting the anesthesiologist in determining optimal ventilation in patients with poorly compliant lungs. Newer anesthesia machines that compensate for breathing circuit compliance like the Aisys anesthesia ventilator systems (GE Healthcare, Madison, WI, USA) and the Apollo anesthesia ventilator (Draeger Medical, Telford, PA, USA) provide accurate measures of delivered VT [104].

Anesthesia ventilators

Traditional anesthesia ventilators combined with a circle anesthesia system have limitations which make it challenging to ventilate pediatric patients accurately [110,111]. The compliance of the breathing system and changes in fresh gas flow interact in a subtle but significant fashion to influence the volume delivered to the patient. When caring for anesthetized pediatric patients, clinicians have used different strategies to ventilate their patients despite the limitations of traditional technology. A common approach is to adjust the ventilator settings based on a clinical assessment that includes observation of chest expansion during inspiration and measurement of inspiratory pressure, as well as monitoring the effectiveness of ventilation with capnography and pulse oximetry or blood gas analysis. Clinical assessment is always important and new anesthesia ventilators are designed to make it even easier to satisfy the ventilation requirements of even the smallest patients. Depending upon the device and the manufacturer, different strategies are employed to overcome the influence of compliance and fresh gas flow on delivered volume.

When using volume controlled ventilation, the goal of modern ventilator designs is to deliver a volume to the patient that is as close as possible to the volume set to be delivered. To achieve this goal, the ventilator must be able to compensate for both the compliance of the breathing system and the influence of fresh gas flow on VT independent of changes in lung compliance. Modern bellows ventilators (e.g., Aestiva and Avance from GE Healthcare, Madison, WI, USA) utilize a flow sensor at the inspiratory limb to control the volume delivered by the ventilator. The ventilator output is controlled by the flow sensor such that the set volume is delivered to the breathing circuit independent of changes in fresh gas flow or the compliance of the system between the ventilator and the flow sensor. Piston anesthesia ventilators (e.g., Fabius GS and Apollo from Draeger Medical, Telford, PA, USA) measure the compliance of the breathing system during the preuse checkout. The compliance measurement is then used to determine how much additional volume must be added to each breath to deliver the set volume to the patient. The influence of fresh gas on delivered volume is eliminated in the piston design by altering the configuration of the circle system and including a valve that prevents fresh gas from entering the patient circuit during mechanical inspiration. In addition, the exhaled volume measurement is corrected using the circuit compliance measurement.

Efforts to improve the design of anesthesia ventilators have been directed toward improving the accuracy of volume ventilation so that the patient reliably receives a VT that is as close as possible to the set VT [104,110,112]. Newer generation anesthesia machine ventilators that compensate for breathing circuit compliance and for fresh gas flow are able to deliver small VTs accurately to the airway under conditions of normal and low lung compliance during volume-controlled ventilation [104].

Specialized problems

Hypoxic gas mixture and inspired CO_2

Infants and children with single ventricle physiology and excess PBF (e.g., those with hypoplastic left heart syndrome) may benefit from a ventilatory strategy designed to increase PVR and diminish PBF. Hypoxic gas mixtures (i.e., $FIO_2 < 0.21$) or inhaled CO_2 have been used to accomplish this. Among neonatal patients with single ventricle physiology, 3% inhaled carbon dioxide improves cerebral oxygen saturation, mean arterial pressure, and oxygen delivery when compared with 17% inspired oxygen [112, 113].

Nitric oxide

Nitric oxide (NO), an endothelium-derived smooth muscle relaxant, has been used in neonates with persistent pulmonary hypertension [114, 115] and in infants and children with pulmonary hypertension related to CHD [116, 117]. NO has also been used in adult and pediatric patients with severe hypoxemic respiratory failure due to acute lung injury [118–121]. Inhaled NO selectively reduces PVR and may decrease intrapulmonary shunting. As a result, oxygenation is improved in patients with acute lung injury due to increased perfusion of relatively well-ventilated lung units [122]. PVR and oxygenation are improved to a similar extent by doses of 11 and 60 ppm in children with acute lung injury [123]. Infants with pulmonary hypertension after cardiac surgery have a decrease in pulmonary artery pressures and a 30% increase in oxygenation from the use of as little as 3–5 ppm of NO, and no further benefit from increasing NO to as high as 80 ppm [124]. However, other studies have failed to show improvements in pulmonary artery pressures, oxygenation, or outcome [125, 126]. Future studies are needed to determine the risks, benefits, optimal duration, and impact on survival of NO in children with severe respiratory disease after heart surgery.

Summary

Neonates, infants, and children with CHD present numerous challenges to the anesthesiologist. These patients commonly have increased myocardial oxygen consumption (e.g., left-to-right shunts, valvar stenosis) and/or decreased myocardial oxygen supply (e.g., cyanosis). CPB has adverse effects on heart and lung function. Less than optimal airway management, oxygenation, and/or ventilation can lead to further impairment of oxygen delivery to the heart and other organs with associated injury or death. Patients undergoing thoracic surgery may require SLV in order to optimize surgical conditions. Accordingly, the pediatric cardiovascular anesthesiologist must have knowledge and expertise in managing the airway and ventilation during cardiothoracic surgery.

References

1. Wheeler M, Coté CJ, Todres ID (2009) Chapter 12: The pediatric airway. In: Coté CJ, Lerman J, Todres ID (eds) A Practice Of Anesthesia For Infants And Children, 4th edn. WB Saunders, Elsevier, Philadelphia, pp. 237–278.
2. Schwartz RE, Stayer SA, Pasquariello CA (1993) Tracheal tube leak test—is there inter-observer agreement? Can J Anaesth 40:1049–1052.
3. Weber TR, Connors RH, Tracy TF, Jr. (1991) Acquired tracheal stenosis in infants and children. J Thorac Cardiovasc Surg 102:29–34.
4. Main E, Castle R, Stocks J, James I, Hatch D (2001) The influence of endotracheal tube leak on the assessment of respiratory function in ventilated children. Intensive Care Med 27:1788–1797.
5. Khine HH, Corddry DH, Kettrick RG, et al. (1997) Comparison of cuffed and uncuffed endotracheal tubes in young children during general anesthesia. Anesthesiology 86:627–631.
6. Murat I (2001) Cuffed tubes in children: a 3-year experience in a single institution. Paediatr Anaesth 11:748–749.
7. Deakers TW, Reynolds G, Stretton M, Newth CJ (1994) Cuffed endotracheal tubes in pediatric intensive care. J Pediatr 125:57–62.
8. Mossad E, Youssef G (2009) Subglottic stenosis in children undergoing repair of congenital heart defects. J Cardiothorac Vasc Anesth 23 February 19 [Epub ahead of print]
9. Dullenkopf A. Gerber AC, Weiss M (2005) Tracheal sealing characteristics of a new paediatric tracheal tube with high volume-low pressure polyurethane cuff. Acta Anaesthesiol Scand 49:232–237.
10. Salgo G, Schmitz G, Henze K, Stutz A (2006) Evaluation of a new recommendation for improved cuff tracheal tube size selection in infants and small children. Acta Anaesthesiol Scand; 50:557–561.
11. Stevenson JG (1999) Incidence of complications in pediatric transesophageal echocardiography: experience in 1650 cases. J Am Soc Echocardiogr 12:527–532.
12. Holzapfel L, Chevret S, Madinier G, et al. (1993) Influence of long-term oro- or nasotracheal intubation on nosocomial maxillary sinusitis: results of a prospective, randomized, clinical trial. Crit Care Med 21:1132–1138.
13. Bos AP, Tibboel D, Hazebroek FW, et al. (1989) Sinusitis: hidden source of sepsis in postoperative pediatric intensive care patients. Crit Care Med 17:886–888.
14. Hickey PR, Hansen DD, Norwood WI, Castaneda AR (1984) Anesthetic complications in surgery for congenital heart disease. Anesth Analg 63:657–664.
15. Elwood T, Stillions DM, Woo DW, Bradford HM, Ramamoorthy C (2002) Nasotracheal intubation: a randomized trial of two methods. Anesthesiology 96:51–53.
16. Mallampati SR, Gatt SP, Gugino LD, et al. (1985) A clinical sign to predict difficult tracheal intubation: a prospective study. Can Anaesth Soc J 32:429–434.
17. American Society of Anesthesiologists Task Force (1993) A Report by the American Society of Anesthesiologists

Task Force on Management of the Difficult Airway. Practice Guidelines for Management of the Difficult Airway. Anesthesiology 78:597–602.

18. Markakis DA, Sayson SC, Schreiner MS (1992) Insertion of the laryngeal mask airway in awake infants with the Robin sequence. Anesth Analg 75:822–824.

19. Park C, Bahk JH, Ahn WS, Do SH, Lee KH (2001) The laryngeal mask airway in infants and children. Can J Anaesth 48:413–417.

20. Marraro GA (2002) Chapter 38: Airway management. In: Bissonnette B, Dalens BJ (eds) Pediatric Anesthesia: Principles and Practice. McGraw-Hill, New York, pp. 778–814.

21. Motoyama EK, Gronert BJ, Fine GF (2006) Chapter 10: Induction of anesthesia, and maintenance of the airway in infants and children. In: Motoyama EK, Davis PJ (eds) Smith's Anesthesia For Infants And Children, 7th edn. Mosby, St. Louis, pp. 347–353.

22. Toursarkissian B, Fowler CL, Zweng TN, Kearney PA (1994) Percutaneous dilational tracheostomy in children and teenagers. J Pediatr Surg 29:1421–1424.

23. Dellinger RP (1990) Fiberoptic bronchoscopy in adult airway management. Crit Care Med 18:882–887.

24. Robles B, Hester J, Brock-Utne JG (1993) Remember the gum-elastic bougie at extubation. J Clin Anesth 5:329–331.

25. Bedger RC, Jr, Chang JL (1987) A jet-stylet endotracheal catheter for difficult airway management. Anesthesiology 66:221–223.

26. Cooper RM, Cohen DR (1994) The use of an endotracheal ventilation catheter for jet ventilation during a difficult intubation. Can J Anaesth 41:1196–1199.

27. Loudermilk EP, Hartmannsgruber M, Stoltzfus DP, Langevin PB (1997) A prospective study of the safety of tracheal extubation using a pediatric airway exchange catheter for patients with a known difficult airway. Chest 111:1660–1665.

28. Hammer GB, Funck N, Rosenthal DN, Feinstein JA (2001) A technique for maintenance of airway access in infants with a difficult airway following tracheal extubation. Paediatr Anaesth 11:622–625.

29. Walker RW, Allen DL, Rothera MR (1997) A fibreoptic intubation technique for children with mucopolysaccharidoses using the laryngeal mask airway. Paediatr Anaesth 7:421–426.

30. Nitahara K, Watanabe R, Katori K, et al. (1999) Intubation of a child with a difficult airway using a laryngeal mask airway and a guidewire and jet stylet. Anesthesiology 91:330–331.

31. Remolina C, Khan AU, Santiago TV, Edelman NH (1981) Positional hypoxemia in unilateral lung disease. N Engl J Med 304:523–525.

32. Heaf DP, Helms P, Gordon I, Turner HM (1983) Postural effects on gas exchange in infants. N Engl J Med 308:1505–1508.

33. Mansell A, Bryan C, Levison H (1972) Airway closure in children. J Appl Physiol 33:711–714.

34. Polgar G, Weng TR (1979) The functional development of the respiratory system from the period of gestation to adulthood. Am Rev Respir Dis 120:625–695.

35. Weatherford DA, Stephenson JE, Taylor SM, Blackhurst D (1995) Thoracoscopy versus thoracotomy: indications and advantages. Am Surg 61:83–86.

36. Mouroux J, Clary-Meinesz C, Padovani B, et al. (1997) Efficacy and safety of videothoracoscopic lung biopsy in the diagnosis of interstitial lung disease. Eur J Cardiothorac Surg 11:22–26.

37. Angelillo-Mackinlay TA, Lyons GA, Chimondeguy DJ, (1996). VATS debridement versus thoracotomy in the treatment of loculated postpneumonia empyema. Ann Thorac Surg 61:1626–1630.

38. Kubota H, Kubota Y, Toyoda Y, (1987). Selective blind endobronchial intubation in children and adults. Anesthesiology 67:587–589.

39. Lammers CR, Hammer GB, Brodsky JB, Cannon WB (1997) Failure to separate and isolate the lungs with an endotracheal tube positioned in the bronchus. Anesth Analg 85:946–947.

40. Cullum AR, English IC, Branthwaite MA. Endobronchial intubation in infancy. Anaesthesia 1973; 28: 66–70.

41. McLellan I (1974) Endobronchial intubation in children. Anaesthesia 29:757–758.

42. Yeh TF, Pildes RS, Salem MR (1978) Treatment of persistent tension pneumothorax in a neonate by selective bronchial intubation. Anesthesiology 49:37–38.

43. Watson CB, Bowe EA, Burk W (1982) One-lung anesthesia for pediatric thoracic surgery: a new use for the fiberoptic bronchoscope. Anesthesiology 56:314–315.

44. Hammer GB, Manos SJ, Smith BM, (1996). Single-lung ventilation in pediatric patients. Anesthesiology 84:1503–1506.

45. Ginsberg RJ (1981) New technique for one-lung anesthesia using an endobronchial blocker. J Thorac Cardiovasc Surg 82:542–546.

46. Lin YC, Hackel A (1994) Paediatric selective bronchial blocker. Paediatr Anaesth 4:391–392.

47. Turner MW, Buchanan CC, Brown SW (1997) Paediatric one lung ventilation in the prone position. Paediatr Anaesth 7:427–429.

48. Borchardt RA, LaQuaglia MP, McDowall RH, Wilson RS (1998) Bronchial injury during lung isolation in a pediatric patient. Anesth Analg 87:324–325.

49. Guyton DC, Besselievre TR, Devidas M, (1997). A comparison of two different bronchial cuff designs and four different bronchial cuff inflation methods. J Cardiothorac Vasc Anesth 11:599–603.

50. Takahashi M, Horinouchi T, Kato M, Hashimoto Y (2000) Double-access-port endotracheal tube for selective lung ventilation in pediatric patients. Anesthesiology 93:308–309.

51. Arndt GA, DeLessio ST, Kranner PW, (1999). One-lung ventilation when intubation is difficult—presentation of a new endobronchial blocker. Acta Anaesthesiol Scand 43:356–358.

52. Hammer GB, Harrison TK, Vricella LA (2002). Single lung ventilation in children using a new paediatric bronchial blocker. Paediatr Anaesth 12:69–72.

53. Kamaya H, Krishna PR (1985) New endotracheal tube (Univent tube) for selective blockade of one lung. Anesthesiology 63:342–343.

54. Karwande SV (1987) A new tube for single lung ventilation. Chest 92:761–763.

55. Gayes JM (1993) Pro: one-lung ventilation is best accomplished with the Univent endotracheal tube. J Cardiothorac Vasc Anesth 7:103–107.

56. Hammer GB, Brodsky JB, Redpath JH, Cannon WB (1998) The Univent tube for single-lung ventilation in paediatric patients. Paediatr Anaesth 8:55–57.

57. Slinger PD, Lesiuk L (1998) Flow resistances of disposable double-lumen, single-lumen, and Univent tubes. J Cardiothorac Vasc Anesth 12:142–144.

58. Kelley JG, Gaba DM, Brodsky JB (1992) Bronchial cuff pressures of two tubes used in thoracic surgery. J Cardiothorac Vasc Anesth 6:190–192.

59. Benumof JL, Gaughan SD, Ozaki G (1992) The relationship among bronchial blocker cuff inflation volume, proximal airway pressure, and seal of the bronchial blocker cuff. J Cardiothorac Vasc Anesth 6:404–408.

60. Brodsky, JB and Mark, JBD (1983) A simple technique for accurate placement of double-lumen endobronchial tubes. Anesth Rev 10, 26–30.

61. Brodsky JB, Macario A, Mark JB (1996) Tracheal diameter predicts double-lumen tube size: a method for selecting left double-lumen tubes. Anesth Analg 82:861–864.

62. Slinger PD (1989) Fiberoptic bronchoscopic positioning of double-lumen tubes. J Cardiothorac Anesth 3:486–496.

63. Benumof JL, Partridge BL, Salvatierra C, Keating J (1987) Margin of safety in positioning modern double-lumen endotracheal tubes. Anesthesiology 67:729–738.

64. Benumof JL, Wahrenbrock EA (1975) Blunted hypoxic pulmonary vasoconstriction by increased lung vascular pressures. J Appl Physiol 38:846–850.

65. Domino KB, Wetstein L, Glasser SA, et al. (1983) Influence of mixed venous oxygen tension (Pvo_2) on blood flow to atelectatic lung. Anesthesiology 59:428–434.

66. Schwarzkopf K, Klein U, Schreiber T, et al. (2001) Oxygenation during one-lung ventilation: the effects of inhaled nitric oxide and increasing levels of inspired fraction of oxygen. Anesth Analg 92:842–847.

67. Fradj K, Samain E, Delefosse D (1999). Placebo-controlled study of inhaled nitric oxide to treat hypoxaemia during one-lung ventilation. Br J Anaesth 82:208–212.

68. Yau KI, Fang LJ, Wu MH (1996) Lung mechanics in infants with left-to-right shunt congenital heart disease. Pediat.Pulmonol 21:42–47.

69. Davies CJ, Cooper SG, Fletcher ME, et al. (1990) Total respiratory compliance in infants and young children with congenital heart disease. Pediatr Pulmonol 8:155–161.

70. Greenspan JS, Davis DA, Russo P, et al. (1996) Infant thoracic surgery: procedure-dependent pulmonary response. J Pediatr Surg 31:878–880.

71. DiCarlo JV, Raphaely RC, Steven JM, et al. (1992) Pulmonary mechanics in infants after cardiac surgery. Crit Care Med 20:22–27.

72. Schindler MB, Bohn DJ, Bryan AC, et al. (1995). Increased respiratory system resistance and bronchial smooth muscle hypertrophy in children with acute postoperative pulmonary hypertension. Am J Respir Crit Care Med 152:1347–1352.

73. Freezer NJ, Lanteri CJ, Sly PD (1993) Effect of pulmonary blood flow on measurements of respiratory mechanics using the interrupter technique. J Appl Physiol 74:1083–1088.

74. Stayer SA, Andropoulos DB, East DL, et al. (2002). Changes in pulmonary mechanics in infants undergoing heart surgery. Anesthesiology 97:A1289 (Abstract).

75. Davis DA, Tucker JA, Russo P (1993) Management of airway obstruction in patients with congenital heart defects. Ann Otol Rhinol Laryngol 102:163–166.

76. Macnaughton PD, Braude S, Hunter DN, (1992). Changes in lung function and pulmonary capillary permeability after cardiopulmonary bypass. Crit Care Med 20:1289–1312.

77. Vincent RN, Lang P, Elixson EM, et al. (1984) Measurement of extravascular lung water in infants and children after cardiac surgery. Am J Cardio 54:161–165.

78. Vincent RN, Lang P, Elixson EM, et al. (1985). Extravascular lung water in children immediately after operative closure of either isolated atrial septal defect or ventricular septal defect. Am J Cardiol 56:536–539.

79. Griese M, Wilnhammer C, Jansen S, Rinker C (1999) Cardiopulmonary bypass reduces pulmonary surfactant activity in infants. J Thorac Cardiovasc Surg 118:237–244.

80. Emhardt JD, Moorthy SS, Brown JW, et al. (1991) Chest radiograph changes after cardiopulmonary bypass in children. J Cardiovasc Surg (Torino) 32:314–317.

81. Kawahito S, Kitahata H, Tanaka K, et al. (2001). Bronchospasm induced by cardiopulmonary bypass. Ann Thorac Cardiovasc Surg 7:49–51.

82. Asimakopoulos G, Smith PL, Ratnatunga CP, Taylor KM (1999) Lung injury and acute respiratory distress syndrome after cardiopulmonary bypass. Ann Thorac Surg 68:1107–1115.

83. Deal C, Osborn JJ, Miller GE, Jr, Gerbode F (1968) Pulmonary compliance in congenital heart disease and its relation to cardiopulmonary bypass. J Thorac Cardiovasc Surg 55:320–327.

84. Rady MY, Ryan T, Starr NJ (1997) Early onset of acute pulmonary dysfunction after cardiovascular surgery: risk factors and clinical outcome. Crit Care Med 25:1831–1839.

85. Gilliland HE, Armstrong MA, McMurray TJ (1999) The inflammatory response to pediatric cardiac surgery: correlation of granulocyte adhesion molecule expression with postoperative oxygenation. Anesth Analg 89:1188–1191.

86. Stayer SA, Andropoulos DB, East DL, et al. (2002). Predictors of duration of mechanical ventilation after congenital heart surgery in infants. Anesthesiology 97:A1224 (Abstract).

87. Guyton AC (1991) Effect of cardiac output by respiration, opening the Chest, and cardiac tamponade. In: Guyton AC, Jones CE, Coleman CE (eds) Circulatory Physiology: Cardiac Output And Its Regulation. WB Saunders, Philadelphia, pp. 378–386.

88. Weber KT, Janicki JS, Shroff S, Fishman AP (1981) Contractile mechanics and interaction of the right and left ventricles. Am J Cardiol 47:686–695.

89. Lumb AB (2000) The pulmonary circulation. In: Lumb AB (ed.) Nunn's Applied Respiratory Physiology. Butterworth-Heinemann, Oxford, pp. 138–162.

90. Malik AB, Kidd BS (1973) Independent effects of changes in H^+ and CO_2 concentrations on hypoxic pulmonary vasoconstriction. J Appl Physiol 34:318–323.

91. Berend N, Christopher KL, Voelkel NF (1982) The effect of positive end-expiratory pressure on functional residual capacity: role of prostaglandin production. Am Rev Respir Dis 126:646–647.

92. Scharf SM, Brown R, Tow DE, Parisi AF (1979) Cardiac effects of increased lung volume and decreased pleural pressure in man. J Appl Physiol 47:257–262.

93. Scharf SM, Brown R, Saunders N, Green LH (1979) Effects of normal and loaded spontaneous inspiration on cardiovascular function. J Appl Physiol 47:582–590.

94. Chang AC, Zucker HA, Hickey PR, Wessel DL (1995) Pulmonary vascular resistance in infants after cardiac surgery: role of carbon dioxide and hydrogen ion. Crit Care Med 23:568–574.

95. Grace MP, Greenbaum DM (1982) Cardiac performance in response to PEEP in patients with cardiac dysfunction. Crit Care Med 10:358–360.

96. Mathru M, Rao TL, El Etr AA, Pifarre R (1982) Hemodynamic response to changes in ventilatory patterns in patients with normal and poor left ventricular reserve. Crit Care Med 10:423–426.

97. Meliones JN, Bove EL, Dekeon MK, et al. (1991) High-frequency jet ventilation improves cardiac function after the Fontan procedure. Circulation 84:III364–III368.

98. Pontoppidan H, Wilson RS, Rie MA, Schneider RC (1977) Respiratory intensive care. Anesthesiology 47:96–116.

99. Stayer SA, Shetty S, Andropoulos DB (2002) Perioperative management of tetralogy of Fallot with absent pulmonary valve. Paediatr Anaesth 12:705–711.

100. Berry CB, Butler PJ, Myles PS (1993) Lung management during cardiopulmonary bypass: is continuous positive airways pressure beneficial? Br J Anaesth 71:864–868.

101. Cogliati AA, Menichetti A, Tritapepe L, Conti G (1996) Effects of three techniques of lung management on pulmonary function during cardiopulmonary bypass. Acta Anaesthesiol Belg 47:73–80.

102. Tusman G, Bohm SH, Tempra A, et al. (2003) Effects of recruitment maneuver on atelectasis in anesthetized children. Anesthesiology 98:14–22.

103. Stayer SA, Andropoulos DB, Bent ST, et al. (2001). Volume ventilation of infants with congenital heart disease: a comparison of Drager, NAD 6000 and Siemens, Servo 900C ventilators. Anesth Analg 92:76–79.

104. Bachiller PR, McDonough JM, Feldman JM (1987) End-tidal P_{CO_2} measurements sampled at the distal and proximal ends of the endotracheal tube in infants and children. Anesth Analg 66(10):959–964.

105. Dreyfuss D, Soler P, Basset G, Saumon G (1988) High inflation pressure pulmonary edema. Respective effects of high airway pressure, high tidal volume, and positive end-expiratory pressure. Am Rev Respir Dis 137:1159–1164.

106. Davis K, Jr, Branson RD, Campbell RS, Porembka DT (1996) Comparison of volume control and pressure control ventilation: is flow waveform the difference? J Trauma 41:808–814.

107. Rappaport SH, Shpiner R, Yoshihara G, et al. (1994) Abraham E. Randomized, prospective trial of pressure-limited versus volume-controlled ventilation in severe respiratory failure. Crit Care Med 22:22–32.

108. Badgwell JM, Swan J, Foster AC (1996) Volume-controlled ventilation is made possible in infants by using compliant breathing circuits with large compression volume. Anesth Analg 82:719–723.

109. Badgewell JM, McLeod ME, Lerman J, et al. (1987) End-tidal P_{CO_2} measurements sampled at the distal and proximal ends of the endotracheal tube in infants and children. Anesth Analg 66:959–964.

110. Stayer SA, Bent ST, Campos CJ (2000) Comparison of NAD 6000 and servo 900C ventilators in an infant lung model. Anesth Analg 90 (2):315–321.

111. Stayer SA, Bent ST, Skjonsby BS, et al. (2000) Pressure control ventilation: three anesthesia ventilators compared using an infant lung model. Anesth Analg 91 (5): 1145–1150.

112. Ramamoorthy C, Tabbutt S, Kurth CD, et al. (2002) Effects of inspired hypoxic and hypercapnic gas mixtures on cerebral oxygen saturation in neonates with univentricular heart defects. Anesthesiology 96:283–288.

113. Tabbutt S, Ramamoorthy C, Montenegro LM, et al. (2001) Impact of inspired gas mixtures on preoperative infants with hypoplastic left heart syndrome during controlled ventilation. Circulation 104:I159–I164.

114. Kinsella JP, Neish SR, Ivy DD, et al. (1993). Clinical responses to prolonged treatment of persistent pulmonary hypertension of the newborn with low doses of inhaled nitric oxide. J Pediatr 123:103–108.

115. Roberts JD, Polaner DM, Lang P, Zapol WM (1992) Inhaled nitric oxide in persistent pulmonary hypertension of the newborn. Lancet 340:818–819.

116. Wessel DL, Adatia I, Giglia TM, et al. (1993) Use of inhaled nitric oxide and acetylcholine in the evaluation of pulmonary hypertension and endothelial function after cardiopulmonary bypass. Circulation 88:2128–2138.

117. Morris K, Beghetti M, Petros A (2000) Comparison of hyperventilation and inhaled nitric oxide for pulmonary hypertension after repair of congenital heart disease. Crit Care Med 28:2974–2978.

118. Rossaint R, Falke KJ, Lopez F, et al. (1993). Inhaled nitric oxide for the adult respiratory distress syndrome. N Engl J Med 328:399–405.

119. Abman SH, Griebel JL, Parker DK, et al. (1994) Acute effects of inhaled nitric oxide in children with severe hypoxemic respiratory failure. J Pediatr 124:881–888.

120. Bigatello LM, Hurford WE, Kacmarek RM, et al. (1994) Prolonged inhalation of low concentrations of nitric oxide in patients with severe adult respiratory distress syndrome. Effects on pulmonary hemodynamics and oxygenation. Anesthesiology 80:761–770.

121. Puybasset L, Stewart T, Rouby JJ, et al. (1994) Inhaled nitric oxide reverses the increase in pulmonary vascular resistance induced by permissive hypercapnia in patients with acute respiratory distress syndrome. Anesthesiology 80:1254–1267.

122. Putensen C, Rasanen J, Downs JB (1994) Effect of endogenous and inhaled nitric oxide on the ventilation-perfusion relationships in oleic-acid lung injury. Am J Respir Crit Care Med 150:330–336.

123. Day RW, Guarin M, Lynch JM, et al. (1996) Inhaled nitric oxide in children with severe lung disease: results of acute and prolonged therapy with two concentrations. Crit Care Med 24:215–221.

124. Gothberg S, Edberg KE (2000) Inhaled nitric oxide to newborns and infants after congenital heart surgery on cardiopulmonary bypass. A dose–response study. Scand Cardiovasc J 34:154–158.

125. Day RW, Hawkins JA, McGough EC, (2000) Randomized controlled study of inhaled nitric oxide after operation for congenital heart disease. Ann Thorac Surg 69: 1907–1912.

126. Curran RD, Mavroudis C, Backer CL, et al. (1995). Inhaled nitric oxide for children with congenital heart disease and pulmonary hypertension. Ann Thorac Surg 60: 1765–1771.

19 Regional anesthesia and postoperative pain management

M. Gail Boltz, M.D.
Lucile Packard Children's Hospital, Stanford University School of Medicine, Stanford, California, USA

Gregory B. Hammer, M.D.
Lucile Packard Children's Hospital, Stanford University School of Medicine, Stanford, California, USA

Dean B. Andropoulos, M.D., M.H.C.M.
Texas Children's Hospital, Baylor College of Medicine, Houston, Texas, USA

Introduction

Treatment of pain following cardiac surgery is the subject of a growing number of publications and presentations given the current trend toward fast-track management of cardiac surgery patients. Tracheal extubation in the operating room (OR) or within a few hours of reaching the intensive care unit has become common practice after the repair of simple cardiac defects [1–6]. This precludes the use of large doses of systemic opioids during and after surgery due to resultant respiratory depression. An alternative approach to the treatment of postoperative pain is therefore required.

Neuraxial anesthesia involves the use of intrathecal or epidural opioids with or without local anesthetic agents. The use of neuraxial anesthesia in combination with general anesthesia for children undergoing cardiac surgery

has been reported to facilitate early tracheal extubation following cardiac surgery in children [7,8]. Reported benefits of neuraxial anesthesia in patients having cardiac surgery include attenuation of the neuroendocrine response to surgical stress, improved postoperative pulmonary function, enhanced cardiovascular stability, and improved postoperative analgesia. To the extent that neuraxial anesthesia facilitates early tracheal extubation in cardiac surgical patients, complications and costs associated with postoperative mechanical ventilation may be reduced. These benefits must, however, be weighed against the adverse effects that may accompany the use of neuraxial anesthesia. These include hypotension, postoperative respiratory depression, and epidural hematoma formation. In this chapter, the benefits and risks of neuraxial anesthesia in infants and children having open-heart surgery are reviewed. In addition, specific techniques currently in use are described.

Anesthesia for Congenital Heart Disease 2nd edition. Edited by
Dean Andropoulos, Stephen Stayer, Isobel Russell and Emad Mossad.
© 2010 Blackwell Publishing.

The benefits of neuraxial anesthesia in cardiac surgery

Adverse physiologic responses which occur during and after cardiac surgery include alterations in circulatory (tachycardia, hypertension, vasoconstriction), metabolic (increased catabolism), immunologic (impaired immune response), and hemostatic (platelet activation) systems [9,10]. Together, these changes are referred to as the "stress response." The stress response associated with cardiac surgery in neonates may be profound and is associated with increased morbidity and mortality. Anand et al. measured the stress response during and after cardiac surgery in 15 neonates anesthetized with halothane and morphine [11]. They found elevated plasma concentrations of epinephrine, norepinephrine, cortisol, glucagon, and beta-endorphin in all patients, accompanied by hyperglycemia and lactic acidemia. The four deaths in the study group occurred in neonates with the greatest stress responses.

Bromage et al. first demonstrated in 1971 that the stress response associated with major abdominal and thoracic surgery could be attenuated with epidural blockade [12]. Since then, several investigators have shown that the use of neuraxial anesthesia during and after cardiac surgery (i.e., intraoperative anesthesia and postoperative analgesia) may decrease the stress response as well as morbidity and mortality [13–20]. Neuraxial anesthesia (intrathecal or epidural blockade) with opioids and/or local anesthetics appears to be more effective in inhibiting the stress response associated with surgery than intravenous (IV) opioids. For example, epidural fentanyl is more effective than IV fentanyl in reducing the stress response after thoracotomy in adults [21]. Epidural morphine administration was shown to attenuate the adverse decrease in triiodothyronine (T3) concentration in children undergoing open-heart surgery compared with general anesthesia alone [18]. Epidural anesthesia with bupivacaine suppresses the increase in serum catecholamines, glucose, and ACTH more effectively than IV fentanyl in infants [19]. Epidural local anesthetics may be more efficacious than opioids in attenuating the stress response [20]. In a study of fetal lambs, total spinal anesthesia completely blocked the stress response to surgical manipulation and cardiopulmonary bypass [22]. Humphries recently evaluated the effects of high spinal anesthesia in infants and children younger than 3 years undergoing cardiac surgery with cardiopulmonary bypass. They compared a high-dose bupivacaine technique delivered during and after surgery through a small spinal catheter with a conventional high-dose opioid technique in a prospective randomized trial of 60 patients [23]. The authors were able to demonstrate virtual elimination of catecholamine responses with spinal anesthesia and improved plasma lactate in the perioperative period compared to opioid-based anesthesia. In addition, their data suggested that spinal anesthesia may moderate the rise in IL-6 after surgery compared to opioid anesthesia either due to better preservation of splanchnic blood flow during bypass or by reducing the adverse sympathetic effects on the heart after cardioplegia and ischemia.

IV anesthetic techniques do not appear to mitigate the stress response. Gruber et al. studied the effects on the stress response of IV fentanyl and midazolam on 45 infants undergoing cardiac surgery [24]. Patients were randomized to receive fentanyl 0.05–0.10 mg/kg with or without midazolam 0.10 mg/kg/h during the surgery. Plasma epinephrine, norepinephrine, cortisol, adrenocortical hormone, glucose, and lactate were measured at five intervals during and after surgery. In all groups, plasma epinephrine, norepinephrine, cortisol, glucose, and lactate concentrations were significantly greater at the completion of surgery than prior to skin incision. The authors concluded that fentanyl-dosing strategies, with or without midazolam, do not prevent a hormonal or metabolic stress response in infants undergoing cardiac surgery.

Additional benefits that may be attributed to neuraxial anesthesia include improved pulmonary function, greater circulatory stability, and reduced pain scores. Several randomized, controlled studies in adults have shown that patients receiving epidural analgesia have better pulmonary function after thoracic surgery than those treated with IV opioids. Thoracic epidural opioids are associated with improved pulmonary function following chest surgery compared with IV opioids [25]. In a study comparing thoracic epidural meperidine to IV meperidine for postoperative analgesia, the patients receiving epidural infusions had significantly greater forced expiratory volumes in 1 second (FEV1) and forced vital capacity (FVC), and were more cooperative with deep breathing maneuvers than those in the IV meperidine group [26]. Thoracic epidural anesthesia may also improve respiratory performance postoperatively by effecting an improvement in diaphragmatic function [27].

Early tracheal extubation is an important factor in reducing ICU length of stay and the duration of hospitalization [4]. Especially in children with single ventricle physiology (e.g., following bilateral cavopulmonary anastomosis or modified Fontan operations), spontaneous ventilation may result in improved hemodynamics by decreasing intrathoracic pressure and thereby increasing pulmonary blood flow [28]. Early tracheal extubation may also obviate or reduce complications associated with mechanical ventilation, including trauma to the lungs and airways, inadvertent dislodgement or malpositioning of the tracheal tube, and adverse hemodynamic changes associated with tracheal suctioning. The cost of mechanical ventilation can be avoided in patients who are extubated in the OR [4]. A number of studies have shown that infants and children can be safely extubated within several hours following the completion of surgery [1,2,29,30]. The majority of reports of early extubation following open-heart surgery in infants and children include a period of 6–8 hours of mechanical ventilation in the ICU after surgery. A limited number of reports describe tracheal extubation in the OR at the completion of surgery.

Early extubation without neuraxial anesthesia

In an early report of tracheal extubation in the OR following congenital heart surgery, Schuller et al. reviewed the records of 209 children who had undergone repair of congenital heart defects [31]. Fifty-two percent of infants between the ages of 3 and 12 months and 88% of patients older than 12 months were extubated in the OR. Four patients were reintubated in the OR or ICU. Inhaled agents were supplemented with low doses of fentanyl to provide anesthesia. Similarly, Burrows et al. reviewed the management of 36 children undergoing repair of secundum atrial septal defects (ASDs) under isoflurane and fentanyl anesthesia [3]. The tracheas of 19 children (53%) were extubated in the OR. Compared to those children receiving postoperative mechanical ventilation, these patients had shorter cardiopulmonary bypass times (24 vs 32 min) and received lower doses of fentanyl (5.9 mcg/kg vs 35.1 mcg/kg).

Laussen et al. reported tracheal extubation in the OR after ASD repair as part of a clinical practice guideline in children [5]. Of 66 children reviewed subsequent to the implementation of the practice guideline, 25 patients (38%) were extubated in the OR, while the remainder received postoperative mechanical ventilation. The children in the early extubation group received less fentanyl (6 mcg/kg vs 27.5 mcg/kg), were more likely to have a respiratory acidosis on admission to the intensive care unit, and had an increased frequency of vomiting in the intensive care unit. Eight children in the early extubation group received caudal morphine 50–75 mcg/kg versus two children in the postoperative mechanical ventilation group. There was no difference in ICU stay nor in clinical outcomes. The patients extubated in the OR had significantly lower hospital charges due to the absence of postoperative mechanical ventilation.

Cray et al. reported the use of propofol with "low-dose" opioid anesthesia to facilitate early tracheal extubation following cardiac surgery in children between the ages of 6 months and 18 years [6]. Isoflurane and fentanyl (up to a maximum dose of 20 mcg/kg) were given prior to and during cardiopulmonary bypass. In patients for whom early tracheal extubation was considered, a propofol infusion was started at 50 mcg/kg/min as well as a morphine infusion at a dose of 10–40 mcg/kg/min. The median time to tracheal extubation was 5 hours. The goal of extubation within 6 hours was achieved in 56 children (62%). Causes for prolonged intubation included bleeding and phrenic nerve palsy. One child was reintubated shortly following extubation due to excessive respiratory depression.

In recent years, even higher risk patients have been extubated in the OR, without neuraxial anesthesia. Vida et al. [32] reported a retrospective series of 100 pediatric patients with subaortic ventricular septal defect (VSD) and pulmonary hypertension who received 10 mcg/kg fentanyl, 1 mg/kg ketorolac, and sevoflurane for anesthesia. 65% of these patients were extubated in the OR, and another 25% were extubated within 6 hours of ICU admission, with only 2 reintubations. Thus, it appears that early extubation is successful without neuraxial anesthesia in many patients.

Neuraxial anesthesia and early extubation

Neuraxial anesthesia techniques have been used to facilitate early tracheal extubation following cardiac surgery, improve postoperative analgesia, and reduce the incidence of side effects caused by IV opioids. Jones et al. reported the use of intrathecal morphine for postoperative analgesia in 56 children undergoing cardiac surgery [33]. Following induction of anesthesia, patients received intrathecal morphine 0.02 or 0.03 mg/kg. Tracheal extubation was performed in all patients after admission to the ICU shortly following the completion of surgery. The duration of analgesia in both groups was similar, with two-thirds of patients requiring no supplemental analgesia for more than 18 hours.

In a retrospective review of pain control in 91 children undergoing cardiac surgery, Shayevitz et al. compared lumbar epidural morphine infusions to IV opioid analgesia [34]. In the epidural analgesia group, lumbar epidural catheters were placed following induction of anesthesia. Preservative-free morphine sulfate was administered in an initial dose of 0.05 mg/kg followed by a continuous infusion of 0.003–0.004 mg/kg/h during and after surgery. Children in the IV analgesia group received an initial dose of fentanyl 0.05 mg/kg IV followed by a continuous infusion of 0.018 mg/kg/h IV during surgery. The fentanyl infusion was reduced to 0.006 mg/kg/h IV postoperatively. Patients in the epidural analgesia group had significantly lower pain scores and received significantly less supplemental analgesia postoperatively than patients in the IV analgesia group.

In a prospective, randomized, controlled study, Rosen and Rosen evaluated the efficacy of caudal epidural morphine compared with IV morphine in 32 children following open cardiac surgery [35]. Patients in the study group received a caudal injection of preservative-free morphine sulfate 0.075 mg/kg in the OR following surgery prior to awakening and tracheal extubation. Children in the control group received IV morphine alone for postoperative analgesia. Supplemental doses of IV morphine were given to children in both groups as needed, prior to which pain scores were recorded. Children having received caudal morphine required significantly less IV morphine and had significantly lower pain scores postoperatively than patients in the control group. The mean duration of complete analgesia in children receiving caudal morphine was 6 hours (range 2–12 h), but decreased analgesic requirements were noted for the entire 24-hour study period.

In another prospective, randomized, controlled study, Hammer, et al. compared postoperative analgesia in children receiving a remifentanil-based anesthetic with or without spinal anesthesia for open-heart surgery [36]. Patients in both groups were extubated in the OR immediately following the completion of surgery. IV fentanyl was administered according to age appropriate pain scores postoperatively. Patients in the spinal anesthesia group received significantly less fentanyl during the initial 8- and 24-hour periods following surgery than those in the control group ($p < 0.01$, $p = 0.02$, respectively). There was a trend toward lower pain scores in patients receiving spinal anesthesia compared with those in the control group ($p = 0.16$, $p = 0.15$, respectively).

In addition to the benefits of improved lung function and pain control, patients receiving neuraxial anesthesia have fewer opioid-related side effects than patients treated with IV opioids. Patients receiving epidural anesthesia have more rapid return of bowel function following surgery compared with those receiving IV analgesics. In a recent review of 16 studies comparing epidural and systemic analgesia with regard to postoperative recovery of gastrointestinal function, all 8 studies with epidural catheter placement above T12 showed more rapid recovery of bowel function when epidural analgesia was used [37]. The use of postoperative thoracic epidural analgesia with bupivacaine and morphine was associated with earlier return of gastrointestinal function and decreased hospital costs due to shortened hospital stay compared with IV morphine patient-controlled analgesia (PCA) [38]. A study comparing epidural versus IV fentanyl analgesia following thoracotomy also reported a lower incidence of nausea, shorter duration of ileus, and earlier hospital discharge in the epidural analgesia group [21].

Caudal anesthesia and analgesia has been utilized to facilitate early extubation even in higher risk patient groups. Heinle et al. [39] reported that in a series of 56 patients younger than 90 days, undergoing surgery with bypass, all of whom received single shot caudal morphine, 50–75 mcg/kg, 45% of patients were extubated in the OR or within 3 hours of ICU admission. Jaquiss et al. [40] reported a series of 68 patients undergoing Fontan opera-

tion, where early extubation is highly desirable because of the effect of positive pressure ventilation on venous return in this physiology. Patients received caudal bupivacaine and morphine at the beginning of the case, and 85% were extubated in the OR.

In the absence of a well-designed, prospective, randomized controlled study of neuraxial analgesia versus standard analgesic techniques, the data reviewed above suggests that successful early extubation, even in some higher risk patients, can be achieved with or without caudal, spinal, or epidural analgesia.

Adverse effects of neuraxial anesthesia for cardiac surgery

Although neuraxial anesthesia offers many benefits, adverse effects may occur. The most serious complications that may be associated with neuraxial anesthesia for cardiac surgery are hypotension, respiratory depression, and epidural hematoma formation.

Systemic arterial hypotension is an undesired effect of intrathecal and epidural local anesthetic blockade. In adults with coronary artery stenosis and myocardial ischemia, local anesthetic-induced blockade of cardiac sympathetic nerve activation alleviates angina and improves coronary blood flow and ventricular function [20,41–43]. However, local anesthetic blockade to upper thoracic dermatomes produces hypotension accompanied by a decrease in coronary artery perfusion [13,44]. In infants and young children, local anesthetic blockade to T3–T5 does not produce significant changes in blood pressure nor heart rate [45]. This may be attributable to decreased sympathetic innervation of the lower extremities and/or immaturity of the sympathetic nervous system in young children. In two recent studies of high spinal blockade in children undergoing open-heart surgery, hemodynamic stability was demonstrated in all patients [7,46].

Respiratory depression may be seen in children following the administration of epidural opioids in doses exceeding 0.05 mg/kg [47]. In a study of children undergoing cardiac surgery and receiving epidural morphine in an initial dose of 0.05 mg/kg followed by a continuous infusion, however, respiratory depression did not occur [34]. Several other studies in children have shown excellent analgesia and no evidence of respiratory depression when the dose of epidural morphine does not exceed 0.05 mg/kg [48–50].

Similarly, doses of intrathecal morphine exceeding 0.02 or 0.03 mg/kg may result in significant respiratory depression following cardiac surgery in children [33]. Intrathecal morphine 0.01 mg/kg has also been associated with respiratory depression postoperatively when combined with midazolam and IV fentanyl 0.02 mg/kg in adult patients undergoing cardiac surgery [51]. However, in a review of children given intrathecal morphine in a dose of 0.02 mg/kg in whom no IV opioids were administered during surgery, no patient had postoperative respiratory depression [52]. In addition, no child required supplemental opioid analgesia for at least 15 hours following surgery. In a recent study comparing intrathecal morphine in doses of 0.005, 0.007, and 0.010 mg/kg in children having open-heart surgery, the trachea of each patient was extubated at the conclusion of surgery and no patient had signs of respiratory depression [53]. Hammer et al. reported results of a study of postoperative respiratory depression in children anesthetized with remifentanil with or without spinal anesthesia for open-heart surgery [54]. The authors found only mild elevation in arterial CO_2 tension in children in both groups following surgery. No patient required intervention for respiratory depression.

Epidural hematoma formation following epidural or spinal anesthesia is a rare but potentially catastrophic complication of neuraxial blockade. In an analysis of 20 series, including more than 850,000 cases of epidural blockade and 650,000 cases of spinal anesthesia in adult patients, only 3 case reports of epidural hematoma were documented [55]. Based on these data, the author estimated the risk of epidural hematoma to be 1:150,000 following epidural anesthesia and 1:220,000 following spinal anesthesia. Unfortunately, it is unknown what the incidence of clotting disorders, use of anticoagulants, or traumatic procedures was in these reports.

In a thorough review of the literature from 1906 through 1994, Vandermeulen et al. found 61 published cases of epidural or subdural hematoma following epidural or spinal anesthesia in adult patients [56]. Of these 61 cases, 42 occurred in patients with impaired coagulation prior to epidural or spinal needle placement, including 25 patients receiving heparin. In 15 patients, the procedure was reported to be difficult and/or traumatic. A clotting disorder or difficult/traumatic needle placement was present in 53 of the 61 cases (87%).

In a series of over 4,000 epidural or spinal anesthetics performed prior to anticoagulation with heparin for vascular surgery, no cases of epidural hematoma were reported [57]. The authors highlighted important precautions that were undertaken in these patients, including delaying surgery for 24 hours in the event of traumatic needle placement, allowing at least 1 hour between needle placement and heparin administration. Other recommended precautions include use of the smallest dose of heparin necessary to achieve therapeutic objectives and removal of epidural catheters only when normal coagulation function has been restored [58]. Although traumatic needle placement may increase the risk of hemorrhage, there is no data to guide the practitioner as to whether or not surgery should be cancelled. Patients must be monitored postoperatively for signs of unexpected motor blockade suggestive of epidural hematoma formation. When epidural analgesia is used following surgery, the minimum effective concentration of local anesthetic should be administered to allow early detection of an epidural hematoma [59]. Epidural hematoma formation has not been reported in a patient following spinal or epidural anesthesia performed prior to cardiopulmonary bypass.

Pediatric data regarding neuraxial hematoma are sparse, but a symptomatic intraspinal hematoma has been reported in a neonate undergoing noncardiac surgery from a caudal epidural catheter threaded to the lumbar level [60]. In the largest series reported to date, 961 pediatric patients undergoing cardiothoracic surgery who received catheter epidural techniques were studied [61]. Caudal, lumbar, and thoracic sites were studied, and heparinized and nonheparinized cases, as well as coarctation of aorta repairs were included. There was a 7.9% incidence of observing blood through the needle or catheter during placement, and 88% of these incidents were with caudal catheters. Surgery apparently was not delayed in these cases, but a median of 90 minutes elapsed between catheter placement and heparinization for caudal catheters, and 183 minutes for thoracic epidurals. No neurological deficits attributable to the epidurals were noted in any patient, including 60 patients undergoing coarctation repair, 3 of whom bled during catheter placement. Rosen et al. [62] reported a case of epidural hematoma in an 18-year-old after aortic valve replacement with a thoracic epidural catheter placed in the OR before bypass. After an uncomplicated surgery and first 48 hours postoperatively, the patient received heparin bolus for thromboprophylaxis and then several hours later a dose of tissue plasminogen activator for an obstructed vascular catheter. Acute back pain and paraplegia ensued, necessitating emergency drainage of the epidural hematoma and restoration of normal neurological functioning.

Despite the paucity of reports of neurological injury with neuraxial techniques, and their benefits to facilitate early extubation and pain control, neuraxial anesthesia for cardiac surgery in children remains a very controversial topic, and awaits large-scale controlled studies [63]. Many anesthesiologists would consider that a simple median sternotomy does not produce severe enough pain in the average patient to justify the risk of major neuraxial techniques when bypass and full heparinization are used.

Neuraxial anesthesia techniques

A variety of neuraxial blockade techniques have been reported in children undergoing cardiac surgery. These include intrathecal (spinal) and epidural techniques utilizing opioids and/or local anesthetics. Epidural approaches include single dose ("single shot") caudals as well as thoracic, lumbar, and caudal catheter techniques.

Intrathecal (spinal) techniques

The use of spinal opioid analgesia as an adjunct to general anesthesia was first described by Mathews and Abrams in 1980 [64]. In this report, 40 adults received intrathecal morphine in a dose of 1.5–4.0 mg prior to surgery. All patients remained comfortable for more than 24 hours. Subsequently, many studies have demonstrated the efficacy of spinal opioids, primarily morphine, in producing analgesia following cardiac surgery in adult patients. These reports have been summarized elsewhere [58]. Although intrathecal morphine alone has not been shown to attenuate the stress response associated with cardiac surgery per se, it may attenuate the stress response in the immediate postoperative period [65].

In order to augment the effects of intrathecal opioids in reducing the stress response and circulatory instability in patients undergoing cardiac surgery, local anesthetics have been used in combination with intrathecal opioids. In adults, however, intrathecal injection of local anesthetics in doses needed to attain high spinal blockade results in hypotension [66]. Young children, on the other hand, do not develop hypotension following high spinal blockade. Finkel et al. studied the hemodynamic effects of spinal anesthesia in children undergoing cardiac surgery [46]. In this study, 30 children between the ages of 7 months and 13 years received intrathecal morphine mixed with tetracaine following induction of general anesthesia and tracheal intubation. The dose of tetracaine was adjusted for age, according to the estimated volume of cerebrospinal fluid. Patients aged 6–12 months received intrathecal tetracaine 2.0 mg/kg, those between the ages of 1 and 3 years received 1.0 mg/kg, and those older than 4 years received 0.5 mg/kg. Tetracaine was mixed with 10% dextrose to yield a 0.5% hyperbaric solution, and all patients received preservative-free morphine in a dose of 0.005–0.010 mg/kg. Patients were placed in a 30° head-down (Trendelenburg) position for a minimum of 10 minutes following administration of the intrathecal solution. Although there was mild slowing of the heart rate in children older than 4 years, there was no clinically significant bradycardia nor hypotension observed. Hammer et al. have also reported hemodynamic stability following intrathecal tetracaine/morphine in children undergoing cardiac surgery [7].

The use of spinal anesthesia in combination with general anesthesia has been reported in children for whom tracheal extubation is planned prior to leaving the OR following open-heart surgery [7]. Surgical procedures included repair of ASD and/or VSD, anomalous pulmonary venous return, aortic or pulmonary valvuloplasty, right

Table 19.1 Dosing regimens for spinal anesthesia

Age (yr)	Tetracaine (mg/kg)	Morphine (mg/kg)
<1	2.0	0.007
1–3	1.0	0.007
4–8	0.5	0.007
>8	0	0.010

ventricle-to-pulmonary artery conduit placement or exchange, bidirectional cavopulmonary shunt, and the modified Fontan procedure. Spinal anesthetic blocks (SABs) were performed immediately after tracheal intubation (i.e., prior to placement of arterial and central venous catheters) in order to maximize the time interval between SAB and heparinization for cardiopulmonary bypass. Patients were placed with the head of the table 30° down for a minimum of 15 minutes following SAB. No IV opioids were administered intraoperatively. The authors' dosing regimen for SAB is shown in Table 19.1.

Epidural techniques

The use of postoperative epidural analgesia in patients undergoing open-heart surgery was first described by Hoar et al. in 1976 [67]. Subsequently, El-Baz and Goldin reported the use of epidural blockade initiated prior to surgical incision [17]. In 1989, Rosen and Rosen first reported the efficacy of epidural morphine analgesia in children undergoing cardiac surgery [35]. Since then, many studies have reported favorable results with epidural anesthesia and analgesia for cardiac surgery [58].

In general, epidural anesthesia is used in patients undergoing open-heart surgery for whom tracheal extubation is planned in the OR following the completion of surgery or shortly thereafter. The epidural technique most commonly used in children is the administration of a single dose of morphine injected into the caudal epidural space. Morphine is favored for caudal epidural administration due to its low lipid solubility and tendency to spread cephalad to thoracic dermatomes [68,69]. Following induction of general anesthesia and tracheal intubation, preservative-free morphine sulfate is injected in a dose of 0.05–0.10 mg/kg into the caudal epidural space via an epidural needle or IV catheter. IV opioids, if administered intraoperatively, are given in restricted doses (e.g., fentanyl 0.01–0.02 mg/kg).

Alternatively, a caudal epidural catheter may be inserted to facilitate continuous administration of morphine during and after surgery. Following an initial dose of epidural morphine 0.04 mg/kg, a continuous infusion is begun in a dose of 0.0075 mg/kg/h. The infusion is continued throughout the intraoperative period and maintained postoperatively for 48–72 hours.

In order to attenuate the stress response associated with cardiac surgery and cardiopulmonary bypass as

(a)

(b)

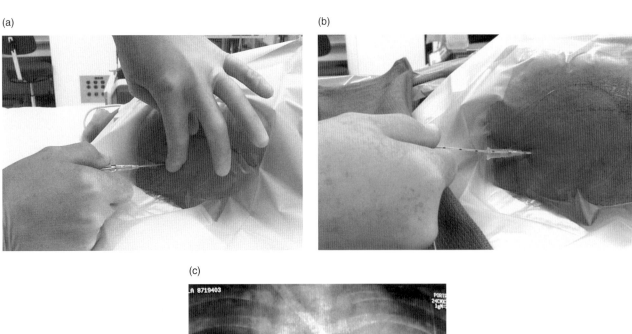

(c)

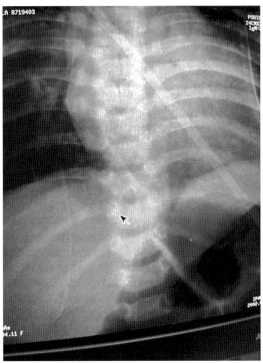

Figure 19.1 Placement of a thoracic epidural catheter via the caudal route. (a) An 18-g angiocatheter is used to access the caudal space. (b) A 20-g epidural catheter is threaded through the angiocatheter, to the low thoracic region. ECG guidance, electrical nerve root stimulation, or ultrasound can be used to determine and guide the location of the catheter tip. (c) Chest radiograph with catheter in low thoracic (T10) region (*arrow*)

well as optimize postoperative analgesia, a combination of epidural opioids and local anesthetic agents may be used. Although local anesthetic agents may spread to thoracic dermatomes when administered via the caudal epidural space, potentially toxic doses of local anesthetics may be required to achieve thoracic analgesia [70,71]. Thoracic epidural blockade may be achieved with greater safety and efficacy by placing the epidural catheter tip in proximity to the spinal segment associated with surgical incision. Segmental anesthesia may then be achieved with

lower doses of local anesthetic than those needed when the catheter tip is distant from the surgical site. In infants, a catheter can be advanced from the caudal to the thoracic epidural space [72]. For example, with the infant in the lateral decubitus position, a 20-gauge epidural catheter may be inserted via an epidural needle or an 18-gauge IV catheter placed through the sacrococcygeal membrane and advanced 16–18 cm to the mid-thoracic epidural space (Figure 19.1). Minor resistance to passage of the catheter may be overcome by simple flexion or extension

(a)

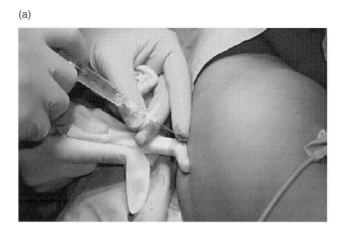

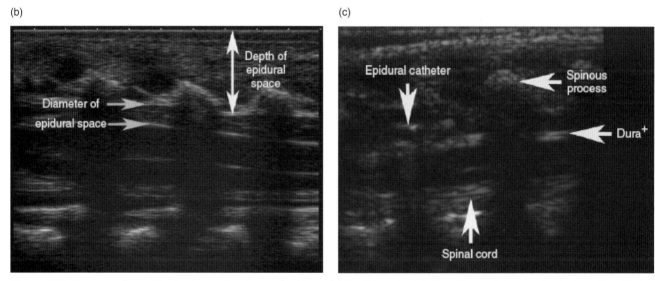

Figure 19.2 Placement of an epidural catheter using ultrasound guidance. (a) Needle insertion is in the midline, and ultrasound probe is positioned in the paramedian longitudinal position. (b) Identification of epidural space. Depth of epidural space is the distance between the skin and the ligamentum flavum. Upper horizontal arrow indicates the ligamentum flavum and lower horizontal arrow indicates the dura. (c) Epidural catheter tip identified in epidural space (*arrow*) (Used with permission from Reference [75])

of the spine. If continued resistance is encountered, no attempt should be made to advance the catheter further, as the catheter may become coiled within or exit the epidural space. A newly described method to guide placement of caudal epidural catheters at thoracic dermatomes is to use the electrocardiogram [73]. All catheters in this report were within two vertebrae of the target. Additional novel methods to place epidural catheters in the desired dermatomal location include epidural nerve root electrical stimulation, and ultrasound guidance [74] (Figure 19.2). Radiographic confirmation of tip location should be undertaken postoperatively. In older children, a thoracic epidural catheter may be inserted directly between T4 and T8 to provide intraoperative anesthesia and postoperative analgesia. As with SAB, epidural catheter placement should be performed immediately following tracheal intubation in order to maximize the time elapsed prior to heparin administration for cardiopulmonary bypass. Hammer et al. reported the use of an initial dose of hydromorphone 0.007–0.008 mg/kg and 0.25% bupivacaine 0.5 mL/kg [7]. Subsequent doses of 0.25% bupivacaine 0.3 mL/kg are administered intraoperatively at approximately 90-minute intervals. No IV opioids are given during surgery. Postoperatively, a continuous infusion of 0.10% bupivacaine and hydromorphone 0.003 mg/mL is administered at a rate of 0.3 mL/kg/h. Intraoperative and postoperative thoracic epidural local anesthetic regimens are listed in Table 19.2. An advantage of epidural catheter compared with "single shot" techniques is that adjustments can be made in dosing postoperatively according to the patient's level of comfort. For example, a "bolus" of epidural anesthetic agents may be given and the infusion rate increased if the

Table 19.2 Local anesthetics dosing regimens for thoracic epidural anesthesia

Intraoperative dosing	Postoperative infusion
Bupivacaine 0.25%: 0.5 mL/kg initial and then 0.3 mL/kg every 90 min	0.1%: 0.15–0.3 mL/kg/h, max dose 0.4 mg/kg/h
Ropivacaine 0.2% 0.5 mL/kg initial and then 0.3 mL/kg every 90 min	0.1%: 0.15–0.3 mL/kg/h, max dose 0.4 mg/kg/h

patient is experiencing pain. Alternatively, the infusion may be decreased if the patient becomes somnolent. Table 19.3 lists suggested regimens for thoracic epidural narcotics.

Ropivacaine is a newer long-acting local anesthetic agent that has the advantage of reduced cardiotoxicity and neurotoxicity compared to bupivacaine [76,77]. It also has less propensity to cause motor blockade in children [78]. Its pharmacokinetics for long-term (2–4 days) infusion via lumbar or low thoracic epidural catheter has been studied, and plasma levels are well within the safe range in children 4 months to 7 years in age undergoing major abdominal surgery [79]. Analgesia was excellent and side effects few with 0.2% ropivacaine infused at 0.4 mg/kg/h. Of note is that starting doses for neonates and young infants younger than 3 months should be reduced by 50% because of reduced clearance of all agents due to renal and hepatic immaturity in this age group.

In a retrospective case-control study of 117 patients undergoing repair of ASD, VSD, or tetralogy of Fallot, 46 of whom received caudal anesthesia consisting of 1 mL/kg of 0.25% bupivacaine and 70–110 mcg/kg of caudal morphine, Leyvi et al. [80] reported that the tetralogy of Fallot patients receiving caudal anesthesia had a higher rate of extubation by 4 hours postoperatively (65% vs 30%), but no differences in ICU or hospital length of stay, or complications. Finally, Diaz et al. [81] reported 15 patients who had thoracic epidural catheter placement to provide analgesia for pediatric bilateral sequential lung transplant patients who underwent thoracosternotomy (clamshell) incision, with full heparinization and bypass. Seven patients had catheters placed preoperatively, and eight postoperatively within 12 hours of ICU admission when international normalized ratio was <1.5, platelet count > 100,000, fibrinogen > 200 mg/dL, and there was no clinical bleeding. Patients received either 0.1% ropivacaine, or 0.125% bupivacaine infusion with 2–5 mcg/kg fentanyl, for a median of 4 days, with catheter removal only when laboratory and clinical parameters noted above were achieved. Median time to extubation was 12 hours, with good to excellent pain relief and no complications.

Treatment of side effects

Side effects related to neuraxial opioids include nausea and vomiting, pruritus, somnolence, respiratory depression, and urinary retention. Nausea and vomiting as well as pruritus appear to be relatively uncommon in infants and are primarily seen in children older than 3 years. These side effects are more common with morphine compared with hydromorphone and fentanyl [82]. Due to greater rostral spread, respiratory depression is also more common when morphine is used compared with hydromorphone [68,82]. Urinary retention is seen most commonly during the initial 24 hours of therapy, during which time the majority of patients have urinary catheters in place. Suggested treatment for side effects related to spinal and epidural opioids is shown in Table 19.4. Most of these patients will initially be cared for in a monitoring unit, but many will be discharged to a ward setting within 24–48 hours, and need appropriate monitoring for respiratory depression and motor blockade while receiving epidural infusions.

Table 19.3 Thoracic epidural narcotics

Agent	Intraoperative bolus (mcg/kg)	Postoperative infusion
Fentanyl (thoracic)	1–2	1–5 mcg/mL: 0.25–1 mcg/kg/h
Hydromorphone (caudal/lumbar)	7–8	10–30 mcg/mL: 2–3 mcg/kg/h
Morphine (caudal/lumbar)	50–75	50 mcg/mL: 4–6 mcg/kg/h

Note: Reduce doses of all agents 50% for infants younger than 3 months; use local anesthetic doses at lower end of range for thoracic epidural catheters.

Adjuncts and alternatives to neuraxial analgesia

Clonidine

In order to decrease the incidence and magnitude of side effects associated with spinal and epidural opioids, a variety of drugs may be used to provide supplemental analgesia. Recently, the use of epidural and intrathecal clonidine to provide postoperative analgesia has been described. Clonidine has been shown to prolong and potentiate the effects of local anesthetics by as much as 50–114% [83–85]. The addition of clonidine in an initial dose of 1–2 mcg/kg followed by a continuous infusion of 0.08–0.12 mcg/kg/h with bupivacaine or ropivicaine appears safe and effective for use in children. Motsch et al. compared caudal

Table 19.4 Treatment for side effects of neuraxial opioid administration

Side effect	Treatment	Comments
Nausea/vomiting	Metoclopromide 0.1–0.2 mg/kg/dose IV Q 6 h Maximum dose: 10 mg	Extrapyramidal reactions may occur but are uncommon
	Droperidol 0.025–0.05 mg/kg IV Q 6 h prn Maximum dose: 1.25 mg	Very sedating; avoid if somnolent
	Diphenhydramine 0.5–1.0 mg/kg IV Q 6 h prn Maximum dose: 50 mg	Very sedating; avoid if somnolent
	Ondansetron 0.1–0.2 mg/kg IV Q 6 h prn Maximum dose: 4 mg	May substitute other 5-HT3 antagonist, e.g., granisetron or dolasetron
	Nalbuphine 0.1 mg/kg IV Q 6 h prn	
	Naloxone 0.001–0.005 mg/kg/hr infusion	Excessive doses may compromise analgesia
	Propofol 0.001–0.010 mg/kg h infusion	
Pruritus	Diphenhydramine 0.5–1.0 mg/kg IV Q 6 h prn Maximum dose: 50 mg	Very sedating; avoid if somnolent
	Nalbuphine 0.1 mg/kg IV Q 6 h prn	
	Naloxone 0.001–0.005 mg/kg/h infusion	Excessive doses may compromise analgesia
Somnolence	Decrease epidural opioid infusion Consider low-dose naloxone infusion (above)	
Respiratory depression	Severe Administer 100% O_2 via facemask Initiate positive pressure ventilation prn Naloxone 0.001–0.010 mg/kg IV Stop epidural infusion Subsequently/Mild–moderate depression Increase F_{IO_2} Reduce epidural opioid infusion Naloxone 0.001–0.005 mg/kg/h infusion	
Urinary retention	Replace urinary catheter prn	

clonidine 5 mcg/kg with 0.175% bupivacaine to 0.175% bupivicaine alone. The authors reported a prolongation of caudal blockade with the addition of clonidine, but some sedation, hypotension, and bradycardia were seen at this dose [86].

Patient controlled analgesia

For patients who are not receiving a regional anesthetic technique to provide postoperative analgesia, systemic opioids are used to treat postoperative pain. Although

Table 19.5 Patient-controlled analgesia regimens

Agent	Bolus dose (mcg/kg)	Continuous rate (mcg/kg/hr)	4-h limit (mcg/kg)
Morphine	15–25	4–15	300
Hydromorphone	3–5	1–3	60
Fentanyl	0.25	0.15	4

Note: Patient should be developmentally normal 6–7 years of age or older; meperidine is contraindicated for patient-controlled analgesia.

intermittent intramuscular and subcutaneous injections have been used widely in the past, these routes of administration are painful and are associated with unpredictable and erratic uptake and distribution. Intermittent IV injections with opioids of short or moderate duration are also associated with periods of excessive sedation and inadequate analgesia. Continuous analgesia may be achieved when opioids are administered by continuous IV infusion with or without "PCA" dosing.

Morphine is commonly used for postoperative analgesia. In neonates younger than 1 month, clearance is reduced and elimination half-life is prolonged, about three times that in adults [87]. For continuous infusions of morphine, a loading dose of 0.025–0.075 mg/kg followed by infusion rates of 0.005–0.015 mg/kg/h result in therapeutic plasma concentrations in neonates [88]. Older infants and children require a loading dose of 0.05–0.10 mg/kg followed by an initial infusion rate of 0.01–0.03 mg/kg/h. In children receiving PCA, dosing in the range of 0.01–0.03 mg/kg with a lockout interval of 6–10 minutes with or without a continuous infusion has been recommended [89]. In children at risk for morphine-induced histamine release, fentanyl (0.0005–0.001 mg/kg/hr ± 0.0005–0.001 mg/kg PCA dose) or hydromorphone (0.003–0.005 mg/kg/h ± 0.003–0.005 mg/kg PCA dose) may be used [88]. PCA dosing regimens are listed in Table 19.5.

The use of methadone, which has a half-life of approximately 19 hours in children older than 1 year, may provide more continuous analgesia than shorter-acting agents [90,91]. For moderate-to-severe pain, intermittent IV doses of methadone between 0.05 mg/kg and 0.08 mg/kg as needed may be given [92].

The side effects that may occur with IV opioid administration are similar to those described with epidural opioids, and may be treated similarly (Table 19.4). With epidural or IV techniques, improved analgesia and a decrease in opioid dosing (and side effects) may be achieved with concomitant administration of nonopioid analgesic agents. Ketamine has been administered in a subhypnotic dose by continuous infusion to achieve sedation and analgesia in adults during mechanical ventilation after major

surgery [93]. In a study by Hartvig, 10 children were given continuous infusions of ketamine supplemented with intermittent doses of midazolam to provide analgesia and sedation after cardiac surgery [94]. Ketamine infusions were administered in doses of 1 and 2 mg/kg/h. Both ketamine infusion regimens provided acceptable analgesia and sedation during and after weaning from mechanical ventilation. Psychomimetic effects were not seen and may have been suppressed by the supplemental use of midazolam. Ketamine infusions can also be used to decrease morphine requirements and may be useful in patients developing signs of spinal cord sensitization [95].

Local anesthetic wound infusions

A recent addition to postoperative analgesia techniques is the use of local anesthetic infusions via a small tunneled multiorifice catheter placed subcutaneously in the surgical wound. Tirotta et al. [96] reported a prospective, randomized, controlled, double-blind study of the infusion of 0.25% bupivacaine or levobupivacaine of 40 pediatric patients undergoing cardiac surgery with bypass. A catheter connected to an elastomeric continuous infusion pump (OnQ Pump, I-Flow Corp., Lake Forest CA, USA) delivered local anesthetic dose predetermined by weight at a maximum of 0.4 mg/kg/h. IV morphine dose was reduced by 50% in the treatment group, and plasma levels of local anesthetic remained well below toxic levels in all patients.

Nonsteroidal anti-inflammatory agents

Nonsteroidal anti-inflammatory drugs (NSAIDs) are commonly used as an adjunct to other forms of analgesia after thoracic surgery, but their use after cardiac surgery is controversial [97]. NSAID use in cardiac surgical patients has been limited by the risks of gastritis, renal impairment, and inhibition of platelet aggregation. NSAIDs exert their antinociceptive action by blocking the peripheral synthesis of prostaglandins through inhibition of the cyclooxygenase enzymes (COX-1 and COX-2). A central mechanism has also been proposed. Inhibition of COX-2 causes gastritis, platelet dysfunction, and renal impairment [98]. Studies evaluating the use of NSAIDs after cardiac surgery have concluded that a morphine-sparing effect is present. In 120 patients scheduled for elective coronary artery bypass surgery, diclofenac, ketoprofen, and indomethacin were compared to placebo. Diclofenac appeared to have the best analgesic effect as evidenced by reducing the need for morphine and other analgesic agents postoperatively [99]. The short-term use of NSAIDs in the postoperative period does not appear to be associated with increased bleeding from the surgical site nor with an increased incidence of gastrointestinal bleeding [100]. In a prospective, randomized trial of ketorolac 0.5 mg/kg Q6H for 48 hours plus morphine, versus morphine alone in 70 pediatric patients undergoing cardiac surgery with bypass, Gupta et al. [101] found that chest tube output was not different between groups. Morphine dosage was also not different, creatinine change was not different between groups, and one patient had gastrointestinal bleeding in the ketorolac group.

Acetaminophen suppositories are a frequently overlooked but effective adjunct to other analgesic methods in infants and children following major surgery. An initial dose of 30–45 mg/kg (maximum dose 1000 mg), followed by 20 mg/kg every 6 hours, for 48–72 hours, has a narcotic sparing effect, with negligible danger of toxicity [102,103]. IV acetaminophen preparations are now available and have been used for postoperative analgesia in children; however, the benefit of this agent in pediatric cardiac surgery has not been studied [104].

Conclusions

The use of epidural and spinal anesthesia in infants and children may attenuate the stress response and thereby decrease morbidity and mortality associated with cardiac surgery. In addition, the use of these neuraxial anesthesia techniques during and after cardiac surgery may result in improved pulmonary function, greater circulatory stability, and better postoperative pain control compared with general anesthesia and postoperative IV opioid analgesia. To the extent that neuraxial anesthesia may facilitate tracheal extubation in the OR immediately following surgery, complications and the expense associated with mechanical ventilation in the postoperative period may be avoided. In those patients who undergo tracheal extubation in the ICU, cost savings may be achieved due to reductions in time of mechanical ventilation and ICU length of stay, as well as earlier resumption of a regular diet.

The risks of epidural and spinal anesthesia in these patients include undesired side effects (nausea and vomiting, pruritus), hypotension, respiratory depression, and epidural hematoma formation. The incidence of side effects does not appear to exceed that associated with IV opioid analgesia. Hypotension, associated with local anesthetic spinal and epidural blockade in adult patients, is uncommon in infants and young children. Postoperative respiratory depression is greatly reduced by avoiding intraoperative opioids and using prudent doses of spinal and epidural opioids.

The risk of epidural hematoma formation is small but finite. This risk can be minimized by employing reasonable safeguards. Appropriate precautions include selecting patients with normal coagulation function prior to

needle placement, abandoning the neuraxial anesthesia technique if needle placement is difficult, and delaying surgery in the event of return of blood via the needle or epidural catheter. The time interval between needle placement and heparin administration should be maximized, allowing for an interval of at least 60 minutes. Epidural catheters should be removed only after normal coagulation function has been restored following surgery.

Future studies may provide additional information regarding the dose–response relationships of neuraxial anesthetic agents in patients undergoing cardiac surgery. Modulation of the stress response in neonates, e.g., utilizing total spinal anesthesia, warrants investigation. In addition, strategies to decrease the incidence of opioid related side effects (e.g., prophylactic antiemetic therapy) may be developed.

References

1. Marianeschi SM, Seddio F, Mcelhinney DB (2000) Fast-track congenital heart operations: a less invasive technique and early extubation. Ann Thorac Surg 69:872–876.
2. Vricella LA, Dearani JA, Gundry SR (2001) Ultra-fast track in elective congenital heart surgery. Ann Thorac Surg 69:865–871.
3. Burrows FA, Taylor RH, Hillier SC (1992) Early extubation of the trachea after repair of secundum-type atrial septal defects in children. Can J Anaesth 39:1041–1044.
4. Turley K, Tyndall M, Turley K, et al. (1995) Radical outcome method. A new approach to critical pathways in congenital heart disease. Circulation 92:II245–II249.
5. Laussen PC, Reid RW, Stene RA (1996) Tracheal extubation of children in the operating room after atrial septal defect repair as part of a practice guideline. Anesth Analg 82:988–993.
6. Cray SH, Holtby HM, Kartha VM (2001) Early tracheal extubation after paediatric cardiac surgery: the use of propofol to supplement low-dose opioid aneaesthesia. Paediatrc Anaesth 11:465–471.
7. Hammer GB, Ngo K, Macario A (2000) A retrospective examination of regional plus general anesthesia in children undergoing open heart surgery. Anesth Analg 90:1020–1024.
8. Peterson KL, DeCampli WM, Pike NA, et al. (2000) Regional anesthesia in pediatric cardiac surgery: report of 220 cases. Anesth Analg 90:1014–1019.
9. Weissman C (1990) The metabolic response to stress: an overview and update. Anesthesiology 73:308–327.
10. Kehlet H (1989) Surgical stress: the role of pain and analgesia. Br J Anaesth 63:189–195.
11. Anand KJS, Hansen DD, Hickey PR (1990) Hormonal-metabolic stress responses in neonates undergoing cardiac surgery. Anesthesiology 73:661–670.
12. Bromage PR, Shibata HR, Willoughby HW (1971) Influence of prolonged epidural blockade on blood sugar and

cortisol responses to operations upon the upper part of the abdomen and thorax. Surg Gynecol Obstet 132:1051–1056.

13. Kirno K, Friberg P, Grzegorczyk A (1994) Thoracic epidural anesthesia during coronary artery bypass surgery: effects on cardiac sympathetic activity, myocardial blood flow and metabolism, and central hemodynamics. Anesth Analg 79:1075–1081.

14. Stenseth R, Bjella L, Berg EM (1994) Thoracic epidural analgesia in aortocoronary bypass surgery, II. Effects on the endocrine metabolic response. Acta Anaesthesiol Scand 38:834–839.

15. Moore CM, Cross MH, Desborough JP (1995) Hormonal effects of thoracic extradural analgesia for cardiac surgery. Br J Anaesth 75:387–393.

16. Fawcett WJ, Edwards RE, Quinn AC (1997) Thoracic epidural analgesia started after cardiopulmonary bypass. Adrenergic, cardiovascular and respiratory sequelae. Anaesthesia 52:294–299.

17. El-Baz N, Goldin M (1987) Continuous epidural infusion of morphine for pain relief after cardiac operations. J Thorac Cardiovasc Surg 93:878–883.

18. Rosen DA, Rosen KR, Matheny JM (1997) Maintenance of T3 levels in children undergoing cardiac surgery. Anesthesiology 87:A1069.

19. Wolf AR, Eyres RL, Laussen PC (1993) Effect of extradural analgesia on stress responses to abdominal surgery in infants. Br J Anaesth 70:654–660.

20. Liu S, Carpenter RL, Neal JM (1995) Epidural anesthesia and analgesia: their role in postoperative outcome. Anesthesiology 82:1474–1506.

21. Salomaki TE, Leppaluoto J, Laitinen JO (1993) Epidural vs. intravenous fentanyl for reducing hormonal, metabolic, and physiologic responses after thoracotomy. Anesthesiology 79:672–679.

22. Fenton KN, Heinemann MK, Hickey PR (1994) Inhibition of the fetal stress response improves cardiac output and gas exchange after fetal cardiac bypass. J Thorac Cardiovasc Surg 107:1416–1422.

23. Humphreys N, Bays, SM, Parry AJ, et al (2005) Spinal anesthesia with an indwelling catheter reduces the stress response in pediatric open heart surgery. Anesthesiology 103:1113–1120.

24. Gruber EM, Laussen PC, Casta A (2001) Stress response in infants undergoing cardiac surgery: a randomized study of fentanyl bolus, fentanyl infusion, and fentanyl-midazolam infusion. Anesth Analg 92:882–890.

25. Guinard JP, Mavrocordatos P, Chiolero R (1992) A randomized comparison of intravenous versus lumbar and thoracic epidural fentanyl for analgesia after thoracotomy. Anesthesiology 77:1108–1115.

26. Slinger P, Shennib H, Wilson S (1995) Postthoracotomy pulmonary function: a comparison of epidural versus intravenous meperidine infusion. J Cardiothorac Vasc Anesth 9:128–134.

27. Mankikan B, Cantineau JP, Berttrand M (1988) Improvement in diaphragmatic function by a thoracic extradural block after upper abdominal surgery. Anesthesiology 68:1379–1386.

28. Penny DJ, Reddington AN (1991) Doppler echocardiographic evaluation of pulmonary blood flow after the Fontan operation: the role of the lungs. Br Heart J 66:372–374.

29. Barash PG, Lescovich F, Katz JD (1980) Early extubation following pediatric cardiac operation: a viable alternative. Ann Thorac Surg 29:228–233.

30. Heard GG, Lamberti JJ, Park SM (1985) Early extubation of the trachea after open heart surgery for congenital heart disease. Crit Care Med 13:830–832.

31. Schuller JL, Bovill JG, Nijveld A (1984) Early extubation of the trachea after open heart surgery for congenital heart disease. Br J Anaesth 56:1101–1108.

32. Vida VL, Leon-Wyss J, Rojas M, et al. (2006) Pulmonary artery hypertension: is it really a contraindicating factor for early extubation in children after cardiac surgery? Ann Thorac Surg 81:1460–1465.

33. Jones SEF, Beasley JM, Macfarlane DWR (1984) Intrathecal morphine for postoperative pain relief in children. Br J Anaesth 56:137–140.

34. Shayevitz JR, Merkel S, O'Kelly SW (1996) Lumbar epidural morphine infusions for children undergoing cardiac surgery. J Cardiothorac Vasc Anesth 10:217–224.

35. Rosen KR, Rosen DA (1989) Caudal epidural morphine for control of pain following open heart surgery in children. Anesthesiology 70:418–421.

36. Hammer GB, Drover D, Jackson E, et al. (2002) Comparison of remifentanil with or without spinal anesthesia for children undergoing open heart surgery. Anesthesiology 96:A1222.

37. Steinbrook RA (1998) Epidural anesthesia and gastrointestinal motility. Anesth Analg 886:837–844.

38. de Leon-Casasola OA, Karabella D, Lema MJ (1996) Bowel function recovery after radical hysterectomies: thoracic epidural bupivacaine-morphine versus intravenous patient-controlled analgesia with morphine—a pilot study. J Clin Anesth 8:87–92.

39. Heinle JS, Diaz LK, Fox LS (1997) Early extubation after cardiac operations in neonates and young infants. J Thorac Cardiovasc Surg 114:413–418.

40. Jaquiss RD, Siehr SL, Ghanayem NS, et al. (2006) Early cavopulmonary anastomosis after Norwood procedure results in excellent Fontan outcome. Ann Thorac Surg 82:1260–1265.

41. Kock M, Blomberg S, Emanuelsson H (1990) Thoracic epidural anesthesia improves global and neuraxial left ventricular function during stress-induced myocardial ischemia in patients with coronary artery disease. Anesth Analg 71:625–630.

42. Blomberg SG (1994) Long term home self-treatment with high thoracic epidural anesthesia in patients with severe coronary artery disease. Anesth Analg 79:413–421.

43. Blomberg S, Curelaru I, Emanuelsson H (1989) Thoracic epidural anesthesia in patients with unstable angina pectoris. Eur Heart J 10:437–444.

44. Sivarajan M, Amory DW, Lindbloom LE (1975) Systemic and regional blood-flow changes during spinal anesthesia in the rhesus monkey. Anesthesiology 43:78–88.

45. Dohi S, Naito H, Takahashi T (1979) Age-related changes in blood pressure and duration of motor block in spinal anesthesia. Anesthesiology 50:319–323.

46. Finkel JC, Boltz MG, Conran AM (1998) Hemodynamic changes during spinal anesthesia in children undergoing open heart surgery. Anesth Analg 86:S400.

47. Krane EJ, Tyler DC, Jacobson LE (1989) The dose response of caudal morphine in children. Anesthesiology 71:48–52.

48. Wolf AR, Hughes D, Hobbs AJ (1991) Combined morphine–bupivacaine caudals for reconstructive penile surgery in children: systemic absorption of morphine and post-operative analgesia. Anaesth Intens Care 19:17–21.

49. Shapiro LA, Jedeikin RJ, Shalev D (1984) Epidural morphine analgesia in children. Anesthesiology 61:210–212.

50. Krane EJ, Jacobson LE, Lynn AM (1987) Caudal morphine for postoperative analgesia in children: a comparison with caudal bupivacaine and intravenous morphine. Anesth Analg 66:647–653.

51. Chaney MA, Furry PA, Fluder EM (1997) Intrathecal morphine for coronary artery bypass grafting and early extubation. Anesth Analg 84:241–248.

52. Tobias JD, Deshpande JK, Wetzell RC (1990) Postoperative analgesia: use of intrathecal morphine in children. Clin Pediatr 29:44–48.

53. Finkel JC, Doyle JM, Conran AM (1997) A comparison of 3 intrathecal morphine doses during spinal anesthesia in children having open heart surgery. Anesthesiology 87:A1052.

54. Hammer GB, Drover D, Jackson E, et al. (2002) Postoperative respiratory depression in children anesthetized with remifentanil with or without spinal anesthesia for open heart surgery. Anesthesiology 96:A1223.

55. Tryba M (1993) Epidural regional anesthesia and low molecular weight heparin: Pro [German]. Anasth Intensivmed Notfallmed Schmertzther 28:179–181.

56. Vandermeulen EP, Van Aken H, Vermylen J (1994) Anticoagulants and spinal-epidural anesthesia. Anesth Analg 79:1165–1177.

57. Rao TLK, El-Etr AA (1981) Anticoagulation following placement of epidural and subarachnoid catheters: an evaluation of neurologic sequelae. Anesthesiology 55:618–620.

58. Chaney MA (1997) Intrathecal and epidural anesthesia and analgesia for cardiac surgery. Anesth Analg 84:1211–1221.

59. Liu SS, Mulry MF (1998) Neuraxial anesthesia and analgesia in the presence of standard heparin. Reg Anesth Pain Med 6 (Suppl. 2):157–163.

60. Bressehan C, Krumpholz R, Jost R, et al. (2001) Intraspinal haematoma following lumbar epidural anesthesia in a neonate. Paediatr Anaesth 11:105–108.

61. Rosen DA, Rosen KR, Gustafson RA, et al 2001) Long-term follow-up in children undergoing cardiothoracic procedures with epidural anesthesia/analgesia. Anesthesiology 95 A1298.

62. Rosen DA, Hawkinberry DW, Rosen KR, et al. (2004) An epidural hematoma in an adolescent patient after cardiac surgery. Anesth Analg 98:966–969.

63. Steven JM, McGowan FX (2000) Neuraxial blockade for pediatric cardiac surgery: lessons yet to be learned. Anesth Analg 90:1011–1013.

64. Mathews ET, Abrams LD (1980) Intrathecal morphine in open heart surgery (correspondence). Lancet 2:543.

65. Vanstrum GS, Bjornson KM, Ilko R (1988) Postoperative effects of intrathecal morphine in coronary bypass surgery. Anesth Analg 67:261–267.

66. Kowalewski RJ, MacAdams CL, Eagle CJ (1994) Anaesthesia for coronary bypass surgery supplemented with subarachnoid bupivacaine and morphine: A report of 18 cases. Can J Anaesth 41:1189–1195.

67. Hoar PF, Hickey PF, Ullyot DJ (1976) Systemic hypertension following myocardial revascularization: A method of treatment using epidural anesthesia. J Thorac Cardiovasc Surg 71:859–864.

68. Bromage PR, Camporesi EM, Durant PAC (1982) Rostral spread of epidural morphine. Anesthesiology 56:431–436.

69. Dahlstrom B (1986) Pharmacokinetics and pharmacodynamics of epidural and intrathecal morphine. Int Anesthesiol Clin 24:29–42.

70. Schulte-Steinberg O, Rahlfs VW (1982) Spread of extradural analgesia following caudal injection in children. Br J Anaesth 49:1027–1034.

71. Satoyoshi M, Kaniyama Y (1984) Caudal anaesthesia for upper abdominal surgery in infants and children: a simple calculation of the volume of local anaesthesia. Acta Anaesthesiol Scand 28:57–60.

72. Bosenberg AT, Bland BA, Schulte-Steinberg O (1988) Thoracic epidural anesthesia via the caudal route in infants. Anesthesiology 69:265–269.

73. Tsui BC, Seal R, Koller J (2002) Thoracic epidural catheter placement via the caudal approach in infants by using electrocardiographic guidance. Anesth Analg 95:326–330.

74. Tsui BC (2006) Innovative approaches to neuraxial blockade in children: the introduction of epidural nerve root stimulation and ultrasound guidance for epidural catheter placement. Pain Res Manag 11:173–180.

75. Willscheke H, Marhofer P, Bosenberg A, et al. (2006) Epidural catheter placement in children: comparing a novel approach using ultrasound guidance and a standard loss-of-resistance technique. Br J Anaesth 97:200–207.

76. Graf BM, Abraham I, Eberbach N, Kunst G, Stowe DR, Martin E (2002) Differences in cardiotoxicity of bupivacaine and ropivacaine are the result of physicochemical and stereoselective properties. Anesthesiology 96:1427–1434.

77. Ladd LA, Chang DH, Wilson KA, Copeland SE, Plummer JL, Mather LE (2002) Effects of CNS site-directed carotid arterial infusions of bupivacaine, levobupivacaine, and ropivacaine in sheep. Anesthesiology 97:418–428.

78. Ivani G, DeNegri P, Conio A, et al. (2002) Comparison of racemic bupivacaine, ropivacaine, and levo-bupivacaine for pediatric caudal anesthesia: effects on postoperative analgesia and motor block. Reg Anesth Pain Med 27:157–161.

79. Hansen TG, Ilett KF, Lim SI, et al. (2000) Pharmacokinetics and clinical efficacy of long-term epidural ropivacaine infusion in children. Br J Anaes 85:347–353.

80. Leyvi G, Taylor DG, Reith E, et al. (2005) Caudal anesthesia in pediatric cardiac surgery: does it affect outcome? J Cardiothorac Vasc Anesth 19:734–738.

81. Diaz LK, Elidemir O, Heinle JS, et al. (2005) Thoracic epidural anesthesia in pediatric lung transplant recipients. Pediatr Crit Care Med 6:392 (Abstract).

82. Goodarzi, M (1999) Comparison of epidural morphine, hydromorphone and fentanyl for postoperative pain control in children undergoing orthopaedic surgery. Paediatr Anaesth 9:419–422.

83. Nishima K, Mikawa K, Shiga M (1999) Clonidine in paediatric anaesthesia. Paediatr Anaesth 9:187–202.

84. Eisenach JC, Hood DD, Curry R (1998) Intrathecal, but not intravenous, clonidine reduces experimental thermal or capsaicin-induced pain and hyperalgesia in normal volunteers. Anesth Analg 87:591–596.

85. De Negri P, Ivani G, Visconti C (2001) The dose–response relationship for clonidine added to a postoperative continuous epidural infusion of ropivicaine in children. Anesth Analg 93:71–76.

86. Motsch J, Bottinger B, Bach A (1997) Caudal clonidine and bupivicaine for combined epidural and general anesthesia in children. Acta Anaesthesiol Scand 41:877–883.

87. Lynn AM, Slattery JT (1987) Morphine pharmacokinetics in early infancy. Anesthesiology 66:136–139.

88. Lynn AM, Opheim KE, Tyler DC (1984) Morphine infusion after pediatric cardiac surgery. Crit Care Med 12:863–866.

89. . Yaster M, Billett C, Monitto C (1997) Intravenous patient controlled analgesia. In: Yaster M (ed.) Pediatric Pain Management and Sedation. Mosby, St. Louis, pp. 89–112.

90. Berde CB, Beyer JE, Bournaki MC, et al. (1991) A comparison of morphine and methadone for prevention of postoperative pain in 3 to 7 year old children. J Pediatr 119:136–141.

91. Berde CB, Sethna NF, Holtzman RS, et al. (1987) Pharmacokinetics of methadone in children and adolescents in the perioperative period. Anesthesiology 67:A519.

92. Berde CB (1989) Pediatric postoperative pain management. Pediatr Clin North Am 36:921–940.

93. Domino EF, Domino ES, Smith RE (1984) Ketamine kinetics in premedicated and diazepam-premedicated subjects. Clin Pharmacol Ther 36:645–653.

94. Hartvig P, Larsson E, Joachimsson P (1993) Postoperative analgesia and sedation following pediatric cardiac surgery using a constant infusion of ketamine. J Cardiothorac Vasc Anesth 7:148–153.

95. Chow TKF, Penberthy AJ, Goodchild CS (1998) Ketamine as an adjunct to morphine in postthoracotomy analgesia: an unintended N-of-1 study. Anesth Analg 87:1372–1374.

96. Tirotta CF, Lagueruela RG, Munro HM, et al. (2005) A continuous incosional infusion of either levobupivacaine 0.25% or bupivacaine 0.25% in pediatric patients. Anesthesiology 103:A1333 (Abstract).

97. Kruger M, McRae K (1999) Pain management in cardiothoracic practice. Surg Clin North Am 79:387–398.

98. Bailey K, Karski J, Zulys V (1994) Safety of indomethacin in the early postoperative period following aortocoronary bypass surgery. Can J Anaesth 41:A41.

99. Hynninen M, Cheng DC, Hossain I (2000) Non-steroidal anti-inflammatory drugs in treatment of postoperative pain after cardiac surgery. Can J Anaesth 47:1182–1187.

100. Laitinen J, Nuutinen LS, Puranen J (1992) Effect of nonsteroidal anti-inflammatory drug, diclofenac, on haemostasis in patients undergoing total hip replacement. Acta Scand 36:486–489.

101. Gupta A, Daggett C, Drant S, et al. (2004) Prospective randomized trial of ketorolac after congenital heart surgery. J Cardiothorac Vasc Anesth 18:454–457.

102. Montgomery CJ, McCormack JP, Reichert CC, et al. (1995) Plasma concentrations after high-dose (45 mg/kg) rectal acetaminophen in children. Can J Anaes 42:982–986.

103. Birmingham PK, Tobin MH, Henthorn TK, et al. (1997) Twenty four hour pharmacokinetics of rectal acetaminophen in children: an old drug with new recommendations. Anesthesiology 87:244–252.

104. Palmer GM, Atkins M, Anderson BJ, et al. (2008) I.V. acetaminophen pharmacokinetics in neonates after multiple doses. Br J Anaesth 101:523–530.

5 Anesthesia for Specific Lesions

20 Anesthesia for left-to-right shunt lesions*

Scott G. Walker, M.D.

Riley Hospital for Children, Indiana University School of Medicine, Indianapolis, Indiana, USA

Introduction

Left-to-right shunt lesions are the most common congenital heart defects, accounting for approximately 50% of

*Portions of this chapter were previously published as Chapter 18: Anesthesia for Left-to-Right Shunt Lesions, by Sabrina T. Bent, M.D., M.S., in *Anesthesia for Congenital Heart Disease*, 1st edn.

Anesthesia for Congenital Heart Disease 2nd edition. Edited by Dean Andropoulos, Stephen Stayer, Isobel Russell and Emad Mossad.
© 2010 Blackwell Publishing.

all lesions. They are defined by a communication between the systemic and pulmonary circulations that allows shunting of well-oxygenated (systemic) blood to the less-oxygenated (pulmonary) circuit. This definition applies whether the associated structures are located on the left or right side anatomically. For instance, a child with a ventricular septal defect (VSD) and ventricular inversion will shunt blood from the right-sided systemic ventricle to the subpulmonic, lower pressure left-sided ventricle. Degree of shunting through a left-to-right shunt lesion may be limited by the size of the defect or the resistance to blood flow on either side. For example, shunting between high-pressure systems like the ventricles through a large VSD is dependent on the ratio of pulmonary vascular resistance (PVR) to systemic vascular resistance (SVR). In contrast, left-to-right shunting through a large atrial septal defect (ASD) occurs primarily during atrial contraction and is dependent on the relative diastolic compliances of the right and left ventricles into which the atria eject.

All left-to-right shunts produce a volume burden on the cardiovascular system, the effects of which vary according to the location of the shunt. Shunting at the level of the great arteries results in increased pulmonary artery blood flow, which increases pulmonary venous return to the left atrium, leading to increased left ventricular end-diastolic volume and left ventricular stroke work by the Frank–Starling mechanism. The left ventricle gradually dilates and hypertrophies, producing increased left ventricular end-diastolic pressure followed by increased left atrial pressure. Shunting at level of the great arteries also produces a decrease in diastolic blood pressure from runoff of blood into the low-pressure pulmonary circuit after closure of the aortic valve. Low diastolic pressures decrease coronary perfusion, potentially creating ischemia from decreased myocardial oxygen delivery in the setting of increased oxygen demand from the hypertrophied ventricle. The final result is pulmonary edema from pulmonary venous congestion and left heart failure. As PVR increases, there is an increased pressure burden on the right ventricle and eventual right heart failure.

Shunting at the atrial or ventricular level, if significant, results in an increased right ventricular volume load in addition to the hemodynamic effects present with shunting at the great artery level. Prolonged exposure of the pulmonary vasculature to increased flow and pressure results in a fixed increase in PVR. When PVR exceeds the SVR, shunt reversal occurs resulting in cyanosis, erythrocytosis, and eventually polycythemia. Eisenmenger's syndrome results when this level of PVR becomes irreversible.

Hemoglobin concentration is another contributing factor to the amount of left-to-right shunting. Elevated blood viscosity, which rises with increasing hemoglobin concentration, increases both PVR and SVR. The net effect is a reduction in left-to-right shunting. The physiologic decline in hemoglobin concentration in the first 3 months of life is thought to have a substantial role in the normal fall of PVR after birth, and may contribute to exacerbation of symptoms related to left-to-right shunting. Figure 20.1 presents a schematic representation of the pathophysiology of the left-to-right shunting lesions.

The normal compensatory mechanisms that maintain systemic cardiac output and myocardial performance in the patient with a left-to-right shunt include the Frank–Starling mechanism, the sympathetic nervous system, and hypertrophy of the myocardium. Manifestations of these compensatory mechanisms include sweating and

tachycardia. Infants are also often tachypneic from decreased lung compliance associated with increased pulmonary blood flow. Tachypnea impairs feeding, and growth failure develops from both decreased caloric intake and increased caloric utilization. Although significant left-to-right shunts induce biventricular failure, infants rarely manifest peripheral edema or jugular venous distension like adults; the most consistent sign of right-sided failure is hepatomegaly.

Anesthetic management for left-to-right shunt lesions should be individualized to the patient, but certain generalities do exist. Premedication with intravenous or oral drugs such as midazolam (0.05–0.1 mg/kg IV or 0.75–1.0 mg/kg PO) can be safely administered for the purpose of decreasing anxiety and providing more controlled induction of anesthesia [1]. Standard American Society of Anesthesiologists (ASA) monitors, along with the use of invasive arterial and central venous pressure monitoring and careful attention to urine output, are recommend for all cases involving cardiopulmonary bypass. Transesophageal echocardiography (TEE), cerebral oximetry, and cerebral blood flow monitoring are also useful monitoring adjuncts (see Chapters 10 and 11 for a more detailed discussion). Patients with severe, poorly controlled congestive heart failure (CHF) may be intolerant to the myocardial depressant effects of inhalational anesthetics, and for this group of patients intravenous anesthesia with fentanyl and midazolam is preferred [2–4]. In most situations, however, inhalation induction with sevoflurane is a viable option when intravenous access is not initially available.

Additional anesthetic issues include avoidance of air bubbles in intravenous lines to prevent paradoxical emboli. The anesthesiologist must be cognizant of the pulmonary vasodilatory effect of oxygen and hypocarbia and manipulate ventilation in order to balance the PVR and SVR. Such measures generally include minimizing the FIO_2 and avoiding hyperventilation (maintaining $PaCO_2$ between 40–50 mm Hg).

Patent ductus arteriosus

The ductus arteriosus is an essential component in normal fetal circulation; it becomes functionally closed within 10–15 hours after birth and permanently closes by thrombosis, intimal proliferation, and fibrosis in the first 2–3 weeks. Functional closure is initiated by several mechanisms including aeration of the lungs, removal of prostaglandins produced in the placenta, increased arterial PO_2, and release of vasoactive substances (bradykinin, thromboxanes, and endogenous catecholamines) [5–7].

Isolated persistent patent ductus arteriosus (PDA) occurs in approximately 1 in 2500 to 1 in 5000 live births.

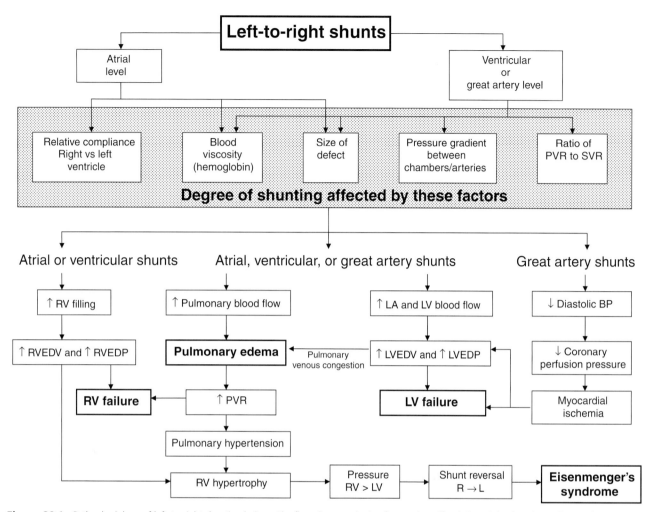

Figure 20.1 Pathophysiology of left-to-right shunting lesions. The flow diagram depicts factors that affect left-to-right shunting at the atrial, ventricular, and great artery level and the pathophysiology produced by these shunts. A large shunt will result in LV failure, RV failure, and pulmonary edema. Increased pulmonary blood flow and pulmonary artery pressures leads to pulmonary hypertension and eventually Eisenmenger's syndrome. These final common outcomes are highlighted in bold lettering. PVR, pulmonary vascular resistance; SVR, systemic vascular resistance; RV, right ventricle; LA, left atrium; LV, left ventricle; BP, blood pressure; RVEDV, right ventricular end-diastolic volume; RVEDP, right ventricular end-diastolic pressure; LVEDP, left ventricular end-diastolic pressure; LVEDV, left ventricular end-diastolic volume (see text for detailed discussion)

The incidence is higher for premature births and PDA is two to three times more common in females than in males [5,8]. PDA is also found as part of other complex congenital heart defects and is usually the source for pulmonary or systemic blood flow in patients with a functional single ventricle before palliative repair.

Anatomy

The ductus arteriosus is a vascular communication between the descending aorta and pulmonary artery. Embryologically, it arises from the distal portion of one of the sixth paired aortic arches [5]. It most commonly originates from the aorta, just distal to the left subclavian artery, and attaches to the left pulmonary artery (Figure 20.2).

Pathophysiology and natural history

The degree of left-to-right shunting depends on several factors, including the size of the PDA and the ratio of PVR and SVR. Ductal dimensions of importance include diameter and length. Larger diameters and shorter lengths produce less resistance, with the potential to allow greater flow. In patients with large PDAs, the diastolic runoff into the pulmonary artery results in lowered aortic diastolic pressure, which may increase the risk of myocardial ischemia, especially in the presence of anemia or lowered SVR.

The consequences of a PDA left untreated depend on many factors. A small PDA may be hemodynamically insignificant and unrecognized. The larger the PDA and left-to-right shunt, the more likely the progression to CHF,

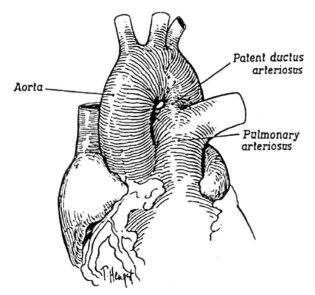

Aorta

Patent ductus
arteriosus

Pulmonary
arteriosus

Figure 20.2 Patent ductus arteriosus (Reproduced with permission from Reference [9])

pulmonary hypertension, and if chronic and/or extreme, reversal of the shunt. In premature infants, PDA is associated with increased morbidity from associated respiratory distress syndrome, necrotizing enterocolitis, and intracranial hemorrhage.

Surgical approaches

In premature newborns, initial management of a PDA is typically pharmacological closure using cyclo-oxygenase inhibitors such as ibuprofen or indomethacin [10]. Surgical treatment is usually reserved for patients who fail medical therapy. Surgical options include posterolateral thoracotomy with ligation or division of the PDA, video-assisted thoracoscopic surgery (VATS), and robotically assisted total endoscopic closure [11]. These approaches have mortality approaching 0% and minimum morbidity; however, mortality rates in premature neonates are slightly higher [6]. Complications of surgical treatment include bleeding, chylothorax, vocal cord paralysis (injury to recurrent laryngeal nerve), pneumothorax, atelectasis, recurrence of patency, and inadvertent ligation of the pulmonary artery or descending aorta [6].

VATS has increasing popularity due to decreased pain, decreased hospital cost (secondary to decreased hospital stay), and avoidance of postthoracotomy syndrome (rib fusion, chest wall deformities, scoliosis, and compromise of pulmonary function). Disadvantages of VATS include intraoperative desaturations and hypercarbia, as well as higher morbidity during the surgical learning curve [12–14]. Use of robotic assistance results in longer surgical times because of increased complexity [15].

Transcatheter closure techniques

Nonsurgical catheter techniques for PDA closure include Gianturco coils, the Gianturco–Grifka vascular occlusion device, and the Amplatzer duct occluder [16–18]. These methods are considered safe, efficacious, and cost effective when compared to surgical closure. Risks of transcatheter approaches include arrhythmias, embolization of the device, and incomplete closure. In addition, there are size limitations in small infants [16–20].

Anesthetic considerations

The anesthetic management for PDA ligation depends on factors such as patient's clinical condition, prematurity, coexisting disease, body weight, and surgical technique. Large volume venous access (which may be a 22- or 24-gauge IV in a premature infant) and forced air-warming devices are recommended. Pulse oximetry of both upper and lower extremities will assist in detecting inadvertent ligation of the descending aorta. For patients with coexisting disease, intra-arterial pressure monitoring provides a method of assessing arterial blood gases, electrolytes, hematocrit, and acid–base status. Whether by cuff or arterial line, blood pressure should be monitored in both an upper and lower extremity and observed carefully before and after ductal occlusion. Proper ductal occlusion will typically be accompanied by an increase in diastolic blood pressure consistent with elimination of pulmonary runoff. Significantly decreased or absent blood pressure in the lower extremity indicates aortic rather than ductal occlusion. A gradient between the systolic pressure in the upper and lower extremities indicates creation of an aortic coarctation.

Although inhaled anesthetics can be safely used for many patients undergoing PDA ligation, neonates are prone to hemodynamic instability with exposure to inhaled anesthetics and benefit from an intravenous anesthetic technique using opioids such as fentanyl and possibly a benzodiazepine along with muscle relaxation.

Neonatal PDA ligation is often performed in the newborn intensive care unit to avoid the additional risks of transport, need for ventilator changes, and hypothermic exposure. High spinal anesthesia, caudal and thoracic epidural techniques have all been described as safe and producing faster recovery [21,22].

Lung isolation improves surgical exposure, especially for VATS surgical techniques, but may require ventilation with 100% inspired oxygen to maintain acceptable oxygenation. Prior to lung isolation, FIO_2 should be minimized and hypocarbia avoided in order maintain pulmonary vascular tone and limit the degree of left-to-right shunting.

Aortopulmonary window

Aortopulmonary window (APW), also know as aortopulmonary septal defect, is a rare anomaly comprising approximately 0.1–0.6% of all congenital heart defects [23,24]. Fifty to eighty percent of patients with APW have associated defects including PDA (72%), right pulmonary artery from aorta (32%), anomalous origin of a coronary artery from the pulmonary artery (23%), VSD (20%), agenesis of the ductus arteriosus (20%), and other lesions [23,25]. Embryologically, APW is thought to originate from nonfusion or malalignment of the aortopulmonary and truncal septi, or complete absence of the aortopulmonary septum [23,26].

Anatomy

The basic anatomical defect in APW consists of a communication between the aorta and the pulmonary artery. Using the Society of Cardiothoracic Surgeons Congenital Heart Surgery Nomenclature and Database Project classification, Type I APW is a proximal defect located just above the sinus of Valsalva, a few millimeters above the semilunar valve. Type II is a distal APW located in the uppermost portion of the ascending aorta. Type III is a total defect involving the majority of the ascending aorta. Intermediate defects, which are neither proximal nor distal, are also designated in this system; these defects are noted for being conducive to device closure because of adequate superior and inferior rims (Figure 20.3) [27,28].

Pathophysiology and natural history

The pressure gradient between the aorta and pulmonary artery will produce significant left-to-right shunting depending on the size of the defect and the relative resistances of the pulmonary and systemic vascular beds. Coexisting cardiac anomalies may alter the pathophysiology. Pulmonary hypertension can develop as early as 12 days of age [29]. Uncorrected APW results in a reported 40% mortality in the first year of life, with a substantial proportion of survivors succumbing to CHF later in childhood [25].

Surgical approaches

A variety of techniques have been described for repair of APW, including ligation and/or division with or without cardiopulmonary bypass, transaortic patch closure, complete separation, and reconstruction of both the aorta and pulmonary artery, and transcatheter closure [28,30–32]. The repair is usually performed via median sternotomy with the use of cardiopulmonary bypass. Surgical repair of

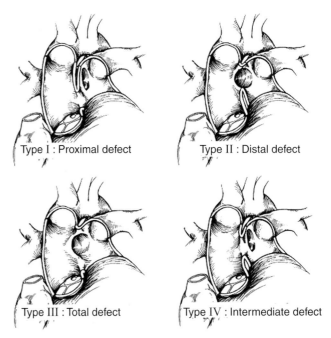

Type I : Proximal defect   Type II : Distal defect

Type III : Total defect   Type IV : Intermediate defect

Figure 20.3 Classification scheme recommended by the Society of Thoracic Surgeons Congenital Heart Surgery Database Committee for aortopulmonary window (see text for further explanation) (Reproduced with permission from Reference [27])

the aortic defect can be accomplished using a pulmonary artery flap with subsequent repair of the pulmonary artery with pericardial patch [33,34]. Care must be taken to explore and repair associated anomalies of the pulmonary and coronary arteries, and to repair coexisting cardiac abnormalities. Actuarial survival after repair of APW is approximately 90% at 1, 5, and 10 years [25]. Transcatheter closure of APW has been reported utilizing the Rashkind double umbrella as well as the Amplatzer occlusion device [31,32].

Anesthetic considerations

The anesthetic management of APW is similar to that of truncus arteriosus. Younger patients may have considerable diastolic runoff from low PVR. Prior to cardiopulmonary bypass, efforts should focus on maintaining pulmonary vascular tone by lowering of the FiO_2 and allowing the oxygen saturation to fall to levels between 80 and 85%, and by maintaining elevated $PaCO_2$, thereby allowing respiratory acidosis to develop. In these cases, surgical snaring of the pulmonary artery prior to bypass may also be helpful. In contrast, patients undergoing later repair are likely to present with elevated PVR, and anesthetic management should include avoiding further increases in PVR.

Regardless of PVR at presentation, all patients with APW are at risk to develop perioperative pulmonary

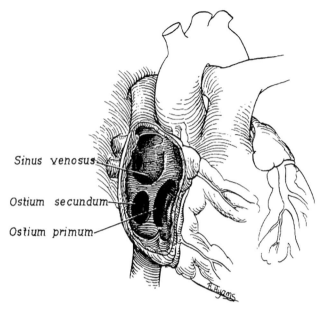

Sinus venosus

Ostium secundum

Ostium primum

Figure 20.4 Composite of major types of atrial septal defect (see text for explanation) (Reproduced with permission from Reference [35]

hypertension. The administration of inhaled nitric oxide as well as other maneuvers described above may be necessary to lower PVR. Those patients exhibiting signs of pulmonary hypertension should initially be maintained under deep sedation with or without neuromuscular blockade during the immediate postoperative periods (see Chapter 27).

Atrial septal defects

The right and left atria are normally divided by the fusion of two septa: the septum primum and the septum secundum. The septum primum develops during the fourth week of gestation and the septum secundum during the fifth week [5]. The septum secundum forms an incomplete partition and leaves an opening called the foramen ovale. The septum primum becomes the valve of the foramen ovale [5]. Five different types of ASDs exist: (i) secundum, (ii) primum, (iii) sinus venosus, (iv) patent foramen ovale (PFO), and (v) coronary sinus (Figure 20.4). Isolated ASDs are more common in females than males by a factor of 2:1. ASDs make up approximately 5–10% of all congenital heart defects with the secundum ASD comprising nearly 80% of all ASDs [6]. A probe PFO is found in approximately 30% of normal adult hearts. ASD may be isolated or associated with other congenital heart defects, where it may be a life-saving communication allowing mixing of blood between the pulmonary and systemic circulations, such as in total anomalous pulmonary venous return, tricuspid atresia, and transposition of the great arteries.

Anatomy

Secundum atrial septal defect

The secundum ASD is contained within the area bordered by the limbus of the fossa ovalis [36]. It results from an abnormal reabsorption of the septum primum or defective formation or shortening of the septum secundum. Combinations of these abnormalities may contribute to large defects.

Primum atrial septal defect

The primum ASD results from abnormalities in formation of the septum primum. It is frequently associated with atrioventricular canal (AVC) defects, especially partial atrioventricular canal (PAVCs) that include a cleft in the anterior leaflet of the left atrioventricular valve. AVC defects are due to abnormalities in fusion of the endocardial cushions.

Sinus venosus atrial septal defect

Sinus venosus defects result from abnormal development of the septum secundum or the sinus venosus (the primitive venous collecting chamber). The most common type is located near the superior vena cava (SVC) orifice and is associated with partial anomalous pulmonary venous return involving the right upper and middle pulmonary veins. Defects near the orifice of the inferior vena cava (IVC) also exist and may involve partial anomalous pulmonary venous return of the right lower pulmonary vein [6].

Patent foramen ovale

PFO results from failure of fusion of the septum primum to the limbus of the septum secundum. Patency of the foramen ovale is normal during fetal life and allows right-to-left shunting of blood in order to bypass the lungs in fetal circulation. Following birth, as PVR decreases and SVR increases, the foramen ovale closes, but may not fuse.

Coronary sinus atrial septal defect

Coronary sinus ASD, also called an unroofed coronary sinus, results from an absence in the wall between the coronary sinus and the left atrium. This allows blood from the left atrium to drain into the right atrium via the coronary sinus. Persistent left SVC is also associated with this defect [36].

Pathophysiology and natural history

The amount of left-to-right shunting at the atrial level is dependent on two factors: the size of the defect and the relative compliance of the right and left ventricles. Shunting occurs primarily during diastole and produces a volume burden on the cardiovascular system that is proportionate to the degree of shunting. Isolated ASDs are usually asymptomatic during infancy and childhood despite the increased volume load on the right ventricle. CHF usually occurs after the second or third decade of life due to chronic right ventricular volume overload. Pulmonary hypertension can occur in up to 13% of unoperated patients younger than 10 years of age; however, progression to Eisenmenger's syndrome is unusual [6]. Risk of arrhythmia is increased with increasing shunt volume and atrial dilation. Patients with a Qp:Qs of 2:1 or less have an 11% incidence of atrial arrhythmia, compared to 38% in those with Qp:Qs of 3:1 or greater [37]. An ASD is sometimes discovered during a neurological work-up for transient ischemic attacks or strokes from paradoxical emboli [36].

Surgical approaches

Surgical repair of an ASD is usually recommended between the ages of 3 and 5 years [38]. Spontaneous closure of small secundum type ASDs occur in up to 87% of infants in the first year of life [6], and controversy exists regarding the closure of small ASDs that are asymptomatic. Conventional surgical treatment involves median sternotomy with the use of cardiopulmonary bypass to perform a primary repair or patch closure, with surgical mortality approaching 0% [6]. Sinus venosus defects are usually repaired using a patch to close the ASD and baffle the anomalous pulmonary veins to the left atrium. Many centers now favor partial sternotomy approaches because of the improved cosmetic result with similar morbidity and mortality to complete sternotomy [39–41]. Postoperative dysrhythmias are reported in 23% of patients, and as many as 2% of patients may need a pacemaker following surgery [6].

Transcatheter closure techniques

Increased use of transcatheter ASD closure in the cardiac catheterization laboratory has dramatically reduced the number of operative repairs. FDA-approved devices include the Amplatzer septal occluder (AGA Medical Corp, Golden Valley, MN, USA), CardioSEAL septal occluder (Nitinol Medical Technologies, Inc., Boston, MA, USA), and the Helex device (WL Gore and Associates, Inc., Flagstaff, AZ, USA) [42]. Nonsurgical transcatheter closure of PFO without an occluding device has also been described, using either radio frequency ablation or su-

ture closure [43,44]. Transcatheter ASD closure is usually performed under general anesthesia with the use of TEE to guide placement. However, intracardiac echocardiography using intravascular two-dimensional imaging may eliminate the need for TEE and reduce the need for general anesthesia [45]. Transcatheter closure is safe, associated with decreased hospital stay, lack of a surgical scar, avoidance of cardiopulmonary bypass, and reduced anesthetic requirements. Limitations to transcatheter closure of ASD include patient size (introducer sheaths may be too large for smaller patients), type of ASD (usually limited to PFO or secundum), and the requirement for an adequate tissue rim to which the device can attach [46].

Anesthetic considerations

Patients with an isolated ASD are generally asymptomatic and do not have pulmonary hypertension. Therefore, the induction of anesthesia can be safely accomplished with either inhalation or intravenous technique. Whenever possible, patients should have an intraoperative TEE performed prior to incision, because transthoracic echocardiographic studies are sometimes unable to exclude the possibility of partial anomalous pulmonary venous return due to difficulty in visualizing all four pulmonary veins. During surgery, TEE can be helpful to assess de-airing of the left heart and adequacy of the repair. Most patients have good myocardial function and do not require inotropic support perioperatively. Maintenance of anesthesia may consist of inhaled agents, intravenous agents, regional anesthesia, or a combination. Regional techniques are favored by some to assist in early extubation [47–49]. Tracheal extubation in the operating room has been shown to decrease patient charges without compromising patient care when compared to extubation in the intensive care unit [50]. Whatever technique is chosen, the primary goals for the uncomplicated ASD patient should include preparation for an early extubation either in the operating room or within the first 4 hours postoperatively.

Ventricular septal defects

VSD is the most common congenital heart defect, occurring in 50% of all children with congenital heart disease and in 20% as an isolated lesion. Reported incidence ranges from 1.56 to 53.2 per 1000 live births [51]. VSD is associated with a variety of inherited conditions, including trisomy 13, 18, and 21 as well as VACTERL (vertebral, vascular, anal, cardiac, tracheoesophageal fistula, renal, and limb anomalies) association and CHARGE (coloboma, heart anomaly, choanal atresia, retardation, and genital and ear anomalies) syndrome [52]. Embryologically, the primitive left ventricle is formed from the ventricular

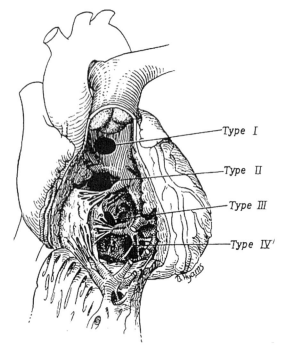

Figure 20.5 Composite of major types of ventricular septal defect. Type I, subarterial; Type II, perimembranous; Type III, inlet or canal type; Type IV, muscular (see text for further explanation) (Reproduced with permission from Reference [53])

portion of the bulbis cordis and the primitive right ventricle is formed from the proximal portion at approximately 23–25 days gestation. Disruption of ventricular septation at a given point during primary morphogenesis is responsible for the four different types of VSD: type I: subarterial; type II: perimembranous; type III: inlet; and type IV: muscular (Figure 20.5) [51,54].

Anatomy

Type I: subarterial ventricular septal defect

The subarterial VSD (also called *subpulmonary* or *infundibular*) is located within the outlet septum, above the crista supraventricularis, and border of the semilunar valves; and comprises approximately 5% of all VSDs. As a result of the location of this defect, a Venturi effect may be produced by the jet of blood flowing through the VSD causing the right or noncoronary aortic cusp of the aortic valve to prolapse toward the defect producing aortic insufficiency [6]. This type of lesion is more common in the Asian population [55].

Type II: perimembranous ventricular septal defect

The perimembranous VSD is a communication adjacent to a portion of the membranous septum and the fibrous trigone of the heart, where the aortic, mitral, and tricuspid valves are in fibrous continuity with the tricuspid, aortic, and mitral valves [6]. These infracristal defects (below the crista supraventricularis) are the most common VSD subtype, occurring in approximately 80%.

Type III: inlet ventricular septal defect

Inlet VSDs (also called *canal type*) are located in the posterior region of the septum beneath the septal leaflet of the tricuspid valve. These defects accounts for approximately 10% of VSDs.

Type IV: muscular ventricular septal defect

Muscular VSDs are located within the muscular portion of the interventricular septum. These defects can be multiple and represent approximately 2–7% of VSDs.

Pathophysiology and natural history

Isolated VSDs produce left-to-right shunting at the ventricular level, predominantly during systole. In contrast to ASDs, in which ventricular dilation is isolated to the right ventricle, the volume load induced by shunting through a VSD affects both ventricles. A VSD is considered "restrictive" when it is small enough that there is a size-related flow limitation across the defect, often indicated by a significant pressure gradient between the left and right ventricles. Flow across a "nonrestrictive" VSD is not limited by size; any pressure gradient between the right and left ventricles is related only to the relative resistances of the pulmonary and systemic vascular beds. Fifteen percent of patients with large VSDs develop pulmonary hypertension that will progress to the development of pulmonary vascular obstructive disease by the age of 20 years [56].

Patients presenting with VSD may be asymptomatic or exhibit signs and symptoms of CHF in varying degrees. The rate and extent of progression of symptomatology depends on the patient age, size of the defect, and the degree of left-to-right shunting. Infants who have nonrestrictive VSDs typically develop symptoms of CHF by 3 months of age because of the physiologic decline in PVR that occurs during early postnatal life. Spontaneous closure of small perimembranous and muscular VSDs occurs in as many as 50% of patients [56–58], and such patients are typically asymptomatic.

Surgical approaches

Surgical repair of VSD is usually by patch closure and occasionally by primary closure using cardiopulmonary bypass via median sternotomy. Perimembranous and inlet VSDs are most commonly repaired via a right atriotomy, which may require detachment of the septal leaflet of the tricuspid valve for exposure. Subarterial VSDs are most commonly repaired via the transpulmonary approach. Midmuscular VSDs are most commonly repaired via right atriotomy, and anterior or apical muscular VSD may be approached using right ventriculotomy. However, the use of right ventriculotomies carries the risks of conduction disturbances and ventricular dysfunction later in life. At our institution, symptomatic patients with lesions that are not approachable via right atriotomy are usually treated with pulmonary artery banding until the patient is larger allowing transatrial repair. Pulmonary artery banding is also utilized for multiple muscular VSDs and in patients that are high-risk candidates for cardiopulmonary bypass. Partial median sternotomies as well as small right anterolateral thoracotomies are advocated by some because of improved cosmetic results [59,60], Video-assisted cardioscopy (VAC) is used in some centers to improve visualization of small intracardiac structures in limited spaces during open-heart surgery for congenital heart repairs. VAC has been successfully utilized for a variety of intracardiac repairs including ASD, VSD, tetralogy of Fallot, double outlet right ventricle (DORV), AVC, and others [41,61–63].

Timing for surgical repair varies depending on age at presentation and severity of signs and symptoms. Patients younger than 6 months of age are repaired if they manifest uncontrollable CHF and failure to thrive. Patients between 6 and 24 months of age undergo repair to treat CHF symptoms or pulmonary hypertension. Patients older than 24 months undergo repair if the Qp:Qs is greater than 2:1. Among patients with subarterial VSD, the presence of aortic insufficiency is an indication for surgical repair to prevent further progression of the valvular insufficiency [64,65]. A defect size of greater than 5 mm is repaired to avoid progression to aortic cusp prolapse and aortic insufficiency, and defects less than 5 mm can be managed conservatively [55].

Mortality for uncomplicated VSD in older patients is less than 1–2% [66]. Mortality for VSD repair in infants during the first year of life is less than 5% [67].

Transcatheter closure techniques

Transcatheter closure of VSDs has been performed successfully for more than 20 years [68–72]. In the USA, the CardioSEAL septal occluder (Nitinol Medical Technologies, Inc., Boston, MA< USA) and the Amplatzer muscular VSD occluder (AGA Medical Corp, Golden Valley, MN, USA) are approved for use by the FDA, and the Amplatzer membranous VSD occluder (AGA Medical Corp, Golden Valley, MN, USA) is undergoing clinical trials [73]. Indications for use of these devices include all types of muscular VSDs, including apical and multiple, as well as perimembranous VSDs. Transcatheter techniques may serve as an adjunct to surgery or an alternative to surgery in selected patients. Intraoperative use of VSD closure devices during cardiopulmonary bypass for defects with difficult surgical closure has been described [74], and postoperative residual VSDs or "Swiss cheese" type muscular VSD may be preferentially treated by this technique. The major limitation in the application of this technique is related to the size of the sheaths necessary for device delivery, precluding use in infancy. Complications of device closure include need for blood transfusion, tricuspid valve regurgitation, and device embolization [68,71]. Heart block is a particular concern following device closure of perimembranous VSDs [73,75].

Anesthetic considerations

Anesthetic management for the patient with VSD is similar to that of ASD. Pulmonary hypertension may develop early, especially in patients with trisomy 21, and preoperative chest X-ray revealing decreased pulmonary vascular markings is indicative of pulmonary hypertension [76–79]. Such patients may respond to the use of inhaled nitric oxide prior to termination of cardiopulmonary bypass and/or in the postoperative period. Right heart failure with decreased cardiac output may result if pulmonary hypertension is not controlled, and may require the use of dopamine, milrinone, dobutamine, or isoproterenol.

Conduction disturbances may be transient or permanent. Atrial-ventricular heart block, formerly reported to occur in up to 10% of patients post-VSD repair [6], is now a rare complication occurring in less than 1% of patients after VSD closure [6]. If heart block develops, treatment with atrioventricular synchronous pacing using temporary pacing wires is indicated. Junctional ectopic tachycardia is sometimes observed in patients younger than 1 year after repair for lesions that involve VSD repair, most commonly after tetralogy of Fallot repair. Treatment includes cooling to 35°C, increasing anesthetic depth, paralysis, procainamide, esmolol, or amiodarone [6].

Intraoperative use of TEE will allow recognition of residual VSDs and intracardiac air, as well as provide an assessment of ventricular volume and function. Small muscular VSDs often become apparent after closure of larger VSDs. Frequently these smaller defects, especially if near the apex, may not be amenable to surgical repair or worth the risk of returning to cardiopulmonary bypass.

Patients with uncomplicated VSDs are good candidates for extubation in the operating room or early after arrival in the intensive care unit.

Atrioventricular canal

Atrioventricular canal results from failure of the endocardial cushions to fuse during the fifth week of fetal development [5]. Four to five percent of congenital heart disease involves defects of the atrioventricular septum, and AVC defects occur in 0.19 in 1000 live births [80,81]. AVC is associated with multiple syndromes and occurs in approximately 20% of persons with trisomy 21. It accounts for 15% of congenital heart defects in persons with Noonan's syndrome and nearly 50% in persons with Ellis–van Creveld syndrome [82].

Anatomy

Anatomically, AVC consists of three basic defects: (i) an ostium primum defect resulting in an interatrial communication, (ii) abnormal atrioventricular valves, and (iii) an inlet VSD resulting in an interventricular communication. Three types of AVC exist: (i) partial, (ii) transitional, and (iii) complete [83].

Partial atrioventricular canal

The PAVC defect consists of an ostium primum ASD and a cleft in the anterior leaflet of the mitral valve, usually resulting in some degree of insufficiency [83]. The tricuspid valve is often abnormal as well, and no VSD or other interventricular communication exists.

Transitional atrioventricular canal

The transitional (also called *intermediate*) atrioventricular canal (TAVC) defect consists of an ostium primum ASD, abnormal atrioventricular valves, and a VSD, often restrictive, just below the atrioventricular valves [83]. Like the PAVC defect, the left atrioventricular valve is usually associated with a cleft and has some degree of insufficiency.

Complete atrioventricular canal

The complete atrioventricular canal (CAVC) defect consists of an ostium primum ASD and a nonrestrictive VSD just below a common atrioventricular valve that bridges both the right and left sides of the heart [83]. The left atrioventricular portion of the valve usually contains a cleft that is insufficient. Three classifications of CAVC defects exist based on the chordal attachments of the anterior bridging leaflet of the common atrioventricular valve and are commonly referred to as Rastelli types A, B, and C [84].

In Rastelli type A CAVC, the anterior bridging leaflet is divided at the septum into right and left components and attached to the crest of the ventricular septum by thin chordae tendinae. Rastelli type B CAVC is rare and characterized by anomalous papillary muscle attachment from the right side of the ventricular septum to the left side of the anterior bridging leaflet. Rastelli type C CAVC is defined by an anterior leaflet that lacks any ventricular septal attachments and "floats" above the septum [83]. The Rastelli type C defect is most common type, and may be associated with other major cardiac or extracardiac anomalies such as tetralogy of Fallot or trisomy 21 [36].

Other variants of AVC also exist, including right or left ventricular dominant types in which one ventricle is hypoplastic. The physiology produced by such lesions is similar to other single ventricle lesions, and the reader is referred to Chapter 24. Many lesions occur in association with AVC, including PDA, tetralogy of Fallot, coarctation of the aorta, subaortic stenosis, left SVC, asplenia, and polysplenia [6].

Pathophysiology and natural history

A left-to-right shunt may occur at the atrial, ventricular, and atrioventricular valvar level, depending on the type of AVC present. This shunting, in addition to atrioventricular valve regurgitation, results in volume overload of both the atria and ventricles. Volume overload soon develops into CHF and may result in pulmonary hypertension as the ratio of pulmonary to systemic blood flow increases. As with other left-to-right shunts, pulmonary hypertension may develop by 1 year of age and eventually lead to Eisenmenger's syndrome [85]. The severity of CHF and symptoms will depend on the degree of left-to-right shunting and the severity of atrioventricular valve regurgitation. Among the forms of AVC, PAVC is the least symptomatic, CAVC the most, and TAVC intermediate. Patients with untreated PAVC may do well through childhood, but have an increased likelihood of developing CHF in adulthood, especially as atrial dysrhythmias develop [36]. The presence of moderate to severe atrioventricular valve regurgitation leads to earlier development of CHF and higher morbidity and mortality if untreated [27]. Those patients with PAVC presenting with CHF in the first year of life should be suspected of having additional lesions, most commonly left-sided obstructive lesions [86]. Patients with CAVC develop CHF, failure-to-thrive, and frequent respiratory infections in the first year of life. During this same interval, 12% of these children will develop irreversible pulmonary hypertension, and a chest radiograph demonstrating black lung fields, indicating decrease pulmonary blood flow, is an ominous sign [76]. Those with trisomy 21 develop pulmonary hypertension earlier and with increased severity as compared to other children; however, this has not manifest as a risk factor in surgical repair or long-term outcome [79,87,88].

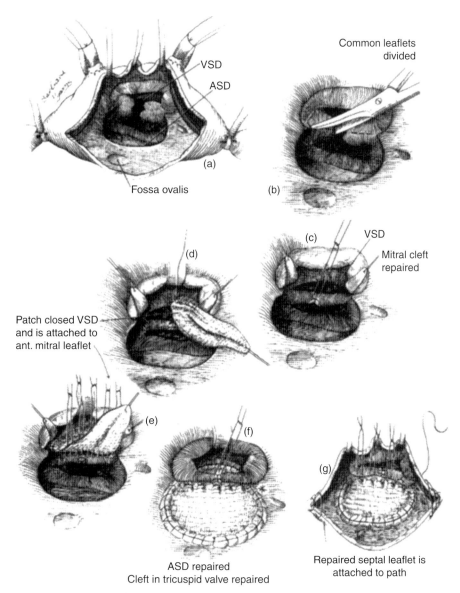

VSD
ASD

Common leaflets
divided

Fossa ovalis

(a)

(b)

(d)

(c)   VSD

Mitral cleft
repaired

Patch closed VSD
and is attached to
ant. mitral leaflet

(e)

(f)

(g)

ASD repaired
Cleft in tricuspid valve repaired

Repaired septal leaflet is
attached to path

Figure 20.6 Single patch technique for repair of complete atrioventricular canal defect (Used with permission from Reference [91])

Surgical approaches

Surgical repair of PAVC is usually performed at age 2–5 years unless there are signs of CHF or other lesions that necessitate earlier repair. Patients with TAVC may be relatively asymptomatic and may tolerate surgical repair at an older age.

Primary complete surgical repair for patients with CAVC is performed between 1 and 6 months of age because it is safe, controls CHF, prevents the development of fixed pulmonary hypertension, and reduces annular dilation (a cause of atrioventricular valvar regurgitation) [86,89,90].

Surgical techniques vary, but generally consist of a right atriotomy with patch closure of the ASD, closure of clefts in the anterior leaflet of the left atrioventricular valve, and closure of the VSD with a patch or, in the case of the TAVC, pledgetted sutures [6,36,89]. A one- or two-patch technique can be used (Figure 20.6). Pulmonary artery banding is reserved for cases of severe respiratory illness, sepsis, or anatomy not suitable for biventricular repair. Presence of associated cardiac anomalies such as tetralogy of Fallot, DORV, left-sided obstructive lesions, and unbalanced AVC (with a hypoplastic ventricle) further complicate the repair and result in higher mortality, especially in those patients with a hypoplastic ventricle [92,93].

Mortality for repair of the PAVC is less than 5%, and the mortality for complete repair of CAVC is between 2.5 and 10.5% [6,90,94–96]. Pulmonary artery banding is associated with mortality near 5% [6,36]. Presence of preoperative pulmonary hypertension and increasing size of the VSD is associated with higher morbidity and mortality among patients undergoing complete repair of CAVC [36,94].

Anesthetic considerations

Anesthetic management of the AVC defects depends primarily on the degree of left-to-right shunting, and the presence and severity of pulmonary vascular hypertension. As with other septal defects, balancing the ratio of PVR to SVR and thereby limiting the amount of pulmonary overcirculation is paramount to successful management, and is usually accomplished by manipulations in FIO_2 and ventilation (see above). TEE is very helpful in detecting residual intracardiac shunts, assessing atrioventricular valvar function, and determining ventricular function and volume following repair.

Surgical placement of left atrial and pulmonary arterial pressure lines may be used to guide management of inotropes, use of nitric oxide, and volume replacement. Persistent elevation and acute increases in pulmonary arterial pressure contribute to right heart failure and increased mortality [6,94]. Pulmonary hypertension develops commonly in these patients and is treated with hyperventilation, 100% oxygen, systemic alkalinization, opioids, and nitric oxide. Increasing the pH is more effective than lowering the PCO_2 in controlling pulmonary pressures and may be accomplished by the administration of sodium bicarbonate. Sildenafil has also been effective in this setting [97].

Most patients require inotropic support upon weaning from cardiopulmonary bypass, and those with residual atrioventricular valve regurgitation and/or VSD benefit from use of milrinone or other afterload reduction. Hypotensive patients who have elevated left atrial pressures should be evaluated for the presence of severe residual left atrioventricular valve regurgitation or stenosis, residual VSD, left ventricular outflow tract obstruction, or left ventricular dysfunction [6]. Intraoperative TEE is essential for initial diagnosis of these conditions, and reinitiation of cardiopulmonary bypass and repair may be necessary.

CAVC repair is associated with conduction abnormalities, especially atrioventricular and sinoatrial nodal dysfunction resulting in complete heart block. In this situation, atrioventricular sequential pacing is necessary to minimize atrioventricular valve regurgitation and to improve cardiac output [6].

Double outlet right ventricle

DORV is a type of ventriculoarterial connection in which both great vessels arise either entirely or predominantly from the right ventricle. This definition, which has been adopted by the Congenital Heart Surgery Nomenclature Database Project, is intended to simplify what is in fact a complex spectrum of defects ranging from morphology that mimics tetralogy of Fallot to that which resembles transposition of the great vessels [98]. DORV comprises approximately 1–1.5% of all patients with congenital heart disease with an incidence estimated at 1 per 10,000 live births [99]. DORV is a bulboventricular malformation that results from failure of proper alignment of the conotruncus with the ventricular septum [99]. Although DORV can occur with an intact ventricular septum, this is extremely rare [100]; almost all patients with DORV also have a VSD.

Characterization of the anatomy of DORV is crucial in understanding the physiologic consequences as well in determining the surgical approach for palliation or correction. Complete characterization of the anatomy will include (i) the relationship of the VSD to the great arteries, (ii) the relationship of the great arteries with respect to one another, (iii) the morphology of the ventricles and their outflow tracts, and (iv) the presence of associated anomalies [100]. Four different anatomic types of DORV are defined on the basis of the relationship of the VSD to the great arteries: (i) subaortic VSD, (ii) subpulmonary VSD, (iii) doubly committed VSD, and (iv) noncommitted VSD [98].

Anatomy

Double outlet right ventricle with subaortic VSD

These lesions represent approximately 51–56% of DORV [100,101] and are characterized by a VSD located beneath the aortic valve. The great vessels may be normally related or transposed. When this defect is associated with pulmonary stenosis, the resulting physiology is similar to that of tetralogy of Fallot [98].

Double outlet right ventricle with subpulmonary VSD

DORV with subpulmonary VSD represents approximately 30% of DORV [101, 102]. Pulmonary stenosis is rare, but subaortic or aortic arch obstructions are common. The VSD is typically nonrestrictive. This lesion often occurs in the form of the *Taussig–Bing* type: with L-malposition of the great arteries in the absence of pulmonary stenosis [98]. The resulting physiology is similar to that of transposition of the great arteries.

Double outlet right ventricle with doubly committed VSD

Doubly committed VSD represents approximately 3–10% of DORV [101–103]. The doubly committed VSD results from the hypoplasia of the infundibular septum and variable degrees of override of the VSD by both great arteries [99].

Double outlet right ventricle with noncommitted VSD

Noncommitted VSD represents approximately 12–17% of DORV [100,101], and the VSD is an apical muscular or membranous-inlet type. The VSD is remote from the great arteries and is frequently associated with AVC defects [99].

Pathophysiology and natural history

The pathophysiology of DORV is dependent on the specific anatomy of the lesion and degree of pulmonary versus aortic blood flow as well as the degree of mixing of pulmonary and systemic venous blood. Consideration of these variables serves to simplify the pathophysiology of DORV into three basic subtypes: VSD, tetralogy of Fallot, and transposition of the great arteries [98].

DORV with a doubly committed or subaortic VSD without pulmonary stenosis produces physiology similar to that of a VSD. Because VSDs in this setting are usually nonrestrictive, the degree of left-to-right shunting will generally depend on the relative ratio of PVR to SVR.

DORV associated with pulmonary stenosis resembles the physiology of tetralogy of Fallot with varying degrees of cyanosis depending on the severity of pulmonic stenosis. These patients have right-to-left shunting across the VSD and may have hypercyanotic spells, polycythemia, and failure to thrive. Although there is a fixed component of obstruction, pulmonary blood flow may vary due to alterations in PVR. Pulmonary stenosis is present in approximately 50% of patients with DORV [99].

DORV with a subpulmonary VSD without pulmonary stenosis usually produces physiology similar to transposition of the great arteries. Streaming of pulmonary venous blood to the pulmonary artery and systemic venous blood toward the aorta results in variable degrees of mixing of oxygenated and deoxygenated blood. Patients can present early with both cyanosis and CHF followed by development of pulmonary vascular occlusive disease if left untreated.

DORV may be associated with other anomalies that further affect pathophysiology, such as multiple VSDs, AVC defects, PDA, aortic arch obstruction, interrupted aortic arch, subaortic stenosis, hypoplastic ventricle, or mitral valve abnormalities [101–106].

Surgical approaches

The surgical approach to DORV varies depending on the type of DORV and the associated anomalies, and the

preoperative delineation of anatomy is crucial to determine the operative strategy. However, echocardiography, angiography, and magnetic resonance imaging may still result in incomplete information due to the complexity and anatomic variations of this lesion [105,107]. Often only intraoperative inspection of the heart by the surgeon leads to the definitive operative plan. Four surgical treatment options generally exist: (i) palliative procedures such as Blalock–Taussig shunts, coarctation repairs, and pulmonary artery banding; (ii) intraventricular repair with a baffle from the left ventricle to the aorta; (iii) intraventricular baffle from the left ventricle to the pulmonary artery followed by arterial switch; and (iv) bidirectional cavopulmonary shunt staged to the Fontan procedure (univentricular heart repair) [101–106].

The overall early mortality for the repair of DORV is approximately 9% [101,102,106]. Ten-year survival is 81–86% [101,102]. Significant risk factors for early mortality include congenital mitral valve anomalies, side-by-side great arteries, multiple VSDs, and age at operation <1 month [101–104]. Among patients with DORV and complex anatomy, Fontan palliation may be the procedure of choice as it has been associated with lower early mortality in this group compared to biventricular repair [101].

Anesthetic considerations

Anesthetic management varies greatly depending on the specific type of DORV and associated anomalies. Management of palliative procedures, such as the modified Blalock–Taussig shunt, is reviewed in Chapter 22. Patients with pulmonary stenosis who present with physiology similar to tetralogy of Fallot should be managed to minimize right-to-left shunting (see Chapter 22). Patients with subpulmonary VSD without pulmonary stenosis who have physiology similar to transposition of the great arteries should be managed as such (see Chapter 23). Subaortic and noncommitted VSDs without pulmonary stenosis produce physiology similar to that of a VSD and should be managed as described earlier in this chapter. Patients with complex DORV and other associated anomalies that proceed through the single ventricle staged palliation to the Fontan procedure are reviewed in Chapter 24. In all patients with DORV, regardless of specific anatomy, intracardiac shunting must be balanced with manipulation of PVR and SVR to optimize systemic cardiac output and oxygen delivery.

Arrhythmias are common, especially with repairs involving baffling and enlargement of the VSD. Ventricular tachyarrhythmias and complete heart block can occur in as many as 9% of patients postoperatively and may require permanent pacing [99,101,102]. Frequently, repair of DORV is complex and requires periods of circulatory arrest. Patients may have residual VSDs, valvar insufficiency, outflow tract obstruction, or ventricular dysfunction. Postoperative TEE and left atrial pressure monitoring are helpful in determining the diagnosis and guiding management.

Truncus arteriosus

Truncus arteriosus is an uncommon congenital heart defect representing less than 3% of all congenital heart defects [6,108–110]. It is defined by the presence of a single great artery arising from the base of the heart that supplies the coronary, pulmonary, and systemic circulations. Embryologically, this defect results from failure of the truncus arteriosus to divide into the aorta and pulmonary artery. Deletion of chromosome 22q11 is present in approximately 11–35% of patients with truncus arteriosus, and this chromosomal abnormality is associated with DiGeorge and velocardiofacial syndromes. Patients with these syndromes also have noncardiac anomalies such as aplasia or hypoplasia of the thymus and/or parathyroid glands (T-cell deficiency), hypocalcemia, palatal abnormalities, speech and learning disabilities, neuropsychological disorders, and craniofacial dysmorphia [111–113]. As many as 77% of patients with 22q11 deletion are immunocompromised [113].

Anatomy

Truncus arteriosus has historically been classified by two main systems. The first and most widely used classification system was described by Collett and Edwards in 1949 and the second by Van Praagh and Van Praagh in 1965 [114,115]. The Collett and Edwards classification is based on the embryologic arrested development of the pulmonary arteries from the sixth aortic arches and categorized into four different subtypes. A modified Van Praagh system was adopted by the Congenital Heart Surgery Nomenclature and Database Project, but the continued value of the classical naming systems was recognized (Figure 20.7) [116]. For the purpose of this chapter, the Collett and Edwards system will be used.

Type I truncus arteriosus

Type I truncus arteriosus accounts for 70% of truncus arteriosus lesions. It is defined by the origin of the main pulmonary artery from the truncus dividing into left and right pulmonary arteries.

Type II truncus arteriosus

Type II truncus arteriosus accounts for 30% and is defined by separate origination of the left and right pulmonary

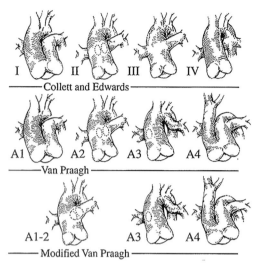

Figure 20.7 Major classification systems for truncus arteriosus. The "A" in the Van Praagh and modified Van Praagh systems indicates presence of a VSD (rare cases of intact ventricular septum are designated with a "B"). Types I and A1 are identical. Types II and III are grouped together as Van Praagh type A2. Types A1 and A2 are grouped together as modified Van Praagh A1–2. Type IV is a variant of tetralogy of Fallot with pulmonary atresia and major aortopulmonary collaterals. Type A3 is unilateral pulmonary artery atresia with collateral supply to the affected lung (left shown). Type A4 involves interrupted aortic arch (see text for full explanation) (Reproduced with permission from Reference [116])

arteries from the posterior surface of the truncus, with the branch pulmonary arteries arising very close to one another.

Type III truncus arteriosus

Type III truncus arteriosus is also characterized by separate origination of the left and right pulmonary arteries, but in this case, the arteries arise from the lateral aspects of the truncus and are widely separated. This type accounts for approximately 1% of cases.

Type IV truncus arteriosus

Type IV is included for historical purposes, but has been rejected as a true form of truncus arteriosus. It is now defined as a variant of tetralogy of Fallot with pulmonary atresia. There is complete absence of the pulmonary arteries in this defect, with bronchial and collateral arteries of the descending aorta providing the blood supply to the lungs.

Truncus arteriosus is most commonly associated with a VSD, but can occur with an intact ventricular septum. The truncal valve may be dysplastic and may have an abnormal number of leaflets, varying between two and six [6,115]. Truncal valve insufficiency is estimated to occur in 25–50% of patients [115]. Anomalies of the coronary arteries may also exist. Additionally, truncus arteriosus is associated with other cardiac anomalies such as aortic arch obstruction, ASDs (62%), right aortic arch (21–36%), aortic arch interruption (11–19%), PDA (18%), aberrant subclavian artery (4–10%), absence of one pulmonary artery (10%), and persistent left SVC (4–9%) [6,108,110].

Pathophysiology and natural history

Truncus arteriosus by definition has a common arterial trunk that provides blood flow to the coronary, pulmonary, and systemic arteries. As PVR falls in the early neonatal period, pulmonary blood flow progressively increases and results in CHF. A variable degree of mixing of the systemic and pulmonary venous blood occurs at the ventricular level through the VSD. The large runoff provided by the pulmonary arteries results in low diastolic pressures, which may be worsened by the presence of truncal valve insufficiency. Low diastolic pressures in the face of increased myocardial work and increased ventricular pressures place the patient at risk of developing myocardial ischemia. Early CHF and increased pulmonary blood flow lead to rapid development of pulmonary vascular occlusive disease in infancy if left untreated.

Patients without surgical treatment have a 74–100% mortality in the first year of life [107–109]. Surgical repair in patients older than 2 years is contraindicated when PVR is greater than 8 Wood units or in the presence of Eisenmenger's syndrome is present [6,108].

Surgical approaches

Definitive surgical repair is usually recommended in the neonatal period, although some centers time surgery on an individual basis, performing repair between 2–3 months of age [108–110,117]. Early repair is indicated due to the rapid development of pulmonary hypertension and high mortality rate in patients in the first year of life if left untreated. Palliative surgery involving pulmonary artery banding has largely been abandoned except for those very few patients who are not suitable candidates for definitive repair [110]. Definitive surgical repair involves removal of the pulmonary arteries from the truncal root and closing the resulting defect either primarily or with a patch. The VSD is usually closed with a patch via a transatrial or transventricular approach. A right ventricle to pulmonary artery connection is provided by a valved homograft. Direct anastomosis of the pulmonary artery with the right ventricle has been described, but may distort the pulmonary arterial architecture. If high right ventricular pressures are anticipated, a small ASD may be created in order to improve cardiac output at the expense of arterial oxygen saturation [6,108,109,117,118]. This ASD creation can be closed at a later date by a transcatheter technique in the cardiac catheterization laboratory. Moderate to severe truncal valve regurgitation is repaired by valvuloplasty, "double-homograft" technique with coronary reimplantation, or mechanical valve implantation [108,119,120]. Valve repair has been successful even in neonates and avoids or delays serial truncal valve replacements [119]. Early mortality after repair of truncus arteriosus is 5–18% [108,109,117,118], and mortality rates are higher in infants who weigh less than 3 kg or have other cardiac anomalies [109,117,120].

Anesthetic considerations

Anesthetic management is dependent on the patient's anatomy and age at presentation. Depending on the severity of CHF, the patient may require preoperative inotropic support, and the induction of anesthesia should be accomplished with drugs that maintain SVR and preserve myocardial function. Ketamine or etomidate, often combined with fentanyl and/or midazolam, may be used to safely attain this goal. If an inhalational induction with sevoflurane is chosen, it should be performed with careful titration and extreme caution. Muscle relaxation may be provided with cisatracurium, vecuronium, or pancuronium. Maintenance of anesthesia often includes high-dose opioids, and total fentanyl doses commonly exceed 50 mcg/kg. Efforts to balance PVR and SVR to make the ratio of Qp:Qs approach 1:1 are essential. Care must be taken to avoid hyperventilation and excessive oxygenation, which lower PVR and may exacerbate pulmonary overcirculation and decrease diastolic blood pressure. Patients with truncal valve insufficiency combined with excessive pulmonary blood runoff will be particularly susceptible to myocardial ischemia, and it may be necessary for the surgeon to temporarily place a vessel snare around the pulmonary artery to limit pulmonary blood flow and increase diastolic blood pressure in the prebypass period. Those patients presenting late in infancy who have developed significant pulmonary hypertension from long-standing pulmonary overcirculation may require increased FIO_2 to maintain oxygen saturations between 80 and 90%. Unless ruled out by a chromosomal evaluation, patients with truncus arteriosus should be assumed to have DiGeorge syndrome and given irradiated blood products due to the high incidence of associated T-cell deficiencies. Upon weaning from cardiopulmonary bypass, most patients require inotropic support, afterload reduction, ventricular volume assessment, and efforts to minimize pulmonary arterial pressures in order to improve right heart function.

Pulmonary hypertension is commonly present after cardiopulmonary bypass. These patients have signs of right heart failure with high central venous pressures, desaturation, tachycardia, hypotension, acidosis, and oliguria

[6]. Management includes hyperventilation, 100% oxygen, correction of acidosis, and nitric oxide as needed. These patients are usually kept sedated and paralyzed for at least 24 hours postoperatively to minimize early pulmonary hypertensive crises. Signs similar to right ventricular dysfunction may also occur from residual VSDs or truncal valve stenosis or regurgitation. VSD closure or right ventricular incision may produce complete right bundle branch block, complete heart block (3–5%), junctional ectopic tachycardia, atrial tachycardias, or atrioventricular block in the postoperative period [65]. After bypass many patients benefit from calcium infusions because of the hypocalcemia associated with DiGeorge syndrome and citrate binding of ionized calcium from administration of blood products.

Partial and total anomalous pulmonary venous return

Partial anomalous pulmonary venous return (PAPVR) is an anomaly in which some, but not all, of the pulmonary veins connect to the right atrium or to one or more of its venous tributaries. In total anomalous pulmonary venous return (TAPVR), all of the pulmonary veins connect anomalously to the right atrium. Although these lesions are sometimes referred to as anomalous pulmonary venous *connections*, use of the term *return* recognizes the fact that the pulmonary veins may be connected normally to the left atrium, but have an ASD anatomically configured to cause abnormal return to the right atrium [121, 122]. In either case, the pathophysiology is that of a left-to-right shunt. Both PAPVR and TAPVR are rare cardiac lesions. Since PAPVR is often asymptomatic, its true incidence is unclear, but it has been reported as an incidental finding on autopsy in approximately 0.6% of the general population [123]. TAPVR represents less than 5% of congenital heart lesions [124–126].

The stage in embryologic development during which errors occur determines the various anatomic subtypes of abnormal pulmonary venous return. At 27–30 days of gestation, the pulmonary veins are derived from the splanchnic plexus that communicates with the cardinal and umbilicovitelline system of veins. Anomalous drainage to the left common cardinal system results in pulmonary venous connections to the coronary sinus or left innominate vein. Drainage to the right common cardinal system results in pulmonary venous connections to the SVC and/or the azygous vein. Drainage to the umbilicovitelline system results in pulmonary venous connection to the portal vein, ductus venous, or IVC. Early atresia of the common pulmonary vein, while primitive pulmonary–systemic venous connections are still present, results in TAPVR. If only the right or left portion of the common pulmonary vein

becomes atretic, persistence of the primitive pulmonary venous–systemic venous connection on that side leads to PAPVR [124].

Both PAPVR and TAPVR can be associated with other cardiac lesions. PAPVR is most commonly associated with sinus venosus type ASDs. Congenital mitral stenosis, DORV, VSD, tetralogy of Fallot, coarctation of the aorta, and PDA have all been described with PAPVR [124]. Nearly 33% of patients with TAPVR have other cardiac anomalies, such as CAVC, hypoplastic left heart syndrome or other single ventricle lesions, PDA, and transposition of the great arteries. Abnormalities of the atrial and visceral situs with the heterotaxy syndrome, asplenia, and polysplenia are also common among patients with TAPVR [124]. Scimitar syndrome consists of either partial or complete anomalous drainage of the right pulmonary veins to the IVC, dextrocardia, and hypoplasia of the right lung. In these patients, the descending vertical vein resembles a scimitar, or Turkish sword, on a frontal chest radiograph [122,124].

Anatomy

Partial anomalous pulmonary venous return

Multiple types of PAPVR exist. The most common is connection of the right pulmonary veins to the right SVC or right atrium that represents approximately 74% of patients. The next most common type is connection of the right pulmonary veins to the IVC. The least common type is connection of the left pulmonary veins to the left innominate vein or to the coronary sinus [124].

Four different types of TAPVR exist based on the location of the anomalous connection: supracardiac, cardiac, and infracardiac (Figure 20.8).

Supracardiac total anomalous pulmonary venous return

Supracardiac connection comprises approximately 55% of cases of TAPVR. In this type, pulmonary venous drainage is to the SVC. In the most common form of this lesion, the two pulmonary veins from each lung converge posterior to the left atrium. A vertical vein then arises from the left side of the confluence and usually passes anterior to the left pulmonary artery and the left mainstem bronchus to drain into the left innominate vein, which then drains to the SVC. Pulmonary venous obstruction is unusual, but may occur as a result of either intrinsic narrowing or extrinsic compression of the vertical vein. Although anomalous connection can occur to the SVC via a right-sided vertical vein, this is much less common [124].

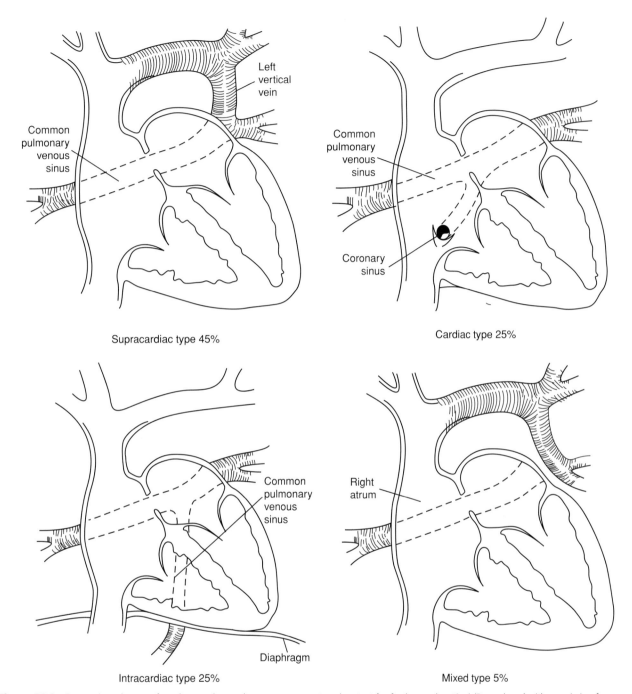

Figure 20.8 Four major subtypes of total anomalous pulmonary venous return (see text for further explanation) (Reproduced with permission from Reference [127])

Cardiac total anomalous pulmonary venous return

The cardiac type of TAPVR accounts for approximately 30% of cases. The pulmonary veins in this type drain into the coronary sinus or right atrium. Obstruction to the pulmonary veins was reported in 22% of patients in a series of TAPVR to the coronary sinus [128].

Infracardiac total anomalous pulmonary venous return

Infracardiac TAPVR comprises approximately 13% of cases, and is commonly referred to as infradiaphragmatic TAPVR [124]. This type of connection usually involves a confluence of pulmonary veins from both lungs posterior to the left atrium. A descending vein then courses anterior to the esophagus through the diaphragm at the esophageal hiatus [129]. In 70–80% of patients, the descending vein then joins the portal venous system at either the splenic or the confluence of the splenic and superior mesenteric veins [129]. Nearly all patients with infracardiac TAPVR have obstructed pulmonary veins. This obstruction, which may be either intrinsic or extrinsic, can occur at any location along the pulmonary venous pathway.

Mixed total anomalous pulmonary venous return

Mixed type TAPVR makes up approximately 2% of cases. This type of TAPVR consists of anomalous connections at two or more levels. The most common connection involves the left pulmonary veins draining into the left innominate vein and the right pulmonary veins draining to the right atrium or the coronary sinus [124]. Pulmonary venous obstruction has also been observed in these types of connections.

Pathophysiology and natural history

PAPVR results in a variable amount of left-to-right shunting that depends on several factors: the number of anomalously draining veins as a percentage of the total pulmonary venous return, the pulmonary lobes or segments from which the anomalous veins originate, the relative resistances of the normally and anomalously drained pulmonary vascular beds, and the compliance of the receiving chambers. The left-to-right shunt leads to increased pulmonary blood flow and enlargement of the right atrium and ventricle as well as dilation of the pulmonary artery [124].

Most patients with an isolated single vein PAPVR and intact atrial septum are asymptomatic and have a normal life expectancy even if left untreated. Those patients with greater than 50% of the pulmonary veins draining anomalously or those with an associated ASD usually remain relatively asymptomatic until the third to fourth decades of life, when progressive symptoms of dyspnea, recurrent bronchitis, hemoptysis, chest pain, and palpitations with supraventricular arrhythmias can occur. These patients may also present with right heart failure or with pulmonary hypertension and cor pulmonale [124].

The pathophysiology of TAPVR depends largely on whether or not pulmonary venous return is obstructed. In the presence of obstructed pulmonary veins, pulmonary venous hypertension exists with associated pulmonary edema. It is commonly confused with intrinsic lung disease when chest radiograph reveals bilateral infiltrates in the absence of cardiomegaly. Pulmonary arteriolar vasoconstriction occurs as a compensatory mechanism to minimize pulmonary edema. As PVR increases, the right ventricular systolic and end-diastolic pressures increase re-

sulting in increased right atrial pressure and right-to-left shunting at the atrial level. Progressive systemic hypoxemia ensues with metabolic acidosis and multisystem organ failure. Left untreated, death occurs in the first few months of life [6,124].

In unobstructed TAPVR, the left-to-right shunt of pulmonary venous blood results in right atrial and ventricular enlargement with pulmonary overcirculation and subsequent right heart failure. The presence or absence of a restrictive interatrial communication is another major determinant in the pathophysiology of TAPVR; 70–80% of infants have only a PFO, which restricts filling of the left atrium and ventricle. This causes tremendous pulmonary overcirculation, right-sided dilation, and minimal left-sided filling, which results in decreased size of the left atrium and ventricle. The abnormal displacement of the interventricular septum along with chronic underfilling of the left ventricle leads to decreased systemic cardiac output. Symptomatic CHF usually develops in the second month of life and may be partially or totally relieved by transvenous balloon atrial septostomy. Patients with an unrestrictive interatrial communication, generally consisting of a secundum type ASD, have a large left-to-right shunt with increased pulmonary blood flow, but if left untreated may not develop signs of right heart failure or pulmonary hypertension until the third or fourth decade of life [124,130].

Surgical approaches

Timing of surgical repair of PAPVR is dependent in part on symptomatology. Patients with a single anomalous pulmonary vein with an intact atrial septum may never require surgical treatment. Surgical therapy is generally reserved for those patients with (i) hemodynamically significant left-to-right shunting with Qp:Qs greater than 2:1; (ii) patients with recurrent pulmonary infections, especially those associated with Scimitar syndrome; (iii) patients having surgical repair of other major cardiac lesions; and (iv) patients with anomalous connections which affect surrounding structures by compression or obstruction [124]. Surgical technique for repair of PAPVR varies depending on the specific anatomy present. The repair can consist of a direct anastomosis of the anomalous veins to the left atrium or an indirect communication may be developed utilizing a patch to baffle the anomalous veins to the left atrium.

Obstructed TAPVR should be corrected emergently at time of diagnosis [131]. Patients with unobstructed TAPVR with restrictive interatrial communications are urgently palliated with blade and/or balloon atrial septostomies. These patients (and those with unobstructed TAPVR and nonrestrictive interatrial communications) can be medically managed for elective surgical repair, usually in the first year of life.

Techniques for surgical repair of TAPVR depend on the specific anatomy involved. In some cases, a period of deep hypothermic circulatory arrest may be necessary. Surgical repair generally includes incision and enlargement of the anomalous pulmonary venous confluence and direct anastomosis with the left atrium. Occasionally, a patch is needed to baffle the veins to the left atrium. So-called "sutureless" techniques have more recently been advocated, which are intended to reduce the risk of acquired pulmonary vein stenosis by using marsupialization of pericardium or pleura to create the atrial anastomosis [132,133].

Operative mortality for repair of asymptomatic PAPVR approaches zero [134], and in older symptomatic patients has been reported as less than 6% [135]. Operative mortality for patients with TAPVR has historically been significantly higher, but the 30-day mortality over a recent decade at Texas Children's Hospital was found to be only 7% [136]. Risk factors for operative mortality in TAPVR include heterotaxy syndrome and single ventricle [136,137].

Anesthetic considerations

The anesthesiologists' first encounter of the patient with PAPVR may be in the cardiac catheterization laboratory when, during attempted transcatheter closure of an ASD, the presence of an anomalous pulmonary vein is discovered, thereby preventing the utilization of the device. However, the first encounter of the patient with TAPVR may be in radiology, because an increasing number of newborns with suspected TAPVR undergo magnetic resonance imaging, which may be superior to echocardiography and angiography in the evaluation of TAPVR [138,139].

Intraoperative considerations for patients with PAPVR are similar to management of ASD. Minimizing pulmonary blood flow by control of ventilation and consideration for early extubation following repair should be the primary goals.

The prebypass management of the patient with obstructed TAPVR generally includes maximizing P_{O_2}, avoiding metabolic acidosis, and maintaining hemodynamic stability with the use of inotropic medications as necessary. TEE is usually contraindicated due to risk of further compression and obstruction to pulmonary veins even in the presence of nonobstructed TAPVR. Perioperative monitoring of central venous, left atrial, and pulmonary arterial pressures is helpful.

After bypass, nitric oxide should be used empirically in the case of obstructed TAPVR and should be readily available in unobstructed TAPVR. Perioperative pulmonary hypertension occurs in as many as 50% of patients, and

is a major risk factor for early mortality [140,141]. Pulmonary hypertensive crises may be avoided by employing hyperventilation, use of 100% oxygen, systemic alkalinization, sedation, paralysis, and nitric oxide. Sildenafil, magnesium sulfate, and prostaglandin E1 have been used in some patients to treat severe pulmonary hypertension [142]. Paradoxical pulmonary hypertension with systemic hypotension has been reported from the postoperative use of nitric oxide in patients with preoperative atrial obstruction and a poorly compliant and dysfunctional left ventricle. This paradoxical pulmonary hypertension is thought to be due to acute increases in pulmonary blood flow and resultant excessive preload to the noncompliant left side [143].

Pulmonary function may be compromised after bypass as a result of two pulmonary insults: (i) preoperative pulmonary edema secondary to pulmonary venous obstruction, and (ii) the inflammatory response from cardiopulmonary bypass. Pulmonary compliance is decreased and a large arterial-to-alveolar gradient develops. Pulmonary gas distribution may be optimized with the use of pressure control ventilation and altering PEEP to improve lung compliance.

Following repair, left atrial filling pressures may be elevated due to the small size and low compliance of the left atrium and ventricle. Accepting low blood pressures while weaning from cardiopulmonary bypass will help avoid overdistending the "unprepared" left side. Careful fluid management, optimization of heart rate and rhythm, and inotropic support will improve cardiac output. Temporary pacing may also be helpful. Perioperative dysrhythmias, especially supraventricular tachycardias, occur in as many as 20% of patients. If tolerated, an inovasodilator like milrinone will decrease left ventricular work and improve cardiac output. It is important to recognize that the Frank–Starling curve is very flat in the small, noncompliant LV, and administration of only a few milliliters of fluid may cause the left ventricle to become overdistended and fail.

Key points for anesthetic management of lesions

Patent ductus arteriosus

1 Avoid air bubbles in intravenous lines due to risk of paradoxical emboli.
2 Critically ill neonates may require a high dose narcotic technique to minimize the stress response to surgery.
3 Lung isolation is usually required for video-assisted surgery to allow adequate surgical exposure.

Aortopulmonary window

1 Patients with pulmonary overcirculation should be managed to maintain pulmonary vascular tone.
2 Surgical snaring of the pulmonary artery can assist in increasing diastolic blood pressure and coronary perfusion.
3 Perioperative pulmonary hypertension frequently requires hyperventilation, 100% oxygen, systemic alkalinization, deep sedation, and paralysis.

Atrial septal defects

1 Avoid air bubbles in intravenous lines due to risk of paradoxical emboli.
2 Tailor anesthetic techniques to allow early extubation.

Ventricular septal defects

1 Maintain pulmonary vascular tone in those patients with pulmonary overcirculation prior to repair.
2 Diagnose and treat possible dysrhythmias, especially heart block.
3 Patients with uncomplicated VSDs should be considered for early extubation.

Common atrioventricular canal

1 Maintaining pulmonary vascular tone is usually necessary during the prebypass interval.
2 Postbypass pulmonary hypertension frequently requires hyperventilation, 100% oxygen, systemic alkalinization, deep sedation, and paralysis.
3 TEE is helpful for postrepair assessments.
4 Inotropic support is frequently required with dopamine and/or milrinone.
5 Diagnose and treat dysrhythmias.

Double outlet right ventricle

1 Patients with physiology associated with pulmonary overcirculation should be managed by maintaining or increasing PVR.
2 Patients with physiology associated with inadequate pulmonary blood flow should be managed to improve pulmonary blood flow.
3 Postbypass pulmonary hypertension frequently requires hyperventilation, 100% oxygen, systemic alkalinization, deep sedation, and paralysis.
4 Diagnose and treat dysrhythmias.
5 Inotropic support is frequently required.

Truncus arteriosus

1 Patients with pulmonary overcirculation should be managed to maintain or increase PVR.
2 Surgical snaring of the pulmonary artery can assist in increasing diastolic blood pressure and coronary perfusion.
3 Perioperative pulmonary hypertension frequently requires hyperventilation, 100% oxygen, systemic alkalinization, deep sedation, and paralysis.
4 High incidence of DiGeorge syndrome may require perioperative calcium infusions and use of irradiated blood products.
5 Inotropic support is frequently required perioperatively.

Partial and total anomalous pulmonary venous return

1 Maximize oxygenation in cyanotic patients with mechanical ventilation, 100% oxygen, hyperventilation, and other maneuvers to decrease PVR.
2 Perioperative pulmonary hypertension frequently requires hyperventilation, 100% oxygen, systemic alkalinization, deep sedation, and paralysis.
3 Avoid use of TEE, which may worsen obstructed pulmonary veins and occlude nonobstructed veins.
4 Avoid overfilling the left heart.
5 Inotropic support is frequently required perioperatively.
6 Diagnose and treat dysrhythmias.

References

1. Levine MF, Hartley EJ, Macpherson BA, et al. (1993) Oral midazolam premedication for children with congenital cyanotic heart disease undergoing cardiac surgery: a comparative study. Can J Anaesth 40: 934–938.
2. Rivenes SM, Lewin MB, Stayer SA, et al. (2001) Cardiovascular effects of sevoflurane, isoflurane, halothane, and fentanyl-midazolam in children with congenital heart disease: an echocardiographic study of myocardial contractility and hemodynamics. Anesthesiology 94: 223–229.
3. Hickey PR, Hansen DD, Wessel DL, et al. (1985) Pulmonary and systemic hemodynamic responses to fentanyl in infants. Anesth Analg 64: 483–486.
4. Gruber EM, Laussen PC, Casta A, et al. (2001) Stress response in infants undergoing cardiac surgery: a randomized study of fentanyl bolus, fentanyl infusion, and fentanyl-midazolam infusion. Anesth Analg 92: 882–890.
5. Moore KL (2008) The Cardiovascular System, the Developing Human: Clinically Oriented Embryology, 8th edn. Saunders/Elsevier, Philadelphia, pp. 285–337.
6. Chang AC, Wells W, Jacobs J, et al. (1998) Shunt lesions. In: Chang AC, Hanley FL, Wernovsky G, Wessel D (eds)

Pediatric Cardiac Intensive Care. Williams & Wilkins, Baltimore, pp. 201–232.

7. Allen HD (2001) Moss and Adams' Heart Disease in Infants, Children, and Adolescents: Including the Fetus and Young Adult, 6th edn. Lippincott Williams and Wilkins, Philadelphia, pp. 746–764.

8. Mullins CE, Pagatto L (1998) Patent ductus arteriosus. In: Garson A Jr, Bricker JT, Fisher DJ, Neish SR (eds) The Science and Practice of Pediatric Cardiology, 3rd edn. Williams & Wilkins, Baltimore, pp. 1181–1197.

9. Cooley DA, Norman JC (1975) Closure of patent ductus arteriosus. In: Cooley DA, Norman JC (eds) Techniques in Cardiac Surgery. Texas Medical Press, Houston, pp. 10–17.

10. Sekar KC, Corff KE (2008) Treatment of patent ductus arteriosus: indomethacin or ibuprofen? J Perinatol 28: S60–S62.

11. Suematsu Y, Mora BN, Mihaljevic T, del Nido PJ (2005) Totally endoscopic robotic-assisted repair of patent ductus arteriosus and vascular ring in children. Ann Thor Surg 80: 2309–2313.

12. Lavoie J, Burrows FA, Hansen DD (1996) Video-assisted thoracoscopic surgery for the treatment of congenital cardiac defects in the pediatric population Anesth Analg 82: 563–567.

13. Shaw AD, Mitchell JB (1998) Anaesthesia for video-assisted thoracoscopic patent ductus arteriosus ligation. Anaesthesia 53: 914–917.

14. Uezono S, Hammer GB, Wellis V, et al. (2001) Anesthesia for outpatient repair of patent ductus arteriosus. J Cardiothorac Vasc Anesth 15: 750–752.

15. Le Bret E, Papadatos S, Folliguet T, et al. (2002) Interruption of patent ductus arteriosus in children: robotically assisted versus videothoracoscopic surgery. J Thorac Cardiovasc Surg 123: 973–976.

16. Lloyd TR, Fedderly R, Mendelsohn AM, et al. (1993) Transcatheter occlusion of patent ductus arteriosus with Gianturco coils. Circulation 88: 1412–1420.

17. Ebeid MR, Gaymes CH, Smith JC, et al. (2001) Gianturco–Grifka vascular occlusion device for closure of patent ductus arteriosus. Am J Cardiol 87: 657–660.

18. Pass RH, Hijazi Z, Hsu DT, et al. (2004) Multicenter USA Amplatzer patent ductus arteriosus occlusion device trial: initial and one-year results. J Am Coll Cardiol 44: 513–519.

19. Prieto LR, DeCamillo DM, Konrad DJ, et al. (1998) Comparison of cost and clinical outcome between transcatheter coil occlusion and surgical closure of isolated patent ductus arteriosus. Pediatrics 101: 1020–1024.

20. Dutta S, Mihailovic A, Benson L, et al. (2008) Thoracoscopic ligation versus coil occlusion for patent ductus arteriosus: a matched cohort study of outcomes and cost. Surg Endosc 22: 1643–1648.

21. Williams RK, Abajian JC (1997) High spinal anaesthesia for repair of patent ductus arteriosus in neonates. Paediatr Anaesth 7: 205–209.

22. Lin YC, Sentivany-Collins SK, Peterson KL, et al. (1999) Outcomes after single injection caudal epidural versus continuous infusion epidural via caudal approach for postoperative analgesia in infants and children undergoing patent ductus arteriosus ligation. Paediatr Anaesth 9: 139–143.

23. Wiggins JW (1998) Aortopulmonary septal defect. In: Garson A Jr, Bricker JT, Fisher DJ, Neish SR (eds) The Science and Practice of Pediatric Cardiology, 2nd edn. Williams & Wilkins, Baltimore, pp. 1199–1205.

24. Tanoue Y, Sese A, Ueno Y, Joh K (2000) Surgical management of aortopulmonary window. Jpn J Thorac Cardiovasc Surg 48: 557–561.

25. Tkebuchava T, von Segesser LK, Vogt PR (1997) Congenital aortopulmonary window: diagnosis, surgical technique and long-term results. Eur J Cardiothorac Surg 11: 293–297.

26. Kutsche LM, Van Mierop LH (1987) Anatomy and pathogenesis of aorticopulmonary septal defect. Am J Cardiol 59: 443–447.

27. Jacobs JP, Quintessenza JA, Gaynor JW, et al. (2000) Congenital Heart Surgery Nomenclature and Database Project: aortopulmonary window. Ann Thorac Surg 69: S44–S49.

28. Backer CL, Mavroudis C (2002) Surgical management of aortopulmonary window: a 40-year experience. Eur J Cardiothorac Surg 21: 773–779.

29. Blieden LC, Moller JH (1974) Aorticopulmonary septal defect. An experience with 17 patients. Br Heart J 36: 630–635.

30. Erez E, Dagan O, Georghiou GP, et al. (2004) Surgical management of aortopulmonary window and associated lesions. Ann Thorac Surg 77: 484–487.

31. Tulloh RM, Rigby ML (1997) Transcatheter umbrella closure of aorto-pulmonary window. Heart 77: 479–480.

32. Sivakumar K, Francis E (2006) Transcatheter closure of distal aortopulmonary window using Amplatzer device. Cong Heart Dis 1: 321–323.

33. Di Bella I, Gladstone DJ (1998) Surgical management of aortopulmonary window. Ann Thorac Surg 65: 768–770.

34. Matsuki O, Yagihara T, Yamamoto F, et al. (1999) As originally published in 1992: new surgical technique for total-defect aortopulmonary window. Ann Thorac Surg 67: 891.

35. . Cooley DA, Norman JC (1975) Closure of atrial septal defect. In: Cooley DA, Norman JC (eds) Techniques in Cardiac Surgery. Texas Medical Press, Houston, pp. 70–79.

36. Vick GW (1998) Defects of the atrial septum including atrioventricular septal defects. In: Garson A Jr, Bricker JT, Fisher DJ, Neish SR (eds) The Science and Practice of Pediatric Cardiology, 2nd edn. Williams & Wilkins, Baltimore, pp. 1141–1179.

37. Sealy WC, Farmer JC, Young WG, et al. (1969) Atrial dysrhythmia and atrial secundum defects. J Thorac Cardiovasc Surg 57: 245–250.

38. Reybrouck T, Bisschop A, Dumoulin M, et al. (1991) Cardiorespiratory exercise capacity after surgical closure of atrial septal defect is influenced by the age at surgery. Am Heart J 122: 1073–1078.

39. Nicholson IA, Bichell DP, Bacha EA, del Nido PJ (2001) Minimal sternotomy approach for congenital heart operations. Ann Thorac Surg 71: 469–472.

40. Khan JH, McElhinney DB, Reddy VM, Hanley FL (1999) A 5-year experience with surgical repair of atrial septal defect employing limited exposure. Cardiol Young 9: 572–576.

41. Black MD, Freedom RM (1998) Minimally invasive repair of atrial septal defects. Ann Thorac Surg 65: 765–767.

42. Taaffe M, Fischer E, Baranowski A, et al. (2008) Comparison of three patent foramen ovale closure devices in a randomized trial (Amplatzer versus CardioSEAL-STARflex versus Helex occluder). Am J Cardiol 101: 1353–1358.

43. Sievert H, Fischer E, Heinisch C, et al. (2007) Transcatheter closure of patent foramen ovale without an implant: initial clinical experience. Circulation 116: 1701–1706.

44. Ruiz CE, Kipshidze N, Chiam PT, Gogorishvili I (2008) Feasibility of patent foramen ovale closure with no-device left behind: first-in-man percutaneous suture closure. Catheter Cardiovasc Interv 71: 921–926.

45. Boccalandro F, Baptista E, Muench A, et al. (2004) Comparison of intracardiac echocardiography versus transesophageal echocardiography guidance for percutaneous transcatheter closure of atrial septal defect. Am J Cardiol 93: 437–440.

46. Marie Valente A, Rhodes JF (2007) Current indications and contraindications for transcatheter atrial septal defect and patent foramen ovale device closure. Am Heart J 153: 81–84.

47. Peterson KL, DeCampli WM, Pike NA, et al. (2000) A report of two hundred twenty cases of regional anesthesia in pediatric cardiac surgery. Anesth Analg 90: 1014–1019.

48. Hammer GB (1999) Regional anesthesia for pediatric cardiac surgery. J Cardiothorac Vasc Anesth 13: 210–213.

49. Humphreys N, Bays SM, Parry AJ, et al. (2005) Spinal anesthesia with an indwelling catheter reduces the stress response in pediatric open heart surgery. Anesthesiology 103: 1113–1120.

50. Laussen PC, Reid RW, Stene RA, et al. (1996) Tracheal extubation of children in the operating room after atrial septal defect repair as part of a clinical practice guideline. Anesth Analg 82: 988–993.

51. Minette MS, Sahn DJ (2006) Ventricular septal defects. Circulation 114: 2190–2197.

52. Baptista MJ, Fairbrother UL, Howard CM, et al. (2000) Heterotrisomy, a significant contributing factor to ventricular septal defect associated with Down syndrome? Hum Genet 107: 476–482.

53. Cooley DA, Norman JC (1975) Closure of ventricular septal defect. In: Cooley DA, Norman JC (eds) Techniques in Cardiac Surgery. Texas Medical Press, Houston, pp. 80–87.

54. Jacobs JP, Burke RP, Quintessenza JA, Mavroudis C (2000) Congenital Heart Surgery Nomenclature and Database Project: ventricular septal defect. Ann Thorac Surg 69: S25–S35.

55. Lun K, Li H, Leung MP, et al. (2001) Analysis of indications for surgical closure of subarterial ventricular septal defect without associated aortic cusp prolapse and aortic regurgitation. Am J Cardiol 87: 1266–1270.

56. Hoffman JI, Rudolph AM, Heymann MA (1981) Pulmonary vascular disease with congenital heart lesions: pathologic features and causes. Circulation 64: 873–877.

57. Moe DG, Guntheroth WG (1987) Spontaneous closure of uncomplicated ventricular septal defect. Am J Cardiol 60: 674–678.

58. Ramaciotti C, Vetter JM, Bornemeier RA, Chin AJ (1995) Prevalence, relation to spontaneous closure, and association of muscular ventricular septal defects with other cardiac defects. Am J Cardiol 75: 61–65.

59. Kadner A, Dave H, Dodge-Khatami A, et al. (2004) Inferior partial sternotomy for surgical closure of isolated ventricular septal defects in children. Heart Surg Forum 7: E467–E470.

60. Wang YQ, Chen RK, Ye WW, et al. (1999) Open-heart surgery in 48 patients via a small right anterolateral thoracotomy. Tex Heart Inst J 26: 124–128.

61. Burke RP, Michielon G, Wernovsky G (1994) Video-assisted cardioscopy in congenital heart operations. Ann Thorac Surg 58: 864–868.

62. Rao V, Freedom RM, Black MD (1999) Minimally invasive surgery with cardioscopy for congenital heart defects. Ann Thorac Surg 68: 1742–1745.

63. Miyaji K, Hannan RL, Ojito J, et al. (2000) Video-assisted cardioscopy for intraventricular repair in congenital heart disease. Ann Thorac Surg 70: 730–737.

64. Ishikawa S, Morishita Y, Sato Y, et al. (1994) Frequency and operative correction of aortic insufficiency associated with ventricular septal defect. Ann Thorac Surg 57: 996–998.

65. Karpawich PP, Duff DF, Mullins CE, et al. (1981) Ventricular septal defect with associated aortic valve insufficiency. Progression of insufficiency and operative results in young children. J Thorac Cardiovasc Surg 82: 182–189.

66. Backer CL, Winters RC, Zales VR, et al. (1993) Restrictive ventricular septal defect: how small is too small to close? Ann Thorac Surg 56: 1014–1018.

67. Hardin JT, Muskett AD, Canter CE, et al. (1992) Primary surgical closure of large ventricular septal defects in small infants. Ann Thorac Surg 53: 397–401.

68. Waight DJ, Bacha EA, Kahana M, et al. (2002) Catheter therapy of Swiss cheese ventricular septal defects using the Amplatzer muscular VSD occluder. Catheter Cardiovasc Interv 55: 355–361.

69. Thanopoulos BD, Rigby ML (2005) Outcome of transcatheter closure of muscular ventricular septal defects with the Amplatzer ventricular septal defect occluder. Heart 91: 513–516.

70. Holzer R, Balzer D, Cao QL, et al;. Amplatzer Muscular Ventricular Septal Defect Investigators (2004) Device closure of muscular ventricular septal defects using the Amplatzer muscular ventricular septal defect occluder: immediate and mid-term results of a U.S. registry. J Am Coll Cardiol 43: 1257–1263.

71. Lock JE, Block PC, McKay RG, et al. (1988) Transcatheter closure of ventricular septal defects. Circulation 78: 361–368.

72. O'Laughlin MP, Mullins CE (1989) Transcatheter occlusion of ventricular septal defect. Cathet Cardiovasc Diagn 17: 175–179.

73. Fu YC, Bass J, Amin Z, et al. (2006) Transcatheter closure of perimembranous ventricular septal defects using

the new Amplatzer membranous VSD occluder: results of the U.S. phase I trial. J Am Coll Cardiol 47: 319–325.

74. Okubo M, Benson LN, Nykanen D, et al. (2001) Outcomes of intraoperative device closure of muscular ventricular septal defects. Ann Thorac Surg 72: 416–423.

75. Sullivan ID (2007) Transcatheter closure of perimembranous ventricular septal defect: is the risk of heart block too high a price? Heart 93: 284–286.

76. Malec E, Mroczek T, Pajak J, et al. (1999) Results of surgical treatment of congenital heart defects in children with Down's syndrome. Pediatr Cardiol 20: 351–354.

77. Hasegawa N, Oshima M, Kawakami H, Hirano H (1990) Changes in pulmonary tissue of patients with congenital heart disease and Down syndrome: a morphological and histochemical study. Acta Paediatr Jpn 32: 60–66.

78. Yamaki S, Horiuchi T, Sekino Y (1983) Quantitative analysis of pulmonary vascular disease in simple cardiac anomalies with the Down syndrome. Am J Cardiol 51: 1502–1506.

79. Chi TPL (1975) The pulmonary vascular bed in children with Down syndrome. J Pediatr 86: 533–538.

80. Andersen HO, de Leval MR, Tsang VT, et al. (2006) Is complete heart block after surgical closure of ventricular septum defects still an issue? Ann Thorac Surg 82: 948–956.

81. Eidem BW, Jones C, Cetta F (2000) Unusual association of hypertrophic cardiomyopathy with complete atrioventricular canal defect and Down syndrome. Tex Heart Inst J 27: 289–291.

82. Marino B, Digilio MC, Toscano A, et al. (1999) Congenital heart diseases in children with Noonan syndrome: an expanded cardiac spectrum with high prevalence of atrioventricular canal. J Pediatr 135: 703–706.

83. Jacobs JP, Burke RP, Quintessenza JA, Mavroudis C (2000) Congenital Heart Surgery Nomenclature and Database Project: atrioventricular canal defect. Ann Thorac Surg 69: S36–S43.

84. Rastelli G, Kirklin JW, Titus JL (1966) Anatomic observations on complete form of persistent common atrioventricular canal with special reference to atrioventricular valves. Mayo Clin Proc 41: 296–308.

85. Newfeld EA, Sher M, Paul MH, Nikaidoh H (1977) Pulmonary vascular disease in complete atrioventricular canal defect. Am J Cardiol 39: 721–726.

86. Giamberti A, Marino B, di Carlo D, et al. (1996) Partial atrioventricular canal with congestive heart failure in the first year of life: surgical options. Ann Thorac Surg 62: 151–154.

87. Lange R, Guenther T, Busch R, et al. (2007) The presence of Down syndrome is not a risk factor in complete atrioventricular septal defect repair. J Thoracic Cardiovasc Surg 134: 304–310.

88. Kado H, Tanoue Y, Fukae K, et al. (2005) Does Down syndrome affect the long-term results of complete atrioventricular septal defect when the defect is repaired during the first year of life? Eur J Cardio Thorac Surg 27: 405–409.

89. Singh RR, Warren PS, Reece TB, et al. (2006) Early repair of complete atrioventricular septal defect is safe and effective. Ann Thorac Surg 82: 1598–1601.

90. Cope JT, Fraser GD, Kouretas PC, Kron IL (2002) Complete versus partial atrioventricular canal: equal risks of repair in the modern era. Ann Surg 236: 514–520.

91. Cooley DA, Norman JC (1975) Techniques in Cardiac Surgery. Texas Medical Press, Houston, pp. 88–93.

92. Redmond JM, Silove ED, De Giovanni JV, et al. (1996) Complete atrioventricular septal defects: the influence of associated cardiac anomalies on surgical management and outcome. Eur J Cardiothorac Surg 10: 991–995.

93. Oshima Y, Yamaguchi M, Yoshimura N, et al. (2001) Anatomically corrective repair of complete atrioventricular septal defects and major cardiac anomalies. Ann Thorac Surg 72: 424–429.

94. Schaffer R, Berdat P, Stolle B, et al. (1999) Surgery of the complete atrioventricular canal: relationship between age at operation, mitral regurgitation, size of the ventricular septum defect, additional malformations and early postoperative outcome. Cardiology 91: 231–235.

95. Hanley FL, Fenton KN, Jonas RA, et al. (1993) Surgical repair of complete atrioventricular canal defects in infancy. Twenty-year trends. J Thorac Cardiovasc Surg 106: 387–394.

96. Stark J, Gallivan S, Lovegrove J, et al. (2000) Mortality rates after surgery for congenital heart defects in children and surgeons' performance. Lancet 355: 1004–1007.

97. Trachte AL, Lobato EB, Urdaneta F, et al. (2005) Oral sildenafil reduces pulmonary hypertension after cardiac surgery. Ann Thorac Surg 79: 194–197.

98. Walters HL, Mavroudis C, Tchervenkov CI, et al. (2000) Congenital Heart Surgery Nomenclature and Database Project: double outlet right ventricle. Ann Thorac Surg 69: S249–S263.

99. Silka MJ (1998) Double-outlet ventricles. In: Garson A Jr, Bricker JT, Fisher DJ, Neish SR (eds) The Science and Practice of Pediatric Cardiology, 2nd edn. Williams & Wilkins, Baltimore, pp. 1505–1523.

100. Troise DE, Ranieri L, Arciprete PM (2001) Surgical repair for double outlet right ventricle and intact ventricular septum. Ann Thorac Surg 71: 1018–1019.

101. Kleinert S, Sano T, Weintraub RG, et al. (1997) Anatomic features and surgical strategies in double-outlet right ventricle. Circulation 96: 1233–1239.

102. Belli E, Serraf A, Lacour-Gayet F, et al. (1998) Biventricular repair for double-outlet right ventricle. Results and long-term follow-up. Circulation 98: II360–II365.

103. Musumeci F, Shumway S, Lincoln C, Anderson RH (1988) Surgical treatment for double-outlet right ventricle at the Brompton Hospital, 1973 to 1986. J Thorac Cardiovasc Surg 96: 278–287.

104. Takeuchi K, McGowan FX, Jr, Moran AM, et al. (2001) Surgical outcome of double-outlet right ventricle with subpulmonary VSD. Ann Thorac Surg 71: 49–52.

105. Cil E, Ozme S, Saraclar M, et al. (1997) The angiocardiographic analysis of 73 patients with double-outlet right ventricle. Turk J Pediatr 39: 27–33.

106. Belli E, Serraf A, Lacour-Gayet F, et al. (1999) Double-outlet right ventricle with non-committed ventricular septal defect. Eur J Cardiothorac Surg 15: 747–752.

107. Beekmana RP, Roest AA, Helbing WA, et al. (2000) Spin echo MRI in the evaluation of hearts with a double outlet right ventricle: usefulness and limitations. Magn Reson Imaging 18: 245–253.

108. Barbero-Marcial ML, Tanamati C (1998) Repair of truncus arteriosus. Adv Card Surg 10: 43–73.

109. Brown JW, Ruzmetov M, Okada Y, et al. (2001) Truncus arteriosus repair: outcomes, risk factors, reoperation and management. Eur J Cardiothorac Surg 20: 221–227.

110. Williams JM, de Leeuw M, Black MD, et al. (1999) Factors associated with outcomes of persistent truncus arteriosus. J Am Coll Cardiol 34: 545–553.

111. Goldmuntz E, Clark BJ, Mitchell LE, et al. (1998) Frequency of 22q11 deletions in patients with conotruncal defects. J Am Coll Cardiol 32: 492–498.

112. Momma K, Ando M, Matsuoka R (1997) Truncus arteriosus communis associated with chromosome 22q11 deletion. J Am Coll Cardiol 30: 1067–1071.

113. Frohn-Mulder IM, Wesby SE, Bouwhuis C, et al. (1999) Chromosome 22q11 deletions in patients with selected outflow tract malformations. Genet Couns 10: 35–41.

114. Collett RW, Edwards JE (1949) Persistent truncus arteriosus: a classification according to anatomical types. Surg Clin North Am 29: 1245–1270.

115. Van Praagh R, Van Praagh S (1965) The anatomy of common aorticopulmonary trunk (truncus arteriosus communis) and its embryologic implications. A study of 57 necropsy cases. Am J Cardiol 16: 406–425.

116. Jacobs ML (2000) Congenital Heart Surgery Nomenclature and Database Project: truncus arteriosus. Ann Thorac Surg 69: S50–S55.

117. Brizard CP, Cochrane A, Austin C, et al. (1997) Management strategy and long-term outcome for truncus arteriosus. Eur J Cardiothorac Surg 11: 687–695.

118. McElhinney DB, Rajasinghe HA, Mora BN, et al. (2000) Reinterventions after repair of common arterial trunk in neonates and young infants. J Am Coll Cardiol 35: 1317–1322.

119. Black MD, Adatia I, Freedom RM (1998) Truncal valve repair: initial experience in neonates. Ann Thorac Surg 65: 1737–1740.

120. Rajasinghe HA, McElhinney DB, Reddy VM, et al. (1997) Long-term follow-up of truncus arteriosus repaired in infancy: a twenty-year experience. J Thorac Cardiovasc Surg 113: 869–878.

121. Edwards JE (1952) Pathologic and developmental considerations in anomalous pulmonary venous connection. Mayo Clin Proc 28: 441–452.

122. Herlong JR, Jaggers JJ, Ungerleider RM (2000) Congenital Heart Surgery Nomenclature and Database Project: pulmonary venous anomalies. Ann Thorac Surg 69: S56–S69.

123. Healey JE Jr (1952) Anatomic survey of anomalous pulmonary veins: their clinical significance. J Thorac Surg 23: 433–444.

124. . Ward KE, Mullins CE (1998) Anomalous pulmonary venous connections, pulmonary vein stenosis, and atresia of the common pulmonary vein. In: Garson A Jr, Bricker JT, Fisher DJ, Neish SR (eds) The Science and Practice of Pediatric Cardiology, 2nd edn. Williams & Wilkins, Baltimore, pp. 1431–1461.

125. Wessels MW, Frohn-Mulder IM, Cromme-Dijkhuis AH, Wladimiroff JW (1996) In utero diagnosis of infradiaphragmatic total anomalous pulmonary venous return. Ultrasound Obstet Gynecol 8: 206–209.

126. Bogers AJ, Baak R, Lee PC, et al. (1999) Early results and long-term follow-up after corrective surgery for total anomalous pulmonary venous return. Eur J Cardiothorac Surg 16: 296–299.

127. Kouchoukos NT, Blackstone EH, Doty DB, Hanley FL, Karp RB (eds) (2003) Kirklin/Barratt-Boyes Cardiac Surgery, 3rd edn. Churchill Livingstone, Philadelphia, pp. 753–779.

128. Jonas RA, Smolinsky A, Mayer JE, Castaneda AR (1987) Obstructed pulmonary venous drainage with total anomalous pulmonary venous connection to the coronary sinus. Am J Cardiol 59: 431–435.

129. Duff DF, Nihill MR, McNamara DG (1977) Infradiaphragmatic total anomalous pulmonary venous return. Review of clinical and pathological findings and results of operation in 28 cases. Br Heart J 39: 619–626.

130. Ward KE, Mullins CE, Huhta JC, et al. (1986) Restrictive interatrial communication in total anomalous pulmonary venous connection. Am J Cardiol 57: 1131–1136.

131. Burroughs JT, Edwards JE (1960) Total anomalous pulmonary venous connection. Am Heart J 59: 913–931.

132. Devaney EJ, Chang AC, Ohye RG, et al. (2006) Management of congenital and acquired pulmonary vein stenosis. Ann Thorac Surg 81: 992–995.

133. Buitrago E, Panos AL, Ricci M (2008) Primary repair of infracardiac total anomalous pulmonary venous connection using a modified sutureless technique. Ann Thorac Surg 86: 320–322.

134. Alsoufi B, Cai S, Van Arsdell GS, et al. (2007) Outcomes after surgical treatment of children with partial anomalous pulmonary venous connection. Ann Thorac Surg 84: 2020–2026.

135. John Sutton MG, Tajik AJ, McGoon DC (1981) Atrial septal defect in patients ages 60 years or older: operative results and long-term postoperative follow-up. Circulation 64: 402–409.

136. Morales DL, Braud BE, Booth JH, et al. (2006) Heterotaxy patients with total anomalous pulmonary venous return: improving surgical results. Ann Thorac Surg 82: 1621–1627.

137. Hancock Friesen CL, Zurakowski D, Thiagarajan RR, et al. (2005) Total anomalous pulmonary venous connection: an analysis of current management strategies in a single institution. Ann Thorac Surg 79: 596–606.

138. Masui T, Seelos KC, Kersting-Sommerhoff BA, Higgins CB (1991) Abnormalities of the pulmonary veins: evaluation with MR imaging and comparison with cardiac angiography and echocardiography. Radiology 181: 645–649.

139. Yoshioka K, Niinuma H, Kawakami T, et al. (2004) Three-dimensional demonstration of total anomalous pulmonary

venous return with contrast-enhanced magnetic resonance angiography. Ann Thorac Surg 78: 2186.

140. Sano S, Brawn WJ, Mee RB (1989) Total anomalous pulmonary venous drainage. J Thorac Cardiovasc Surg 97: 886–892.

141. Lincoln CR, Rigby ML, Mercanti C, et al. (1988) Surgical risk factors in total anomalous pulmonary venous connection. Am J Cardiol 61: 608–611.

142. Lin SC, Teng RJ, Wang JK (1996) Management of severe pulmonary hypertension in an infant with obstructed total anomalous pulmonary venous return using magnesium sulfate. Int J Cardiol 56: 131–135.

143. Rosales AM, Bolivar J, Burke RP, Chang AC (1999) Adverse hemodynamic effects observed with inhaled nitric oxide after surgical repair of total anomalous pulmonary venous return. Ped Cardiol 20: 224–226.

21

Anesthesia for left-sided obstructive lesions

James P. Spaeth, M.D. and Andreas W. Loepke, M.D., Ph.D.

Cincinnati Children's Hospital Medical Center, University of Cincinnati School of Medicine, Cincinnati, Ohio, USA

Introduction

Left-sided obstructive lesions of the heart may occur at various anatomic levels, ranging from a bicuspid aortic valve with minimal hemodynamic compromise to aortic atresia and hypoplastic left heart syndrome with profound hemodynamic derangements. These derangements in systemic flow may occur due to obstruction at multiple levels, such as seen in patients with Shone's complex, or from circumscribed obstructions at a single level, such as in hypertrophic cardiomyopathy, coarctation of the aorta, interrupted aortic arch, subvalvar, valvar, or supravalvar aortic stenosis. An understanding of the level and degree of the obstruction is important for optimal anesthetic management.

Aortic valve stenosis

Anatomy

The normal aortic valve has three leaflets and an area of $2\,cm^2/m^2$ body surface area. Although by some estimates,

Anesthesia for Congenital Heart Disease 2nd edition. Edited by Dean Andropoulos, Stephen Stayer, Isobel Russell and Emad Mossad.
© 2010 Blackwell Publishing.

isolated congenital valvar aortic stenosis occurs in only approximately 1 per 10,000 births [1], it is associated with other cardiac lesions in more than 5% of children suffering from congenital heart disease and presents with three to four times higher prevalence in males [2]. Valvar aortic stenosis may be associated with aortic coarctation or with hypoplasia of the ascending aorta due to decreased antegrade blood flow in the fetus. Aortic stenosis has also been described as part of Hunter's, Hurler's, and Turner's syndrome. In this disease, structural variations from the customary tricuspid contour of the aortic valve are common and result in a bicuspid or monocuspid appearance of the valvular apparatus, whose formation starts during weeks 5–7 of embryonic development [3–5]. The diseased valve leaflets are gelatinously or myxomatously malformed and the commissures are often partially fused, leaving a reduced aortic orifice, which can be located eccentrically. Left-ventricular myocardial hypertrophy is commonly observed, but nonhypertrophied left-ventricular dilation has also been reported [6].

Pathophysiology and diagnosis

The age of diagnosis, clinical presentation, treatment modality, and timing of intervention depend not only on the degree of valvular obstruction, but also on concomitant cardiac lesions and left-ventricular size and function. The diagnosis is typically made using transthoracic echocardiography, which provides comprehensive information regarding valve anatomy, annular size, aortic root diameter, and ventricular function. Continuous wave mean Doppler gradients adequately predict the peak-to-peak transvalvular gradient as measured during cardiac catheterization, whereas peak instantaneous Doppler gradients slightly overestimate the transvalvular gradient [7, 8]. However, depressed left-ventricular function can lead to an incorrectly diminished gradient. A Doppler peak systolic instantaneous gradient of less than 50 mm Hg is generally considered indicative of mild aortic stenosis, with peak-to-peak transvalvular gradients of less than 25–30 mm Hg. Many of these patients remain asymptomatic throughout childhood and adolescence. Severe aortic stenosis, on the other hand, signified by a peak instantaneous Doppler gradient of greater than 65–75 mm Hg and peak-to-peak gradients of more than 50–60 mm Hg usually presents during the first week of life [4]. In the most severe form of aortic stenosis, systemic blood flow and coronary perfusion can often be dependent on retrograde blood flow via a patent ductus arteriosus. After spontaneous ductal closure, affected neonates frequently present with symptoms of significant congestive heart failure, metabolic acidosis, and mitral valve insufficiency, quickly progressing to cardiogenic shock. Aggressive hemodynamic, respiratory, and metabolic resuscitation as well as immediate treatment with prostaglandin E1 are essential to reestablish adequate systemic perfusion. In infants with a less dramatic presentation, left-ventricular stroke volume is often maintained for extended periods of time. Normal ventricular wall tension is maintained by concentric ventricular hypertrophy; however, increased left-ventricular systolic and end-diastolic pressures can result in impaired subendocardial perfusion and ischemia. In severe cases, this malperfusion leads to the replacement of myocardium by fibrous tissue, termed endocardial fibroelastosis, further impairing ventricular performance and diminishing survival [9–11].

Surgical and interventional approaches

Treatment options and timing for intervention depend on the acuity of the clinical presentation and the concomitant cardiac abnormalities. Patients with mild aortic stenosis can be followed conservatively, whereas neonates suffering from critical aortic stenosis require immediate intervention. Important consideration needs to be given to the size and adequacy of the left ventricle to determine the patient's suitability for a one- or a two-ventricle repair [12]. Anatomic characteristics guiding this decision include patient age, aortic valve size, degree of endocardial fibroelastosis, presence of tricuspid regurgitation, aortic root diameter (ROOT), long-axis dimension of the left ventricle relative to the long axis of the heart (LAR), body surface area (BSA), and mitral valve area (MVA) [10,11]. The Rhodes' score, which can be used to predict outcome, can be calculated according to the formula:

$$\text{Score} = 14.0(\text{BSA}) + 0.943(\text{ROOT}) + 4.78(\text{LAR})$$
$$+ 0.157(\text{MVA}) - 12.03$$

A Rhode's score greater than −0.35 predicts with approximately 90% probability that a neonate would survive a two-ventricle repair. The risk for mortality increases when the left-ventricular long axis to heart long-axis ratio is 0.8 or less, the indexed aortic root diameter is 3.5 cm/m^2 or less, or the indexed mitral valve area is 5.75 cm^2/m^2 or less. If prior to intervention the left-ventricular size is considered inadequate to proceed with a biventricular repair, neonates may need to follow a single-ventricle palliation pathway (discussed in Chapter 25).

Given an adequate left-ventricular size, the majority of pediatric cardiac centers currently favor percutaneous balloon valvuloplasty as the first treatment option for severe, ductal-dependent congenital aortic stenosis. Using a retrograde approach, the balloon sheath is most commonly advanced from the femoral, umbilical, or carotid arteries. However, femoral vascular complications are not uncommon using this technique [13]. An alternative, antegrade approach can be used, in which the balloon is

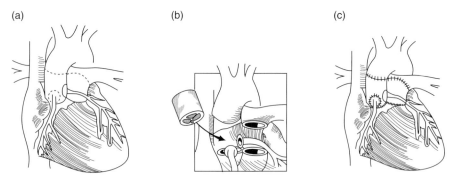

Figure 21.1 The Ross procedure (pulmonary autograft). (a) Incisions on the aorta, pulmonary artery, and the coronary buttons. (b) Pulmonary autograft and reimplantation of the coronary arteries. (c) Completed operation with a right ventricle to pulmonary artery conduit to replace the native pulmonary valve (Reproduced and used with permission from Reference [21])

usually inserted from the femoral or umbilical veins, via the foramen ovale, into the left atrium and ventricle. If left-ventricular function is adequate, administration of a bolus of adenosine (0.3–0.5 mg/kg), rapid right-ventricular overdrive pacing (rate of 220–240/min), or an infusion of esmolol (200 mcg/kg bolus followed by titrated infusion) during balloon dilation prevents forceful ventricular contraction against the balloon-occluded left-ventricular outflow tract and ejection of the balloon from the aortic position. In order to avoid postinterventional aortic valve insufficiency, the selected balloon size usually does not exceed the diameter of the aortic root. Using these techniques, severe aortic valve insufficiency is usually avoided in greater than 80% of patients early after intervention, and the 5-year mortality typically remains below 20% [13–17]. If the left ventricle is of borderline size, significant aortic insufficiency would disqualify patients from single-ventricle palliation.

Some congenital heart surgeons prefer primary surgical valvotomy of the severely stenotic aortic valve. Advantages of this open approach include direct inspection and commissurotomy of the valve, and the ability to address concomitant cardiac lesions such as patent ductus arteriosus, ventricular septal defect, or aortic coarctation during the same procedure. However, the need for cardiopulmonary bypass can increase morbidity for the patient. Historical case series demonstrated an operative mortality of 0–18%, 5-year survival of 60–100%, and aortic valve competency in greater than 95% of patients [14,18–20].

More recently, the Ross procedure, an aortic valve replacement using a pulmonary autograft combined with placement of a homograft in the pulmonary position, has gained popularity (Figure 21.1). It can also be combined with enlargement of the left-ventricular outflow tract, also termed the Ross–Konno procedure. These procedures can be performed in neonates and infants, but have more commonly been carried out in childhood or adolescence. Compared with prosthetic valve replacement, the Ross procedure avoids the need for anticoagulation. Long-term outcomes have been favorable, with greater than 75% freedom from reoperation up to 10 years postoperatively [21–24]. Allograft or prosthetic valve replacement is usually reserved for adolescent patients after completion of the majority of their somatic growth, if they are candidates for chronic anticoagulation.

Experimental treatment options for critical aortic stenosis or aortic atresia include fetal transcatheter valvuloplasty [25]. The rationale for intervention, despite the risks for both mother and fetus, is to avoid single-ventricle palliation by preventing the natural progression of severe aortic stenosis to hypoplastic left heart syndrome. The treatment is based on the assumption that alleviating the restricted blood flow across the aortic valve will lead to improved growth and function of the left ventricle, thereby allowing a postnatal, biventricular repair. However, at present, fetal interventions for aortic stenosis remain highly controversial [26,27].

Anesthetic considerations

Neonates with critical aortic stenosis can present with significant metabolic derangement and hemodynamic instability. Anesthetic management is directed toward meeting the increased oxygen requirement of the hypertrophied left-ventricular myocardium and optimizing cardiac output. Physiologic goals include maintenance of preload, afterload, and contractility. A normal or, to some extent, decreased heart rate is preferred. Bradycardia, however, is not well tolerated in neonates, whose cardiac output is heart rate-dependent given their fixed stroke volume, even without aortic stenosis. A sudden decrease in systemic vascular resistance with concomitant, compensatory tachycardia can quickly lead to myocardial ischemia and rapid deterioration of the patient's status. Vasoconstrictors, such as phenylephrine, can be used in this clinical situation. Dysrhythmias are not uncommon during cardiac catheterization and should be treated aggressively.

Inotropic support with a medication such as epinephrine may be required if myocardial function becomes depressed, but must be used with caution given its ability to increase heart rate and myocardial oxygen requirement. In unstable patients, a high-dose opioid technique will facilitate both balloon valvuloplasty and surgical valvotomy.

Subvalvar aortic stenosis

Anatomy

Subvalvular aortic stenosis (subAS) is a fixed obstruction occurring within the left-ventricular outflow tract and accounts for approximately 1% of patients with congenital heart disease. Patients with subAS usually become symptomatic after infancy, with a higher male predilection of 2:1–3:1 [28]. Most commonly, the anatomic correlate of the left-ventricular outflow tract obstruction is either a thin, discrete membrane of endocardial or fibrous tissue, or a fibromuscular ridge emanating from the crest of the interventricular septum. Less common manifestations include a circumferential, fibromuscular ring that originates from the anterior mitral valve leaflet, or a diffuse, tunnel-like fibromuscular obstruction. Other rare causes of subAS include anomalous attachments of mitral valve leaflets or mitral chordae. A variety of congenital heart lesions may exist in association with subAS and include bicuspid valves, aortic stenosis, ventricular septal defect, and aortic coarctation (Table 21.1).

Pathophysiology and diagnosis

SubAS can occasionally present in infancy as part of Shone's complex or following the surgical closure of a ventricular septal defect, but more commonly, the diagnosis is not made before the end of the first year of life. Patients usually present with complaints of orthopnea, dyspnea on exertion, or exertional angina and syncope. A systolic ejection murmur is present, most notable in the left, second and third parasternal spaces, and a carotid artery thrill can be palpated in a significant number of patients. The diagnosis is confirmed by color Doppler echocardiography, which allows assessment of the degree of the stenosis, biventricular enlargement and function, and concomitant mitral and aortic regurgitation. Cardiac catheterization is usually only needed to assess patients with serial obstructions or a tunnel-like stenosis. Since the severity of the subaortic stenosis (SAS) increases with age, progression of the left-ventricular outflow tract obstruction may lead to left-ventricular diastolic dysfunction and pulmonary venous hypertension. Moreover, abnormal blood flow across the aortic valve can lead to thickening of the valve leaflets, causing valvar aortic stenosis, left-ventricular hypertrophy, damage to the aortic valve, and subsequent aortic insufficiency.

Surgical approaches

Currently, surgery is favored as an early intervention and indicated for LVOT peak pressure gradients exceeding 40 mm Hg, and consists of fibromuscular resection with or without myectomy through an aortotomy (Figure 21.2). A study comparing early and late surgery in 83 patients with subAS found that the LVOT gradient was successfully reduced in both groups, but that the late surgery group had a much higher recurrence rate at 5 and 10 years (28 and 57%) compared to the early surgery group (6 and 0%) [31]. Failure to intervene early also increases the risk of developing aortic regurgitation, which does not necessarily improve following subaortic resection. Transcutaneous balloon dilation is usually ineffective, due to only temporary relief of the stenosis. Surgical complications include newly developed or worsened aortic insufficiency and postoperative atrioventricular heart block. In patients with tunnel-type subAS, an aortoventriculoplasty (Konno procedure), or, in the presence of aortic insufficiency, an aortic root replacement with a prosthetic valve or Ross–Konno procedure may be required.

Anesthetic considerations

Anesthetic management of subvalvar stenosis aims at maintaining the oxygen requirements of the myocardium and other end organs. Accordingly, the goal is to decrease myocardial oxygen demand and maintain both preload and afterload while maintaining or allowing a slightly decreased heart rate. In this regard, the anesthetic management of the patient with subAS is very similar to that for valvar aortic stenosis.

Table 21.1 Concurrent congenital anomalies in patients with subvalvar aortic stenosis

Lesions	Percentage of patients
Bicuspid valves	40
Aortic stenosis	28
Ventricular septal defect	24
Coarctation of aorta	12
Patent ductus arteriosus	12
Atrial septal defect	4

Source: Adapted from Reference [29].

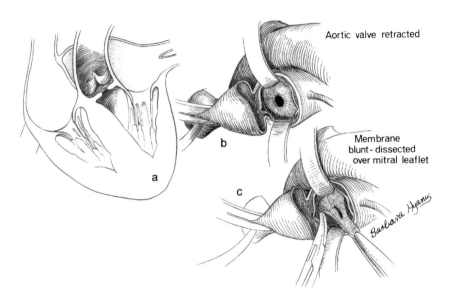

Aortic valve retracted

Membrane
blunt-dissected
over mitral leaflet

b

a

c

Barbara Hyams

Figure 21.2 Surgical repair of subaortic stenosis (Reproduced and used with permission from Reference [30])

Supravalvar aortic stenosis

Anatomy and morphology

Supravalvar aortic stenosis is the least common fixed-obstructive lesion of the LVOT, accounting for less than 0.05% of congenital heart disease. However, caused by abnormalities in the elastin gene (ELN), supravalvar aortic stenosis occurs in up to two-thirds of patients with Williams–Beuren syndrome, also known as Williams syndrome, and as part of familial supravalvar aortic stenosis [32–35]. The outflow tract obstruction frequently arises as a concentric narrowing of the ascending aorta at the superior margin of the sinuses of Valsalva, creating a typical hourglass deformity of the aorta. Other manifestations include a diffuse narrowing along the entire ascending aorta or a fibrous semicircular membrane at the sinotubular junction. Coronary artery involvement, which is common in children with Williams syndrome, may include a reduction of the left coronary artery ostial size, ostial obstruction by fusion of the aortic cusp to the supravalvar ridge, or diffuse narrowing of the left coronary artery (Figure 21.3).

Pathophysiology and diagnosis

Supravalvar aortic stenosis is a progressive disease, usually diagnosed after infancy, but may present earlier in life in patients with Williams syndrome. Its underlying mechanism is an elastin arteriopathy, leading to a lack of elastic tissue in the walls of large arteries, increased amounts of collagen, and hypertrophy of smooth muscle cells [36]. Accordingly, pulmonary artery stenosis is also observed in over 30% of patients suffering from Williams

syndrome, which can lead to biventricular hypertrophy [35]. Supravalvar aortic stenosis may also be associated with a bicuspid aortic valve and aortic valvar stenosis in up to 50% of patients [37]. Concentric left-ventricular hypertrophy can lead to myocardial ischemia, which is exacerbated by concomitant coronary artery stenosis. The risk of sudden death may only be slightly increased in patients with sporadic supravalvar aortic stenosis, but is significantly higher in patients suffering from Williams syndrome, compared with the general population [38,39].

A low-pitched, crescendo–decrescendo, systolic murmur is commonly heard at the base of the heart, radiating to the right carotid artery. The diagnosis of supravalvar aortic stenosis is routinely made using two-dimensional echocardiography, and Doppler echocardiography can be used to determine the pressure gradient across the ascending aorta. Electrocardiograms usually show left ventricular hypertrophy with special attention given to potential ischemic ECG changes. Patients with Williams syndrome, occurring in approximately 1 in 20,000 live births, are easily recognized due to their characteristic facial dysmorphisms; common features include a wide mouth with full lips, micrognathia, dental malocclusion, widely spaced teeth, a short nose with a flat nasal bridge, and a long philtrum. They may also suffer from arterial hypertension, hypercalcemia with nephrolithiasis, esotropia, a hoarse voice, joint hyperelasticity, and sensorineural hearing loss. Although patients often exhibit cognitive impairment, they commonly have a characteristic desire for conversation and company with a lack of social inhibition [35,40]. The suspected diagnosis of Williams syndrome can be verified even in neonates who do not yet exhibit the characteristic features, using genetic testing for karyotype and the fluorescent in situ hybridization (FISH) test for the 7q11.23 elastin gene deletion.

(a)

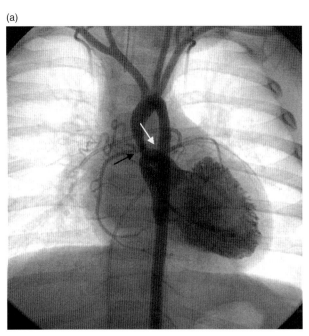

(b)

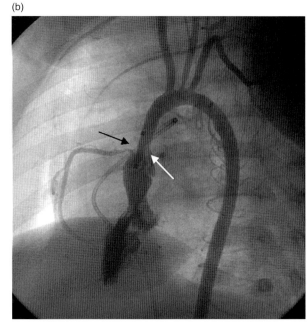

Figure 21.3 Representative angiogram of a patient with Williams syndrome, demonstrating supravalvar aortic stenosis (*black arrow*) and left coronary artery ostial stenosis (*white arrow*). (a) Anteroposterior view. (b) Lateral view. Peak systolic gradient during catheterization was 70 mm Hg (Angiograms courtesy of Robert Beekman, M.D.)

Surgical and interventional approaches

Infants with a peak pressure gradient of less than 20 mm Hg across the supravalvar stenosis often remain stable and do not require intervention; however, a peak instantaneous pressure gradient of greater than 75 mm Hg is usually an indication for surgical intervention. Surgical techniques for repair of supravalvar stenosis include patch aortoplasty (Figure 21.4), complete excision of the stenotic ring with end-to-end anastomosis, or the Ross or Ross–Konno procedures [37,41]. Significant coronary ostial obstruction may be relieved by a patch enlargement of the coronary os, excision of the obstructing aortic leaflet, or by coronary artery bypass grafting [42]. Concomitant pulmonary artery stenosis in many patients with Williams syndrome is frequently addressed by balloon dilation of the right-ventricular outflow tract stenosis prior to surgical repair of the LVOT obstruction.

Anesthetic considerations

Supravalvar aortic stenosis shares many of the pathophysiological characteristics and anesthetic management requirements of valvar and subvalvar stenosis. However, due to the potential combination of supravalvar aortic stenosis, left-ventricular hypertrophy, right-ventricular outflow tract obstruction, and coronary artery disease, patients with Williams syndrome can be at significantly increased risk for anesthesia-related complications. Ac-

cordingly, several reports have described perioperative fatalities in these patients, ranging from events during anesthesia induction or intubation, to postoperative complications [38,43–48]. The majority of these reported events

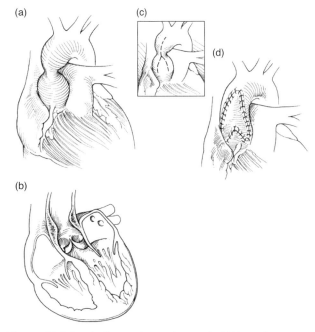

Figure 21.4 Repair of supravalvar aortic stenosis. (a) External appearance. (b) Coronal plane view of the defect. (c) Inverted Y incision in the ascending aorta. (d) Placement of an autologous pericardial patch (Reproduced and used with permission from Reference [21])

403

seemed to be caused by myocardial ischemia. Maintaining afterload at slightly elevated levels is therefore paramount to preserve coronary perfusion pressure. Volatile anesthetics must be used with caution due to their myocardial depressive and vasodilatatory effects. High-dose opioid techniques may be more appropriate and intramuscular premedication with ketamine may facilitate establishing intravenous access. However, significant increases in heart rate, such as potentially resulting from the administration of ketamine or vagolytic agents, are not well tolerated and need to be treated aggressively. It must be emphasized that the coronary arteries are frequently significantly involved, being partially obstructed or "hooded" from the abnormal surrounding connective tissue in the aorta, and that the degree of coronary obstruction often does not correlate with the severity of the supravalvar aortic stenosis. Other anesthetic complications, such as difficult mask ventilation or difficult tracheal intubation, may arise to the concomitant facial deformities in this syndrome. Moreover, the potential development of abnormal skeletal muscle tissue with lipid deposits may lead to an increased sensitivity to muscle relaxants, thus warranting close monitoring of neuromuscular blockade [49]. Additional sources of perioperative morbidity include the patients predisposition to renal insufficiency and arterial hypertension, which need to be appropriately addressed in the anesthetic plan.

Hypertrophic cardiomyopathy

Hypertrophic cardiomyopathy (HCM) is an autosomal dominant disease that occurs in about 1 in 500 live births (about 0.2% of the population) [50]. The annual mortality in tertiary care centers is 3–4% overall and up to 6% in children, while in the unselected population the mortality rate may be less than 1% [51]. HCM is most commonly caused by mutations in genes encoding proteins of the myocardial sarcomere, and in fact, over 50 mutations causing the disease have been identified, making it one of the most widespread genetic diseases of the myocardium. Depending on the specific mutation, abnormalities in the protein may lead to ineffective contraction of the sarcomere and the development of myocyte hypertrophy. A mutation on the β-myosin heavy chain leads to HCM in approximately one-third of cases [51].

Anatomy and pathophysiology

The characteristic gross morphologic feature in HCM is a hypertrophied and nondilated left ventricle, and the absence of other disease processes capable of causing this degree of hypertrophy (e.g., aortic stenosis). There is significant heterogeneity in regard to the location and degree of cardiac hypertrophy, and in fact, even first-degree rel-

atives with familial HCM often exhibit different patterns of hypertrophy [52, 53]. Myocardial hypertrophy may occur in the anterior, posterior, and/or basal regions of the ventricular septum, and in the ventricular free wall. The hemodynamic severity is dependent on the particular region where hypertrophy is most prominent: significant hypertrophy of the anterior region of the ventricular septum compared with the posterior septum more commonly causes subaortic outflow obstruction [54]. The histology of the left ventricle is remarkable for disarray of the hypertrophied cardiac muscle cells, myocardial scarring, and thickened walls in small intramural coronary arteries causing luminal narrowing [54, 55]. Although fiber disarray is present even in normal hearts, the extent to which this happens in the heart with HCM is significantly increased [56]. A minority of patients may progress to a secondary phase characterized by wall thinning in areas of previous hypertrophy, enlargement of cavity size, and impairment of ventricular function; a phenomenon likely related to myocardial ischemia and necrosis [57].

The most common finding in the patient with HCM is a hyperdynamic left ventricle with abnormal diastolic relaxation and compliance; left-ventricular outflow tract obstruction is present in no more than 25% of patients [54]. The degree of outflow tract obstruction is a dynamic process and may be reduced or abolished by decreasing myocardial contractility, increasing preload, and increasing afterload. The dynamic obstruction is increased during periods of increased ventricular contractility or sympathetic stimulation, as for instance, with exercise. The outflow tract gradient is felt to be caused in part by anterior movement of the mitral valve toward the ventricular septum during early systole, and more likely to occur in the setting of a hypertrophied anterior septum [54]. Anterior movement of the mitral valve may interfere with optimal valve closure causing mitral regurgitation, occurring more commonly in the setting of left-ventricular outflow tract obstruction. The combination of severe left-ventricular hypertrophy, left-ventricular outflow tract obstruction, and abnormalities of the intramural coronary arteries all place these patients at increased risk for myocardial ischemia and ventricular arrhythmias.

Diagnosis and treatment

Most patients with HCM and neonates, in particular, often remain asymptomatic for a long period of time. Many patients are not diagnosed until they present with symptoms of congestive heart failure, cardiac rhythm disturbances, or following a near-death cardiac event [51]. HCM has become the leading cause of sudden cardiac death in young athletes today, usually occurring in individuals older than 35 years [58, 59]. Even when the diagnosis is made prior to a catastrophic event, the clinical course of the disease is inconsistent and dependent on whether the HCM is obstructive or nonobstructive. If obstructive, more than 25% of infants will develop symptoms of congestive heart failure manifested by feeding intolerance or failure to thrive [60]. Adult patients with HCM are at substantial risk for the development of atrial fibrillation, which can cause significant hemodynamic impairment due to its negative effects on ventricular preload [61].

Echocardiography is extremely helpful in determining the extent, location, and severity of the disease. Quantitative echocardiographic findings in patients with HCM include increased left-ventricular wall thickness, decreased left-ventricular end-diastolic cavity size, and increased left-ventricular fractional shortening [60]. Other important findings include the presence and severity of left-ventricular outflow tract obstruction, systolic anterior motion of the mitral valve, and mitral regurgitation [62].

Treatment modalities for HCM include medical therapy, surgical therapy, and the use of pacing and/or implantable cardioverter-defibrillators. Aggressiveness of therapy in any given patient depends on the risk factors for morbidity and mortality. Identified risk factors for patients with HCM include family history of sudden death or syncope, extreme septal hypertrophy, and left-ventricular outflow tract obstruction [63,64]. Asymptomatic patients with HCM may not require any therapy. When medical therapy is initiated, it usually consists of either a β-blocker or calcium-channel blocker, and can be guided by treadmill exercise testing or patient symptoms [51]. Another treatment option is dual-chamber pacing, which has been used as an alternative to surgery with mixed results. Although pacing has been shown to be of benefit in some patients, randomized-controlled trials showing long-term improvement in outcomes are lacking. For patients at high risk for sudden death, such as those with documented sustained VT/VF, significant family history of sudden death, or a high-risk mutation, many centers will now place an implantable cardioverter-defibrillator [51].

Indications for surgical management include a left-ventricular outflow gradient >50 mm Hg and significant symptoms such as dyspnea, angina, or syncope unresponsive to medical therapy. Septal myectomy is an effective treatment in both pediatric and adult patients [63,65]. In pediatric patients with HCM undergoing septal myectomy at the Mayo Clinic over a 28-year period, there were no early deaths and survival at 5 and 10 years was 97 and 95%, respectively. Late follow-up was remarkable for 96% of patients in NYHA functional class I or II [63]. The surgery approach is commonly transaortic, and often technically challenging in the smaller child. Transesophageal echocardiography (TEE) can be used to aid in the assessment of intracardiac anatomy before resection and adequacy of resection following myectomy. Despite an excellent surgical result with minimal residual left-ventricular

outflow gradient, these children remain at risk for cardiac arrhythmias and sudden death [63].

Anesthetic management

Patients with HCM are at significant risk for cardiac complications during anesthesia and surgery. Although there are few studies looking at the pediatric population with HCM, one adult study was remarkable for 40% of patients having at least one adverse cardiac event [66]. Predictors of adverse outcome included major surgery and duration of surgery. To avoid hemodynamic instability, anesthetic management should be tailored toward maintaining preload and afterload, decreasing myocardial contractility, and avoiding tachycardia. Maintenance of normovolemia prior to induction is vital, and if necessary an intravenous catheter should be inserted prior to surgery. While halothane meets many of the hemodynamic goals and has been well tolerated in such cases, it is no longer widely available [67]. Sevoflurane and desflurane, on the other hand, may cause significant increases in heart rate and reductions in systemic vascular resistance, and should be used with caution. High-dose opioid anesthesia provides stable hemodynamics and maintenance of a normal to low heart rate. Remifentanil, a short-acting potent opioid administered by continuous infusion, may be an excellent choice when extubation of the trachea following surgery is planned. For patients not already on β-blocker therapy, esomolol can be used in the perioperative period to control heart rate and reduce cardiac contractility.

Depending on the procedure and severity of HCM, arterial vascular access and central venous access may be indicated. Patients with a critical LVOT gradient may benefit from preinduction placement of an arterial line for close monitoring of systemic blood pressure during the anesthetic induction. However, one must carefully judge whether the increased anxiety and pain caused by the procedure might precipitate an adverse event. The placement of a central venous line for this disease state is not a trivial occurrence, and the patient must be closely monitored for the occurrence of an atrial dysrhythmia. Rapid treatment of dysrhythmias is important as hemodynamics may deteriorate swiftly. Central venous pressure may be significantly elevated in the patient with HCM due to the hypertrophied noncompliant ventricle.

Pompe disease

HCM can present in infancy without sarcomeric protein gene mutations, such as in infants of insulin-dependent diabetic mothers or in patients with Pompe disease. This glycogen storage disease type II (GSD-II) is a rare autosomal recessive disorder occurring in 1 out of 40,000 live births, in which lysosomal glycogen accumulates in

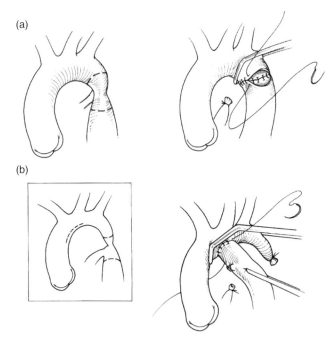

Figure 21.5 Two surgical approaches for repair of coarctation of the aorta. (a) Resection of coarctation with end-to-end anastomosis. (b) End-to-side, or aortic arch advancement technique (Reproduced and used with permission from Reference [21])

both cardiac and skeletal muscle because of a deficiency of acid α-glucosidase [68, 69]. Children presenting with the infantile form of this disease exhibit a severe HCM, and untreated often die in the first year of life from respiratory or cardiac complications. Therapy with long-term intravenous recombinant α-glucosidase has been shown to lead to significant resolution of the cardiac hypertrophy and skeletal muscle weakness [70] (Figure 21.5). To facilitate treatment, infants now commonly present to the operating room for central line placement. Infants presenting for surgery prior to therapy with recombinant human α-glucosidase are at high risk for anesthetic complications [71]. In a retrospective review, 6% of patients with infantile-onset Pompe disease receiving anesthetics developed an arrhythmia or cardiac arrest soon after induction of anesthesia [72]. Two-thirds of these events were attributed to the use of sevoflurane or propofol. Adaptation of the anesthetic technique to maintain systemic blood pressure is critical in these patients.

Coarctation of the aorta

Anatomy

Coarctation of the aorta denotes a narrowing of the aortic lumen just distal to the opening of the left subclavian artery at the point of insertion of the ductus arteriosus.

Although usually presenting as a discrete narrowing, the coarctation can also be a long-segment stenosis or be associated with hypoplasia of the transverse aortic arch. Up to 8% of all congenital cardiac patients have an aortic coarctation, which is more prevalent in males than females by a 1.5:1 ratio [2,73]. The etiology of the coarctation is a folding of the medial tissue of the aortic wall such that it encroaches upon the aortic lumen. When the coarctation is severe with limited anterograde flow from the transverse arch, blood flow to the distal aorta may be entirely dependent on a patent ductus arteriosus. If the coarcted segment remains uncorrected for sufficient time, collateral blood flow will develop thus allowing for adequate perfusion distal to the aortic obstruction. Other congenital cardiac anomalies are present in about one-half of patients with aortic coarctation and include ventricular septal and atrioventricular canal defects, valvar aortic stenosis, and SAS.

Pathophysiology and diagnosis

The neonate with a severe coarctation generally presents in the first few weeks of life with congestive heart failure, left-ventricular systolic dysfunction, and in some cases cardiogenic shock. The closure of the ductus arteriosus causes an acute increase in left-ventricular afterload, elevation of LVEDP, reduction in stroke volume, pulmonary venous congestion, and pulmonary artery hypertension [2]. The infant with a less severe coarctation may exhibit tachypnea and failure to thrive. The asymptomatic child with an unrecognized coarctation is at increased risk for developing systemic hypertension proximal to the coarctation and subsequent left-ventricular failure. Over 90% of untreated patients with coarctation of the aorta die by the age of 50 [74]. Even with surgical repair, patients with aortic coarctation demonstrate an increased predilection for hypertension, coronary artery disease, stroke, heart failure, and ruptured aortic and cerebral aneurysms. Over 50% of patients have arterial hypertension at long-term follow-up, which is not necessarily related to the presence of a recurrent stenosis [75].

The diagnostic feature of aortic coarctation is a systolic and mean blood pressure difference between the upper extremities and lower extremities of greater than 10 mm Hg. Transthoracic echocardiography [76] using a suprasternal long-axis view typically shows a localized narrowing ("posterior shelf") just distal to the left subclavian artery, and Doppler analysis aids in assessing the severity of the coarctation. Evaluating the heart for other associated lesions is important. Magnetic resonance imaging and CT angiography with three-dimensional reconstruction are other modalities used to image the aortic arch, and are more commonly utilized in older children and adults where imaging by transthoracic echocardiography is more likely suboptimal. A study comparing transthoracic echocardiography and CT angiography demonstrated a greater sensitivity of CT angiography compared with Doppler echocardiography for diagnosis of coarctation (100% vs 87.5%) [77]. Drawbacks to these modalities include the use of ionizing radiation with CT angiography, and the necessity for anesthesia or sedation for MRI in younger children.

Surgical and interventional approaches

Therapeutic options for aortic coarctation include surgery, balloon dilation, and placement of endovascular stents. However, there currently exists considerable uncertainty regarding the optimal long-term treatment strategy. At the present time, neonates are thought to have a superior outcome with surgical repair, while patients 6 months or older may benefit from balloon dilatation with or without stenting as the initial therapy [78]. A retrospective study comparing balloon angioplasty and surgery for initial therapy of neonatal coarctation showed that over 80% of patients receiving balloon angioplasty subsequently required surgery or repeat balloon dilation, while less than 20% of patients undergoing surgery required reintervention [79]. The options for surgical repair include a subclavian flap aortoplasty, a resection of the narrowed portion of the aorta with a traditional end-to-end anastomosis, an aortic arch advancement technique (extended end-to-end or end-to-side reconstruction), or tube graft interpositioning. The aortic arch advancement technique is used when transverse arch hypoplasia is present, and requires proximal extension of the anastomosis onto the underside of the transverse arch up to the level of the innominate artery [80] (Figure 21.5). This approach requires placement of a cross-clamp just distal to the innominate artery, placing the patient at risk for cerebral hypoperfusion. Perioperative complications from surgical repair of coarctation include recurrent laryngeal nerve or phrenic nerve injury, chylothorax, bleeding, and rarely paraplegia (0.4%) [81].

Restenosis after surgical repair of aortic coarctation is not uncommon, with an incidence varying widely depending on the surgical technique, age of patient at time of repair, definition of recurrence, and length of follow-up [82]. A study examining long-term complications in a cohort of patients up to 27 years after repair found a restenosis rate of 11%, with restenosis defined as a systolic brachial-ankle blood pressure difference of greater than 20 mm Hg [75]. Earlier studies showed a high incidence of recoarctation if the operation was performed in the first 3 years of life; the recurrence rate was <3% if performed afterward [83]. Current surgical techniques emphasizing aggressive excision of ductal tissue and the use of an extended end-to-end anastomosis in the setting of arch hypoplasia may lead to a lower incidence of resteno-

sis. Because of the significant incidence of hypertension and other long-term sequelae following coarctation repair, many centers aggressively treat even mild recurrent stenosis in the interventional catheterization suite.

Balloon angioplasty and stenting

The use of balloon angioplasty for initial treatment of discrete aortic coarctation in children 1 year and older provides excellent hemodynamic results [76,78,84]. Reluctance to use this approach in some centers is related to concerns about restenosis and aneurysm formation, which occur in 10–20% and 5–10% of patients respectively [85]. Approximately 25% of children undergoing an initial balloon angioplasty will require a reintervention within 2 years [76,78]. This is compared to patients undergoing surgical repair who rarely require reintervention. Balloon angioplasty is generally accepted as the first-line therapy for restenosis following surgical repair of aortic coarctation, providing excellent immediate and long-term results [82,86,87]. In approximately 80% of cases, the residual systolic pressure gradient can be reduced to less than 20 mm Hg. Repeat balloon angioplasty or surgery is required in about 25% of patients due to restenosis [82]. Complications related to balloon angioplasty include femoral artery thrombosis, aortic rupture, and stroke. The risk of femoral artery injury is greater in the smaller child. An increased mortality risk has been reported for patients undergoing angioplasty for recurrent coarctation versus native coarctation [86].

Balloon-expandable endovascular stents provide an effective therapy for treatment of native or recurrent coarctations occurring after surgery or balloon angioplasty [88–91] (Figure 21.6). In a study of 565 procedures from multiple institutions, 97.9% of patients had a successful reduction in the coarctation gradient at the time of the procedure [88]. Stents have been successfully used to treat patients with both discrete coarctation and transverse arch hypoplasia. Intermediate follow-up in patients receiving stents shows that the incidence of restenosis is reduced compared to balloon angioplasty [89–91]. Stents allow for future redilation to a larger size to accommodate the growth of the child. This therapy is limited by the need for a large sheath (8–9 Fr) in the femoral artery, and is thus not utilized in some centers until a child reaches a certain size. Endovascular stents have been placed in smaller children using the carotid artery, thus requiring a surgical procedure to place a sheath in this vessel. Complications related to stent placement include aneurysm formation, aortic dissection, stent migration, balloon rupture, femoral artery injury, and stroke, and may occur in as many as 15% of patients [88].

(a)

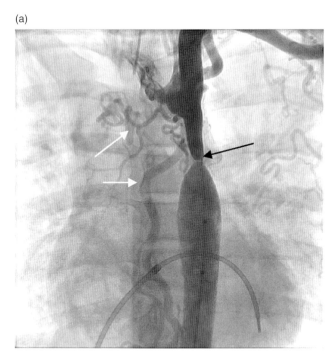

(b)

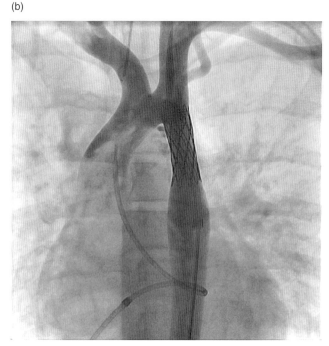

Figure 21.6 (a) Angiograms of a 12-year-old patient with a native aortic coarctation (*black arrow*) and a long, moderately hypoplastic isthmus before placement of a stent. Note multiple arterial collaterals (*white arrows*). (b) Angiogram after stent placement. The systolic gradient was reduced from 30 to 3 mm Hg following stent placement (Angiograms courtesy of Robert Beekman, M.D.)

Anesthetic considerations

The medical management of infants with severe coarctation consists of inotropic support and diuretics. In infants younger than 1 month, intravenous prostaglandin is utilized to open the ductus arteriosus. Intubation may be necessary to decrease the work of breathing and reduce left-ventricular demand. Metabolic acidosis should be corrected to improve left-ventricular function.

The anesthetic management of the patient presenting for surgical repair of a coarctation of the aorta should include a right-sided upper extremity arterial catheter in addition to the usual anesthetic monitors. The placement of the intra-arterial catheter ensures that blood pressure will be monitored during the phase of the operation when the left subclavian artery and/or aorta may be clamped or compressed. The use of cerebral near-infrared spectroscopy (NIRS) for continuous monitoring of cerebral oxygenation allows the anesthesiologist to identify cerebral hypoperfusion related to aortic cross-clamp position or inadequate cardiac output [92]. Central venous access may be indicated for initiation of inotropic support.

Induction of anesthesia can be accomplished either by intravenous or inhalational anesthesia; however, in the child with significant ventricular dysfunction an opioid-based induction may be preferable. The surgical repair is usually performed through a left thoracotomy and lung

retraction can impact ventilation. Close monitoring of arterial blood gases for adequacy of ventilation is vital. Inadequate ventilation causing severe acidosis in a critically ill neonate can worsen cardiac function and lead to cardiac arrest. There have been reports that infants with a core temperature greater than 38°C are at increased risk for spinal cord ischemia. Many centers choose to allow the child to cool to about 35°C in order to protect against this complication [93]. The application of the cross-clamp can cause upper body hypertension. The blood flow to the lower body and spinal cord is reliant on collateral flow that can vary depending on the anatomy of collateral blood vessels and on arterial pressure. It is possible that the failing ventricle may be unable to mount an appropriate blood pressure, in which case an inotropic agent may need to be administered [94]. If myocardial function is adequate, volatile anesthetics can be used to limit arterial hypertension during aortic cross-clamp. However, following completion of the vascular anastomosis, the dose of volatile anesthetic is usually reduced and fluid boluses may be administered in anticipation of systemic hypotension following release of the aortic cross-clamp.

The early postoperative period is often complicated by the onset of hypertension, which may be exacerbated in the setting of poor pain control. Greater than one-half of patients who undergo repair of a coarctation experience significant increases in blood pressure for up to 2 weeks

[95]. It has been postulated that the increase in blood pressure may be secondary to stimulation of the sympathetic system distal to the anastomotic site, with the subsequent increases in plasma renin activity. Untreated hypertension can result in mesenteric arteritis [96]. Hypertension in the acute perioperative period is usually treated with infusions of sodium nitroprusside or esmolol. Some centers utilize continuous epidural analgesia for control of pain following coarctation repair. Purported benefits of this technique compared with intravenous opioid therapy include better pain and blood pressure control.

Interrupted or hypoplastic aortic arch

Anatomy

An interrupted aortic arch (IAA) exists in about 1% of patients with congenital malformations of the heart. The interruption may be divided into three anatomical variants: type A, which is characterized by a location just distal to the left subclavian artery (25% of IAA); type B, located in the space between the left subclavian artery and the left common carotid artery (70% of IAA); and type C between the innominate and left common carotid arteries (5% of IAA) [97,98] (Figure 21.7). The majority of patients with a type B IAA have DiGeorge syndrome (22q11 deletion) [100]. Common features in the infant with DiGeorge syndrome include hypocalcemia, an absent thymus, and anomalies of the ears, face, and palate.

All types of IAA have a high incidence of associated congenital cardiac anomalies. A ventricular septal defect is most prevalent and present in greater than 90% of type B interruptions and more than 50% of type A interruptions [101]. Other cardiac defects include bicuspid aortic valve, truncus arteriosus, transposition of the great arteries, and double outlet right ventricle [102]. Left-ventricular outflow tract obstruction has been reported to occur in as many as 57% of patients with IAA, and is more commonly

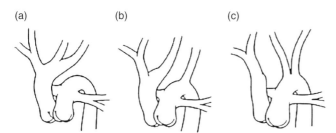

Figure 21.7 Interrupted aortic arch. (a) Type A: interruption between the left subclavian artery and the ductus arteriosus. (b) Type B: interruption between the left carotid and left subclavian arteries. (c) Type C: interruption at the proximal aortic arch between the innominate and left carotid arteries (Reproduced and used with permission from Reference [21])

associated with a type B interruption and anomalous right subclavian artery [103,104].

Pathophysiology and diagnosis

Neonates suffering from IAA often remain asymptomatic initially after birth, but over the course of a few days or weeks can become precipitously ill following closure of the ductus arteriosus. As the duct constricts, blood flow to the lower body becomes compromised, drastically increasing the risk of shock. Congestive heart failure may develop as a greater proportion of blood flow is directed to the pulmonary circulation. Rapid diagnosis accompanied by initiation of prostaglandin therapy, treatment of metabolic acidosis, and myocardial support may be lifesaving. Fetal echocardiography has led to improvements in early diagnosis and a reduction in the number of neonates presenting with circulatory collapse.

The diagnosis of IAA can usually be established with transthoracic echocardiography, and cardiac catheterization is usually not indicated. Magnetic resonance imaging has also been used to delineate complex arch anatomy. Careful evaluation for additional cardiac anomalies including the presence of left-ventricular outflow tract obstruction is important.

The use of prostaglandins, inotropic support, and diuretics is standard prior to surgical repair. The prognosis for survival without surgical intervention is poor, with as many as 90% of patients dying within the first year of life [105]. Those who survive past the first year develop a collateral circulation that allows for adequate lower-body perfusion despite the aortic interruption [106].

Surgical approaches

Surgical strategies for treatment have varied. A two-stage repair involving initial repair of the aortic arch through a left thoracotomy accompanied by pulmonary artery banding allows for palliation without the use of cardiopulmonary bypass. This approach results in limited exposure of the proximal aorta and does not allow the surgeon to address other coexisting lesions such as LVOT obstruction. A primary one-stage repair using a midline sternotomy and cardiopulmonary bypass is now favored. This approach provides optimal exposure for aortic arch repair, and the ability to close the VSD and address other associated lesions. A recent multicenter study suggested that surgical approaches other than direct anastomosis with patch augmentation of the IAA may increase the risk for future aortic arch reintervention [107]. However, one center recently reported that 100% of patients required no arch reintervention at 5 years after direct anastomosis without patch augmentation when the descending thoracic aorta was circumferentially mobilized, ductal tissue

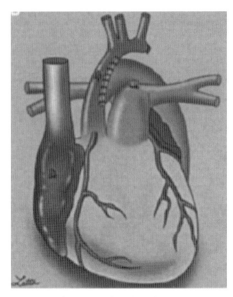

Figure 21.8 Repair of Interrupted aortic arch using an aortic arch advancement technique without a patch (Reproduced and used with permission from Reference [99])

aggressively excised, and a wide anastomosis made between the descending aorta and the posterior aspect of the distal ascending aorta [99] (Figure 21.8).

Until the last decade, major aortic arch surgery required the use of deep hypothermia with circulatory arrest, a technique shown to adversely impact long-term neurodevelopmental outcomes [108]. Many centers now use antegrade cerebral perfusion and myocardial perfusion during arch repair providing continuous delivery of oxygen to the brain and minimizing myocardial ischemic time (see Chapter 7). Over the next decade, studies should elucidate whether these techniques improve survival and reduce long-term morbidities.

IAA continues to be associated with significant mortality during the perioperative period and subsequent long-term follow-up. A study reporting outcomes from 33 institutions between 1987 and 1997 found an overall survival of 59% at 16 years after initiation of study entry [107]. Other studies found an overall perioperative mortality rate for procedures done since 1990 of 12%, compared to an overall mortality rate of 42% prior to 1985 [109, 110]. One-month survival of >92% following IAA repair has been reported at a number of centers [104,99]. Risk factors reported to be associated with increased mortality include low birth weight, type B IAA, other major associated cardiac anomalies, DiGeorge syndrome, LVOT obstruction, and an episode of circulatory collapse prior to repair [102,107,99]. Several studies have questioned whether LVOT obstruction is a risk factor for increased operative mortality [104,99].

Anesthetic considerations

Intravenous access will have been established in children with IAA scheduled for surgery. Induction of general anesthesia is therefore usually accomplished with an opioid and benzodiazepine in combination with a nondepolarizing muscle relaxant such as pancuronium. Inhaled anesthetic agents can be safely used as long as blood pressure is closely monitored and maintained. Management of ventilation following anesthetic induction and intubation is aimed toward optimizing systemic cardiac output. The use of a low inspired FIO_2 and avoidance of hyperventilation reduces pulmonary overcirculation. The use of cerebral NIRS can help guide anesthetic management during this period.

The optimal position for placement of the arterial catheter requires careful consideration in the infant with IAA. The right subclavian artery may originate in an anomalous fashion from the descending aorta, especially in a type B IAA with associated SAS [111]. In one study, 15 of 49 patients with type B IAA had a coexisting anomalous right subclavian artery [104]. In some cases, the left subclavian artery may be utilized during the surgical repair. The use of an umbilical artery catheter is ideal for this procedure. Central venous access is helpful for the infusion of inotropic agents and monitoring of intracardiac pressures. This can be accomplished by either percutaneous catheterization or placement of intracardiac lines by the surgeon prior to separating from cardiopulmonary bypass. Echocardiography using a pediatric TEE probe can effectively guide inotropic and fluid management, determine the adequacy of VSD closure, and assess the left-ventricular outflow tract for any evidence of obstruction. Two intravenous catheters should be placed as significant blood loss may occur following separation from cardiopulmonary bypass. The use of deep hypothermia places the infant at higher risk for significant bleeding after cardiopulmonary bypass; red blood cells, platelets, and cryoprecipate should be available. In the case of the infant with DiGeorge syndrome, the use of irradiated blood is necessary to avoid graft versus host reactions [112].

Separation from cardiopulmonary bypass usually requires inotropic support and close monitoring of serum calcium levels. The infant with DiGeorge syndrome is prone to hypocalcemia and may benefit from a calcium infusion. Once the hemodynamics are stabilized and the bleeding is controlled, sternal closure may be attempted. Inotropic support, fluid management, and ventilation may need to be adjusted at this time. The patient should be closely monitored for pulmonary hypertension following repair, and if present, may benefit from inhaled nitric oxide. Should sternal closure result in unacceptable instability due to a reduction in cardiac output or pulmonary function, a Goretex patch may be placed over the open chest for subsequent closure in 1–3 days.

Shone's anomaly

Anatomy

Shone's anomaly consists of a supravalvar mitral ring, parachute deformity of the mitral valve, SAS, and coarctation of the aorta, and was first described by Shone and colleagues in 1963. This complex of lesions causes multilevel left heart obstruction and is variable in regard to the presence and severity of each lesion [113, 114]. The parachute mitral valve describes a mitral valve deformity where two mitral valve leaflets are supported by only one papillary muscle and the chordae are usually shortened and thickened. Because the mitral leaflets are pulled together in proximity, the mitral valve can become stenotic. The supravalvar ring is a ridge of connective tissue arranged circumferentially on the atrial side of the mitral leaflets. Although this ring does not cause severe obstruction in the majority of cases, fibrous tissue can obtrude into the mitral inflow tract causing obstruction. Although not classically considered part of Shone's anomaly, "typical" congenital mitral stenosis with a small annulus size has been noted in 25% to 50% of patients with Shone's anomaly in two published series [115, 116]. SAS is caused by either a discrete membranous thickening in the outflow tract or by a more complex long-segment "tunnel" stenosis. The coarctation is usually located in the descending aorta in proximity to the left subclavian artery.

In 30 consecutive patients with Shone's anomaly, 73% had a supravalvar mitral ring, 87% a parachute mitral valve, 87% had SAS, and 97% had coarctation of the aorta. Additional lesions also present in these patients were a bicuspid aortic valve (61%) and ventricular septal defect (67%) [114].

Cor triatriatum must also be considered in the setting of left-sided obstructive disease. The anomaly is characterized by the pulmonary venous return entering an accessory left-sided chamber that connects with the left atrium through a slender passageway. The left atrial appendage and fossa ovalis are always distal to the obstructing membrane. In contrast, a supravalvar stenosing ring, when present as part of Shone's complex, has a left atrial appendage in connection to the upper portion of left atrium and proximal to the stenosing formation [117].

Pathophysiology and diagnosis

Patient symptoms depend on the atomic location of the most critical areas of obstruction. As many as two-thirds of patients with Shone's anomaly may present in the neonatal period with an aortic coarctation [116]. Assessment of the hemodynamic significance of lesions causing obstruction of the mitral valve or subaortic region is very challenging in the context of a ductal-dependent systemic circulation. Following repair of aortic coarctation, these infants are followed closely for signs of congestive heart failure often related to mitral valve abnormalities. SAS is rarely significant in the neonatal period but can rapidly progress during infancy [31]. Those patients with a high degree of SAS will develop left-ventricular hypertrophy.

Echocardiography and cardiac catheterization with angiography are the primary diagnostic modalities for detecting and defining the extent of the Shone's anomaly [118]. The presence of markedly elevated pulmonary vascular resistance at cardiac catheterization increases perioperative risk and worsens long-term outcome. It is extremely important to be aware of all levels of obstruction since the intraoperative repair of one obstruction may often reveal other less critical stenoses that now impede blood flow. Failure to recognize all levels of obstruction leads to increased perioperative risk for the patient.

Surgical approaches

The surgical repair generally consists of resection of the supravalvar ring, fenestration of the tensor apparatus, repair or replacement of the mitral valve, and resection of any encroaching muscular tissue in the LVOT. Early mitral valve repair is advocated whenever possible allowing for continued annular growth and avoidance of anticoagulation, and should occur before pulmonary hypertension develops [116]. When SAS is caused by a discrete membranous lesion, resection is performed through a transaortic approach and accompanied by ventricular septal myectomy, which is felt to reduce the incidence of recurrence [119]. A long-segment "tunnel" type of SAS is commonly corrected with an aortoventriculoplasty (Konno procedure). Depending on the degree of aortic valvular obstruction, a Ross–Konno operation may be necessary to optimally relieve the obstruction [120, 121]. Intraoperative TEE is important for anatomic assessment before cardiopulmonary bypass and then following surgical repair. Surgical and long-term outcomes for Shone's anomaly depend on the age of presentation, severity of mitral valve disease, need for multiple surgical procedures, and presence of pulmonary hypertension [2,114–116].

Anesthetic considerations

The medical management of these patients depends on the location of the critical stenosis. Neonates with coarctation of the aorta will require prostaglandins to maintain patency of the ductus arteriosus and appropriate ventilatory strategies aimed at reducing pulmonary overcirculation. Children with dynamic LVOT obstruction may require β-blockers to improve intracavitary laminar blood flow. Congestive heart failure is usually treated with diuretics and may require inotropic support, while pulmonary hypertension before or after surgery may require a phosphodiesterase-inhibitor (such as milrinone) and nitric oxide [122,123].

The anesthetic management of the patient with Shone's anomaly requires an appreciation for all levels of stenosis and knowledge of the location of the dominant lesion. A patient with predominantly mitral stenosis needs sufficient preload to maintain left atrial pressure, and a normal to slow heart rate to optimize ventricular filling during diastole. In the patient primarily suffering from SAS and left-ventricular hypertrophy, arterial blood pressure needs to be maintained for optimal myocardial perfusion. An anesthetic plan carefully tailored to meet these hemodynamic goals is vital for optimal outcome.

Mitral stenosis

Anatomy

Mitral stenosis is most often observed as a component of a complex left-sided malformation syndrome, i.e., Shone Anomaly. Isolated congenital mitral stenosis is a rare lesion, occurring in well less than 1% of infants with congenital heart disease and a normal-sized left ventricle [124]. The anatomical complexity of the mitral valve and its supporting apparatus, the papillary muscles and chordae tendinae, have led to several complicated schemes to describe abnormalities of the mitral valve [124,125,126]. One functional classification of mitral stenosis anatomy divides this lesion into type A, with a normal papillary muscle, which includes commissural fusion, a valvular or supravalvular ring, or and obstructive left superior vena cava [126]. Type B mitral stenosis consists of an abnormal papillary muscle, producing a parachute, or a hammock mitral valve.

Pathophysiology and diagnosis

Depending on the degree of mitral stenosis, a progressive elevation in left atrial pressure can lead to pulmonary venous, and then pulmonary arterial hypertension. This can result in interstitial pulmonary edema, "cardiac asthma," frequent respiratory infections, tachypnea, poor feeding, poor growth in the infant. Significant pulmonary hypertension will be accompanied by elevated right-ventricular pressures and possibly poor function, or hypertrophy. Left-sided cardiac output will be restricted by restriction of blood flow into the left ventricle. Tachy-

cardia shortens diastolic filling time and can severely depress systemic cardiac output. Hypovolemia reduces left-ventricular end-diastolic volume and pressure, worsening the functional mitral stenosis. In patients with elevated pulmonary artery pressure and resistance, maneuvers to reduce PVR may conversely worsen the obstructive symptoms by promoting increased pulmonary blood flow in the face of a fixed downstream obstruction, worsening the patient's pulmonary symptoms. The often-dilated left atrium predisposes to atrial arrhythmias such as atrial flutter, atrial fibrillation, or atrial tachycardia.

Anatomical diagnosis of mitral stenosis is often based solely on echocardiographic findings. Three-dimensional echocardiography is particularly useful in defining the morphological complexity of the mitral valve, and is gaining more widespread use [127]. Decisions about intervening are often made on the basis of increasing clinical symptomatology such as frequent respiratory infections and failure to thrive.

Surgical approaches

As a general principal, most congenital heart surgeons adopt a conservative approach, repairing the valve in mitral stenosis whenever possible [128]. There are a number of techniques employed, including resection of a supravalvar ring, commissurotomy, division or reconstruction of the papillary muscle, reconstruction of the chordae tendinae, and many others [126,128]. The main goal of surgery is to reduce the mitral stenosis without producing mitral regurgitation; the surgeon will often perform a test of the repair with the aorta cross-clamped by rapidly instilling saline solution through the repaired valve to produce a normal end-diastolic volume. Retention of this volume in the left ventricle signifies lack of significant mitral regurgitation. After separating from bypass, TEE is critical in assessing the adequacy of repair and the need to return to bypass to improve the surgery. Because of the potential morbidity from anticoagulation and the need for future replacement with growth in a child, mitral valve replacement is only performed as a last resort, when attempts at repair have failed. Interventional catheter approaches to dilate a stenotic mitral valve have also been performed successfully [129].

Anesthetic considerations

Hemodynamic goals in mitral stenosis include maintaining a low-normal heart rate to enhance diastolic filling time for the left ventricle, and maintaining preload to minimize functional stenosis across the valve. Preserving ventricular contractility and afterload are important goals of any technique. Maintaining normal sinus rhythm is critical, so prompt recognition and treatment of atrial dysrhythmias is important. With severe mitral stenosis, the patient will have significant pulmonary hypertension and care must be taken not to induce a pulmonary hypertensive crisis, i.e., large catecholamine surge from inadequate anesthetic depth. On the other hand, acutely lowering PVR with excessive FIO_2 and hyperventilation will promote excessive pulmonary blood flow, often leading to worsening pulmonary function due to the fixed downstream obstruction at the level of the mitral valve.

During surgical repair, the left side of the heart will by necessity be opened, and there is the potential for retention of significant air in the heart during weaning from bypass. Some surgeons will insufflate CO_2 into the surgical field to improve the dissolution of any retained gas in the left side of the heart [130]. Prolonged cardiac de-airing maneuvers, assisted by TEE, may be required.

After bypass, a left atrial and possibly a pulmonary artery catheter may be placed by the surgeon. It is important to realize that pulmonary artery pressures may not be immediately reduced, and treatment with adequate depth of anesthesia and analgesia, milrinone, nitric oxide, high FIO_2, and mild hyperventilation may be required for hours or days. Left atrial pressure should decrease with successful mitral valve repair in the face of normal left-ventricular function. Transesophageal echocardiography is crucial to assess the immediate results of the surgical repair.

Cor triatriatum

Cor triatriatum is a rare anomaly seen in about 0.1% of patients with congenital heart disease, consisting of a membrane or diaphragm in the left atrium, functionally dividing it into two chambers, where the pulmonary veins enter superior to the membrane [131]. Blood flows from the upper to the lower left atrial chamber through one or more orifices, and the patient's symptoms and presentation depend on the degree of restriction of blood flow through these orifices, and can range from completely asymptomatic, to severely restricted blood flow resulting in severe left atrial hypertension, pulmonary venous and arterial hypertension, and low cardiac output similar to that seen in severe mitral stenosis. Pulmonary symptoms such as wheezing are prominent and may be the only presenting complaint [132]. Most patients present in the first year of life, and 24–80% have associated cardiac anomalies such as anomalous pulmonary venous drainage, left SVC, or hypoplastic left heart syndrome. Surgical approach consists of resecting the membrane in the left atrium and repairing associated defects. Anesthetic considerations are identical to those for the patient with mitral stenosis.

Key points for anesthetic management of lesions

Aortic valve stenosis

1 Neonates may present in shock and need resuscitation before catheter or surgical intervention.
2 Physiologic goals include maintaining preload, afterload, and contractility at high-normal levels in neonates.
3 In older patients with preserved myocardial function, maintain normal to below normal contractility.
4 Normal or decreased heart rate preferred; bradycardia is not tolerated in the neonate.
5 During and after balloon angioplasty, prepare to resuscitate the patient from profound myocardial depression, bradycardia, ventricular fibrillation, or asystole.

Subvalvar aortic stenosis

1 Management goals are similar to valvar aortic stenosis.
2 Maintain preload and afterload at high-normal levels.
3 Maintain heart rate and contractility at low-normal levels.

Supravalvar aortic stenosis

1 Many patients have Williams syndrome; this syndrome is associated with many case reports of death during induction of anesthesia due to myocardial ischemia from coronary insufficiency.
2 Williams syndrome patients have a defect in the elastin gene; coronary artery involvement is frequently present, and not proportional to the degree of supravalvar aortic stenosis.
3 Maintain afterload at higher than normal levels to promote coronary perfusion.
4 Maintain heart rate at low-normal levels, and contractility at low-normal levels.
5 Maintain preload at high-normal levels.
6 Avoid anesthetic techniques that produce the potentially fatal combination of decreased preload, and decreased afterload, i.e., large doses of propofol or volatile anesthetics.

Hypertrophic cardiomyopathy

1 Anesthetic goals include maintaining preload and afterload at high-normal levels, decreasing myocardial contractility, and avoiding tachycardia.

2 Consider perioperative short acting β-blocker therapy to decrease contractility.

3 Use caution in advancing a guidewire into the heart during central venous catheterization; arrhythmias, including atrial tachycardia and premature ventricular contractions are not well tolerated and may lead to myocardial ischemia and deterioration to ventricular fibrillation.

Coarctation of the aorta

1 The neonate with critical coarctation may present in shock, with decreased myocardial function. These patients may require resuscitation before surgery or catheter intervention, and will require PGE_1 infusion to maintain ductal patency.

2 A right arm arterial line is required for monitoring during surgery.

3 Maintaining myocardial contractility, and high-normal blood pressure in the aorta proximal to the cross-clamp during surgical repair is important to provide perfusion pressure to the spinal cord and subdiaphragmatic viscera.

4 High blood pressure during aortic cross-clamping can be controlled with volatile anesthetics.

5 Cooling the patient to 35°C may confer additional protection to the spinal cord and vital organs during cross-clamping.

Interrupted or hypoplastic aortic arch

1 Neonates are dependent on PGE_1 infusion for ductal patency before surgery.

2 Use low FIO_2 and high-normal $PaCO_2$ to prevent pulmonary overcirculation.

3 Use right arm arterial catheter for monitoring; however, a significant percentage of IAA patients have an aberrant right subclavian artery whose origin is distal to the interruption. Consult with the surgeon and use NIRS for monitoring.

4 Beware of hypocalcemia in patients with IAA and DiGeorge syndrome.

Shone's anomaly

1 Management goals should be directed at the site of the most critical stenosis.

2 Maintain myocardiac contractility, and beware of pulmonary hypertension in the neonate, or patients with significant left-sided obstruction.

3 When a proximal obstruction is repaired, i.e., supravalvar mitral stenosis, the most critical level of obstruction may move distally, i.e., aortic stenosis or coarctation of aorta.

Mitral stenosis/cor triatriatum

1 Hemodynamic goals include slow–normal heart rate, maintenance of normal sinus rhythm, and maintaining adequate preload, and afterload.

2 Severe obstruction from these lesions can result in significant left atrial hypertension, and pulmonary venous and arterial hypertension, which may need to be managed during surgery, i.e., with nitric oxide postbypass.

3 In severe obstruction prebypass, nitric oxide and other maneuvers to decrease PVR can worsen the problems because they do not address the anatomic obstruction.

References

1. Pradat P, Francannet C, Harris JA, Robert E (2003) The epidemiology of cardiovascular defects, part I: a study based on data from three large registries of congenital malformations. Pediatr Cardiol 24: 195–221.
2. Fedderly RT (1999) Left ventricular outflow obstruction. Pediatr Clin North Am 46: 369–384.
3. Maron BJ, Hutchins GM (1974) The development of the semilunar valves in the human heart. Am J Pathol 74: 331–344.
4. Eroglu AG, Babaoglu K, Saltik L, et al. (2006) Echocardiographic follow-up of congenital aortic valvular stenosis. Pediatr Cardiol 27: 713–719.
5. Stadler TW (2006) Cardiovascular system. In: Sadler TW, Langman J, Leland J (eds) Langman's Medical Embryology, 10th edn. Lippincott Williams & Wilkins, Philadelphia, pp. 159–194.
6. Drury NE, Veldtman GR, Benson LN (2005) Neonatal aortic stenosis. Expert Rev Cardiovasc Ther 3: 831–843.
7. Currie PJ, Hagler DJ, Seward JB, et al. (1986) Instantaneous pressure gradient: a simultaneous Doppler and dual catheter correlative study. J Am Coll Cardiol 7: 800–806.
8. Vlahos AP, Marx GR, McElhinney D, et al. (2008) Clinical utility of Doppler echocardiography in assessing aortic stenosis severity and predicting need for intervention in children. Pediatr Cardiol 29: 507–514.
9. Gundry SR, Behrendt DM (1986) Prognostic factors in valvotomy for critical aortic stenosis in infancy. J Thorac Cardiovasc Surg 92: 747–754.
10. Rhodes LA, Colan SD, Perry SB, et al. (1991) Predictors of survival in neonates with critical aortic stenosis. Circulation 84: 2325–2335.
11. Lofland GK, McCrindle BW, Williams WG, et al. (2001) Critical aortic stenosis in the neonate: a multi-institutional study of management, outcomes, and risk factors. Congenital Heart Surgeons Society. J Thorac Cardiovasc Surg 121: 10–27.
12. Corno AF (2005) Borderline left ventricle. Eur J Cardiothorac Surg 27: 67–73.
13. Egito ES, Moore P, O'Sullivan J, et al. (1997) Transvascular balloon dilation for neonatal critical aortic stenosis: early and midterm results. J Am Coll Cardiol 29: 442–447.

14. McCrindle BW, Blackstone EH, Williams WG, et al. (2001) Are outcomes of surgical versus transcatheter balloon valvotomy equivalent in neonatal critical aortic stenosis? Circulation 104: I152–I158.
15. Reich O, Tax P, Marek J, et al. (2004) Long term results of percutaneous balloon valvoplasty of congenital aortic stenosis: independent predictors of outcome. Heart 90: 70–76.
16. McElhinney DB, Lock JE, Keane JF, et al. (2005) Left heart growth, function, and reintervention after balloon aortic valvuloplasty for neonatal aortic stenosis. Circulation 111: 451–458.
17. Han RK, Gurofsky RC, Lee KJ, et al. (2007) Outcome and growth potential of left heart structures after neonatal intervention for aortic valve stenosis. J Am Coll Cardiol 50: 2406–2414.
18. Gildein HP, Kleinert S, Weintraub RG, et al. (1996) Surgical commissurotomy of the aortic valve: outcome of open valvotomy in neonates with critical aortic stenosis. Am Heart J 131: 754–759.
19. Hawkins JA, Minich LL, Tani LY, et al. (1998) Late results and reintervention after aortic valvotomy for critical aortic stenosis in neonates and infants. Ann Thorac Surg 65: 1758–1762.
20. Alexiou C, Langley SM, Dalrymple-Hay MJ, et al. (2001) Open commissurotomy for critical isolated aortic stenosis in neonates. Ann Thorac Surg 71: 489–493.
21. Chang AC, Hanley FL, Wernovsky G, Wessel DL (1998) Left ventricular outflow tract obstruction. In Pediatric Cardiac Intensive Care, 1st edn. Lippincott Williams & Wilkins, Philadelphia, pp. 233–256.
22. Alphonso N, Baghai M, Dhital K, et al. (2004) Midterm results of the Ross procedure. Eur J Cardiothorac Surg 25: 925–930.
23. Kouchoukos NT, Masetti P, Nickerson NJ, et al. (2004) The Ross procedure: long-term clinical and echocardiographic follow-up. Ann Thorac Surg 78: 773–781.
24. Raja SG, Pozzi M (2004) Ross operation in children and young adults: the Alder Hey case series. BMC Cardiovasc Disord 4: 3.
25. Tworetzky W, Wilkins-Haug L, Jennings RW, et al. (2004) Balloon dilation of severe aortic stenosis in the fetus: potential for prevention of hypoplastic left heart syndrome: candidate selection, technique, and results of successful intervention. Circulation 110: 2125–2131.
26. Kleinman CS (2006) Fetal cardiac intervention: innovative therapy or a technique in search of an indication? Circulation 113: 1378–1381.
27. Pavlovic M, Acharya G, Huhta JC (2008) Controversies of fetal cardiac intervention. Early Hum Dev 84: 149–153.
28. Singh GK (2000) Subvalvular aortic stenosis. Curr Treat Options Cardiovasc Med 2: 529–535.
29. Tentolouris K, Kontozoglou T, Trikas A, et al. (1999) Fixed subaortic stenosis revisited. Congenital abnormalities in 72 new cases and review of the literature. Cardiology 92: 4–10.
30. Cooley DA, Norman JA (1975) Techniques in Cardiac Surgery. Texas Medical Press, Houston, pp. 129–137.
31. Brauner R, Laks H, Drinkwater DC, Jr., et al. (1997) Benefits of early surgical repair in fixed subaortic stenosis. J Am Coll Cardiol 30: 1835–1842.
32. Williams JC, Barratt-Boyes BG, Lowe JB (1961) Supravalvular aortic stenosis. Circulation 24: 1311–1318.
33. Beuren AJ, Apitz J, Harmjanz D (1962) Supravalvular aortic stenosis in association with mental retardation and a certain facial appearance. Circulation 26: 1235–1240.
34. Ewart AK, Morris CA, Atkinson D, et al. (1993) Hemizygosity at the elastin locus in a developmental disorder, Williams syndrome. Nat Genet 5: 11–16.
35. Pober BR, Johnson M, Urban Z (2008) Mechanisms and treatment of cardiovascular disease in Williams–Beuren syndrome. J Clin Invest 118: 1606–1615.
36. Stamm C, Friehs I, Ho SY, et al. (2001) Congenital supravalvar aortic stenosis: a simple lesion? Eur J Cardiothorac Surg 19: 195–202.
37. McElhinney DB, Petrossian E, Tworetzky W, et al. (2000) Issues and outcomes in the management of supravalvar aortic stenosis. Ann Thorac Surg 69: 562–567.
38. Bird LM, Billman GF, Lacro RV, et al. (1996) Sudden death in Williams syndrome: report of ten cases. J Pediatr 129: 926–931.
39. Wessel A, Gravenhorst V, Buchhorn R, et al. (2004) Risk of sudden death in the Williams–Beuren syndrome. Am J Med Genet 127A: 234–237.
40. Ingelfinger JR, Newburger JW (1991) Spectrum of renal anomalies in patients with Williams syndrome. J Pediatr 119: 771–773.
41. Chard RB, Cartmill TB (1993) Localized supravalvar aortic stenosis: a new technique for repair. Ann Thorac Surg 55: 782–784.
42. Thistlethwaite PA, Madani MM, Kriett JM, et al. (2000) Surgical management of congenital obstruction of the left main coronary artery with supravalvular aortic stenosis. J Thorac Cardiovasc Surg 120: 1040–1046.
43. Conway EE, Jr, Noonan J, Marion RW, Steeg CN (1990) Myocardial infarction leading to sudden death in the Williams syndrome: report of three cases. J Pediatr 117: 593–595.
44. van Son JA, Edwards WD, Danielson GK (1994) Pathology of coronary arteries, myocardium, and great arteries in supravalvular aortic stenosis. Report of five cases with implications for surgical treatment. J Thorac Cardiovasc Surg 108: 21–28.
45. Horowitz PE, Akhtar S, Wulff JA, et al. (2002) Coronary artery disease and anesthesia-related death in children with Williams syndrome. J Cardiothorac Vasc Anesth 16: 739–741.
46. Monfared A, Messner A (2006) Death following tonsillectomy in a child with Williams syndrome. Int J Pediatr Otorhinolaryngol 70: 1133–1135.
47. Odegard KC, DiNardo JA, Kussman BD, et al. (2007) The frequency of anesthesia-related cardiac arrests in patients with congenital heart disease undergoing cardiac surgery. Anesth Analg 105: 335–343.
48. Burch TM, McGowan FX Jr, Kussman BD, et al. (2008 Dec) Congenital supravalvular aortic stenosis and sudden death associated with anesthesia: what's the mystery? Anesth Analg 107 (6): 1848–1854.

49. Lashkari A, Smith AK, Graham JM, Jr. (1999) Williams–Beuren syndrome: an update and review for the primary physician. Clin Pediatr 38: 189–208.

50. Maron BJ, Gardin JM, Flack JM, et al. (1995) Prevalence of hypertrophic cardiomyopathy in a general population of young adults. Echocardiographic analysis of 4111 subjects in the CARDIA Study. Coronary Artery Risk Development in (Young) Adults. Circulation 92: 785–789.

51. Spirito P, Seidman CE, McKenna WJ, Maron BJ (1997) The management of hypertrophic cardiomyopathy. N Engl J Med 336: 775–785.

52. Maron BJ, Gottdiener JS, Epstein SE (1981) Patterns and significance of distribution of left ventricular hypertrophy in hypertrophic cardiomyopathy. A wide angle, two dimensional echocardiographic study of 125 patients. Am J Cardiol 48: 418–428.

53. Ciro E, Nichols PF, 3rd, Maron BJ (1983) Heterogeneous morphologic expression of genetically transmitted hypertrophic cardiomyopathy. Two-dimensional echocardiographic analysis. Circulation 67: 1227–1233.

54. Maron BJ, Bonow RO, Cannon RO, et al. (1987) Hypertrophic cardiomyopathy. Interrelations of clinical manifestations, pathophysiology, and therapy (1). N Engl J Med 316: 780–789.

55. Maron BJ, Wolfson JK, Epstein SE, Roberts WC (1986) Intramural ("small vessel") coronary artery disease in hypertrophic cardiomyopathy. J Am Coll Cardiol 8: 545–557.

56. St John Sutton MG, Lie JT, Anderson KR, et al. (1980) Histopathological specificity of hypertrophic obstructive cardiomyopathy. Myocardial fibre disarray and myocardial fibrosis. Br Heart J 44: 433–443.

57. Maron BJ, Bonow RO, Cannon RO, et al. (1987) Hypertrophic cardiomyopathy. Interrelations of clinical manifestations, pathophysiology, and therapy (2). N Engl J Med 316: 844–852.

58. Maron BJ, Savage DD, Wolfson JK, Epstein SE (1981) Prognostic significance of 24 hour ambulatory electrocardiographic monitoring in patients with hypertrophic cardiomyopathy: a prospective study. Am J Cardiol 48: 252–257.

59. Maron BJ (2007) Hypertrophic cardiomyopathy and other causes of sudden cardiac death in young competitive athletes, with considerations for preparticipation screening and criteria for disqualification. Cardiol Clin 25: 399–414.

60. Bryant RM (1999) Hypertrophic cardiomyopathy in children. Cardiol Rev 7: 92–100.

61. Robinson K, Frenneaux MP, Stockins B, et al. (1990) Atrial fibrillation in hypertrophic cardiomyopathy: a longitudinal study. J Am Coll Cardiol 15: 1279–1285.

62. Shah PM, Taylor RD, Wong M (1981) Abnormal mitral valve coaptation in hypertrophic obstructive cardiomyopathy: proposed role in systolic anterior motion of mitral valve. Am J Cardiol 48: 258–262.

63. Minakata K, Dearani JA, O'Leary PW, Danielson GK (2005) Septal myectomy for obstructive hypertrophic cardiomyopathy in pediatric patients: early and late results. Ann Thorac Surg 80: 1424–1429.

64. Maron MS, Olivotto I, Betocchi S, et al. (2003) Effect of left ventricular outflow tract obstruction on clinical outcome in hypertrophic cardiomyopathy. N Engl J Med 348: 295–303.

65. Ommen SR, Maron BJ, Olivotto I, et al. (2005) Long-term effects of surgical septal myectomy on survival in patients with obstructive hypertrophic cardiomyopathy. J Am Coll Cardiol 46: 470–476.

66. Haering JM, Comunale ME, Parker RA, et al. (1996) Cardiac risk of noncardiac surgery in patients with asymmetric septal hypertrophy. Anesthesiology 85: 254–259.

67. Reitan JA, Wright RG (1982) The use of halothane in a patient with asymmetrical septal hypertrophy: a case report. Can Anaesth Soc J 29: 154–157.

68. Gutgesell HP, Speer ME, Rosenberg HS. (1980) Characterization of the cardiomyopathy in infants of diabetic mothers. Circulation 61: 441–450.

69. Slonim AE, Bulone L, Ritz S, et al. (2000) Identification of two subtypes of infantile acid maltase deficiency. J Pediatr 137: 283–285.

70. Klinge L, Straub V, Neudorf U, Voit T (2005) Enzyme replacement therapy in classical infantile Pompe disease: results of a ten-month follow-up study. Neuropediatrics 36: 6–11.

71. Ing RJ, Cook DR, Bengur RA, et al. (2004) Anaesthetic management of infants with glycogen storage disease type II: a physiological approach. Paediatr Anaesth 14: 514–519.

72. Wang LY, Ross AK, Li JS, et al. (2007) Cardiac arrhythmias following anesthesia induction in infantile-onset Pompe disease: a case series. Paediatr Anaesth 17: 738–748.

73. Campbell M, Polani PE (1961) The aetiology of coarctation of the aorta. Lancet 1: 463–468.

74. Campbell M (1970) Natural history of coarctation of the aorta. Br Heart J 32: 633–640.

75. Hager A, Kanz S, Kaemmerer H, et al. (2007) Coarctation Long-term Assessment (COALA): significance of arterial hypertension in a cohort of 404 patients up to 27 years after surgical repair of isolated coarctation of the aorta, even in the absence of restenosis and prosthetic material. J Thorac Cardiovasc Surg 134: 738–745.

76. Rodes-Cabau J, Miro J, Dancea A, et al. (2007) Comparison of surgical and transcatheter treatment for native coarctation of the aorta in patients > or = 1 year old. The Quebec Native Coarctation of the Aorta study. Am Heart J 154: 186–192.

77. Hu XH, Huang GY, Pa M, et al. (2008) Multidetector CT angiography and 3D reconstruction in young children with coarctation of the aorta. Pediatr Cardiol 29: 726–731.

78. Fletcher SE, Nihill MR, Grifka RG, et al. (1995) Balloon angioplasty of native coarctation of the aorta: midterm follow-up and prognostic factors. J Am Coll Cardiol 25: 730–734.

79. Fiore AC, Fischer LK, Schwartz T, et al. (2005) Comparison of angioplasty and surgery for neonatal aortic coarctation. Ann Thorac Surg 80: 1659–1664.

80. van Heurn LW, Wong CM, Spiegelhalter DJ, et al. (1994) Surgical treatment of aortic coarctation in infants younger than three months: 1985 to 1990. Success of extended end-to-end arch aortoplasty. J Thorac Cardiovasc Surg 107: 74–85.

81. Brewer LA, 3rd, Fosburg RG, Mulder GA, Verska JJ (1972) Spinal cord complications following surgery for coarctation

of the aorta. A study of 66 cases. J Thorac Cardiovasc Surg 64: 368–381.

82. Yetman AT, Nykanen D, McCrindle BW, et al. (1997) Balloon angioplasty of recurrent coarctation: a 12-year review. J Am Coll Cardiol 30: 811–816.

83. Beekman RH, Rocchini AP, Behrendt DM, Rosenthal A (1981) Reoperation for coarctation of the aorta. Am J Cardiol 48: 1108–1114.

84. Massoud Iel S, Farghly HE, Abdul-Monem A, et al. (2008) Balloon angioplasty for native aortic coarctation in different anatomic variants. Pediatr Cardiol 29: 521–529.

85. Fawzy ME, Awad M, Hassan W, et al. (2004) Long-term outcome (up to 15 years) of balloon angioplasty of discrete native coarctation of the aorta in adolescents and adults. J Am Coll Cardiol 43: 1062–1067.

86. Hellenbrand WE, Allen HD, Golinko RJ, et al. (1990) Balloon angioplasty for aortic recoarctation: results of Valvuloplasty and Angioplasty of Congenital Anomalies Registry. Am J Cardiol 65: 793–797.

87. Siblini G, Rao PS, Nouri S, et al. (1998) Long-term follow-up results of balloon angioplasty of postoperative aortic re-coarctation. Am J Cardiol 81: 61–67.

88. Forbes TJ, Garekar S, Amin Z, et al. (2007) Procedural results and acute complications in stenting native and recurrent coarctation of the aorta in patients over 4 years of age: a multi-institutional study. Catheter Cardiovasc Interv 70: 276–285.

89. Hamdan MA, Maheshwari S, Fahey JT, Hellenbrand WE (2001) Endovascular stents for coarctation of the aorta: initial results and intermediate-term follow-up. J Am Coll Cardiol 38: 1518–1523.

90. Marshall AC, Perry SB, Keane JF, Lock JE (2000) Early results and medium-term follow-up of stent implantation for mild residual or recurrent aortic coarctation. Am Heart J 139: 1054–1060.

91. Suarez de Lezo J, Pan M, Romero M, et al. (1999) Immediate and follow-up findings after stent treatment for severe coarctation of aorta. Am J Cardiol 83: 400–406.

92. Farouk A, Karimi M, Henderson M, et al. (2008) Cerebral regional oxygenation during aortic coarctation repair in pediatric population. Eur J Cardiothorac Surg 34: 26–31.

93. Crawford FA, Jr, Sade RM (1984) Spinal cord injury associated with hyperthermia during aortic coarctation repair. J Thorac Cardiovasc Surg 87: 616–618.

94. Hosking MP, Beynen F (1989) Repair of coarctation of the aorta in a child after a modified Fontan's operation: anesthetic implications and management. Anesthesiology 71: 312–315.

95. Fixler DE (1988) Coarctation of the aorta. Cardiol Clin 6: 561–571.

96. Rocchini AP, Rosenthal A, Barger AC, et al. (1976) Pathogenesis of paradoxical hypertension after coarctation resection. Circulation 54: 382–387.

97. Celoria GC, Patton RB (1959) Congenital absence of the aortic arch. Am Heart J 58: 407–413.

98. Sell JE, Jonas RA, Mayer JE, et al. (1988) The results of a surgical program for interrupted aortic arch. J Thorac Cardiovasc Surg 96: 864–877.

99. Morales DL, Scully PT, Braud BE, et al. (2006) Interrupted aortic arch repair: aortic arch advancement without a patch minimizes arch reinterventions. Ann Thorac Surg 82: 1577–1583.

100. Rauch A, Hofbeck M, Leipold G, et al. (1998) Incidence and significance of 22q11.2 hemizygosity in patients with interrupted aortic arch. Am J Med Genet 78: 322–331.

101. Bailey WW (1994) Interrupted aortic arch. Adv Card Surg 5: 97–114.

102. Oosterhof T, Azakie A, Freedom RM, et al. (2004) Associated factors and trends in outcomes of interrupted aortic arch. Ann Thorac Surg 78: 1696–1702.

103. Scott WA, Rocchini AP, Bove EL, et al. (1988) Repair of interrupted aortic arch in infancy. J Thorac Cardiovasc Surg 96: 564–568.

104. Fulton JO, Mas C, Brizard CP, et al. (1999) Does left ventricular outflow tract obstruction influence outcome of interrupted aortic arch repair? Ann Thorac Surg 67: 177–181.

105. Schumacher G, Schreiber R, Meisner H, et al. (1986) Interrupted aortic arch: natural history and operative results. Pediatr Cardiol 7: 89–93.

106. Wong CK, Cheng CH, Lau CP, et al. (1989) Interrupted aortic arch in an asymptomatic adult. Chest 96: 678–679.

107. McCrindle BW, Tchervenkov CI, Konstantinov IE, et al. (2005) Risk factors associated with mortality and interventions in 472 neonates with interrupted aortic arch: a Congenital Heart Surgeons Society study. J Thorac Cardiovasc Surg 129: 343–350.

108. Bellinger DC, Jonas RA, Rappaport LA, et al. (1995) Developmental and neurologic status of children after heart surgery with hypothermic circulatory arrest or low-flow cardiopulmonary bypass. N Engl J Med 332: 549–555.

109. Schreiber C, Mazzitelli D, Haehnel JC, et al. (1997) The interrupted aortic arch: an overview after 20 years of surgical treatment. Eur J Cardiothorac Surg 12: 466–469.

110. Serraf A, Lacour-Gayet F, Robotin M, et al. (1996) Repair of interrupted aortic arch: a ten-year experience. J Thorac Cardiovasc Surg 112: 1150–1160.

111. Menahem S, Brawn WJ, Mee RB (1991) Severe subaortic stenosis in interrupted aortic arch in infancy and childhood. J Card Surg 6: 373–380.

112. Van Mierop LH, Kutsche LM (1986) Cardiovascular anomalies in DiGeorge syndrome and importance of neural crest as a possible pathogenetic factor. Am J Cardiol 58: 133–137.

113. Shone JD, Sellers RD, Anderson RC, et al. (1963) The developmental complex of "parachute mitral valve," supravalvular ring of left atrium, subaortic stenosis, and coarctation of aorta. Am J Cardiol 11: 714–725.

114. Bolling SF, Iannettoni MD, Dick M, et al. (1990) Shone's anomaly: operative results and late outcome. Ann Thorac Surg 49: 887–893.

115. Brauner RA, Laks H, Drinkwater DC, et al. (1997) Multiple left heart obstructions (Shone's anomaly) with mitral valve involvement: long-term surgical outcome. Ann Thorac Surg 64: 721–729.

116. Brown JW, Ruzmetov M, Vijay P, et al. (2005) Operative results and outcomes in children with Shone's anomaly. Ann Thorac Surg 79: 1358–1365.

117. Goel AK, Saxena A, Kothari SS (1998) Atrioventricular septal defect with cor triatriatum: case report and review of the literature. Pediatr Cardiol 19: 243–245.

118. Macartney FJ, Scott O, Ionescu MI, Deverall PB (1974) Diagnosis and management of parachute mitral valve and supravalvar mitral ring. Br Heart J 36: 641–652.

119. van Son JA, Schaff HV, Danielson GK, et al. (1993) Surgical treatment of discrete and tunnel subaortic stenosis. Late survival and risk of reoperation. Circulation 88: II159–II169.

120. Misbach GA, Turley K, Ullyot DJ, Ebert PA (1982) Left ventricular outflow enlargement by the Konno procedure. J Thorac Cardiovasc Surg 84: 696–703.

121. Reddy VM, Rajasinghe HA, Teitel DF, et al. (1996) Aortoventriculoplasty with the pulmonary autograft: the "Ross–Konno" procedure. J Thorac Cardiovasc Surg 111: 158–165.

122. Colucci WS (1989) Myocardial and vascular actions of milrinone. Eur Heart J 10 (Suppl C): 32–38.

123. Deb B, Bradford K, Pearl RG (2000) Additive effects of inhaled nitric oxide and intravenous milrinone in experimental pulmonary hypertension. Crit Care Med 28: 795–799.

124. Mitruka SN, Lamberti JJ (2000) Congenital Heart Surgery Nomenclature and Database Project: mitral valve disease. Ann Thorac Surg 69 (4 Suppl): S132–S146.

125. Carpentier A, Branchini B, Cour JC, et al. (1976) Congenital malformations of the mitral valve in children. Pathology and surgical treatment. J Thorac Cardiovasc Surg 72: 854–866.

126. Chauvaud S (2004) Surgery of congenital mitral valve disease. J Cardiovasc Surg (Torino) 45: 465–476.

127. Bharucha T, Roman KS, Anderson RH, Vettukattil JJ (2008) Impact of multiplanar review of three-dimensional echocardiographic data on management of congenital heart disease. Ann Thorac Surg 86: 875–881.

128. Fraser CD (1998) Technical considerations for valve repair in patients with congenital heart disease. Curr Opin Cardiol 13: 96–104.

129. Fawzy ME, Stefadouros M, El Amraoui S, et al. (2008) Long-term (up to 18 years) clinical and echocardiographic results of mitral balloon valvuloplasty in children in comparison with adult population. J Interv Cardiol 21: 252–259.

130. Martens S, Neumann K, Sodemann C, et al. (2008) Carbon dioxide field flooding reduces neurologic impairment after open heart surgery. Ann Thorac Surg 85: 543–547.

131. Alphonso N, Nørgaard MA, Newcomb A, et al. (2005) Cor triatriatum: presentation, diagnosis and long-term surgical results. Ann Thorac Surg 80: 1666–1671.

132. Pisanti A, Vitiello R (2000) Wheezing as the sole clinical manifestation of cor triatriatum. Pediatr Pulmonol 30: 346–349.

22 Anesthesia for right-sided obstructive lesions

Michael L. Schmitz, M.D. and Sana Ullah, M.D.

Arkansas Children's Hospital, University of Arkansas for Medical Sciences, Little Rock, Arkansas, USA

Introduction

Right-sided obstructive congenital heart disease (CHD) encompasses a set of heart defects that can present with a wide range of clinical signs and symptoms. Some minimally affected teenagers or adults present only with vague complaints of exercise intolerance or fatigue. At the other extreme, right-sided obstructive CHD can be immediately apparent in the neonate who manifests severe cyanosis or congestive heart failure (CHF). All lesions of this category have the potential for right-to-left shunting of blood flow. The severity of the disease depends upon the degree of structural malformation of the heart and great vessels.

Congenital malformations that impede blood flow through the right heart can occur at a single or combination of critical anatomical areas. These include the right atrioventricular valve (AV), the outflow tract of the right ventricle (RV), the pulmonary valve (PV), and the main pulmonary artery (MPA) and/or branch pulmonary arteries. Commonly, congenital malformations affect several of these critical areas simultaneously, such as in the tetralogy of Fallot (TOF). Malformations can occur directly as a result of aberrant movement of tissues during development, or indirectly as a result of impaired flow hemodynamics due to malaligned structural anatomy. Often the resultant congenital heart deformity is a combination of both processes.

Patients with obstructive right-sided congenital heart anomalies can present in the neonatal period with either cyanosis or CHF. Right-sided lesions, which have potential for right-to-left shunting, can produce cyanosis, such as with right-to-left shunt through an atrial septal defect (ASD) or patent foramen ovale (PFO) in severe Ebstein's anomaly or through a ventricular septal defect (VSD) in TOF. The shunt direction can vary, becoming right-to-left as right-sided pressures exceed those in the comparable

Anesthesia for Congenital Heart Disease 2nd edition. Edited by Dean Andropoulos, Stephen Stayer, Isobel Russell and Emad Mossad. © 2010 Blackwell Publishing.

left-sided chamber, providing a "pop-off" mechanism for right-sided obstructive hypertension. Neonates with restrictive right-to-left communications or without anatomical potential for shunt develop congestive right heart failure. Infants with obstructive right-sided lesions such as critical pulmonary stenosis (PS) or pulmonary atresia (PA) can be ductal dependent, achieving pulmonary flow either in part or entirely from a patent ductus arteriosus (PDA). Unless patency is maintained by exogenous prostaglandin, increasing cyanosis can occur when the ductus arteriosus begins to close shortly after birth.

The physiology of right-sided obstructive defects and the changes that occur with surgical intervention in the context of perioperative anesthetic care are described in this chapter for:
• Ebstein's anomaly
• Tetralogy of Fallot
• PS with intact ventricular septum
• PA with intact ventricular septum
• PA and ventriculoseptal defect with multiple aortopulmonary collateral arteries (MAPCAs)

Other right-sided obstructions such as those that result in a single functional ventricle (e.g., tricuspid atresia) are covered elsewhere in this book.

Ebstein's anomaly

Anatomy

Ebstein's anomaly is by far the most common congenital malformation of the tricuspid valve (TV). The earliest description of TV malformation was by Ebstein in 1866

[1]. Ebstein's anomaly is present in only about 0.3–0.7% of patients with CHD and occurs in approximately 1 in 20,000 live births [2]. Other tricuspid anomalies such as TV stenosis, TV insufficiency (TI), and various malformations of leaflets, chordae tendinae, and papillary muscles are much less common [3].

Ebstein's anomaly consists of (i) a downward displacement of septal and posterior leaflet attachments at the junction of the inlet and trabecular portions of the RV, (ii) an "atrialized" portion of the RV between the tricuspid annulus and the attachment of the posterior and septal leaflets, and (iii) a malformed RV chamber (Figure 22.1). The dysplastic characteristics of the anomaly are quite variable in functional severity, leading to a wide range of functional presentations from infancy to adulthood.

The position, size, and shape of the posterior and septal leaflets are inconsistent. Posterior and septal leaflets can insert at varying distances below the AV annulus or can be closely adherent to the ventricular wall rather than displaced in one-third of patients. Shortened chordae often attach to papillary muscles that can be deformed. Over one-third of the hearts have an ASD, while most of the remaining two-thirds contain a PFO [6]. The anterior leaflet is attached at the AV annulus superior to the other leaflets, but it is always abnormal. It is often large and redundant, shaped like a sail, with abnormal attachments to the border of the inlet and trabecular portions of the RV. The anterior leaflet and/or the chordae can act as a barrier to blood flow from the atrium/atrialized RV to the trabecular RV. The aperture between the atrialized and trabecular portions of the RV can be restricted to slits or perforations in the anterior leaflet. As a result of the distally displaced valves, the trabecular portion of the RV is often very small,

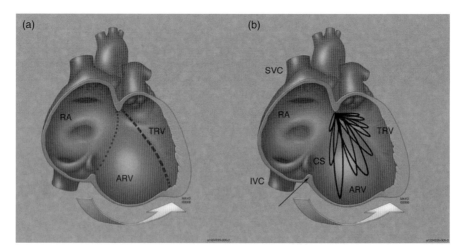

Figure 22.1 (a) Normal proximal tricuspid attachments at the atrioventricular junction (*circle dotted line*) and the direction of the hinge line in Ebstein's malformation (*square dotted line*). The displacement of the orifice of the valve is rotational (*flat arrow*). ARV, atrialized right ventricle; RA, right atrium; TRV, true right ventricle. (b) The location of the functional orifice of the abnormal valve (black ovals) as observed in the series of hearts examined by Schreiber et al. [4]. CS, coronary sinus; IVC, inferior vena cava; SVC, superior vena cava (Reproduced with permission from Reference [5])

lacking an inlet chamber. The walls of the RV can be normal, or thin with impaired contractile function [2,3,6].

The RV wall above the line of insertion of the distally displaced leaflets functions as part of the right atrium (RA), but is anatomically ventricular. This inlet portion of the RV is often thin and dilated. Although it is exposed to atrial pressures, this atrialized RV manifests electrical conduction of an abnormal ventricular pattern. In some cases, the wall of the inlet portion is so thin that it moves paradoxically during ventricular systole, dilating with RA contraction. The RA is dilated, sometimes massively.

Left ventricular geometry can be compromised by the abnormal position of the interventricular septum, resulting in a small left ventricle (LV) chamber. In addition, mitral valve prolapse can occur because the chordae tendinae of the normally situated mitral valve leaflets are altered in shape and size by the LV distortion [7].

Pathophysiology and natural history

The effects of TV dysfunction ultimately determine the manifestation of Ebstein's anomaly in the developing heart as TI can impair adequate development of other portions of the right heart. In utero, severe TI might result in such diminished forward flow through the RV and PA that RVOT obstruction and PS or even PA occurs. The volume load on the RV can create a grossly dilated RV that impairs LV function. The massive TI can produce a huge, ballooned RA. The symptomatic neonate with Ebstein's anomaly generally shows rapid improvement of hemodynamics in the postnatal period due to gradual reduction of pulmonary vascular resistance (PVR) [8].

The neonatal clinical presentation of Ebstein's anomaly varies greatly depending upon the extent of the downward displacement of the TV leaflets and the consequences of severe TI to the rest of the heart. If the ASD is unrestrictive, the infant will be cyanotic until PVR falls in the postnatal period to near adult levels, but cardiac output (CO) might be sufficient. A restrictive ASD can result in low CO due to impairment of LV function due to malposition and paradoxical motion of the interventricular septum. Noncompaction of the LV, a phenomenon of arrested morphologic development of the LV that results in large trabeculations and intratrabecular recesses and poor function, is sometimes associated with Ebstein's anomaly, causing systolic and diastolic dysfunction, ventricular arrhythmias, and an increased risk for systemic emboli [9].

Ebstein's cases with lesser anatomical aberration can have no signs during the neonatal period and only mild to moderate signs and symptoms later in childhood. Unless the foramen ovale is not patent, there is little exercise intolerance. Ultimately, CHF might develop from long-term effects of TI and when it does, it is often a harbinger

Table 22.1 Major electrophysiologic abnormalities in Ebstein's anomaly

Intra-atrial conduction disturbance; right atrial P wave abnormalities, PR interval prolongation

Atrioventricular nodal conduction: PR interval prolongation
Infranodal conduction
   Intra- or infra-His conduction abnormalities
   Right bundle branch block
   Bizarre second QRS attached to preceding normal QRS

Type B Wolff–Parkinson–White preexcitation
Supraventricular tachycardia
Atrial fibrillation or flutter
Arrhythmogenic atrialized right ventricle
Deep Q waves in leads V_{1-4} and in inferior leads

Source: Reproduced with permission from Reference [2].

of death within a few years. If there is cyanosis, the more severe the cyanosis in the child or young adult, the poorer the prognosis is. Without surgical intervention, death from Ebstein's anomaly that presents in late childhood, adolescence, or young adulthood is usually secondary to CHF in the second or third decades of life.

Ebstein's anomaly is often complicated by life-threatening arrhythmias that further reduce function in an anatomically impaired heart. Paroxysmal supraventricular tachycardia can occur in up to 20–25% of children, but other electrophysiological abnormalities are also common (Table 22.1). To make matters worse, accessory pathways are more difficult to ablate with Ebstein's anomaly than with hearts with normal anatomy, and the recurrence rate postablation is higher [9].

Surgical approach

The natural history of the disease varies with its severity, and accordingly, the management of Ebstein's anomaly is based on its severity and the age at which surgical intervention is necessary. The size of the trabecular portion of the RV usually determines whether the patient is eligible for a two-ventricular, one-and-a-half-ventricular, or single-ventricular repair/palliation. For the neonate, further consideration is given to the degree of RVOT obstruction and the transitional decline of PVR from prenatal to near adult levels. Cardiac transplantation is generally reserved for the most severely afflicted infants, and perhaps those with significant LV dysfunction [8].

The first TV replacement was performed in 1963 as valvuloplasty techniques were rapidly evolving. Large numbers of patients have survived with a valvuloplasty technique described by Danielson et al. [10] which includes a reduction atrioplasty and ablation of accessory conduction pathways. Many variations of Danielson's technique, TV repair, and plication of RV have been

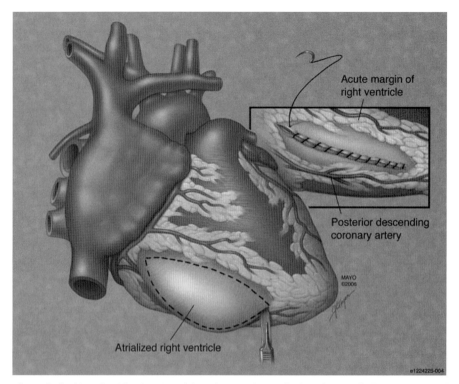

Figure 22.2 Resection of a markedly thinned atrialized portion of the right ventricle, usually the inferior wall. The resection (or plication) is performed from the base toward the apex and parallel to the coronary arteries. Inset: completed suture line is parallel to the long axis of the heart. The acute margin of the right ventricle is effectively brought close to the posterior descending coronary artery (Reproduced with permission from Reference [5])

described in the last two decades [9]; a representation of the wide anatomical variation found in Ebstein's anomaly. More recent techniques include (i) cone reconstruction of the TV and RV plication as described by da Silva et al. [11], and (ii) approximation of the ventricular septum or septal leaflet to the anterior leaflet by drawing the RV free wall toward the interventicular septum with suture, avoiding an RV incisional plication (Figure 22.2), followed by approximation of the TV leaflets and reduction of the TV orifice as described by Dearani et al. [5] (Figures 22.3–22.5).

Dysrhythmias are often problematic after surgical repair of Ebstein's anomaly, and temporary pacing wires placed on the RA and RV during surgery might be useful in some patients for monitoring of rhythm postoperatively or pacing. For teenaged and adult patients with preoperative dysrhythmias, intermediate follow-up postrepair indicates substantial reduction of dysrhythmia in survivors who did not require placement of pacemakers [12]. Outcomes analysis [13] has shown a hospital mortality of 10% (largely due to acute postoperative RV failure), but a long-term actuarial survival of 75% at 10 years for children and adults (no infants). High-risk patients (severely impaired RV function, difficult TV repair, and/or permanent atrial fibrillation) seem to benefit from a cavopulmonary anastomosis.

Surgical intervention is infrequently necessary in the infant and child unless tricuspid incompetence results in progressive right heart failure. Moderate CHF due to TI can be managed with digoxin in combination with diuretic therapy. Dysrhythmias are medically controlled. Teenagers and young adults do well with TV replacement as progressive valvular deterioration can preclude valvuloplasty. Children who survive infancy have a greater likelihood of undergoing successful valvuloplasty or prosthetic TV replacement. For the child with an RV capable of adequate right CO, resection of redundant atrialized RV tissue and realignment of TV leaflets or placement of a prosthetic TV have all provided reasonable surgical outcomes. In one recent study of 52 young children undergoing repair, survival at 5, 10, and 15 years was 92%, 90%, and 90%, respectively, and freedom from reoperation for recurrent TI was 91%, 80%, and 68%, respectively [14].

Although severe TV dysplasia in the neonate is often not reparable with surgical valvuloplasty, some infants can do well with an aggressive two-ventricular repair that includes reconstruction of a monocuspid TV from the anterior leaflet, ventriculorrhaphy, reduction atrioplasty, subtotal closure of the ASD, and repair of other associated defects [15]. In the early 1990s, the Starnes procedure (right ventricular exclusion via pericardial patch

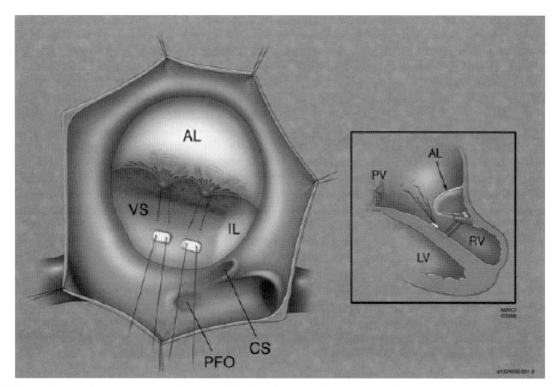

Figure 22.3 Basic principles of a current technique for repair of the tricuspid valve in Ebstein's anomaly. The maneuvers are designed to progressively bring the leading edge of the anterior leaflet (AL) closer to the ventricular septum (VS), or septal leaflet, in order to optimize leaflet coaptation and establish competence of the valve. The base of the intact major papillary muscle(s), which arise from the free wall of the right ventricle, is moved toward the ventricular septum at the appropriate level with pledgeted horizontal mattress sutures. CS, coronary sinus; IL, inferior leaflet; PFO, patent foramen ovale. Inset: coronal view of the right ventricle (RV) and right atrium demonstrating a small dimple effect that occurs in the anterior free wall of the right ventricle after this maneuver is completed. LV, left ventricle; PV, pulmonary valve (Reproduced with permission from Reference [5])

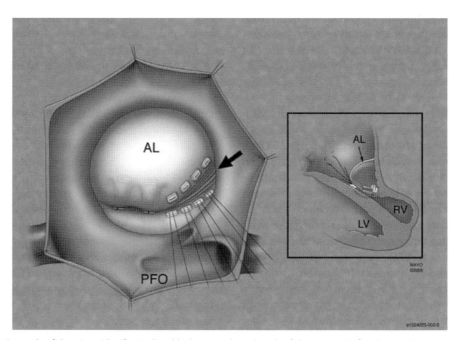

Figure 22.4 The inferior angle of the tricuspid orifice is closed by bringing the right side of the anterior leaflet down to the septum and plicating the nonfunctional inferior leaflet in the process (*arrow*). Inset: after all of the mattress sutures are secured, improved proximity of the leading edge of the anterior leaflet with the ventricular septum is noted. AL, anterior leaflet; LV, left ventricle; PFO, patent foramen ovale; RV, right ventricle (Reproduced with permission from Reference [5])

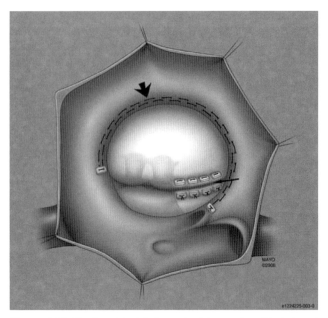

Figure 22.5 Plication of the inferior angle of the annulus with pledgeted mattress sutures (*arrow*). An anterior purse string annuloplasty (*arrowhead*) may be performed to further narrow the tricuspid annulus. This annuloplasty may begin at the anteroseptal commissure, anterior to the membranous septum, and ends beyond the inferoseptal commissure, adjacent to the coronary sinus. Alternatively, the annuloplasty can be performed posterolaterally to reduce the size of the annulus, which also brings the free wall closer to the septum (Reproduced with permission from Reference [5])

closure of the TV, reduction atrioplasty ± RV plication, and modified Blalock–Taussig shunt [mBTS]) was proposed for prostaglandin E1 (PGE_1) dependent neonates with Ebstein's anomaly and physiologic PA, converting the cardiac physiology effectively to that of the single-ventricular system [16]. There have been many reported modifications to this procedure since that time, but the basic elements include placing a fenestrated patch over the TV orifice (to allow RV decompression from filling via the thebesian veins), creating a nonrestrictive ASD, and providing for pulmonary blood flow (PBF) with an aortopulmonary shunt [8]. Sano et al. [17] have taken this concept further with the RV exclusion operation that also includes excision of the RV free wall with subsequent primary closure or closure with a polytetraflouroethylene patch, removing much of the potentially arrhythmogenic RV that could impair LV function. Survival for the most severe neonatal forms of Ebstein's anomaly treated with aggressive neonatal surgery has improved, but is still much lower than for other complex congenital heart lesions. Two large, recent, single center series report hospital survival rates of 70%/ [18] and 73% [15].

Patients with a severely hypoplastic or poorly functioning RV might ultimately require a single-ventricle repair with cavopulmonary anastomosis or Fontan circulation. However, there are instances when a hypoplastic or small RV is still capable of ejecting partial CO to the pulmonary arteries. These patients might benefit from a one-and-a-half-ventricular repair, allowing the diminutive RV to pump part of the systemic venous return to the lungs. The venous drainage of the upper body returns by passive flow via a cavopulmonary anastomosis to the pulmonary circulation, and ranges from one-third to one-half of the systemic venous return. In brief, the one-and-a-half-ventricle repair includes valvuloplasty, possible repair of the ASD, and creation of a cavopulmonary anastomosis. A small ASD can be left if there is an anticipated need for a "pop-off" for systemic venous return to the "half" pulmonary ventricle. The pulmonary arteries must be of adequate size, and PVR must be low for successful implementation.

Advantages exist in utilizing a semifunctional pulmonary ventricle. Preservation of some pulsatile flow to the PA might reduce the risk of development of MAPCAs. Also, a hypoplastic pulmonary ventricle might be able to respond to increased demand by increasing CO beyond what might result with a Fontan circulation [19]. Van Arsdell et al. [20] have proposed that the one-and-a-half-ventricular repair might be of benefit to the patients with Ebstein's anomaly who have a partial RV outflow tract (RVOT) obstruction due to billowing of the anterior leaflet.

Reported mortality with the one-and-a-half-ventricular repair for all lesions (including Ebstein's anomaly) is variable between 0 and 12% [21, 22]. Long-term outcomes have not been compared to the Fontan procedure, but the one-and-a-half-ventricle repair seems not to have the short-term and intermediate-term complications of cyanosis, chronic atrial dysrhythmias, and protein-losing enteropathies associated with the Fontan physiology [21, 22]. However, an increase in perioperative effusions and chylothorax has been found. Other complications have included chronically increased superior vena cava (SVC) pressure, early-morning periorbital edema, and one instance of an SVC aneurysm. Another instance is reported of development of pulmonary arteriovenous fistulas with a one-and-a-half-ventricle repair in combination with the classic Glenn procedure [21].

Decision making for the type of surgical repair or palliation relies on two critical assessments: the morphology of the TV and the size of the pumping chamber of the pulmonary ventricle. Valvuloplasty is preferred in infants and young children due to the need to upsize valves as the child grows. The teenager who has reached near adult size might do better with a prosthetic valve as the native valve might have incurred much damage due to abnormal dynamics over time. Patients with less than adequate pumping chambers will generally present for definitive surgical management in infancy or early childhood.

Perioperative anesthetic management

Preoperative care

Given the variability in presentation, the preanesthetic evaluation of the infant or child with Ebstein's anomaly must include an assessment of the severity of the disease. Specifically, the patient is evaluated for symptoms of fatigue, dyspnea, and if there have been signs of cyanotic episodes, or if cyanotic episodes have been becoming more frequent or severe. One can assess exercise tolerance for an individual child by asking about the child's ability to play with the same vigor as the child's healthy peers. For an infant, one can focus questions for the caretakers on usual baby activities and growth; poor feeding ability, failure to thrive, and/or signs of dyspnea, irritability, cyanosis, or diaphoresis are indicative of a poorly functioning heart. A history of syncope, chest pain, and palpitations suggests dysrhythmia in the older child.

With Ebstein's anomaly, physical examination might be notable for triple or quadruple heart sounds, often with a soft, high-pitched systolic murmur. A soft, scratchy mid-diastolic murmur heard best at the left sternal border and apex might be present. The second heart sound is widely split with little respiratory variation due to delayed emptying of the RV. With failure, the child can be diaphoretic, tachypneic, and irritable with rales present on chest auscultation and hepatomegaly on abdominal palpation. The chest roentgenogram can reveal moderate to severe cardiomegaly with a large RA and diminished pulmonary vascular markings. The heart often has a globular shape. Electrocardiogram (ECG) usually suggests RA hypertrophy, an increased PR interval, and complete or incomplete right bundle branch block. Interestingly, the preexcitation patterns of Wolff–Parkinson–White syndrome are seen in 10–15% of individuals. Two-dimensional echocardiography is usually diagnostic, revealing a large tricuspid orifice complete with apical displacement of the septal leaflet of the TV. Cardiac catheterization is seldom indicated and can be complicated by induction of tachyarrhythmias. Magnetic resonance imaging (MRI) is being used more frequently to measure displacement of the TV leaflets and to estimate the functional size of the RV [22].

The cyanotic neonate benefits from a reduction in PVR. Prevention of atelectasis with adequate tidal volumes while minimizing airway pressure in the intubated infant is beneficial. Nitric oxide might be useful for encouraging PBF in the neonate with marginal heart function and could help distinguish between functional and anatomic obstructions to PBF. Often, PGE_1 is necessary in the early neonatal period to augment pulmonary arterial blood flow by maintaining the PDA. However, a large PDA can cause high output cardiac failure with what is known as a "cir-

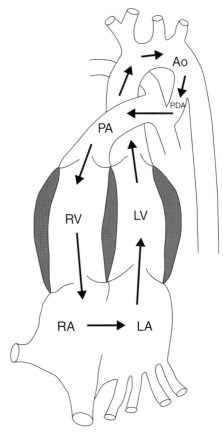

Figure 22.6 Circular shunt: aortic blood enters the lower pressure pulmonary artery (PA) via the patent ductus arteriosus (PDA). Pulmonary insufficiency allows blood to continue retrograde into the right ventricle (RV), right atrium (RA), left atrium (LA), left ventricle (LV), and then again to the aorta (Ao).

cular shunt." In this circumstance, generous blood flow from the aorta flows through the PDA into the PA, but follows the course of least resistance retrograde sequentially through the PV, RV, RA, ASD or PFO, LA, LV, and again into the aorta with minimal perfusion of the pulmonary capillary bed (Figure 22.6). Discontinuation of the PGE_1 reduces this shunt by allowing the PDA to become smaller, increasing afterload and reducing high output failure [9].

Anxiolysis can be accomplished with midazolam, either given orally (0.5–0.75 mg/kg up to 15–20 mg) or intravenously (0.1–0.15 mg/kg up to 2–4 mg). Infants who manifest stranger fear (approximately 9 months of age and older) might also benefit from such sedation.

Intraoperative care

For infants and children with mild-to-moderate disease, an inhalational induction with nitrous oxide and sevoflurane can provide a smooth transition to the anesthetized state. Lowered CO or small right-to-left shunt at the atrial level can slow an inhalational induction. Alternatively, intravenous induction with ketamine (1–4 mg/kg) or thiopental (4 mg/kg) can provide reasonable induction hemodynamics. For patients with moderate to severe TV pathology, intravenous induction with glycopyrrolate and ketamine (1–4 mg/kg) or etomidate (0.2–0.3 mg/kg) allows stable hemodynamics in most instances without excessive myocardial depression or reduced afterload. Since these patients are dependent upon adequate preload, increases in vascular compliance due to anesthetic-induced vasodilation need to be met with intravenous volume replacement such as with 5% albumin. Choices of muscle relaxant depend upon the expected duration of the procedure and the need for rapid sequence or modified rapid sequence induction techniques. Pancuronium, a long-acting muscle relaxant, is sufficient for most cases and provides vagolysis via ganglionic blockade for a sustained increase in baseline heart rate. The maintenance technique is often narcotic based (fentanyl 10–20 µg/kg prior to CPB and 25–50 µg/kg, total) with low-dose isoflurane (e.g., 0.4%) prior to onset of cardiopulmonary bypass (CPB). Lower doses of fentanyl and a higher minimum alveolar concentration (MAC) of a halogenated agent such as isoflurane, sevoflurane, or desflurane can be used with patients who have sufficient cardiac reserve to tolerate the myocardial depressant effects of the halogenated agents. (Myocardial [23,24] and neurological [24,25] preconditioning and delayed preconditioning [26] have been demonstrated in vitro and in animal models when administered near 1 MAC prior to a significant ischemic event.) For repeat sternotomy, plasmin binding inhibitor antifibrinolytic drugs such as ε-aminocaproic acid or tranexamic acid can reduce blood loss during the pre- and post-CPB period.

Five-lead ECG with an ability to display multiple lead tracings is useful in monitoring changes in rhythm both during the pre- and postrepair periods. Other than standard monitoring, near-infrared spectroscopy is useful for monitoring brain oxygenation during periods of cannulation and CPB. Transcranial Doppler flow velocity gives insight into changes in cerebral blood flow within the clinical context and provides extremely sensitive detection of gas or particulate emboli entering the cerebral circulation. Intraoperative transesophageal echocardiography (TEE) allows one to check for clearance of air bubbles in the heart prior to coming off CPB and rapidly assess the function of the TV in the immediate post-CPB period.

Patients with severely dilated right hearts are at high risk for potentially lethal ventricular arrhythmias postrepair. Prior to separation from CPB, a prophylactic intravenous infusion of an antiarrhythmic drug such as lidocaine or amiodarone can lend some protection against ventricular arrhythmias. Patients who have undergone a right-ventricular plication as part of the repair are at added risk for ventricular arrhythmias. Inotropic drugs that promote forward flow in the right heart (e.g., milrinone 0.3–0.5 µg/kg/min or dobutamine 5 µg/kg/min) can improve hemodynamics for hearts with preexisting myocardial dysfunction after separating from CPB. Generous RV filling pressures might be needed to maintain adequate preload with a poorly functioning ventricle.

Postoperative care

At the end of surgery, patients are transported to the intensive care unit (ICU) equipped to care for the postoperative pediatric cardiac patient with continuous monitoring for rhythm and arterial blood pressure. Pain can be well controlled with opioid infusions such as morphine sulfate (20–80 mcg/kg/h, depending on the need for sedation beyond analgesia). Patients with minimal preexisting myocardial dysfunction can be weaned from mechanical ventilation and extubated in the operating room or within hours of arrival in the ICU. For others, it is prudent to allow the patient to emerge more slowly from narcotic sedation and inotropic support in order to assess the remodeled tricuspid competency and allow more time for recovery of myocardial function. Midazolam (0.1–0.2 mg/kg/h) can be added simultaneously with narcotic analgesic infusion to provide sedation for patients who need longer myocardial recover times and remain intubated and ventilated beyond the operative day.

As stated above, dysrhythmias are common in the immediate postoperative period after repair of Ebstein's anomaly, and can persist as a late complication of repair. Supraventricular tachycardia, junctional rhythm, or intermittent AV block can complicate recovery. Risk for ventricular arrhythmias and sudden death persists through the first postoperative month. Those patients who demonstrate perioperative ventricular tachycardia or ventricular fibrillation are likely at greatest risk [27]. Patients with intermittent AV block or junctional rhythm might benefit from temporary pacing to enhance CO in the immediate postoperative period. As myocardial edema subsides, return of functional conduction pathways might allow return of normal sinus rhythm. As mentioned above, intravenous amiodarone or lidocaine might be helpful in the early postoperative period, and switching to oral amiodarone for several months might be warranted for high-risk individuals.

In the early postoperative period, echocardiography often shows poor coaptation of the TV leaflets. This finding is likely due to post-CPB dysfunction of the papillary muscle bundles (possibly of ischemic etiology) as the leaflet coaptation often improves with subsequent echocardiographic examinations.

Tetralogy of Fallot

Anatomy

Representing 10% of all congenital heart defects, TOF is the most common form of cyanotic heart disease. The French physician Etienne Fallot, as far back as 1888, first published the most comprehensive clinical and anatomical description, based on numerous postmortem studies. Classic TOF consists of four abnormalities (the "tetrad"): (i) a large unrestrictive VSD, (ii) RVOT obstruction, (iii) overriding of the aorta above the RVOT, and (iv) RV hypertrophy (Figure 22.7). Embryologically, TOF is believed to result from incomplete rotation and faulty partitioning of the conotruncus during septation resulting in the conus septum developing too far anteriorly, producing two unequal sized vessels: a large aorta and a smaller pulmonary trunk.

The VSD is perimembranous, large (usually the same diameter as the aorta), and unrestrictive. The cardiac conduction tissue lies in close proximity to the margins of the VSD and might be damaged during repair, producing temporary or permanent heart block. Additional muscular VSDs might also be present. The aortic outflow overrides the VSD and thus has a biventricular origin, receiving a variable amount of blood from the RV depending

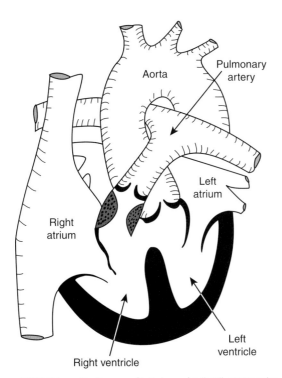

Figure 22.7 Schematic diagram of tetralogy of Fallot illustrating the infundibular stenosis (*stippled area*), ventricular septal defect, overriding aorta, and right ventricular hypertrophy.

on the degree of RVOT obstruction. In 25% of TOF patients, the aortic arch is right-sided, with mirror image branching of the head vessels. Other associated rare vessel abnormalities include an aberrant origin of the ipsilateral subclavian artery from the descending aorta and an isolated origin of the left subclavian artery from the PA. These abnormalities might have implications when selecting the surgical approach for the placement of palliative shunts.

Coronary abnormalities occur in 5–12% of patients with TOF. Failure to detect these preoperatively can have serious consequences for a successful outcome if they are injured in the surgical repair. The most common abnormality consists of a left anterior descending artery that originates from the right coronary artery and crosses the RVOT inferiorly. This arrangement makes it very susceptible to damage if the transannular incision is carried too far inferiorly across the RVOT. Indeed, an alternative surgical approach might be needed in relieving the subpulmonary obstruction, or alternatively a RV to PA conduit might be required. Other coronary anomalies include a right coronary artery originating from the left coronary artery and a left coronary artery originating from the PA. Precise definition of the coronary anatomy might be possible with echocardiography alone [28]. If there is still uncertainty, aortic root or selective coronary angiography can be used, but it is sometimes a risky procedure in an unpalliated patient due to the danger of a severe hypercyanotic spell caused by cardiac catheter manipulations.

Other lesions that might be associated with TOF include left SVC, AV septal defect, PDA, ASD, and interrupted inferior vena cava. All of these might require modifications to the surgical repair such as an additional venous drainage cannula in the left SVC.

Two important variants of TOF are PA/VSD, and the absent PV syndrome. With PA/VSD, there is complete obstruction to RV outflow and hypoplasia of the central and peripheral pulmonary arteries. The MPA might be absent or the branch PAs might be nonconfluent or stenosed. Pulmonary blood supply is usually via MAPCAs. The surgical correction of this lesion is very different from that of classic TOF and is discussed later in this chapter [29,30]. Absent PV syndrome is characterized by combined PV stenosis and insufficiency (PI), which in utero produces increased pulsatile PBF, causing massive enlargement of the main and branch PAs. This also results in a characteristic feature of airway compression and tracheobronchomalacia. These babies typically present in the neonatal period with severe respiratory distress, cyanosis, and air trapping. Tracheal intubation with high levels of positive end-expiratory pressure (PEEP) and prone positioning might be useful in keeping the airways open. An additional risk factor in causing airway obstruction, which we have witnessed on several occasions, is insertion of the transesophageal echocardiographic probe in preparation for surgery. Infants with significant lung disease require urgent surgical intervention. However, even after repair, respiratory symptoms commonly persist due to the underlying intrinsic airway abnormalities, and such patients might need long-term ventilation.

In TOF, the RVOT obstruction usually has dynamic and fixed components. The dynamic component consists of hypertrophied infundibulum and muscle bundle fibers. The hypertrophy occurs in response to the increased pressure load on the RV. Fixed components of the obstruction occur at the valvular and supravalvular level. The PV is frequently thickened, dysplastic, and often bicuspid. There is usually some degree of PA hypoplasia in all patients. There might also be localized narrowing of the main and branch PAs. Atresia or discontinuity of the main and branch PAs can occur, further complicating surgical correction, as restoration of continuity or augmentation of the pulmonary arteries is required.

There is a weak association of familial inheritance of TOF. Indeed, TOF is associated with major extracardiac malformations, and might occur as part of a syndrome. Some examples are the VACTERL association (vertebral, vascular, anal, cardiac, tracheoesophageal fistula, renal, and limb anomalies), DiGeorge syndrome, velocardiofacial syndrome, and CHARGE association (coloboma, heart anomaly, choanal atresia, retardation, and genital and ear anomalies). Recent genetic studies have shown that TOF is associated with chromosome 22q11 deletion ("catch 22 syndrome"). This chromosomal abnormality is also responsible for DiGeorge syndrome, velocardiofacial syndrome, and conotruncal anomaly face syndrome. In one study of TOF patients, prevalence of 22q11 deletion was 13%. This deletion is considered to be the most common genetic cause of TOF-associated syndromes [31].

Pathophysiology and natural history

The clinical manifestation of TOF ranges from extreme cyanosis at one end of the spectrum, because of profound right-to-left shunting through the VSD, to normal saturation for patients who have minimal RVOT obstruction. The latter group is referred to as "pink tets" because of the absence of cyanosis. They might even show signs of CHF from pulmonary over circulation. The severity of symptoms correlates primarily with the degree of RVOT obstruction, as this determines the amount of shunting of desaturated blood into the systemic circulation. Detrimental effects of RV hypertrophy, a response to the high afterload (systemic and pulmonary) include (i) RV diastolic dysfunction requiring high filling pressures to maintain CO; (ii) increased difficulty for surgical repair of the VSD and resection of the RVOT muscle bundles due to a

thickened, stiff ventricle; and (iii) a lessened ability to protect the hypertrophied RV during aortic cross-clamping, which might contribute to postoperative RV dysfunction. To limit the progression of ventricular hypertrophy, most centers now undertake surgical correction in early infancy.

With a nonrestrictive VSD and equalization of RV and LV pressures, the major determinant of the degree of shunting (and hence, cyanosis) is the balance of systemic vascular resistance (SVR) and PVR. A fall in SVR (hypovolemia, acidosis, hypoxia), and/or an increase in PVR (infundibular spasm) will favor right-to-left shunting and worsening cyanosis. Acute severe RVOT obstruction occurs during a hypercyanotic or "tet spell," which can result in syncope or stroke. These spells can occur spontaneously, but are usually precipitated by crying, agitation, pain, defecation, injury, or fright, conditions that increase sympathetic activity and cardiac contractility, resulting in infundibular spasm. If not treated aggressively, resulting hypoxia and acidosis will further reduce SVR, leading to more right-to-left shunting. Induction of anesthesia can be particularly challenging and hazardous if intravenous access is unavailable. The anesthesiologist must be well prepared to treat such an episode. The goal of treatment is to use maneuvers (described later in this chapter) to reverse the amount of right-to-left shunting. "Tet spells" in patients who are conscious are usually accompanied by hyperventilation due to hypoxemia and metabolic acidosis. Older children with unrepaired TOF (rare in the current era) would adopt a squatting posture during a spell to alleviate discomfort. Squatting increases intraabdominal pressure, thereby increasing RV preload, allowing the RVOT to open, and increasing PBF. Squatting also increases SVR, increasing blood pressure in the left atrium (LA), reducing or eliminating right-to-left atrial shunting.

The presenting clinical features depend on the degree of RVOT obstruction. Prenatal diagnosis is possible with ultrasonography. Genetic screening for 22q11 deletion is often offered after prenatal ultrasonic diagnosis. In the neonate, cyanosis and a heart murmur will lead to further diagnostic evaluation. In newborns with critical PS and ductal-dependent PBF, the clinical presentation might be delayed until the ductus arteriosus closes. Then, the infant might develop sudden severe cyanosis during a "tet spell."

Physical findings are not specific for TOF. Cardiac auscultation reveals a crescendo–decrescendo systolic murmur best heard at the upper left sternal border. The intensity of the murmur will decrease during a hypercyanotic spell due to diminished PBF. Clubbing is a relatively late finding in chronically cyanotic patients. The ECG usually shows RV hypertrophy and right axis deviation. The chest radiograph will show a characteristic "boot-shaped" heart, reflecting RV hypertrophy and a concave upper left heart border from a small or absent MPA. The diagnosis is confirmed by echocardiography. Other important echocardiographic information includes (i) the degree of RVOT obstruction, (ii) the size and location of VSDs, (iii) definition of coronary anatomy, (iv) additional cardiac pathology such as arch sidedness and ASD, and (v) biventricular function.

Survival beyond the fourth decade is very rare in untreated patients. Mortality is usually a result of hypoxemia and its hematological consequences, endocarditis, or brain abscess. Even children who are completely palliated show delayed growth and development due to the associated noncardiac conditions. With complete repair in early infancy or childhood, over 85% of patients are expected to survive to adulthood [32].

Surgical approach

All patients diagnosed with TOF require some form of intervention. In some centers, balloon dilation of the RVOT is used as an alternative to a systemic artery-to-PA shunt placement [33, 34]. Advantages of this technique include avoiding a sternotomy or thoracotomy and distortion of the PA anatomy from shunt placement.

The optimal timing for surgery and complete versus staged repair are the subjects of ongoing debate, although most centers now favor total repair in early infancy [35–41]. Other factors that influence these decisions are the institution's capability for providing perioperative critical care to patients with complex CHD and specific anatomical features that are contraindications to complete early repair. Examples of unfavorable anatomy include the presence of coronary abnormalities such as the left anterior descending artery arising from the right coronary artery and crossing the RVOT, the presence of multiple VSDs, and inadequate PA anatomy. In these cases, it is reasonable to place a palliative shunt and allow the baby to grow, facilitating eventual complete repair on a bigger patient. This two-stage repair subjects the baby to additional surgical procedures with attendant risks and complications: (i) potential injury to the recurrent laryngeal and phrenic nerves, (ii) inadequate or excessive PBF requiring shunt revision, (iii) potentially fatal shunt thrombosis, (iv) distortion of the PA at the shunt site, and (v) the need for a second sternotomy [42]. However, there are problems with doing a complete repair in the neonatal period. In addition to the usual risks of performing a complex cardiac repair on small babies and the effects of CPB on immature organ systems, the surgical procedure is much more challenging due to the patient's small size. Although most centers perform the repair using a transatrial–transpulmonary approach, smaller patients might need a ventriculotomy to facilitate repair.

Surgical palliation

The aim of palliation, using a systemic artery-to-PA anastomosis, is to provide a stable source of PBF until complete repair can be accomplished. The "classic" Blalock–Taussig shunt (BTS), an end-to-side anastomosis of the subclavian artery to the PA to alleviate cyanosis, was first performed in 1944. Potts and Waterston later described shunts using direct anastomosis between the aorta and PA. However, despite providing good palliation, their size was difficult to control, and they were also extremely difficult to take down during subsequent complete repair and thus were largely abandoned. The most common palliative procedure in the current era is the "modified" BTS using an interposition graft between a branch of the brachiocephalic trunk (usually the subclavian artery) and the ipsilateral PA (Figure 22.8). There are several advantages of the mBTS: (i) it preserves blood flow to the arm; (ii) it can placed on either side, although most are done on the right because the pulmonary anastomosis can be placed more centrally allowing easier control of the shunt during subsequent repair; and (iii) it avoids excessive PBF when appropriately sized. An alternative procedure is to place a central shunt between the ascending aorta and the MPA using graft material. The central shunt is useful when the vascular anatomy precludes placement of an mBTS.

Surgical repair

Lillehei performed the first successful complete repair of TOF in 1954. The goals of repair, then as now, are (i) maximal relief of RVOT obstruction, (ii) VSD closure, and (iii) preservation of RV function in the short and long term. The surgical technique has been well described [43]. After cardioplegic arrest, the repair is done using a transatrial–transpulmonary approach. Right ventriculotomy is avoided, if possible, to preserve RV function [44]. The PV is examined through a longitudinal incision in the MPA, and if necessary, a valve commissurotomy is performed. The RVOT is exposed through the RA and TV and resection of the infundibular septum is carried out. The RVOT and MPA size are assessed using Hegar dilators, and if judged inadequate, the MPA incision is extended down toward the annulus onto the RV free wall. A transannular patch can then be used to augment the size of the RVOT. A monocusp valve might be placed in the RVOT to limit PI. The VSD is closed using a patch, and the ASD, if present, is also closed. Some surgeons prefer to leave a small atrial communication as a "pop off" valve in case of RV dysfunction postoperatively. This will maintain LV preload at the expense of some cyanosis. In patients who have a coronary artery crossing the RVOT, a transatrial–transpulmonary repair is still feasible if the transannular incision is limited. Many of these patients,

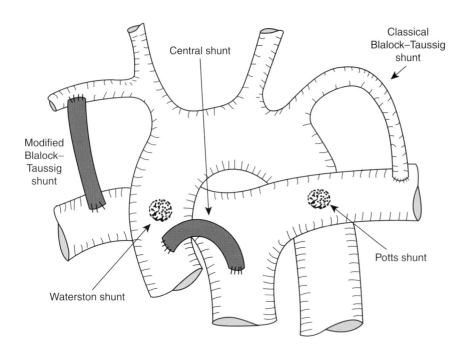

Figure 22.8 Diagram showing the various types of shunts used to increase pulmonary blood flow. The modified Blalock–Taussig shunt and central shunts are the only shunts used in the modern era.

however, will require a valved RV–PA conduit to avoid damage to the coronary artery.

The immediate adequacy of repair is assessed using several techniques. Immediate preoperative and intraoperative TEE is very useful in demonstrating gradients across the RVOT, showing residual VSDs, and assessing valves and ventricular function [45,46]. The RV:LV pressure ratio can be measured, less than 0.75 being considered acceptable. However, these pressure measurements in the early post-CPB period do not reflect measurements made at follow-up, and might lead to unnecessary revisions of the repair [47]. Blood gas measurements from the vena cava and the PA can also be used to detect residual shunts.

Long-term surgical complications

Despite excellent survival, many patients have residual sequelae from surgical repair: residual intracardiac shunts, TI, PA stenoses, and aneurysmal dilatation of the RVOT might need surgical intervention. Chronic PI leads to progressive volume overload of the RV producing ventricular dysfunction, reduced exercise tolerance and increased incidence of arrhythmias. Many of these patients present for PV replacement, and the indications and timing of this procedure are well discussed in a recent review article [48]. Cardiac MRI is becoming increasingly utilized in making volumetric and functional assessments of the RV and predicting clinical outcomes [49]. Another recent development is percutaneous PV replacement in patients who do not have aneurysmal dilation of the RVOT [50]. The valve is harvested from bovine jugular vein and mounted inside

a nitinol expandable stent, and is delivered intravenously. See Chapter 27 for a more detailed discussion.

Perioperative anesthetic management

Unrepaired patients who do not have a palliative shunt might develop a "tet spell" at any time during the pre-CPB period. Worsening cyanosis and hypoxemia leading to cardiovascular collapse can occur without prompt and aggressive treatment. Particularly vulnerable periods are during anesthetic induction and before surgical stimulation, when reduced sympathetic tone causes a fall in the SVR leading to increased right-to-left shunting. Manipulation of the heart and great vessels by the surgeon might also result in sudden right-to-left shunting. The primary goal of management of a spell is to correct the hypoxemia by relieving the infundibular spasm and reversing the shunt. Some or all of the following maneuvers can be employed:

1 Increase inspired oxygen. This does not relieve the spasm but helps reduce hypoxic pulmonary vasoconstriction.
2 Phenylephrine, 5–10 mcg/kg and titrated to effect to increase SVR.
3 Volume infusion to support the blood pressure and increase right heart filling that helps to open up the RVOT.
4 Abdominal compression and placing the child in a knee–chest position can increase the SVR.
5 Esmolol, 50 mcg/kg and titrated to effect by its negative inotropic effect can help to relieve the infundibular spasm. Propranolol (0.1 mg/kg given slowly) also works but is slower in onset.

6 Increasing the depth of anesthesia with a volatile agent will help the infundibular spasm through its negative inotropic effect. Although halothane has been traditionally used for this purpose, a recent echocardiographic study showed that sevoflurane has less effect on the SVR index than halothane or isoflurane at 1.5 MAC [51] and therefore might also be a good choice. Isoflurane is a poor choice because it is a potent vasodilator and also causes tachycardia, which increases contractility. Although morphine is frequently recommended for the treatment of "tet spells" in conscious patients, it produces too much vasodilation under anesthesia and therefore is not recommended.

7 If all these measures fail and the patient continues to deteriorate, the chest might have to be opened quickly, and the aorta might need to be compressed to reverse the shunting. In redo sternotomies, extracorporeal membrane oxygenation (ECMO) might be used as rescue therapy.

Perioperative anesthetic management for surgical palliation

Many patients who require surgical palliation are critically ill due to severely reduced PBF. They might be mechanically ventilated and on prostaglandin infusion to maintain ductal patency. If intravenous access is available, anesthesia can be induced with a combination of ketamine and fentanyl and maintained with low concentrations of a volatile agent. It is important to maintain adequate SVR to limit right-to-left shunting through the VSD; in this regard, sevoflurane is a good choice as this has the least effect on SVR [51]. The myocardial depressant effect of volatile agents is also useful in limiting infundibular spasm. Low SVR is treated with fluid boluses and phenylephrine. Inotropic agents are best avoided, as these will worsen infundibular spasm by increasing heart rate and contractility. If there is no intravenous access, induction can be carried out rapidly and smoothly with sevoflurane. An alternative is to use intramuscular ketamine and rocuronium in unstable patients who might not tolerate the vasodilation from volatile agents. Central venous access is obtained for the infusion of fluids and vasoactive agents. A radial arterial line is placed on the side opposite to that of the planned mBTS in order to get a true assessment of the blood pressure because after the shunt is opened there might be significant "steal" from the ipsilateral subclavian artery. A femoral arterial line can also be placed as long as care is taken to observe for evidence of distal lower extremity ischemia.

Most mBTS are performed via a thoracotomy. The median sternotomy approach is used for central shunt placement if the surgeon feels that the patient will not tolerate lung retraction or side clamping of the PA, and there is a possibility that CPB might be required. Low-dose heparin (100 units/kg) is administered prior to shunt placement. Lung retraction can severely impair oxygenation and ventilation, and intermittent reinflation might be required. Similar hypoxemia can occur during partial clamping or obstruction of the MPA during the construction of the anastomosis. This is usually managed with fluids, vasopressors, and ventilation adjustments to reduce PVR. For central shunts, partial clamping of the ascending aorta is required, sometimes poorly tolerated in the presence of LV dysfunction for which inotropic support with dopamine is helpful. Once the shunt is open, oxygen saturation often improves immediately. However, blood pressure can drop significantly due to diastolic runoff, requiring volume infusion and vasopressor support. If the diastolic pressure becomes very low, coronary flow can be reduced. Ventilation and inspired oxygen are adjusted to mimic spontaneous, nonanesthetized blood oxygen, and carbon dioxide levels for an accurate assessment of the shunt flow. An oxygen saturation of near 80–85% is optimal as this estimates balanced pulmonary and systemic blood flow. A high saturation suggests pulmonary overcirculation and the shunt size might have to be reduced. Conversely, a low saturation suggests inadequate PBF, and a larger diameter shunt might be needed. In cases of persistent hypoxemia after apparently uneventful shunt placement via a thoracotomy, it is important to rule out the possibility of endobronchial intubation because failure to do so might lead to unnecessary shunt revision or even sternotomy.

Postoperative care for surgical palliation

After chest closure, the patient is transferred to the cardiac ICU and kept on a ventilator for 12–24 hours. Increased PBF can cause the patient to become acutely unstable due to pulmonary edema or pulmonary hemorrhage (which can be unilateral). Diastolic hypotension can cause myocardial ischemia, requiring close monitoring and treatment. Other complications include injury to the phrenic and recurrent laryngeal nerves, Horner's syndrome, chylothorax, and shunt thrombosis. Briefly disconnecting the patient from the ventilator and auscultating the end of the endotracheal tube can clinically confirm patency of the shunt. The murmur is transmitted via the tracheal tube due to the proximity of the shunt to the bronchus. When it is determined that there is no excessive postsurgical bleeding, a low-dose heparin infusion is started (8–10 units/kg/h) to maintain shunt patency. After enteral intake has begun, patients are prescribed low-dose aspirin until the time of complete repair. Platelet transfusions are generally avoided for patients undergoing shunt placement due to the risk of shunt thrombosis.

Perioperative anesthetic management for surgical repair

There are additional considerations for complete repair using CPB. The anesthetic induction strategy is similar to that for shunt placement. Generally, we utilize a total fentanyl dose of 20–50 mcg/kg and administer inhalational agents to supplement anesthesia. The lower dose of fentanyl usually allows for extubation within 4–8 hours after surgery. A ketamine infusion has been shown to provide more hemodynamic stability by preserving SVR in the pre-CPB period when compared with isoflurane [52]. A TEE probe is placed if patient size permits. If TEE is not possible or unavailable, epicardial echocardiography can be performed post-CPB to assess repair. In addition to routine monitors, brain oxygen saturation trends can be followed with near-infrared spectroscopy. Other neurological monitoring modalities include electroencephalography and transcranial Doppler, and are discussed in Chapter 10.

During the rewarming phase of CPB, preparations are made for weaning from CPB. The following problems should be anticipated:

1 RV dysfunction might result, especially if the transannular incision was extended down along the RV free wall. The mainstays of treatment are fluid loading to higher filling pressures, inotropic support, and reduction of RV afterload. Dopamine at 5 mcg/kg/min is started when rewarming commences. Milrinone can also be added to help RV function and reduce PVR. Due to RV hypertrophy and diastolic dysfunction, high filling pressures might be needed to maintain CO. An RA and/or an LA pressure line might very useful in optimizing preload. Ventilation is adjusted to reduce PVR prior to weaning.

2 Arrhythmias and heart block are common after VSD repairs because of the close proximity of the conduction system. Epicardial pacing might be needed to accomplish weaning from CPB. In most instances, heart block is a transient phenomenon due to the edema around the VSD patch. If it does not resolve after 7–10 days, permanent pacing might be required. Junctional ectopic tachycardia occurs in approximately 10% of patients after surgery, and is an important cause of morbidity, mortality, and increased ICU stay. The usual onset is 12–24 hours after surgery, and is characterized by heart rates above 170/min and AV dissociation. The loss of AV synchrony can produce serious hemodynamic deterioration. Possible risk factors include long bypass times, high inotropic requirements, and surgery close to the AV node. Treatment consists of sedation, normalization of electrolytes, especially magnesium, cooling to 34–35°C, and intravenous amiodarone [53]. Overdrive pacing can also be used to reestablish AV synchrony.

3 Post-CPB bleeding is usually due to the extreme hemodilution and the effects of CPB on platelet function, and might require transfusion of multiple component blood products. The use of antifibrinolytics such as ε-aminocaproic acid or protease inhibitors such as aprotinin (withdrawn from the market by the manufacturer at the time of writing) can reduce post-CPB bleeding and minimize the use of blood products. See Chapter 12.

4 A residual VSD might be present. Due to the low resistance RVOT, this will place an excessive volume load on the LV, and will be poorly tolerated. A defect larger than 3 mm requires further hemodynamic evaluation by quantifying the shunt and measurement of left atrial pressure, to decide whether to return to CPB. Two-thirds of the defects less than 3 mm detected by intraoperative TEE are not detectable by the time of hospital discharge [54].

Other important complications include residual RVOT obstruction, which might require revision, and TI. Due to PI and high RV cavity pressure, the patient poorly tolerates TI.

Postoperative care for surgical repair

Once the chest is closed, the patient is transferred to the ICU. Analgesia is provided with a continuous infusion of morphine at 20–40 mcg/kg/h, supplemented with intermittent boluses of midazolam for sedation. Hemodynamically stable patients with minimal bleeding are good candidates for early extubation, usually within 4 hours. After the patient is extubated, analgesia can be reliably provided with a combination of acetaminophen and a nonsteroidal anti-inflammatory agent such as ibuprofen.

Pulmonary stenosis with intact ventricular septum

Anatomy

PS with intact ventricular septum (PA/IVS) is a relatively common malformation, accounting for 8–10% of congenital heart defects. PS can be valvular, subvalvular, or supravalvular. In valvular PS, the PV is dome-shaped with a centrally placed orifice. The RV is usually normal in dimension with the exception of the infundibular hypertrophy that occurs as a result of outflow obstruction. Valvular PS is frequently associated with Noonan's syndrome. Although isolated subvalvular PS is rare, obstruction can occur within the RV cavity due to abnormal hypertrophied muscle bands that run between the ventricular septum and the anterior wall, effectively dividing the RV cavity into a proximal high-pressure chamber and a distal low-pressure chamber ("double-chambered RV"). Supravalvular PS involving the MPA can be seen with congenital rubella and Williams' syndrome. There is often poststenotic dilation of the MPA and sometimes the LPA as well. The etiology of the defect is unknown, but there is likely a genetic factor as the incidence in the defect in siblings of the affected patient is 2–4%.

Pathophysiology and natural history

In its most severe manifestation, PS/IVS presents in the neonatal period with cyanosis and right heart failure. However, most children develop signs and symptoms more slowly, depending on the severity of the PS and the relative sizes of a PFO or ASD. Many patients are initially identified by the presence of a harsh systolic ejection murmur and perhaps a thrill over the PV auscultation area. There is often poststenotic dilation of the MPA and branch PAs that can be visible on chest roentgenogram. Radiographic cardiomegaly is a late sign, coincident with signs of failure. The ECG often shows right axis deviation, prominent P waves, and evidence of RV hypertrophy. Echocardiography with Doppler evaluation of the valve gradient can be used to measure the severity of the lesion; serial measurement is used for follow-up studies. Cardiac catheterization, in addition to its value in obtaining further measurements, can also be used to perform balloon valvuloplasty.

Surgical approach

Symptomatic patients and those with severe gradients and impending RV failure are treated primarily with balloon valvuloplasty, which has replaced surgery as the first line treatment. Balloon valvuloplasty can be used repeatedly for recurrent PV stenosis. The incidence of PI after balloon valvuloplasty is 80% but is usually mild in clinical severity. Surgical repair can be attempted with or without CPB via a median sternotomy approach. With the CPB-assisted technique, a transverse incision is made in the MPA. Fused valve leaflets are incised. The annulus can be enlarged with Hegar dilators. Subvalvular obstruction in the infundibular region can be excised. Rarely, a transannular patch might be needed. A right atriotomy is used to close a PFO or ASD and an infundibular resection through the TV if needed. Surgical pulmonary valvotomy can also be performed off CPB via a transventricular approach through a purse string suture in the anterior RV. Hegar dilators are inserted in increasing diameters across the valve. The CPB pump can be kept primed and on standby for this approach. With either surgical technique, residual valve gradients can be measured utilizing needle pressure transducers.

Perioperative anesthetic management

Ensuring effective inotropic therapy, ensuring adequate diuresis, and correcting metabolic acidosis and electrolyte abnormalities medically optimizes the patient with CHF prior to surgery. Neonates with critical PS should be stabilized with PGE_1 and taken for cardiac catheterization without delay. Most patients will be eligible for elective repair.

After CPB, the RV filling pressures must be adequate while avoiding high PA pressure to enhance forward right-sided CO. Pulmonary vasodilators begun in the early postoperative course or in the late CPB period might increase pulmonary flow and reduce RV afterload. Although most patients tolerate PI that results from either open or closed pulmonary valvotomy, inotropic support is often needed to assist the transient RV dysfunction that is frequently present after anterior right ventriculotomy with the closed approach. Inotropic support is used judiciously in patients that might have a dynamic subvalvular obstructive component due to infundibular hypertrophy, but might be needed to achieve adequate RV function for a few days after repair. Residual infundibular hypertrophy often resolves with time after the valvular obstruction is relieved.

Pulmonary atresia with intact ventricular septum

Anatomy

Unlike PS/IVS, PA/IVS does not have a familial association. The defect comprises approximately 1.0–1.5% of congenital heart defects. Although the etiology of the defect is unknown, the inciting event appears to be severe intrauterine RVOT obstruction, leading to maldevelopment of the TV, RV, and coronary arteries. The degree of abnormality varies with the gestational age at which the RVOT obstruction occurs. Patients with a diminutive RV, small TV, and extensive RV to coronary artery communications would be presumed to have incurred PA at an earlier stage of gestational development. Multiple morphologic abnormalities occur with this lesion, all of them proximal to the PV (in contrast to PA with VSD in which the major associated defects occur distal to the valve). There is almost always a PFO or secundum ASD, restrictive in 5–10%. The TV is usually smaller than normal, but can range from extremely stenotic to the dilated annulus of Ebstein's anomaly (5–10%). The RA is dilated proportionately to the degree of TI. The RV is hypertrophic with reduced size of the cavity.

In about 50% of cases, there are endothelial-lined blind channels within the RV myocardium known as sinusoids.

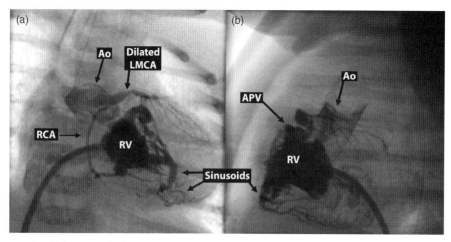

Figure 22.9 Pulmonary atresia with intact ventricular septum in a 1-day-old infant. A National Institutes of Health (NIH) catheter has been placed prograde into the right ventricle (RV) via a hypoplastic tricuspid valve for a contrast hand injection. There is mild tricuspid regurgitation. Numerous coronary sinusoids from the RV cavity to both right (RCA) and left coronary arteries are demonstrated. Contrast faintly opacifies the aorta (Ao) retrograde through a dilated left main coronary artery (LMCA). (a) Frontal view. (b) Lateral view. RV outflow tract ends at the atretic pulmonary valve (APV) (Courtesy of Eudice E. Fontenot, MD, University of Arkansas for Medical Sciences & Arkansas Children's Hospital, Little Rock, AR, USA)

These sinusoids are in direct communication with the RV cavity and can form coronary artery to RV fistulae. The prevalence of these sinusoids is inversely proportional to the diameter of the TV, RV cavity size, and magnitude of TI, but directly proportional to RV systolic pressure. In the least affected individuals, RV blood might be sent as part of a dual supply of blood to small areas of myocardium in tandem with normal aortocoronary flow. But approximately 20% of patients with PA/IVS have an absence of anterograde aortocoronary flow, a finding confirmed with either cardiac catheterization (Figure 22.9) or more recently, 64-slice computed tomography [55]. In these patients, the coronary bed is perfused with desaturated systemic venous blood directly from the RV and, therefore, the myocardium can be chronically ischemic. In the most affected, aortocoronary connections will be absent and solely an RV-dependent coronary circulation will supply the RV myocardium [56]. Sometimes the PV is seemingly intact, but with fused commissures. Most often, there is a fibrous tissue at the ventriculoarterial junction. The pulmonary arteries usually have normal branching and can be hypoplastic in about 6% of cases. There is almost always a PDA. The LA is enlarged and hypertrophic, sometimes exhibiting fibroelastosis. Subaortic stenosis might also be present due to bulging of the ventricular septum into the LV from RV hypertension [57].

Pathophysiology and natural history

Untreated, PA/IVS results in death in 50% of neonates, and in 85% of infants by 6 months of age. Fetuses with small, hypertrophied ventricles often survive to birth; those with dilated RVs and severe TI can die of fetal hydrops. In the presence of moderate to severe TI, RV pressure will remain low and sinusoids and coronary fistulae will not develop. Alternatively, if TI is mild or nil, the RV will hypertrophy and remain small, developing systolic hypertension. The increased flow across the foramen ovale in utero causes a volume overload of the left heart, resulting in neonatal LV hypertrophy and dilation, and potential aortic root dilation.

The affected newborn is dependent upon the PDA and is resuscitated with PGE$_1$. Generally, the left heart functions normally and CO is maintained with the presence of an adequate PDA. If there is LV hypertrophy from septal hypertrophy/LV outflow tract obstruction, there might be coronary fistulae and resulting myocardial ischemia. Effectively, the newborn manifests a single ventricle physiology. TI is common, partly because of the RVOT obstruction and, in approximately one-third of cases, due to structural abnormalities of the TV. Over 90% of patients will present with cyanosis and a ductal flow murmur within the first 3 postnatal days. The ECG reveals small RV forces and often a large P wave, indicative of RA enlargement. Chest roentgenogram often shows decreased to normal pulmonary vascular markings, depending on the amount of ductal flow. The cardiac silhouette is normal unless RA and RV enlargement occur due to severe TI. Echocardiography can define the RVOT, RV dimensions, the TV, and the PDA. RV pressure can be derived from Doppler measurement of the TI. Ventricular function can be assessed, but dependency of coronary blood flow cannot be determined solely with echocardiography. Cardiac catheterization is essential in all cases to define major stenoses and fistulae in the coronary anatomy. Balloon pulmonary vavluloplasty can be employed, but rarely serves to avoid subsequent surgical repair [58].

Surgical approach

In the early 1960s, palliative shunts and closed pulmonary valvotomies were done. However, survival was dismal given that an estimated 2.5% of patients survived to 3 years of age. RV outflow procedures were combined with systemic artery-to-PA shunts in the 1970s. Since that time, repair techniques have varied among surgeons, partly based on the spectrum of anatomic dysmorphology and partly on the individual surgical outcome experiences. Current corrective procedures include (i) neonatal RVOT patch augmentation with continued infusion of PGE_1 (average of 6 days), (ii) neonatal RVOT patch augmentation with concurrent systemic artery-to-PA shunt, and (iii) pulmonary valvotomy (open or closed) and a systemic artery-to-PA shunt. Success rates in achieving ultimate biventricular repair have varied from 40–60%. However, all congenital heart surgeons avoid RV decompression if there is a complete dependency of myocardial blood supply on the RV. In such cases, initial palliation usually consists only of placing a systemic artery-to-PA shunt. Some surgeons have maintained RV-dependent coronary perfusion during CPB by pressurizing the RV with a second arterial cannula via the RA with bicaval venous cannulation [59]. Different surgeons manage patients with partial RV dependency for myocardial blood supply variably, but regional LV wall motion abnormalities can worsen after RV decompression [57].

The major determinants of the most appropriate surgical approach for a particular patient are (i) the degree of RV and TV hypoplasia, (ii) presence of RV-dependent coronary circulation, and (iii) the degree of TI. The surgical options include (i) complete biventricular repair with later closure of the interatrial communication, (ii) biventricular repair with allowable mixing of blood at the atrial level (ASD/PFO left open, or surgically adjustable ASD [60]), but using the RV to pump blood to the lungs, (iii) one-and-a-half-ventricular repair using a cavopulmonary anastomosis to reduce RV load, (iv) ultimate modified Fontan procedure, and (v) cardiac transplantation (last resort) [57,61].

Reddy and Hanley [57] outline the goals of initial surgical therapy as (i) minimize mortality, (ii) promote growth of the RV such that chances are improved for a later two-ventricular repair, and (iii) minimize the need for non-definitive later surgeries. They point out that (i) survival after systemic artery-to-PA shunt is at least as successful as any other initial surgical procedure, (ii) the RV will not grow if it is not decompressed and RVOT relief will be needed if two-ventricular repair is thought to be possi-

ble later, and (iii) the ultimate functional potential of the RV is often unclear in the neonate with PA/IVS. The initial procedure often determines the final repair/palliation outcome (Figure 22.10).

Perioperative anesthetic management

Given the variety of surgical options available for this particular lesion, general considerations are outlined. For any patient with a small hypertrophic, hypertensive RV, RV filling pressures must be maintained such that the RV cavity does not collapse, causing it to be an ineffective pump. This is especially important after RV outflow obstruction is relieved with the biventricular repair. Inotropic RV support is often essential as RV dysfunction is present after CPB in the presence of increased afterload of an unadjusted pulmonary vascular circulation. Minimizing ventilation pressures and vasodilating the pulmonary vasculature with drugs such as milrinone or dobutamine might reduce RV afterload. With severe pulmonary hypertension, nitric oxide is useful in the immediate postrepair period to aid in pulmonary vasodilation until the vascular bed adjusts to the increased flow. Also, pulmonary edema causes oxygenation difficulties and bronchospasm after the acute increase in pulmonary flow. The one-and-a-half-ventricular repair requires a balance of adequate preload to a partially unloaded RV and maintenance of low PVR for upper body passive venous return to the pulmonary vasculature. Along with the ventilation and pharmacological maneuvers, positioning patients with the head up 30° will aid in augmenting upper body venous return to the pulmonary vascular bed. When RV function becomes adequate to support work of breathing, spontaneous respiration in an extubated patient will generate a relative negative intrathoracic pressure that aids in increasing PBF.

With palliative aortopulmonary shunt placement, consideration is given to continued balance of pulmonary and systemic parallel circulations. Low CO in the postoperative period might occur secondary to unrecognized RV-dependent coronary circulation or from a "circular shunt." The latter occurs in patients who have had a transannular patch and a systemic artery-to-PA shunt. Because the transannular patch produces free PI, blood ejected from the LV flows through the systemic artery-to-PA shunt and enters the RV in a retrograde fashion. If there is significant TI, blood flows back into the RA and then into the LA through the interatrial communication (Figure 22.6). This flow effectively "steals" blood from the systemic circuit and might lead to hypoperfusion of the distal organs and metabolic acidosis. Conservative measures such as raising the PVR and reducing the SVR might be helpful, but often surgery is needed to revise the shunt and treat TI.

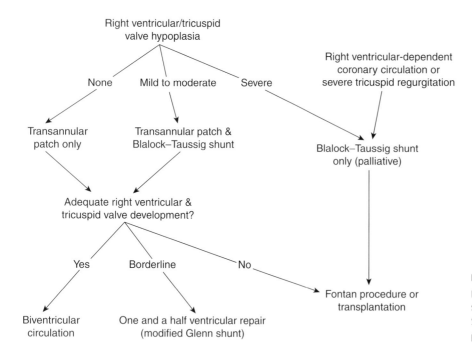

Figure 22.10 Consensus approach to pulmonary atresia with intact ventricular septum as described by the Congenital Heart Surgeons' Society (CHSS) (Reproduced with permission from Reference [62])

Sedation with benzodiazepines and pain control with opioid infusions such as morphine are balanced with the patient's condition, the anticipated duration of mechanical ventilation, and time needed for pulmonary vascular adjustment/RV recovery.

Pulmonary atresia/ventriculoseptal defect/multiple aortopulmonary collateral arteries

Anatomy

In its simplest form, with normal pulmonary vasculature, this lesion can be considered an extreme variation of TOF. However in most cases, there is great morphologic variability regarding PA architecture and sources of PBF, posing major challenges for corrective surgery. With PA, there is no continuity between the RV and the pulmonary trunk. The VSD is usually large and malaligned. The PAs can be normal in size or have varying degrees of hypoplasia to even complete absence. The LPA and RPA can be confluent or nonconfluent. An additional major source of PBF is derived from multiple collateral arteries arising from the aorta or its major branches. A given lung segment can be supplied solely from the true PAs, solely from the aortopulmonary collaterals, or from both. A classification system has been proposed, based on the morphology of the PAs and MAPCAs, which can be useful in surgical decision making (Figure 22.11).

Pathophysiology and natural history

The great variability in the sources of PBF determines the natural history and management options of this lesion. Excessive PBF through the collateral arteries will produce pulmonary congestion and a clinical picture of CHF. Moderate stenoses of the collateral arteries can result in a balanced PBF with arterial saturation around 80% and minimal symptoms. Severe stenoses of the collateral arteries or a ductal-dependent circulation will lead to inadequate PBF, cyanosis, and hypoxemia. Patients with a balanced blood flow can even survive to adulthood with minimal symptoms, but eventually LV failure will ensue from chronic left-to-right shunting and volume overload.

Although the diagnosis of PA/VSD/MAPCAs can be made with echocardiography, virtually all patients require cardiac catheterization to delineate the true PA architecture and collateral artery anatomy in order to plan the optimal surgical approach. Magnetic resonance angiography with three-dimensional reconstruction of the images is also becoming increasingly useful in delineating the complex anatomy [64] (Figure 22.12).

Surgical approach

Based on the different morphological subgroups, a clinical decision-making algorithm is a useful way to summarize the management of this complex condition (Figure 22.13). The ultimate goal of surgery is to achieve a biventricular repair by (i) constructing a pulmonary vascular bed from the different sources of PBF, capable of receiving the

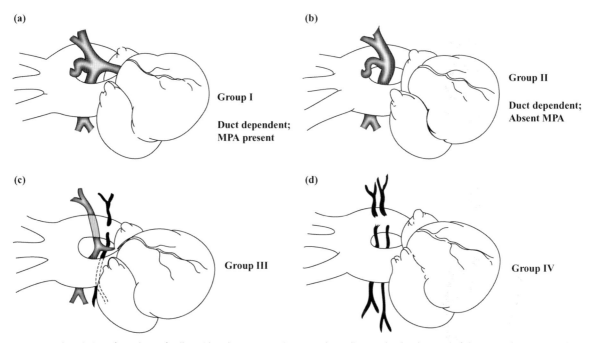

Figure 22.11 Much variation of tetralogy of Fallot with pulmonary atresia occurs depending on the development of the true pulmonary arteries and aortopulmonary collateral arteries. (a) Group I: simple valvar or infundibular atresia. (b) Group II: absence of the main pulmonary artery although there is continuity of the branch pulmonary arteries. Pulmonary artery blood flow is duct dependent. (c) Group III: hypoplastic true pulmonary arteries with multiple aortopulmonary collateral arteries. (d) Group IV: true pulmonary arteries are absent and all pulmonary blood supply is from multiple aortopulmonary collateral arteries (Reproduced with permission from Reference [63])

entire RV output without imposing too a high ventricular afterload, (ii) restoring continuity between the RV and the reconstructed pulmonary vascular bed, and (iii) closing the VSD. It might not be possible to achieve all these goals in all patients. An inadequate pulmonary vascular bed will eventually cause RV failure due to chronic increased afterload: an important factor for a successful outcome is the postrepair RV pressure, which should optimally be 50% or less than systemic pressure. Therefore, in patients with hypoplastic native PAs, the initial surgical priority is establishing increased blood flow through these arteries to promote their growth. This is achieved either by an RV–PA conduit, or an aortopulmonary shunt (variously described as a central shunt, Melbourne shunt [66], or aortopulmonary window [67]). The pulmonary vascular bed is then reconstructed by a procedure known as "unifocalization" in which as many of the aortopulmonary collateral arteries as possible are detached from the aorta and anastomosed to the central pulmonary arterial tree to provide a vascular bed for unobstructed blood flow from the RV (Figure 22.14). This centralization of multiple sources of PBF can be done in a single-stage midline approach (including VSD closure, if feasible) or as a multistage procedure involving sequential bilateral thoracotomies, followed by a definitive intracardiac repair through a median sternotomy. However, some centers are obtaining good results with a single-stage unifocalization and repair, and this approach does have many advantages [29]. It avoids subjecting the patient to multiple surgeries, which, if performed via thoracotomies, can make subsequent procedures extremely hazardous (especially lung transplants) due to increased adhesions and the potential for massive bleeding. Additionally, serious neurological injury can occur during CPB-assisted unifocalization because increased runoff into the pulmonary circuit can result in cerebral hypoperfusion despite apparently adequate pump flows. Obviously, a single-stage approach will not be applicable in all patients, and this group will need a systemic artery-to-PA shunt or a conduit from the RV to the PA to allow growth before definitive repair. Reddy *et al.* [30], in their series of 85 patients, were able to complete one-stage unifocalization and intracardiac repair in 56 patients. In 23 patients, single-stage unifocalization was done, but the VSD was left open. Six patients required staged unifocalization through sequential thoracotomies. There were six early and seven late deaths.

Perioperative anesthetic management

The anesthetic management will vary according to whether a staged approach to unifocalization via

(a)   (b)

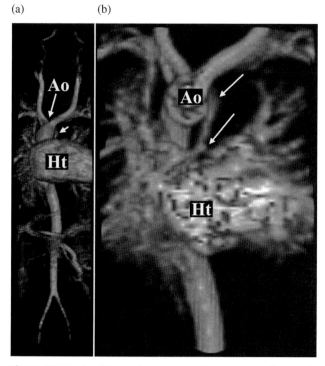

Figure 22.12 Gadolinium-enhanced magnetic resonance angiogram of a 3-day-old, 2.5-kg infant with tetralogy of Fallot, pulmonary atresia, and multiple aortopulmonary collateral arteries. (a) Anterior–posterior view demonstrating a right aortic arch (Ao) and no visible pulmonary artery originating from the heart (Ht). *Short arrow* shows a large collateral artery originating from the left side of the aortic arch. (b) Same view, but with ascending aorta removed. *Upper arrow* shows same large collateral artery descending to supply tiny branch pulmonary arteries (*lower arrow*) (Courtesy of S. Bruce Greenberg, MD, University of Arkansas for Medical Sciences & Arkansas Children's Hospital, Little Rock, AR, USA).

thoracotomy or one-stage unifocalization with intracardiac repair is being contemplated. The general principles for induction, maintenance, and monitoring are similar to those described above for TOF repair. There are several major anesthetic challenges for unifocalization via a thoracotomy including difficulties with oxygenation and ventilation from one-lung anesthesia, hemodynamic instability, bleeding, and metabolic acidosis [68]. In the older child, lung separation with either a double-lumen tube or a bronchial blocker will greatly facilitate surgical exposure and minimize lung contusion from surgical retraction (see Chapter 18). Extensive intrapulmonary and major airway bleeding from multiple vascular anastomoses will also compromise ventilation. Major blood loss should be anticipated, and large-bore intravenous access is essential. Warming of fluids before transfusion will reduce the chance of hypothermia.

Finally, thoracotomies are extremely painful, and a thoracic epidural will provide excellent postoperative anal-

gesia. However, the benefits of epidural anesthesia need to be balanced against the potential risk of neurological damage from catheter placement in an anesthetized child. Other alternatives include (i) local anesthetic infusion via a cutaneous multiorifice catheter either aligned within the wound or placed percutaneously. For the percutaneous approach, the catheter is inserted through an intercostal space caudal to the chest tube site and thoracotomy incision and into the extradural space; or (ii) multiple intercostal single injection rib blocks (see Chapter 19).

One-stage unifocalization (with or without definitive repair) is carried out via a median sternotomy or bilateral transsternal thoracotomy ("clamshell" incision). As many MAPCAs as possible are mobilized, ligated, and unifocalized without CPB. As each MAPCA is ligated, the arterial saturation will decrease because a proportion of the PBF is being eliminated. At the point at which the patient nears compromise from arterial desaturation (70–75%), CPB (with moderate hypothermia and a beating heart) is initiated and the rest of the unifocalization is completed. As mentioned above, it is vital to control as many of the MAPCAs as possible prior to initiating CPB to prevent cerebral hypoperfusion due to increased runoff into the pulmonary circulation. After placement of a valved conduit between the RV and the MPA to restore continuity, the feasibility of VSD closure is then assessed. This is a critical step because if the VSD is closed, and the "new" pulmonary vascular bed is inadequate to receive all of the CO, RV failure will rapidly ensue. One approach is to perform an intraoperative pulmonary flow study to estimate the resistance of the new vascular bed [69]. This is accomplished by perfusing the lungs with the equivalent of one CO, and if the mean PA pressure is less than 30 mm Hg, the VSD is closed. If the RV pressure is unacceptably high after VSD closure, a fenestration can be created in the VSD that can be closed later with a catheter-delivered device.

Several major problems can be anticipated post-CPB:

1 RV dysfunction can result and is usually secondary to increased afterload due to an inadequate pulmonary vascular bed. The mainstays of therapy are optimization of preload, inotropic support with and manipulation of ventilation to lower PVR (see Chapter 18). Inhaled nitric oxide might also be helpful as a pulmonary vasodilator in this setting.

2 Intrapulmonary bleeding due to multiple vascular suture lines, systemic anticoagulation, and the effects of CPB can occur.

3 Lung reperfusion injury due to increased blood flow to many previously underperfused lung segments can manifest as pulmonary edema, bronchospasm, and difficulties with ventilation and oxygenation. Frequent endotracheal suctioning, fiberoptic bronchoscopy,

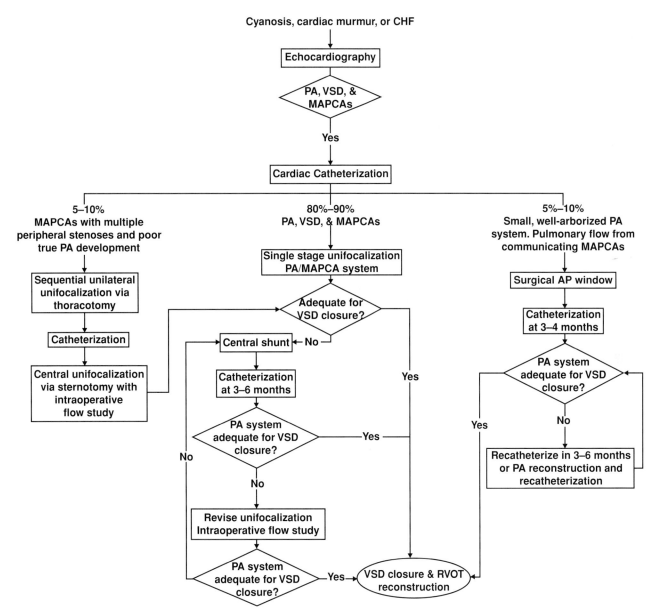

Figure 22.13 Algorithm for decision making for patients with pulmonary atresia (PA), a ventriculoseptal defect (VSD), and multiple aortopulmonary collateral arteries (MAPCAs). CHF, congestive heart failure; AP, aortopulmonary; RVOT, right ventricular outflow tract (Reproduced with permission from Reference [65])

bronchodilators, and PEEP will be helpful in managing this problem. In general, these patients are not good candidates for early extubation.

4 Bleeding from multiple suture lines is often substantial will require appropriate blood component therapy.

Postoperatively, these patients will benefit from sedation with benzodiazepines and aggressive pain control to minimize systemic and pulmonary hypertension.

Summary

Right-sided obstructive congenital heart lesions present in many different ways. Depending upon the severity of the structural anomalies, patients can present in widely divergent patterns, from the ductal-dependent, cyanotic neonate in CHF to the minimally affected young adult with mild to moderate exercise tolerance. All right-sided

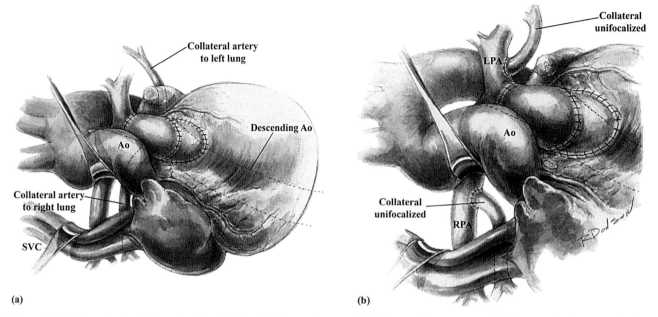

(a)　　　　　　　　　　　　　　　　　(b)

Figure 22.14 View of unifocalization of collateral arteries to the true pulmonary arteries via a median sternotomy. (a) As the aorta (Ao) is retracted to the left, a collateral artery to the right lung is seen posterior to the transverse sinus. (b) One collateral artery has been unifocalized to the true right pulmonary artery (RPA) and another collateral artery has been unifocalized to the left pulmonary artery (LPA) (Reproduced with permission from Reference [63])

obstructive CHD is characterized by the nearly universal presence of a septal defect that has the potential for right-to-left intracardiac shunt. An understanding of the physiology of the defect and effects of the proposed surgical intervention as well as the potential complications are essential for the meticulous and well-planned perioperative anesthetic management of such patients.

Key points

Ebstein's anomaly

1 Patients with extreme cardiomegaly or perioperative ventricular arrhythmias should receive prophylactic antiarrhythmic treatment, such as amiodarone.
2 Patients with poorly functioning RVs might be dependent upon high filling pressures to maintain adequate CO.

Tetralogy of Fallot

1 Hypercyanotic spells are treated with oxygen, phenylephrine, intravenous fluid, and esmolol.
2 During BT shunt placement, difficulties might be encountered with oxygenation and ventilation, and later hypotension after the shunt is open.
3 Postoperative ventilation is recommended for 12–24 hours after BT shunt placement because of the risk of pulmonary edema.

4 A thoracic epidural catheter via the caudal route provides excellent analgesia after thoracotomy.
5 Following complete repair, RV dysfunction, heart block, arrhythmias, and bleeding should be anticipated.

PS or atresia with intact ventricular septum, and PA with ventricular septal defects and major aortopulmonary collaterals

1 Inotropes are used cautiously with patients with PS/IVS when there is a component of dynamic infundibular stenosis such that outflow obstruction is not worsened.
2 Small hypertrophic RVs require meticulous attention to preload to maintain function.
3 An RV-dependent coronary circulation requires maintenance of RV intracavitary pressure to prevent myocardial ischemia.
4 After repair of PA/IVS and PA/VSD, severe RV dysfunction is often present due to the high afterload of an insufficient pulmonary vasculature: inotropic support, mechanical ventilation adjustment to minimize airway pressures, and pulmonary vasodilators are helpful.
5 Enhanced postrepair lung perfusion might result in pulmonary edema, intrapulmonary bleeding, bronchospasm, and difficulties with oxygenation.
6 Antifibrinolytic agents might be useful for minimizing bleeding after unifocalization of MAPCAs.

References

1. Schiebler GL, Gravenstein JS, Van Mierop JL (1968) Ebstein's anomaly of the tricuspid valve. Translation of the original description with comments. Am J Cardiol 22:867–873.
2. Perloff JK (2003) Ebstein's anomaly of the tricuspid valve. In: Perloff JK (ed.) The Clinical Recognition of Congenital Heart Disease, 5th edn. Saunders, Philadelphia, pp. 194–215.
3. Carpentier A (1993) Malformations of the tricuspid valve and Ebstein's anomaly. In: Stark J, de Leval M (eds) Surgery for Congenital Heart Defects, 2nd edn. Saunders, Philadelphia, pp. 615–622.
4. Schreiber C, Cook A, Ho SY et al. (1999) Morphologic spectrum of Ebstein's malformation: revisitation relative to surgical repair. J Thorac Cardiovasc Surg 117:148–155.
5. Dearani JA, O'Leary PW, Danielson GK (2006) Surgical treatment of Ebstein's malformation: state of the art 2006. Cardiol Young 16(Suppl 3):12–20.
6. Anderson KR, Zuberbuhler JR, Anderson RH, et al. (1979) Morphologic spectrum of Ebstein's anomaly of the heart: a review. Mayo Clin Proc 54:174–180.
7. Celermajer DS, Dodd SM, Greenwald SE, et al. (1992) Morbid anatomy in neonates with Ebstein's anomaly of the tricuspid valve: pathophysiologic and clinical implications. J Am coll Cardiol 19:1049–1053.
8. Jaquiss RDB, Imamura M (2007) Management of Ebstein's anomaly and pure tricuspid insufficiency in the neonate. Thorac Cardiovasc Surg 19:258–263.
9. Paranon S, Acar P (2008) Ebstein's anomaly of the tricuspid valve: from fetus to adult. Heart 94:237–243.
10. Danielson GK (1994) Ebstein's anomaly of the tricuspid valve. In: Mavrouidis C, Backer CL (eds) Pediatric Cardiac Surgery. Mosby, Philadelphia, pp. 413–424.
11. Da Silva JP, Baumgratz JF, da Fonseca L, et al. (2007) The cone reconstruction of the tricuspid valve in Ebstein's anomaly. The operation: early and midterm results. J Thorac Cardiovasc Surg 133:215–223.
12. Chauvaud SM, Brancaccio G, Carpentier AF (2001) Cardiac arrhythmia in patients undergoing surgical repair of Ebstein's anomaly. Ann Thorac Surg 71:1547–1552.
13. Chauvaud S (2000) Ebstein's malformation. Surgical treatment and results. Thorac Cardiovasc Surg 48:200–203.
14. Boston US, Dearani JA, O'Leary PW, et al. (2006) Tricuspid valve repair for Ebstein's anomaly in young children: a 30-year experience. Ann Thorac Surg 81:690–696.
15. Knott-Craig CJ, Goldberg SP, Overholt ED, et al. (2007) Repair of neonates and young infants with Ebstein's anomaly and related pathology. Ann Thorac Surg 84:587–592.
16. Starnes VA, Pitlick PT, Bernstein D, et al. (1991) Ebstein's anomaly appearing in the neonate. A new surgical approach. J Thorac Cardiovasc Surg 101:1082–1087.
17. Sano S, Ishino K, Kawada M, et al. (2002) Total right ventricular exclusion procedure: an operation for isolated congestive right heart failure. J Thorac Cardiovasc Surg 123:640–647.
18. Reemsten BL, Fagan BT, Wells WJ, et al. (2006) Current surgical therapy for Ebstein anomaly in neonates. J Thorac Cardiovasc Surg 132:1285–1290.
19. Marcelletti CF, Iorio FS (1998) Workshop on "one and one-half" ventricular repairs. Ann Thorac Surg 66:615.
20. Van Arsdell GS, Williams WG, Maser CM, et al. (1996) Superior vena cava to pulmonary artery anastomosis: an adjunct to biventricular repair. J Thorac Cardiovasc Surg 112:1143–1149.
21. Van Arsdell GS, Williams WG, Freedom RM, et al. (1998) A practical approach to $1\frac{1}{2}$ ventricle repairs. Ann Thorac Surg 66:678–680.
22. Quinonez LG, Dearani JA, Puga FJ, et al. (2007) Results of the 1.5-ventricle repair for Ebstein anomaly and the failing right ventricle. J Thorac Cardiovasc Surg 133:1303–1310.
23. Hanouz JL, Zhu L, Lemoine S, et al. (2007) Reactive oxygen species mediate sevoflurane- and desflurane-induced preconditioning in isolated human right atria *in vitro*. Anesth Analg 105:1534–1539.
24. Chiari PC, Bienengraeber MW, Weihrauch D, et al. (2005) Role of endothelial nitric oxide synthase as a trigger and mediator of isoflurane-induced delayed preconditioning in rabbit myocardium. Anesthesiology 103:74–83.
25. Wang L, Traystman RJ, Murphy SJ (2008) Inhalational anesthetics as preconditioning agents in ischemic brain. Curr Opin Pharmacol 8:104–110.
26. Sang H, Cao L, Qiu P, et al. (2006) Isoflurane produces delayed preconditioning against spinal cord ischemic injury via release of free radicals in rabbits. Anesthesiology 105:953–960.
27. Pierard LA, Henrad L, Demoulin JC (1985) Persistent atrial standstill in familial Ebstein's anomaly. Br Heart J 54:594–597.
28. Need LR, Powell AJ, del Nido PJ, Geva T (2000) Coronary echocardiography in tetralogy of Fallot: diagnostic accuracy, resource utilization and surgical implications over 13 years. J Am Coll Cardiol 36:1371–1377.
29. Reddy VM, Liddicoat JR, Hanley FL (1995) Midline one-stage complete unifocalization and repair of pulmonary atresia with ventricular septal defect and major aortopulmonary collaterals. J Thorac Cardiovasc Surg 109:832–844; discussion 844–845.
30. Reddy VM, McElhinney DB, Amin Z, et al. (2000) Early and intermediate outcomes after repair of pulmonary atresia with ventricular septal defect and major aortopulmonary collateral arteries: experience with 85 patients. Circulation 101:1826–1832.
31. Maeda J, Yamagishi H, Matsuoka R, et al. (2000) Frequent association of 22q11.2 deletion with tetralogy of Fallot. Am J Med Genet 92:269–272.
32. Murphy JG, Gersh BJ, Mair DD, et al. (1993) Long-term outcome in patients undergoing surgical repair of tetralogy of Fallot. N Engl J Med 329:593–599.
33. Arab SM, Kholeif AF, Zaher SR, et al. (1999) Balloon dilation of the right ventricular outflow tract in tetralogy of Fallot: a palliative procedure. Cardiol Young 9:11–16.
34. Kohli V, Azad S, Sachdev MS, et al. (2008) Balloon dilation of the pulmonary valve in premature infants with tetralogy of Fallot. Pediatr Cardiol 29:946–949.
35. Van Arsdell GS, Maharaj GS, Tom J, et al. (2000) What is the optimal age for repair of tetralogy of Fallot? Circulation 1029(Suppl III):123–129.

36. Dodge-Khatami A, Tulevski II, Hitchcock JF, et al. (2001) Neonatal complete correction of tetralogy of Fallot versus shunting and deferred repair: Is the future of the right ventriculo-arterial junction at stake, and what of it? Cardiol Young 11:484–490.

37. Hirsch JC, Mosca RS, Bove EL (2000) Complete repair of tetralogy of Fallot in the neonate: results in the modern era. Ann Surg 232:508–514.

38. Pigula FA, Khalil PN, Mayer JE, et al. (1999) Repair of tetralogy of Fallot in neonates and young infants. Circulation 100(Suppl II):157–161.

39. Reddy VM, Liddicoat JR, McElhinney DB, et al. (1995) Routine primary repair of tetralogy of Fallot in neonates and infants less than three months of age. Ann Thorac Surg 60:S592–S596.

40. Caspi J, Zalstein E, Zucker N, et al. (1999) Surgical management of tetralogy of Fallot in the first year of life. Ann Thorac Surg 68:1344–1349.

41. Fraser CD, McKenzie DE, Cooley DA (2001) Tetralogy of Fallot: surgical management individualized to the patient. Ann Thorac Surg 71:1556–1563.

42. Gladman G, McCrindle BW, Williams WG, et al. (1997) The modified Blalock–Taussig shunt: clinical impact and morbidity in Fallot's tetralogy in the current era. J Thorac Cardiovasc Surg 114:25–30.

43. Jonas RA (2004) Tetralogy of Fallot with pulmonary stenosis. In: Jonas RA (ed.) Comprehensive Surgical Management of Congenital Heart Disease. Arnold, London, pp. 279–300.

44. Stellin G, Milanesi O, Rubino M, et al. (1995) Repair of tetralogy of Fallot in the first six months of life: transatrial versus transventricular approach. Ann Thorac Surg 60:S588–S591.

45. Xu J, Shiota T, Ge S, et al. (1996) Intraoperative transesophageal echocardiography using high-resolution biplane 7.5 MHz probes with continuous-wave Doppler capability in infants and children with tetralogy of Fallot. Am J Cardiol 77:539–542.

46. Joyce JJ, Hwang EY, Wiles HB, et al. (2000) Reliability of intraoperative transesophageal echocardiography during tetralogy of Fallot repair. Echocardiography 17:319–327.

47. Kaushal SK, Radhakrishnans, Dagar KS, et al. (1999) Significant intraoperative right ventricular outflow tract gradients after repair for tetralogy of Fallot: to revise or not to revise? Ann Thorac Surg 68:1705–1713.

48. Geva T (2006) Indications and timing of pulmonary valve replacement after tetralogy of Fallot repair. Semin Thorac Cardiovasc Surg Pediatr Card Surg Ann 9:11–22.

49. Knauth AL, Gauvreau AJ, Powell AJ, et al. (2008) Ventricular size and function assessed by cardiac MRI predict major adverse clinical outcomes late after tetralogy of Fallot repair. Heart 94:211–216.

50. Khambadkone S, Bonhoeffer P (2006) Percutaneous pulmonary valve implantation. Semin Thorac Cardiovasc Surg Pediatr Card Surg Ann 9:23–28.

51. Rivenes SM, Lewin MB, Stayer SA, et al. (2001) Cardiovascular effects of sevoflurane, isoflurane, halothane, and fentanyl-midazolam in children with congenital heart disease: an echocardiographic study of myocardial contractility and hemodynamics. Anesthesiology 94:223–229.

52. Tugrul M, Camci E, Pembeci K, et al. (2000) Ketamine infusion versus isoflurane for the maintenance of anesthesia in the prebypass period in children with tetralogy of Fallot. J Cardiothorac Vasc Anesth 14:557–61.

53. Andreasen JB, Johnsen SP, Ravn HB (2008) Junctional ectopic tachycardia after surgery for congenital heart disease in children. Intensive Care Med 34:895–902.

54. Yang S, Novello R, Nicolson S, et al. (2000) Evaluation of ventricular septal defect repair using intraoperative transesophageal echocardiography: frequency and significance of residual defects in infants and children. Echocardiography 17:681–684.

55. Saltik L, Bayrak F, Guneysu T, et al. (2008) Right ventricle-dependent coronary circulation demonstrated with 64-slice computed tomography. Eur Heart J 29:1018.

56. Eisses MJ, Jimenez N, Permut L, et al. (2008) Absent aortocoronary connections in a neonate with pulmonary atresia and an intact ventricular septum. J Cardiothorac Vasc Anesth 22:98–101.

57. Reddy VM, Hanley FL (1996) Pulmonary atresia with intact ventricular septum: early palliation, subsequent management, and possible role of fetal surgical intervention. In: Baue AE, Geha AS, Hammond GL, Laks H, Naunheim KS (eds) Glenn's Thoracic and Cardiovascular Surgery. Appleton & Lange, Stamford, pp. 1315–1332.

58. Hirata Y, Chen JM, Quaegebeur JM, et al. (2007) Pulmonary atresia with intact ventricular septum: limitations of catheter-based intervention. Ann Thorac Surg 84:574–580.

59. Kawaraguchi Y, Taniguchi A, Otomo T, et al. (2006) Anesthetic management of bidirectional cavopulmonary shunt in a patient with pulmonary atresia with intact ventricular septum associated with sinusoidal communications. J Anesth 20:220–222.

60. Laks H, Pearl JM, Drinkwater DC, et al. (1992) Partial biventricular repair of pulmonary atresia with intact ventricular septum. Use of an adjustable atrial septal defect. Circulation 86:II59–II66.

61. Takayama H, Sekiguchi A, Chikada M (1995) Pulmonary atresia with intact ventricular septum: long-term results of "one and a half ventricular repair." Updated in 2001. Ann Thorac Surg 72:2178–2179.

62. Yuh DD, Reitz BA (2002) Consensus approach to pulmonary atresia with intact ventricular septum as described by the Congenital Heart Surgeons' Society (CHSS). In: Yuh DD, Reitz BA (eds) Congenital Cardiac Surgery. McGraw-Hill, Inc., New York, p. 99.

63. Jonas RA (2004) Tetralogy of Fallot with pulmonary atresia. In: Jonas RA (ed.) Comprehensive Surgical Management of Congenital Heart Disease. Arnold, London, pp. 441–451.

64. Geva T, Greil GF, Marshall AC, et al. (2002) Gadolinium enhanced three-dimensional magnetic resonance angiography of pulmonary blood supply in patients with complex pulmonary stenosis or atresia: comparison with x-ray angiography. Circulation 106:473–478.

65. MacDonald MJ, Hanley FL (2007) Pulmonary atresia with ventricular septal defect and major aortopulmonary collaterals. In: Yuh DD, Vricella LA, Baumgartner WA (eds) The

Johns Hopkins Manual of Cardiothoracic Surgery. McGraw-Hill Medical, New York, p. 1143.

66. Duncan BW, Mee RBB, Prieto LR, et al. (2003) Staged repair of tetralogy of Fallot with pulmonary atresia and major aortopulmonary collateral arteries. J Thorac Cardiovasc Surg 126:694–702.

67. Rodefeld MD, Reddy VM, Thompson LD, et al. (2002) Surgical creation of aortopulmonary window in selected patients with pulmonary atresia with poorly developed aortopulmonary collaterals and hypoplastic pulmonary arteries. J Thorac Cardiovasc Surg 123:1147–1154.

68. Hayashi Y, Takaki O, Uchida O, et al. (1993) Anesthetic management of patients undergoing bilateral unifocalization. Anesth Analg 76:755–759.

69. Reddy VM, Petrossian E, McElhinney DB, et al. (1997) One stage unifocalization in infants: When should the ventricular septal defect be closed? J Thorac Cardiovasc Surg 113:858–866.

23 Anesthesia for transposition of the great vessels

Kathryn Rouine-Rapp, M.D.

Moffitt-Ling Hospitals, University of California, San Francisco, California, USA

Introduction

Transposition of the great arteries (TGA) is found in about 5% of patients with congenital heart disease and is thought to be an alteration in conotruncal development of the heart [1,2]. Nomenclature for this defect has been discussed by several groups and exists as an international pediatric and congenital cardiac code, but its use is inconsistent [3]. This chapter uses nomenclature established by members of the Society of Thoracic Surgeons and the European Association for Cardiothoracic Surgery [4]. Three general categories of TGA are described: TGA with intact ventricular septum (IVS), TGA with ventricular septal defect (VSD), and TGA with VSD and left-ventricular outflow tract obstruction (LVOTO). In this chapter, TGA refers to a physiologically uncorrected defect. Another defect, congenitally corrected transposition of the great arteries (ccTGA), is discussed separately using the nomenclature established by the aforementioned groups.

D-Transposition of the great arteries

Anatomy

In TGA, also termed *transposition of the great vessels*, the distinguishing feature is an abnormal connection between the ventricles and great vessels known as discordant ventriculoarterial connections, or VA discordance. The atria most commonly are normal in orientation and connections between the atria and ventricles also are normal (atrioventricular or AV concordance). In the presence of VA discordance, the aorta arises from the morphologic right ventricle (RV) and the pulmonary artery (PA) arises from the morphologic left ventricle (LV).

In the normal heart, the position of the aorta is posterior and to the right of the pulmonary trunk. There is a subpulmonary muscular infundibulum and the annulus of the aortic valve is in fibrous continuity with the mitral valve annulus [5]. In TGA, the aorta most often is

Anesthesia for Congenital Heart Disease 2nd edition. Edited by
Dean Andropoulos, Stephen Stayer, Isobel Russell and Emad Mossad.
© 2010 Blackwell Publishing.

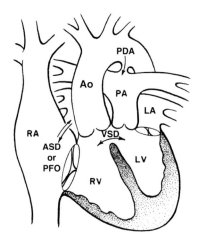

Figure 23.1 Basic anatomy and sites of mixing between the systemic and pulmonary circulation in transposition of the great arteries. Ao, Aorta; ASD, atrial septal detect; LA, left atrium; LV, left ventricle; PA, pulmonary artery; PDA, patent ductus arteriosus; PFO, patent foramen ovale; RA, right atrium; RV, right ventricle (Reproduced with permission from Reference [8])

anterior and to the right of the pulmonary trunk. There is a subaortic muscular infundibulum in most patients and the pulmonary valve is in fibrous continuity with the mitral valve [6, 7] (Figure 23.1). Typical anatomic characteristics in TGA include normal intracardiac attachments of the tricuspid and mitral valves and a PA diameter that equals or often exceeds that of the aorta.

Other terms are used to define TGA and include d-TGA and complete transposition. The term d-TGA commonly is used to define the aorta as anterior and to the right of the pulmonary trunk. This term is misleading because four additional aortic positions have been described and the letter "d" refers to cardiac loop formation that occurs during development of the heart [2,7].

Transposition of the great arteries with intact ventricular septum

Up to 85% of patients with TGA are in the category of TGA with IVS. Additional findings include a persistent patent foramen ovale (PFO) and in 50% of patients, a persistent patent ductus arteriosus (PDA) [4,9–11]. A right aortic arch is present in up to 4% of these patients, i.e., the aorta arches over the right mainstem bronchus, lies to the right of the trachea and esophagus, and descends on the right. In this aortic variation, the first branch off the aorta is the left innominate artery [4,12]. A comparable number who undergo surgical correction have tricuspid valve abnormalities [4].

Transposition of the great arteries with ventricular septal defect

Another category of TGA is TGA with VSD. An estimated 10–25% of patients undergoing surgical correction have a VSD [10,13]. It is the most common defect associated with TGA, and although most are perimembranous, the size, location, and hemodynamic significance of the VSD can vary as they do in the normal heart [6,14]. In addition, abnormalities of the aorta can occur in association with TGA and VSD. Up to 20% of patients in this category have a right aortic arch and of the 5% of patients with TGA who have interrupted aortic arch and coarctation of the aorta, most have TGA and VSD [4].

Although considered part of the cardiac malformation known as double-outlet RV, the Taussig–Bing malformation is discussed here because when VA discordance exists it can be similar physiologically to TGA with VSD [15]. Taussig–Bing malformation occurs when malalignment of the infundibular septum and interventricular septum increases until the VSD becomes subpulmonic and both great vessels, typically side-by-side in location, arise predominantly from the RV. Blood "streams" from the LV to the PA and RV to the aorta. Aortic arch obstruction is relatively common in patients with Taussig–Bing malformation [16].

Transposition of the great arteries with ventricular septal defect and left ventricular outflow tract obstruction

A third category of TGA is TGA with VSD and LVOTO. Anatomic LVOTO is rare in TGA with IVS but a functional form of LVOTO may occur when the RV systemic pressure load shifts the IVS into the LV. Up to 30% of patients with TGA and VSD have anatomic LVOTO. In some classification systems LVOTO, particularly when limited to the pulmonary valve, is known as pulmonary stenosis. LVOTO can be diffuse or discrete and can occur at several levels along the outflow tract of the LV. Causes include pulmonary annular hypoplasia, pulmonary valve stenosis, and subvalvar obstruction from abnormal attachments of the mitral valve apparatus, redundant tricuspid valve tissue that migrates into the LVOT through a VSD, and a membranous ring or fibromuscular tunnel that causes a fixed stenosis [4].

Coronary artery anatomy

Coronary artery anatomy is variable in patients with TGA. In the normal heart, the coronary arteries almost always arise from the aortic sinuses of Valsalva that face or are adjacent to the pulmonary trunk. The usual aortic sinuses of Valsalva are defined as right, left, and noncoronary.

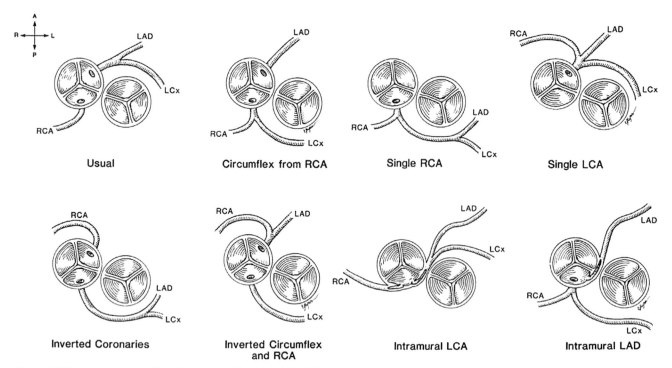

Figure 23.2 Coronary patterns found in patients with transposition of the great arteries. LAD, left anterior descending; LCA, left coronary artery; LCx, left circumflex; RCA, right coronary artery (Reproduced with permission from Reference [18])

In addition, one commissure from the aortic and one from the pulmonary valve are in direct alignment, whereas direct commissural alignment is absent in about 13% of pathologic specimens from patients with TGA [7]. Similarly, in patients with TGA, the coronary arteries most often arise from the aortic sinuses of Valsalva that face the pulmonary trunk, but the epicardial course of the coronary arteries frequently is abnormal [6]. Many classification systems exist to define coronary artery anatomy in patients with TGA but the Leiden classification system appears most commonly in surgical literature and is used here [4,17]. In this classification system, the sinuses of Valsalva from which the coronary arteries originate are renamed sinus 1 and sinus 2. The usual coronary artery patterns found in patients with TGA are shown in Figure 23.2. Most often, the left and right coronary arteries arise from sinus 1 and sinus 2, respectively, and are described as 1 LCx and 2R. About 5% of patients have a coronary artery that is intramural and provides a challenge for arterial switch reconstruction, although alteration in operative technique can lead to satisfactory results [19].

Abnormal (i.e., non-1 LCx and 2R) coronary patterns are seen more commonly in TGA with VSD and have been used in some published series as predictors of postoperative morbidity and mortality [10,16,17,20,21]. In other published series, coronary artery pattern showed no effect on survival but did predict the need for reoperation in patients with TGA, VSD, and aortic arch obstruction [22, 23].

Physiology and natural history

In the normal infant, several physiologic changes occur following birth and lung expansion that are relevant to review prior to a discussion of abnormal physiology. Changes relevant to this discussion are summarized in Table 23.1. For a more detailed discussion the reader is referred to Chapters 4 and 5.

In normal infants, following birth, pulmonary and systemic blood circulates in series. Thus, deoxygenated blood from the systemic circulation enters the right atrium (RA), RV, and then enters the pulmonary circulation via the PA. After crossing the pulmonary capillary bed, oxygenated blood from the pulmonary circulation enters the left atrium (LA) via the pulmonary veins, flows into the LV then exits via the aorta, and ultimately returns as deoxygenated blood to the RA. In the infant with TGA, the pulmonary and systemic blood circulates in parallel rather than in series. Deoxygenated blood from the systemic circulation enters the RA then RV and returns to the systemic circulation via the aorta. Oxygenated blood from the pulmonary circulation enters the LA, the LV and returns to the pulmonary circulation via the PA. Thus, mixing between the systemic and pulmonary circulations is essential for survival in infants with TGA. Although mixing may occur

Table 23.1 Summary of physiologic changes in the normal neonate following birth and lung expansion

Pulmonary vascular resistance	Decreases
Pulmonary artery pressure	Decreases
Pulmonary blood flow	Increases
Pulmonary venous return	Increases
Left atrial pressure	Increases with increase in pulmonary venous return
Right atrial pressure	Decreases with loss of blood flow from placenta
Patent foramen ovale	Functional closure at birth following decrease in right atrial pressure and increase in left atrial pressure
	Anatomic fusion in 80% of infants at about 1 yr
	Can reopen if right atrial pressure increases
Patent ductus arteriosus	Functional closure within 12–15 h of birth
Left-ventricular volume load	Increases
Left-ventricular pressure load	Increases due to loss of low resistance placenta and closure of patent ductus arteriosus

at several levels including the atrial level (ASD), ventricular level (VSD), or arterial level (PDA), the amount of mixing of systemic and pulmonary venous blood at the atrial level is an important determinant of hemoglobin oxygen saturation and the severity of the clinical picture [24] (Figure 23.1). The most common clinical finding in an infant with TGA is cyanosis (arterial partial pressure of oxygen 25–40 mm Hg). The degree of cyanosis varies among infants with TGA but neonates with TGA and IVS or a restrictive PFO or ASD usually have more pronounced cyanosis at birth. In these neonates, supplemental oxygen may increase pulmonary blood flow thus increase arterial oxygen saturation but cyanosis persists in most. Infants with TGA and IVS but with a large PDA and better mixing are less likely to develop cyanosis but are more likely to develop congestive heart failure.

Blood flow through a PDA may improve arterial oxygen saturation but infants, especially smaller infants without adequate interatrial mixing, can develop pulmonary venous congestion and are at risk for preoperative death or sudden death at birth following premature closure of a PFO [25, 26]. Others can develop acidosis and cardiovascular collapse and require resuscitation with mechanical ventilation, prostaglandin E_1 to maintain patency of the ductus arteriosus, and a procedure to provide interatrial mixing. One such procedure is known as a balloon atrial septostomy (BAS) and can be performed in the cardiac catheterization laboratory or at the bedside using echocardiographic guidance. Developed by Rashkind and Miller

in 1966, this procedure uses a balloon septostomy catheter introduced via percutaneous venous access into the RA, through the PFO, and into the LA where it is inflated and then pulled downward to tear the inferior fossa ovalis and enlarge the ASD [27]. In infants younger than 1 month, the atrial septum tends to be thin so it can be torn by the inflated balloon, providing improvement of interatrial mixing and hemoglobin oxygen saturation, relief of pulmonary venous congestion, and subsequent decompression of the LV. Poor results after BAS suggest pulmonary hypertension [28]. Even with good results following BAS, cerebral emboli occur preoperatively and survival without surgical intervention is bleak [29, 30].

Infants with TGA and VSD often have mixing of blood at the atrial and ventricular levels. Interatrial mixing tends to be from the LA to RA and interventricular mixing tends to be from the RV to LV but bidirectional shunting is possible at both levels. Thus, these infants are less likely to develop cyanosis and more likely to develop congestive heart failure. Although many infants are symptomatic during the neonatal period, clinical symptoms of congestive heart failure may develop around 4–6 weeks of life when pulmonary vascular resistance reaches its postnatal nadir. Infants with TGA and IVS or VSD with aortic obstruction are prone to develop early pulmonary vascular disease due to excess pulmonary blood flow [31].

Nearly all infants with TGA and LVOTO have a VSD. The pulmonary blood flow, enhanced by flow across the VSD, is limited by the LVOTO, so that the balance between the pulmonary and systemic blood flow is determined by the degree of LVOTO. The reduction of pulmonary blood flow caused by the obstruction exacerbates the cyanosis found in infants with TGA; however, cyanosis can occur later in infancy when LVOTO is not severe and may be evident only when the infant is crying or feeding [24].

Options for surgical correction

Prior to the 1950s, up to 90% of infants with a diagnosis of TGA died within the first year of life [32]. Early surgical therapy was palliative and began when Blalock and Hanlon created a defect in the atrial septum to provide interatrial mixing of blood [33]. Physiologic correction of TGA was achieved in 1959 by Senning who redirected systemic venous blood to the LV then PA and pulmonary venous blood to the RV then aorta using autologous atrial flaps. This procedure was called the Senning operation or baffle and later was modified by Mustard who created a large interatrial baffle of pericardium to redirect systemic and pulmonary venous return. The Senning and Mustard procedures were the predominant surgical approaches until the 1980s. After good early results, many patients developed late complications largely due to retention of the discordant VA connection. Late complications

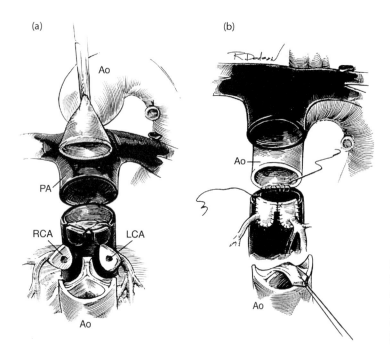

Figure 23.3 (a, b) Arterial switch operation. Aorta and pulmonary artery are transected and translocated. Coronary arteries have been excised with surrounding tissue "buttons" and reimplanted in the neoaorta site. Ao, aorta; LCA, left coronary artery; PA, pulmonary artery; RCA, right coronary artery (Reproduced with permission from Reference [38])

include atrial tachyarrhythmias, baffle leaks and obstructions, failure of the systemic RV, RV dyssynchrony, and systemic (tricuspid) AV valve regurgitation [34–37]. In 1975, Jatene performed the first arterial switch operation (ASO), a procedure that provided anatomic and physiologic correction of TGA through translocation of the great vessels and coronary arteries (Figure 23.3). Initially only infants with TGA and VSD underwent successful ASO [39,40]. Older infants with TGA and IVS were at risk preoperatively for regression of LV myocardial mass and at risk postoperatively for the LV to fail as the systemic ventricle when presented with a sudden increase in pressure load [20]. Thus, the initial stage of ASO for infants with TGA and IVS became placement of a pulmonary artery band (PAB) to increase LV mass in response to an increase in LV pressure load, so-called LV "retraining" [41]. Subsequently the ASO was performed on neonates within the first week of life before regression of LV myocardial mass, with good early and late results [42,43]. The upper age limit before significant regression of the LV myocardium contributes to failure after ASO is unknown and may be as late as 3 months of age [44,45]. Currently when patients are diagnosed later in infancy with TGA and IVS, the initial surgical procedure may be PAB placement for LV "retraining." These patients often require concurrent placement of an arterial to PA shunt to provide adequate pulmonary blood flow [46]. Infants undergoing placement of a PAB prior to ASO may be at increased risk to develop aortic valve insufficiency due to progressive dilation of the neoaortic root [47].

Other patients who may undergo PAB placement as the initial step in a staged conversion to ASO include older children or adults who have systemic RV dysfunction or systemic (tricuspid) AV valve regurgitation following a Senning or Mustard operation [48]. In this group, successful anatomic correction to ASO is more likely in younger patients [49].

Infants with TGA and VSD with LVOTO require a different surgical approach predicted by the nature of the LVOTO, but many can undergo successful ASO [50]. Other procedures may be required in patients with more complex TGA and VSD with LVOTO and a detailed discussion of such surgical techniques can be found in textbooks of cardiothoracic surgery [51]. Overall, ASO remains the surgical option of choice for TGA with IVS, VSD, and in the minority of suitable candidates, VSD with LVOTO.

Anesthetic considerations

Two-dimensional echocardiography provides noninvasive imaging to diagnosis and define features of TGA, thus cardiac catheterization is reserved for selected infants who have associated intracardiac or extracardiac abnormalities [51]. Review of the echocardiogram by the anesthesiologist should include evaluation of patterns of shunting, presence and location of associated defects, coronary artery connections, atrioventricular valve abnormalities, and evaluation of biventricular size and function [52].

Preoperative evaluation of an infant scheduled to undergo surgical correction of TGA includes careful assessment of hemodynamic status, level of inotropic support, cardiac arrhythmias, intravenous access including peripheral, peripherally inserted central catheters (PICC), central or umbilical catheters, intra-arterial access, laboratory values (including measurement of serum lactate), chest X-ray, electrocardiogram, ventilatory status and airway issues, and status of noncardiac organ systems [53, 54]. The anesthesiologist should be aware of risk factors for preoperative or postoperative mortality in infants with TGA. Risk factors for preoperative mortality include restrictive PFO or ASD, persistent pulmonary hypertension, low birth weight, prematurity, and time of diagnosis [25,44,55]. Infants with a prenatal diagnosis of TGA by fetal echocardiography, feasible as early as 18 weeks gestational age, are less likely than infants with a postnatal diagnosis to develop hemodynamic compromise, an important predictor of preoperative and postoperative mortality [11,44,55]. Evaluation of the infant with TGA and IVS frequently includes assessment of adequacy of interatrial mixing following BAS. In addition, infants receiving prostaglandin E_1 intravenous therapy to maintain patency of the ductus arteriosus, especially in doses exceeding 0.05 mcg/kg/min, should be assessed for side effects including apnea, hypotension, fever, CNS excitation, and decreased intravascular volume. Patency of the ductus arteriosus and associated reduction of systemic blood flow and hypotension can lead to a decrease in blood flow to the bowel and contribute to the development of necrotizing enterocolitis in some of these infants [56]. Assessment of the infant with TGA and VSD includes evaluation for signs of pulmonary overcirculation and congestive heart failure including increased heart rate, cardiomegaly, decreased skin temperature, diaphoresis, low body weight, tachypnea, intercostal and substernal retraction, and prolonged capillary refill.

Intraoperatively, routine monitors are placed prior to induction of anesthesia. Options for induction of anesthesia in the unusual infant presenting for ASO without intravenous access include inhalation or intramuscular delivery of induction agent. More often, these infants will undergo an intravenous induction using an opioid. The safety and efficacy of opioid-based anesthesia for cardiac surgery in infants has been established for many years [57]. However, opioids alone have had inconsistent effects on stress hormone release and outcome in neonates who undergo cardiac surgery [58, 59]. Thus, a balanced opioid-based anesthetic that includes an anesthetic vapor may control hemodynamic and stress responses better in these infants [50,60,61]. For a more detailed discussion of anesthetic agents and their cardiovascular effects, refer to Chapter 6. A catheter placed in an umbilical artery preoperatively provides reliable intraoperative monitoring of arterial blood pressure. Other options for invasive monitoring of arterial blood pressure include placement of a catheter via percutaneous puncture of the radial or femoral artery or an incision to provide direct cannulation of an artery. Ventilation should be adjusted to maintain normocarbia. A catheter placed in the umbilical vein preoperatively provides reliable monitoring of central venous pressure when positioned in the inferior vena cava or RA. Central line placement may be difficult in infants less than 4 kg and more successful when ultrasound guidance is used to locate the vessel [62,63]. A PICC line placed following ICU admission provides a reliable port for intravenous access and withdrawal of venous blood and central venous pressure monitoring [64]. In some centers, surgeons place intracardiac lines before weaning from cardiopulmonary bypass (CPB) that can be used to monitor intracardiac pressures and infuse inotropes.

Following placement of the lines, gastric contents are suctioned and a transesophageal echocardiography (TEE) probe is placed. Pediatric biplane probes have been placed in infants as small as 2.9 kg; however, the anesthesiologist should monitor for hemodynamic compromise or a change in peak airway pressures during probe placement and manipulation and remove the probe if problems occur [65]. In the infant with TGA, TEE can be used following bypass to detect residual defects, assess regional and global ventricular function, valvular function, evaluate neoaortic valve regurgitation, and detect a gradient at the supravalvar anastomotic sites of the great arteries [66]. Regional wall motion abnormalities (RWMA) may be detected after bypass and although functional implications remain unknown, RWMA that persist in multiple myocardial segments at completion of ASO correlate with myocardial ischemia [67,68].

Antifibrinolytic agents are used in many centers where neonates undergo ASO and include aminocaproic acid and tranexamic acid. These agents and coagulation-related issues are discussed in detail in Chapter 12. The conduct of CPB is unique to each institution but may include a flow rate of up to 200 mL/kg/min and avoidance of low flow or circulatory arrest, infant temperature of 28–32°C, use of blood cardioplegia, and modified ultrafiltration immediately following termination of CPB. For a complete discussion of CPB and modified ultrafiltration, refer to Chapter 7. Following separation from CPB, TEE and left atrial pressure (LAP) monitoring can help assess global and regional LV function and may indicate inadequate myocardial perfusion or compromised LV performance. Arrhythmias may develop, although sinus rhythm persists in most of these neonates [69].

Most of these patients will require inotropic support, often in the form of dopamine at 3–10 mcg/kg/min, epinephrine at 0.03–0.05 mcg/kg/min, or milrinone at 0.25–0.75 mcg/kg/min. Many centers add nitroglycerine infusion at 1–2 mcg/kg/min to maximally dilate coronary arteries and reduce preload, and calcium chloride infusion to normalize ionized Ca^{++}, which is important to myocardial contractility in the newborn. There are several considerations unique to the ASO which deserve mention. Although uncommon, obstruction to translocated coronary arteries can be a significant problem after ASO. Signs of this problem include global myocardial dysfunction, detected clinically and with echocardiography [68]; RWMA do not appear to be as common in neonates. Ventricular arrhythmias in neonates are uncommon; when these occur after ASO and persist, a coronary artery problem must be ruled out. Neonates with TGA/IVS often undergo rapid deconditioning of the LV after birth, making them intolerant of either excessive afterload or preload. Overdistention of the LV is not tolerated, because excessive myofibril length places them too far to the right on the Starling curve. Increased afterload (hypertension) is also not tolerated. Thus, the hemodynamic goals for the ASO patient postbypass should be to achieve adequate cardiac output with the lowest possible LAP. In many patients, an LAP of 4–6 mm Hg with systolic blood pressure in the 50–75 range achieves these goals. If the LV is overdistended (high and increasing LAP in the face of decreasing systemic pressure and cardiac output), diuretics can be used, or if the situation is deteriorating quickly, removing blood from the central venous catheter until the LAP has decreased is effective. Some of these patients are so sensitive to intravascular and intracardiac volume that removing and reinfusing as little as 3–5 cc of blood for blood gases may cause significant changes in LAP and systemic blood pressure.

Infusion of blood products to achieve hemostasis, hemodynamic instability, and edema of the myocardium and lungs following a long period of CPB can preclude chest closure at the end of the operation. A narcotic infusion may be continued during transport and postoperatively in these neonates as they are not suitable for early extubation [53]. Care should be taken during transport to the intensive care unit to maintain conditions present in the operating room. Specifically the anesthesiologist should prevent major changes in ventilation, tracheal extubation, interruption of delivery of intravenous inotropes, loss of body temperature, and sudden changes in hemodynamics.

Congenitally corrected transposition of the great arteries

ccTGA is a rare congenital heart defect. It is a type of TGA with AV discordance in addition to VA discordance; hence it has AV–VA or double discordance (defined below). There are three main anatomic types with two ventricles, but this discussion is limited to the most common anatomic type found in 94% of pathologic specimens [70]. This common anatomic type consists of the usual atrial arrangement (atrial situs solitus), left-right reversal of the AV connection, TGA, and a very high prevalence of Ebstein-like inferior displacement toward the cardiac apex and

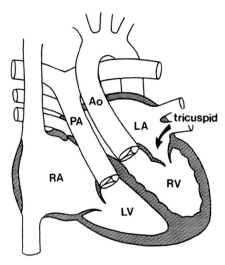

Figure 23.4 Congenitally corrected transposition of the great arteries. Ao, aorta; LA, left atrium; LV, left ventricle; PA, pulmonary artery; RA, right atrium; RV, right ventricle; tricuspid, systemic (tricuspid) atrioventricular valve (Reproduced with permission from Reference [71])

dysplasia of the systemic (tricuspid) AV valve and systemic RV dysplasia (Figure 23.4). Other terms used to define this lesion include corrected transposition, ventricular inversion, l-transposition, double discordance, physiologically corrected transposition, discordant transposition, and inverted transposition [72]. The terminology atrial situs solitus, AV–VA discordance, and congenitally corrected TGA are used here. In the presence of AV–VA discordance, the LV receives blood from the RA then empties into the PA, and the RV receives blood from the LA then empties into the aorta. This provides a physiologic correction so that oxygenated pulmonary venous blood passes to the systemic circulation and deoxygenated systemic venous blood to the pulmonary circulation [72]. Associated malformations occur in up to 98% of patients and include VSD, LVOTO (often multilevel), abnormalities of the systemic (tricuspid) AV valve, abnormalities of the systemic RV, and AV conduction system abnormalities [70,72].

Physiology and natural history

The age at presentation and clinical course of patients with ccTGA is determined by the combination and severity of associated cardiac defects. Patients without associated defects are unusual, more likely to survive to adulthood, but often develop systemic (tricuspid) AV valve regurgitation, impaired systemic RV function, and rhythm disturbance after the age of 50 years [73]. Patients with associated defects may die as infants and children or live a shortened lifespan, and exhibit a spectrum of symptoms that ranges from none to cyanosis or heart failure [73, 74]. Patients with cyanosis most often have a VSD and LVOTO that cause decreased pulmonary blood flow and a right-to-left shunt, thus they may have undergone a palliative surgical procedure such as placement of an arterial to PA shunt to increase pulmonary blood flow. Patients with systemic RV failure tend to become symptomatic earlier, have a VSD with a left-to-right shunt, and have abnormalities of the systemic (tricuspid) AV valve [75]. Extracorporeal membrane oxygenation or a ventricular assist device may be needed to treat failure of the systemic ventricle prior to surgery or cardiac transplant [76,77]. Patients may have a combination of cyanosis and heart failure and complete heart block, and are at increased risk to develop infective endocarditis [74,75].

Options for surgical correction

Although optimal surgical management is controversial, the conventional option for complete surgical repair of patients with ccTGA is to repair the intracardiac-associated defects and leave the systemic (tricuspid) AV valve and systemic RV connected to the aorta. Thus, surgical procedures include VSD closure, alone or with relief of LVOTO, systemic (tricuspid) AV valve repair or replacement, and pacemaker placement. Preoperative systemic AV valve regurgitation and associated systemic RV dysfunction, present in many patients, can be an important risk factor for death after conventional surgical repair [75,77,79]. Perioperative mortality ranges from 4 to 16%, and 5- and 10-year survival estimates are 71–85% and 68–85%, respectively [80–82]. In some patients, survival decreases to 60% 15 years following conventional surgical repair [79]. Postoperatively, the systemic AV valve often develops regurgitation, even without surgical manipulation. This may be due to a change in geometry or increase in blood flow through the valve following surgical correction of an associated intracardiac defect [78,80]. RV dysfunction develops postoperatively in up to 55% of these patients, especially in patients with a high preoperative pulmonary to systemic blood flow ratio [75,78,80]. Intrinsic abnormalities of the cardiac conduction system are present in these patients and cause additional postoperative morbidity; specifically, the development of complete heart block in up to 24% of patients [82].

Concern about progressive dysfunction of the systemic AV valve and RV in patients with ccTGA led to the development of anatomic correction for these patients and the "double-switch" operation, i.e., a combination of the Senning and ASO procedures so that the mitral valve and LV become the systemic AV valve and ventricle [83] (Figure 23.5). Before the LV can become the systemic ventricle, some patients must undergo preoperative placement of a PAB to provide an increase in LV pressure and mass, i.e., "retraining" of the LV. Placement of a PAB is not risk free and may be less successful in patients post-

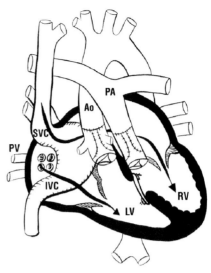

Figure 23.5 Senning and arterial switch operation (double switch). Ao, aorta; IVC, inferior vena cava; LV, left ventricle; PA, pulmonary artery; RV, right ventricle; SVC, superior vena cava (Reproduced with permission from Reference [75])

puberty [71,84,85]. In addition, placement of a PAB can increase the risk of death or LV dysfunction following a double-switch operation [86]. Overall, the Senning and ASO procedures are indicated in patients with systemic RV deterioration and systemic AV (tricuspid) valve regurgitation. Patient selection criteria include a competent mitral valve and good LV function, balanced ventricular and AV valve sizes, no major AV valve straddling, translocatable coronary arteries, LV/RV pressure ratio >0.7, and unobstructed connections to both great vessels [83,71]. A conceptually similar procedure has been performed successfully on patients with ccTGA and VSD with obstructed connection to the PA, incorporating the Senning and Rastelli (insertion of a valved conduit between the RV and PA) procedures [87]. Presently, the perioperative mortality for Senning and ASO ("double-switch") procedures is 7–12%, and survival after 2–7 years is 55–91% [88,86,89,90]. Postoperative venoatrial obstruction and arrhythmias may limit the application of this procedure, as in prior patients who underwent Senning or Mustard operation for TGA [89,90]. Long-term results of this procedure are variable but anatomic findings support the opinion that it may be a better surgical option in selected patients [70].

Anesthetic considerations

Careful preoperative assessment of these patients includes a thorough history and physical examination and review of baseline cardiac anatomy, presence of associated intracardiac defects, prior surgery performed and residual defects, and evaluation for signs and symptoms of cyanosis and heart failure. It is important to note the presence and degree of systemic (tricuspid) AV valve regurgitation, the status of systemic RV function, and any cardiac conduction system abnormalities. Functional status and mass of the LV must be evaluated in patients who have undergone PAB placement for LV "retraining."

Preoperatively, patients can be quite ill. Some can be dependent on a ventilator and inotropes, while others have complete heart block and are dependent on a pacemaker [87]. Although rare, older patients can have angina and abatement of symptoms with nitrate therapy but normal coronary artery anatomy [75].

Anesthetic management of the patient with systemic AV valve regurgitation and systemic RV dysfunction is aimed at decreasing RV pressure load by careful control of arterial blood pressure. Care should be taken to prevent sudden increases in arterial blood pressure in response to stimulation from tracheal intubation, placement of invasive monitoring lines, or surgical stimulation.

After completion of the Senning and ASO, TEE is used to detect venoatrial obstruction, assess biventricular function, detect residual defects, assess valvular function, evaluate neoaortic valve regurgitation, and detect a gradient at the supravalvar anastomotic sites of the great arteries [66]. Intracardiac lines can be used to measure RAP and LAP to evaluate RV and LV function and deliver inotropes. Bleeding can be brisk and coagulation defects as expected from a long period of CPB. These patients are not candidates for early extubation and those in whom the LV is unable to function well as the systemic ventricle can require extracorporeal support postoperatively.

Key points for the anesthetic management of transposition of the great vessels

Transposition of the great arteries

Prerepair
1   Assure adequate mixing of systemic and pulmonary venous blood (may require BAS or PGE-1 for ductal patency)
2   Confirm adequate left-ventricular mass and function to sustain systemic circulation (may require a period of PAB for LV "retraining")
3   Evaluate coronary anatomy
Postrepair (ASO)
1   Manage coagulopathy and bleeding from extended suture lines
2   Assess RWMA (may require inotropic support or revision of coronary translocation)
3   Early diagnosis and treatment of arrhythmias

Congenitally corrected transposition of the great arteries

Prerepair
1   Assess the systemic RV function and the ventricular mass and function of the LV (may require a preparation procedure of PAB for LV "retraining")
2   Evaluate for systemic AV (tricuspid) regurgitation
3   Examine EKG and evaluate for conduction abnormalities
4   Determine coronary anatomy
Postrepair (double-switch – ASO and Senning)
1   Manage coagulopathy and bleeding from extended suture lines
2   Assess RWMA (may require inotropic support or revision of coronary translocation)
3   Early diagnosis and treatment of arrhythmias

References

1. Hoffman JI, Christianson R (1978) Congenital heart disease in a cohort of 19,502 births with long-term follow-up. Am J Cardiol 42: 641–647.
2. Sadler TW (2000) Cardiovascular system. In: Sadler TW (ed.) Langman Medical Embryology. Lippincott Williams & Wilkins, Philadelphia, pp. 208–259.
3. Jacobs JP, Franklin RCG, Wilkinson JL, et al. (2006) The nomenclature, definition and classification of discordant atrioventricular connections. Cardiol Young 16 (Suppl 3): 72–84.
4. Jaggers JJ, Cameron DE, Herlong JR, et al. (2000) Congenital heart surgery nomenclature and database project: transposition of the great arteries. Ann Thorac Surg 69 (4 Suppl): S205–S235.
5. Anderson RH, Becker AE (1992) Cardiac anatomy. In: Anderson RH, Becker AE (eds) The Heart Structure in Health and Disease. Gower Medical Publishing, London, 1.1–1.41.
6. Anderson RH, Becker AE (1992) Anomalies of the ventricles and the subsystems. In: Anderson RH, Becker AE (eds) The Heart Structure in Health and Disease. Gower Medical Publishing, London, pp. 7.1–7.30.
7. Massoudy P, Baltalarli A, de Leval MR, et al. (2002) Anatomic variability in coronary arterial distribution with regard to the arterial switch procedure. Circulation 106: 1980–1984.
8. Garson A, Bricker JT (1998) Transposition of the great arteries. In: Garson A, Bricker JT, Fisher DJ, Neish SR (eds) The Science and Practice of Pediatric Cardiology, 2nd edn. Williams & Wilkins, Baltimore, pp. 1470–1503.
9. Waldman JD, Paul MH, Newfeld EA, et al. (1977) Transposition of the great arteries with intact ventricular septum and patent ductus arteriosus. Am J Cardiol 39: 232–238.
10. Serraf A, Lacour-Gayet F, Bruniaux J, et al. (1993) Anatomic correction of transposition of the great arteries in neonates. J Am Coll Cardiol 22: 193–200.

11. Brown JW, Park HJ, Turrentine MW (2001) Arterial switch operation: factors impacting survival in the current era. Ann Thorac Surg 71: 1978–1984.

12. Knight L, Edwards JE (1974) Right aortic arch. Types and associated cardiac anomalies. Circulation 50: 1047–1051.

13. Losay J, Touchot A, Serraf A, et al. (2001) Late outcome after arterial switch operation for transportation of the great arteries. Circulation 104 (Suppl I): I-121–I-126.

14. Serraf A, Bruniaux J, Lacour-Gayet F, et al. (1991) Anatomic correction of transposition of the great arteries with ventricular septal defect: experience with 118 cases. J Thorac Cardiovasc Surg 102: 140–147.

15. Artrip JH, Sauer H, Campbell DN, et al. (2006) Biventricular repair in double outlet right ventricle: surgical results based on the STS-EACTS International Nomenclature classification. Eur J Cardiothorac Surg 29: 545–550.

16. Walters HL, Mavroudis C, Tchervenkov CI, et al. (2000) Congenital heart surgery nomenclature and database project: double outlet right ventricle. Ann Thorac Surg 69: S249–S263.

17. Gittenburger-de Groot A, Sauer U, Oppenheimer-Dekker A, et al. (1983) Coronary arterial anatomy in transposition of the great arteries: a morphologic study. Pediatr Cardial 4 (Suppl 1): 15–24.

18. DiDonato RM, Castaneda AR (1995) Anatomic correction of transposition of the great arteries at the arterial level. In: Sabiston DC, Spencer FC (eds) Surgery of the Chest, 6th edn. WB Saunders Co., Philadelphia, pp. 1592–1604.

19. Asou T, Karl TR, Pawade A, et al. (1994) Arterial switch: translocation of the intramural coronary artery. Ann Thorac Surg 57: 461–465.

20. Kirklin JW, Blackstone EH, Tchervenkov CI, et al. (1992) Clinical outcomes after the arterial switch operation for transposition. Circulation 86: 1501–1515.

21. Pasquali SK, Hasselblad V, Li JS, et al. (2002) Coronary artery pattern and outcome of arterial switch operation for transposition of the great arteries. Circulation 106: 2575–2580.

22. Qamar ZA, Goldberg CS, Devaney EJ, et al. (2007) Current risk factors and outcomes for the arterial switch operation. Ann Thorac Surg 84: 871–878; discussion 878–879.

23. Gottlieb D, Schwartz ML, Bischoff K, et al. (2008) Predictors of outcome of arterial switch operation for complex D-transposition. Ann Thorac Surg 85: 1698–1702; discussion 1702–1703.

24. Karl TR (2006) Transposition of the great arteries. In: Nichols DG, Cameron DE (eds) Critical Heart Disease in Infants and Children. Mosby Year Book, St. Louis, pp. 500–530.

25. Soongswang J, Adatia I, Newman C, et al. (1998) Mortality in potential arterial switch candidates with transposition of the great arteries. J Am Coll Cardiol 32: 753–757.

26. Berry LM, Padbury J, Novoa-Takara L (1998) Premature "closing" of the foramen ovale in transposition of the great arteries with intact ventricular septum: rare cause of sudden neonatal death. Pediatr Cardiol 19: 246–248.

27. Rashkind WJ, Miller WW (1966) Creation of an atrial septal defect without throracotomy: a palliative approach to complete transposition of the great arteries. JAMA 196: 991–992.

28. Kumar A, Taylor GP, Sandor GG, et al. (1993) Pulmonary vascular disease in neonates with transposition of the great arteries and intact ventricular septum. Br Heart J 69: 442–445.

29. Kidd BSL (1976) The fate of children with transposition of the great arteries following balloon atrial septostomy. In: Kidd BSL, Rowe RD, (eds) The Child with Congenital Heart Disease After Surgery. Futura Publishing Co, Mount Kisco, pp. 153–164.

30. McQuillen PS, Hamrick SE, Perez MJ, et al. (2006) Balloon atrial septostomy is associated with preoperative stroke in neonates with transposition of the great arteries. Circulation 113: 280–285.

31. Newfeld EA, Paul MM, Muster AJ, et al. (1974) Pulmonary vascular disease in complete transposition of the great arteries: a study of 200 patients. Am J Cardiol 34: 75–82.

32. Liebman J, Cullum L, Belloc NB (1969) Natural history of transposition of the great arteries, Anatomy and birth and death characteristics. Circulation 40: 237–262.

33. Blalock A, Hanlon CR (1950) The surgical treatment of complete transposition of the aorta and the pulmonary artery. Surg Gynecol 90: 1.

34. Trusler GA, Williams WG, Duncan KF, et al. (1987) Results with the mustard operation in simple transposition of the great arteries 1963–1985. Ann Surg 206: 251–260.

35. Williams WG, Trusler GA, Kirklin JW, et al. (1988) Early and late results of a protocol for simple transposition leading to an atrial switch (mustard) repair. J Thorac Cardiovasc Surg 95: 717–726.

36. Gelatt M, Hamilton RM, McCrindle BW, et al. (1997) Arrhythmia and mortality after the mustard procedure: a 30-year single-center experience. J Am Coll Cardiol 29: 194–201.

37. Chow PC, Liang XC, Lam WW, et al. (2008) Mechanical right ventricular dyssynchrony in patients after atrial switch operation for transposition of the great arteries. Am J Cardiol. Mar 15; 101: 874–881.

38. Castaneda AR, Jonas RA, Mayer JE (1994) Transposition of the great arteries. In: Castaneda AR, Jonas RA (eds) Cardiac Surgery of the Neonate and Infant. WB Saunders Co, Philadelphia, pp. 420–421.

39. Jatene AD, Fones VF, Paulista PP, et al. (1976) Anatomic correction of transposition of the great vessels. J Thorac Cardiovasc Surg 72: 364–370.

40. Yacoub MH, Radley-Smith R, Hilton CJ (1976) Anatomical correction of complete transposition of the great arteries and ventricular septal defect in infancy. Br Med J 1 (6018): 1112–1114.

41. Yacoub MH, Radley-Smith R, Maclaurin R (1977) Two stage operation for anatomical correction of transposition of the great arteries with intact interventricular septum. Lancet 1 (8025): 1275–1278.

42. Lupenetti FM, Bove EL, Minich LL, et al. (1992) Intermediate-term survival and functional results after arterial repair for transposition of the great arteries. J Thorac Cardiovasc Surg 103: 421–427.

43. Wernovsky G, Mayer JE, Jonas RA, et al. (1995) Factors influencing early and late outcome of the arterial switch operation for transposition of the great arteries. J Thorac Cardiovasc Surg 109: 289–302.

44. Foran JP, Sullivan ID, Elliott MJ, et al. (1998) Primary arterial switch operation for transposition of the great arteries with intact ventricular septum in infants older than 21 days. J Am Coll Cardiol 31: 883–889.

45. Däbritz S, Engelhardt W, von Bernuth G, et al. (1997) Trial of pulmonary artery banding: a diagnostic criterion for "one-stage" arterial switch in simple transposition of the great arteries beyond the neonatal period. Eur J Cardiothorac Surg 11: 112–116.

46. Lacour-Gayet F, Piot D, Zoghbi J, et al. (2001) Surgical management and indication of left ventricular retaining in arterial switch for transposition of the great arteries with intact ventricular septum. Eur J Cardiothoracic Surg 20: 824–829.

47. Schwartz ML, Gauvreau K, del Nido P, et al. (2004) Long-term predictors of aortic root dilation and aortic regurgitation after arterial switch operation. Circulation 110 (11 Suppl 1): II128–II132.

48. Cochrane AD, Karl TR, Mee RB (1993) Staged conversion to arterial switch for late failure of the systemic right ventricle. Ann Thorac Surg 56: 854–861.

49. Winlaw DS, McGuirk SP, Balmer C, et al. (2005) Intention-to-treat analysis of pulmonary artery banding in conditions with a morphological right ventricle in the systemic circulation with a view to anatomic biventricular repair. Circulation 111: 405–411.

50. Sohn YS, Brizard CP, Cochrane AD, et al. (1998) Arterial switch in hearts with left ventricular outflow and pulmonary valve abnormalities. Ann Thorac Surg 66: 842–848.

51. Spray TL (1998) Transposition of the great arteries. In: Kaiser LR, Kron IL, Spray TL (eds) Mastery of Cardiothoracic Surgery. Lippincott-Raven Publishers, Philadelphia, pp. 785–799.

52. Silverman NH (1993) Ventriculoarterial discordance (transposition of the great arteries). In: Pediatric Echocardiography, 1st edn. Williams & Wilkins, Baltimore, pp. 245–278.

53. Laussen PC, Wessel DL (1989) Anesthesia for congenital heart disease. In: Gregory GA (ed.) Pediatric Anesthesia, 4th edn. Churchill Livingstone, New York, pp. 467–539.

54. Freed DH, Robertson CM, Sauve RS, et al. (2006) Intermediate-term outcomes of the arterial switch operation for transposition of great arteries in neonates: alive but well? J Thorac Cardiovasc Surg 132: 845–852.

55. Bonnet D, Coltri A, Butera G, et al. (1999) Detection of transposition of the great arteries in fetuses reduces neonatal morbidity and mortality. Circulation 99: 916–918.

56. Hoffman JIE (1996) The circulatory system. In: Rudolph AM, Hoffman JIE, Rudolph CD (eds) Rudolph's Pediatrics, 20th edn. Appleton & Lange, Stamford, 20.6.3, pp. 1462–1464.

57. Hickey PR, Hansen DD (1984) Fentanyl- and sufentanil-oxygen-pancuronium anesthesia for cardiac surgery in infants. Anesth Analg 63: 117–124.

58. Anand KJ, Hickey PR (1992) Halothane-morphine compared with high-dose sufentanil for anesthesia and postoperative analgesia in neonatal cardiac surgery. N Engl J Med 326: 1–9.

59. Gruber EM, Laussen PC, Casta A, et al. (2001) Stress response in infants undergoing cardiac surgery: a randomized study of fentanyl bolus, fentanyl infusion, and fentanyl-midazolam infusion. Anesth Analg 92: 882–890.

60. Crean P, Koren G, Goresky G, et al. (1986) Fentanyl-oxygen versus fentanyl-N$_2$O/oxygen anaesthesia in children undergoing cardiac surgery. Can Anaesth Soc J 33: 36–40.

61. Duncan HP, Cloote A, Weir PM, et al. (2000) Reducing stress responses in the pre-bypass phase of open heart surgery in infants and young children: a comparison of different fentanyl doses. Br J Anaesth 84: 556–564.

62. Hayashi Y, Uchida O, Takaki O, et al. (1992) Internal jugular vein catheterization in infants undergoing cardiovascular surgery: an analysis of the factors influencing successful catheterization. Anesth Analg 74: 688–693.

63. Asheim P, Mostad U, Aadahl P (2002) Ultrasound-guided central venous cannulation in infants and children. Acta Anaesthesiol Scand 46: 390–392.

64. Tan LH, Hess B, Diaz LK, et al. (2007) Survey of the use of peripherally inserted central venous catheters in neonates with critical congenital cardiac disease. Cardiol Young 17: 196–201.

65. Muhiudeen Russell IA, Miller-Hance WC, Silverman NH (1998) Intraoperative transesophageal echocardiography for pediatric patients with congenital heart disease. Anesth Analg 87: 1058–1076.

66. Stevenson JG, Sorensen GK, Gartman DM, et al. (1993) Transesophageal echocardiography during repair of congenital cardiac defects: identification of residual problems necessitating reoperation. J Am Soc Echocardiogr 6: 356–365.

67. Balaguru D, Auslender M, Colvin SB, et al. (2000) Intraoperative myocardial ischemia recognized by transesophageal echocardiography monitoring in the pediatric population: a report of 3 cases. J Am Soc Echocardiogr 13: 615–618.

68. Rouine-Rapp K, Rouillard KP, Miller-Hance W, et al. (2006) Segmental wall-motion abnormalities after an arterial switch operation indicate ischemia. Anesth Analg 103: 1139–1146.

69. Rhodes LA, Wernovsky G, Keane JF, et al. (1995) Arrhythmias and intracardiac conduction after the arterial switch operation. J Thorac Cardiovasc Surg 109: 303–310.

70. Van Praagh R, Papagiannis J, Grunenfelder J, et al. (1998) Pathologic anatomy of corrected transposition of the great arteries: medical and surgical implications. Am Heart J 135: 772–785.

71. Karl TR, Weintraub RG, Brizard CP, et al. (1997) Senning plus arterial switch operation for discordant (congenitally corrected) transposition. Ann Thorac Surg 64: 495–502.

72. Wilkinson JL, Cochrane AD, Karl TR (2000) Congenital heart surgery nomenclature and database project: corrected (discordant) transposition of the great arteries (and related malformations). Ann Thorac Surg 69: S236–S248.

73. Presbitero P, Somerville J, Rabajoli F, et al. (1995) Corrected transposition of the great arteries without associated defects in adult patients: clinical profile and follow up. Br Heart J 74: 57–59.

74. Connelly MS, Liu PP, Williams WG, et al. (1996) Congenitally corrected transposition of the great arteries in the adult: functional status and complications. J Am Coll Cardiol 27: 1238–1243.

75. Lundstrom U, Bull C, Wyse RKH, et al. (1990) The natural and "unnatural" history of congenitally corrected transposition. Am J Cardiol 65: 1222–1229.

76. Devaney EJ, Charpie JR, Ohye RG, et al. (2003) Combined arterial switch and Senning operation for congenitally corrected transposition of the great arteries: patient selection and intermediate results. J Thorac Cardiovasc Surg 125: 500–507.

77. Gregoric ID, Kosir R, Smart FW, et al. (2005) Left ventricular assist device implantation in a patient with congenitally corrected transposition of the great arteries. Tex Heart Inst J 32: 567–569.

78. Acar P, Sidi D, Bonnet D, et al. (1998) Maintaining tricuspid valve competence in double discordance: a challenge for the paediatric cardiologist. Heart 80: 479–483.

79. Shin'oka T, Kurosawa H, Imai Y, et al. (2007) Outcomes of definitive surgical repair for congenitally corrected transposition of the great arteries or double outlet right ventricle with discordant atrioventricular connections: risk analyses in 189 patients. J Thorac Cardiovasc Surg 133: 1318–1328, 1328.e1–4.

80. Sano T, Riesenfeld T, Karl TR, et al. (1995) Intermediate-term outcome after intracardiac repair of associated cardiac defects in patients with atrioventricular and ventriculoarterial discordance. Circulation 92 (Suppl II): II-272–II-278.

81. McGrath LB, Kirklin JW, Blackstone EH, et al. (1985) Death and other events after cardiac repair in discordant atrioventricular connection. J Thorac Cardiovasc Surg 90: 711–728.

82. Termignon JL, Leca F, Vouhe PR, et al. (1996) "Classic" repair of congenitally corrected transposition and ventricular septal defect. Ann Thorac Surg 62: 199–206.

83. Yamagishi M, Imai Y, Hoshino S, et al. (1993) Anatomic correction of atrioventricular discordance. J Thorac Cardiovasc Surg 105: 1067–1076.

84. Poirier NC, Mee RB (2000) Left ventricular reconditioning and anatomical correction for systemic right ventricular dysfunction. Semin Thorac Cardiovasc Surg Pediatr Card Surg Annu 3: 198–215.

85. Helvind MH, McCarthy JF, Imamura M, et al. (1998) Ventriculo-arterial discordance: switching the morphologically left ventricle into the systemic circulation after 3 months of age. Eur J Cardiothorac Surg 14: 173–178.

86. Quinn DW, McGuirk SP, Metha C, et al. (2008) The morphologic left ventricle that requires training by means of pulmonary artery banding before the double-switch procedure for congenitally corrected transposition of the great arteries is at risk of late dysfunction. J Thorac Cardiovasc Surg 135: 1137–1144, 1144.e1–2.

87. Ilbawi MN, DeLeon SY, Backer CL, et al. (1990) An alternative approach to the surgical management of physiologically corrected transposition with ventricular septal defect and pulmonary stenosis or atresia. J Thorac Cardiovasc Surg 100: 410–415.

88. Friedberg DZ, Nadas AS (1970) Clinical profile of patients with congenital corrected transposition of the great arteries: a study of 60 cases. N Engl J Med 282: 1053–1059.

89. Yagihara T, Kishimoto H, Isobe F, et al. (1994) Double switch operation in cardiac anomalies with atrioventricular and ventriculoarterial discordance. J Thorac Cardiovasc Surg 107: 351–358.

90. Reddy VM, McElhinney DB, Silverman NH, et al. (1997) The double switch procedure for anatomical repair of congenitally corrected transposition of the great arteries in infants and children. Eur Heart J 18: 1470–1477.

24 Anesthesia for the patient with a single ventricle

Laura K. Diaz, M.D., Susan C. Nicolson, M.D. and James M. Steven, M.D.

The Children's Hospital of Philadelphia, University of Pennsylvania School of Medicine, Philadelphia, Pennsylvania, USA

Introduction

In the early 1970s, Fontan [1] and Kreutzer [2] independently introduced operative treatment of tricuspid atresia that resulted in nearly normal systemic arterial oxygen saturation and normal volume work for the single ventricle. This procedure, subsequently referred to as the Fontan operation, created a series circulation that requires the single ventricle to pump fully saturated blood only to the systemic circulation, thereby reducing the pressure and volume work to that of a normal systemic ventricle. The systemic venous drainage passes directly through the pulmonary vascular bed without benefit of a pumping chamber. The child's pulmonary vascular resistance (PVR) must

be low to maintain the pulmonary circulation and the cardiac output (CO) on which it depends. Since that time, the principle of the Fontan operation has been applied to the full spectrum of cardiac lesions with one functional ventricle. Suitable physiology for ultimate repair by a modification of the Fontan procedure is predicated on carefully planned appropriately timed and executed palliative operations designed for the specific patient's single ventricle physiology. This chapter illustrates these principles using hypoplastic left heart syndrome (HLHS), the most common congenital cardiac malformation where there is only one developed ventricle. HLHS represents the fourth most common defect presenting in the neonatal period and accounts for 7.5% of the newborns with congenital heart disease sufficiently significant to require early therapeutic intervention. Recent work by Hinton and colleagues has demonstrated a high heritability component to HLHS, suggesting HLHS as a severe form of valve malformation

Anesthesia for Congenital Heart Disease 2nd edition. Edited by Dean Andropoulos, Stephen Stayer, Isobel Russell and Emad Mossad. © 2010 Blackwell Publishing.

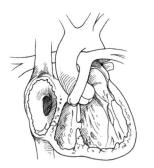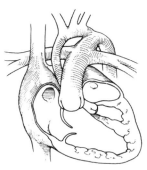

Figure 24.1 Basic anatomical features of tricuspid atresia (*left*) and hypoplastic left heart syndrome (*right*). In tricuspid atresia, pulmonary blood flow depends on the degree of hypoplasia of the pulmonary valve and artery. In hypoplastic left heart syndrome, there may be atresia or stenosis of the aortic and mitral valves, but all variants have a small or nonexistent left ventricle and a hypoplastic ascending aorta (Reproduced and used with permission from Reference [4])

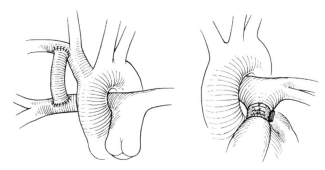

Figure 24.2 Right modified Blalock–Taussig shunt (*left*). A 3–4 mm Goretex® graft is sewn between the right subclavian or innominate artery and the right pulmonary artery. Pulmonary artery banding (*right*). An umbilical tape or similar material is placed around the main pulmonary artery to limit pulmonary blood flow (Reproduced and used with permission from Reference [5])

with inheritance as a complex trait and emphasizing the importance of screening first degree relatives of HLHS patients [3].

A variety of anatomic lesions may be classified as producing single ventricle anatomy or physiology, also referred to as a univentricular heart (Figure 24.1). Most of these lesions have both atrioventricular valves committed to a single systemic ventricular chamber, or atresia/severe stenosis of one of the atrioventricular valves. Many of these hearts actually have two ventricles, although one of the ventricles is typically small with minimal contribution to cardiac ejection, thus functionally considered a single ventricle. Finally, some patients have two ventricles of normal size that cannot be separated because a ventricular septal defect (VSD) is remote from either great vessel, or due to straddling of the atrioventricular valve attachments over the VSD. Additionally, some very large intraventricular communications cannot be septated.

After assessing the details of the cardiac anatomy, the initial approach to the single ventricle patient involves determining the degree of pulmonary blood flow (PBF) and whether the pulmonary circulation is dependent on the ductus arteriosus. Patients with ductal dependent circulation will require a reliable source of PBF, which is accomplished by creation of a systemic-to-pulmonary shunt. The most commonly performed shunt is a modified Blalock–Taussig (BT) shunt, in which a Goretex® tube graft connects the subclavian to the pulmonary artery (PA) (Figure 24.2). Some single ventricle patients will have unrestricted flow to both the PA and aorta. Such patients usually develop progressive congestive heart failure as the PVR decreases in infancy, requiring PA banding to limit PBF and protect the pulmonary circulation from high flow and pressure that can eventually cause irreversible pulmonary hypertension rendering the patient unsuitable for Fontan completion (Figure 24.2). Finally, an occasional sin-

gle ventricle patient will have a combination of pathologic abnormalities (such as a restrictive VSD with pulmonary stenosis) providing the appropriate amount of PBF and obviating the need for neonatal surgical intervention (see Table 24.1).

Pathophysiology of hypoplastic left heart syndrome

The left ventricle is a nonfunctional structure in the child with HLHS. Pulmonary venous return must be routed to the right atrium through a stretched foramen ovale, an atrial septal defect (ASD), or rarely by total anomalous pulmonary venous connection (Figure 24.3). Systemic and pulmonary venous returns mix in the right atrium. The right ventricle (RV) supplies both the systemic

Table 24.1 Initial surgical strategy for single ventricle patients

Anatomy	Surgical intervention
2 Semilunar Valves of adequate size, normal aortic arch	Pulmonary artery band
1 Semilunar valve, normal aortic arch	BT shunt
1 Semilunar valve, hypoplastic aortic arch	Aortic arch reconstruction with BT shunt, or Norwood procedure
2 Semilunar valves, aortic stenosis	Damus, Kaye, Stanzel with BT shunt (possible aortic arch reconstruction) or palliative arterial switch
2 Semilunar valves with pulmonary stenosis	No initial intervention required

BT, Blalock–Taussig.

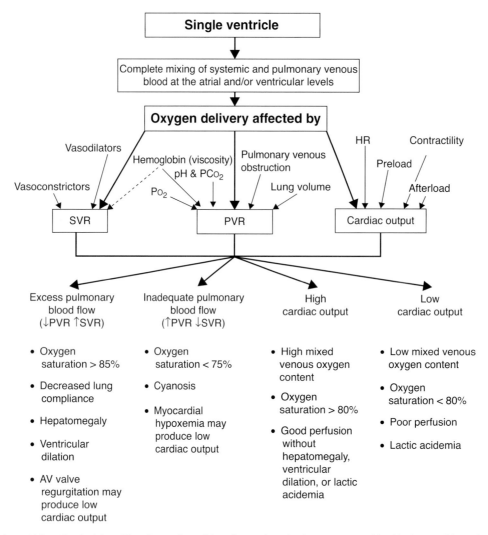

Figure 24.3 Single ventricle pathophysiology. There is complete mixing of systemic and pulmonary venous blood in the ventricle, and oxygen delivery is affected by the balance between the systemic vascular resistance (SVR), the pulmonary vascular resistance (PVR), and the cardiac output. Optimal oxygen delivery is provided by a balance between the SVR and PVR, and maintaining good cardiac output. AV valve, atrioventricular valve; HR, heart rate

and pulmonary circulations in a parallel fashion, since the main PA gives rise to the branch pulmonary arteries as well as the systemic circulation via the ductus arteriosus. Blood flows retrograde from the ductus arteriosus through the transverse aortic arch to its branches, and through the ascending aorta to the coronary arteries. Flow to the lower body is antegrade from the ductus arteriosus via the descending aorta. Ductal closure results in inadequate systemic and coronary perfusion, leading to progressive metabolic acidemia, ischemia, and death.

Although uncommon, ductal narrowing will result in reduced systemic blood flow. The compensatory increase in RV pressure necessary to provide sufficient systemic perfusion may cause an increased pulmonary (Qp) to systemic blood flow (Qs) ratio (Qp:Qs), thereby mimicking the findings of unrestrictive PBF. With the pulmonary and

systemic arteries connected in parallel, the Qp:Qs depends on a delicate balance between the pulmonary and the systemic vascular resistance (SVR).

Stage I reconstruction (Norwood operation)

In 2003, Sano reported improvement in Stage I survival in a small number of patients at one institution when PBF was provided by an RV–PA shunt rather than via a BT shunt [6]. While some centers have demonstrated improvement in Stage I morbidity and mortality and a decrease in interstage death (ISD) with the RV–PA shunt [5,7,8], others have found no difference. All reported studies are significantly limited in interpretation due to selection bias, nonrandomization, historical controls, inadequate number of subjects, and short-term follow-up. A prospective randomized multicenter trial sponsored by the US National Institutes of Health and the Pediatric Heart Network has recently been completed (www.pediatricheartnetwork.org). This study compares risk stratified 1-year survival and freedom from transplant between the two shunts in over 500 patients with publication of results anticipated in 2010.

Theoretical advantages of the RV–PA shunt include higher diastolic pressure and decreased likelihood of thrombosis in a larger conduit. The use of the RV–PA shunt raises other concerns, however, which include increased ventricular volume load, diminished PA growth, and potential for late arrhythmias and cardiac dysfunction secondary to the ventriculotomy. The principal theoretical advantage of the BT shunt is better PA growth. Concerns with the BT shunt include a lower diastolic pressure, which may compromise coronary blood flow and predispose to shunt thrombosis. The basic surgical approach is illustrated in Figure 24.4.

Preoperative management

Much of the preoperative management of neonates with HLHS entails optimizing the condition of the cardiovascular and other organ systems. The key to management of HLHS perioperatively rests with the ability to assess and manipulate systemic perfusion and Qp:Qs. While clinicians have traditionally relied on estimates based upon systemic oxygen saturation, data from Rychik and colleagues comparing the accuracy of Doppler flow patterns in the aorta to other methods of estimating Qp:Qs reveal a weak correlation between systemic oxygen saturation and measured Qp:Qs [10]. Although cumbersome for routine evaluations, Doppler flow patterns are substantially more accurate and precise in evaluation of Qp:Qs. When available, the addition of data to quantify systemic output and Qp:Qs, such as mixed venous oxygen saturation [11,12] or Doppler aortic flow patterns, has greatly improved the assessment and appropriate intervention in neonates with HLHS. This information assumes even greater importance in the volatile physiology exhibited in the early postoperative period.

In the preoperative period, neonates with HLHS who have been stabilized and who are not impaired by other vital organ system dysfunction are initially assumed to be able to maintain a satisfactory Qp:Qs balance. The goal for such patients is to allow spontaneous ventilation via a natural airway, and the majority of neonates are able to meet this objective.

The most common imbalance of Qp:Qs typically manifests itself with signs of inadequate systemic output and relative excess in PBF. These signs might include hypotension, lactic acidosis, and diminished urine output in the context of relatively high systemic oxygen saturation. Once assured of an adequate circulating intravascular volume, oxygen carrying capacity, and a nonrestrictive

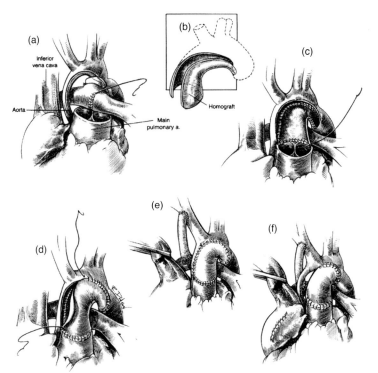

Figure 24.4 The Norwood Stage I palliation for hypoplastic left heart syndrome. (a) Incision of hypoplastic ascending aorta and preparation of the native pulmonary valve to become the neoaortic valve. (b) Cutting of a homograft patch to augment the neoaorta. (c,d) Construction of the neoaorta. (e,f) Completion of the Blalock–Taussig shunt and final anatomy (Reproduced and used with permission from Reference [9])

patent ductus arteriosus, therapeutic measures are often directed at increasing PVR. In order to obtain selective constriction of the pulmonary vasculature, clinicians have employed gas mixtures that either reduced alveolar P_{O_2} [13], promoting hypoxic pulmonary vasoconstriction, or increased alveolar P_{CO_2} [14] to achieve constriction via local effects on pH or tissue CO_2 [15]. Either of these ambient gas manipulations can be accomplished by placing the infant in a hood supplemented with nitrogen or carbon dioxide, respectively. Controversy persists as to the comparative efficacy of these strategies [16]. Caution must be used when altering the inspired gas mixtures in neonates breathing spontaneously while receiving PGE_1 by infusion. Mild hypoventilation can result in significant hypoxemia in neonates breathing an F_{IO_2} below 0.21. Although increased inspired carbon dioxide has been shown to improve oxygen delivery in the anesthetized neonate under conditions of controlled ventilation [17], the increased oxygen consumption associated with carbon dioxide induced tachypnea in the spontaneously breathing patient might negate the benefits observed in the anesthetized patient.

Anatomic variables can have a major impact upon the observed physiology. Some restriction to pulmonary venous return, such as occurs with left-to-right flow across the foramen ovale, is desirable as it tends to balance pulmonary and systemic resistance, and thus Qp:Qs. Infants who lack that restriction, such as those with an ASD or unrestrictive anomalous pulmonary venous return, tend to exhibit high Qp:Qs. In contrast, those who have severely obstructed pulmonary venous return, such as the few who present with an intact atrial septum and no alternative decompressing vein, have an extremely low Qp:Qs. Despite therapeutic maneuvers designed to lower PVR and promote PBF, these infants exhibit marked hypoxemia that requires urgent intervention to decompress pulmonary venous return in order to have any hope of survival.

Preoperative evaluation and stabilization should also include a survey of other vital organ systems for congenital or acquired abnormalities. Our series of 102 newborns with HLHS indicates that approximately 15% have some genetic syndrome or significant noncardiac malformation [18]. The magnitude and distribution of acquired vital organ dysfunction usually relates to circulatory instability at the time of diagnosis. Infants who have suffered a profound or protracted shock state at the time of diagnosis can demonstrate a wide spectrum of injury to renal, central nervous system (CNS), cardiac, gastrointestinal, or hepatic systems [19,20]. These derangements may necessitate a delay in operative intervention to permit recovery.

HLHS is increasingly being diagnosed in utero, allowing for planned management at delivery and optimally yielding greater stability through controlled circumstances. A study of patients with critical left heart obstructive lesions including HLHS showed greater hemodynamic stability and a lower incidence of preoperative neurological events in those patients with prenatal diagnosis [21].

HLHS with obstruction of pulmonary venous outflow

Management changes significantly in the context of an infant with extremely high PVR and very low Qp:Qs, such as the infant with an intact atrial septum. Despite transient hemodynamic and metabolic stability that might ensue with aggressive maneuvers designed to lower PVR and promote PBF, these infants exhibit marked hypoxemia that requires urgent intervention and decompression of the pulmonary venous return in order to have any hope of survival. Our approach to these patients is delivery via Caesarean section adjacent to a hybrid room capable of surgical and/or catheter-based intervention. In most patients, the immediate intervention involves stenting of the interatrial septum with planned completion of Stage I palliation following a period of assessment and recuperation. Between 2006 and the present this management strategy has resulted in survival to hospital discharge following Stage I in 6 of 10 patients. If tolerated hemodynamically, a higher dose of opioid affords the advantage of blunting the response that any noxious stimulus might have on PVR. Substantial ventilation with high F_{IO_2} is typically necessary to achieve marginal gas exchange. When systemic oxygenation falls below a threshold value, temporizing measures designed to diminish metabolic demand deserve strong consideration, such as surface cooling of particularly vulnerable organs (e.g., CNS). The use of sodium bicarbonate to address metabolic acidemia in the face of extremely limited PBF offers limited benefit, and may even pose hazard as the elimination of carbon dioxide following bicarbonate hydrolysis is severely impaired. Thus, bicarbonate administration will often result in a shift from metabolic to respiratory acidemia with little change in pH and the attendant prospect of highly undesirable increase in PVR.

Intraoperative management

Although the vast majority of neonates presenting for Stage I reconstruction (e.g., Norwood or Sano operation) receive an intravenous induction of anesthesia, virtually any anesthetic agent can be used for this purpose with careful attention to the hemodynamic consequences of the technique selected. We prefer the phenylpiperidine-based synthetic opioids (e.g., fentanyl) because they blunt the endogenous catecholamine response to noxious stimuli at doses that are usually tolerated hemodynamically [22–24]. However, even with these hemodynamically "neutral" agents, large doses may result in significant cardiovascular changes, such as bradycardia and hypotension. These observations suggest that the neonate with HLHS requires some endogenous catecholamine release to sustain satisfactory hemodynamics. Unfortunately, this threshold dose that separates "sufficient" from "excessive" varies between patients, necessitating individual titration to arrive at the optimal dose.

Although clinical research conducted nearly two decades ago popularized the view that very large doses of opioid analgesics should be administered perioperatively to effect stress hormone suppression in neonates undergoing cardiac surgery [25], recent efforts to duplicate these findings have not confirmed the original results [26]. The latter demonstrated that very large doses of fentanyl did not completely suppress release of endogenous catecholamines, even in combination with benzodiazepine infusions. Additionally, outcome measures were no different in any of the study groups. We typically employ total intraoperative fentanyl doses between 10 and 20 mcg/kg followed by a fentanyl infusion (1–2 mcg/kg/h) begun postoperatively in the cardiac intensive care unit (CICU) with the target being tracheal extubation on the first postoperative day.

Management of the airway and ventilation assumes great importance during induction of anesthesia. Given the propensity for the majority of neonates with HLHS to exhibit excessive PBF, the anesthesiologist must take care not to employ ventilatory maneuvers that lower PVR, such as hyperventilation with high concentrations of oxygen. In an infant with typical HLHS physiology, one might initiate manual ventilation with air or a low concentration of supplemental oxygen. The extent to which the anesthesiologist adjusts FIO_2 prior to laryngoscopy would depend upon the magnitude of hemodynamic response to the initiation of controlled ventilation. Infants who demonstrate significant reduction in systemic arterial pressure despite low FIO_2 may not tolerate prolonged exposure to high FIO_2 without deleterious hemodynamic consequences. Means of increasing PVR, as discussed previously, should be available in the operating room. We favor inspired CO_2 for several reasons. It tends to augment systemic arterial pressure immediately and does not require neutralization of all safety systems designed to avoid delivery of a hypoxic gas mixture. Also, as a gas of some historical importance in anesthesia delivery systems, it is available with flow meters in appropriate clinical ranges. Tabbutt et al., in a clinical comparison of intubated, paralyzed, and anesthetized neonates with HLHS, demonstrated that inspired CO_2 proved consistently more effective than hypoxic gas mixtures at increasing indices of systemic output, including systemic arterial pressure and oxygen delivery [17].

Intraoperative monitoring consists of continuous invasive arterial pressure in addition to standard cardiovascular, respiratory, and temperature monitors. Whenever possible umbilical arterial lines are utilized in patients during first stage surgery in order to preserve access for future interventions. In order to minimize the hazard of thrombosis in the central thoracic veins in all single ventricle patients, we employ direct transthoracic atrial lines in lieu of percutaneous jugular or subclavian central venous pressure catheters. In addition, an umbilical venous catheter positioned in the orifice of the superior vena cava (SVC) at the time of surgery serves as a valuable monitor of mixed venous oxygen saturation, enabling more precise assessment of systemic CO and Qp:Qs [11,12,17].

At the termination of cardiopulmonary bypass (CPB), the physiologic goals are identical to those expressed preoperatively, although the proclivities are quite different. The pulmonary circulation now resides at either the distal end of a restrictive prosthetic systemic-to-pulmonary shunt or an RV–PA tube graft (Sano modification—Figure 24.5). A variety of subtleties in the technical execution of either shunt, relief of atrial obstruction, and preexisting condition of the pulmonary circulation can render the ultimate physiology somewhat unpredictable. Technical issues of graft insertion, proper graft size (particularly in the neonate under 2.0 kg), and the ability to delineate the etiology of insufficient PBF on termination of CPB introduce additional complexities in a number of patients where a Sano modification has been performed.

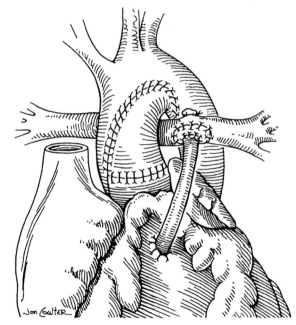

Figure 24.5 The Sano modification of the Norwood Stage I operation. Instead of a right modified Blalock–Taussig shunt, pulmonary blood flow is provided by a right ventricle to pulmonary artery conduit, usually a 5-mm Goretex® graft (Reproduced and used with permission from Reference [5])

Measures to assure a clear airway and complete reexpansion of the pulmonary parenchyma are performed in the terminal phases of rewarming on bypass. The magnitude of reduction in the mean systemic arterial pressure that occurs with trial opening of the shunt during the terminal phase on CPB can provide qualitative insights as to what PVR one might expect in the early postbypass period. Initial ventilatory support should be adjusted accordingly. In general, we begin with a pattern of ventilation designed to result in low-normal $PaCO_2$ and an FIO_2 between 0.6 and 1, recognizing that adjustments become necessary in all patients as indicated by the individual infant's physiology. In addition, the physiology typically demonstrates dynamic change over time, requiring continuous surveillance and further adjustment. Assuming a technically satisfactory repair and no unusual risk factors, PVR typically falls in the first few hours after surgery.

Despite a perfect technical result, the Norwood operation does not result in any reduction of the volume or pressure burden placed on the single ventricle, as the physiology of parallel systemic and pulmonary circulations with a Qp:Qs of unity remains the objective throughout the postoperative period. Yet the heart incurs the cost of insults related to cessation of coronary perfusion, CPB, and deep hypothermic circulatory arrest (DHCA). This may account for the cardiovascular frailty exhibited by these infants in the early postoperative period. However, in the absence of major deficiencies in myocardial protection or persistent anatomic residua such as significant aortic arch obstruction, coronary compromise, or valvular insufficiency, myocardial dysfunction can usually be ameliorated with relatively modest doses of inotropic agents (e.g., dopamine at 3–5 mcg/kg/min) and vasodilation. In a postoperative time course characteristic of many major cardiac interventions in neonates and young infants, myocardial performance may deteriorate in the first 6–12 hours postoperatively before it begins to improve. As a result, we routinely take measures to reduce metabolic demands by provision of continuous neuromuscular relaxant (pancuronium 0.035–0.1 mg/kg/h) and opioid (fentanyl 1–2 mcg/kg/h) infusions. Infants demonstrating increased SVR during rewarming on CPB often receive a loading dose of milrinone at that time. Zuppa et al. described the pharmacokinetics of milrinone in 16 neonates with HLHS given a loading dose of milrinone on CPB at the time of rewarming [27]. These investigators recommended a loading dose of 100 μg/kg, followed by initiation of an infusion of 0.2 μg/kg/min within 90 minutes of the bolus dose to achieve and maintain plasma concentrations similar to those reported in other therapeutic settings. No data exist to guide bolus and/or infusion doses when milrinone is begun after termination of CPB.

Modified ultrafiltration (MUF) conducted immediately following CPB has been demonstrated to exert beneficial effects upon hematocrit, hemodynamics, hemostasis, pulmonary function, and CNS recovery [28–32]. Perioperative weight gain is reduced significantly as are certain inflammatory mediator levels. Whenever possible, we conduct MUF at the termination of CPB following Stage I reconstruction. Occasionally, the position of the bypass cannulae or the continuous flux of blood through the MUF circuit results in unfavorable hemodynamic changes precluding completion of the filtration. In 99 consecutive patients undergoing Stage I between September 2000 and August 2002, all tolerated the hemodynamic perturbations of MUF [33].

Stage I reconstruction requires substantial suture lines in creation of the neoaorta, thus rapid restoration of normal hemostasis represents an important early postoperative objective. Following completion of MUF, and once satisfied with the technical and physiologic result of the repair, heparin effect is reversed with protamine. Given the risk factors that jeopardize platelet number and function, including deep hypothermia and profound dilution of circulating volume on CPB [34], replacement of blood loss with fresh whole blood (<48-h old) restores hemostasis more effectively than other blood products [35]. Fresh whole blood replacement also serves to minimize donor exposure to these patients who are anticipated to require a minimum of three open-heart surgical interventions. Despite the theoretical advantages of fresh whole blood, other studies have not demonstrated a benefit of this strategy versus reconstituted whole blood [36]. In addition, fresh whole blood is not available in the great majority of institutions. A recent publication demonstrated that a reconstituted fresh whole blood bypass prime, consisting of packed red blood cells, fresh frozen plasma, and platelets from the same donor, less than 7 days old, followed by a second such unit given after bypass, reduced bleeding in infants undergoing surgery compared to standard blood component therapy [37]. Should these measures fail to achieve adequate hemostasis despite elimination of all surgical bleeding sites, laboratory testing should be conducted to direct component therapy at those elements of the hemostatic pathway most likely to be impaired: platelet and fibrinogen replacement.

No systematic data have been published specifically examining procoagulant medications in infants undergoing Stage I reconstruction, and only sparse data exists examining neonates as a group. Antifibrinolytic therapies have demonstrated efficacy in infants and children following heart surgery, but data in neonates continues to be very limited [38–41]. The lysine analogs epsilon aminocaproic acid (EACA) and tranexamic acid (TA) appear to have comparable efficacy [38,41], and extensive experience implying safety, although there are insufficient pediatric follow-up data to validate their safety scientifically. Their benefit is probably most notable in high-risk patient populations, such as cyanotic patients undergoing extensive operations. While aprotinin, a serine protease inhibitor that acts as an antifibrinolytic agent with anti-inflammatory properties, has demonstrated effectiveness comparable to other antifibrinolytics in infants and children [35], this agent was voluntarily removed from the market when it was linked to greater 5-year mortality following coronary bypass grafting [42]. Recombinant activated Factor VII (rFVIIa) has been used as rescue therapy in infants and children, including neonates undergoing Stage I reconstruction, following cardiac surgery when conventional correction of postoperative coagulopathy with blood product transfusions fails to control hemorrhage [43,44]. While rFVIIa can be effective in controlling intractable hemorrhage, caution is warranted, as systematic studies of safety and efficacy have not been conducted [39]. Among procoagulant therapies, rFVIIa is uniquely capable of producing a hypercoagulable state that poses risks to certain surgical repair elements such as prosthetic shunts.

Prompt control of hemostasis resulting in reduced transfusion requirement can be associated with a reduced need for reexploration for bleeding. Reexploration in patients younger than 2 years undergoing complex surgery at our institution, which includes all single ventricle patients, was reduced from 3 to 0.8% following adoption of the routine use of fresh whole blood. Cardiac tamponade can easily occur from a small quantity of mediastinal blood accumulated in the early postoperative period before bleeding has completely ceased. Continuous removal is essential because blockage easily occurs in the relatively small mediastinal drainage tubes of these neonates. A technique of active, continuous aspiration of accumulating blood from the mediastinum has virtually eliminated this complication [45].

Common problems in the early postbypass period

Excessive hypoxemia represents one of the more commonly encountered problems in the early postbypass period. Although inadequate Qp:Qs becomes the assumed cause, factors that impair systemic oxygen delivery thereby reducing mixed venous oxygen saturation are now known to be more common than previously believed [10–12,46]. One typically observes a progressive increase in systemic oxygen saturation during MUF, e.g., probably due to the impact that hemoconcentration and the resulting increased oxygen delivery have upon mixed venous oxygen saturation. Thereafter, measures directed at maintaining hematocrit above 40–45% may alleviate excessive demands placed upon the recovering heart to increase systemic output. The distinction between systemic hypoxemia due to low Qp:Qs, low pulmonary venous oxygen saturation, or low mixed venous saturation is a critical one, as the therapies are diametrically different. Measures designed to reduce PVR will impose a further volume load on a heart already struggling to provide marginal systemic perfusion. Patients demonstrating low SVO_2 are better served with therapies that promote systemic output, such as inotropic agents or vasodilators.

Similarly, those with low pulmonary venous oxygen saturation require a strategy of ventilatory support designed to reduce atelectasis and promote gas exchange in impaired alveoli. Unfortunately, the latter diagnosis is rarely made definitively in the operating room or cardiac ICU, as blood sampling from the pulmonary veins presents logistic challenges. Intraoperatively, expectant measures directed at expansion of the lungs and maintenance of normal functional residual capacity (FRC) usually suffice to avoid pulmonary vein desaturation. Among the three etiologies of persistent systemic hypoxemia, this was believed to be the least common, but a recent series found pulmonary vein desaturation in as many as 30% of patients [47].

When systemic hypoxemia occurs due to low Qp:Qs, other manifestations provide supporting evidence. Trial opening of the systemic-to-pulmonary artery shunt during the latter phases of rewarming on CPB fails to demonstrate significant drop in the mean systemic arterial pressure and early postbypass hemodynamics reveal a relatively narrow pulse pressure and/or high diastolic pressure. A substantial discrepancy exists between arterial and end-tidal CO_2 measurements. These suggestive pieces of inferential evidence can be confirmed by aortic Doppler flow analysis or calculation of a Fick ratio using oxygen saturation determinations. Most commonly, diminished PBF reflects a subtle technical aspect of the arch reconstruction, innominate artery dimension, or the BT shunt. However, certain patient subsets exhibit profound abnormalities in the pulmonary vasculature that result in excessive PVR elevations. Neonates with HLHS routinely demonstrate extremely high and volatile PVR when born with severe pulmonary venous obstruction due to intact atrial septum without alternative decompressing veins. Even the typical HLHS anatomic constellation is associated with marked abnormalities in the number and muscularization of the pulmonary vasculature by pathologic examination [48]. Hypotheses attribute these changes to chronic fetal pulmonary venous obstruction [49]. One can speculate that these changes become more extreme in the context of the marked obstruction caused by HLHS with intact atrial septum. Fetal echocardiography has confirmed alteration in pulmonary venous flow pattern in relation to the magnitude of restriction at the atrial septum [50].

In the context of hypoxemia due to low Qp:Qs, interventions fall into three categories: technical, pulmonary vasodilation, and systemic vasoconstriction. In the subgroup of patients expected to have unusually elevated PVR, modifications in surgical technique might entail placement of a larger shunt or shunt interposition between a larger systemic vessel (e.g., aorta) and pulmonary arteries. Pulmonary vasodilator therapy includes the strategies one might employ in any patient demonstrating elevated PVR, such as oxygen, moderate hyperventilation, normothermia, alkali, and nitric oxide [51–53]. Should those measures prove insufficient to result in adequate PBF, the focus might be expanded to include measures designed to increase the driving pressure across the shunt, using higher doses of inotropic infusions or even vasoconstrictors. The latter necessitates careful monitoring to avoid jeopardizing perfusion to other vital organs.

Depressed myocardial performance represents another potential problem in the early postbypass period. As mentioned previously, some degree of myocardial dysfunction typically occurs following this Stage I palliation as there is no hemodynamic benefit achieved to offset the cost of CPB and an ischemic interval. When this dysfunction becomes more significant than usual, specific causes should be sought. Even in the context of the typical conduct of stage I reconstruction, the consequences of aortic atresia make routine myocardial protection measures, such as the infusion of cardioplegia solutions, challenging. Thus inadequate myocardial preservation represents one potential cause for persisting or excessive myocardial depression.

Technical considerations represent the predominant cause of myocardial dysfunction following this complex intervention. One of the most intricate aspects of this procedure is the reconstruction of an aortic arch in such a way that the small ascending aorta, which principally serves to provide coronary flow, is not compromised. This subtle finding may not become evident until the cardiac volume is restored in anticipation of terminating CPB. Residual hemodynamic derangement represents another potential cause of myocardial dysfunction. Given that under the best of circumstances, one emerges from the Norwood operation with no appreciable hemodynamic benefit, one would expect a result with newly imposed volume or pressure loads to be poorly tolerated. Examples of such findings would include residual aortic arch obstruction, atrioventricular valve dysfunction, and/or semilunar valve obstruction or regurgitation.

Metabolic disturbances can also result in significant myocardial dysfunction. A fragile RV struggling to cope with significantly increased volume output demands at systemic pressure is perhaps more susceptible to what might otherwise be modest metabolic disturbances. As such, one should track and address those variables that have impact upon myocardial performance, such as ionized calcium and lactic acidosis. The rapid administration of blood products, e.g., which contain calcium-binding drugs, high levels of potassium and lactic acid, as well as other vasoac-

tive mediators, can result in an acute, profound deterioration in cardiac performance in the early postoperative period. In our experience, myocardial performance will deteriorate when the arterial pH falls below 7.3 and may contribute to further reduction in Qs. The administration of intravenous bicarbonate, calculated to completely eliminate the base deficit, often exerts a beneficial effect on both myocardial performance and Qs. In addition to the inherent cardiac sensitivity, inescapable anatomic peculiarities accentuate this vulnerability. Blood carrying the transfused products from the systemic venous circulation enters the RV and is directed immediately to the reconstructed aorta, whereby the first branch is the coronary circulation. Thus constituents of the transfused blood (e.g., citrate, potassium, lactate) infused into the venous circulation arrives at the coronary arteries with greater speed and concentration than might have occurred had they been dissipated over the course of the pulmonary vasculature before entering the aorta. This effect is further accentuated if central venous catheters are employed to infuse the blood product. We abide by a protocol whereby blood transfused via central lines or rapidly through peripheral catheters is either less than 7 days of age or washed packed cells.

Arrhythmias most commonly occur as manifestations of the problems described previously. When they become manifest early in the process of rewarming on CPB, coronary insufficiency represents the most common cause, particularly if the arrhythmia is ventricular in origin. Metabolic disturbances produce the same qualitative rhythm changes seen in normal hearts, although the manifestations might be more extreme. Given the predominantly extracardiac nature of the Norwood procedure, acquired heart block rarely follows this operation unless it existed preoperatively. On rare occasions, a patient presents with HLHS and a primary arrhythmia, such as Wolf–Parkinson–White syndrome.

Excessive PBF may complicate the early postoperative period; however, this diagnosis should be entertained cautiously. In many instances, the apparent excess PBF really reflects a relative imbalance with respect to significantly diminished systemic CO (Qs). The latter should be specifically excluded and addressed before invoking extreme measures to restrict PBF. Of course, subtle technical differences in the conduct of the operation can result in an anatomic propensity to an excessive Qp:Qs, and this can, in turn, jeopardize systemic perfusion. Such patients typically exhibit an extremely wide pulse pressure or low diastolic pressure reflecting pulmonary "runoff." If myocardial performance otherwise appears robust, the specific measures employed to increase PVR preoperatively are appropriate in this setting. In most patients, this condition dissipates as the infant recovers from surgery. Should the problem persist beyond the first postoperative day, a cardiac catheterization should be considered to evaluate the need for further surgical intervention aimed at diminishing PBF.

The subset of patients who demonstrate inability to separate from CPB or refractory cardiac dysfunction postoperatively may benefit from utilization of extracorporeal membrane oxygenation (ECMO) as a support strategy. Ungerleider and colleagues have advocated the routine use of mechanical ventricular assistance in all patients following Stage I reconstruction, reporting 89% survival to hospital discharge [54]. More recently a retrospective review of patients who required nonelective institution of ECMO either in the operating room or CICU revealed a 38.8% survival to hospital discharge. Significantly, all patients with acute shunt thrombosis were early survivors. Risk factors for mortality in this patient population included longer CPB time, need for institution of ECMO <24 hours postoperatively, cannulation via the chest, and longer duration of ECMO support [55].

The volume work of the single ventricle after Stage I reconstruction is equal to the sum of the systemic and PBF (Qp + Qs). After a period of maturation of the pulmonary vasculature, systemic venous return may be directed to the pulmonary arteries, thus placing the two circulations in series. When Fontan's operation was uniformly undertaken 12–18 months after Stage I, an operative mortality of 16–40% occurred [56]. The most common cause of early death was low CO associated with tachycardia, low systolic and diastolic blood pressures, and high ventricular end-diastolic pressures. The majority of patients with signs of low CO demonstrated echocardiographic evidence of an abrupt change in ventricular geometry that resulted in a small, thick-walled cavity with a low diastolic volume when compared to the preoperative state. Although systolic shortening appeared normal, the ventricular compliance was diminished. The physiologic result was impaired diastolic function of the ventricle resulting in increased end-diastolic pressure. The resulting increase in pulmonary venous pressure impeded PBF, thereby reducing systemic output. Retrospective analysis of the data available preoperatively proved insufficient to predict those children who would develop physiologically important reduction of ventricular compliance associated with rapid contraction of end-diastolic volume following single-stage Fontan.

Outcomes

Since the introduction of a viable reconstructive strategy for patients with HLHS, outcomes have improved dramatically. Centers with the greatest experience in staged reconstruction typically report survival from the Norwood operation between 86 and 93% in patients with "standard" risk [57–60]. Stasik et al. evaluated 111 patients operated

on at a single institution between May 2001 and April 2003 and found weight <2.5 kg at time of operation and noncardiac abnormalities to be independent risk factors using multivariate analysis. Patients with either of these risk characteristics had a hospital survival of 52% compared to 86% in those with standard risk [61]. Gaynor and colleagues assessed 158 neonates who underwent the Norwood procedure between January 1998 and June 2001 and identified the following risk factors: birth weight of less than 2–2.5 kg, presence of a genetic syndrome or noncardiac anomaly, additional cardiac risk factors including obstruction to pulmonary venous return, tricuspid regurgitation, severe ventricular dysfunction, and preoperative shock. Survival was improved (86% vs 66%) in those patients without risk factors [18].

Generally accepted risk factors include prematurity, low birth weight, noncardiac anomalies, and severely restrictive inter-atrial communication in utero. Aortic atresia was initially believed to be an independent risk factor that has subsequently been refined to those with associated mitral stenosis [55], possibly linked to a subset with LV–coronary fistulae [58]. Alone or in combination, these risk factors can result in substantial reduction in survival rates from the Norwood operation to between 53 and 79%. This finding has generated interest in developing alternative strategies for high-risk subpopulations, such as fetal interventions and the hybrid procedures described below [58,62–65]. Fetal intervention to relieve severe inter-atrial restriction has shown promise in small series [58], with 6-month survival 69% versus 38% in those who had this obstruction addressed immediately after birth, although the small numbers in this series did not have sufficient statistical power. This benefit may relate to interrupting the development of "arterialization" of the pulmonary veins, which creates sustained increases in PVR [57]. While these superb results have been sustained across a group of centers for whom HLHS is a common diagnosis, an international survey of institutions treating HLHS revealed that nearly 70% see fewer than 20 cases each year [66] and the results from lower volume institutions have not been systematically reported.

The observation that HLHS survivors of the Norwood operation exhibit significant mortality between discharge and superior cavopulmonary anastomosis (SCPA) has given rise to much speculation prompting alterations in the nature of Stage I reconstruction and interstage timing. In various series, this interstage mortality ranges from 5 to 18% [58,67–70]. Although the reasons for this interstage mortality are unknown, speculation exists that a contributing mechanism is acute coronary insufficiency exacerbated by diastolic runoff through the BT shunt. Significant reductions in coronary perfusion have been demonstrated in neonates following Norwood operation lending credence to this hypothesis [71]. In order to improve diastolic coronary flow characteristics, several centers returned to a revised RV–PV conduit as proposed by Sano [58,67–70,72]. While some series have suggested reduction in interstage mortality [58,67], the finding has not been consistently observed [69,73]. A multi-institutional trial is currently underway to examine this potential benefit against theoretical disadvantages of the Sano modification, e.g., diminished PBF and vascular development, regurgitant volume into the RV, and arrhythmogenic hazard of right ventriculotomy [74].

Feeding difficulties are widely prevalent among neonates following Stage I procedures [74,75]. When compared to a group of neonates following arterial switch operation for transposition of the great arteries, Stage I survivors took twice as long to achieve full enteral caloric intake [75]. In part, this finding probably relates to the underlying physiology that leaves Stage I survivors with a significant residual ventricular volume load. In addition, they are more likely to have postoperative vocal cord paresis and gastroesophageal reflux. As a result, only 25% in some series are able to consume all their necessary calories orally [75], although the figure is closer to 80% in others [73,76]. Even hybrid procedure survivors required feeding gastrostomy in 15% [62], corroborating the contribution of underlying physiology. An intriguing observation in preoperative magnetic resonance imaging (MRI) studies has revealed a subtle brain underdevelopment of the operculum, an area associated with feeding and swallowing [57]. More serious gastrointestinal complications, such as necrotizing enterocolitis, are more likely as well. Depending upon the sensitivity of diagnostic criteria, as many as 18% of infants following Stage I reconstruction meet Bell Stage I criteria for necrotizing enterocolitis [76]. These tend to be infants under 3 kg and those with higher PRISM scores.

Hybrid procedure

Despite continuing improvements in the perioperative management of infants with HLHS, certain populations of patients remain at high risk and demonstrate a more significant level of morbidity and mortality during and after surgical Stage I palliation [77]. In general, these risk factors include birth weight <2.5 kg, gestational age <34 weeks, ascending aortic size <2 mm, poor ventricular function, severe tricuspid regurgitation, restrictive atrial septum, and the presence of additional cardiac or noncardiac anomalies [65,78]. Continuing advancements in interventional cardiology techniques have facilitated the development of alternative therapeutic strategies for these subpopulations of patients; due to the utilization of both surgical and interventional catheterization procedures, these interventions are known as "hybrid" procedures. Advan-

tages of hybrid procedures include the avoidance of CPB and/or DHCA in the neonatal period, as well as the provision of an extended waiting period for infants who either require cardiac transplantation or who may be eligible for biventricular repair.

Physiologic goals of a hybrid procedure include the provision of unobstructed systemic flow through the ductus arteriosus, protection of the pulmonary vascular bed, and assurance of adequate intra-atrial communication for left heart decompression. These objectives are achieved by placement of right and left PA bands to optimize balance between the pulmonary and systemic circulations, along with stenting of the ductus arteriosus for provision of unobstructed systemic flow. If atrial intervention is necessary, unobstructed atrial communication can be achieved either via balloon angioplasty, blade septostomy, or placement of an atrial stent. Modifications to the hybrid procedure continue to occur as newer devices become available, such as internal self-expanding nitinol flow restrictors which can be utilized in place of external, surgically placed PA bands, allowing all components of the hybrid procedure to be accomplished in the catheterization laboratory [79].

As with surgically palliated patients interstage mortality continues to be an issue. Close echocardiographic monitoring for tricuspid valve regurgitation and/or RV dysfunction as indicators for obstruction at the atrial level or through the PDA stent has been advocated and reinterventions in the catheterization laboratory are not infrequently required to relieve such obstructions [80]. The most concerning and potentially life-threatening complication involves the development of reverse or preductal coarctation, which can result in diminished coronary and cerebral perfusion occurring either secondary to uncovered ductal tissue that remains capable of closure, or as a result of placement of the ductal stent. Once recognized additional placement of a retrograde stent is utilized to address proximal arch obstruction [81].

At the age of 3–6 months, aortic reconstruction, along with removal of the PA bands, ductal and atrial stents, repair of the pulmonary arteries (if necessary), atrial septectomy, and superior cavopulmonary connection (SCPA) is performed in a comprehensive second-stage surgical procedure. Patients subsequently progress to Fontan procedure completion either via surgical approach or placement of a covered stent via catheter intervention [82].

Although reported survival statistics for high-risk patients do not appear to vary significantly from those achieved via traditional Stage I palliation [64], Galantowicz and colleagues recently reported overall survival of 82.5% in a cohort of 62 patients without known high-risk characteristics, with 15 patients having completed the Fontan procedure [62]. With continuing experience and technical modifications, the hybrid procedure may allow increased survival opportunity for high-risk patients and those awaiting cardiac transplantation or the potential for biventricular repair.

Initial management for other univentricular heart malformations

Although HLHS represents the most common anatomic constellation resulting in a single functional ventricle, many other forms exist (e.g., tricuspid atresia). In fact, these malformations may formerly have appeared to be more common than HLHS because they survive without the need for complex reconstructive surgery in the neonatal period and hence were much more prevalent during childhood before Stage I reconstruction was developed as a viable option for neonates with HLHS.

The management of other single ventricle malformations strives for the same physiologic goals as Stage I: balanced Qp:Qs, unobstructed flow from the single ventricle to the systemic circulation, and conditions in the pulmonary circulation that promote the fall in PVR that normally occurs with maturation. The latter typically entails assurance that no resistance to pulmonary venous return exists and pulmonary arterial flow is subjected to an anatomic restriction that limits Qp:Qs ratio to unity. For example, tricuspid atresia variants may require a range of interventions in the neonatal period, depending on their anatomy. Those with ductal-dependent PBF will require a systemic-to-pulmonary artery shunt to provide a balanced Qp:Qs. Variants with associated VSD may have adequate PBF without a shunt. A small subgroup with tricuspid atresia and a large VSD may exhibit excessive PBF requiring a PA band to achieve a Qp:Qs of 1.

Evolution of staged approach to Fontan

Many programs have adopted a systematic staged approach to the Fontan operation for all patients with univentricular hearts in an effort to reduce the volume load of the ventricle as early as possible and to minimize the impact of rapid changes in ventricular geometry and diastolic function that accompany primary Fontan [83]. Two options have gained acceptance as the first step of the staged Fontan: bidirectional Glenn [84] or hemi-Fontan [85]. The SVC is divided and anastomosed to the undivided pulmonary arteries, creating a bidirectional cavopulmonary (Glenn) shunt (Figure 24.6). This source of PBF may be exclusive if the previous shunt is ligated, or additive if they are not. When previous sources are occluded, it provides the same physiologic benefit as hemi-Fontan and can be performed without bypass. During hemi-Fontan, all systemic-to-pulmonary artery

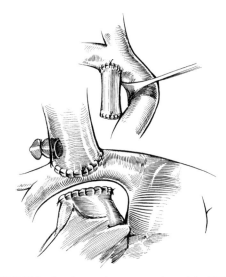

Figure 24.6 Bidirectional cavopulmonary anastomosis (or bidirectional Glenn shunt). *Top*, the previous right modified Blalock–Taussig shunt is divided and ligated, and (*bottom*) the superior vena cava is anastomosed to the right pulmonary artery (Reproduced and used with permission from Reference [86])

shunts are ligated, and PBF is achieved exclusively via an SVC–PA anastomosis. Certain technical features of the hemi-Fontan make it, in our opinion, a more logical step in the process of eventual completion of the Fontan. First, it enables elimination of stenosis or distortion of the branch pulmonary arteries and their confluence. Second, the normal relation of the SVC to the right atrium is preserved. As bypass is needed, other coexisting anatomical risk factors can be addressed. Thirdly, it simplifies execution of the Fontan itself.

Interstage evaluation and interventions

Interstage death refers to infants who die following hospital discharge after the Norwood procedure and prior to admission for planned Stage II reconstruction. ISD rates are unchanged in most centers over time and remain between 4 and 15%. Because of the improvement in out-of-hospital survival for the neonatal surgery, ISD constitutes an increasing percentage of the overall mortality in the current era. In an attempt to identify the risk factor(s) for ISD, Hehir conducted a retrospective case control study of 368 consecutive neonates undergoing the Norwood procedure between January 1998 and August 2005 in a single center [87]. Intact atrial septum and older age at time of operation were independent risk factors using multivariate analysis. The heterogeneous nature of events resulting in death makes it unlikely that a single medical or surgical intervention will impact ISD. Ghanayem demonstrated a marked reduction in ISD (15.8–0%) with the initiation of standardized home surveillance that monitored two physiological variables daily: arterial oxygen saturation and body weight. When a derangement in either variable was identified (13 of 24 patients), early Stage II was undertaken. Outcomes for Stage II at an earlier age (3.7 vs 5.2 months of age) and beyond were no different between the two groups [88].

Superior cavopulmonary anastomosis

Preoperative assessment

The conversion from a circulation based upon complete mixing and parallel perfusion of both the systemic and pulmonary vascular beds via an arterial shunt to a "series" circulation where PBF becomes a diversion of systemic venous return requires certain preconditions. In essence, the flow of blood through the pulmonary circulation must be free of significant impediments in order that systemic venous pressure does not reach physiologically unacceptable levels. These potential impediments take three forms: elevated PVR, atrioventricular valve dysfunction, and diminished ventricular compliance. Elevated PVR encompasses two distinct mechanisms: the size of the major branches or the state of the arteriolar resistance vessels. In patients with HLHS, one must also confirm that no obstruction to flow exists at the remnant of the atrial septum. With the caveat that systemic venous pressures of 16 mm Hg or less are generally tolerated without significant sequelae, while those 20 mm Hg and over are associated with a variety of morbidities, very small differences distinguish those who do well with the operation from those who have a poor outcome. Candidates for SCPA have routinely undergone cardiac catheterization prior to surgery, but more recently noninvasive methods of assessing the anatomy and physiology such as cardiac MRI have been successfully utilized in patients who do not require catheter-based interventions before surgery [89,90]. Knowledge of PVR, ventricular end-diastolic pressure, AV valve function, and any residual obstruction at the atrial septum remnant is desirable prior to surgical intervention. In addition, anatomic information about the PA architecture is obtained via contrast injection to evaluate for the presence of accessory venous communications between the superior venous drainage and the heart or inferior vena cava (IVC) (e.g., left SVC to coronary sinus). Postoperatively, such vessels could serve as a mechanism by which upper body venous return is diverted to the heart without passing through the pulmonary circulation, thereby resulting in unanticipated levels of hypoxemia.

These data can be used to estimate the SVC pressure on completion of SCPA. Recognizing that this formula requires several assumptions that render it an oversimplification, one can estimate the postoperative SVC pressure

as follows:

$$P_{SVC} = \left(\frac{(P_{PA} - P_{PV})(Q_{PA} : Q_{SA})}{Q_{PB} : Q_{PB}} \right) + P_{LA}$$

Where P_{SVC} and P_{LA} represent the pressure determinations in the SVC postoperatively, and the left atrium, respectively.

Where P_{PA} and P_{PV} are the preoperative pressures in the PA and vein, respectively.

Where $Q_{PB}:Q_{SB}$ and $Q_{PA}:Q_{SA}$ are the Qp:Qs ratios before and after SCPA, respectively.

In infants approximately 6 months of age, we estimate the proportion of venous return coming from the upper body to be roughly equal to that from the lower body, although SVC flow may comprise as much as 60–70% of the total venous return in some. In other words, $Q_{PB}:Q_{SB}$ approximates 0.5–0.7. For example, assuming the following hemodynamics measured preoperatively: $P_{PA} = 17$, $P_{PV} = 8$, Qp:Qs = 1.5, and $P_{LA} = 8$, the P_{SVC} postoperatively = $\left(\frac{(17-8)(0.5)}{1.5} \right) + 8 = 11$].

Unfortunately, several of the assumptions limit this sort of calculation to the level of a crude estimate. P_{PA} is notoriously difficult to measure accurately when the only source of PBF is a systemic–pulmonary shunt. Catheters placed across the shunt probably alter PBF while they are present, while PV wedge pressures to estimate P_{PA} have a variety of limitations, particularly if PVR is elevated. The ventricular compliance is dynamic as well, particularly in the context of significant changes in ventricular volume and pressure loading conditions. In addition, the imposition of CPB and an ischemic interval have a negative impact on ventricular compliance, albeit a transient one if the operation proceeds according to plan. Finally, the Qp:Qs determinations depend upon PVR, which might be altered by the medications employed to sedate an infant for catheterization. Despite all the limitations, however, this estimate does help to predict problem patients as well as the type of problem they might encounter, whether PVR, ventricular compliance, or AV valve function.

Preoperative assessment should also incorporate an evaluation of other vital organ systems with a history of primary or secondary dysfunction. For patients receiving anticoagulant medications or functional platelet inhibitors, plans for the cessation of those therapies must be formalized. Careful history regarding the child's response to sedative medications should also be elicited.

Intraoperative management

Infants typically return for SCPA between 4 and 8 months of age. Given their developmental stage and prior hospital experiences, many will manifest separation anxiety when taken from the parents. Thus, unless they have some contraindication, sedative premedication is administered orally prior to surgery. Although a variety of sedative potions are available, we prefer pentobarbital 4 mg/kg given orally because of its potency and duration of action. When administered 45–60 minutes in advance, a high proportion of patients will be sleeping. This serves to allay parental anxiety and also facilitates induction with a volatile inhaled anesthetic agent, if that is the planned technique.

Anesthesia can be induced with a variety of intravenous or inhaled agents. Unless the preoperative evaluation has revealed myocardial dysfunction or significant unusual hemodynamic loading conditions (e.g., arch obstruction, AV valve insufficiency), these infants generally tolerate nearly normal doses of anesthetic agents without manifesting untoward cardiovascular effects. We usually employ a combination of inhaled anesthetic, opioid, and muscle relaxant. Most commonly, the total opioid administered for the case is the equivalent of fentanyl 5–10 mcg/kg, with the desired goal sufficient emergence from the anesthetic effect to permit tracheal extubation on arrival to the cardiac ICU.

Although these infants at the time of anesthetic induction have the same anatomy and physiology as the newborn following Stage I, subtle changes have occurred in the intervening months that make them significantly more resilient. Maturation and compensatory mechanisms in myocardial development render the heart more capable of managing the excess volume load of a parallel circulation. In addition, through differential growth, the shunt is more restrictive, protecting the infant from excessive acute volume loads irrespective of manipulations that lower PVR significantly. Finally, the baseline PVR is low, so even extreme measures cannot produce a substantial reduction in PVR from baseline values, therefore any Qp:Qs change is comparably small. Nevertheless, we try to minimize any additional volume burden that might be placed on the ventricle prior to CPB and planned ischemia by minimizing supplemental oxygen delivery and ventilating to normocapnia.

All standard noninvasive monitors are applied for induction. An intra-arterial catheter is placed for continuous monitoring following tracheal intubation. The site selected for this catheter varies according to a variety of considerations related to congenital or acquired vascular anomalies. The placement of a BT shunt may have compromised the ipsilateral subclavian artery. In addition, previous monitoring and catheterization sites may not be available. There are also a variety of aortic arch branching patterns some of which result in stenosis of the subclavian supply. Noninvasive arterial pressure measurement on all four extremities provides the data necessary to identify the appropriate site(s). Cannulation of the central veins via the jugular or subclavian is avoided out of concern for the implications of thrombosis in those vessels.

Unlike Stage I, the SCPA provides significant hemodynamic benefit. With occlusion of the shunt, the circulations are no longer connected in parallel, thereby reducing the volume output demand for the RV to that necessary to perfuse the systemic circulation alone. PBF becomes a diversion for venous return from the upper body, effecting a "series" circulation of a pump and two resistors. Since the volume of blood flow to the upper body is at least as great as that to the lower body at 6 months of age, the mixture of oxygenated and deoxygenated blood remains 1:1, or higher. Thus, the expected systemic oxygen saturation tends to increase slightly, but the heart need only accomplish half the volume work (Qs) to accomplish this. Most patients exhibit robust hemodynamics on completion of this procedure. Although we usually infuse low-dose dopamine (1–3 mcg/kg/min) via the atrial catheter, it may not be necessary in many patients. Infants exhibiting substantial diastolic dysfunction or valvular regurgitation may benefit from an inodilator such as milrinone. When anticipated on the basis of preoperative information, a loading dose may be administered during rewarming on CPB.

The strategy for managing PVR changes dramatically as well. With PBF now relying upon "passive" venous return (i.e., no pump to propel blood through the pulmonary circulation), measures designed to minimize the impediments to PBF assume paramount importance. Since medical therapies are limited in their capacity to produce reliable, substantial improvement in ventricular compliance or AV valve function, attention is focused on minimizing PVR. Shortly before the termination of CPB, the tracheal tube should be cleared of secretions and the lungs completely reexpanded, as PVR will be minimized at normal FRC. Both atelectasis and alveolar overdistension increase PVR. A tidal volume designed to achieve a low-normal $PaCO_2$ at a respiratory rate no greater than 20 is selected. Doppler flow studies have demonstrated that PBF occurs preferentially during the expiratory phase of positive-pressure ventilation in patients following cavopulmonary anastomosis, thus we strive to limit rate and inspiratory time to no greater than 1 second [91,92]. Positive end-expiratory pressure (PEEP) is only applied judiciously to preserve normal FRC, based upon investigations in Fontan patients demonstrating significant reduction in cardiac index mediated by an increase in PVR at PEEP values over 6 mm Hg [93]. Ventilatory strategies producing $PaCO_2$ of 45–50 mm Hg will increase cerebral blood flow, thus increasing PBF through the direct SVC–PA connection. This strategy will not only increase systemic and cerebral oxygen saturation, but also increases systemic oxygen delivery [94,95]. In some instances of significant hypoxemia despite optimizing other measures, nitric oxide inhalation can be used to lower PVR.

Immediately following termination of CPB, MUF is instituted. MUF offers significant benefit to patients following cavopulmonary anastomosis [96]. Postoperative blood loss and the proportion of patients demonstrating significant pleural and pericardial effusions are both significantly reduced. Other investigators have shown benefits in pulmonary function across a wider spectrum of patients that may prove particularly crucial in this population.

Infants for SCPA represent a high-risk group for postoperative bleeding. They have several risk factors that tend to exacerbate bleeding, including age less than 2 years, reoperation, hypoxemia, frequent use of aspirin, and in some, deep hypothermic bypass management. Upon completion of MUF, heparin effect is rapidly reversed with protamine. Fresh whole blood, if available, comprises the preferred product for blood replacement following protamine administration. As described previously, this product provides restoration of all hemostatic elements, including platelets, and thereby limits donor exposures as well. In the vast majority, SCPA can be performed while limiting patient exposure to a single blood donor.

Specific problems in the immediate postoperative period

Hypoxemia of greater magnitude than anticipated represents the most common postoperative problem encountered by patients following SCPA. In some instances, this may represent a manifestation of hypovolemia and diminished PBF, while in others it might reflect the mechanical ventilation strategy. In the latter circumstance, PaO_2 should rise as ventilatory support is tapered. In the absence of improvement with manipulation of intravascular volume or ventilation, diagnostic evaluation is indicated to search for connections that enable venous return from the upper body to bypass the pulmonary circulation and enter the heart or lower body venous system (e.g., an unrecognized left SVC draining to the coronary sinus). Often these collateral vessels can be occluded using transcatheter coil embolization, but the hemodynamic impact of occlusion should be tested with a balloon catheter prior to definitive embolization.

Although the incidence of myocardial dysfunction is significantly lower following SCPA, it does occur. In the absence of significant hemodynamic causes (e.g., aortic arch obstruction, AV valve regurgitation), one must suspect an issue with myocardial protection or coronary perfusion. Despite their young age, some infants have developed extremely thick ventricular walls, particularly in the context of a high Qp:Qs and residual aortic arch obstruction. Adequate protection for these ventricles requires meticulous technique. Even under optimal circumstances, the compliance of these hearts may not return to normal for an extended period postoperatively. While dysfunctional dilated hearts seem to respond to increasing inotropic support, no medical regimen has proven consistently beneficial to the thick-walled ventricle operating at low end-diastolic volume.

Sinus node dysfunction represents the most common rhythm disturbance following SCPA, especially with the hemi-Fontan operation. Approximately 15% of infants will have periods of junctional rhythm in the early postoperative period. Over 80% return to sinus rhythm in the ensuing days or weeks. Temporary epicardial pacing is employed when the hemodynamics appear impaired by heart rate.

Outcomes

Outcomes following SCPA have been excellent in experienced centers, with operative survival over 96% [58,73,97,98]. While some infants who have had a Sano modification of Stage I may require an earlier SCPA [73], this intervention can be performed at 4 months without discernable difference in mortality, morbidity, or ultimate suitability for Fontan operation [73,98]. This observation has led some to advocate for earlier SCPA routinely as a means to reduce interstage mortality [99].

The total morbidity and mortality following a hybrid approach in the neonatal period may be higher through the "Comprehensive Stage 2," since this entails aortic arch reconstruction, as well as the SCPA with the potential for PA repair as well. Depending upon criteria used for hybrid approach (i.e., standard vs. high-risk) and the experience of the center, mortality ranges from 8 to 22% [63,64,81]. However, most case series are quite small to date and further experience with this approach is necessary before concluding which approach is superior.

Completion of Fontan

The basic surgical approach is illustrated in Figure 24.7. Precise timing of the completion requires weighing several considerations, each of which is incompletely understood. At a minimum, the interval between the two stages of the Fontan must permit restoration of optimal ventricular compliance at the new end-diastolic dimension. In the absence of a diagnostic tool sensitive or specific enough to evaluate this process, many have arbitrarily established a minimal interval of 9–12 months. Despite its hemodynamic resilience, hemi-Fontan anatomy and physiology does pose risks that may provide compelling reasons not to extend this interval inordinately. These children are subject to the risk of paradoxical emboli returning via the IVC, as well as the consequences of hypoxemia, which

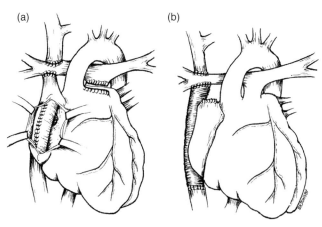

Figure 24.7 Modern variations of the Fontan operation. (a) The lateral tunnel Fontan, where a conduit is fashioned inside the right atrium. (b) The extracardiac Fontan, where a Goretex® tube is used to connect inferior vena cava and hepatic venous blood to the pulmonary artery. A fenestration can be created with both modifications (Modified and used with permission from Reference [100])

accelerate with age. Diversion of the IVC blood away from the pulmonary circulation may predispose the child to development of pulmonary arteriovenous malformations.

Preoperative assessment

In preparation for Fontan operation, the same considerations apply as discussed for SCPA; however, the implications are more significant. Unlike the patient following SCPA, the Fontan operation leaves the child's CO nearly totally dependent upon PBF. Whereas impediments to PBF following SCPA might result in lower systemic oxygenation, they produce low CO after Fontan operation. Clinical experience suggests that infants and young children are far more tolerant of hypoxemia than diminished CO.

Although candidates for Fontan operation have traditionally undergone cardiac catheterization preoperatively, an increasing number now are evaluated only via cardiac MRI studies [101]. One can use the catheterization data gathered to predict systemic venous pressure following Fontan operation in much the same way we described for SCPA. A fenestration is often created connecting systemic and pulmonary venous return, in order to ameliorate early postoperative morbidity and provide a pathway that sustains ventricular preload under conditions that might impede PBF [101,102]. Apart from coronary sinus return and whatever flow might cross the fenestration created in the IVC to PA pathway, all systemic venous return traverses the pulmonary circulation. Thus, one would estimate the Qp:Qs following fenestrated Fontan operation to reach 0.9 or higher. As an example, in a child catheterized in prepa-

ration for Fontan operation, the following determinations were made:

$$Qp : Qs = 0.6, \ P_{PA} = 12, \ P_{LA} = 8$$

Estimation of the systemic venous pressure (which should equal the PA pressure) would be calculated as:

$$P_{SVC} = P_{IVC} = P_{PA} = \left(\frac{(12 - 8)(0.9)}{0.6} \right) + 8 = 14 \, \text{mmHg}$$

An interval assessment should include both cardiac and noncardiac problems and interventions. Knowledge regarding previous experiences with sedation and anesthesia exerts significant influence on management options. Finally, a plan should be devised in conjunction with the patient's cardiologist for the perioperative management of any cardiac drugs, anticoagulants, or other medical regimens.

Intraoperative management

Patients most commonly present for Fontan operation between 15 months and 3 years of age. At this developmental age, they will demonstrate significant separation anxiety. We prefer to alleviate their anxiety with either pentobarbital (4 mg/kg p.o, maximum dosage 120 mg) or midazolam (0.5 mg/kg given orally, maximum dosage 10 mg). The history of each child's response to previous sedatives assumes importance in governing the decision as to which regimen to employ.

As with infants for SCPA, anesthesia for Fontan operation can be induced with a variety of intravenous or inhaled agents. Unless the preoperative evaluation has revealed myocardial dysfunction or significant unusual hemodynamic loading conditions (e.g., aortic arch obstruction, AV valve insufficiency), these infants generally tolerate the qualitative hemodynamic effects of anesthetic agents in a manner that is similar to normal children, although inhalation induction is slower due to the right-to-left shunting bypassing the lungs and delaying anesthetic uptake [103]. We usually employ a combination of inhaled anesthetic, opioid, and muscle relaxant, most commonly limiting the total opioid administered to the equivalent of fentanyl 10–15 mcg/kg. Our goal is sufficient emergence from the anesthetic effect to permit tracheal extubation on arrival in the cardiac ICU, assuming that the child is normothermic, exhibits appropriate hemodynamics, and has no significant ongoing bleeding.

All standard noninvasive monitors are applied for induction. The considerations for invasive arterial monitoring site selection remain as described for the SCPA. Similarly, the philosophy regarding systemic venous pressure monitoring and postoperative transthoracic monitoring catheters in the PA and common atrium remains consistent.

The immediate benefits from Fontan operation are limited to improved systemic oxygenation at the expense of higher IVC pressure. Volume and pressure loading conditions for the single ventricle do not change in response to this procedure. Nevertheless, this relatively brief operation is well tolerated by the majority of children, particularly the intracardiac lateral tunnel technique. The details of immediate postbypass management are identical to those following SCPA. Management includes meticulous ventilation designed to minimize PVR, low-dose inotropic support, MUF, and rapid restoration of hemostasis with protamine and fresh whole blood. As noted previously, PEEP is employed only as necessary to preserve normal FRC.

Specific problems in the immediate postoperative period

Unlike the manifestations of diminished PBF following SCPA anastomosis, in which reduction in systemic oxygen saturation occurs, the same phenomenon after Fontan operation will cause reduced CO. The signs of the latter tend to be far more insidious and ambiguous. These patients require the utmost vigilance to maintain adequate intravascular volume during the process of rewarming and blood loss in the early postoperative period. Conduit or baffle fenestration tends to ameliorate some of the early postoperative hemodynamic instability. When fenestrated, the IVC conduit allows some blood to shunt from systemic venous to pulmonary venous system, acting to preserve ventricular preload despite diminished PBF [101,102].

Hypoxemia usually indicates some communication from systemic venous system to the atrium. A modest degree of hypoxemia frequently occurs related to flow through a planned fenestration and the coronary sinus, which normally enters the atrium on what is functionally the pulmonary venous side. Systemic oxygen saturation less than 85–90% suggests more flow across the fenestration than usual, extremely low mixed venous oxygen saturation, or an additional venous channel diverting blood around the pulmonary circulation. Alternatively, pulmonary arteriovenous malformations, such as those described following Glenn operation, may account for the hypoxemia. Distinguishing these prospects may require cardiac catheterization.

Myocardial dysfunction typically follows the same differential described previously for SCPA. In the absence of a hemodynamic cause, one must conclude that it reflects inadequate myocardial preservation, coronary perfusion, or a metabolic process. In the absence of remediable causes (e.g., hypocalcemia), supportive measures represent the mainstay of therapy.

Arrhythmias can arise immediately following Fontan operation. While heart block is uncommon, junctional rhythms occur in a quarter of the patients. If the escape rate is sufficiently low to have a deleterious impact on overall hemodynamics, epicardial atrial or atrioventricular pacing usually proves beneficial. In the current era, tachyarrhythmias are less common in the early postoperative period, but more likely to have a significantly negative hemodynamic impact when they occur. Doppler interrogations of PBF patterns suggest that flow is most brisk during diastole under normal circumstances [104], perhaps explaining the intolerance of tachyarrhythmias. Alternatively, unfavorable hemodynamics may serve to provoke tachyarrhythmias.

Outcomes

As with SCPA, operative mortality following Fontan operation in the current era is less than 2% in experienced centers [58,98,105], and HLHS is no longer an independent predictor of adverse outcome following Fontan operation [106]. Nevertheless, significant morbidity and late mortality can occur following this procedure, including deteriorating ventricular function, arrhythmias, thrombotic events, and protein-losing enteropathy (PLE). In a cohort of 330 patients evaluated a median of 8 years following Fontan operation, the freedom from death or transplant at 5 and 10 years was 95 and 93%, respectively. Overall parental assessment of their child's health was excellent (57%) or good (38%), cardiac performance was New York Heart Association functional Class I or II (87%), and school performance was above average (30%) or average (40%). Parents also reported that their children had either slight (53%) or significant (12%) limitations to their physical activity [107].

Sequelae of the Fontan operation include arrhythmias, thrombotic events, and PLE. Arrhythmias occur in 25–50%, although a far smaller number require therapeutic intervention. Although proposed as a means to reduce atrial suture lines and thus proclivity to late rhythm disturbances, extracardiac conduit techniques have not demonstrated selective benefit to date [108]. Thromboembolic events are estimated to occur in approximately 10% [57,109], probably due to flow characteristics of the Fontan circulation as well as underlying abnormalities of coagulation factors [110]. PLE represents one of the least understood complications, occurring in as many as 25% of patients in some centers. A large multicenter review of more than 3000 patients found an overall incidence of 3.8% presenting a median of 2.7 years after Fontan completion. PLE has proven extremely recalcitrant to medical or surgical interventions and is associated with 50% mortality within 5 years. Typically, PLE resolves with transplantation, although there have been reports of late recurrence [111].

Anesthesia for patients with single ventricle for noncardiac surgery

During the course of their lives a substantial portion of children with single ventricle physiology will require one or more noncardiac surgical interventions. These procedures span a wide range of complexity and urgency. As such, this section cannot serve as a comprehensive guide to all possible scenarios but instead outlines general concepts to serve as a framework for patient care.

It is our impression that a carefully administered anesthetic, appropriate for age and surgical procedure, is tolerated provided the unique ventilatory and circulatory requirements of these patients are consistently met. When possible, one might defer elective major noncardiac surgery until the infant has recovered from SCPA. At this stage of the reconstructive sequence, hemodynamic performance tends to be most resilient, as the single ventricle is no longer operating with the excess volume load (Qp + Qs) required to sustain a parallel circulation, nor is the CO entirely dependent upon PBF, as occurs following completion of the Fontan [85,112,113]. An additional consideration arises when major blood loss is anticipated. Both the SCPA and Fontan operation result in significant increases in venous pressure, potentially promoting blood loss. One has to weight the risks entailed in managing such a patient functioning with the volume load of a parallel circulation against the impact that elevated venous pressure would have on blood loss. Unfortunately, many interventions will not wait for optimum hemodynamic stability. Urgent and emergency surgery often transpires when hemodynamics are least favorable. Whatever the timing, a clear understanding of each patient's anatomy and physiology constitutes the foundation of any perioperative plan. These details can usually be obtained most succinctly from the child's cardiologist. When a considerable interval has elapsed since the cardiologist has evaluated the patient, they must be included in the preoperative assessment plans.

Between July 2005 and June 2008, 445 neonates, infants, and children with HLHS and comparable single ventricle lesions underwent noncardiac surgery at the Children's Hospital of Philadelphia. Noncardiac surgery was performed at every stage of care, including 12 patients who either had native anatomy or had undergone a hybrid procedure. Of the remaining 332 patients, 150 had noncardiac surgery between SCPA and Fontan and 182 after Fontan completion. Procedures ranged in complexity from simple, superficial procedures ($n = 321$; 72%) to highly complex surgeries such as major intracavitary, CNS, craniofa-cial, or spinal instrumentation ($n = 124$; 28%). Emergency surgery accounted for 12% of the cases.

Intraoperative management

Anesthetic management varies depending upon the physiologic state of the patient and the magnitude of the planned intervention. As a starting point, the perioperative plan entails the same components that would be included for any child undergoing the same intervention. The plan is modified according to the cardiac physiology and constraints it imposes. For superficial procedures in a hemodynamically sound patient, no special monitoring is necessary. On the other hand, a neonate with single ventricle and a perforated viscus requires invasive monitoring to track hemodynamic, ventilatory, and metabolic changes and all the therapies available as outlined previously to manipulate cardiac function and the vascular beds.

Similarly, induction and maintenance of anesthesia are governed by perioperative expectations, the qualitatively predictable hemodynamic effects of anesthetic agents, and the cardiovascular state of the child. For superficial procedures in a well-compensated child with one ventricle, short-acting agents that enable a prompt recovery are appropriate. The plan needs to be adjusted in response to more extensive interventions or hemodynamically compromised patients.

Postoperative management

Postoperative surveillance also ranges from that which would be used for any child of similar age having a given procedure through admission to an ICU. While some added degree of caution is warranted, patients with one ventricle can have outpatient surgery when they are healthy and the procedure permits. If, however, any aspect of the child's condition would render them vulnerable to the routine consequences of anesthesia and surgery, hospital admission should be considered. These include, but are not limited to, nausea, vomiting, pain, and inability to take fluids or medications orally. If one could envision a dramatic or life-threatening physiologic change during the perioperative period, surveillance in a cardiac ICU is advisable. In the Children's Hospital of Philadelphia series discussed above, 58% of the children had day surgery, while another 19% had "same day" surgery in which they were admitted from home on the day of their procedure.

Outcomes

Taken together, the overall 3–5-year survival in surgically managed HLHS is between 70 and 80% [58,73,97]. In more recent cohorts of "standard" risk patients, survival may even be higher. Although early results are mixed, the long-term impact of innovations such as the Sano modification and hybrid approaches remains to be determined. At present, the morbidity and mortality following Fontan operation does not appear to be significantly different for children with HLHS compared to other single ventricle malformations, as noted above. Routine staging of the Fontan procedure, baffle fenestration, and use of MUF results in both low mortality (<1% for both SCPA and Fontan completion) and morbidity for all patients regardless of anatomic subset of univentricular heart.

The one possible exception to that finding is neurodevelopmental outcome. In a recent study of Fontan patients comparing those with HLHS to other single ventricle patients, median full scale IQ was 94 compared to 107, respectively [114]. Infants with HLHS exhibit a unique confluence of predisposing factors and potential for acquired injury. In an autopsy series, 29% of infants with HLHS exhibited congenital CNS abnormalities and 36% were microcephalic [115]. While autopsy series may introduce bias, a series of 129 live patients with HLHS confirmed that 12% were microcephalic and the population was skewed such that 81% were in the lowest 5 deciles [116]. In addition, microcephaly was associated with a smaller ascending aorta, suggesting a relationship to cerebral perfusion in utero. Given this predisposition, there is also evidence supporting diminished cerebral perfusion in the pre- and postoperative period [117]. While studies of early survivors of HLHS reconstructive surgery showed marked cognitive impairment, the magnitude of impairment has diminished in more recent survivors [117–119], although patients with known or suspected genetic syndromes or younger gestational ages still perform poorly [120]. A substantial percentage (18–28%) also demonstrates attention problems, anxiety, and depression. Many (33–55%) also demonstrate some degree of gross or fine motor deficit [73,120]. Interestingly, similar neurocognitive findings have been described in HLHS patients following cardiac transplantation [121].

Heart transplantation for single ventricle malformations

Although cardiac transplantation has been performed in selected patients with single ventricle malformations in late childhood and adolescence for progressive ventricular dysfunction, this strategy gained widespread notoriety when it was advocated for neonates with HLHS. In 1986, Bailey described successful allotransplantation methods for HLHS [122]. The most recent International Society for Heart and Lung Transplantation data reveal approximately 400 pediatric heart transplants occurring yearly, with roughly one-quarter occurring in infants younger than 1 year [123]; unfortunately, however, in excess of 1000 children are born with HLHS each year in the USA alone

[124]. A multicenter study of the fate of infants awaiting cardiac transplantation demonstrated that although the number of infants with unpalliated HLHS listed for cardiac transplantation continued to decrease each year, 25% of these patients died while awaiting transplantation despite the fact that their mean time to transplantation was 1.5 months, significantly less than other subgroups studied [125]. The group of patients awaiting transplantation will also continue to grow as children with HLHS who have failed surgical palliation are referred for cardiac replacement or "rescue transplantation" [122]. In a review of 417 infants and children transplanted at Loma Linda over 20 years, while over one-third of patients studied were primarily transplanted for HLHS, 9 patients had previously undergone surgical palliative procedures for HLHS [126]. Extending this therapy generally would likely result in an increase in both waiting time to transplantation and pretransplant mortality, although increased utilization of hybrid procedures may allow more prolonged waiting periods in neonates with an increased margin of survival. Additionally, increasing experience and success with ABO-incompatible infant and pediatric cardiac transplantation may also assist in enlarging the list of potential donors for patients who require transplantation [126].

While 10-year survival rates of 76% have recently been reported in a cohort of patients who underwent cardiac transplantation as infants, concerns regarding both long-term survival and quality of life for recipients continue to persist. Of 31 survivors of infant cardiac replacement, 3 have undergone retransplantation, 6 have significant renal insufficiency, 5 have acquired posttransplant lymphoproliferative disease, and 5 have been diagnosed with coronary artery disease [127]. For the relatively small proportion of neonates with HLHS who are currently listed for transplantation, the waiting period can extend as long as 6 months and the mortality as high as 30% during that interval [125,128]. Extending this therapy generally would likely result in an increase in both the waiting time and pretransplant mortality. Consideration needs to be given to the long-term impact of this decision. Chronic immunosuppression and rejection limit 12-year survival to 50% in all pediatric heart recipients and infants with congenital heart malformations fare even less well [129]. Beyond the initial year, mortality in pediatric transplant recipients is approximately 3% per year, whereas comparable mortality following Fontan operation is <1% per year [130,131].

Summary

The anesthesia management for patients with single ventricle encompasses a wide spectrum of care. Careful assessment and planning entails a comprehensive understanding of the typical physiology at each stage of the reconstructive sequence, the specific condition of each patient with respect to that physiology, and the impact that the proposed procedure will likely have. Armed with that knowledge, an anesthesiologist can design a plan taking into account the qualitatively predictable effects of anesthetic agents, airway and ventilatory manipulations, and cardiovascular drugs. This plan is titrated to achieve the desired effects in each patient. No absolute formulas exist. Rather, absolute needs, expectations, capabilities, and goals vary between institutions, clinicians, and patients. Optimal results entail carefully orchestrated interactions among anesthesiologists, surgeons, cardiologists, and intensivists.

References

1. Fontan F, Baudet E (1971) Surgical repair of tricuspid atresia. Thorax 26: 240–248.
2. Kreutzer G, Galindez E, Bono H, et al. (1973) An operation for the correction of tricuspid atresia. J Thorac Cardiovasc Surg 66: 613–621.
3. Hinton RB, Jr, Martin LJ, Tabangin ME, et al. (2007) Hypoplastic left heart is heritable. J Am Coll Cardiol 50: 1590–1595.
4. Wernovsky G, Bove EL (1998) Single ventricle lesions. In: Chang AC, Hanley FL, Wernovsky G, Wessel DL (eds) Pediatric Cardiac Intensive Care. Williams & Wilkins, Baltimore, pp. 271–287.
5. Pizarro C, Malec E, Maher KO, et al. (2003) Right ventricle to pulmonary artery conduit improves outcome after stage I Norwood for hypoplastic left heart syndrome. Circulation 108 (Supp 1): II155–II160.
6. Sano S, Ishino K, Kawada M, et al. (2003) Right ventricle–pulmonary artery shunt in first-stage palliation of hypoplastic left heart syndrome. J Thorac Cardiovasc Surg 126: 504–510.
7. Malec E, Januszewska K, Kolcz J, et al. (2003) Right ventricle-to-pulmonary artery shunt versus modified Blalock–Taussig shunt in the Norwood procedure for hypoplastic left heart syndrome—influence on early and late haemodynamic status. Eur J Cardiothorac Surg 23: 728–733.
8. Azakie A, Martinez D, Sapru A, et al. (2004) Impact of right ventricle to pulmonary artery conduit on outcome of the modified Norwood procedure. Ann Thorac Surg 77: 1727–1733.
9. Castaneda AR, Jonas RA, Mayer JE, Hanley FL (1994) Hypoplastic left heart syndrome. In: Castaneda AR, Jonas RA, Mayer JE, Hanley FL (eds) Cardiac Surgery of the Neonate and Infant. W.B. Saunders Co., Philadelphia, pp. 363–385.
10. Rychik J, Bush DM, Spray TL, et al. (2000) Assessment of pulmonary/systemic blood flow ratio after first-stage palliation for hypoplastic left heart syndrome: development of a new index with the use of Doppler echocardiography. J Thorac Cardiovasc Surg 102: 81–87.
11. Rossi AF, Sommer RJ, Lotvin A, et al. (1994) Usefulness of intermittent monitoring of mixed venous oxygen saturation after stage I palliation for hypoplastic left heart syndrome. Am J Cardiol 73: 1118–1123.
12. Riordan CJ, Locher JP, Santamore WP, et al. (1997) Monitoring systemic venous oxygen saturations in hypoplastic left heart syndrome. Ann Thorac Surg 63: 835–837.
13. Day RW, Barton AJ, Pysher TJ, et al. (1998) Pulmonary vascular resistance of children treated with nitrogen during early infancy. Ann Thorac Surg 65: 1400–1404.
14. Jobes DR, Nicolson SC, Steven JM, et al. (1992) Carbon dioxide prevents pulmonary overcirculation in hypoplastic left heart syndrome. Ann Thorac Surg 54: 150–151.
15. Chang AC, Zucker HA, Hickey PR, et al. (1995) Pulmonary vascular resistance in infants after cardiac surgery: role of carbon dioxide and hydrogen ion. Crit Care Med 23: 568–754.
16. Wessel DL (1996) Commentary: simple gases and complex single ventricles. [letter; comment]. J Thorac Cardiovasc Surg 112: 665–667.
17. Tabbutt S, Ramamoorthy C, Montenegro LM, et al. (2001) Impact of inspired gas mixtures on preoperative infants with hypoplastic left heart syndrome during controlled ventilation. Circulation 104: I159–I164.
18. Gaynor JW, Mahle WT, Cohen MI, et al. (2002) Risk factors for mortality after the Norwood procedure Eur J Cardiothorac Surg 22: 82–89.
19. Hebra A, Brown, MF, Hirschl RB, et al. (1993) Mesenteric ischemia in hypoplastic left heart syndrome. J Pediatr Surg 28: 606–611.
20. McElhinney DB, Hedrick HL, Bush DM, et al. (2000) Necrotizing enterocolitis in neonates with congenital heart disease: risk factors and outcomes. Pediatrics 106: 1080–1087.
21. Eapen RS, Rowland DG, Franklin WH (1998) Effect of prenatal diagnosis of critical left heart obstruction on perinatal morbidity and mortality. Am J Perinatology 15: 237–242.
22. Hansen DD, Hickey PR (1986) Anesthesia for hypoplastic left heart syndrome: use of high-dose fentanyl in 30 neonates. Anesth Analg 65: 127–132.
23. Hickey PR, Hansen DD, Wessel DL, et al. (1985) Blunting of stress responses in the pulmonary circulation of infants by fentanyl. Anesth Analg 64: 1137–1142.
24. Hickey PR, Hansen DD (1991) High-dose fentanyl reduces intraoperative ventricular fibrillation in neonates with hypoplastic left heart syndrome. J Clin Anesth 3: 295–300.
25. Anand KJ, Hickey PR (1992) Halothane-morphine compared with high-dose sufentanil for anesthesia and postoperative analgesia in neonatal cardiac surgery. N Engl J Med 326: 1–9.
26. Gruber EM, Laussen PC, Casta A, et al. (2001) Stress response in infants undergoing cardiac surgery: a randomized study of fentanyl bolus, fentanyl infusion, and fentanyl-midazolam infusion. Anesth Analg 92: 882–890.
27. Zuppa AF, Nicolson SC, Wernovsky G, et al. (2002) The effect of cardiopulmonary bypass and modified ultrafiltration on plasma pharmacokinetics of milrinone in neonates with HLHS. Crit Care Med 30: A-155 (Abstract).
28. Naik SK, Knight A, Elliott MJ (1991) A successful modification of ultrafiltration for cardiopulmonary bypass in children. Perfusion 6: 41–50.

29. Elliott MJ (1993) Ultrafiltration and modified ultrafiltration in pediatric open-heart operations [Review]. Ann Thorac Surg 56: 1518–1522.

30. Bando K, Turrentine MW, Vijay P, et al. (1998) Effect of modified ultrafiltration in high-risk patients undergoing operations for congenital heart disease. Ann Thorac Surg 66: 821–827.

31. Davies MJ, Nguyen K, Gaynor JW, et al. (1998) Modified ultrafiltration improves left ventricular systolic function in infants after cardiopulmonary bypass. J Thorac Cardiovasc Surg 115: 361–369.

32. Skaryak LA, Kirshbom PM, DiBernardo LR, et al. (1995) Modified ultrafiltration improves cerebral metabolic recovery after circulatory arrest. J Thorac Cardiovasc Surg 109: 744–751.

33. Gaynor JW, Kuypers M, van Rossem M, et al. (2005) Haemodynamic changes during modified ultrafiltration immediately following the first stage of the Norwood reconstruction. Cardiol Young 15 (1): 4–7.

34. Kern FH, Morana NJ, Sears JJ, et al. (1992) Coagulation defects in neonates during cardiopulmonary bypass. Ann Thorac Surg 54: 541–546.

35. Manno CS, Hedberg KW, Kim HC, et al. (1991) Comparison of the hemostatic effects of fresh whole blood, stored whole blood, and components after open-heart surgery in children. Blood 77: 930–936.

36. Mou SS, Giroir BP, Molitor-Kirsch EA, et al. (2004) whole blood versus reconstituted blood for pump priming in heart surgery in infants. N Engl J Med 351: 1635–1644.

37. Gruenwald CE, McCrindle BW, Crawford-Lean L, et al. (2008) Reconstituted fresh whole blood improves clinical outcomes compared with stored component blood therapy for neonates undergoing cardiopulmonary bypass for cardiac surgery: a randomized controlled trial. J Thorac Cardiovasc Surg 136: 1442–1449.

38. Eaton MP (2008) Antifibrinolytic therapy in surgery for congenital heart disease. Anesth Analg 106: 1087–1100.

39. Jaggers J, Lawson JH (2006) Coagulopathy and inflammation in neonatal heart surgery: mechanisms and strategies. Ann Thorac Surg 81: S2360–S2366.

40. Reid RW, Zimmerman AA, Laussen PC, et al. (1997) The efficacy of tranexamic acid versus placebo in decreasing blood loss in pediatric patients undergoing repeat cardiac surgery. Anesth Analg 84: 990–996.

41. Chauhan S, Das SN, Bisoi A, et al. (2004) Comparison of epsilon aminocaproic acid and tranexamic acid in pediatric cardiac surgery. J Cardiothorac Vasc Anesth 18: 141–143.

42. Mangano DT, Miao Y, Vuylsteke A, et al. (2007) Mortality associated with aprotinin during 5 years following coronary artery bypass graft surgery. JAMA 297: 471–479.

43. Tobias JD, Berkenbosch JW, Russo P (2003) Recombinant factor VIIa to treat bleeding after cardiac surgery in an infant. Pediatr Crit Care Med 4: 49–51.

44. Pychynska-Pokorska M, Moll JJ, Krajewski W, et al. (2004) The use of recombinant coagulation factor VIIa in uncontrolled postoperative bleeding in children undergoing cardiac surgery with cardiopulmonary bypass. Pediatr Crit Care Med 5: 246–250.

45. Jobes DR, Nicolson SC, Pigott JD, Norwood WI (1988) An enclosed system for continuous postoperative mediastinal aspiration. Ann Thorac Surg 45: 101–102.

46. Hoffman GM, Ghanayem NS, Kampine JM, et al. (2000) Venous saturation and the anaerobic threshold in neonates after the Norwood procedure for hypoplastic left heart syndrome. Ann Thorac Surg 70: 1515–1520.

47. Taeed R, Schwartz SM, Pearl JM, et al. (2001) Unrecognized pulmonary venous desaturation early after Norwood palliation confounds Qp:Qs assessment and compromises oxygen delivery. Circulation 103: 2699–2704.

48. Haworth SG (1984) Pulmonary vascular disease in different types of congenital heart disease. Implications for interpretation of lung biopsy findings in early childhood. Br Heart J 52: 557–571.

49. Haworth SG, Reig L (1977) Structural study of pulmonary circulation and of heart in total anomalous pulmonary venous return in early infancy. Br Heart J 39: 80–92.

50. Better DJ, Apfel HD, Zidere V, et al. (1999) Pattern of pulmonary venous blood flow in the hypoplastic left heart syndrome in the fetus. Heart 81: 646–649.

51. Morray JP, Lynn AM, Mansfield PB (1988) Effect of pH and P_{CO_2} on pulmonary and systemic hemodynamics after surgery in children with congenital heart disease and pulmonary hypertension. J Pediatr 113: 474–479.

52. Russell IA, Zwass MS, Finerman JR, et al. (1998) The effects of inhaled nitric oxide on postoperative pulmonary hypertension in infants and children undergoing surgical repair of congenital heart disease. Anesth Analg 87: 46–51.

53. Atz AM, Wessel DL (1997) Inhaled nitric oxide in the neonate with cardiac disease. Semin Perinatol 21: 441–455.

54. Ungerleider RM, Shen I, Yeh T, et al. (2004) Routine mechanical ventricular assist following the Norwood procedure-improved neurologic outcome and excellent hospital survival. Ann Thorac Surg 77: 18–22.

55. Ravishankar C, Dominguez TE, Kreutzer J, et al. (2006) Extracorporeal membrane oxygenation after Stage I reconstruction for hypoplastic left heart syndrome. Pediatr Crit Care Med 7: 319–323.

56. Norwood WI, Jacobs ML, Murphy JD (1992) Fontan procedure for hypoplastic left heart syndrome. Ann Thorac Surg 54: 1025–1029.

57. Glatz JA, Fedderly RT, Ghanayem NS, et al. (2008) Impact of mitral stenosis and aortic atresia on survival in hypoplastic left heart syndrome. Ann Thorac Surg 85: 2057–2062.

58. Rychik J (2005) Hypoplastic left heart syndrome: from in utero diagnosis to school age. Semin Fetal Neonatal Med 10: 553–566.

59. Pigula FA, Vladimiro V, del Nido P, et al. (2007) Contemporary results and current strategies in the management of hypoplastic left heart syndrome. Semin Thorac Cardiovasc Surg 19: 238–244.

60. Tweddell JS, Ghanayem NS, Mussatto KA, et al. (2007) Mixed venous oxygen saturation monitoring after stage I palliation for hypoplastic left heart syndrome. Ann Thorac Surg 84: 1301–1311.

61. Stasik CN, Goldberg CS, Bove EL, et al. (2006) Current outcomes and risk factors for the Norwood procedure. J Thorac Cardiovasc Surg 131: 412–417.

62. Galantowicz M, Cheatham JP, Phillips A, et al. (2008) Hybrid approach to hypoplastic left heart syndrome: intermediate results after the learning curve. Ann Thorac Surg 85: 2063–2071.

63. DiBardino DJ, McElhinney DB, Marshall AC, et al. (2008) A review of ductal stenting in hypoplastic left heart syndrome: bridge to transplantation and hybrid stage I palliation. Pediatr Cardiol 29: 251–257.

64. Pizarro C, Derby CD, Baffa JM, et al. (2008) Improving the outcome of high-risk neonates with hypoplastic left heart syndrome: hybrid procedure or conventional surgical palliation? Eur J Cardiothorac Surg 33: 613–618.

65. Gutgesell HP, Lim DS (2007) Hybrid palliation in hypoplastic left heart syndrome. Curr Opin Cardiol 22: 55–59.

66. Wernovsky G, Ghanayem N, Ohye RG, et al. (2007) Hypoplastic left heart syndrome: consensus and controversies in 2007. Cardiol Young 17 (Suppl 2): 75–86.

67. Tabbutt S, Dominguez TE, Ravishankar C, et al. (2005) Outcomes after the stage I reconstruction comparing the right ventricle to pulmonary artery conduit with the modified Blalock–Taussig shunt. Ann Thorac Surg 80: 1582–1591.

68. Reemtsen BL, Pike NA, Starnes VA (2007) Stage I palliation for hypoplastic left heart syndrome: Norwood versus Sano modification. Curr Opin Cardiol 22: 60–65.

69. Ghanayem NS, Jaquiss RDB, Cava JR, et al. (2006) Right ventricle-to-pulmonary artery conduit versus Blalock–Taussig shunt: a hemodynamic comparison. Ann Thorac Surg 82: 1603–1610.

70. Ohye RG, Devaney EJ, Hirsch JC, et al. (2007) The modified Blalock–Taussig shunt versus the right ventricle-to-pulmonary artery conduit for the Norwood procedure. Pediatr Cardiol 28: 122–125.

71. Donnelly JP, Raffel DM, Shulkin BL, et al. (1998) Resting coronary flow and coronary flow reserve in human infants after repair or palliation of congenital heart defects as measured by positron emission tomography. J Thorac Cardiovasc Surg 115: 103–110.

72. Sano S, Ishino K, Kado H, et al. (2004) Outcome of right ventricle-to-pulmonary artery shunt in first-stage palliation of hypoplastic left heart syndrome: a multi-institutional study. Ann Thorac Surg 78: 1951–1958.

73. Ballweg JA, Dominguez TE, Ravishankar C, et al. (2007) A contemporary comparison of the effect of shunt type in hypoplastic left heart syndrome on the hemodynamics and outcome at stage 2 reconstruction. J Thorac Cardiovasc Surg 134: 297–303.

74. Alsoufi B, Bennetts J, Verma S, et al. (2007) New developments in the treatment of hypoplastic left heart syndrome. Pediatrics 119: 109–117.

75. Davis D, Davis S, Cotman K, et al. (2008) Feeding difficulties and growth delay in children with hypoplastic left heart syndrome versus d-Transposition of the great arteries. Pediatr Cardiol 29: 328–333.

76. Jeffries HE, Wells WJ, Starnes VA, et al. (2006) Gastrointestinal morbidity after Norwood palliation for hypoplastic left heart syndrome. Ann Thorac Surg 81: 982–987.

77. Griselli M, McGuirk SP, Stumper O, et al. (2006) Influence of surgical strategies on outcome after the Norwood procedure. J Thorac Cardiovasc Surg 131: 418–426.

78. Ashburn DA, McCrindle BW, Tchervenkov CI, et al. (2003) Outcomes after the Norwood operation in neonates with critical aortic stenosis or aortic valve atresia. J Thorac Cardiovasc Surg 125: 1070–1082.

79. Boucek MM, Mashburn C, Chan KC (2005) Catheter-based interventional palliation for hypoplastic left heart syndrome. Semin Thorac Cardiovasc Surg Pediatr Card Surg Annu 72–77.

80. Akinturk H, Michel-Behnke I, Valeske K, et al. (2007) Hybrid transcatheter-surgical palliation; basis for univentricular or biventricular repair: the Giessen experience. Pediatr Cardiol 28: 79–87.

81. Galantowicz M, Cheatham JP (2005) Lessons learned from the development of a new hybrid strategy for the management of hypoplastic left heart syndrome. Pediatr Cardiol 26: 190–199.

82. Crystal MA, Yoo S, Mikailian H, et al. (2006) Catheter-based completion of the Fontan circuit. Circulation 114: e5–e6.

83. Penny DR, Lincoln C, Shone DR, et al. (1992) The early response of the systemic ventricle during transition to the Fontan circulation: an acute cardiomyopathy? Cardiol Young 2: 78–84.

84. Lamberti JJ, Spicer RL, Waldman JD, et al. (1999) The bidirectional cavopulmonary shunt. J Thorac Cardiovasc Surg 100: 22–29.

85. Douville EC, Sade RM, Fyfe DA (1991) Hemi-Fontan operation in surgery for single ventricle: a preliminary report. Ann Thorac Surg 51: 893–899.

86. Castaneda AR, Jonas RA, Mayer JE, Hanley FL (1994) Single-ventricle tricuspid atresia. In: Castaneda AR, Jonas RA, Mayer JE, Hanley FL (eds) Cardiac Surgery of the Neonate and Infant. W.B. Saunders Co., Philadelphia, pp. 249–272.

87. Hehir DA, Dominquez TE, Ballweg JA, et al. (2008) Risk factors for interstage death after stage 1 reconstruction of hypoplastic left heart syndrome and variants. J Thorac Cardiovasc Surg 136: 94–99.

88. Ghanayem NS, Hoffman GM, Mussatto KA, et al. (2003) Home surveillance program prevents interstage mortality after the Norwood procedure. J Thorac Cardiovasc Surg 126: 1367–1377.

89. Muthurangu V, Taylor AM, Hegde SR, et al. (2005) Cardiac magnetic resonance imaging after stage I Norwood operation for hypoplastic left heart syndrome. Circulation 112: 3256–3263.

90. Brown DW, Gauvreau K, Powell AJ, et al. (2007) Cardiac magnetic resonance versus routine cardiac catheterization before bidirectional Glenn anastomosis in infants with functional single ventricle. Circulation 116: 2718–2725.

91. Donofrio MT, Jacobs ML, Spray TL, et al. (1998) Acute changes in preload, afterload, and systolic function after superior cavopulmonary connection. Ann Thorac Surg 65: 503–508.

92. Fyfe DA, Kline CH, Sade RM, et al. (1991) The utility of transesophageal echocardiography during and after Fontan operations in small children. Am Heart J 122: 1403–1415.

93. Williams DB, Kiernan PD, Metke MP, et al. (1984) Hemodynamic response to positive end-expiratory pressure following right atrium-pulmonary artery bypass (Fontan procedure). J Thorac Cardiovasc Surg 87: 856–861.

94. Li J, Hoskote A, Hickey C, et al. (2005) Effect of carbon dioxide on systemic oxygenation, oxygen consumption, and blood lactate levels after bidirectional superior cavopulmonary anastomosis. Crit Care Med 33: 984–989.

95. Mott AR, Alomrani A, Tortoriello TA, et al. (2006) Changes in cerebral saturation profile in response to mechanical ventilation alterations in infants with bidirectional superior cavopulmonary connection. Pediatr Crit Care Med 7: 346–350.

96. Koutlas TC, Gaynor JW, Nicolson SC, et al. (1997) Modified ultrafiltration reduces postoperative morbidity after cavopulmonary connection. Ann Thorac Surg 64: 37–42.

97. Bove EL, Ohye RG, Devaney EJ (2004) Hypoplastic left heart syndrome: conventional surgical management. Semin Thorac Cardiovasc Surg 7: 3–10.

98. Jaquiss RDB, Siehr SL, Ghanayem NS, et al. (2006) Early cavopulmonary anastomosis after Norwood procedure results in excellent Fontan outcome. Ann Thorac Surg 81: 982–987.

99. Graham TP (2007) The year in congenital heart disease. J Am Coll Cardiol 50: 368–377.

100. Stayer SA, Andropoulos DB, Russell IA (2003) Anesthetic management of the adult patient with congenital heart disease. Anesthesiol Clin North America 21: 653–673.

101. Bridges ND, Lock JE, Castaneda AR (1990) Baffle fenestration with subsequent transcatheter closure. Modification of the Fontan operation for patients at increased risk. Circulation 82: 1681–1689.

102. Laks H, Pearl JM, Haas GS, et al. (1991) Partial Fontan: advantages of an adjustable interatrial communication. Ann Thorac Surg 52: 1084–1094.

103. Huntington JH, Malviya S, Voepel-Lewis T, et al. (1999) The effect of a right-to-left intracardiac shunt on the rate of rise of arterial and end-tidal halothane in children. Anesth Analg 88: 759–762.

104. Frommelt PC, Snider AR, Meliones JN, et al. (1991) Doppler assessment of pulmonary artery flow patterns and ventricular function after the Fontan operation. Am J Cardiol 68: 1211–1215.

105. Meyer DB, Zamora G, Wernovsky G, et al. (2006) Outcomes of the Fontan procedure using cardiopulmonary bypass with aortic cross-clamping. Ann Thorac Surg 82: 1611–1620.

106. Gaynor JW, Bridges ND, Cohen MI, et al. (2002) Predictors of outcome after Fontan operation: is hypoplastic left heart syndrome still a risk factor? J Thorac Cardiovasc Surg 123: 237–245.

107. Mitchell ME, Ittenbach RF, Gaynor JW, et al. (2006) Intermediate outcomes after the Fontan operation in the current era. J Thorac Cardiovasc Surg 131: 172–180.

108. Fiore AC, Turrentine M, Rodenfeld M, et al. (2007) Fontan operation: a comparison of lateral tunnel with extracardiac conduit. Ann Thorac Surg 83: 622–630.

109. Schultz AH, Wernovsky G (2005) Late outcomes in patients with surgically treated congenital heart disease. Semin Thorac Cardiovasc Surg 8: 145–156.

110. Odegard KC, McGowan FX, Zurakowski D, et al. (2003) Procoagulant and anticoagulant factor abnormalities following the Fontan procedure: increased factor VIII may predispose to thrombosis. J Thorac Cardiovasc Surg 125: 1260–1267.

111. Mertens L, Hagler DJ, Sauer U, et al. (1998) Protein-losing enteropathy after the Fontan operation: an international multicenter study. J Thorac Cardiovasc Surg 115: 1063–1073.

112. Nicolson SC, Steven JM, Kurth CD, et al. (1994) Anesthesia for noncardiac surgery in infants with hypoplastic left heart syndrome following Hemi-Fontan operation. J Cardiothorac Vasc Anesth 8: 334–336.

113. Karl HW, Hensley FA, Cyran SE, et al. (1990) Hypoplastic left heart syndrome: anesthesia for elective noncardiac surgery. Anesthesiology 72: 753–757.

114. Goldberg CS, Schwartz EM, Brunberg JA, et al. (2000) Neurodevelopmental outcome of patients after Fontan operation: a comparison between children with hypoplastic left heart syndrome and other functional single ventricle lesions. J Pediatr 137: 646–652.

115. Glauser TA, Rorke LB, Weinberg PM, et al. (1990) Congenital brain anomalies associated with the hypoplastic left heart syndrome. Pediatrics 85: 984–990.

116. Shillingford AJ, Ittenback RF, Marino BS, et al. (2007) Aortic morphometry and microcephaly in hypoplastic left heart syndrome. Cardiol Young 17: 189–195.

117. Mahle WT, Wernovsky G (2004) Neurodevelopmental outcomes in hypoplastic left heart syndrome. Semin Thorac Cardiovasc Surg 7: 39–47.

118. Shillingford AJ, Wernovsky G (2004) Academic performance and behavioral difficulties after neonatal and infant heart surgery. Pediatr Clin N Am 51: 1625–1639.

119. Wernovsky G, Newburger J (2003) Neurologic and developmental morbidity in children with complex congenital heart disease. J Pediatrics 142: 6–8.

120. Tabbutt S, Nord AS, Jarvik GP, et al. (2008) Neurodevelopmental outcomes after staged palliation for hypoplastic left heart syndrome. Pediatrics 121: 476–483.

121. Ilke L, Hale K, Fashaw L, et al. (2003) Developmental outcome of patients with hypoplastic left heart syndrome treated with heart transplantation. J Pediatr 142: 20–25.

122. Bailey LL, Nehlsen-Cannarella SL, Doroshow RW, et al. (1986) Cardiac allotransplantation in newborns as therapy for hypoplastic left heart syndrome. N Eng J Med 315: 949–951.

123. Kirk R, Edwards LB, Aurora P, et al. (2008) Registry of the International Society for Heart and Lung Transplantation: eleventh official pediatric heart transplantation report—2008. J Heart Lung Transplant 27: 970–977.

124. Botto L, Correa A, Erickson JD (2001) Racial and temporal variations in the prevalence of heart defects. Pediatrics 107: E32.

125. Chrisant MR, Naftel DC, Drummond-Webb J, et al. (2005) Fate of infants with hypoplastic left heart syndrome listed for cardiac transplantation: a multicenter study. J Heart Lung Transplant 24: 576–82.

126. Jacobs JP, Quintessenza JA, Chai PJ, et al. (2006) Rescue cardiac transplantation for failing staged palliation in patients with hypoplastic left heart syndrome. Cardiol Young 16: 556–562.

127. Dionigi B, Razzouk AJ, Hasaniya NW, et al. (2008) Late outcomes of pediatric heart transplantation are independent

of pre-transplant diagnosis and prior cardiac surgical intervention. J Heart Lung Transplant 27: 1090–1095.

128. Roche SL, Burch M, O'Sullivan J, et al. (2008) Multicenter experience of ABO-incompatible pediatric cardiac transplantation. Am J Transplant 8: 208–215.

129. Gandhi SK, Canter CE, Kulikowska A, et al. (2007) Infant heart transplantation ten years later—where are they now? Ann Thorac Surg 83: 169–172.

130. Jenkins PC, Flanagan MF, Sargent JD, et al. (2001) A comparison of treatment strategies for hypoplastic left heart syndrome using decision analysis. J Am Coll Cardiol 38: 1181–1187.

131. Boucek MM, Faro A, Novick RJ, et al. (2001) The registry of the International Society for Heart and Lung Transplantation: fourth official pediatric report—2000. J Heart Lung Transplant 20: 39–52.

25 Anesthesia for miscellaneous cardiac lesions

Maria Markakis Zestos, M.D.
Detroit Children's Hospital, Wayne State University School of Medicine, Detroit, Michigan, USA

Dean B. Andropoulos, M.D., M.H.C.M.
Texas Children's Hospital, Baylor College of Medicine, Houston, Texas, USA

Introduction

This chapter discusses the anatomy, pathophysiology, surgical approach, and anesthetic management of two groups of rare lesions: vascular rings and anomalies of the coronary arteries. Mitral regurgitation (MR) and anesthetic considerations for pericardial effusion and tamponade are then reviewed.

Vascular rings

Vascular rings are a variety of anomalies of the aortic arch and its branches, which result in compression of the trachea and/or esophagus. These lesions are rare, accounting for less than 1% of all congenital heart defects. Although patients may be asymptomatic, respiratory or feeding problems in infancy are common.

Anesthesia for Congenital Heart Disease 2nd edition. Edited by
Dean Andropoulos, Stephen Stayer, Isobel Russell and Emad Mossad.
© 2010 Blackwell Publishing.

Anatomy

Vascular rings were first described in 1737 by Hommel [1] who described a double aortic arch. Bayford [2] reported the first case of retroesophageal right subclavian artery in 1794. However, it was not until 1945 that a vascular ring was successfully divided by the pioneering efforts of Robert Gross [3].

Vascular rings [4,5] encompass many different vascular anomalies, all of which result from the abnormal regression of the aortic arch complex. The majority (60%) of all vascular rings are of the double aortic arch variety, which results from the persistence of the fourth aortic arch. Many variations in the arrangement of the aorta and its branches exist, and can result in complete or partial rings.

Of the many different anatomies, (i) double aortic arch and (ii) right aortic arch with aberrant left subclavian artery are the most common. In double aortic arch, the right aortic arch passes to the right of the esophagus to join the left-sided descending aorta, to form a complete vascular ring that encircles both the trachea and the esophagus (Figure 25.1). Two other varieties of vascular ring include (iii) right aortic arch with mirror image branching and

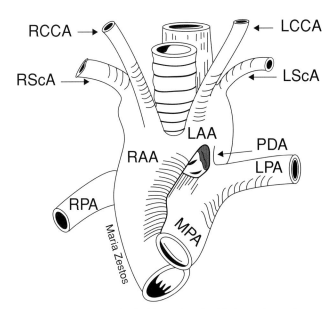

Figure 25.1 Drawing of a double aortic arch with the trachea and esophagus encircled by the vascular ring. LAA, left aortic arch; LCCA, left common carotid artery; LPA, left pulmonary artery; LScA, left subclavian artery; MPA, main pulmonary artery; PDA, patent ductus arteriosus; RAA, right aortic arch; RCCA, right common carotid artery; RPA, right pulmonary artery; RScA, right subclavian artery.

left ligamentum arteriosus, and (iv) left aortic arch with retroesophageal right subclavian artery.

Intracardiac lesions are rarely seen with double aortic arch but are often present in cases of (v) left aortic arch with right descending aorta. The left arch crosses behind the esophagus, and a right ligamentum arteriosus completes the ring.

Partial vascular rings or "slings" may also occur. For example, (i) an aberrant right subclavian artery of an otherwise normal arch may pass to the right behind the esophagus with resultant dysphagia. Other partial rings that have been described include (ii) ductus arteriosus sling and (iii) compression of the lower trachea from severe malrotation of the heart. In the latter two, dividing the ductus arteriosus relieves the compression.

Finally, with the pulmonary artery sling, the left pulmonary artery arises from the proximal right pulmonary artery, and passes behind the trachea [6]. The ligamentum arteriosum completes the vascular ring by compressing the trachea anteriorly.

Pathophysiology and natural history

Symptoms are usually prominent in patients with a tightly obstructed ring as is seen in double aortic arch. Infants often present with respiratory distress, stridor, and swallowing difficulties within the first 6 months of life. Subcostal retractions can be seen in severe obstruction. Recur-

rent respiratory difficulty or dysphagia in a young infant should raise the question of the presence of a vascular ring. However, the diagnosis of vascular ring in infants without associated anomalies is often delayed months to years after onset of symptoms [7,8]. Aortoesophageal fistula have been described in adults and in infants [9,10]. Partial vascular rings may be asymptomatic if there is little tracheoesophageal compression. Older infants and adults with undiagnosed vascular rings have presented with acute esophageal foreign body impaction [11], unsuccessfully treated asthma [12], and progressive dyspnea on exertion [13].

Radiographic studies play a crucial role in delineating vascular causes of airway obstruction [14]. A plain chest X-ray may show the presence of a right-sided aortic arch, a retrotracheal opacity, tracheal narrowing, or tracheal compression. The combination of frontal and lateral views shows at least one abnormality in every patient [15]. A barium esophagram can be useful revealing indentation, which is usually diagnostic [5]. Bronchoscopy or esophagoscopy, though unnecessary and rarely done, may reveal a pulsating mass compressing the esophagus or trachea. Computed tomography (CT) and magnetic resonance imaging (MRI) are the preferred methods of diagnosis. They have been shown to be diagnostically accurate, eliminating the need for other studies. MRI is often preferred because it can identify anatomic details of structures including better visualization of atretic part of the ring without radiation exposure [16,17]. However, multislice CT has resulted in excellent images for diagnosis. Echocardiography is used liberally by some centers to evaluate the presence of a congenital heart anomaly that may be present in up to 20% of children with symptomatic vascular rings.

Surgical approaches

Delayed treatment may result in tracheobronchial damage in symptomatic patients [18]. Surgery, however, is not indicated if symptoms are mild or absent. Because of the persistence of symptoms after successful division of the vascular ring, many physicians reserve surgical repair for children with major symptoms or proven compression and respiratory symptoms [19]. Best exposure is provided by the left thoracotomy approach through the fourth intercostal space [4]. If coexisting cardiac anomalies require repair, a median sternotomy may be used. The arch, including the retroesophageal component is dissected out completely. Care must be given to the identification and division of the ring without compressing blood flow to the descending aorta or carotid arteries. In double aortic arch, the nondominant arch is divided and sutured at its distal end close to the junction with the descending aorta. The ligamentum arteriosus is also divided in all cases.

The trachea and esophagus are dissected and freed of all strands or bands of tissue that may add to the constriction. On occasion, the descending aorta is suspended to the rib periosteum to keep it away from the esophagus. If the vascular ring is of the right aortic arch type, the division of the left ligamentum arteriosus opens the ring and relieves the constriction.

On rare occasion, right thoracotomy may be indicated. This is the case in double aortic arch with a smaller non-dominant right aortic arch, as well as the case of left aortic arch with a retroesophageal subclavian artery and right ligamentum arteriosus.

Video-assisted thoracoscopic division of vascular rings has been described [20,21]. This approach is limited by decreased vascular exposure and the reduced ability for direct vascular control. The safety of thoracoscopic approach is increased if there is an absence of blood flow and atresia of the ring structure undergoing division.

The pulmonary artery sling is usually repaired via median sternotomy with cardiopulmonary bypass [6]. The left pulmonary artery is removed from its origin on the right pulmonary artery, brought in front of the trachea, and reimplanted on the main pulmonary artery.

Anesthetic considerations and approach

With any surgery involving dissection and ligation of large vascular structures, there is a potential for significant and rapid blood loss, necessitating adequate and reliable intravenous access. Induction of anesthesia is straightforward in the less symptomatic patient. However, children with significant airway compression are at risk for complete airway obstruction and benefit from an inhalation induction with the maintenance of spontaneous ventilation. In these symptomatic patients, paralysis should be administered only after the ability to assist with positive pressure ventilation has been ascertained. These patients may also require a smaller than expected endotracheal tube size. Neuraxial opioids and/or local anesthetics, either by single shot caudal, or continuous techniques, may greatly facilitate pain relief, early extubation, and pulmonary toilet (see Chapter 19). In addition to standard monitors, an arterial catheter should be placed in most of these patients because of the potential for hemodynamic and respiratory instability. In the case of an aberrant subclavian artery, site of the arterial catheter should be chosen after discussion of the surgical approach with the surgeon. Central venous catheterization should be considered for extensive surgery, poor vascular access, or anticipated hemodynamic instability. Consideration should also be given to monitoring the cerebral circulation with near-infrared spectroscopy and/or transcranial Doppler ultrasound in cases where cerebral blood flow may be compromised, e.g., clamping and reimplantation of a carotid artery that

arises from an aberrant subclavian artery. Finally, some of these operations may be facilitated by single lung ventilation to improve surgical exposure and lessen movement of vascular structures with ventilation (see Chapter 18 for a discussion of the available techniques).

Postoperative airway management and pain control

Asymptomatic patients can be extubated at the end of the case. Respiratory symptoms may worsen in symptomatic patients during the first postoperative week, occasionally necessitating intubation for adequate pulmonary toilet. For these infants, continuous positive airway pressure with humidified gas via nasal prongs may also be helpful. Good postoperative analgesia is essential to encourage deep breathing and lung expansion. This can be facilitated with epidural analgesia, intercostal rib blocks, or adequate intravenous opioid administration.

Anomalies of the coronary arteries

Abnormalities can exist in the number, origin, and termination of the coronary arteries. The number of coronary arteries can vary from one to four, often occurring in association with other congenital defects. Coronary artery fistulas have also been described [22]. A single coronary artery may be associated with myocardial ischemia, myocardial infarction, or sudden death [23]. Coronary arteries may have an anomalous origin from the aorta, the innominate artery, the carotid artery, the left anterior descending artery, or, most commonly, from the pulmonary arteries [24,25].

Anatomy

Anomalous origin from the aorta

If the left main coronary artery arises from the right aortic sinus, it courses between the ascending aorta and the pulmonary artery where compression can occur, leading to myocardial infarction or sudden death. Variations in the aortic origin of the coronary arteries often occur in association with congenital heart defects. In 7% of patients with tetralogy of Fallot, the left anterior descending artery originates from the right coronary artery, crossing over the right ventricular outflow tract where it can easily be injured during surgical repair. In patients with transposition of the great arteries, the right coronary artery and the circumflex artery often originate from the posterior sinus. Anomalous aortic origin of a coronary artery with an interarterial course is thought to have a possible genetic link [26].

Anomalous origin from the pulmonary artery

When both coronary arteries originate from the pulmonary artery in an otherwise structurally normal heart, survival is rare beyond the first few months of life. The presence of intracardiac or extracardiac lesions that increase pulmonary artery pressure and oxygen saturation may increase the survival.

Anomalous origin of the left anterior descending coronary artery, or the circumflex coronary artery from the pulmonary artery has also been reported [27]. Both lesions can result in ischemia and should be surgically repaired with aortic reimplantation or aortocoronary bypass graft.

Anomalous origin of the right coronary artery from the pulmonary artery

Occasionally, the right coronary artery arises from the pulmonary artery [28]. Blood usually flows via collaterals from the enlarged left coronary artery to the right coronary artery and then into the pulmonary artery, creating a coronary artery–pulmonary artery fistula. Although a relatively benign condition, death from ischemia can occur and surgical correction is recommended. Surgical repair involves aortic reimplantation of the right coronary artery. This repair is straightforward because of the anterior origin of the anomalous artery and its close proximity to the aorta.

Anomalous origin of the left coronary artery from the pulmonary artery

Anomalous origin of the left coronary artery from the pulmonary artery (ALCAPA) [29] is the most studied of this class of defects and was first described in 1908. ALCAPA occurs in 1 in 300,000 live births and usually occurs as an isolated lesion. The left coronary artery usually arises from the left posterior sinus of the pulmonary artery. The right coronary artery is usually enlarged, with a normal origin from the aorta. Numerous collaterals of variable size and number course over the right ventricular outflow tract, or through the interventricular septum, connecting the two coronary arteries. ALCAPA is one of the most common causes of myocardial ischemia and infarction in children. The left ventricle is usually enlarged and hypertrophied. Endocardial fibrosis and scarring can occur in infancy. Fibrosis may also involve the papillary muscles of the mitral valve and may cause variable degrees of valvular incompetence.

Pathophysiology and natural history

The physiologic changes produced by ALCAPA worsen after delivery. In utero, when the pulmonary artery pres-sure and oxygen saturation nearly equal the systemic pressure and oxygen saturation, left ventricular myocardial perfusion and oxygenation are adequate. Myocardial ischemia develops soon after birth as pulmonary vascular resistance falls, causing a marked decrease in left coronary artery perfusion pressure. The infant's survival is dependent on the extent of collateral formation from the right coronary artery to the left coronary artery. These intercoronary collaterals, however, also allow the flow of blood from the right coronary artery via the left coronary artery system into the pulmonary artery and are often referred to as coronary artery fistulization. This coronary artery "steal" causes lower perfusion pressure and results in myocardial damage.

Typical presentation includes profuse sweating, tachycardia, tachypnea, dyspnea, coughing, wheezing, pallor, and failure to thrive. In some infants, atypical chest pain upon eating and crying has been mistaken for colic [30]. One should have a high index of suspicion of ALCAPA in any infant with global myocardial dysfunction. However, about 10% of patients with ALCAPA with good collateral flow do not develop myocardial ischemia until adolescence or adulthood [31]. Adults have presented with malignant ventricular arrhythmias [32], shortness of breath with exercise [31], cardiac murmur [33], and cardiac arrest during exercise [34]. Although the most common cause of sudden death in young competitive athletes is hypertrophic cardiomyopathy, 13% of deaths in these athletes involve anomalous coronary artery origin [35]. All older patients with asymptomatic ALCAPA had multiple unusual color flow Doppler signals within the ventricular septum, representing septal coronary collaterals [36].

Physical examination reveals evidence of congestive heart failure, cardiomegaly, and the murmur of mitral insufficiency. The chest X-ray consistently shows massive cardiomegaly. Bronchial compression by the enlarged heart can result in atelectatic changes in the left lung.

The electrocardiogram (ECG) is abnormal in all patients, showing evidence of ischemia, infarction, and left ventricular hypertrophy. ECG findings have been described that are present in all patients with ALCAPA but absent from most patients with myocarditis and cardiomyopathy. These ECG criteria are (i) Q-wave depth >3 mm, (ii) Q-wave width >30 ms, and (iii) a QR pattern in one of the following leads: I, aVL, V5–V7 [37]. Multislice cardiac CT is also useful for diagnosing congenital coronary abnormalities [38,39].

Echocardiography can demonstrate the anatomic origin of the ALCAPA and provides an assessment of the degree of left ventricular impairment. Studies show a significant enlargement of the right coronary artery and a dilated left ventricle with global hypokinesia. Pulse and color flow Doppler imaging can directly visualize the anomalous origin as well as the reversal of flow from the ALCAPA into the pulmonary artery [25]. Preliminary data evaluating PET perfusion images suggest its clinical utility to assess myocardial perfusion in the pediatric population [40]. Cardiac catheterization is not routinely performed unless ALCAPA is suspected but cannot be visualized by echocardiography. When performed, aortography can show filling of the left coronary artery thru collaterals from the dilated right coronary artery and can exclude other anomalies.

The need for early surgical repair of all infants with AL-CAPA is essential in even asymptomatic infants because of the extremely poor survival with medical management. Ninety percent of undiagnosed or medically treated infants die within the first year of life. Sudden death frequently occurs in untreated older children and adults. Thus, surgical correction is indicated in all patients with ALCAPA.

Surgical approaches

Surgical treatment for ALCAPA is directed toward correcting the "coronary steal" phenomenon, and increasing left ventricular myocardial perfusion and function. This can be accomplished by either reconstituting a two-coronary system or by simply ligating the fistulous flow. Restoring a two-coronary circulation is preferred, and when possible, direct coronary–aortic reimplantation is performed [41]. Scarred myocardium or free wall aneurysm is not addressed at the time of initial surgery.

Simple ligation of the ALCAPA eliminates the "steal" phenomenon, and in the past had been recommended as the procedure of choice in critically ill infants but has a prohibitive mortality rate ranging from 20 to 50% [42]. A single coronary artery system is less physiologic with greater risk of postoperative complications, a higher early postoperative mortality, and a higher potential for atherosclerosis as well as late sudden death.

Surgical reconstitution of a two-coronary artery system results in greater recovery of left ventricular function and is now the standard surgical procedure [43,44]. Direct coronary aortic reimplantation is an excellent procedure because it is simple, does not require prosthetic material, and is expected to provide excellent late results. However, it often requires creative surgical technique to obtain sufficient length and correct angling of the coronary artery to the aorta (Figure 25.2). This is difficult when the anomalous vessel originates from the left posterior wall of the pulmonary trunk. If mobilization and reimplantation will compromise the vessel, the left subclavian artery may be anastomosed to the left coronary artery (Figure 25.3). This procedure may be done without cardiopulmonary bypass but is not feasible if the left main coronary artery is short in length [46].

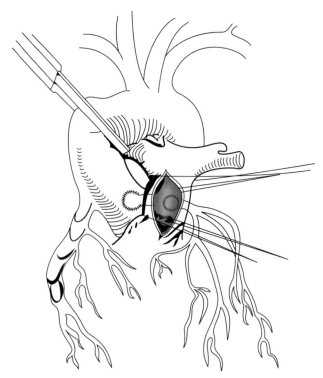

Figure 25.2 Direct aortic reimplantation of anomalous left coronary artery from the pulmonary artery. The anomalous ostium is excised with a button of pulmonary artery wall. This button is then implanted into the left lateral side of the ascending aorta. The resulting defect is closed with a pericardial patch (Reproduced with permission from Reference [45])

A saphenous vein bypass graft may also be used, but requires deep hypothermia (18°C) with total circulatory arrest. The small vein caliber and the incidence of late graft occlusion limit the utility of the saphenous vein graft in infants. Alternatively, an aortocoronary bypass graft with a free segment of the subclavian artery may be used. An end-to-side retroaortic coronary bypass graft construction with a free segment of the left subclavian artery is applicable in the majority of infants. More recently, the left internal mammary artery (LIMA) has been used but long-term results are lacking with ALCAPA [47,48].

Newer techniques utilize the pulmonary artery as a conduit graft from the left coronary artery to the aorta. This is useful for cases where the left coronary artery arises from the left posterior sinus. The Takeuchi procedure [49] uses a flap derived from the anterior wall of the pulmonary trunk to create a coronary tunnel inside the pulmonary trunk between a surgically created aortopulmonary window and the left coronary ostium (Figure 25.4). The opening in the pulmonary trunk is then patched with pericardium. Late complications have been reported with the Takeuchi procedure. Tashiro et al. has described left coronary angioplasty using pulmonary trunk without prosthetic material, which is expected to yield excellent late

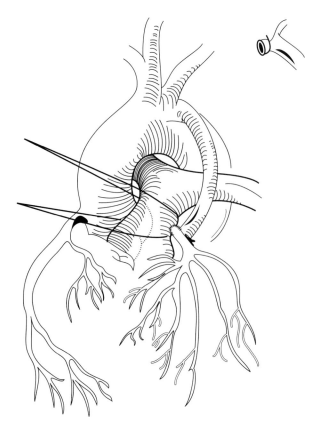

Figure 25.3 Left subclavian artery–left coronary artery anastomosis for the management of anomalous origin of the left coronary from the pulmonary artery. The anomalous vessel is also ligated at its origin (Reproduced with permission from Reference [45])

results. This procedure combines left coronary angioplasty, side-to-side anastomosis of the aorta with the newly created left coronary artery and direct anastomosis of the transected pulmonary artery [50]. To date, no difference has been shown in the long-term left ventricular function or late mortality among the various surgical techniques which reestablish a two-coronary circulation [51,52]. Orthotopic heart transplantation for ALCAPA has also been described [53].

There have been conflicting opinions as to the necessity for the repair of mitral incompetence in these patients. Some surgeons recommend mitral annuloplasty at the time of the initial operation [54]. However, the vast majority of regurgitant valves gradually improve within 6 months by serial echocardiography without annuloplasty [44]. Even severe MR has been reported to regress fully after reperfusion alone in 62% of cases [55]. Many surgeons now feel that mitral valve repair is not generally necessary at the time of the initial operation [56]. In some patients, the persistence or recurrence of MR may signify a significant coexistent coronary stenosis. Patients who have significant obstruction in their left coronary artery will have residual MR and may require not only mitral valve repair, but also revascularization of the left coronary artery [56].

Anesthetic considerations and approach

Infants with ALCAPA are often critically ill with little cardiac reserve and significant ischemia. More severe preoperative MR is associated with increased perioperative mortality [57]. Adequate monitoring, including a multi-lead ECG, arterial pressure monitoring, and central venous access for drug administration and assessment of volume status are essential. Induction should be a gradual one to avoid major swings in blood pressure. A gentle and rapid laryngoscopy is also critical. Fluid administration is titrated to assure adequate preload for maintenance of cardiac output while avoiding pulmonary edema. Measures to mildly increase pulmonary vascular resistance such as normocapnia and decreasing F_{IO_2} to the lowest level tolerated can help minimize the coronary steal phenomenon.

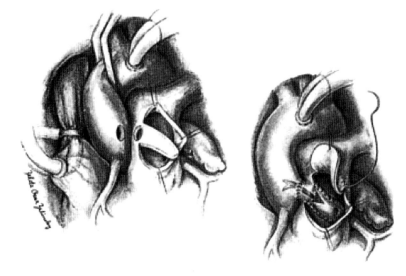

Figure 25.4 The Takeuchi procedure is shown through a median sternotomy with cardiopulmonary bypass and cross-clamped aorta. A tunnel for coronary flow (*arrow*) has been created between the aorta and the anomalous left coronary artery by means of a flap of pulmonary artery wall. The pulmonary wall is then reconstructed with pericardium (Reproduced with permission from Reference [42])

Inotropic agents can improve cardiac function, but can also increase heart rate and myocardial oxygen consumption and worsen the ischemia. The cardiovascular depressant effects of volatile anesthetics are often poorly tolerated, and an opioid technique may be preferred.

If repair requires the use of cardiopulmonary bypass, significant postbypass inotropic support may be needed, e.g., dopamine, dobutamine, or epinephrine. Nitroglycerin is often used to improve coronary perfusion. Decreasing the afterload of the left ventricle is also desirable and can be accomplished with an inodilator (milrinone) or a vasodilator (sodium nitroprusside). Mechanical support of the left ventricle with a left ventricular assist device (LVAD) may be required in some patients who are unable to be weaned from cardiopulmonary bypass [58]. This may be more common in the younger infant with poor collateralization of coronary blood flow and acute myocardial infarction. Postoperative pain control with intravenous narcotic is adequate. Most patients are kept intubated and ventilated postoperatively to allow time for ventricular recovery.

Normalization of left ventricular function occurs substantially after restoration of a two-coronary circulation, although this may take as long as 2 years, and some degree of chronic impairment may persist. Even in the group requiring LVAD support, a high survival rate and good long-term recovery can be achieved.

The optimal follow-up method after ALCAPA repair is controversial, with ECG, Holter monitoring, stress-thallium scanning, and cardiac catheterization all showing equivocal results. Serial echocardiography can be useful to assess the left ventricular function, the severity of mitral insufficiency and the patency of the revascularized left coronary artery flow. Long-term survivors of ALCAPA repair show regional impairment of myocardial flow reserve that may contribute to impaired exercise performance [59]. However, even under stress testing, the normal growth of the heart has not been found to compromise the anastomosis. Patients with ALCAPA that survive the perioperative period have an excellent prognosis for functional recovery of the left ventricle regardless of their preoperative state [60]. Subclinical changes suggestive of ischemia may occur despite patent neocoronary ostia [61].

Mitral regurgitation

Anatomy

MR rarely occurs as an isolated lesion in congenital heart disease. Rather, it usually occurs as a component of another lesion, such as complete or partial atrioventricular canal defect, mitral valve prolapse, myocardial or papillary muscle infarction such as that seen with the ALCAPA

syndrome (see above), connective tissue disorder such as Marfan's Syndrome, rheumatic disease, endocarditis, or Kawasaki disease [62,63].

Pathophysiology and natural history

In the normal mitral valve, the leaflets are asymmetric, with the anterior leaflet spanning one-third of the annulus, and the C-shaped posterior leaflet two-thirds. The anterior leaflet inserts into the anterolateral papillary muscle, and the posterior leaflet into the posteromedial papillary muscle. The papillary muscles insert into the left ventricular free wall in the normal mitral valve; the anterior leaflet is normally perfused by the left coronary artery and the posterior leaflet by branches of both left and right coronary arteries [64]. Valve competency depends on the large posterior leaflet overlapping the anterior leaflet during systole, and thus complete coaptation is necessary. Any process interfering with this coaptation, be it a cleft in the posterior leaflet, annular dilation from left ventricular infarction, or severe dysfunction, may cause MR.

The clinical severity and symptoms of MR can be classified as mild, moderate, or severe [65]. In the patient with chronic MR, the patient may be asymptomatic. As MR worsens, both left atrium and left ventricle dilate, resulting in enlargement of the mitral annulus, and creating a vicious cycle of worsening MR as the annulus dilates. Resting heart rate increases, and as left atrial pressures increase, pulmonary venous, capillary, and finally pulmonary artery hypertension can occur. This results in tachypnea, pulmonary edema, poor feeding, and diaphoresis in infants, and may result in atrial arrhythmias such as atrial fibrillation. The enlarged left atrium may cause compression of the left mainstem bronchus in infants. Obstructive airways disease and frequent infections occur in infants with moderate to severe MR. Physical examination in moderate to severe MR often reveals a diaphoretic, tachypneic patient, with resting tachycardia and an increased precordial impulse. The left ventricular apex may be displaced laterally, and the second heart sound intensity may be increased with pulmonary hypertension. A holosystolic, high-frequency murmur is heard at the apex, radiating to the axilla. A low-pitched diastolic rumble is heard with moderate or severe MR. The presence of a third heart sound indicates severe MR. Chest radiograph reveals cardiomegaly, with left atrial and left ventricular enlargement, and varying degrees of increase pulmonary vascular markings. The left lower lobe may have atelectasis due to left atrial enlargement and compression of left-sided bronchi. Medical treatment includes the use of diuretics, digoxin, and afterload reduction provided by angiotensin-converting enzyme inhibitors. Acute MR, such as that seen with acute infarction of a papillary muscle or left ventricle from ALCAPA, is often very poorly tolerated, with rapid development of pulmonary edema and respiratory and circulatory decompensation. Indications for surgical intervention include uncontrolled congestive heart failure resulting in failure to thrive, progressive enlargement of left atrium and ventricle despite medical management, or atrial arrhythmias or persistent airway symptoms.

Echocardiographic diagnosis is essential to define the anatomy underlying the MR, and its severity. Various schema for grading echocardiographic severity have been devised; generally, when there is flow reversal in the pulmonary veins, the MR is considered significant. A regurgitant fraction can be calculated. Another indicator of severity of MR is the diameter of the regurgitant jet at the level of the orifice [66]. Cardiac catheterization is infrequently required for MR, but a regurgitant fraction can often be calculated angiographically, with a 20% regurgitant fraction considered mild MR, 20–40% moderate, 40–60% moderately severe, and >60% severe. The left atrial pressure is elevated with a large A wave [67].

Surgical approaches

Surgical approaches include annuloplasty with a prosthetic DeVega or Carpentier ring, suturing the cleft in the mitral valve, resection of a portion of the posterior leaflet, repairing or foreshortening a ruptured or damaged chordae tendinae, or mitral valve replacement [68]. Mitral valve repair is preferred in most centers in growing children, because of the need for anticoagulation with prosthetic valves, and the need for repeated replacement until growth is complete [68]. Surgical repair of congenital mitral valve can be performed with low mortality and satisfactory valve function [69]. The surgery is done via midline sternotomy with cardiopulmonary bypass, and is often approached through an incision in the left atrium. The exact surgical approach is often not determined until the surgeon inspects the anatomy. After the repair of the valve, appropriate annular size may be tested by passing a Hegar dilator of appropriate size for the patient's body surface area, and competence of the valve by injecting saline rapidly through the valve orifice into the left ventricle and noting competence while the heart is flaccid, which often predicts residual regurgitation.

Anesthetic considerations

The optimal hemodynamic state for a patient with moderate or severe MR consists of afterload reduction, adequate preload and contractility, and high–normal heart rate. Faster heart rates lead to less diastolic filling time, and less time for ejection, which will lead to a smaller regurgitant fraction, i.e., more forward stroke volume and cardiac output. Afterload reduction will encourage forward flow as well, and adequate preload is necessary for forward flow to be normal [70]. Contractility should be maintained at normal levels to ensure ejection of the large stroke volumes seen in this lesion. A number of anesthetic regimens can be used to meet these goals, but high-dose synthetic narcotics will need to be combined with a vagolytic agent such as pancuronium to maintain high heart rates. Ketamine may not be desirable because this agent usually elevates systemic vascular resistance. Volatile agents are acceptable as long as they do not unduly depress contractility and they maintain heart rate; thus, isoflurane, desflurane, or sevoflurane is preferable to halothane in this lesion [71].

Monitoring consists of standard monitors, arterial and central catheters, and transesophageal echocardiography (TEE), which is critical to reconfirm the preoperative findings, and most importantly, to assess the adequacy of surgical repair [66]. In addition, since the left side of the heart is opened for mitral valve surgery, TEE is critical to assess adequacy of intracardiac de-airing before the aortic cross-clamp is removed and before the patient is weaned from cardiopulmonary bypass [72]. Carbon dioxide is insufflated into the surgical field in some centers when the left side of the heart is open to air to decrease the number and size of air bubbles in the heart [73]. A left atrial catheter is often placed transthoracically by the surgeon during rewarming on bypass, in order to measure left-sided filling pressures after bypass. Transcranial Doppler ultrasound is used in some centers to detect cerebral emboli, along with near-infrared cerebral oximetry. Inotropic support is often required after cardiopulmonary bypass, and phosphodiesterase inhibitors such as milrinone are often used because of their vasodilating effects on both pulmonary and systemic circulations, and effects on both systolic and diastolic ventricular function.

Assessment of the postoperative repair and hemodynamics after bypass includes left atrial pressure measurement, both the absolute number (may be elevated in both residual MR, or in mitral stenosis), and the presence or absence of a large V wave (present in MR, not at prominent in mitral stenosis or left ventricular dysfunction.), which signifies residual MR. Once again, the TEE is crucial to determine the presence of residual MR, or the occasional creation of mitral stenosis, signified by elevated mitral valve inflow velocities or abnormal inflow patterns (see Chapter 11). These patients usually are not at great risk for postoperative bleeding because the suture lines are low pressure atrial sutures. Length of postoperative ventilation depends entirely on the patient's pre- and postoperative condition; some older patients with preserved ventricular function may be candidates for early extubation.

Pericardial effusion and tamponade

The pericardium is composed of visceral and parietal layers, and forms an avascular fibrous sac that surrounds the heart and extends a short distance onto the great vessels [74,75]. Collagen and connective tissue fibers form the fibrosa, and is compliant under normal conditions of low fluid volume and stretch, but when fluid in the pericardial sac increases significantly, the steep portion of the pressure–volume curve may be reached, and intrapericardial pressures increase greatly, and create tamponade physiology. The pericardium is opened and partially removed for most cardiac surgeries, but the closed mediastinal space still has limited reserve to accumulate blood and fluid, especially in small infants.

Symptomatic pericardial effusion and tamponade may be seen in a number of clinical settings, both postsurgical, and in medical conditions [76]. Acute postoperative hemorrhagic tamponade is obviously a life-threatening emergency, but mediastinal bleeding and tamponade physiology may develop more slowly, over hours to several days postoperatively [77]. Other causes of pericardial effusion and tamponade include cardiac perforation from cardiac catheterization or central venous catheter placement [78], chylous pericardial effusion after surgery, acute viral or bacterial infections, trauma, postpericardiotomy syndrome, malignancy, congestive heart failure, renal failure, and inflammatory and autoimmune disorders [79] and pericardial cysts [80].

Cardiac tamponade occurs when fluid, blood, or blood clots fill the pericardial space or mediastinum and increase pressure enough to significantly affect cardiac output. Beck's triad consists of hypotension, elevated systemic venous pressure, and a small quiet heart on auscultation [81]. Clinically, patients with tamponade physiology have dyspnea, tachycardia, distended neck veins, narrow pulse pressure, and pulsus paradoxus in the presence of a pericardial effusion. Tamponade physiology develops as right and left atrial, and biventricular end-diastolic pressures equalize as the cardiac chambers compete for restricted space [79]. Diastolic filling and thus stoke volume becomes restricted, and the sympathetic nervous system compensates by increasing contractile state, ejection fraction, and heart rate. Inspiration lowers intrathoracic pressure and promotes venous inflow into the right ventricle, which fills but this shifts the interventricular septum to the left, restricting left ventricular filling. The negative intrathoracic pressure also decreases pressure in the pulmonary veins, and in combination with elevated left ventricular diastolic pressure, this also inhibits left ventricular filling, and thus stroke volume decreases greatly during inspiration, creating pulsus paradoxus. Interestingly, pulsus paradoxus detected on the pulse oximeter plethysmographic wave-

form correlates well with clinical cardiac tamponade in pediatric patients [82]. Of note, positive pressure ventilation, atrial septal defect, severe left ventricular dysfunction, hypertrophic cardiomyopathy, and aortic insufficiency all reduce or eliminate pulsus paradoxus.

Aside from clinical signs and symptoms, echocardiography is the most important diagnostic tool in pericardial effusion and tamponade syndromes [83]. The size and location of the effusion can be defined, as well as its consistency—serous or bloody versus fibrous or clots. In addition, tamponade physiology can be confirmed by detecting reduced mitral valve and pulmonary vein inflow during inspiration. The echocardiogram can also direct the physician to the best and safest location for pericardiocentesis, or open drainage.

In a patient with tamponade physiology, the induction of general anesthesia, muscle relaxation, tracheal intubation, and positive pressure ventilation are fraught with danger, and cardiac arrest and death occurs in this scenario. The patient is often barely compensating, and only the combination of maximal sympathetic stimulation and negative intrathoracic pressure during spontaneous respiration are allowing enough stoke volume to maintain barely adequate cardiac output. Any upset in this balance can result in cardiac arrest. Anesthetic agents may remove sympathetic stimulation, and the institution of positive pressure ventilation may increase intrathoracic pressure to the point that systemic and pulmonary venous return essentially cease. The ideal situation would be to drain some of the fluid under local anesthesia so that ventricular filling and cardiac output can improve to the point that the patient can tolerate anesthetic induction for a definitive procedure. This is often possible in the adult or cooperative older child or teenager, but not in the infant or toddler. In this situation, ketamine, despite its potential for direct myocardial depression, is usually well tolerated, while maintaining spontaneous ventilation until some fluid can be drained.

If general anesthesia must be induced, the cardiologist or surgeon responsible for the drainage of the fluid must be present, prepared to emergently access the pericardial or mediastinal space, either by needle, or incision. Echocardiographic guidance is essential for pericardiocentesis, where the pericardial space is not being accessed under direct vision. All equipment and cross-matched blood must also be readily available, and in some instances it is prudent to have the subxyphoid area sterilely prepared and draped for immediate incision if hemodynamic collapse occurs on induction. An adequate period of preoxygenation is essential. Intravascular volume loading is recommended because it may maximize venous return, and is unlikely to worsen the situation acutely. Etomidate would appear to be the preferable agent for rapid intravenous induction of anesthesia because of its lack of negative inotropic effect on the myocardium [84,85]. Ketamine would be a possible choice, but again has direct negative effects on the myocardium [86]. If the patient is not at high risk for gastric aspiration, it may be preferable to induce anesthesia and keep the patient breathing spontaneously or gently assisted, if possible, until some of the fluid can be drained. Succinylcholine may need to be avoided because of its propensity to cause bradycardia. Tracheal intubation should be rapid, and positive pressure ventilation extremely gentle, or avoided for as long as possible. Preparations should be made for a full resuscitation, including epinephrine and atropine. In the event of hemodynamic collapse, drainage of the pericardial space must proceed immediately while resuscitative efforts are made. Draining the fluid normally allows the patient to recover enough cardiac output to continue the procedure at a more controlled pace.

Drainage of the pericardium or mediastinum can be accomplished by pericardiocentesis, where the space is accessed under echocardiographic guidance with a needle, then a guidewire, and finally a catheter is placed for drainage. Injection of agitated saline as echocardiographic contrast medium may assist in localizing the pericardial space [87]. This is normally performed by a cardiologist, and should be performed in a location where full resuscitative resources, including personnel, are available. A subxyphoid pericardial window for drainage is frequently performed by the surgeon, with a mediastinal drain left in place for several days. Occasionally, as in the case of constrictive pericarditis, with impending tamponade, a pericardial stripping must be done with full sternotomy. Acute postoperative tamponade from mediastinal bleeding is heralded by low blood pressure and poor systemic perfusion accompanied by elevated central venous and left atrial pressures. Mediastinal tube drainage may be increased, or may have decreased greatly, giving the team the false sense of security. A widened mediastinum may be seen on chest radiograph, and this can be confused with low cardiac output due to myocardial dysfunction. Echocardiography, if time permits, will exclude the latter diagnosis. The sternum must be reopened immediately at the bedside in the intensive care unit in cases of impending cardiac arrest. A more controlled reexploration may be undertaken in the operating room, if time permits.

Reported complications for pericardiocentesis in pediatric patients range from death from cardiac perforation and tamponade to pneumopericardium, to ST segment changes from coronary artery lacerations [88,89]. Higher complication rates are seen with younger patients under the age of 2 years, inexperienced operators, and lack of echocardiographic guidance, making the latter essential. Hand-held portable ultrasound technology has progressed to the point where this may be a viable option in any hospital setting [90].

Summary of management

Vascular rings

- Reliable vascular access is essential because of the potential for significant and rapid blood loss. Arterial line for most; consider central line.
- An inhalation induction should be performed with maintenance of spontaneous ventilation until the ability to assist with positive pressure ventilation has been ascertained.
- Patients may require a smaller-than-expected endotracheal tube size, and single lung ventilation may be desirable
- Minimally symptomatic patients can be extubated at the end of the case.
- Good postoperative analgesia is essential using epidural analgesia, intercostal rib blocks, or adequate intravenous opioids.

Anomalies of the coronary arteries

- Infants with ALCAPA are often critically ill with little cardiac reserve and significant myocardial ischemia.
- Adequate monitoring, including a multilead ECG, arterial pressure monitoring, and central venous access for drug administration and volume assessment are essential.
- Induction should be gradual to avoid major swings in blood pressure. A gentle and rapid laryngoscopy is also critical.
- Fluid administration is titrated to assure adequate preload for maintenance of cardiac output while avoiding pulmonary edema.
- Measures to mildly increase pulmonary vascular resistance such as normocapnia can help minimize the coronary steal phenomenon.
- Inotropic agents can improve cardiac function, but can also increase heart rate and myocardial oxygen consumption and worsen the ischemia.
- The cardiovascular depressant effects of volatile anesthetics are often poorly tolerated, and an opioid technique may be preferred.
- After cardiopulmonary bypass, significant inotropic, inodilator, and coronary and systemic vasodilator support may be needed.
- Most patients are kept intubated and ventilated postoperatively to allow time for ventricular recovery.
- Mechanical support of the left ventricle with an LVAD may be required in some patients who are unable to be weaned from cardiopulmonary bypass.
- Severe preoperative mitral insufficiency and ventricular dysfunction often result in postoperative hemodynamic instability and increased perioperative mortality.

Mitral regurgitation

- The optimal hemodynamic state for a patient with moderate of severe MR consists of afterload reduction, adequate preload and contractility, and high–normal heart rate.
- High-dose synthetic narcotics will need to be combined with a vagolytic agent such as pancuronium.
- Volatile agents are acceptable as long as they do not unduly depress contractility and they maintain heart rate; halothane may not be desirable.
- TEE and left atrial pressure monitoring are crucial to determine the presence of residual MR, or the occasional creation of mitral stenosis.

Pericardial effusion and tamponade

- Patients with tamponade physiology have dyspnea, tachycardia, distended neck veins, narrow pulse pressure, and pulsus paradoxus.
- Induction of general anesthesia, muscle relaxation, tracheal intubation, and positive pressure ventilation may precipitate cardiovascular collapse.
- Drainage of a small amount of the pericardial fluid with sedation (ketamine) and local anesthesia should be performed if possible.
- Etomidate is the preferred drug for induction of general anesthesia.
- Personnel and equipment for immediate drainage and resuscitation must be immediately available.
- Echocardiographic guidance is essential for closed procedures not under direct vision, i.e., pericardiocentesis.

References

1. Hommel, cited by Turner W (1962) On irregularities of the pulmonary artery, arch of the aorta and the primary branches of the arch with an attempt to illustrate their mode of origin by a reference to development Br Foreign Med Chir Rev 173 (30): 461.
2. Bayford D (1974) An account of a singular case of deglutition. Memoirs Med Soc London 2: 275.
3. Gross RE (1945) Surgical relief for tracheal obstruction from a vascular ring. N Engl J Med 233: 586–590.
4. Kouchoukos NT, Blackstone EH, Doty DB, et al. (2003) Vascular ring and sling. In: Kirklin JW, Barrat-Boyes BG (eds) Cardiac Surgery: Morphology, Diagnostic Criteria, Natural History, Techniques, Results and Indications, 3rd edn. Churchill Livingstone, New York, pp. 1415–1437.
5. Chun K, Colombani PM, Dudgeon DL, et al. (1992) Diagnosis and management of congenital vascular rings: a 22-year experience. Ann Thorac Surg 53: 597–603.
6. Chang AC, Hanley FL (1998) Rings and slings. In: Chang AC (ed.) Pediatric Cardiac Intensive Care. Williams & Wilkins, Baltimore, pp. 322–324.
7. Bakker DA, Berger RM, Witsenburg M, et al. (1999) Vascular rings: a rare cause of common respiratory symptoms. Acta Paediatr 88: 947–952.
8. Hickey EJ, Aftab K, Anderson D, et al. (2007) Complete vascular ring presenting in adulthood: an unusual management dilemma. J Thorac Cardiovasc Surg 134 (1): 235–236.
9. Massaad J, Crawford K (2008) Double aortic arch and nasogastric tubes: a fatal combination. World J Gastroenterol 14 (16): 2590–2592.
10. Heck HA, Jr, Moore HV, Lutin WA, et al. (1993) Esophageal-aortic erosion associated with double aortic arch and tracheomalacia. Experience with 2 infants. Tex Heart Inst J 20: 126–129.
11. Pumberger W, Voitl P, Gopfrich H (2002) Recurrent respiratory tract infections and dysphagia in a child with an aortic vascular ring. South Med J 95: 265–268.
12. Parker JM, Cary-Freitas B, Berg BW (2000) Symptomatic vascular rings in adulthood: an uncommon mimic of asthma. J Asthma 37: 275–280.
13. Grathwohl KW, Afifi AY, Dillard TA, et al. (1999) Vascular rings of the thoracic aorta in adults. Am Surg 65: 1077–1083.
14. Berdon WE (2000) Rings, slings, and other things: vascular compression of the infant trachea updated from the mid-century to the millennium—the legacy of Robert E. Gross, MD, and Edward B. D. Neuhauser, MD. Radiology 216: 624–632.
15. Pickhardt PJ, Siegel MJ, Gutierrez FR (1997) Vascular rings in symptomatic children: frequency of chest radiographic findings. Radiology 203: 423–426.
16. Becit N, Bilgehan E, Karaca Y (2008) Tracheoesophageal compression associated with symmetrical double aortic arch. Tex Heart Inst J 35 (2): 209–210.
17. Beekmann RP, Hazekamp MG, Sobotka MA, et al. (1998) A new diagnostic approach to vascular rings and pulmonary slings: the role of MRI. Magn Reson Imaging 16: 137–145.
18. Alsenaidi K, Gurofsky R, Karamlou T, et al. (2006) Management and outcomes of double aortic arch in 81 patients. Am J Pediatr 118 (5): 1336–1341.
19. Zani A, Morini F, Paolantonio P, et al. (2008) Not all symptoms disappear after vascular ring division. Pediatr Cardiol 29: 676–678.
20. Woods RK, Sharp RJ, Holcomb GW 3rd, et al. (2001) Vascular anomalies and tracheoesophageal compression: a single institution's 25-year experience. Ann Thorac Surg 72: 434–439.
21. Burke RP, Chang AC (1993) Video-assisted thoracoscopic division of a vascular ring in an infant: a new operative technique. J Card Surg 8: 537–540.
22. Ceresnak S, Gray RG, Altmann K, et al. (2007) Coronary artery fistulas: a review of the literature and presentation of two cases of coronary fistulas with drainage into the left atrium. Congenit Heart Dis 2 (3): 208–213.
23. Said SA, Lam J, Van Der Werf T (2006) Solitary coronary artier fistulas: a congenital anomaly in children and adults. A contemporary review. Congenit Heart Dis 1 (3): 63–76.
24. Kaushal SK, Radhakrisnan S, Dagar KS, et al. (1998) Anomalous origin of the left anterior descending coronary artery from the pulmonary artery. J Thorac Cardiovasc Surg 116: 1078–1080.

25. Fernandes ED, Kadivar H, Hallman G, et al. (1992) congenital malformations of the coronary arteries: the Texas Heart Institute experience. Ann Thorac Surg 54: 732–740.

26. Brothers JA, Stephens P, Gaynor W, et al. (2008) Anomalous aortic origin of a coronary artery with an interarterial course. Should family screening be routine? JACC 51 (21): 2062–2064.

27. Alexi-Meskishvili V, Dähnert I, Hetzer R, et al. (1998) Origin of the circumflex coronary artery from the pulmonary artery in infants. Ann Thorac Surg 66: 1406–1409.

28. Radke PW, Messmer BJ, Haager PJ, et al. (1998) Anomalous origin of the right coronary artery: preoperative and postoperative hemodynamics. Ann Thorac Surg 66: 1444–1449.

29. Kouchoukos NT, Blackstone EH, Doty DB, et al. (2003) Congenital anomalies of the coronary arteries. In: Kirklin JW, Barrat-Boyes BG (eds) Cardiac Surgery: Morphology, Diagnostic Criteria, Natural History, Techniques, Results and Indications, 3rd edn. Churchill Livingstone, New York, pp. 1240–1263.

30. Mahle WT (1998) A dangerous case of colic: anomalous left coronary artery presenting with paroxysms of irritability. Pediatr Emerg Care 14: 24–27.

31. Noda R, Sasao H, Kyuma M, et al. (2001) Cardiac imaging in a patient with anomalous origin of the left coronary artery from the pulmonary artery—a case report. Angiology 52: 567–571.

32. Frapier JM, Leclercq F, Bodino M, et al. (1999) Malignant ventricular arrhythmias revealing anomalous origin of the left coronary artery in two adults. Eur J Cardiothorac Surg 15: 539–541.

33. Fierens C, Budts W, Denef B, et al. (2000) A 72 year old woman with ALCAPA. Heart 83: E2.

34. Nielsen HB, Perko M, Aldershvile J, et al. (1999) Cardiac arrest during exercise: anomalous left coronary artery from the pulmonary trunk. Scand Cardiovasc J 33: 369–371.

35. Maron BJ, Shirani J, Poliac LC, et al. (1996) Sudden death in young competitive athletes. Clinical, demographic, and pathological profiles. JAMA 276: 199–204.

36. Frommelt MA, Miller E, Williamson J, et al. (2002) Detection of septal coronary collaterals by color flow Doppler mapping is a marker for anomalous origin of a coronary artery from the pulmonary artery. J Am Soc Echocardiogr 15: 259–263.

37. Johnsrude CL, Perry JC, Smith EO, et al. (1995) Differentiating anomalous left main coronary artery originating from the pulmonary artery in infants from myocarditis and dilated cardiomyopathy by electrocardiogram. Am J Cardiol 75: 71–74.

38. Girish R (2006) Multislice cardiac computed tomographic images of anomalous origin of the left coronary artery from the pulmonary artery (ALCAPA). Heart 92: 2.

39. Coche E, Muller P, Gerber B (2006) Anomalous origin of the left main coronary artery from the amin pulmonary artery (ALCAPA) illustrated before and after surgical correction on ECG-gated 40-slice computed tomography. Heart 92: 1193.

40. Chhatriwalla AK, Prieto LR, Brunken RC, et al. (2008) Preliminary data on the diagnostic accuracy of Rubidium-82 cardiac PET perfusion imaging for the evaluation of ischemia in a pediatric population. Pediatr Cardiol 29: 732–738.

41. Vouhé PR, Tamisier D, Sidi D, et al. (1992) Anomalous left coronary artery from the pulmonary artery: results of isolated aortic reimplantation. Ann Thorac Surg 54: 621–627.

42. Backer CL, Stout MJ, Zales VR, et al. (1992) Anomalous origin of the left coronary artery. A twenty-year review of surgical management. J Thorac Cardiovasc Surg 103: 1049–1058.

43. Alsoufi A, Sallehuddin A, Bulbul Z, et al. (2008) Surgical strategy to establish a dual-coronary system for the management of anomalous left coronary artery origin from the pulmonary artery. Ann Thorac Surg 86: 170–176.

44. Lange R, Vogt M, Hörer J, et al. (2007) Long-term results of repair of anomalous origin of the left coronary artery from the pulmonary artery. Ann Thorac Surg 83: 1463–1471.

45. Arciniegas E (1985) Coronary artery anomalies. In: Arciniegas E (ed.) Pediatric Cardiac Surgery. Year Book Medical Publishers, Chicago, pp. 389–402.

46. Montigny M, Stanley P, Chartrand C, et al. (1990) Postoperative evaluation after end-to-end subclavian-left coronary artery anastomosis in anomalous left coronary artery. J Thorac Cardiovasc Surg 100: 270–273.

47. Mavroudis C, Backer CL, Muster AJ, et al. (1996) Expanding indications for pediatric coronary artery bypass. J Thorac Cardiovasc Surg 111: 181–189.

48. Mavroudis C, Backer CL, Duffy CE, et al. (1999) Pediatric coronary artery bypass for Kawasaki, congenital, post arterial switch, and iatrogenic lesions. Ann Thorac Surg 68: 506–512.

49. Takeuchi S, Imamura H, Katsumoto K, et al. (1979) New surgical method for repair of anomalous left coronary artery from pulmonary artery. J Thorac Cardiovasc Surg 78: 7–11.

50. Tashiro T, Todo K, Haruta Y, et al. (1993) Anomalous origin of the left coronary artery from the pulmonary artery: new operative technique. J Thorac Cardiovasc Surg 106: 718–722.

51. Lenzi AW, Solarewicz L, Wanderley SF, et al. (2008) Analysis of the Takeuchi procedure for the treatment of anomalous origin of the left coronary artery from the pulmonary artery. Arq Bras Cardiol 90 (3): 167–171.

52. Dua R, Smith JA, Wilkinson JL, et al. (1993) Long-term follow-up after two coronary repair of anomalous left coronary artery from the pulmonary artery. J Card Surg 8: 384–390.

53. Nair KK, Zisman LS, Lader E, et al. (2003) Heart transplant for anomalous origin of left coronary artery from pulmonary artery. Ann Thorac Surg 75 (1): 282–284.

54. Isomatsu Y, Imai Y, Shin'oka T, et al. (2001) Surgical intervention for anomalous origin of the left coronary artery from the pulmonary artery: The Tokyo Experience. J Thorac Cardiovasc Surg 121: 792–797.

55. Turley K, Szarnicki RJ, Flachsbart KD, et al. (1995) Aortic implantation is possible in all cases of anomalous origin of the left coronary artery from the pulmonary artery. Ann Thorac Surg 60: 84–89.

56. Huddleston CB, Balzer DT, Mendeloff EN (2001) Repair of anomalous left main coronary artery arising from the pulmonary artery in infants: long-term impact on the mitral valve. Ann Thorac Surg 71: 1985–1989.

57. Schwartz ML, Jonas RA, Colan SD (1997) Anomalous origin of left coronary artery from pulmonary artery: recovery of left ventricular function after dual coronary repair. J Am Coll Cardiol 30: 547–553.

58. del Nido PJ, Duncan BW, Mayer JE, et al. (1999) Left ventricular assist device improves survival in children with left ventricular dysfunction after repair of anomalous origin of

the left coronary artery from the pulmonary artery. Ann Thorac Surg 67: 169–172.

59. Singh TP, Di Carli MF, Sullivan NM, et al. (1998) Myocardial flow reserve in long-term survivors of repair of anomalous left coronary artery from pulmonary artery. J Am Coll Cardiol 31: 437–443.

60. Stern H, Sauer U, Locher D, et al. (1993) Left ventricular function assessed with echocardiography and myocardial perfusion assessed with scintigraphy under dipyridamole stress in pediatric patients after repair for anomalous origin of the left coronary artery from the pulmonary artery. J Thorac Cardiovasc Surg 106: 723–732.

61. Davis JA, McBride MG, Seliem MA, et al. (2007). Evaluation of myocardial ischemia following surgical repair of anomalous aortic origin of a coronary artery in a series of pediatric patients. J Am Coll Cardiol 50 (21): 2078–2082.

62. Davachi F, Moller JH, Edwards JE (1971) Diseases of the mitral valve in infancy: anatomic analysis of 55 cases. Circulation 43: 565–579.

63. Mc Enany MT, English TA, Ross DN (1973) The congenitally cleft posterior mitral valve leaflet. An antecedent to mitral regurgitation. Ann Thorac Surg 16: 281.

64. Ranganathan M, Lam JHC, Wigle ED, et al. (1970) Morphology of the human mitral valve. II: the valve leaflets. Circulation 41: 459–467.

65. Braunwald E. Ross RS, Morrow AG, et al. (1961) Differential diagnosis of mitral regurgitation in childhood: clinical pathological conference at the National Institutes of Health. Ann Intern Med 54: 1223–1242.

66. Lee HR, Montenegro LM, Nicolson SC, et al. (1999) Usefulness of intraoperative transesophageal echocardiography in predicting the degree of mitral regurgitation secondary to atrioventricular defect in children. Am J Cardiol 83: 750–753.

67. Sandler H, Dodge HT, Hay RE, et al. (1963) Quantitation of valvular insufficiency in man by angiocardiography. Am Heart J 65: 501.

68. Raghuveer G, Calderone CA, Hills CB, et al. (2003) Predictors of prosthesis survival, growth, and functional status following mechanical mitral valve replacement in children aged

69. Oppido G, Davies B, McMullan DM, et al. (2008) Surgical treatment of congenital mitral valve disease: midterm results of a repair-oriented policy. J Thorac Cardiovasc Surg 135 (6): 1313–1321.

70. Harshaw CW, Munro AB, McLaurin LP, et al. (1975) Reduced systemic vascular resistance as therapy for severe mitral regurgitation of valvular origin. Ann Intern Med 83: 312.

71. Rivenes SM, Lewin MD, Stayer SA, et al. (2001) Cardiovascular effects of sevoflurane, isoflurane, halothane, and fentanyl-midazolam in children with congenital heart disease: an echocardiographic study of myocardial contractility and hemodynamics. Anesthesiology 94: 223–229.

72. Dalmas JP, Eker A, Girard C, et al. (1996) Intracardiac air clearing in valvular surgery guided by transesophageal echocardiography. J Heart Valve Dis 5: 553–557.

73. Webb WR, Harrison LH, Jr, Helmcke FR, et al. (1997) Carbon dioxide field flooding minimized residual intracardiac air after open heart operations. Ann Thorac Surg 64: 1489–1491.

74. Spodick DH (1992) Macrophysiology, microphysiology, and anatomy of the pericardium: a synopsis. Am Heart J 124: 1046–1051.

75. Little WC, Freeman GL (2006) Pericardial disease. Circulation 113: 1622–1632.

76. Kühn B, Peters J, Marx GR, et al. (2008) Etiology, management and outcome of pediatric pericardial effusions. Pediatr Cardiol 29: 90–94.

77. Bramlet MT, Hoyer MH (2008) Single pediatric center experience with multiple device implantation for complex secundum atrial septal defects. Catheter Cardiovasc Interv 72 (4): 531–537.

78. Nowlen TT, Rosenthal GL, Johnson GL, et al. (2002) Pericardial effusion and tamponade in infants with central catheters. Pediatrics 110: 137–142.

79. Altman CA (1998) Pericarditis and pericardial diseases. In: Garson A, Bricker JT, et al. (eds) The Science and Practice of Pediatric Cardiology, 2nd edn. Williams & Wilkins, Baltimore, pp. 1795–1814.

80. Tanoue Y, Fujita S, Kanaya Y, et al. (2007) Acute cardiac tamponade due to a bleeding pericardial cyst in a 3-year-old child. Ann Thorac Surg 84: 282–284.

81. Beck CS (1935) Two cardiac compression triads. JAMA 104: 714–716.

82. Tamburro RF, Ring JC, Womback K (2002) Detection of pulsus paradoxus associated with large pericardial effusions in pediatric patients by analysis of the pulse-oximetry waveform. Pediatrics 109: 673–677.

83. Tsang TS, El-Najdawi EK, Sewarg JB, et al. (1998) Percutaneous echocardiographically guided pericardiocentesis in pediatric patients: evaluation of safety and efficacy. J Am Soc Echocardiogr 11: 1072–1077.

84. Sarkhar M, Odegard KC, McGowan FX, et al. (2001) Hemodynamic responses to an induction does of etomidate in pediatric patients. Anesthesiology 95: A1263.

85. Sprung J, Ogletree-Hughes ML, Moravec CS (2000) The effects of etomidate on the contractility of failing and nonfailing human heart muscle. Anesth Analg 91: 68–75.

86. Sprung J, Schuetz SM, Stewart RW, Moravec CS (1998) Effects of ketamine on the contractility of failing and nonfailing human heart muscles in vitro. Anesthesiology 88: 1202–1210.

87. Muhler EG, Engelhardt W, von Bernuth G (1998) Pericardial effusions in infants and children: injection of echo contrast medium enhances the safety of echocardiographically-guided pericardiocentesis. Cardiol Young 8: 506–508.

88. Fowler NO, Manitsas GT (1973) Infectious pericarditis. Prog Cardiovasc Dis 16: 323–336.

89. Zahn EM, Houde C, Benson L, et al. (1992) Percutaneous pericardial catheter drainage in childhood. Am J Cardiol 70: 678–680.

90. Osranek M, Bursi F, O'Leary OW, et al. (2003) Hand-carried ultrasound-guided pericardiocentesis and thoracentesis. J Am Soc Echocardiogr 16: 480–484.

26 Anesthesia for cardiac and pulmonary transplantation

Glyn D. Williams, M.B.Ch.B., F.F.A. and
Chandra Ramamoorthy, M.B., B.S., F.F.A.
Lucile Packard Children's Hospital, Stanford University School of Medicine, Stanford, California, USA

Sharma Anshuman, M.D., F.F.A.R.C.S.I., M.B.A.
St. Louis Children's Hospital, Washington University School of Medicine, St. Louis, Missouri, USA

Heart transplantation

Over 100,000 heart and lung transplantations have been reported to the Scientific Registry of the International Society for Heart and Lung Transplantation (ISHLT) [1] since Christian Barnard performed the first human heart transplant on December 3, 1967 [2]. Nearly half of the centers reporting to the ISHLT perform >10 heart transplants per year. The number of reported pediatric recipients has remained stable during the last decade despite improved survival, in part because of limited donor organ availability (Figure 26.1) [3]. Infancy is the commonest age for children to undergo heart transplantation (Figure 26.2).

Anesthesia for Congenital Heart Disease 2nd edition. Edited by
Dean Andropoulos, Stephen Stayer, Isobel Russell and Emad Mossad.
© 2010 Blackwell Publishing.

Organ transplantation in the USA is sanctioned by congressional mandate through the Nation Organ Transplant Act (NOTA). An Organ Procurement and Transplant Network (OPTN) was created and is administered by the United Network for Organ Sharing (UNOS). UNOS has three recipient status categories for patients listed for heart transplantation: Status IA, IB, and II, with Status IA indicating the sickest patients who are in urgent need of transplantation for survival. A 2006 OPTN policy change in the sequence of heart allocation decreased wait list deaths among heart transplant candidates.

Indications for heart transplantation

Indications for heart transplantation were recently updated [4]. Heart transplantation is generally indicated when expected survival is less than 1 or 2 years and/or when there is unacceptable quality of life secondary to

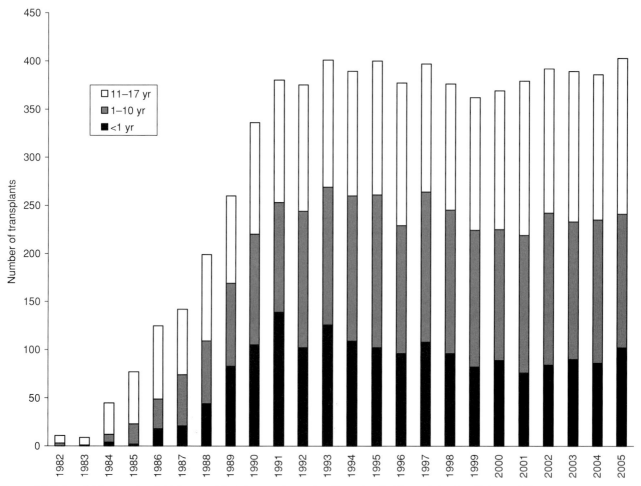

Figure 26.1 Age distribution of pediatric heart recipients by year of transplant (Reproduced with permission from Reference [3])

irreparable cardiac diseases. As survival rates have improved, often the dilemma is no longer whether to transplant, but rather when to do it [5]. Premature transplantation results in exposure of the recipient to the hazards of transplantation and immunosuppression. Excessive delay may result in death without transplantation or the development of high-risk comorbidities such as renal dysfunction, malnutrition, and elevated pulmonary vascular resistance (PVR).

Indications for heart transplantation in children vary with age (Table 26.1). The majority of transplantations in infants are for congenital heart disease (CHD), whereas cardiomyopathy is the predominant indication in older children [3].

Cardiomyopathies

Dilated cardiomyopathies have diverse etiology, including viral myocarditis, drugs (e.g., adriamycin), abnormalities of fatty acid, amino acid, glycogen and mucopolysaccharide metabolism, mitochondria and genetic disorders,

chronic arrhythmia, and coronary artery abnormality [6]. Predictors of poor outcome include a family history of cardiomyopathy, syncope, ventricular arrhythmia or near-death episode, left ventricular end-diastolic pressure greater than 25 mm Hg, and left ventricular ejection fraction less than 30%.

Table 26.1 Diagnosis in pediatric heart transplant recipients

	Age		
	<1 yr (%)	1–10 yr (%)	11–17 yr (%)
Congenital	64.1	37.2	25.3
Myopathy	30.1	52.2	61.6
Retransplant	0.7	5.9	6.6
Malignancy	0.5	0.2	0.2
Coronary artery disease	0.3	0.9	0.9
Other	4.3	3.5	5.4

Source: Reproduced with permission from Reference [3].

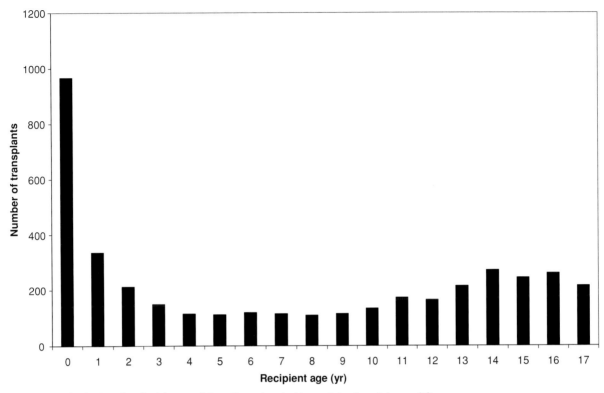

Figure 26.2 Age distribution of pediatric heart recipients (Reproduced with permission from Reference [3])

Hypertrophic cardiomyopathies include several genotypes. Risk factors for sudden death include marked left ventricular wall thickness, family history of sudden death, and nonsustained ventricular tachycardia.

Restrictive cardiomyopathies result in diastolic dysfunction. These uncommon disorders generally have a poor prognosis and are associated with myocardial infiltrative processes such as amyloidosis, hemochromatosis, glycogen storage disease, mucopolysaccharidosis, sarcoidosis, and endomyocardial fibrosis. Elevated PVR is often present and predicts poor outcome.

Congenital heart disease

This group includes children with end-stage heart failure after surgery for single- or two-ventricle physiology and patients with complex congenital heart variants with no option of palliative surgery. The number of children undergoing transplantation for HLHS has diminished greatly because survival rates after staged reconstruction now exceed 80% and the significant mortality (up to 30%) while waiting for transplantation is avoided [7].

Other indications

Although rare, there are children who may require cardiac transplantation for unresectable cardiac tumors and other diseases such as Kawasaki's syndrome.

Recipient evaluation

A detailed assessment of patients is required to determine their suitability for heart transplantation (Table 26.2). Factors that may exclude patients from consideration include severe central nervous system, liver or kidney dysfunction, pulmonary infarction, pulmonary hypertension, morbid obesity, and some infections, malignancies, or chromosomal abnormalities. Prediction of mortality after transplantation was more accurate when multiple high-risk criteria were included in the assessment of potential recipients [9].

Assessment of cardiopulmonary function usually includes cardiac catheterization and, in some cases, MRI and CT cardiac imaging. The recipient's cardiac anatomy has to be accurately delineated because abnormal cardiovascular anatomy influences surgical technique during harvesting and transplantation. Hemodynamic measurements are required, especially determination of PVR. Transplantation in patients with PVR in excess of 5 Wood U/m² or a transpulmonary gradient greater than 15 mm Hg is potentially contraindicated because it is associated with acute right heart failure and increased mortality. The upper limit of PVR associated with successful cardiac transplantation has not been established in children.

All patients with pulmonary hypertension have PVR measured at baseline conditions and during administration of oxygen, nitric oxide (NO), and/or other pulmonary

Table 26.2 Routine precardiac transplant evaluation

History and physical examination
 Age, height, weight, body surface area
 Diagnoses
 Past medical history
 Medications
 Allergies
 Immunization record

Laboratory data
 Liver and kidney function tests
 Urine analysis
 Glomerular filtration rate
 Prothrombin time/INR/partial thromboplastin time
 Complete blood count and differential
 PPD skin test
 Serologies for human immunodeficiency virus, hepatitis,
 cytomegalovirus, Epstein–Barr virus, *Toxoplasmosis gondii*, syphilis
 ABO type
 Panel reactive antibody

Cardiomyopathy workup
 Thyroid function tests
 Blood lactate, pyruvate, ammonia, acyl carnitine
 Urine organic acids, acyl carnitine
 Skeletal muscle biopsy
 Karyotype

Cardiopulmonary data
 Cardiac catheterization
 Echocardiogram
 Radionuclide angiography
 Endomyocardial biopsy
 Electrocardiogram
 Chest radiograph
 Pulmonary function tests
 Vo_{2max}

Psychosocial evaluation
 Possible relocation
 Long-term supportive care
 Parental substance abuse
 History of neglect or abuse

Consultations as required
 Dental services
 Other services

It may be necessary to repeat some tests if the patient's medical status changes over time.
INR, international normalized ratio; PPD, purified protein derivative.
Source: Reproduced with permission and adapted from Reference [8].

vasodilator therapy. When the response is marginal, repeat values after 1–2 weeks of inotropic support, afterload reduction, and pulmonary vasodilation may demonstrate improvement. Experienced institutions may accept children with PVR as high as 8–12 Wood U/m^2 if it is reactive. Patients whose PVR does not respond to ther-

apy may be candidates for heterotopic heart transplantation, heart–lung, domino heart, or lung transplantation. Children with restrictive cardiomyopathy are particularly prone to marked elevation of PVR, which may contribute to the poor prognosis in these patients and make cardiac transplantation problematic. NO appears to be a good agent to demonstrate reversibility of PVR in these patients [10].

Radionuclide angiography is useful for assessing systemic ventricular dysfunction in patients with complex cardiac morphology. Endomyocardial biopsy can identify acute myocarditis and myocardial infiltrates. Pulmonary function tests may be indicated for older children with chronic lung disease. Evaluation of patients with cardiomyopathy should include a metabolic workup because potential etiologic factors include mitochondrial disorders, and genetic studies if indicated by phenotypic appearance or family pedigree.

Infectious disease and immune system evaluation is essential. The child's immunization status should be updated if necessary. Tests are performed for latent infections such as cytomegalovirus or Epstein–Barr virus that may become clinically significant during immunosuppression.

Donor matching is based on ABO typing. The candidate's blood is also screened for antibodies against sera of random blood donors and, if reactive, a serum crossmatch with the donor is performed.

There is an increased risk for graft dysfunction, acute cellular and antibody-mediated allograft rejection, and chronic rejection/coronary artery vasculopathy (CAV) after heart transplantation in patients sensitized to human leukocyte antigens (HLA). The number of heart transplant candidates allosensitized to HLA antigens has increased in recent years because of exposure to blood products, homograft material used in surgical palliation of CHD, use of ventricular assist and mechanical support devices, and patients requiring retransplantation. Determinations of panel reactive antibody (PRA) are done to delineate a patient's potential for sensitization to donor HLA antigens. Patients with a reaction to >10% of antigens (either Class I or II) are generally considered to be allosensitized. However, this is allosensitivity to a *"random"* donor; having a positive crossmatch with the *actual* donor (HLA antibody toward donor alloantigens) at the time of transplant has been clearly demonstrated to increase the risk for poor outcome after transplant. Donor-directed HLA antibodies are associated with rejection-related mortality from cellular and antibody-mediated acute rejection and CAV. Patients with PRA >10% pretransplant and a positive crossmatch are at high risk for graft loss from hyperacute rejection and early acute cellular rejection, which in turn increases the risk of CAV.

Allosensitized patients may be excluded from heart transplant, restricted to certain donors, or experience prolonged waiting times. Some transplant programs require a prospective negative donor-specific crossmatch for patients with PRA screens >10%. However, this approach is problematic because of the donor shortage and some patients have antibodies to many HLA antigens. Therefore, perioperative management protocols for HLA-sensitized children have been developed and include pretreatment of sensitized patients (using treatments such as intravenous immune globulin, cyclophosphamide, mycophenolate mofetil (MMF), and rituximab), intraoperative plasma exchange, and posttransplant plasmapheresis and T- and B-cell suppression [11–15].

Heart transplantation requires long-term immunosuppression, frequent invasive procedures, and lifelong medical care. Patients have to live close to the hospital during the initial months after surgery and temporary relocation of the family may be necessary. Prolonged periods of stressful hospitalization are likely. A stable social situation is essential for success and psychosocial evaluation is an important aspect of the pretransplantation process.

Recipient pretransplant management

Mean waiting period from acceptance for heart transplantation to actual surgery currently is about 3 months but varies with the child's age, blood group, and list status. Approximately 20% of children with cardiomyopathy and 30% of those with end-stage CHD die waiting for a donor heart [16, 17].

Aggressive medical management to achieve stabilization is required and includes supplemental oxygen, diuretics, inotropic support (e.g., dobutamine, dopamine, phosphodiesterase inhibitors), arrhythmia therapy, and mechanical ventilation. Children with chronic heart failure often receive digoxin, diuretics including spironolactone, angiotensin-converting enzyme inhibitors and β-blockade therapy (e.g., metoprolol, carvedilol). Patients with severe left ventricular dilation may need anticoagulation, preferably coumadin, to prevent the development of intracardiac thrombi and systemic embolization. Amiodarone is often chosen for treating arrhythmia. Implantable defibrillators have been effective in pediatric patients large enough for these devices. Biventricular pacing is an experimental modality showing promise.

Patients with refractory myocardial failure require mechanical circulatory support as a bridge to cardiac transplantation. Extracorporeal life support is the only FDA-approved modality available for small children and can be used for at least 2 weeks with acceptable survival and hospital discharge rates. Renal insufficiency requiring dialysis decreases the likelihood of survival [18]. Other complications include sepsis, bleeding, and neurological injury. The Berlin Heart EXCOR is suitable for patients of all ages but is currently only available in USA under a compassion-

ate use exemption [19]. Other ventricular assist devices and intraaortic balloon pumps are usually reserved for older adolescents but have been employed successfully in younger children weighing about 15 kg. Partial left ventriculectomy has been used to improve clinical status and act as a biological bridge to heart transplantation in children with end-stage dilated cardiomyopathy [20]. Patients with CHD may require interventional catheterization procedures such as stent placement or balloon dilation, or pulmonary artery banding surgery to achieve balance between systemic and pulmonary blood flow.

Donor management

Once the diagnosis of brain or cardiac [21] death is established and parental/guardian consent obtained, the donor's specifics are checked for possible match with patients listed by UNOS for transplant. Because of the shortage of suitable organ donors and the high morality rate on the waiting list, most centers use a liberal donor screening strategy. The age distribution of pediatric heart donors is similar to that of heart recipients [3]. Echocardiography is useful for assessment of donor heart function. Widespread malignancy or infection in the prospective donor are exclusion criteria, but cardiac resuscitation and chest trauma are not necessarily contraindications provided the donor's hemodynamics have been stabilized and inotropic agents are no longer needed or are at minimal doses. Usually the donor should be 80–160% of the recipient's weight, but the upper limit may be extended for neonates or for recipients with pulmonary hypertension. Attempts to limit donor heart ischemia time are important but may be hampered by transport issues. Many centers prefer the period to be less than 6 hours, especially if the recipient has increased PVR, although successful outcomes after graft ischemia times of up to 9 hours have been reported. The anesthetic management of a pediatric organ donor is beyond the scope of this chapter [22, 23].

Surgical technique

There are two methods for performing heart transplantation: orthotopic, in which the recipient heart is excised and replaced in the correct anatomical position by the donor heart, and heterotopic, in which the donor heart is placed in the right side of the chest alongside the recipient organ and anastomosed so as to allow blood flow through either or both hearts. The majority of transplants in children have been of the orthotopic type.

The orthotopic approach of Lower and Shumway [24] has been employed for many years in cases where anatomy is straightforward. This technique avoids individual systemic and pulmonary venous anastomoses but results in capacious atrial chambers, comprising donor and recipient components, which contract asynchronously. It has been suggested that atrial contribution to cardiac output (CO) may be superior with near to total cardiac transplantation. A small cuff of left atrial tissue is left in place, incorporating all pulmonary veins, and the entire right atrium is removed. Bicaval anastomoses are then performed. This technique results in more normal anatomical result. A meta-analysis found superiority of the bicaval technique in comparison with the biatrial procedure for early atrial pressure, perioperative mortality, tricuspid valve regurgitation, and sinus rhythm [25], although others found no difference in longer-term survival [26].

Cardiac transplantation for children with congenital malformations can be more complex technically. Deep hypothermic circulatory arrest may be employed in patients requiring extensive vascular reconstruction.

Anesthetic management

Precardiopulmonary bypass period

Children listed for heart transplantation have little or no cardiac reserve and can be extremely sensitive to the perturbations induced by anesthesia and surgery. For children with CHD, the precardiopulmonary bypass (pre-CPB) anesthetic management for heart transplantation differs little from that for nontransplant cardiac surgery and requires a good appreciation of the patient's particular pathophysiology. The physiological consequences of cardiac failure are discussed in Chapter 5. Briefly, children with end-stage cardiac dysfunction have a chronically activated sympathetic nervous system and an impaired response to β-agonists. Reduced renal perfusion triggers the renin–angiotensin system, resulting in increased vasoconstriction, venoconstriction, and intravascular volume, which increase preload, afterload, and perpetuate cardiac failure. Cardiac β_1-receptors are downregulated and there is a partial uncoupling of cardiac β_1-receptors from adenylate cyclase resulting in decrease β_1-receptor sensitivity. The contractile response to direct β-adrenergic inotropes is impaired. Since tissue norepinephrine levels are decreased, indirect-acting agents such as ephedrine may be less effective. Brain natriuretic peptide (BNP), a potent natriuretic and vasodilator, is a diagnostic and prognostic marker in patients with congestive heart failure. It is released from ventricular myocytes in response to myocardial wall stretch and increased transmural pressure [27].

A dysfunctional, dilated heart is exquisitely sensitive to changes in preload, afterload, heart rate (HR), and contractility. Systolic and diastolic function is impaired and high mean atrial pressure is required to ensure adequate filling. Chronic elevated left atrial pressure results in

elevated PVR and right ventricular dysfunction. Any decrease in preload results in decreased HR with a decline in CO. Conversely, an increase in HR decreases the diastolic filling time that reduces end-diastolic volume and stroke volume. Small increases in afterload result in comparatively large increases in end-systolic volume with a large decrease in stroke volume and CO.

Prior to surgery, young infants and children with uncompensated heart failure are usually already in intensive care, and may have invasive lines in situ and be on ventilator support. More stable patients may have been called in from home for the transplantation surgery and could have eaten recently. Several hours usually elapse before surgery but therapy to modify gastric pH and volume and the application of continuous cricoid pressure during induction might be required. Communication between the transplant surgeons, anesthesiologists, operating room staff, and donor procurement team is vital in order to coordinate care and ensure graft ischemia time is minimized.

The advisability of premedication and the method of anesthesia induction depend upon the patient's age, cardiac lesion, and cardiopulmonary function. Establishing invasive hemodynamic monitoring prior to induction of anesthesia may not always be feasible and so it is imperative to institute noninvasive patient monitoring prior to the administration of medications that alter hemodynamic and/or respiratory function. Anesthesia- or surgery-induced changes in HR, preload, afterload, or contractility may precipitate hemodynamic decompensation. Meticulous airway management is vital as hypoxia and hypercarbia aggravate PVR and may further depress CO. Rapid sequence induction may be poorly tolerated in patients with minimal cardiorespiratory reserve. A wide variety of anesthetic agents have been used successfully. The desirable and detrimental cardiovascular effects of anesthetic agents are reviewed in Chapter 6. In children with CHD, a fentanyl/midazolam/muscle relaxant anesthetic technique was reported to preserve cardiac index better than volatile agents, provided HR was maintained [28]. Etomidate has minimal effect on hemodynamics; propofol decreases systemic vascular resistance. Nitrous oxide has myocardial depressant and pulmonary vasoconstrictor properties and is best avoided. Ketamine supports the circulation by indirectly stimulating catecholamine release. This may be blunted in children with dilated cardiomyopathy and impaired β-agonist responses and the drug's direct myocardial depressant effects may then predominate.

Monitoring during surgery does not differ from that used for pediatric open-heart surgery. Some authorities avoid inserting catheters into the right internal jugular vein because the vessel will later be accessed repeatedly for endomyocardial biopsies. Transesophageal echocardiography (TEE) is useful for evaluation of heart anatomy and function, mural thrombus, intracardiac air, and early posttransplant cardiac function. When pulmonary artery pressure monitoring is indicated, many institutions prefer to place a catheter directly into the pulmonary artery rather than use a pulmonary artery flotation catheter. The value of antifibrinolytics for primary heart transplantation is uncertain but administration should be considered in children who have previously undergone median sternotomy.

Cardiopulmonary bypass period

The management on CPB is similar to that in children undergoing cardiac surgery. Ultrafiltration during CPB may benefit the patient by removing excess free water, hemoconcentrating red cells and coagulation factors, and modulating the inflammatory response.

Postcardiopulmonary bypass period

Issues of concern include denervated donor heart, global ischemia–reperfusion injury, elevated PVR, arrhythmia, hemostasis, and hyperacute rejection.

The transplanted heart is functionally denervated. The recipient atrial remnant remains innervated but no electrical impulses cross the suture line so the donor atrium is responsible for the patient's HR. There are two P waves on the electrocardiogram (ECG), representing activity of the transplanted and native sinoatrial nodes. Resting HR is higher than normal because vagal tone is absent and the normal beat-to-beat variations in response to respiration are lost, as are the normal responses of the heart to alterations in body position and carotid body massage. The donor heart cannot abruptly increase HR and CO in response to stress because the baroreceptor reflex is disrupted. The attenuated HR response to stress means the anesthesiologist must be particularly vigilant to ensure the child does not become too lightly anesthetized. With the loss of the baroreceptor reflex, the patient with the denervated heart may initially show an exaggerated response to hypovolemia with a marked decrease in mean blood pressure, and then a delayed exaggerated hypertensive and tachycardia response, due to endogenous catecholamine release. The Frank–Starling (pressure–volume) relationship remains intact and compensates for hypovolemia and hypotension by increasing stroke volume secondary to an increased venous return. Therefore, it is important to maintain adequate preload, especially if vasodilators are administered. Innervation of the peripheral vasculature is preserved, and changes in peripheral vascular resistance may still occur in response to alterations in sympathetic outflow from the vasomotor center due to signals from stretch receptors in the great vessels.

Drugs such as atropine, glycopyrrolate, neostigmine, and pancuronium that act on the heart through vagal or sympathetic neuromechanisms usually will not affect HR. However, there are case reports of profound bradycardia and hypotension following glycopyrrolate–neostigmine administration [29, 30]. α- and β-Adrenergic receptors remain intact and inotropes such as epinephrine and isoproterenol will cause appropriate responses from the heart.

The donor organ is subjected to ischemia–reperfusion injury and patients usually require inotropic support for separation from CPB. Left-ventricular diastolic dysfunction is common and characterized by a restrictive ventricular filling pattern, with a reduced preload reserve and a relatively fixed stroke volume. Sinoatrial node dysfunction is relatively common. Dopamine or isoproterenol are often selected and epicardial atrioventricular pacing can be instituted if necessary to achieve the desired HR. Temporary pacing wires are advisable. Arrhythmias are quite common in the early postoperative period, usually premature atrial or premature ventricular contractions. Compression of intrathoracic structures may be problematic during closure of sternotomy, particularly if the donor heart is relatively oversized [31].

It is important to preserve donor right ventricular function by keeping PVR normal. Catecholamine release is reduced by ensuring the patient remains adequately anesthetized. Ventilation is facilitated by muscle relaxants and normocarbia is maintained. Elevations in central venous pressure with low or normal left atrial pressure and reduced mean arterial pressure might be related to right ventricular failure. Elevated pulmonary artery pressures can be discerned by echocardiography and measured invasively. Additional measures to control PVR may be necessary, including pulmonary vasodilator therapy such as NO [32], prostacyclin, phosphodiesterase inhibitors, and isoproterenol.

More extreme hypocapnia may help, but also causes cerebral vasoconstriction and leftward shift of the oxygen dissociation curve. Cerebral oximetry monitoring using near-infrared spectroscopy is helpful. If the patient's CO remains inadequate despite maximal drug therapy, mechanical right ventricular assist, or extracorporeal membrane oxygenation (EMCO) may be employed [33].

Blood loss during heart transplantation can be considerable and is associated with increased morbidity and mortality. Blood products are cytomegalovirus matched, leukoreduced, and irradiated but coagulation management is no different from that for other open-heart surgeries in children (see Chapter 12). For infants, some centers wash packed red blood cells to reduce the potassium load. Citrate-induced hypocalcemia impairs contractility and coagulation; this may be minimized by initiating a calcium infusion (calcium chloride 10–30 mg/kg/h). Rapid platelet transfusion may aggravate PVR.

PART 5 Anesthesia for specific lesions

Intraoperative immunosuppression regimens are institutional specific. The Stanford protocol is daclizumab (1 mg/kg) and methyl prednisolone (15 mg/kg) intravenously once hemostasis is achieved after CPB.

Immunosuppression

Pediatric heart transplant provides a unique immunological opportunity, because the development of the immune system extends not only into infancy, but continues throughout childhood. T-cell responses and phenotype are naive compared with adults, with decreased expression of integrins and adhesion molecules. Younger age at time of transplantation is associated with better long-term survival and lower frequency of rejection compared with older children [34]. Infants and young children (up to 5 yr of age) have undergone transplantation across ABO barriers without developing clinical rejection. Proposed immune mechanisms include B-cell tolerance and accommodation (absence of humoral rejection despite expression of antigens on the graft's vascular endothelium and the circulation of corresponding antibodies in the recipient) [35].

Immunosuppressive therapies can be categorized by their actions into (i) broad spectrum immunosuppressants: corticosteroids; (ii) calcineurin inhibitors: cyclosporine and tacrolimus; (iii) antiproliferative agents: MMF and azathioprine; (iv) antibodies against inter-leukin-2 (IL-2): basiliximab and daclizumab; (v) target of rapamycin protein (TOR) inhibitors: sirolimus; (vi) mono- and polyclonal T-cell antibodies: OKT3, antithymocyte globulin (ATG), antilymphocyte globulin; and (vii) non-drug therapies: total lymphoid irradiation, photopheresis, and plasmapheresis.

Choice of immunosuppressives is largely guided by institutional experience and the recipient's clinical profile, rejection history, and comorbid associations. Typical clinical use of these agents is summarized below [36]. Be aware of the potential for drug interactions because heart transplant recipients receive many different medications.

Induction therapy: induction therapy has been used to reduce the need for calcineurin antagonists and potentially favorably alter the immune environment. Agents commonly used are polyclonal antibody preparations and IL-2 receptor antagonists. The proportion of patients receiving induction therapy has been steadily increasing, and >60% of patients transplanted during 2006 received induction therapy (Figure 26.3). Despite the popularity of induction therapy, no significant effect of induction therapy on survival, CAV, or incidence of rejection was seen in the pediatric population [3]. Only OKT3 was negatively associated with the frequency of rejection but it has neurological effects, prominent first dose "cytokine release syndrome" and may increase the risk of lymphoproliferative disorders (PTLDs). IL-2 blockers (e.g., daclizumab) are well tolerated.

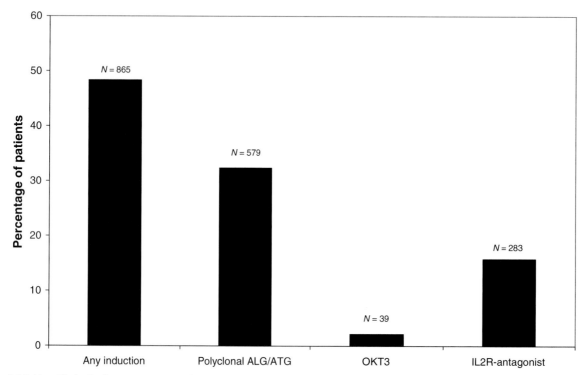

Figure 26.3 Use of induction immunosuppression (Reproduced with permission from Reference [3])

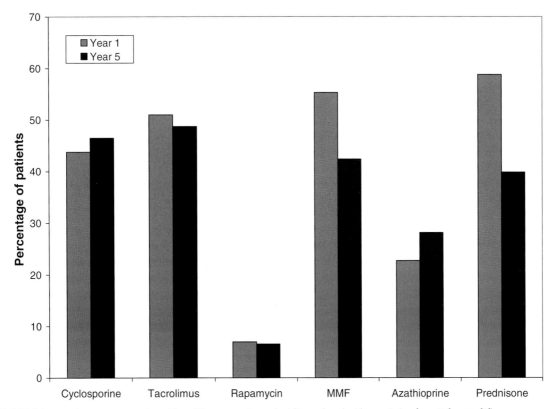

Figure 26.4 Maintenance immunosuppression at 1 and 5 years posttransplant (Reproduced with permission from Reference [3])

Maintenance therapy: the objective is to prevent acute and chronic rejection while minimizing the adverse effects of immunosuppression. All regimens involve a calcineurin inhibitor. Adjunct therapy may include an antiproliferative agent or TOR inhibitor. Often, corticosteroids are also administered, although many programs attempt to limit or avoid their long-term use.

In recent years, cyclosporine and tacrolimus have been used in a similar percentage of patients and MMF has largely replaced azathioprine use early after transplant (Figure 26.4). There is a trend to shift patients who are 5 years posttransplant from cyclosporine-based regimens to tacrolimus-based regimens [3].

Calcineurin inhibitors

Overall survival of transplanted patients increased from 40 to 70% after the introduction of cyclosporine (Sandimmune, Neoral) in 1982. Cyclosporin binds to cyclophilin within the cytoplasm of T cells; this complex inhibits calcineurin phosphatase, thus interfering with the transcription of key cytokines required for T-cell activation and proliferation. Microemulsified formulation of cyclosporin provides better bioavailability and lower rejection rates than the original preparation that had unpredictable absorption. Therapeutic drug monitoring is essential be-

cause the therapeutic window is narrow and other drugs influence drug levels. Cyclosporine trough levels are usually maintained in the range of 100–300 ng/mL. Adverse effects may be dose related and include toxicity of renal, hepatic and neurological systems, hypertension, hyperlipidemia, hirsutism, and gingival hyperplasia.

Tacrolimus (Prograf, FK506) binds to a different cytosolic binding protein (FK-binding protein) and has been particularly effective as a rescue treatment in cases where recurrent rejection has occurred with cyclosporine. Overall patient survival does not differ between the two agents but there appears to be less rejection with tacrolimus and an improved adverse effects profile with respect to hypertension, dyslipidemia, and long-term renal function [3,37,38]. Like cyclosporine, the therapeutic window is narrow and blood levels can be affected by other medications. Trough levels are maintained in the range of 5–15 ng/mL.

Antiproliferative agents

Antiproliferative agents such as azathioprine (Imuran) and MMF (CellCept) inhibit lymphocyte proliferation and one of these agents may be added to calcineurin inhibitor therapy. The choice of either MMF or azathioprine did not have an impact on rejection rate within the first year in the pediatric heart transplant population [3].

Azathioprine is a purine antagonist that inhibits T and B cells. Bone marrow depression is common and dosing is guided by the white blood cell count. MMF converts to mycophenolic acid, an inhibitor of purine synthesis. Lymphocytes are suppressed because they lack a salvage pathway. Absorption is variable and dosing may be guided by blood levels. Gastrointestinal side effects rather than bone marrow depression are the usual dose-limiting factor.

Sirolimus

Proliferation signal or mammalian target of rapamycin inhibitors, everolimus and sirolimus (rapamycin), are newer agents that provide attractive options for use in heart transplantation because they are immunosuppressive and antiproliferative. TOR inhibitors work synergistically with calcineurin inhibitors and thus permit the minimization of calcineurin inhibitors without compromising efficacy. This approach is advantageous for the majority of heart transplant recipients and might provide particular benefit in specific cases, such as patients with cardiac allograft vasculopathy, malignancies and renal dysfunction, or in patients intolerant to other immunosuppressive agents. Sirolimus may inhibit the process of CAV. Adverse effects include hyperlipidemia, wound-healing complications, and proteinuria [39].

Corticosteroids

Corticosteroids are nonspecific anti-inflammatory agents that were widely used in the precyclosporine era. Nowadays, they are mainly used in combination with other immunosuppressives. Many centers try to minimize the dose and duration of corticosteroid therapy. Side effects are myriad and include higher infection risk, diabetes mellitus, bone demineralization, and coronary artery disease. Rejection risk may increase when steroids are withdrawn.

Rejection therapy

High-dose corticosteroid, usually methyl prednisolone, is first line therapy for acute rejection. Recurrent moderate rejection can usually be controlled with enhanced maintenance therapy (tacrolimus, sirolimus) and corticosteroids. Other agents such as polyclonal anti-T antibodies are reserved for severe rejection that is refractory or causing hemodynamic compromise.

Chronic rejection is manifest as coronary vasculopathy. There are no proven therapies that can halt or reverse this process and retransplantation is the most suitable option for advanced diffuse disease. It remains controversial whether statins affect progression of allograft vasculopathy or aid in its prevention in children [40].

Outcome following heart transplantation

2007 ISHLT data show that overall survival was approximately 40% for patients up to 20 years after transplantation (Figure 26.5) [3]. The infant age group has a complex survival curve, with higher early mortality but lower late mortality. Once beyond the first year posttransplant, infants fare significantly better than older children (Figure 26.6), perhaps reflecting the impact of immunological aspects of development on transplant survival.

Risk factors for 1-year mortality were analyzed for the population of patients transplanted between 1995 and 2005. Being on ECMO at the time of transplant represented the highest risk for 1-year mortality. CHD and retransplantation were also important. The severity of medical illness, reflected by the need for ventilation or hospitalization, increased relative risk. The year of transplantation was a risk factor. The continuous factors having a significant effect on mortality in the first year included donor age, creatinine, weight ratio, pediatric center transplant volume, and bilirubin. For serum creatinine >1, there was a small but highly significant effect of increasing mortality as creatinine increased. For weight ratio and donor age, the relationship was parabolic, with increasing risk at the extremes. Risk of mortality declined linearly with increasing pediatric transplant volume.

Acute rejection was the leading cause of death during the first 3 years posttransplant but was displaced thereafter by CAV, which accounted for 35% of all deaths. The percentage of patients dying from infection (7%) or lymphoma (8%) did not increase with late follow-up.

Outcome for retransplant recipients is influenced by the time interval between initial and repeat transplantation. At 1 year, actual survival was about 60% for patients retransplanted within 1 year of the initial transplant, whereas 1-year survival was almost 90% for those retransplanted 5 years after the first transplant.

Rejection

Rejection is defined by the Pediatric Heart Transplant Study Group as the clinical decision to intensify immunosuppression in association with either histopathology or dysfunction [41]. Four clinical types are described (Table 26.3). Hyperacute rejection is rare and manifests soon after transplantation. It is mediated by preformed recipient cytotoxic antibodies against donor heart antigens and often leads to intractable heart failure. On average, pediatric heart transplant recipients have two acute rejection episodes during the first 3 years after transplantation, although about one-third remains rejection-free. Acute cellular rejection is fatal in <10% of episodes; however, it is the commonest cause of death between 30 days and 3 years after heart transplantation. Acute rejection that

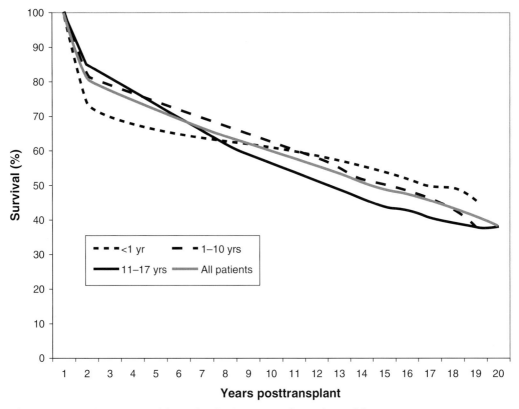

Figure 26.5 Kaplan–Meier survival (1/1982–6/2005) (Reproduced with permission from Reference [3])

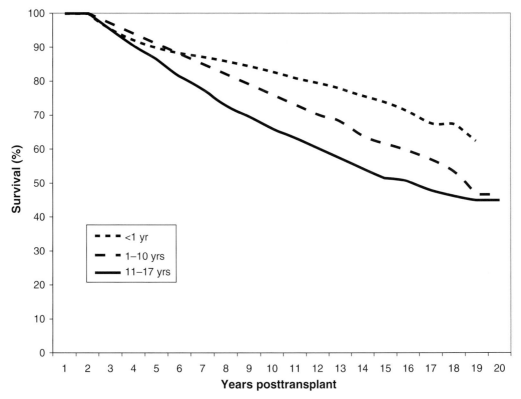

Figure 26.6 One-year conditional Kaplan–Meier survival (1/1982–6/2005) (Reproduced with permission from Reference [3])

Table 26.3 Cardiac rejection—types, mechanism, and timing

Type of rejection	Mechanism	Approximate onset after transplant
Hyperacute	Preformed antibodies	Minutes to hours
Acute cellular	T-cell mediated	Anytime (often first 3–6 mo)
Acute humoral	Antibodies	Days to weeks
Chronic (CAV)	Both humoral and cellular	After first year

CAV, chronic allograft vasculopathy.
Source: Reproduced with permission from Reference [42].

occurs more than 2 years after transplantation is linked to poor compliance with therapy and carries a poor long-term prognosis.

Clinical evidence of rejection ranges from no symptoms to tachycardia, tachypnea, lethargy, irritability, poor feeding, fever, hepatomegaly, new murmur, gallop rhythm, and new-onset arrhythmias. Endomyocardial biopsy remains the "gold standard" for the diagnosis of acute allograft rejection. Specimens are graded for rejection on the basis of the numbers of infiltrating lymphocytes and the presence of myocyte injury [41]. Endomyocardial biopsy is expensive, invasive, technically challenging in small children, and carries small risks of cardiac perforation and tricuspid valve damage. Further, "biopsy negative" acute graft dysfunction can occur.

The use of echocardiography as a noninvasive method of diagnosing acute rejection is unresolved. Indices of systolic and diastolic dysfunction are reportedly useful but have disadvantages [43–45].

Surveillance for late rejection is controversial. In adults, there is strong evidence that intravascular ultrasound findings at 1 year are a powerful predictor of subsequent mortality, nonfatal cardiac events, and the development of angiographic coronary disease. However, experience in children is limited. Hence regular monitoring by multiple modalities is recommended because no single test is reliable [46,47].

Graft atherosclerosis

The long-term decline in patient survival is primarily due to a CAV characterized by concentric smooth muscle and intimal hyperplasia. CAV is a diffuse disease that begins in the distal, small vessels and eventually involves the intramyocardial and epicardial arteries. It is immune-mediated and interacts with nonimmune risk factors such as dyslipidemia and hypertension [48]. ISHLT reports an incidence of graft CAV of about 17% at 10 years posttransplant—much lower than that reported for adults.

The risk of developing CAV was inversely related to recipient age—infant recipients had the lowest risk of vasculopathy. When the risk of CAV was stratified by donor ischemic time, a significant inverse relationship with ischemic time was evident. A strong association existed between early rejection and CAV at 1 and 3 years posttransplant [3].

Infection

Infection is a significant cause of morbidity and mortality, particularly in the first 6 months after transplantation when immunosuppression is greater [3]. The most common types of serious infection are bacterial (60%), cytomegalovirus (18%), other viral (13%), fungal (7%), and protozoal (2%) [49]. Bacterial, protozoal, and fungal infections commonly involve the respiratory tract or sternal wound. Viral infections increase the risk of graft rejection and Epstein–Barr virus is associated with lymphoproliferative disease.

At 5-year follow-up, infant recipients had higher occurrence rates of severe and chronic infections compared with older recipients and the infections were more resistant to treatment. Additionally, the incidence of autoimmune disorders (commonly autoimmune cytopenias) was noteworthy [50].

Malignancy

Although there is an increased risk of malignancy in children after heart transplantation, the risk is extremely low. Freedom from malignancy was >90% in 10-year survivors; almost all malignancies were lymphatic in origin. Many posttransplant PTLDs respond to reduction in immunosuppression.

Other complications

ISHLT follow-up data on complications up to 10 years after transplantation is shown in Table 26.4. Acute renal dysfunction may occur in the immediate postoperative period, probably because the cumulative deleterious effects of a chronic low CO, CPB, and nephrotoxic drugs such as the calcineurin inhibitors. Renal dysfunction increased from 6% at 1 year to 17% at 10 years. However, the need for renal transplant was seen in only 1% by 10 years and freedom from severe renal dysfunction was approximately 90% at 9 years [3]. Risk factors for chronic renal insufficiency included pretransplant dialysis, hypertrophic cardiomyopathy, African American race and previous transplant. Adjusted risk of death in those who developed chronic renal insufficiency was ninefold higher than in those who did not [51].

Table 26.4 Post-heart transplant morbidity. Cumulative prevalence in survivors within 10 yr posttransplant (follow-ups: April 1994 to June 2006)

Outcome	Within 10 yr (%)
Hypertension	72.3
Renal dysfunction	17.4
Abnormal creatinine <2.5 mg/dL	13.2
Creatinine >2.5 mg/dL	1.6
Chronic dialysis	1.6
Renal transplant	1.1
Hyperlipidemia	38.2
Diabetes	4.5
Coronary artery vasculopathy	16.7

Source: Reproduced with permission from Reference [3].

The percentage of recipients with hypertension increased over time to 72% at 10 years posttransplantation. The only medication significantly associated with hypertension was prednisone. Hyperlipidemia also increased steadily to 38% at 10 years after transplantation. Whether abnormal cholesterol values should be treated empirically with statins or whether target ranges for intervention should be established remains controversial. Although pravastatin or atorvastatin in pediatric heart transplant recipients has resulted in significant improvements in lipid profiles, their role in preventing or reducing CAV is unclear.

Serious gastrointestinal complications have been reported in 18% of recipients (median posttransplant follow-up was 3 yr). Complications included (in order) pancreatitis, cholecystitis, recurrent abdominal infection, malignancy, and intestinal pneumatosis. Half of the patients with complications required abdominal surgery [52].

Children with CHD who required extensive reconstruction of vessels during transplantation may develop stenoses at anastomotic sites (e.g., aorta, pulmonary veins). This can usually be relieved by interventional catheterization techniques but some cases may require surgery.

Quality of life

Most pediatric recipients are rapidly rehabilitated and full-time attendance at school is achieved in almost all patients within a few months of transplantation. Approximately 50% of children do not require hospitalization in the first year after transplantation. Rejection and infection are the major causes for hospitalization. The functional status of survivors is excellent. The percentage of survivors without functional limitation was 93% at 1 year and 95% at 5 years and 10 years. Less than 1% required total assistance. Preadolescent children exhibited "catch-up" growth in height and weight after transplantation. Failure of linear growth was correlated with steroid requirements [3].

Formal exercise testing reveals that maximum capacity for physical work and peak HR are only approximately two-thirds of predicted. A longitudinal assessment found low-peak aerobic capacity and diastolic dysfunction [53], although perhaps less so in infants [54].

A review of cognitive and psychological outcomes after pediatric heart transplantation found that recipients generally functioned within the normal range on most measures of cognitive function [55]. About 20% experienced significant symptoms of psychological distress during the first year after transplantation [56]. Posttraumatic stress disorder seems to be relatively common in parents of pediatric heart transplant recipients [57].

Evidence indicates that children with CHD should be considered separately because they have significantly lower scores on IQ and neurodevelopmental tests when compared with a normative sample [58].

Heterotopic and heart–lung transplantation

Potential recipients with elevated fixed PVR may be eligible for heterotopic heart transplantation or heart–lung transplantation. Actuarial survival rates of 83% (1 yr) and 66% (5 yr) have been reported; however, experience is limited [59]. Heart–lung transplantation experience is also limited, but survival rates reported are 67% (1 yr) and 41% (5 yr), equivalent to those of adults. Domino heart transplant surgery has been employed to provide "preconditioned" donor hearts to infants urgently in need of heart transplantation [60].

Retransplantation

Retransplantation currently accounts for less than 5% of heart transplantations [3]. Indications for retransplantation are (i) chronic severe CAV with symptoms of ischemia or heart failure or asymptomatic moderate or severe left ventricular dysfunction or (ii) chronic graft dysfunction with symptoms of progressive heart failure in the absence of active rejection. Patients with graft failure due to acute rejection with hemodynamic compromise, especially <6 months posttransplant, are regarded as inappropriate candidates for retransplantation [61].

Anesthetic management of children who have undergone heart transplantation

Patients may present for surgery because of complications from cardiac transplantation (e.g., infection, malignancy, drug adverse effects), or the indication for surgery may be unrelated to heart transplantation. Successful anesthetic management requires consideration of the patient's medical status, the physiology of the transplanted heart, and the implications of immunotherapy. These have been discussed above.

Future prospects

Donor shortage remains a frustrating problem. Options such as a totally implantable pediatric artificial heart, xenotransplantation, clinical application of stem cell biology, and transplantation across ABO barriers remain frontiers in pediatric heart transplantation. Immunosuppression in the future may be modified on the basis of recipient genetic risk factors [62].

The two main posttransplant morbidities that have steadily increased are CAV and renal failure. Prevention, monitoring, and treatment of CAV are major challenges. Less nephrotoxic immunosuppressive regimens are being studied [63,64].

Retransplantation as an indication for transplant has been slowly increasing in North America, but is almost nonexistent elsewhere in the world. Questions remain about retransplantation for pediatric recipients who become adults. The demand for second heart transplant, or perhaps kidney transplantation, may be substantial. Pediatric management strategies that could allow multidecade survival with less morbidity and reduced demand for retransplantation require evaluation.

A US national conference identified the following research priorities for pediatric solid organ transplantation: Firstly, young children present a unique immunological environment that may lead to tolerance; therefore, including young children in immunosuppression withdrawal and tolerance trials may increase the potential benefits of these studies. Secondly, adolescence poses significant barriers to successful transplantation. Nonadherence may be insufficient to explain poorer outcomes. More studies focused on identification and prevention of nonadherence, and the potential effects of puberty are required. Thirdly, the relatively naive immune system of the child presents a unique opportunity to study primary infections and alloimmune responses. Finally, relatively small numbers of transplants performed in pediatric centers mandate multicenter collaboration. Investment in registries and tissue and DNA repositories will enhance productivity [65].

Lung transplantation

Introduction

Since 1989, lung transplantation has been offered as a lifesaving and life-extending treatment for children suffering from the end-stage lung disease. Compared to adults, the experience with pediatric lung transplantation has been modest. Annually, less than 100 patients younger than 18 years receive lung transplant surgery for a variety of indications. So far more than 1500 children have undergone cadaveric or living-related lung or heart and lung transplantation. The total number of lung transplants and the number of centers performing these procedures has remained consistent over the last decade [66]. According to the last ISHLT report, less than 10 pediatric centers report performing more than five transplant surgeries per year. The results of pediatric lung transplantation, although comparable to adults, are poorer than other solid organ transplant surgeries. Many challenges such as a wide variety of medical condition, donor–recipient match, and development and growth of the transplanted organs are unique for pediatric patients.

These children undergo multiple surgical and diagnostic interventions and frequently require sedation or general anesthesia. Thus, it is vital for the anesthetic team to be familiar with the issues related to various pediatric pulmonary diseases, conduct of lung transplant surgery, and long-term consequences from the lung transplant surgery.

Indications, contraindications, and listing criteria in children

Generally, lung transplant surgery is considered for children with any end-stage lung disease for which there is no medical treatment. The most common indications differ by age (Table 26.5). Overall and for the older children, cystic fibrosis remains the most common indication for lung transplant surgery. For infants and neonates, pulmonary vascular disease, with or without CHD, predominates as the cause for listing for lung transplantation [67]. Many other pediatric lung diseases can cause irreversible pulmonary failure and need transplantation. These include common as well rare disorders like interstitial lung disease, bronchiolitis obliterans (BO), bronchopulmonary dysplasia, and diseases of surfactant metabolism.

Cystic fibrosis: cystic fibrosis remains the most common indication for the pediatric lung transplantation. Respiratory failure is the commonest cause of death in these children. Many variables, like rate of decline in forced expiratory volumes in 1 second (FEV$_1$), elevated PCO_2 (>50 mm Hg.), falling PO_2 (<55 mm Hg), deteriorating nutritional status, frequency of hospitalizations and the six minute walk test, are considered before listing the patient for lung transplant [67]. In a recent review of cystic fibrosis patients, need for pretransplant mechanical ventilation was predictor of poor 1-year survival after lung transplantation [68]. Expected improvement in the quality of life also influences the decision to list the patient for

Table 26.5 Indications for pediatric lung transplantation (transplant: January 1990 to June 2006)

Diagnosis	Age			
	< 1 yr	1–5 yr	6–11 yr	12–17 yr
Cystic fibrosis		3 (3.7%)	107 (54.9%)	441 (69%)
Primary pulmonary hypertension	10 (16.1%)	18 (22.2%)	23 (11.8%)	53 (8.3%)
Re-transplant (obliterative bronchiolitis post-lung transplant)		6 (7.4%)	8 (4.1%)	22 (3.4%)
Congenital heart disease	19 (30.6%)	8 (9.9%)	2 (1.0%)	5 (0.8%)
Idiopathic pulmonary fibrosis		7 (8.6%)	6 (3.1%)	23 (3.6%)
Obliterative bronchiolitis (without transplant)		5 (6.2%)	9 (4.6%)	21 (3.3%)
Re-transplant (no bronchiolitis obliterans)	3 (4.8%)	1 (1.2%)	7 (3.6%)	16 (2.5%)
Interstitial pneumonitis	6 (9.7%)	11 (13.6%)	1 (0.5%)	5 (0.8%)
Pulmonary vascular disease	7 (11.3)	4 (4.9%)	6 (3.1%)	1 (0.2%)
Eisenmenger's syndrome	1 (1.6%)	5 (6.2%)	5 (2.6%)	6 (0.9%)
Pulmonary fibrosis other	1 (1.6%)	1 (1.2%)	4 (2.1%)	11 (1.7%)
Surfactant B deficiency	9 (14.5%)	2 (2.4%)		
Chronic obstructive disease/emphysema		1 (1.2%)	2 (1.0%)	5 (0.8%)
Bronchopulmonary dysplasia	1 (1.6%)	2 (2.5%)	6 (3.1%)	
Bronchiectasis			3 (1.5%)	4 (0.6%)
Other	5 (8.1%)	7 (8.6%)	6 (3.1%)	26 (4.1%)

Source: Reproduced with permission from Reference [66].

lung transplantation. Many of these children have significant comorbidities from cystic fibrosis like diabetes, severe malnourishment, and osteoporosis. Prior to the transplant surgery, many children suffering from cystic fibrosis undergo surgical intervention for sinusitis, nasal polyps, meconium ileus, etc.

Pulmonary hypertension: pulmonary vascular disease resulting in pulmonary hypertension is the most common reason for lung transplant in younger children. A diverse group of diseases with varied etiologies can result in irreversible pulmonary hypertension. In the recent years, the medical treatment of pulmonary arterial hypertension has improved significantly with drugs like endothelin receptor antagonists (bosentan), phosphodiesterase inhibitors (sildenafil), and prostacyclin and its analogs. These drugs have been shown to reduce the pulmonary arterial pressure and reverse the histological changes in the pulmonary vascular architecture secondary to the long-standing pulmonary hypertension. The full impact of these drugs on the models used to predict the life expectancy in patients with pulmonary hypertension is yet to be fully evaluated. Pulmonary hypertension resulting from congenital and veno-occlusive diseases like pulmonary vein stenosis and alveolar capillary dysplasia are usually unresponsive to the medical therapy.

Disorders of surfactant metabolism: various genetic conditions, e.g., protein B deficiency, surfactant protein C deficiency, and other mutations that cause abnormal surfactant formation, usually present immediately after birth with severe respiratory failure. These infants require significant ventilatory support or ECMO support. Most of these children require lung transplantation within few weeks of their births.

Miscellaneous disorders: lung transplant surgery has been performed in children for variety of other indications like bronchopulmonary dysplasia, congenital diaphragmatic hernia, hemosiderosis, BO, and pulmonary dysmaturity.

The criteria for listing children for lung transplant surgery are based on the natural history of the disease, functional status, and expected improvement in the quality of life. Generally, a clear diagnosis with a life expectancy of less than 2 years is necessary for listing the child for the lung transplant. However, it is hard to develop survival models for the relatively rare disease.

Active malignancy, sepsis, tuberculosis, neuromuscular disease, multiple organ failure, and acquired immunodeficiency syndrome are considered as absolute contraindications for any transplant surgery. Children colonized with multidrug resistant organisms like *Burkholderia cenocepacia*, have been shown to have poor survival rates after lung transplant surgery and most centers consider this as a strong relative contraindication for lung transplant surgery. Liver disease secondary to the cystic fibrosis is not an absolute contraindication for lung transplant. Some of these patients have been listed for combined liver–lung transplant surgery and have done unexpectedly well with good survival rates. A compromised left ventricular function is also considered as an absolute contraindication in some centers. Other factors that influence the decision to list the child for transplant surgery are history of non-compliance with medical treatment, severe uncontrolled diabetes, severe osteoporosis, etc.

Donor selection, availability and the new lung allocation system

Like other organ transplant surgeries, donor availability has been a limiting factor. Only about 15% of the cadaveric donors have lungs that are considered acceptable for transplantation [69]. In compliance with the final rule, the OPTN implemented a new lung allocation system that used medical urgency as the primary determinant of organ allocation and discouraged the use of waiting time. Under this system, a lung allocation score is calculated for every patient older than 12 years. Multiple variables like age, functional status, forced vital capacity (FVC), and oxygen requirement are used in calculating the lung allocation score. The new policy also mandates that the donor lungs from pediatric donors be preferentially given to pediatric patients [70]. Recent data from adult and pediatric patients suggest that since the implementation of new lung allocation system, waiting time has decreased and the annual number of lung transplant surgeries performed, has increased [70]. Preliminary observations suggest that since May 2005 waiting list mortality in the pediatric and adult patients has diminished; however, the long-term impact of this new allocation system on early posttransplant mortality and long-term survival is still being evaluated. Children younger than 12 years still receive organs on the basis of the waiting time accrued on the transplant list.

Donor lungs are selected after thorough medical screening and multiple laboratory tests. In younger children, comparable age and height (<20% discrepancy) are considered acceptable for matching lung volume. An ideal donor is younger than 55 years, nonsmoker, and has no history of cardiopulmonary or significant neurological disease. The donor lungs should produce good gaseous exchange ($PaO_2 > 350$ mm Hg with FIO_2 of 1.0) on moderate amount of ventilatory support. The chest X-ray and bronchoscopy should rule out any significant infection, consolidation, and tumor. Ideally, the donor lungs are accepted only if the ischemic time is expected to be less than 6 hours. To increase the number of potential donors, many centers have advocated using "marginal" donors (see Table 26.6) [71]. Donors with mild lung pathology that is considered to be reversible with aggressive therapy fall in this category. Most of these criteria are subjective and soft criteria like surgeon's preference, recipient's state of health, etc., also influence the decision to transplant. Many biochemical markers in the bronchoalveolar lavage fluid from the donor lungs, e.g., IL-8, IL-6, and IL-1b, are being evaluated as predictors of early and late graft dysfunction [72]. Additionally, using donation after cardiac death lungs is another option that has been being considered to alleviate organ shortage [73].

The process of harvest includes systemic heparinization of the donor and infusion of prostaglandin E_1 into the

Table 26.6 Summary of donor selection criteria and extended criteria

Indicator	Ideal donor	Marginal donor	Unsuitable
Age	<55	55–65	>65
PaO_2/FIO_2	>350	300–200	<150
Smoking history	None	<20 pack years	>20 pack years
Chest X-ray	Clear	Mild changes	Dense consolidations, collapse
Ventilation	<5 days	>5 days	>5 days
Microbiology	Negative Gram stain	Positive culture	Resistant organism
Ischemic times	<4–6 h	6–8 h	>8 h

Source: Reproduced with permission from Reference [71].

main pulmonary artery. A number of preservation solutions have been tried but currently Euro-Collins solution is used by most centers. Lungs are inflated with FIO_2 of less than 0.4 to an airway pressure less than 20 cm of H_2O. Lungs are removed en bloc with descending aorta, left atrial cuff, main pulmonary artery (PA), and thoracic aorta.

Anesthetic management

After being listed for lung transplantation, most children will be seen in the anesthesia clinics and undergo extensive evaluation including ECG, echocardiogram, pulmonary function testing arterial blood gases, and complete metabolic panel. Children with pretransplant diagnosis of pulmonary hypertension also undergo a diagnostic cardiac catheterization where response of pulmonary vascular bed to oxygen and NO is noted and cardiac anatomy is defined.

At the time of surgery, these patients are at various degrees of end-stage lung disease. A large number of children are living at home with minimal oxygen supplementation. At the other end of the spectrum are neonates and infants, who are usually critically ill at the time of surgery. Almost all the neonates and infants, who received lung transplant surgery at our institution, were on chronic ventilatory or extracorporeal hemodynamic support prior to their surgery.

Like other solid organ transplants, time of surgery is unpredictable. Anesthesiologists are required to evaluate, anesthetize, and obtain the vascular access in these critically ill patients in a relatively short period of time. Most children carry a hospital given pager and have been anticipating the surgery for a long period of time. They are often excited and frightened at the same time. Anxiolytics such as midazolam can be safely given to most children.

One must be careful in administering sedatives to unintubated children with severe pulmonary hypertension in the absence of proper monitoring.

Standard NPO guidelines are followed to minimize the risk of aspiration and contamination of the new lungs. The choice of induction agent and muscle relaxant is largely guided by the patient's condition and hemodynamics. Propofol and etomidate are safe in children with cystic fibrosis and other hemodynamically stable patients but ketamine may be the preferred drug for inducing children with high pulmonary pressures. Ketamine has been shown to have a minimal effect on PVR in children. Anesthetic depth is maintained with opioids, benzodiazepines, and supplemented with inhalational agents.

Anesthesiologist must ensure that the nonanesthetic drugs like immunosuppressants and preoperative antibiotics are delivered on time. For children with pulmonary hypertension, selective vasodilators like NO and prostacylins must be maintained throughout the prebypass period to avoid rebound pulmonary hypertension.

Most often, pediatric lung transplants are performed with the assistance of CPB and lung isolation is not required. The extensive nature of the surgery and the use of CPB mandate the need of invasive monitoring with arterial and central venous catheters. At our institution, continuous monitoring of pulmonary pressure with PA catheter is limited to adolescents with the pretransplant diagnosis of pulmonary hypertension. The 7 Fr sheath is placed preoperatively and catheter is advanced to the pulmonary artery after the patient has been weaned off the bypass machine. When continuous monitoring of PA pressures is indicated in smaller children, a catheter can be placed directly into the pulmonary artery by the surgeon. Lung transplant surgery is a Class 1 indication for performing intraoperative TEE. TEE is used to monitor the right ventricular pressures, ventricular function, and to rule out pulmonary venous obstruction in the postbypass period.

The surgery is performed through a transsternal, clamshell incision. A meticulous dissection is carried out to ensure the adequate exposure prior to the initiation of CPB. Adhesions in the thoracic cavity from infections and previous surgeries can cause substantial bleeding. Antifibrinolytic drugs like tranexamic acid help in reducing the blood loss, though the effect of these drugs in younger children is not well studied. Adequate ventilation and oxygenation during the prebypass period is another challenge that the anesthesia team has to deal with. Frequent suctioning of copious secretions is needed to effectively ventilate cystic fibrosis patients. Many children with end-stage lung disease are chronic CO_2 retainers. Ventilation during prebypass period should be adjusted to maintain normal pH levels. Overzealous correction of hypercarbia often results in severe respiratory alkalosis leading to reduced cerebral blood flow and potentially causes cerebral ischemia.

Use of cardiopulmonary bypass

Use of CPB is an issue of much debate in the adult lung transplant surgery. There are several factors that make the use of CPB necessary for the lung transplant surgery in children. CPB allows the resection of both diseased lungs simultaneously, thus minimizing the risk of cross-contamination of the new lungs. Many of these children are physically too small to accommodate even the smallest double lumen tube. Other children like those with significant pulmonary hypertension and neonates are often too tenuous to tolerate single lung ventilation for any length of time. In addition, use of CPB provides stable hemodynamics during the extensive surgical dissection, greatly simplifies the anesthetic and surgical management, and consequently reduces lung ischemic times.

Use of CPB, however, comes with its own risks. Generation of inflammatory mediators and activation of complement cascade during CPB contribute to ischemic–reperfusion injury to the implanted lungs. The data from the adult patients suggest that there is a higher incidence of graft dysfunction associated with the use of CPB [74]. This observation, however, may reflect the fact that in the adult patients CPB is more frequently used in patients with pulmonary hypertension, a pretransplant diagnosis, independently associated with poorer outcome.

Surgical technique

During CPB, the patient is cooled to 32°C and surgery is performed without arresting the heart. Use of aortic cross-clamp is necessary when the surgery involves a simultaneous correction of a coexisting intracardiac defect. After establishing CPB, both lungs are removed by ligating and dividing pulmonary arterial, pulmonary venous, and bronchial connections. In most recipients, the tracheobronchial tree is usually colonized with multiantibiotic resistant bacteria. In order to reduce the bacterial load on the new lungs, tracheal stump of the recipient is irrigated with concentrated solution of antibiotics like tobramycin. While the pneumonectomies are being performed, a second surgical team simultaneously prepares the donor lungs. The implantation of the new lungs is initiated with the end-to-end bronchial anastomosis. Since bronchial blood supply is compromised during the procedure, peribronchial tissue is wrapped around the anastomotic site to enhance healing. Vascular supply to the new lungs is established by anatomizing donor pulmonary artery to the native main pulmonary artery. The pulmonary veins are reconnected to the recipient's left atrium en bloc, using donor's atrial cuff. This method not only reduces the surgical time, but also minimizes the risk of developing pulmonary vein stenosis.

Before weaning off the bypass machine, ventilation is resumed. Ventilator parameters are guided by the donor weight. Careful adjustments to tidal volume and airway pressures are made so that all atelectatic areas are expanded but not over-distended. Volutrauma caused by over-distension of the new lungs can increase endothelial permeability and potentiate primary graft dysfunction (PGD). If areas of atelectasis persist, flexible bronchoscopy should be performed to rule out obstruction of the bronchial anastomosis. A thorough intraoperative TEE exam is done to evaluate right ventricular function and right ventricular pressure is estimated. Blood flow should be measured in the pulmonary artery distal to the anastomosis and in the pulmonary veins. Inotropic support and selective pulmonary vasodilator therapy with NO is initiated when high right-sided pressures are measured along with significant right ventricular dysfunction.

Many pretransplant factors like younger age, nutritional status, and rejection influence the need for postoperative ventilation. After initial perfusion scan and diagnostic bronchial biopsies have been performed, most children can be extubated within few hours of the surgery. Infants and neonates tend to have a more protracted course with prolonged ventilatory needs when compared to the older children with cystic fibrosis (average 24 vs 3 days) [75]. This difference can be explained by their poor preoperative status, frequent airway complications, and associated cardiac anomalies. Postoperative pain relief is usually accomplished by patient-controlled analgesia and narcotic infusions. Regional anesthesia with epidural catheter has been frequently used in adult and older children who do not require systemic heparinization. Epidural catheters can also be placed in the postoperative periods once coagulation parameters have normalized.

Primary graft failure

Persistent hypoxemia after CPB often signals the onset of acute graft failure. PGD remains a major contributing factor to early and possibly delayed mortality after pediatric lung transplantation. A large, retrospective, single center, study involving adult and pediatric patients observed a significant difference in the early mortality. Generally, the PGD, also known as ischemic–reperfusion injury or acute lung injury, is defined by poor oxygenation in the immediate and early postoperative period. The incidence of PGD appears to be similar in adults and children (22% vs 23%) [76]. Since 2004, ISHLT has implemented a common system grading the severity of the reperfusion injury. This system is based on PaO_2/FIO_2 ratio and chest X-ray findings (Table 26.7) [77]. Other reversible causes of hypoxemia such as inadequate ventilation and right ventricular

Table 26.7 International Society of Heart and Lung Transplantation (ISHLT) recommendations for grading of primary graft dysfunction

Grade	PaO_2/FiO_2 ratio	Radiological infiltrates consistent with pulmonary edema
0	>300	−
1	>300	+
2	200–300	+
3	<200	+

Source: Reproduced with permission from Reference [77].

dysfunction with right-to-left shunt must be ruled out first before the diagnosis of PGD is made.

Vascular endothelium makes up a vast portion of the lung parenchyma. Unlike other organ transplants, oxygen is readily available to the metabolically active endothelium immediately after the onset of ischemic period. This allows production of free radicals during ischemic period itself, making lungs more susceptible to graft failure than other solid organs. The time course of this complication suggests two distinct but complementary mechanisms. The first phase, seen immediately after the reperfusion, is initiated by the donor macrophage-induced release of superoxide anions, inflammatory cytokines, mast cell degranulation, and complement activation. All these humoral and cellular mediators damage the integrity of the vascular endothelium causing movement of fluid to the interstitial and alveolar space [78]. Clinically, this presents as progressive hypoxemia with copious, pink frothy secretions that are not amenable to the conventions treatment methods like diuresis and institution of PEEP. The initial release of inflammatory cytokine induces the recruitment of recipient's neutrophils to the injury site within a few hours after initial injury and starts the delayed phase of PGD. During the delayed phase, neutrophils produce reactive superoxide anions and hydroxyl ions and greatly amplify the initial injury, causing further damage to the pulmonary endothelium. Neutrophils also produce elastase and block the blood flow in the capillaries, resulting in the architectural damage to the lung tissue.

Data from the adult patients has linked multiple donor factors to the genesis of PGD. These factors included female sex, African American race, age (<21 or >45 yr), and history of smoking. Ischemic times longer than 6 hours were associated with higher early mortality rates. Many preventive measures have been employed to reduce the incidence of PGD. These measures include prophylactic use of prostaglandins and preservation solutions like Euro-Collins and low-potassium dextran. Other empirical measures like retrograde perfusion, avoidance of barotrauma, and use of surfactant are also helpful in reducing the incidence of PGD. Experimental evidence suggests that rapid

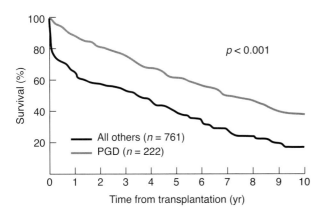

Figure 26.7 Survival after lung transplantation, stratified by the presence or absence of primary graft dysfunction (Reproduced with permission from Reference [76])

reperfusion with high flows and high pulmonary artery pressures may be associated with a higher incidence of reperfusion injury [79].

PGD is associated with a protracted postoperative course and significantly higher early mortality. A retrospective study that included adult and pediatric patients reported significantly higher overall mortality in patients who developed primary graft failure (28.8% vs 4.2%) (see Figure 26.7) [76]. A positive correlation between severe early primary graft failure and bronchiolitis obliterans (BO) BO has also been shown [80]. Huddleston et al. noted that the incidence of BO is lower in children who received lungs with shorter ischemic time [75].

Once PGD develops, patients are managed with aggressive cardiopulmonary support involving mechanical ventilation, inotropes, and occasionally with the use of ECMO. Early use of NO tends to reduce the early mortality. In most patients PGD resolves over several days. Children who need ECMO support are expected to have significantly higher mortality.

The preventive strategies to reduce the incidence of PGD are mainly focused on improving the preservation techniques, reducing ischemic time, improving donor management, and minimizing barotrauma. Surgeons routinely allow ejection of small amount of blood into the pulmonary artery immediately after establishing vascular supply to the first lung. Empirical evidence suggests that the prophylactic use of pulmonary vasodilators like prostaglandin E_{11} and prostacyclin may reduce the incidence and severity of the reperfusion injury. Prophylactic role of NO, however, is less clear. In a small group of patients, Thabut et al. were able to demonstrate a marked decrease in the incidence of allograft dysfunction. In this study, prophylactic use of NO alone or with pentoxifylline, improved hemodynamics, reduced total duration of postoperative mechanical ventilation, and reduced early mortality [81]. Ardehali et al., in a prospective study in lung

transplant patients, observed a significant improvement gas exchange and reduced pulmonary arterial pressures in patients with established PGD. However, in this study, prophylactic use of NO failed to reduce the incidence of PGD [82].

Physiological changes and growth of the transplanted lungs

Denervation of lungs is a consequence of the transplant surgery but this produces few clinically significant effects on airway reflexes, mucociliary movement and bronchial hyperreactivity [83]. The lack of afferent stimuli to the respiratory center in transplanted patients results in poor coordination between thoracic and abdominal muscles—a frequently observed finding in immediate postoperative period. Adult lung transplant patients show a subnormal increase in the minute ventilation with carbon dioxide challenge [84]. Loss of lymphatic drainage makes the transplanted lungs more susceptible to interstitial edema, increased water content, and lower compliance [85].

Serial pulmonary function tests, radiological findings, histological evidence, and clinical examination suggest that donor lungs from younger infants and neonates continue to grow after the surgery. This growth occurs both in lung parenchyma and larger airway and it mirrors the somatic growth of the recipient. Cohen et al. observed that functional reserve capacity increases along with the somatic growth. This increase accompanies a similar increase in the FEV_1, suggesting that the growth in the lungs results from increase in the number of alveoli and not from mere distension of existing alveoli [86]. The lobar lungs transplanted from mature living related donors also demonstrate a similar growth patterns. However, morphometeric studies suggest that number of alveoli in these lobar lungs remain constant and the observed growth in lung volume results primarily from alveolar distension [87]. The measurement of diffusing capacity for carbon monoxide (DLCO) provides an estimate of gas exchange surface area. Serial measurements of DLCO support the opinion that the increase in lung volume seen after mature lobes is secondary to hyperinflation.

Surveillance

These children are closely monitored for rejection, infection, growth, and BO. Pulmonary function tests, bronchopulmonary lavages, and transbronchial biopsies are performed at frequent intervals. Older children can cooperate to perform spirometric test and the values of FEV_1, FVC, and flow–volume loops can be serially measured with reasonable accuracy. After the transplant surgery, most children show immediate improvement in their pulmonary function tests (Figure 26.8). In infants and younger

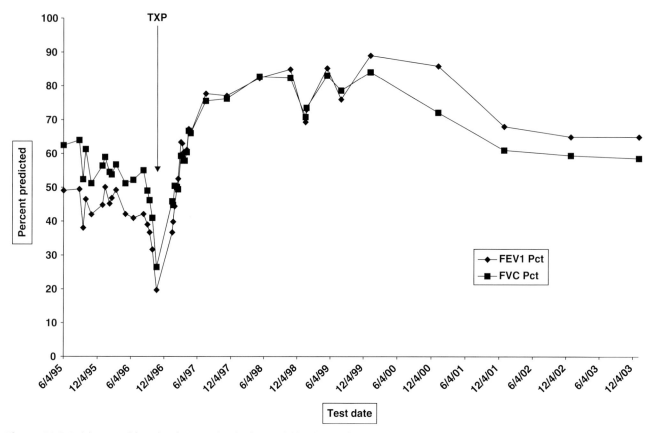

Figure 26.8 Serial FEV₁ and forced vital capacity (FVC) values in child with cystic fibrosis

children (less than 2 yr of age) serial values of peak expiratory flow rates are measured at different values of function residual capacities. Peak expiratory flow rate is measured by rapid inflation, followed by a rapid deflation. This is achieved by using mask inflation followed by a rapid external thoracoabdominal compression. These tests are noninvasive but are physically stimulating and are adversely affected by active patient resistance. Consequently, most of the children require deep sedation and/or general anesthesia for these tests. Any deterioration in the baseline values is further investigated by transbronchial biopsy, bronchoalveolar lavage, and open-lung biopsy.

Surgical complications

Airway complications

The blood supply to the donor bronchus and bronchial anastomosis is compromised during the lung transplant surgery. Inadequate blood supply can result in poor healing at the anastomotic site and other airway complications like airway stenosis, development of granulation tissue, tracheomalacia, and rarely airway dehiscence. Surgical techniques like the use of peribronchial tissue around the anastomotic site and use of smaller segment of donor

bronchus can minimize the incidence of these complications. In a single center study involving 239 transplant surgeries, Choong et al. [88] reported that 13% of children needed surgical interventions for their airway complications. Preoperative bacterial and fungal infections, longer ischemic times, and prolonged mechanical ventilation were identified as significant risk factors. In this study, younger age of the patient was not identified as an independent risk factor for developing airway stenosis. However, infants may have a higher incidence of developing tracheomalacia and dynamic obstruction of major airways. Most patients with tracheobronchomalacia show significant improvement without any surgical interventions, but may need prolonged mechanical ventilation [89]. Usually airway complications are diagnosed within first 3 months of surgery. Airway stenosis is usually treated successfully with repeated mechanical balloon dilatation through a rigid bronchoscope. Children with recurrent airway stenosis after repeated balloon dilations may require mechanical stents to maintain airway patency.

Vascular complications

Vascular complications are rare, mostly presenting in the form of obstruction to the blood flow in pulmonary veins.

Significant pulmonary venous obstruction presents immediately after weaning off bypass or in the immediate postoperative period. Clinical signs include persistent hypoxemia, pink frothy secretions in the airway along with increased pulmonary aerial pressures. Perfusion scans are routinely performed in all transplant patients within hours after their lung transplant surgery, to rule out any undiagnosed discrepancy of pulmonary flow to either lung. If pulmonary venous obstruction is suspected, a definitive diagnosis can be made during cardiac catheterization. Any significant obstruction to pulmonary blood flow requires an urgent treatment either with surgical correction or placement of a stent in the cardiac catheterization lab.

Nerve injuries

Nerves that lie adjacent to the bronchopulmonary tissue are frequently injured during the transplant surgery. Huddleston reported a 22% incidence of phrenic nerve injury in children [90]. The resulting diaphragmatic paralysis is usually a transient phenomenon but can prolong the need the mechanical ventilation and intensive care stay. Injury to the vagus nerve frequently leads to gastroesophageal reflux and gastric paresis. Severe gastric paresis and resulting recurrent silent aspiration has been implicated in deteriorating graft function and resulting BO. The incidence of severe gastroesophageal reflux is as high as 50% [91]. Younger patients are especially susceptible to this injury and most neonatal and infant lung recipients require Nissen fundoplication after their transplant surgery. Patients with deteriorating pulmonary function have been shown to benefit from surgical treatment of gastroesophageal reflux [92,93]. Injury to the recurrent laryngeal nerve (mostly left) and resulting vocal cord dysfunction is seen in 10% children. Most of these children will recover without any residual vocal cord defects [90].

Arrhythmias

A large atrial suture line is a potential source for generating abnormal depolarization and repolarization. Clinically significant atrial flutter requiring medical treatment is seen in about 11% of pediatric patients. Supraventricular tachycardia and atrial fibrillation are also seen [94]. Most arrhythmias are amenable to medical treatment alone.

Common medical complications

Immunosuppressive therapy, side effects, and drug interactions

Transplanted lungs contain large surface of endothelial tissue and other immunologically active cells making lungs more susceptible to rejection when compared to the other solid organs. Pediatric lung transplant recipients are given higher doses of immunosuppressant drugs. Use of induction therapy with PKT3, ATG, or IL2 receptor blockers like daclizumab has increased in the recent years [66]. Most children are given triple drug therapy including calcineurin inhibitor (cyclosporine or tacrolimus), cell cycle inhibitors like azathioprine or MMF, and prednisone. Chronic use of these drugs causes complications like compromised renal function, hypertension, hypercholesteremia, hirsutism, osteoporosis, and others. About 30% children have clinically significant renal dysfunction but many others demonstrate subclinical renal dysfunction with borderline serum creatinine levels. Since a large number of these children are at risk of developing renal failure, nephrotoxic drugs like NSAIDS should be avoided even if renal function is normal. Cystic fibrosis patients, because of the unreliable gastric absorption and hepatic clearance are at risk for developing acute toxicity from oral medications like cyclosporine. In fact, the high incidence of central nervous complications like seizures, headache, and stroke has been attributed to acute increases in plasma levels of cyclosporine. Hepatic enzymes like P450 metabolize commonly used immunosuppressant drugs. Drugs that are commonly used during surgery, e.g., metochopramide and barbiturates, induce P450 enzyme, resulting in dangerously low levels of cyclosporine.

Opportunistic infections

Physiological consequences of denervation, e.g., poor cough effort, poor mucociliary clearance of secretions and anastomotic stenosis, contribute to these patients tendency to get frequent infections. High-degree immunosuppression is needed after lung transplantation and also adds to the risk of bacterial and viral infections. Bacterial infections are most common but fungal and viral infections tend to have higher mortality. CMV, adenovirus, Epstein–Barr, and influenza are the common viral infections.

Posttransplant lympho-proliferative disorder

Posttransplant PTLD mostly results from B-cell proliferation is commonly seen in patients with T-cell depletion. The incidence of PTLD is 8.2% at 5 years and is mostly related to Epstein–Barr virus infection [95]. The hyperplasia of the lymphatic tissue is seen in intrathoracic tissue as lung nodules, mediastinal lymphadenopathy. It can also present in extra-thoracic tissues like tonsillar hypertrophy, cerebral, and visceral masses. Most children will respond to reduction in immunosuppression but chemotherapy may be needed in a few unresponsive patients.

Graft rejection

Recurrent graft rejections are more common after lung transplantation compared to other solid organ transplant surgeries. Infants and younger children appear to be somewhat protected and suffer from fewer episodes of acute rejection [96,34]. This discrepancy can be explained by their relatively immature immune system. The clinical picture of rejection is a nonspecific deterioration in the functional status or pulmonary function parameters. These clinical findings are further investigated by transbronchial or open-lung biopsy. Once the diagnosis of acute rejection is made, these episodes are treated aggressively with a course of intravenous drugs like high-dose steroids ATG, and tacrolimus.

Obliterative bronchiolitis and bronchiolitis obliterans syndrome

Bronchiolitis obliterans syndrome (BOS) remains the Achilles heel of the lung transplant surgery. It continues to be a major challenge for the long-term success after pediatric lung transplantation. Roughly half the surviving children develop bronchiolitis obliterans (BO) by 5 years after their lung transplant surgery [95]. A number of factors, like duration of the ischemic time, number of rejections, and age of the recipient at the time of surgery, appear to influence the incidence of the disease. In a retrospective analysis, children with total ischemic time of less than 2 hours had significantly lower incidence of BO, when compared to a similar group of patients with longer ischemic time (20% vs 52%) (see Figure 26.9) [97]. In general, patients transplanted with mature living donor lobes tend to have shorter ischemic times. This may also explain a lower incidence of BO in these patients [98]. The incidence of BO is also lower in smaller children (age less than 3 yr at the time of transplant). This presumably is related to a lower incidence compared to the older children (0.2 episodes compared to 1.95) [75]. At our center,

children who received simultaneous lung and liver transplant had a significantly lower incidence of acute rejection and BO [99]. Bronchiolitis obliterans (BO) is a histological diagnosis reflecting inflammatory and fibroproliferative changes in the bronchioles of children with chronic graft dysfunction. Since the histological diagnosis is difficult to make, a corresponding clinical syndrome, known as BOS, is used to describe a nonspecific, significant, progressive, and nonreversible decline in airflow. For older children, a 20% decrease in the baseline FEV_1 is a reliable indicator for BOS. The exact mechanism of BO is still not known but recent research suggests that a number of immune-mediated and immune-independent mechanisms are responsible. Alloimmune-mediated mechanisms cause injury by acute rejection, cellular lymphocytic bronchiolitis, activation of humoral immune system, and autoimmune dysfunction. A number of immunity-independent mechanisms like infections, aspiration, ischemia, and primary graft failure also appear to contribute to this irreversible and mostly progressive deterioration of the pulmonary architecture [100]. Injury caused by these mechanisms induces a significant fibrotic reaction, remodeling, and abnormal angiogenesis. So far, there is no effective treatment for BOS. Enhanced immunosuppression is the cornerstone of currently used therapies, though none of the methods have been able to show a consistent benefit to all patients. Azathioprine, a macrolide antibiotic, has been tried to reduce airway neutrophilia in the transplanted lungs. Antireflux surgery may also prevent or even reverse the decline in pulmonary function in some patients. Statins like pravastatins, because of their ability to induce apoptosis in fibroblasts, may hold some promise in treating BOS. Retransplantation is considered in relatively few patients; however, risk of postsurgical death within 1 year is high.

Living donor lobar lung transplant

Living donor lobar lung transplant (LDLLT) is considered as an acceptable alternative to cadaveric lung transplant in few patients who are not expected to survive to receive cadaveric lungs or patients who are listed for retransplantation. In this procedure, lower lobes from two healthy living related donors are transplanted into a single recipient. In order to provide adequate lung volume to the recipient and provide at least 50% of the predicted lung volume, this procedure has been primarily used for children or small adults. LDLLT presents a serious ethical dilemma of subjecting two healthy adults to a procedure with potential of serious complications (10–20%) and inevitable 15–20% reduction in pulmonary function. There has been a recent decline in the number of center performing living-related lung transplants. Only three centers have reported significant experience with living-related transplant surgeries.

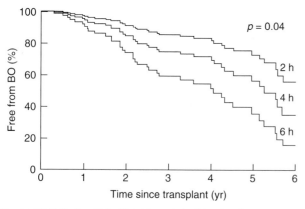

Figure 26.9 Kaplan–Meier life table analysis of freedom from bronchiolitis obliterans when the patients were segregated according to the organ ischemic time. BO, bronchiolitis obliterans (Reproduced with permission from Reference [97])

Since these surgeries are done in a more controlled environment, ischemic times are shorter. As a result, incidence of PGD and bronchiolitis is low [98]. Recently, Date et al. reported a very encouraging 87.6% 5-year survival rate from LDLLT in 43 adult and pediatric patients [101].

Mortality and long-term survival

Overall, lung transplant recipients do not live as long as the recipients of other solid organ transplant. Survival after pediatric lung transplantation remains similar to that reported in adults, with a median survival of 4.3 years. It appears that children who were transplanted after 2002 have much better survival rates (81–58% at 1 and 4 yr) [66]. Single center data from St Louis Children's Hospital suggests that infants have higher early mortality (25% vs 4.9%) but have significantly better long-term outcome than children older than 11 years (survival half-life of 6.5 vs 4.5 years) [66,75]. PGD is the leading cause of early mortality and accounts for 62% of early deaths. BO, infection, and PTLD are usually responsible for the poor long-term outcome. Pretransplant diagnosis of pulmonary hypertension and children undergoing repeat transplant appear to have relatively poorer outcome.

So far no prospective studies analyzing the benefit to pediatric patients have been conducted. Recently Liou et al. [102] performed Cox's proportional hazards test in cystic fibrosis children, using transplant surgery as a time-dependent covariate. Authors observed that based on the recent data from the OPTN database, children with a 5-year life expectancy less than 50% at the time of transplant showed no difference from the nontransplanted group with a similar severity of disease. Among 127 children with a 5-year predicted survival greater than 50%, transplanted group showed a substantial decrease in posttransplant survival when compared to the control nontransplant group. It was concluded that benefit from lung transplantation for cystic fibrosis patients could no longer be assumed. However, the study did not include impact of the recent changes in the lung allocation system and authors were unable to comment on the improvements in the quality of life in cystic fibrosis children after transplant surgery. Another limitation of the study was that it included covariates obtained 2–3 years prior to the surgery and did not account for the medical condition of the patient at the time of transplant. Three previously published studies, using similar statistical methods, have suggested marked improvement in average survival with lung transplantation [103, 104]. Future studies are needed to clarify the potential benefit that lung transplant surgery can provide to children with cystic fibrosis and other diseases leading to end-stage pulmonary failure.

References

1. Hertz MI, Aurora P, Boucek MM, et al. (2007) Registry of the International Society for Heart and Lung Transplantation: introduction to the 2007 annual reports—100,000 transplants and going strong. J Heart Lung Transplant 26:763–768.
2. Barnard CN (1967) The operation. A human cardiac transplant: an interim report of a successful operation performed at Groote Schuur Hospital, Cape Town. S Afr Med J 41:1271–1274.
3. Boucek MM, Aurora P, Edwards LP, et al. (2007) Registry of the International Society for Heart and Lung Transplantation: tenth official pediatric heart transplantation report—2007. J Heart Lung Transplant 26:796–807.
4. Canter CE, Shaddy RE, Bernstein B, et al. (2007) Indications for heart transplantation in pediatric heart disease: a scientific statement from the American Heart Association Council on Cardiovascular Disease in the Young; the Councils on Clinical Cardiology, Cardiovascular Nursing, and Cardiovascular Surgery and Anesthesia; and the Quality of Care and Outcomes Research Interdisciplinary Working Group. Circulation 115:658–676.
5. Kirklin JK, Naftel DC, Caldwell RL, et al. (2006) Should status II patients be removed from the pediatric heart transplant waiting list? A multi-institutional study. J Heart Lung Transplant 25:271–275.
6. Fricker FJ, Addonizio L, Bernstein D, et al. (1999) Heart transplantation in children: indications. Pediatr Transplant 3:333–342.
7. Jenkins PC, Flanagan MF, Sargent JD, et al. (2001) A comparison of treatment strategies for hypoplastic left heart syndrome using decision analysis. J Am Coll Cardiol 38:1181–1187.
8. Boucek MM, Shaddy RE (2001) Pediatric heart transplantation. In: Allen HD, Gutgesell HP, Clark EB, Driscoll DJ (eds) Moss and Adams' Heart Disease in Infants, Children, and Adolescents Including the Fetus and Young Adult, 6th edn. Lippincott, Williams & Wilkins, Philadelphia, 395–407.
9. Davies RR, Russo MJ, Mital S, et al. (2008) Predicting survival among high-risk pediatric cardiac transplant recipients: an analysis of the United Network for Organ Sharing database. J Thorac Cardiovasc Surg 135:147–155.
10. Kimberling MT, Balzer DT, Hirsch R, et al. (2002) Cardiac transplantation for pediatric restrictive cardiomyopathy: presentation, evaluation and short-term outcome. J Heart Lung Transplant 21:455–459.
11. Pollock-BarZiv SM, den Hollander N, Ngan BY, et al. (2007) Pediatric heart transplantation in human leukocyte antigen sensitized patients: evolving management and assessment of intermediate-term outcomes in a high-risk population. Circulation 116 (11 Suppl): I172–I178.
12. Holt DB, Lublin DM, Phelan DL, et al. (2007) Mortality and morbidity in pre-sensitized pediatric heart transplant recipients with a positive donor crossmatch utilizing perioperative plasmapheresis and cytolytic therapy. J Heart Lung Transplant 26:876–882.

13. Feingold B, Bowman P, Zeevi A, et al. (2007) Survival in allosensitized children after listing for cardiac transplantation. J Heart Lung Transplant 26:565–571.

14. Stastny P, Lavingia B, Fixler DE, et al. (2007) Antibodies against donor human leukocyte antigens and the outcome of cardiac allografts in adults and children. Transplantation 84:738–745.

15. Wright EJ, Fiser WP, Edens RE, et al. (2007) Cardiac transplant outcomes in pediatric patients with pre-formed anti-human leukocyte antigen antibodies and/or positive retrospective crossmatch. J Heart Lung Transplant 26:1163–1169.

16. Morrow WR (2000) Cardiomyopathy and heart transplantation in children. Curr Opin Cardiol 15:216–223.

17. Mital S, Addonizio LJ, Lamour JM, et al. (2003) Outcome of children with end-stage congenital heart disease waiting for cardiac transplantation. J Heart Lung Transplant 22:147–153.

18. Gajarski RJ, Mosca RS, Ohye RG, et al. (2003) Use of extracorporeal life support as a bridge to pediatric cardiac transplantation. J Heart Lung Transplant 22:28–34.

19. Kirklin JK (2008) Mechanical circulatory support as a bridge to pediatric cardiac transplantation. Semin Thorac Cardiovasc Surg Pediatr Card Surg Annu 80–85.

20. Hsu R, Chien C, Wang S, et al. (2002) Nontransplant cardiac surgery as a bridge to heart transplantation in pediatric dilated cardiomyopathy. Tex Heart Inst J 29:213–216.

21. Boucek MM, Mashburn C, Dunn SM, et al. (2008) Pediatric heart transplantation after declaration of cardiocirculatory death. N Engl J Med 359:709–714.

22. Sarti A (1999) Organ donation. Paediatr Anaesth 9:287–294.

23. Ullah S, Zabala L, Watkins B, et al. (2006) Cardiac donor organ management. Perfusion 21:93–98.

24. Lower RR, Shumway NE (1960) Studies on orthotopic homotransplantation of the canine heart. Surg Forum 11:18–25.

25. Schnoor M, Schäfer T, Lühmann D, et al. (2007) Bicaval versus standard technique in orthotopic heart transplantation: a systematic review and meta-analysis. J Thorac Cardiovasc Surg 134:1322–1331.

26. Weiss ES, Nwakanma LU, Russell SB, et al. (2008) Outcomes in bicaval versus biatrial techniques in heart transplantation: an analysis of the UNOS database J Heart Lung Transplant 27:178–183.

27. Shaw SM, Fildes J, Yonan N, et al. (2007) Does brain natriuretic peptide interact with the immune system after cardiac transplantation? Transplantation 84:1377–1381.

28. Rivenes SM, Lewin MB, Stayer SA, et al. (2001) Cardiovascular effects of sevoflurane, isoflurane, halothane, and fentanyl–midazolam in children with congenital heart disease: an echocardiographic study of myocardial contractility and hemodynamics. Anesthesiology 94:223–229.

29. Sawasdiwipachai P, Laussen PC, McGowan FX, et al. (2007) Cardiac arrest after neuromuscular blockade reversal in a heart transplant infant. Anesthesiology 107:663–665.

30. Backman SB (2008) Anticholinesterase drugs and the transplanted heart Anesthesiology 108:965.

31. Lin C, Chan K, Chou Y, et al. (2002) Transesophageal echocardiography monitoring of pulmonary venous obstruction induced by sternotomy closure during infant heart transplantation. Br J Anaesth 88:590–952.

32. Dietl W, Bauer M, Podesser BK (2006) Nitric oxide in cardiac transplantation. Pharmacol Rep 58 (Suppl): 145–152.

33. Mitchell MB, Campbell DN, Bielefeld MR, et al. (2000) Utility of extracorporeal membrane oxygenation for early graft failure following heart transplantation in infancy. J Heart Lung Transplant 19:834–839.

34. Ibrahim JE, Sweet SC, Flippin M, et al. (2002) Rejection is reduced in thoracic organ recipients when transplanted in the first year of life. J Heart Lung Transplant 21:311–318.

35. Rochea SL, Burch M, O'Sullivana J, et al. (2008) Multicenter experience of ABO-incompatible pediatric cardiac transplantation. Am J Transplant 8:208–215.

36. Reddy SC, Laughlin K, Webber SA, (2003) Immunosuppression in pediatric heart transplantation: 2003 and beyond. Curr Treat Options Cardiovasc Med 5:417–428.

37. Chan M, Pearson GJ (2007) New advances in antirejection therapy. Curr Opin Cardiol 22:117–122.

38. Patel JK, Kobashigawa JA (2007) Tacrolimus in heart transplant patients: an overview. Biodrugs 21:139–143.

39. Zuckermann A, Manito N, Epailly E, et al. (2008) Multidisciplinary insights on clinical guidance for the use of proliferation signal inhibitors in heart transplantation. J Heart Lung Transplant 27:141–149.

40. Pahl E (2007) Statins in the prevention of transplant coronary artery disease: in pediatric heart recipients. Pediatr Transplantation 11:459–460.

41. Stewart S, Winters GL, Fishbein MC, et al. (2005) Revision of the 1990 working formulation for the standardization of nomenclature in the diagnosis of heart rejection. J Heart Lung Transplant 24:1710–1720.

42. Law YM (2007) Pathophysiology and diagnosis of allograft rejection in pediatric heart transplantation. Curr Opin Cardiol 22:66–71.

43. Leonard GTJr, Fricker FJ, Pruett D, et al. (2006) Increased, myocardial performance index correlates with biopsy-proven rejection in pediatric heart transplant recipients. J Heart Lung Transplant 25:61–66.

44. Behera SK, Trang J, Feeley BT, et al. (2008) The use of Doppler tissue imaging to predict cellular and antibody-mediated rejection in pediatric heart transplant recipients. Pediatr Transplant 12:207–214.

45. Mondillo S, Maccherini M, Galderisi M (2008) Usefulness and limitations of transthoracic echocardiography in heart transplantation recipients. Cardiovasc Ultrasound 6:2.

46. Schmauss D, Weis M (2008) Cardiac allograft vasculopathy: recent developments. Circulation 117:2131–2141.

47. Maiers J, Roger Hurwitz R (2008) Identification of coronary artery disease in the pediatric cardiac transplant patient. Pediatr Cardiol 29:19–23.

48. Labarrere CA, Nelson DR, Park JW (2001) Pathologic markers of allograft arteriopathy: insight into the pathophysiology of cardiac allograft chronic rejection. Curr Opin Cardiol 16:110–117.

49. Schowengerdt KO, Naftel DC, Seib PM, et al. (1997) Infections after pediatric heart transplantation: results

from a multi-institutional study. J Heart Lung Transplant 16:1207–1216.

50. Kulikowska A, Boslaugh SE, Huddleston CB, et al. (2008) Infectious, malignant, and autoimmune complications in pediatric heart transplant recipients. J Pediatr 152:671–6777.

51. Lee CK, Christensen LL, Magee JC, et al. (2007) Pre-transplant risk factors for chronic renal dysfunction after pediatric heart transplantation: a 10-year national cohort study. J Heart Lung Transplant 26:458–465.

52. Rakhit A, Nurko S, Gauvreau K, et al. (2002) Gastrointestinal complications after pediatric cardiac transplantation. J Heart Lung Transplant 21:751–759.

53. Davis JA, McBride MG, Chrisant MR, et al. (2006) Longitudinal assessment of cardiovascular exercise performance after pediatric heart transplantation. J Heart Lung Transplant 25:626–633.

54. Abarbanell G, Mulla N, Chinnock R, et al. (2004) Exercise assessment in infants after cardiac transplantation. J Heart Lung Transplant 23:1334–1338.

55. Todaro JF, Fennell EB, Sears SF, et al. (2000) Review: cognitive and psychological outcomes in pediatric heart transplantation. J Pediatr Psychol 25:567–576.

56. Simons LE, Anglin G, Warshaw BL, et al. (2008) Understanding the pathway between the transplant experience and health-related quality of life outcomes in adolescents. Pediatr Transplant 12:187–193.

57. Young GS, Mintzer LL, Seacord D, et al. (2003) Symptoms of posttraumatic stress disorder in parents of transplant recipients: incidence, severity, and related factors. Pediatrics 111:725–731.

58. Wernovsky G, Newburger J (2003) Neurologic and developmental morbidity in children with complex congenital heart disease. J Pediatr 142:6–8.

59. Khagani A, Santini F, Dyke CM, et al. (1997) Heterotopic cardiac transplantation in infants and children. J Thorac Cardiovasc Surg 113:1042–1049.

60. Astora TL, Galantowiczb M, Phillips A, et al. (2007) Domino heart transplantation involving infants. Am J Transplant 7:2626–2629.

61. Johnson MR, Aaronson KD, Canter CF, et al. (2007) Heart retransplantation. Am J Transplant 7:2075–2081.

62. Di Filippo S, Zeevi A, McDade KK, et al. (2006) Impact of TGF-b1 gene polymorphisms on acute and chronic rejection in pediatric heart transplant allografts. Transplantation 81:934–939.

63. Rockx M, Haddad H (2007) Use of calcium channel blockers and angiotensin-converting enzyme inhibitors after cardiac transplantation. Curr Opin Cardiol 22:128–132.

64. Cantarovich M (2007) Renal protective strategies in heart transplant patients. Curr Opin Cardiol 22:133–138.

65. Bartosh SM, Ryckman FC, Shaddy R, et al. (2008) A national conference to determine research priorities in pediatric solid organ transplantation. Pediatr Transplant 12:153–166.

66. Aurora P, Edwards LB, Christie J, et al. (2008) Registry for the International Society for Heart and Lung transplantation: eleventh official pediatric lung and heart/lung transplantation report—2008. J Heart Lung Transplant 27:978–983.

67. Aurora P, Carby M, Sweet S (2008) Selection of cystic fibrosis patients for lung transplantation. Curr Opin Med 14:589–594.

68. Elizur A, Sweet S, Huddleston CB, et al. (2007) Pre-transplant mechanical ventilation increases short-term morbidity and mortality in pediatric patients with cystic fibrosis. J Heart Lung Transplant 26:17–31.

69. Ware LB, Wang Y, Fang X, et al. (2002) Assessment of lungs rejected for transplantation and implications for donor selection. Lancet 360:619–620.

70. Egan TM, Murray S, Bustami RT, et al. (2006) Development of the new lung allocation system. Am J Transplant 6:1212–1227.

71. Botha P, Rostron AJ, Fisher AJ, et al. (2008) Current strategies in donor selection and management. Semin Thorac Cardiovasc Surg 20:143–151.

72. Kaneda H, Waddlee TK, Liu M, et al. (2005) Dynamic changes in cytokine gene expression during cold ischemia predicts outcome after lung transplantation in humans. J Heart Lung Transplant 24 (Suppl 2): S1–S79.

73. Steen S, Ingemansson R, Eriksson L, et al. (2007) First human transplantation of nonacceptable donor lung after reconditioning ex vivo. An Thorac Surg 83:2191–2194.

74. Gammie JS, Cheul LJ, Pham SL, et al. (1998) Cardiopulmonary bypass is associated with early allograft dysfunction but not death after transplantation. J Thorac Cardiovasc Surg 115:990–997.

75. Huddleston CB, Sweet SC, Mallory GB, et al. (1999) Lung transplant in very young infants. J Thorac Cardiovasc Surg 118:796–804.

76. Meyers BF, de la Morene M, Sweet S, et al. (2005) Primary graft dysfunction and other selected complications of lung transplantation: a single center experience of 983 patients. J Heart Lung Transplant 129:1421–1429.

77. Christie JD, Carby M, Bag R, et al. (2005) Report of the ISHLT working group on primary lung graft dysfunction part II: definition. A consensus statement of the International Society of Heart and Lung Transplantation. J Heart Lung Transplant 24:1454–1459.

78. Carter YM, Gelman AE, Kreisel D (2008) Pathogenesis, management and consequences of primary graft dysfunction. Semin Thorac Cardiovasc Surg 20:165–172.

79. Pierre AF, Decampos KN, Liu M, et al. (1998) Rapid reperfusion causes stress failure in ischemic rat lungs. J Thorac Cardiovasc Surg 116:932–942.

80. Daud SA, Yusen RD, Meyers BF, et al. (2007) Impact of immediate primary lung allograft dysfunction on bronchiolitis obliterans syndrome. Am J Respir Crit Care Med 175:507–513.

81. Thabut G, Brugiere O, Leseche G, et al. (2001) Preventive effect of inhaled nitric oxide and pentoxifylline on ischemia/reperfusion injury after lung transplantation. Transplantation 71:1295–1300.

82. Ardehali A, Laks H, Levine M, et al. (2001) A prospective trial of inhaled nitric oxide in clinical transplantation. Transplantation 72:112–115.

83. Kimoff JR, Cheong TH, Cosio MG, et al. (1990) Pulmonary denervation in humans. Effects on dyspnea and

ventilatory patterns during exercise. Am Rev Respir Dis 142:1034–1040.

84. Conrad I, Peggy S, Skaturd JB, et al. (1995) The Breuer-Hering reflex in humans. Effects of pulmonary denervation and hypocapnia. Am J Resip Crit Care Med 152:1747–1751.
85. Ling Z, Bernadette E, Grad DI, et al. (1999) Airway vascular changes in lung allograft recipients. J Heart Lung Transplant 18:231–238.
86. Cohen AH, Mallory GB, Ross K, et al. (1999) Growth of lungs after transplantation in infants and children younger than three years of age. Am J Respir Crit Care Med 159:1747–1751.
87. Duebener LF, Takahashi Y, Wada H, et al. (1999) Do mature pulmonary lobes grow after transplantation into immature recipient? Ann Thorac Surg 68:1165–1170.
88. Choong CK, Sweet SC, Bell J, et al. (2006) Bronchial airway anastomotic complications after pediatric lung transplantation: incidence, causes, management and outcome. J Thorac Cardiovasc Surg 131:198–203.
89. Kadtis AG, Gondor M, Nixon PA, et al. (2000) Airway complications following pediatric lung and heart and lung transplantation. Am J Respir Crit Care Med 162:310–309.
90. Huddleston CB (1996) Surgical complication in children. Semin Thorac Cardiovasc Surg 8:296–304.
91. Sodhi SS, Guo J, Maurer AH, et al. (2002) Gastroparesis after combined heart and lung transplantation. J Clin Garstroenterol 3:34–39.
92. Hadjiliadis D, Duane DR, Steele MP, et al. (2003) Gastroesophageal reflux disease in lung transplant recipients. Clin Trasnplant 17:362–368.
93. Davis RD, Jr, Lau CL, Eubanks S, et al. (2003) Improved lung allograft function after fundoplication in patients with gastro-esophageal reflux disease undergoing lung transplantation. J Thorac Cardiovasc Surg 125:533–542.

94. Gandhi SK, Bromberg Bi, Schuessler RB, et al. (1996) Left sided atrial flutter: characterization of a novel complication of pediatric lung transplantation in an acute canine model. J Thorac Cardiovasc Surg 112:992–1001.
95. Dishop MK, Mallory GB, White FW (2008) Pediatric lung transplantation: perspectives for the pathologist. Ped Dev Pathol 11:85–105.
96. Wells A, Faro A (2006) Special considerations in pediatric lung transplantation. Semin Resp Crit Med 27:552–560.
97. Huddleston CB, Bloch JB, Sweet SC, et al. (2002) Lung transplantation in children. Ann Surg 236:270–276.
98. Kozower BD, Sweet SC, de la Morena M, et al. (2006) Living donor lobar grafts improve pediatric lung retransplant survival. J Thorac Cardiovasc Surg 131:1142–1147.
99. Faro A, Ross S, Huddleston CB, et al. (2007) Lower incidence of bronchiolitis obliterans in pediatric liver–lung transplant recipients with cystic fibrosis. Transplant 87:1435–1439.
100. Sato M, Keshavjee S (2008) Bronchiolitis obliterans syndrome: alloimmune-dependent and -independent injury with aberrant tissue remodeling. Semin Thorac Cardiovasc Surg 20:173–182.
101. Date H, Yamane M, Toyooka S, et al. (2008) Current status and potential of living-donor lobar lung transplantation. Front Biosci 13:1433–1439.
102. Liou TG, Adler FR, Cox DR, et al. (2007) Lung transplantation and survival in children with cystic fibrosis. N Engl J Med 357:2143–2152.
103. Aurora P, Whitehead B, Wade A, et al. (1999) Lung transplantation and life extension in children with cystic fibrosis. Lancet 354:1591.
104. Liou TG, Cahill BC (2008) Pediatric lung transplantation for cystic fibrosis. Transplanation 86:636–637.

6 Anesthesia Outside the Cardiac Operating Room

27 Anesthesia for the cardiac catheterization laboratory

Philip D. Arnold, B.M., F.R.C.A.
Alder Hey Hospital, Royal Liverpool Children's NHS Trust, Liverpool, United Kingdom

Helen M. Holtby, M.B. B.S., F.R.C.P.C.
The Hospital for Sick Children, University of Toronto Faculty of Medicine, Toronto, Canada

Dean B. Andropoulos, M.D., M.H.C.M.
Texas Children's Hospital, Baylor College of Medicine, Houston, Texas, USA

Introduction

The use of catheters to investigate cardiac function dates back to the nineteenth century. Three early twentieth century pioneers won the Nobel Prize for Medicine in 1956 (Werner Forssmann, Andre Cournand, and Dickin-

Anesthesia for Congenital Heart Disease 2nd edition. Edited by Dean Andropoulos, Stephen Stayer, Isobel Russell and Emad Mossad.
© 2010 Blackwell Publishing.

son Richards). Forssmann's efforts cost him his job at the time, but Cournand and Dickinson went on to use right heart catheterization in a systematic effort to understand cardiac function. For many years, cardiac catheterization was the primary method for obtaining both anatomical and physiological data.

Interventional catheterization was first described in 1954 by Rubio-Alvarez [1] for the treatment of pulmonary stenosis. Subsequently, Rashkind and Miller described balloon atrial septostomy for palliation of transposition of the great vessels [2]. The number and scope of transcatheter interventions has increased dramatically in both adults and children.

Anesthetic involvement in cardiac catheterization dates to the early 1950s. General anesthesia and sedation techniques are described using a variety of agents, including thiopentone, propofol, ketamine, meperidine, barbiturates, and antihistamines [3,4]. In 1958 Smith et al. at the Hospital for Sick Children (HSC) in Toronto described the "CM3" mixture for sedation (chlorpromazine, Demerol, and promethazine) [5]. This intramuscular sedative cocktail was widely used, but has been superseded by shorter-acting intravenous regimens for obvious reasons. The use of general anesthesia for the care of children is widespread, though not universal. More recently, it has been recognized that there is an important role for anesthesiologists during cardiac catheterization of adults, for both congenital and acquired heart disease [6,7].

General issues

Other noninvasive imaging techniques have supplanted cardiac catheterization for evaluation of anatomy and function. It is still required to resolve the anatomy in complex patients and also to make hemodynamic measurements. If meaningful data is to be obtained on which to base critical decisions on the child's treatment, close cooperation between the anesthesiologist and cardiologist is required.

As the number of diagnostic catheterizations has diminished, the use of cardiac catheters for therapeutic purposes has increased steadily [8,9]. At the HSC, interventional catheterizations currently outnumber diagnostic studies by almost two to one. Interventional procedures are done as an alternative to surgery and as an adjunct to surgical treatment. They are used in situations where surgical results are poor, or to avoid the use and complications of cardiopulmonary bypass. During interventional catheterization, the focus is on treatment, not precise diagnosis, and maintenance of *baseline* hemodynamics is less critical. Some procedures are associated with marked hemodynamic disturbance and are performed in high-risk patients. The potential for serious complications is high. The need for mechanical support of the circulation is unusual but certainly not unheard of, and it is important to have systems and protocols in place for the instigation of mechanical support in the facility [10]. Children also undergo catheterization whilst on extracorporeal membrane oxygenation [11]. Individuals caring for patients need familiarity with the issues around the instigation and maintenance of mechanical support.

Electrophysiology (EP) procedures include delineation and transcatheter ablation of abnormal conducting pathways and implantation of pacemakers. The majority of patients presenting for EP studies are adolescents with well-tolerated supraventricular tachycardia (SVT). Anesthetic and sedative drugs have effects on cardiac conduction. Particular agents should be chosen to minimize this effect. Some arrhythmias are sympathetically mediated so that successful anxiolysis can be counterproductive. On occasion, mental arithmetic quizzes or general knowledge tests can be useful to provoke mild anxiety in otherwise cooperative patients.

Environment

The cardiac catheterization laboratory can be inhospitable for the anesthesiologist, and the "locals" do not always speak the same language [7]. It is often remote from the operating room (OR), of necessity not brightly illuminated and filled with equipment that makes access to the patient difficult. Newer hybrid suites are larger in size and contain equipment for both catheter interventions and surgery, including circulatory support backup with extracorporeal membrane oxygenation or standard cardiopulmonary bypass (Figure 27.1). It can be difficult to see and understand what is happening to the patient. Temperature control is often limited. Patients may be transferred some distance to recovery or intensive care facilities and the anesthesiologist must be satisfied that the patient is in a stable condition prior to transfer. Monitoring, oxygen, resuscitation equipment and drugs, and sufficient personnel should accompany the patient, if this is the case.

The design of new facilities and renovations of existing laboratories should include input from the anesthesiologists who care for patients undergoing cardiac catheterization. The design and workflow issues are very complex, and many centers are installing magnetic resonance imaging (MRI) suites in the immediate area. There are published standards for workplace safety around both radiation and magnets, but the actual logistics and daily experience of moving patients and personnel through the area need to be addressed in a thoughtful way. There is increasing recognition of the importance of ergonomic design, but very little published to date [12,13]. Competing "airspace" with suspended equipment (e.g., lights, injectors, echocardiography or ultrasound booms, magnetic stereotactic equipment, and also gas columns and gas lines) can make the functional space very small regardless of the dimensions of the room. The movement of biplane fluoroscopy arms and their "parking place" frequently encroaches on the space at the head of the table.

If procedures requiring cardiopulmonary bypass or combined "hybrid" type procedures are planned then attention needs to be paid to air exchange, OR standards, and appropriate numbers of gas, suction, and electrical outlets as well as anesthetic gas scavenging. Space for a

(a)

(b)

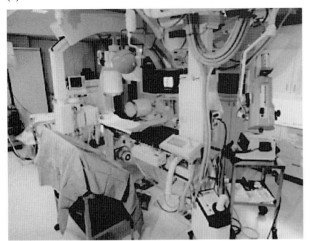
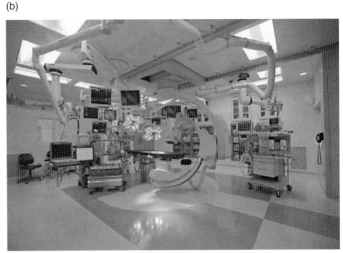

Figure 27.1 The catheter laboratory can be an inhospitable place for both anesthetist and patient. X-ray and hemodynamic monitoring equipment limits access to the patient. (a) Standard cardiac catheterization laboratory. (b) Hybrid catheterization/operating suite (Courtesy Nationwide Children's Hospital, Columbus, OH, USA)

heart–lung machine adjacent to the patient, and not likely to be struck by a rotating C-arm is also a consideration.

It is important for medical personnel to recognize their limitations when looking at design drawings, and for the architects and engineers to understand the full range of medical activity, including catastrophes. Concrete examples include X-ray tables which will indeed support the 150-kg individual but not when they require CPR, or the practical difficulties of going in and out of an MRI suite with magnetic strip ID badges.

Whenever possible, recovery areas should be immediately proximate and meet all the existing standards for OR recovery areas. The issues regarding safety in an area where there is considerable traffic of patients and personnel, as well as ferrous material, in close proximity to a strong magnetic field also need to be addressed in a very particular way. Movement of patients from the catheter suite to the MRI table should be undertaken with a formal process, and checklists are helpful to heighten awareness. The use of checklists in improving safety has been well documented, although it is not without detractors [14].

Radiation exposure of both the patient and staff is a hazard during cardiac catheterization. Nonstochastic effects such as erythema and cataracts are a direct result of cellular injury and are dose related. Stochastic effects are the result of injury to DNA. The risk of injury is increased with increasing dose (amount of energy absorbed); however, the magnitude of effect is not dose related. Exposure is measured in rem or sieverts (1 rem = 1 mSv). Background exposure in Canada is 2 rem/yr. The risk of a fatal cancer is increased by 0.04% per rem of lifetime exposure and no level of radiation exposure can be considered safe [15]. In a 2006 study examining chromosomal damage in

patients with congenital heart disease (CHD), there was clear evidence that cardiac catheterization was associated with long-term chromosomal damage [16].

The patient is inevitably exposed directly to X-rays. In a pediatric study evaluating exposure during both diagnostic and therapeutic procedures, average dose was 4.6 and 6 rem, respectively [17]. The younger patients tend to have higher exposures. Exposure during cinefluoroscopy may be as high as 10–20 rem/min. Digital cineangiography reduces exposure by over 50% compared to conventional techniques.

Staff is inevitably exposed to radiation. The maximum radiation exposure recommended for medical workers is 5 rem/yr. Ideally exposure should be much lower than this (0.12 rem/yr). Health care workers in catheterization facilities have been identified as having higher exposures [18]. Dose limitation relies on time, distance, and barriers. Radiation dose is reduced with distance from the source according to the inverse square law. Barriers include protective clothing ("lead" aprons, thyroid collar, and protective eye glasses) and "plexiglas" screens. The threshold for cataracts may be reached in a few years without appropriate protection [19].

Anesthetic considerations

In 1958 Smith described a satisfactory state for pediatric cardiac catheterization to be one in which there is (a) freedom from pain, (b) absence of restlessness, (c) no respiratory depression, and (d) sedation light enough to allow a normal response to a selective ether test [5]. While selective ether tests are no longer conducted, the requirements for cardiac catheterization today are broadly similar: a comfortable, still patient whose hemodynamic findings accurately reflect their physiology. General anesthesia is not essential to achieve these aims. However, cardiac catheterization for children often involves interventions and procedures can be prolonged. Most children will not tolerate this without some pharmacological support. The benefits of general anesthesia or sedation should be considered in relation to the individual patient and procedure. Small infants with limited cardiovascular reserve who are undergoing a catheter-based intervention deserve the undivided attention of an individual with the skills to manage both general anesthesia, cardiac pathophysiology, and possible complications: for the most part, this means a pediatric anesthesiologist [20].

Sedation may be administered without an anesthesiologist. Who does what, to whom, and when remain controversial [21]. Recognition that adverse events occur in association with this practice has lead to a series of guidelines being produced. The most recently revised guidelines are those of the American Academy of Pediatrics [22] and makes reference to earlier guidelines from the American Society of Anesthesiologists (ASA) [23]. Sedation to a depth that no response or only reflex withdrawal can be produced is defined as general anesthesia. The distinction between deep sedation and anesthesia is often arbitrary. In the UK no distinction is made between the two [24]. The ASA guidelines specify that the individual supervising the sedation must be able to rescue the patient if the level of sedation is deeper than intended. Lack of anesthetic personnel may mean that deep sedation supervised by a nonanesthesiologist is preferable to no sedation. There are small case studies suggesting that these practices are acceptable but no large-scale outcomes have been reported. This situation does not provide optimum care for children. An appropriate care plan for a child undergoing diagnostic catheterization should be based on the child's medical and psychosocial needs.

Poor outcome during sedation has been associated with inadequate preoperative assessment and inadequate monitoring [25]. Assessment of patients undergoing cardiac catheterization, whether under sedation or general anesthesia, should be comparable to that of a patient undergoing any other operative procedure, and should involve a careful assessment of the severity and complexity of CHD. The standards for monitoring have been established in most developed countries are widely available and should be adhered to. A means of monitoring adequacy of ventilation and the airway is mandatory. Oxygen masks or nasal cannulae can be adapted to allow monitoring of end-tidal carbon dioxide in spontaneously breathing children [26].

Access to the airway is limited during the procedure and intubation of the trachea and control of ventilation will provide the safest option in most patients. In some clinical situations, however, it is desirable to avoid positive pressure ventilation (e.g., during diagnostic procedures in patients with Fontan physiology, or restrictive RV). Total intravenous anesthesia (TIVA) with either propofol or ketamine can be achieved in many patients without specific support of the airway, though care and close observation is required. The laryngeal mask airway (LMA) is well tolerated and allows "hands free" maintenance of the airway, with the use of a flexible LMA avoiding obstruction of X-ray equipment. Intubation of the trachea does require a deeper plane of anesthesia and may be associated with higher arterial carbon dioxide concentration unless ventilation is supported. Newer ventilators and anesthetic machines provide more varied modes of ventilation, such as pressure support and synchronized intermittent mandatory ventilation modes which can be useful. Patients at risk of ventilatory failure, including neonates of low birth weight, should have their airway secured by endotracheal intubation at the beginning [27]. Endotracheal intubation is also preferable when transesophageal echo is to be used. Continuous monitoring of the adequacy of the airway and ventilation is mandatory with any of these techniques.

Infiltration of local anesthetics at vascular access sites is simple and if performed correctly should not complicate subsequent access. Toxicity due to lidocaine has been described during cardiac catheterization but only in association with massive overdose [28]. Central blockade may be considered if access is to be confined to the groin. Caudal anesthesia is associated with almost no hemodynamic changes in infants and may avoid the need for sedation [29]. However, the need for heparin during the procedure is a consideration. Topicalization of the skin has been reported, but it was not found to be useful in reducing the need for sedation or in reducing hemodynamic changes [30].

Complications

In a current report of complications in a large series over 12 years [31], there were 25 deaths (0.23%) and an overall incidence of 7.3% complications, of which the majority were vascular injury. Serious complications include arrhythmias, vascular damage at access sites, bleeding, perforation or rupture of vessels or the heart, cardiac tamponade, vascular thrombosis, air embolus, catheter fragment embolus, valvular incompetence, allergy to contrast medium or drugs, stroke, and brachial plexus injury [32]. Risk factors for complications are lower patient age or size and the particular intervention performed. The era of the procedure is also significant. Severe pulmonary hypertension has a significant risk of mortality [33].

Arrhythmias are most often caused by mechanical stimulation and will respond to withdrawal of the catheter. Contributory factors such as electrolyte disturbance, hypercarbia, and excessive catheter manipulation within the heart should be minimized. Pacing can be instituted to treat heart block or SVT. Equipment for defibrillation must be immediately available. Other causes of arrhythmia should be considered including cardiac ischemia, drugs, coronary air emboli, and direct damage to the myocardium or conducting system. Most arrhythmias, including heart block, are transient.

Catheters used for interventional procedures have a larger diameter than those used during diagnostic studies and the risk of vascular damage at the site of insertion is increased, as is the risk of damage to heart structures. Complications such as perforation of the heart or vessels or valvular incompetence may require urgent surgical intervention. Blood should be immediately available and interventional procedures in children should only be conducted in hospitals where facilities for cardiac surgery exist [15,34,35]. In the event of sudden blood loss, rapid transfusion and arterial monitoring are possible via vascular access sheaths placed for the catheterization. During balloon angioplasty, it may be possible for the cardiologist to tamponade the rupture by reinflation of the balloon; however, emergency surgical repair will often be required.

Thrombosis and thromboembolization may occur at any site where the vascular endothelium is disrupted. Heparin is given in a dose of 50–150 units/kg after arterial cannulation, when the systemic circulation is entered and during procedures that inevitably cause damage to the vascular endothelium. Protamine may be used to reverse the effects of heparin but is not routinely required.

Serious complications occur in 0.7–3.3% of EP studies in children [36,37]. This is similar to diagnostic catheterization; however, the patients are generally older and have less systemic illness. Complications are related to vascular access, catheter manipulation, or the use of radio frequency (RF) energy. During RF ablation, a portion of the endocardium and myocardium is destroyed. The Radiofrequency Ablation Registry provides data on complication rates for RF ablation. This includes a mortality rate of 1 in 500, complete heart block in 1%, and valvular regurgitation in 0.5% [38]. Complications are higher in patients with CHD and heart block is more common when the abnormal pathway is close to the normal conducting system. Coronary artery injury has been demonstrated in animal models of RF ablation [38].

Diagnostic catheterization

Advances in other imaging techniques, most notably echocardiography and MRI, coupled with the invasive

Table 27.1 Normal cardiac catheterization data

	Pressure in mmHg		Oxygen saturation (%)
	Newborns	Older children	
Right atrium			60–80
a wave	3–8	5–10	
v wave	2–6	4–8	
Mean	0–4	2–6	
Right ventricle			65–75
Systolic	65–80	15–25	
End diastolic	2–7	3–8	
Pulmonary artery			65–75
Systolic	65–80	15–25	
Diastolic	35–50	8–12	
Mean	40–70	10–16	
PA wedge			95–100
a wave	6–10	8–14	
v wave	7–11	10–17	
Mean	5–8	7–13	
Left atrium			95–100
a wave	4–7	6–12	
v wave	6–12	8–15	
Mean	3–6	5–10	
Left ventricle			95–100
Systolic	65–80	90–120	
End diastolic	3–7	2–5	
Aorta			95–100
Systolic	65–80	90–120	
Diastolic	45–60	60–75	
Mean	55–65	70–90	
Flows	L/min/m^2 BSA		
Pulmonary (Op)	3.5–5.0	3.5–5.0	
Systemic (Qs)	3.5–5.0	3.5–5.0	
Resistances	Woods units x m^2 BSA		
Pulmonary (Rp)	8–10	1–3	
Systemic (Rs)	10–15	15–30	

BSA, body surface area; PA, pulmonary artery.

nature of cardiac catheterization and radiation exposure mean that careful consideration is given to the indications for diagnostic catheterization. Current indications are:

- To measure central and peripheral intravascular pressures and derive hemodynamic information such as pulmonary vascular resistance (PVR) and systemic vascular resistance (SVR), shunt fractions and cardiac output (see Tables 27.1 and 27.2). The most common situation for this type of investigation is in preparation for the Fontan procedure.
- To define cardiac and vascular anatomy: poor windows can defeat the most expert echocardiographer and

Table 27.2 Hemodynamic calculations Performed during cardiac catheterization.

Flows

Pulmonary:

$$Q_P = \frac{Vo_2}{(S_{PV}o_2 - S_{PA}o_2) \times Hgb \times 1.34 \times 10}$$

Systemic:

$$Q_S = \frac{Vo_2}{(S_{A}oo_2 - S_{MV}o_2) \times Hgb \times 1.34 \times 10}$$

Effective pulmonary:

$$Q_{EP} = \frac{Vo_2}{(S_{PV}o_2 - S_{MV}o_2) \times Hgb \times 1.34 \times 10}$$

Resistances

Pulmonary:

$$R_P = \frac{\overline{PAP} - \overline{LAP}}{Q_P}$$

Systemic:

$$R_S = \frac{\overline{AoP} - \overline{RAP}}{Q_S}$$

Shunts

Pulmonary to systemic:

$$\frac{Q_P}{Q_S} = \frac{S_{Ao}o_2 - S_{MV}o_2}{S_{PV}o_2 - S_{PA}o_2}$$ (a flow ratio)

Left to right: $Q_P - Q_{EP}$ (absolute flow)

Right to left: $Q_P - Q_{EP}$ (absolute flow)

Ao, Aorta; *AoP*, Aortic pressure; *LAP*, Left atrial pressure; MV, Mixed venous; PA, Pulmonary artery; *PAP*, Pulmonary artery pressure; PV, Pulmonary vein; Q_{EP}, Effective pulmonary flow; Q_P, Pulmonary flow; Q_v Systemic flow; *RAP*, Right atrial pressure; R_P, Pulmonary vascular resistance; R_S, Systemic vascular resistance; *S*, Saturation. VO2, oxygen consumption

certain anatomical features are difficult to visualize. This occurs in a minority of cases and usually implies either complex anatomy or complicating factors in the patient such as lung disease. MRI is a second choice, but may be contraindicated for related (e.g., incompatible implants) or other reasons.

- To evaluate myocardial function and to assess the effects of drugs and respiratory interventions on the cardiovascular system, such as is performed during investigation of patients with pulmonary hypertension.
- Endocardial biopsies, coronary artery angiography, and assessment of myocardial function are part of the routine surveillance of patients following heart transplantation. Endocardial biopsy is also diagnostic in cases of cardiomyopathy and viral myocarditis.

Diagnostic studies are also an integral part of transcatheter interventional procedures.

Anesthetic considerations

The anesthesiologist's role in the cardiac catheterization laboratory is to provide care such that patient emerges from the procedure with minimal psychological or physiological trauma, and the cardiologist emerges with meaningful data on which to base decisions about the child's future treatment. All sedative and general anesthetic agents have hemodynamic effects and all depress respiration: this in turn influences the results of the investigation. It is important that the anesthesiologist has a clear understanding of the information being sought in the investigation and that the cardiologist has some under-

standing of the effects of sedatives on the cardiovascular system.

More than 30% of children with CHD have reparative surgery in the neonatal period and more than 50% are operated on in the first year of life. The majority of children come to surgery without cardiac catheterization; the necessary information is acquired by echocardiography. By elimination, a majority of patients presenting for diagnostic cardiac catheterization are either infants presenting with some complexity of their condition or postoperative patients. There is a larger population of older, well children presenting for interventional catheterization.

Postoperative patients and parents are often understandably anxious when returning to hospital. There are benefits from premedication even with parental presence at induction of anesthesia [39]. Midazolam 0.5–0.75 mg/kg is a safe and effective oral premedication for children with CHD and has the advantage of a rapid onset [40,41]. The most common sequelae of cardiac surgery for CHD are arrhythmias and myocardial dysfunction. Recurrent laryngeal and phrenic nerve palsy are recognized complications of cardiac surgery and result in limited respiratory reserve, as does congestive heart failure. Feeding difficulties and gastroesophageal reflux are also common. In addition, 25% of children with CHD have other congenital anomalies. Craniofacial, airway, and intrathoracic anomalies are a major cause for concern. The combination of a patient with a challenging airway, limited cardiac reserve, and difficult vascular access in an area of the hospital often some distance from colleagues epitomizes the challenge for the pediatric anesthesiologist in the cardiac catheterization laboratory.

Procedure

The routine approach to diagnostic catheterization in patients with biventricular hearts is via the femoral vein using the Seldinger technique. Upper vein (internal jugular or subclavian) access is required to evaluate the pulmonary arteries following cavopulmonary or hemi-Fontan procedures. If necessary, the femoral artery is also accessed using a similar technique. After dilatation and placement of an appropriate sheath, catheters are advanced through the circulation and pressure and oxygen saturation measurements are made in sequence. Appropriate oxygen saturation measurements will allow the detection of shunts, and calculations of shunt fraction in combination with measurements or estimates of oxygen consumption will allow calculation of cardiac output and pulmonary blood flow (see Tables 27.1 and 27.2 for normal data, and calculations). The use of high-inspired concentration of oxygen at this stage will introduce errors due to dissolved oxygen and pulmonary vasodilatation. It also introduces error into the measurement of oxygen consumption using respiratory mass spectroscopy.

Vascular access can be extremely difficult in children who have had prolonged hospitalization. Venous thrombosis (and the attendant complications) is being increasingly recognized as a source of morbidity in children [42].

Particular concerns during cardiac catheterization of neonates and infants include airway management, limited cardiovascular reserve, hypothermia, and changes in intravascular volume. Hypovolemia can arise from extensive blood sampling during the procedure or as a result of blood loss during catheter placement or exchange. It is difficult to monitor blood loss during cardiac catheterization. The use of check-flow valves markedly reduces bleeding from the sheath. Hypervolemia is also a concern as fluid is routinely administered through the sheath and catheters. Extensive angiographic studies result in the administration of significant amounts of contrast and this should be limited.

Anesthetic techniques

Oral or intramuscular sedation is inappropriate for cardiac catheterization, as the dose cannot be titrated to response and action may be greatly prolonged in infants [43,44]. Periods of excess sedation and of inadequate sedation are common. These techniques have been largely superseded by use of shorter-acting agents with rapid onset [45]. Table 27.3 summarizes agents in common use. Many of these agents have steep dose-response curves and need to be carefully titrated to achieve a predetermined end point. The results of excess sedation are predictable; loss of airway reflexes, respiratory depression, and cardiovascular compromise. Specific antagonists exist for some groups of drugs; however, initial management should be support of the airway and ventilation. In a critical incidence analysis of adverse sedation events, no correlation could be found between particular agents or mode of administration and outcome [25,43]. Combinations of two agents may be useful in specific situations: narcotics and sedatives may be of value for painful procedures and use of benzodiazepines will reduce the incidence of hallucination with ketamine.

The effects of sedative and analgesic drugs on the heart are variable. Inhalational anesthetics cause peripheral vasodilatation, varying degrees of myocardial depression,

Table 27.3 Suitable agents for sedation during cardiac catheterization

Agent	Suggested dose	Comments
Midazolam	Oral 0.25–1.0 mg/kg i.v. bolus 50–150 µg/kg Infusion: 1–2 µg/kg/min	After iv bolus 4 min before peak effect Steeper dose response curve than diazepam
Ketamine	1–2 mg/kg Infusion 50–75 µg/kg/min	Psychic disturbances in 5–30% Prolonged recovery time
Propofol	1–2 mg/kg Infusion: 100–200 µg/kg/min	High risk of loss of airway reflexes
Nitrous oxide	Up to 50%	Seldom adequate as sole agent, useful adjunct during skin infiltration
Morphine	0.05 mg/kg	Risk of respiratory depression and nausea. Prolonged action
Fentanyl	1 µg/kg	
Alfentanil	20 µg/kg then 0.5 µg/kg/min	Much smaller doses required after Fontan procedure
Remifentanil	0.05–0.15 µg/kg/min	High potential for apnea
Etomidate	0.1–0.3 mg/kg i.v. bolus then 25–50 µg/kg/min in infusion	Transient adrenal suppression, pain and thrombophlebitis; excellent maintenance of baseline hemodynamics
Dexmedetomidine	0.5–1 mcg/kg slow IV infusion induction, then 0.3–0.7 mcg/kg/hr maintenance	Hypotension, bradycardia, ?contraindicated for EP studies

and have effects on sinus node function and on cardiac conduction tissue. Sevoflurane has less direct myocardial depressant effect than halothane, but in normal children the concomitant fall in SVR and lack of change in heart rate resulted in no change in cardiac index [46]. Isoflurane preserves contractility, increases heart rate, and decreases SVR in children with CHD [47]. However, greater myocardial depression occurs in neonates [48]. Qp:Qs ratio was not changed from baseline in patients with atrial septal defect (ASD) or ventricular septal defect (VSD) older than 6 months, with isoflurane, sevoflurane, or a fentanyl/midazolam anesthetic [49].

Intravenous agents such as propofol, midazolam, and ketamine are all used for sedation and general anesthesia. Propofol has been studied in children with CHD undergoing cardiac catheterization and has been shown to decrease SVR resulting in significant changes in Qp:Qs calculations [50]. In patients with elevated PVR, propofol causes pulmonary vasodilation [51]. It also causes varying degrees of bradycardia [52]. Midazolam can be given orally, nasally, or intravenously. It has widespread use as an oral premedication in children, and the use of oral midazolam and ketamine has been used for cardiac catheterization. However, intravenous supplementation was required quite frequently and airway obstruction was also reported [45]. A bolus dose of midazolam, given to children following repair of CHD, caused hypotension and a fall in cardiac output [53]. Ketamine causes sympathetic stimulation, salivation, and bad dreams. It has negative inotropic effects on isolated myocardium, but this is masked in the intact patient due to the well-recognized sympathomimetic effects. Ketamine increases oxygen consumption (VO_2), which is a potential source of error in hemodynamic calculations unless VO_2 is actually measured [54]. Etomidate has been used for induction of anesthesia in children with CHD and end-stage cardiomyopathy, but there is little published data regarding its use during cardiac catheterization [55,56]. There are several recent articles and animal studies detailing concerns about N-methyl-D-aspartate receptor inhibitors and some inhalational agents (e.g., ketamine, etomidate, isoflurane) causing adverse effects on the developing brain [57]. A recent editorial and related articles suggest that there is insufficient evidence to make substantive changes in practice, but it may be that with limited evidence to support the use of an agent, it may be more prudent to pursue a strategy of pharmacological conservatism [58–61]. Dexmedetomidine is a newer sedative drug with centrally mediated, α_2 agonist effects. It reduces sympathetic tone, increases parasympathetic tone, and causes sedation, anxiolysis, and mild analgesia with minor hemodynamic effects. This agent is not FDA approved for use in infants and children. The single series report of its off-label use in cardiac catheterization concluded that it was not suitable as a single agent

despite the theoretical attractiveness of the pharmacodynamic profile. [62]. There are editorial reviews of its use in CHD both pro and con [63,64]. There are some potentially troubling side effects including seizure, adverse effects on PVR, and hypertension. Two recent publications raise concerns about its use in patients with conduction defects: in a case report, a patient suffered intractable bradycardia and hypotension attributed to dexmedetomidine, and in the study by Hammer et al. the authors concluded that it should not be used for electrophysiological studies, and that caution should be exercised in patients at risk from heart block or bradycardia [65,66].

The use of short-acting intravenous narcotics such as alfentanil and remifentanil for sedation of spontaneously breathing children has also been reported [67,68]. These drugs are generally associated with good hemodynamic stability. The problems of respiratory depression (apnea and airway obstruction) and vomiting limit the usefulness of these agents unless the airway is controlled. The use of remifentanil with sevoflurane and positive pressure ventilation is associated with a decrease in heart rate and arterial blood pressure [69].

Respiratory manipulations will also affect hemodynamics. A switch from positive to negative pressure (cuirass) ventilation increased cardiac output by 11% in healthy children, 28% in postoperative cardiac patients, and 54% in patients with a Fontan circulation [70, 71]. A similar increase in cardiac output has been demonstrated on extubation of postoperative Fontan patients [72]. If the child has a large left-to-right shunt then the effect of breathing high concentrations of oxygen are twofold: firstly it is necessary to consider the contribution of dissolved oxygen when calculating pulmonary blood flow using the Fick equation, and secondly the high oxygen levels will likely decrease pulmonary vascular resistance acutely increasing the Qp:Qs ratio. Similarly, changes in arterial carbon dioxide tension or pH will affect pulmonary blood flow. From the perspective of deriving meaningful hemodynamic data, the ideal may be a patient spontaneously breathing room air; however, this must be seen in the context of the individual patient. If spontaneous ventilation results in airway obstruction, CO_2 retention, or atelectasis, these are also potent sources of error in the study [73]. Small changes in pulmonary vein saturation make large changes in shunt fraction.

The patient with pulmonary hypertension

Primary pulmonary hypertension is rare in children as in adults. However, children with CHD and large left-to-right shunts are at risk of acquired pulmonary hypertension if their cardiac anomaly is not dealt with in a timely fashion. Infants with outflow obstruction to the pulmonary vascular bed, e.g., mitral stenosis, pulmonary vein obstruction, are also at risk.

When surgery is planned for children with pulmonary hypertension, it is important to carefully assess vascular reactivity, as this is crucial in deciding whether or not the lesion is operable. These investigations more than any other require teamwork on the part of the anesthesiologist and cardiologist. Children with severe pulmonary hypertension are at risk of sudden death, and require careful anesthetic management [33]. Children whose pulmonary vascular bed is labile can appear inoperable if improperly managed.

Pulmonary hypertension ultimately results in right ventricular failure. The thin-walled RV responds to pressure loading by dilating and becoming hypertrophied. This reduces right coronary blood flow rendering the subendocardial region vulnerable to ischemia. The dilated RV interferes with LV geometry and function causing increased left ventricular end-diastolic pressure and decreased stroke volume. Sudden increases in PVR may result in the interventricular septum bowing out into the left ventricular outflow tract, causing subartic stenosis and further jeopardizing coronary perfusion. Tricuspid regurgitation can also occur. Acute changes in pulmonary artery pressure (PAP) and PVR are particularly poorly tolerated and cause reduction in cardiac output, arrhythmias, and death.

The intimate relationship between PVR, alveolar oxygenation, and carbon dioxide means that the first principle of anesthetic management of the child with pulmonary hypertension is meticulous attention to the airway and to gas exchange. Hypercarbia or hypoxia will cause an elevation in PVR. Details such as ineffective bag and mask ventilation, or too large a leak around the endotracheal tube, can result in life-threatening acute increases in PAP in vulnerable children. This is particularly important if there is no intracardiac shunt (e.g., patent foramen ovale, secundum ASD).

The rationale behind the management of children undergoing investigation of pulmonary hypertension is to establish the baseline hemodynamic values and then intervene to assess the reactivity of the pulmonary vascular bed. This also provides data against which the effects of therapy can be measured. Decisions are based on the lowest value of PVR that can be attained.

At HSC all young children receive general anesthesia with muscle relaxants and endotracheal intubation. Premedication with oral midazolam is routine. Cautious inhalation induction with sevoflurane is been used if vascular access is difficult. This avoids the inevitable agitation due to multiple attempts at venipuncture. However, intravenous access is obtained at the earliest moment. The patient is ventilated with air and oxygen at FIO_2 as close

to 21% as can be tolerated and the pH and PCO_2 are maintained within normal limits, while intracardiac pressures and saturation are measured on both left and right side of the heart. The patient is then hyperventilated until the PCO_2 is 30 mm Hg on 70% oxygen and all measurements are repeated. Patients who do not respond to hyperoxia and hypocarbia are given 40 ppm nitric oxide and the study repeated. In selected patients, oral sildenafil is then given followed by inhaled prostacyclin and the measurements are repeated. Oxygen consumption is measured using mass spectrometry and calculations of PVR and pulmonary vascular resistance index (PVRI) are made at each stage and Qp:Qs calculated if relevant. The outcomes and complications of anesthesia and pulmonary hypertension in children were reported from a single center by Carmasino et al. [33]: the mortality is high: 7–10% in patients whose PAP is higher than systemic blood pressure regardless of anesthetic strategy. All the major complications occurred during cardiac catheterization.

Endocardial biopsy

Endocardial biopsy is used in the routine surveillance of patients after cardiac transplant, in the assessment of patients with suspected rejection of the transplanted heart, and in the diagnosis of myocarditis and cardiomyopathy. The latter two groups are more likely to have myocardial dysfunction. When seen preoperatively, all patients should be questioned as to symptoms of heart failure or arrhythmia, and reports of preoperative echocardiograms and EKGs inspected. The procedure is usually performed by canulation of right internal jugular vein. The biopsy catheter is passed into the heart and samples of endocardium taken for histology. Stress testing, coronary angiogram, and ultrasound examination of the coronaries may be performed during the same procedure. There is a higher risk of perforation in dilated cardiomyopathy and in small infants due to the thin RV wall.

Interventional cardiology

Anesthetic considerations

The range of patients presenting for interventional procedures includes those with asymptomatic disease presenting for day case procedures to critically ill neonates undergoing procedures associated with marked hemodynamic disturbance (Table 27.4). The anesthetic approach should be tailored to the individual patient and it is important that the anesthesiologist appreciates the nature of the procedure to be performed. Sedation techniques may be appropriate on occasions; however, transcatheter

Table 27.4 Indications for transcatheter interventional procedures

	Class I: Generally agreed indication	Class II: May be indicated	Class III: Not indicated
Balloon dilation of cardiac valves	Pulmonary stenosis Congenital aortic stenosis Rheumatic mitral stenosis	Discrete subaortic stenosis Dysplastic pulmonary valve Congenital mitral stenosis Prosthetic conduits Pulmonary stenosis with complex heart disease	Infundibular pulmonary stenosis Fibromuscular subaortic stenosis HOCM Supravalvar aortic stenosis
Balloon angioplasty	Recoarctation of aorta Systemic venous stenosis Pulmonary artery stenosis	Systemic-to-PA shunts Native coarctation (> 7 months) PDA	Pulmonary vein stenosis
Stent placement	PA stenosis SVC/IVC stenosis Baffle obstruction following atrial switch	Stenotic RV-to-PA conduit Stenotic AP collaterals Coarctation of aorta PDA	Pulmonary vein stenosis
Balloon atrial septostomy	TGA TAPVC Tricuspid atresia Mitral atresia Pulmonary atresia (IVS)	HLHS with highly restrictive ASD	Interrupted IVC Infants older than 6 weeks
Blade atrial septostomy	As above in infants > 6 weeks old	As above > 6 weeks Pulmonary hypertension with increased RAP	Interrupted IVC
ASD closure devices	Secundum ASD or PFO < 20 mm, rim of >5 mm Fenestrated Fontan	None	Primum ASD Sinus venosus ASD
Other closure devices	Symptomatic PDA Asymptomatic PDA with heart murmur AP collaterals	"Silent" PDA	PDA with irreversible pulmonary obstructive disease
Coil occlusion	AP collaterals (dual supply) Small PDA (< 4mm) Surgical shunts Pulmonary AV fistula Venovenous connections	Moderate PDA (4–7 mm) Coronary AV fistula	AP collaterals (without dual supply) PDA >7 mm

AP aortopulmonary; ASD atrial septal defect; AV arteriovenous; HLHS hypoplastic left heart syndrome; HOCM hypertrophic obstructive cardiomyopathy; IVC inferior vena cava; IVS intact ventricular septum; PA pulmonary artery; PDA patent ductus arteriosus; PFO patent foramen ovale; RA right atrium; RAP, right atrial pressure; RV right ventride; SVC superior vena cava; TAPVC total anomalous pulmonary venous connection; TGA transposition of the great arteries.
Data from Allen HD, Beekman RH IIIrd, Garson A, Jr *et al.* Pediatric therapeutic cardiac catheterization: A statement for healthcare professionals from the Council on Cardiovascular Disease in the Young, American Heart Association, *Circulation* 1998; 97:609–25.
Source: Used with permission from Reference [34].

interventions raise a number of specific concerns. The airway should be controlled during procedures associated with a high risk of hemodynamic instability, or of serious complications likely to require further interventions or resuscitation. Aortic valvotomy, dilatation of severe pulmonary stenosis, and closure of VSD should be considered absolute indications for general anesthesia and tracheal intubation. Transesophageal echo is used during many procedures and necessitates tracheal intubation.

Patient movement or coughing during device or balloon placement may have disastrous consequences and some interventions, e.g., pulmonary angioplasty, may induce coughing. A combination of sedation techniques with an additional bolus of an intravenous anesthetic, such a ketamine, to ensure stillness during interventions has been described [74]. It is not clear what advantage is offered by this technique over general anesthesia with control of the airway.

Interventional cardiology techniques

Valvotomy

The technique used for balloon dilatation of stenotic aortic, pulmonary, mitral, or bioprosthetic valves is essentially similar. First a catheter is introduced past the stenosis and pressures are measured proximal and distal to the stenosis. A wire is positioned across the valve and the catheter is withdrawn. The wire is used to guide a balloon catheter into position across the stenotic valve and to stabilize the balloon. The size of balloon used is selected relative to the valve annulus. The purpose of the procedure is not to dilate the valve annulus but to separate the fused valve leaflets. Larger balloons improve the reduction in gradient but increase the risk of regurgitation. During inflation the valve is completely obstructed. Sustained single inflations are avoided. When a balloon is inflated across a stenotic valve, a "waist" is seen at the site of stenosis. Short inflations are repeated until this waist disappears [75].

Angioplasty

Vascular angioplasty involves the inflation of a balloon across an area of vascular stenosis. The technique is similar to balloon valvotomy and results in tearing of the endothelium and subsequent healing by scar formation and reendothelialization. The technique may be applied to native blood vessels or to stenotic surgical conduits. Established indications are recurrent aortic coarctation, systemic venous stenosis, and pulmonary artery stenosis. Complications include rupture of the vessel, dissection, late aneurysm formation, thrombosis, and restenosis.

Endovascular stents

Modification of balloon angioplasty by the placement of endovascular stents has been applied to pulmonary artery stenosis, systemic venous stenosis, and aortic coarctation [76] (Figure 27.2). The placement of endovascular stents improves initial success, reduces the incidence of recurrence, and may reduce late aneurysm formation. The stents used are deployed over a balloon. When in position the balloon is inflated to dilate the stent and the vessel. The balloon is then withdrawn leaving the stent in situ.

Limitations of the technique are the large size of catheters required to deploy stents and that stents may narrow over time, due to endothelial proliferation. There are also absolute limits to the dilation of a stent. Large catheters increase the risk of damage to vascular and cardiac structures, especially thrombosis of the femoral vessels. Further complications are malposition or embolization of the stent. There are a myriad technical improvements under investigation including drug-eluting stents, which are in commercial use, and bioabsorbable stents, which would "disappear" after a period of time.

Closure of shunts

A number of devices are available to close intravascular shunts. For smaller shunts, the most commonly deployed are helical wire coils available in different diameters and lengths. More complex devices are required for larger vessels and for closure of intracardiac connections. The most commonly used devices have a double umbrella design. They are deployed with the two sides of the "umbrella" on either side of the shunt. Complications are malposition or embolization of the device, vascular occlusion, myocardial perforation, hemolysis, and vascular trauma. The larger devices require large catheters to deploy them and may not be suitable for use in small infants.

Treatment of specific lesions

Pulmonary valvotomy

Percutaneous balloon pulmonary valvotomy has now been performed for over 20 years. It is indicated when the transvalvular gradient is greater than 50 mm Hg with a normal cardiac output and is the treatment of choice for

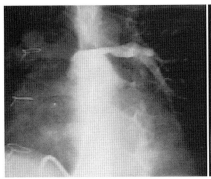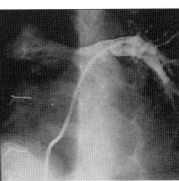

Figure 27.2 In the left-hand image, contrast has been injected into the left pulmonary artery to demonstrate a profound stenosis. In the right-hand image, the stenosis has been dilated and an endovascular stent deployed

isolated pulmonary valve stenosis. It is also useful therapy in selected patients with pulmonary atresia, and tetralogy of Fallot. Immediate results are excellent with most patients not requiring further intervention for 10 years.

Neonates with critical pulmonary stenosis are critically ill and profoundly cyanosed. The pulmonary circulation is dependent on flow from the ductus arteriousum (DA) as there is minimal flow through the pulmonary valve. The majority of infants will be mechanically ventilated because of profound hypoxia and the use of prostaglandin (PgE$_1$) infusion to maintain ductal patency. The open ductus and minimal flow through the pulmonary valve means that inflation of the balloon often does not cause further hemodynamic compromise. Acute complications in 10–30% of patients have been reported [77,78]. The RV is pressure overloaded by the pulmonary stenosis and will not immediately recover after relief of the outflow obstruction. Continuation of PgE$_1$ infusion maintains pulmonary flow during this period. Size of the valve annulus, tricuspid valve size, and ventricular volume are predictors of outcome [79].

In older infants, in whom the DA is closed, inflation of the balloon leads to complete obstruction of the right ventricular outflow tract (RVOT) and greater hemodynamic upset. Cardiac output decreases dramatically resulting in significant hypotension. This usually improves on deflation of the balloon, but if ventricular dilatation has occurred this may not be the case. Bolus epinephrine and occasionally more prolonged inotropic support may be required.

A modification of the technique is used for treatment of pulmonary atresia with intact ventricular septum. Patients present in a similar way to neonates with critical pulmonary stenosis. RF energy is used to perforate the membrane. As the pulmonary valve is absent and the atretic membrane destroyed, pulmonary insufficiency is inevitable. The risk of inadvertent perforation of the RVOT is higher during this procedure.

Pulmonary arterial angioplasty

Pulmonary artery stenosis may be congenital or acquired, often following surgery. Congenital stenosis is seen either in association with other abnormalities with reduced pulmonary blood flow (such as tetralogy of Fallot), as branch stenosis in association with William's syndrome or congenital rubella, or as an isolated stenosis at the site of insertion of the DA. Stenosis may occur after any surgery involving manipulation of pulmonary arteries, particularly shunt formation or pulmonary artery banding. The site of stenosis may be any point in the pulmonary vascular bed and multiple sites are not uncommon. Two-thirds are confined to proximal vessels. The right ventricular pressure is raised when the stenoses affect the main pulmonary artery or when multiple peripheral stenoses are present. If the stenosis affects only one branch pulmonary artery or the peripheral pulmonary arteries, then the PAP may be normal at rest. There is limited data available on the long-term outcomes of endovascular stents in infants, but it is a safe technique with good intermediate outcomes [80].

Surgery may be used for proximal PA stenosis, but surgical treatment of peripheral PA stenosis is difficult. Angioplasty is initially successful in 50% but restenosis is common and long-term benefits are seen in less than 35% of patients [81,82]. In a large series published in 1992, the mortality was 1–2% and the risk of serious complications 5% [82]. Complications include vessel rupture, hemoptysis, paradoxical embolism, balloon rupture, aneurysm formation, air embolism, and unilateral pulmonary edema. The use of cutting balloons has increased the effectiveness of treatment [83–85].

The use of endovascular stents reduces the incidence of initial failure and restenosis. When positioned in a stenotic PA, the large catheter may increase the degree of obstruction resulting in worsening hypoxia and right ventricular failure. Children with RV hypertrophy from peripheral pulmonary stenosis may also deteriorate hemodynamically as a result of tricuspid regurgitation from the catheter.

Patients in whom pulmonary blood flow is dependent on cavopulmonary shunts have a limited capacity to tolerate any obstruction to pulmonary blood flow. Obstruction can occur at the site of the venous to pulmonary artery anastomosis, at the site of previous surgery, or at a remote site. Angioplasty, commonly with placement of stents, may be used to relieve the obstruction. When required in the early postoperative period the patient's condition is often poor.

Patients with William's syndrome often have multiple peripheral stenoses of the pulmonary arteries and associated supravalvular aortic stenosis and coronary artery stenosis. In a series of 39 procedures, the mortality rate was 7.7% [86]. High right ventricular pressure was a predictor of mortality and the creation of an ASD in these patients may have been beneficial. Out of 22 patients initially managed with deep sedation without endotracheal intubation, 3 required intubation.

Percutaneous pulmonary valve implantation

Percutaneous pulmonary valve implantation is a relatively new procedure that is still considered experimental in many countries, but will likely be performed with increasing frequency and is the prototype for other valve placements in the interventional catheterization laboratory. This procedure is performed in patients with previous RVOT surgery, most commonly (95%) in patients with an RV–PA conduit that has either become stenotic, has significant pulmonary regurgitation, or both. Tetralogy of Fallot (60%), previous Ross procedure (10%), and truncus arteriosus (10%) are the predominant diagnoses [87]. Inclusion criteria are that the patient must meet surgical criteria for valve placement, including RV pressure $^2/_3 - ^3/_4$ systemic, or severe pulmonary insufficiency, and outflow tract dimensions 14–22 mm in two dimensions. In addition, the patient weight needs to be greater than 20 kg, with median patient age 18–22 years for this procedure. Under general endotracheal anesthesia, a 21-Fr sheath is used to access a femoral vein, and the valve mounted inside a balloon expandable stent (Figure 27.3) is crimped inside the sheath, and threaded along a guidewire to the correct position under conventional biplane fluoroscopic guidance. The valve is then reexpanded to its final diameter with enough force to prevent migration or paravalvular leak [88]. In a recent series, 6 of 152 patients (3.9%) required emergency surgery, including homograft

rupture in 2 patients, dislodged stented valve in 2 patients, occlusion of right pulmonary artery in 1 patient, and occlusion of left main coronary artery in 1 patient. All 6 patients survived but one had neurological sequelae from prolonged resuscitation after homograft rupture [89]. Significant hemodynamic instability and blood loss will occur in some patients, and surgical and OR backup plans should be in place for these procedures. Immediate hemodynamic results are favorable, with a significant reduction in RV pressure and relief of severe PI, and long-term freedom from reoperation 84% at 50 months postprocedure.

Aortic valvotomy

Balloon dilatation of isolated aortic valve stenosis is indicated when the transvalvular gradient is greater than 70 mm Hg or is greater than 50 mm Hg with symptoms, or when ECG evidence of ischemia is seen. Neonates may have much smaller gradients despite severe stenosis, as flow across the aortic valve will be minimal. Untreated severe stenosis caries a 19% risk of sudden death [75,90].

In a series of 630 dilatations, the immediate outcome was suboptimal (failure or major morbidity) for 17% of patients and procedural mortality was 1.9% [91]. Major complications, including aortic regurgitation, vascular damage, and perforation of heart or great vessels, occurred in 6.3% of patients. Age less than 3 months, high gradient, the use of small balloon sizes, and the presence of an aortic coarctation predicted poor outcome. The procedure is essentially palliative. However, in a recent single center study with up to 17 years of follow-up, two-thirds of patients had a decade of freedom form surgical intervention. The authors acknowledge that there may be selection bias in their findings. Nonetheless, this is a worthwhile result [92]. The valve may be damaged by use of an oversized balloon causing dilation of the valve annulus or by inadvertent puncture of the valve leaflet. The latter complication may be reduced by use of an antegrade approach to the valve via the atrial septum (puncturing the septum if the foramen ovale is closed). This approach also eliminates the risk of damage to the femoral artery, passage of the wire across the stenotic valve is simplified, and less hemodynamic compromise occurs. Should severe aortic insufficiency occur, coronary blood supply is compromised and urgent surgical repair may be required. The mortality in this situation is high [93].

Neonates present significant challenges, for both immediate and long-term management. The decision making can be complex [94] (i.e., single- vs two-ventricle patient) and there is often considerable hemodynamic instability and risk of sudden death from myocardial ischemia and arrhythmia. The systemic and coronary circulations are dependent on right ventricular flow through the DA and the LV is greatly hypertrophied with poor

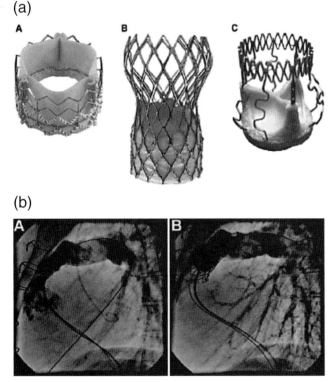

Figure 27.3 (a) Examples of percutaneous heart valves delivered via transcatheter route. Valves A and C are made of bovine pericardium; B is a xenograft valve. Other materials include bovine jugular vein (Reproduced and used with permission from Reference [88]). (b) Lateral angiogram before (A) and after (B) percutaneous pulmonary valve placement in a patient with right ventricle to pulmonary artery homograft obstruction and regurgitation. Note resolution of pulmonary regurgitation and larger homograft diameter, as well as stent in (B) (Reproduced with permission from Reference [87])

compliance. Initial resuscitation includes mechanical ventilation, PgE$_1$, and cautious use of inotropes. Inflation of the balloon across the aortic valve will lead to transient complete obstruction of coronary flow. A narcotic-based anesthetic technique reduces cardiac work and minimizes after-load reduction and tachycardia. Care must be taken to maintain preload, as any reduction in cardiac output will lead to further ischemia. Inotropes, vasopressors, and a defibrillator should be immediately on hand. A more recent study detailed 13% early mortality, with the presence of endocardial fibroelastosis as a significant risk factor [95].

Older infants may present with severe degrees of aortic stenosis [96]. They have heart failure and are at risk of ischemia and arrhythmia. Cardiovascular compromise during balloon inflation is inevitable but on deflation of the balloon prompt return of cardiac output is to be expected. The incidence of arrhythmia is higher than during other interventional procedures. The use of rapid ventricular pacing to decrease cardiac output can be helpful and is associated with good technical conditions and stable hemodynamics [97]. As with neonates, there is a risk of arterial damage and of aortic regurgitation. The latter may require surgical intervention. The need for the patient to be still during positioning of the balloon and the risk of hemodynamic compromise or complications must be considered and at the HSC; it is normal to provide general endotracheal anesthesia for this group. Older patients may present with progressive aortic stenosis or with restenosis.

Coarctation of aorta

Angioplasty is applied to both native and recurrent coarctation of the aorta [98,99,100]. The indications are resting hypertension proximal to the coarctation with a gradient of >20 mm Hg or presence of multiple collaterals (Figure 27.4). The best results are obtained when there is a short discrete coarctation with an otherwise normal arch. Initial success with native coarctation is greater than for recurrent coarctation; however, there is a high incidence of late aneurysm formation (2–6%) and of restenosis (7–12%). In neonates, recoarctation rates are high. In older children with native coarctation, the role of angioplasty is controversial [34]. Surgery for recurrent coarctation is more difficult and recoarctation is an accepted indication for angioplasty. Use of endovascular stents may reduce both restenosis and aneurysm formation, but the risk of damage to the femoral artery and the failure of stents to grow with the patient limit the use of this technique. The anesthesiologist can be thankful that the controversy centers around medium- and long-term outcomes. In the majority of cases, perioperative complication is unusual, especially with use of covered stents. Adult patients may present with recoarctation or with aneurysm formation.

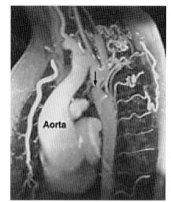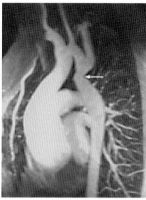

Figure 27.4 On the left-hand side is an MRI image of a coarctation of the aorta prior to dilation. There is a tight narrowing of the aorta (*arrow*) and numerous collaterals. Postballoon dilation (right-hand side), the degree of narrowing is reduced and the collaterals are no longer present

Complications occur in 5% of procedures and include aortic rupture or dissection, stroke, femoral artery damage, thrombosis, and late aneurysm formation [101]. Mortality for the procedure is 0.7%. Patients often have significant collaterals and this limits hemodynamic compromise during balloon inflation. As with surgical repair, hypertension after dilatation should be anticipated. The procedure is generally well tolerated, but the risk of serious sequelae is significant.

Closure of atrial septal defect and ventricular septal defect

Selected ASDs are suitable for device closure. The technique is unsuitable for ostium primum defects or for large defects. A rim of septal tissue is required to allow the device to be anchored. At 1 year, 5–10% of patients have significant residual leaks [102,103]. Complications are uncommon and include embolization of the device, encroachment on AV valves, obstruction of pulmonary or systemic veins, perforation of the heart or great vessels, and air emboli. Generally the procedure is well tolerated. The procedure is usually performed with general endotracheal anesthesia due to the use of transesophageal echo and the need for a still patient. Increasingly, endovascular and transthoracic echocardiography guidance is employed. ASD devices are also used to close Fontan fenestrations, if spontaneous closure has not occurred.

Transcatheter closure of a VSD is a more complex procedure with greater risk of serious complications [104]. It is usual to initially cross the defect from the left side. This wire is then snared from the right heart and brought out so that a continuous connection is made through the venous system and right heart, through the VSD into the left heart and out through the aortic valve and arterial system. The device is then deployed via the right heart, avoiding passage of a large catheter through the femoral artery and aortic valve. Complications include blood loss, arrhythmia, atrioventricular or aortic valve regurgitation, and cardiac arrest. In one early series, 50% of patients were admitted to intensive care following the procedure [105]. General anesthesia and control of the airway is required due to the high risk of cardiovascular instability, the length of the procedures, and the use of transesophageal echocardiography. The likelihood of complications, and periprocedural hemodynamic instability depend in part on the patient population: the elective closure of a congenital defect is much more straightforward than the management of an adult with an acute VSD as a result of a septal wall infarct.

Closure of extracardiac connections

Connections between the systemic and pulmonary circulations may occur in isolation (patent ductus arteriousum [PDA]), in association with CHD (aortopulmonary connections with pulmonary atresia), as a result of palliation of cyanotic heart disease (venovenous connection after cavopulmonary connection) or as surgically created shunts [106].

Often, naturally occurring lesions are closed by embolization with helical wires. Choice of anesthetic technique will depend on the patient's physiology. Cyanosed patients with a cavopulmonary connection and multiple collaterals may not tolerate positive pressure ventilation. Older patients presenting with large PDAs may have significant pulmonary hypertension and be at risk of right heart failure.

A specific concern is the embolization of the device into the pulmonary or systemic circulation. If the device enters the systemic circulation, it may enter the cerebral vessels placing the patient at risk of neurological injury. Often the device can be retrieved via the catheter, but open retrieval may be required in some cases.

Atrial septostomy

Balloon atrial septostomy was first described in 1966 [107]. The objective is to open a nonrestrictive connection between left and right atria to allow bidirectional mixing of blood. It has most widely been used for the initial palliation of transposition of the great arteries and in this situation the improvement in the patients condition may be dramatic. Further indications are total anomalous pulmonary venous drainage, atrioventricular valve atresia, and pulmonary atresia with intact ventricular septum.

The technique involves the passage of balloon-tipped catheter across the foramen ovale into the left atrium. The balloon is inflated and withdrawn across the septum, tearing the atrial septum. This procedure is repeated until the

inflated balloon can be withdrawn without resistance. The procedure can be performed at the patient's bedside using echocardiographic guidance. A modification of the procedure is applied to older infants. At 1 month of age, the atrial septum is too thick to be torn by the balloon alone. A catheter with a retractable blade is used to initiate the tear. Indications are similar to balloon atrial septostomy.

Complications include arrhythmia, perforation of the heart, balloon rupture, and embolization and damage to heart structures. Patients are frequently in a very poor condition. They are often extremely hypoxic, acidotic, and may have pulmonary edema. They will generally require ventilation and PgE_1 infusion. There is significant risk of life-threatening arrhythmia due to catheter manipulation in an irritable myocardium. Another group of patients who may require intervention to the interatrial septum are hypoplastic left heart syndrome (HLHS) patients who have undergone a "hybrid procedure." These patients can develop myocardial ischemia and demonstrate significant hemodynamic changes as a result of the reduction in left atrial pressure, and subsequent increase in pulmonary blood flow (see below).

"Hybrid procedures"

At the present time, this term most frequently refers to treatment of HLHS using a combination of surgical and transcatheter interventions as part of a single procedure. It can (and probably will, over time) be applied to any scenario where there is both an open and a transcatheter intervention. This procedure has been used by some centers as the primary therapy for HLHS, and there are theoretical advantages for employing this strategy, including the avoidance of cardiopulmonary bypass in the neonatal period, and a reduction in blood product exposure in children whose treatment path is aimed toward transplantation. There is no clear survival advantage at the present time, but there is evidence that hospital and intensive care length of stay is reduced [108–111].

The current approach consists of a median sternotomy, bilateral pulmonary artery bands, and stenting of the PDA, which is done via a sheath placed through the RVOT (Figure 27.5a). The sheath is secured with a purse string suture controlled by the surgeons, while the coronary stent (or two) is deployed by the cardiologist. There are opportunities for rapid blood loss, there can be obstruction of retrograde aortic flow and thus coronary and cerebral ischemia, and at the HSC we have seen a significant incidence of atrial tachycardia. Late stent occlusion and migration also occurs, contributing to interval mortality. At HSC we have placed shunts from the main pulmonary artery to the innominate artery to prevent sudden death from stent migration in patients with aortic atresia. Flow through the shunt is in the reverse direction to

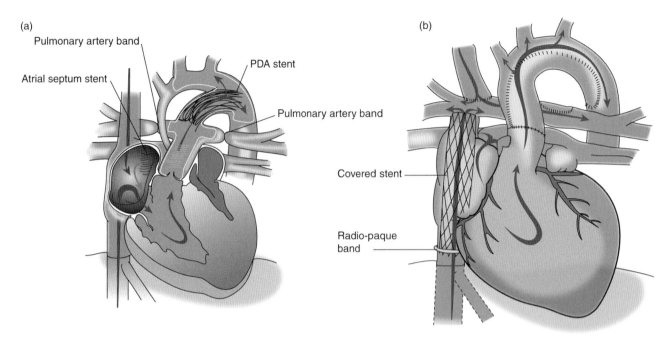

Figure 27.5 (a) Hybrid palliation in a neonate for hypoplastic left heart syndrome. Note stents in patent ductus arteriosus and bilateral pulmonary artery banding. (b) Hybrid completion of Fontan operation. Note covered stent delivered via internal jugular route to complete cavopulmonary connection (see text for further details) (Reproduced and used with permission from Reference [108])

conventional Blalock–Taussig shunts [110–112]. Despite the intuitive appeal of avoiding cardiopulmonary bypass and a lengthy procedure, these patients often demonstrate a hemodynamic profile that is actually worse than standard operative therapy over the first 36–48 hours. In a comparison study of 6 hybrid versus 13 standard Norwood stage I patients, the hybrid patients had higher Qp:Qs, lower mean arterial pressure, lower cardiac index, and higher serum lactates than standard stage I palliation [111]. These patients often need inotropic support, and careful ventilatory management and monitoring to balance Qp:Qs during and after the hybrid procedure, just as in the standard surgical approach. However, they improve more quickly than babies who have undergone cardiopulmonary bypass.

Galantowicz et al. have reported intermediate term outcomes comparable with conventional staged surgical palliation for HLHS. Of 40 patients undergoing hybrid stage I, 36 survived for the comprehensive stage II procedure, 52% were extubated in the OR, and 85% within 24 hours. Of these 36 patients, 33 (92%) survived stage II, and 15 patients have undergone stage III repair (Fontan completion) with no mortality. Overall interstage mortality was 5%, and catheter or surgical reintervention rate 36%. ICU and hospital length of stay, and hospital charges compare favorably to standard approaches [109]. Thus, the proof of concept for the hybrid approach to HLHS seems valid, and it is likely that this approach may be applied to other scenarios. One theoretical advantage of avoiding the by-

pass exposure in the neonatal period, but shifting it to a few months later, is that the brain in full-term neonates has immature features compared to the normal neonate, and has a high incidence of both pre- and postoperative brain injury, especially white matter injury [113]. Older infants have a lower incidence of brain injury after surgery with cardiopulmonary bypass [114]. This approach needs to be validated with well-matched controlled studies.

The optimum approach to the atrial septum in this patient population is also unclear. At the Hospital for Sick Children, Toronto, the infants are closely followed by transthoracic echocardiography, and oxygen saturation monitoring to ascertain the transatrial gradient. If there is significant desaturation (<70%) in combination with a transatrial gradient then balloon septostomy is undertaken. Other centers describe routine septostomy prior to discharge from hospital. Close attention needs to be paid during and immediately after balloon septostomy because of the potential for poorly tolerated atrial arrhythmias, and also the development of pulmonary edema, systemic hypotension, and myocardial ischemia.

After a comprehensive stage II procedure that includes aortic arch reconstruction, removal of PA banding, and bidirectional cavopulmonary connection, the patient can undergo a conventional Fontan operation, or a percutaneous transcatheter Fontan completion using a polytetrafluoroethylene-covered stent delivered via the internal jugular approach, which has been facilitated during the stage I comprehensive repair by placement of a radiopaque band to mark the IVC–RA junction, and a radiopaque marker to mark the blind pouch on the floor of the right pulmonary artery [108] (Figure 27.5b).

Electrophysiology studies and radio frequency or cryoablation

The purpose of an EP study is to identify the mechanism of the patient's arrhythmia by recording signals from electrodes placed within the heart. Use of fluoroscopy and reference to anatomic landmark allows localization of the abnormal pathways and foci responsible for the arrhythmia. Ablation of the abnormal pathway is initially successful in 91% of patients with a recurrence rate of 23% [38,115].

The majority of children presenting for EP investigation and treatment are otherwise healthy, have functionally normal hearts, and present with well-tolerated SVT. A minority will have either life-threatening arrhythmia or arrhythmia complicating CHD. A few children have cardiomyopathy as a cause or result of the arrhythmia. This is in contrast to the adult population, who more frequently present with ventricular arrhythmia complicating ischemic heart disease. Anesthetic concerns include the length of the procedure, poor access to the patient and the possibility of anesthetic agents altering the EP of the heart, and occasionally poor cardiac function. The effect of anesthetic agents on the ability to study the arrhythmia is dependent on the mechanism of the arrhythmia.

Pathogenesis of arrhythmia

The most common mechanism of tachycardia is reentry. This requires a circuit composed of connected pathways with different conduction velocities and refractory periods (see Figure 27.6). Preexcitation syndromes are a subgroup of patients with reentry tachycardia, in whom one arm of the circuit is the patient's atrioventricular node and the other is a congenital muscular pathway between atrium and ventricle. Tachycardia arises when depolarization occurs in the circuit while one limb is refractory and the other is able to conduct. The depolarization continues around the circuit and reaches the previously refractory pathway, which is now able to conduct. The circle is therefore perpetuated [116].

A second mechanism is altered automaticity. During normal sinus rhythm, only the sinoatrial node independently generates rhythmic impulses through spontaneous depolarization of the basement membrane. Other cells demonstrate this activity but at a slower rate and will only control the heart rate if the sinus node is not functioning or conduction is blocked. When cells

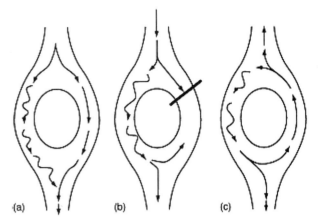

Figure 27.6 Reentry tachycardia requires a circuit with two limbs of different conduction velocities and refractory periods. The left-hand limb of the circuit in the figures has a shorter refractory period and slower conduction velocity (*curved arrows*). In (a) neither pathway is refractory, and the impulse is conducted over both limbs. In (b) a premature impulse travels over the left-hand pathway; however, the right-hand pathway is refractory from previous conduction. If the right-hand pathway is no longer refractory by the time the impulse reaches the distal end of the circuit, it is conducted in a retrograde fashion via the right-hand pathway and the reentry rhythm is perpetuated (c).

are damaged and subjected to extrinsic factors (electrolyte disturbance, hypoxia, hypercarbia, high wall tension, ischemia, and high catecholamine levels), spontaneous depolarization may be accelerated. This leads to rapid repetitive depolarization of a single focus: ectopic tachycardia.

Electrophysiology techniques

Figure 27.7 demonstrates typical electrode catheter position during an EP study for investigation of SVT. The catheters have multiple electrodes along their length. An electrode placed across the tricuspid valve can be positioned to record an EKG from the His bundle. Further electrodes are typically placed high within the right atrium, at the apex of the RV and "roaming" electrodes can be placed elsewhere in the right heart. Potentials from the left heart can be recorded via an electrode within the coronary sinus or from electrodes placed directly within the left heart (via puncture of the atrial septum or retrograde passage through the aortic valve).

Figures 27.8 and 27.9 demonstrate typical EKGs recorded during an EP study. In order to identify the mechanism of the arrhythmia, periods of pacing and programmed stimulation are undertaken. Pacing, commonly via the high right atrium and ventricular apex, allows arrhythmia to be provoked or terminated, permits measurement of EP properties of the conduction system and allows for ventricular pacing should complete heart block

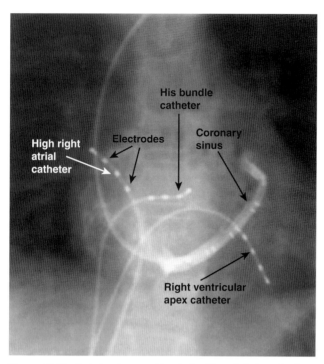

Figure 27.7 Typical catheter position during EP study for investigation of supraventricular tachycardia. Catheters have multiple electrodes along their length. Catheters are positioned across the tricuspid valve to record signal from the His bundle, in the ventricular apex, in the high right atrium, and within the coronary sinus. In this image, contrast has been injected into the coronary sinus

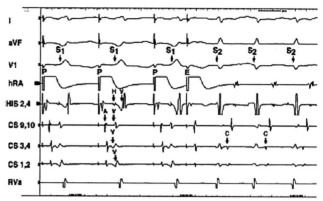

Figure 27.8 Simultaneous surface EKG and intracardiac electrocardiograms are shown. Three paced beats (P) are delivered via the high right atrial catheter followed by a premature stimulus (E) resulting in supraventricular tachycardia (SVT). For each beat, the CS 9,10 lead demonstrates three signals: an artifact corresponding to the pacing stimuli, a signal from depolarization of adjacent atrial muscle (A), followed by a signal from the adjacent ventricle (V). The His bundle depolarization (H) coincides with depolarization of the ventricular septum adjacent to the electrode. During paced rhythm, ventricular depolarization (V) occurs earliest in the CS 3,4 electrode (an electrode in the center of the coronary sinus catheter), indicating proximity to the accessory pathway. The preexcitation (delta wave) seen on the surface EKG (S_1) is confirmed by depolarization of CS 3,4 prior to His bundle depolarization (H). Following initiation of SVT, the morphology of the surface QRS becomes normalized indicating activation via the normal conducting system (S_2). Earliest retrograde activation of atrial muscle is seen on the CS 3,4 electrode confirming the position of the accessory pathway

occur (a rare complication). Drugs may be used to further refine the study. Adenosine will block normal AV conduction exposing a concealed abnormal pathway. Isoprenaline will increase sinoatrial rate, speed atrioventricular node conduction, reduce refractory periods, and increase automaticity of other contractile tissue.

Radio frequency ablation and cryoablation

Destruction of abnormal pathways and automatic foci abolishes the arrhythmia. This is most often accomplished by delivering RF energy to ablate the area. In the treatment of preexcitation syndromes, a specialized catheter is positioned along the atrioventricular ring then adjusted to record the earliest conduction via the abnormal pathway. When delivering RF energy, the size of lesion created is controlled by measurement of the temperature generated at the catheter tip and time of exposure. A further EP study is conducted following attempted ablation to test for residual or additional pathways. The ablation of an abnormal atrial focus is potentially more difficult as reference to anatomical landmarks and obtaining a stable electrode position is less certain.

Indications for RF ablations have recently been discussed [38]. Arrhythmia in patients younger than 4 years, in the absence of CHD, may resolve spontaneously and indications are thus limited to life-threatening arrhythmia not controlled by antiarrhythmic drugs. A small

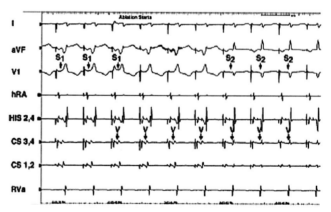

Figure 27.9 Surface EKG and intracardiac electrocardiograms are shown from the same patient as Figure 28.8. Ventricular depolarization (V) is earliest in CS 3,4 and preexcitation is demonstrated on the surface EKG (S_1). As radio frequency energy is delivered, preexcitation is lost with normalization of the surface QRS morphology (S_2) and ventricular depolarization on CS3,4 occurs later in the cardiac cycle

series has described the successful use of RF ablation to treat life-threatening tachycardia in children younger than 18 months; however, the risks in this group are higher [117]. Arrhythmia in older children are less likely to resolve and the indications for ablation are wider. Indications include failure of medical treatment, risk of sudden death, and a patient's preference for ablation rather than long-term treatment with antiarrhythmic drugs. Cryoablation, the freezing abnormal foci, is also used in the pediatric EP laboratory with increasing frequency.

Arrhythmia in patients with congenital heart disease

Patients with CHD may present with arrhythmia in a number of circumstances [118]. Ebstein's anomaly is associated with accessory pathways and preexcitation, atrial dilation is often associated with arrhythmia, and suture lines or scars can act as substrates for reentry or automatic arrhythmia. The latter is especially true following extensive atrial surgery, such as Mustard's procedure or classical Fontans. These patients may have poor reserve to tolerate tachycardia and placement of intracardiac electrodes may be complex. In a series of 139 patients, RF ablation was possible in 66% of studies with a recurrence of 11% at 2 years. No significant morbidity was caused by the procedure [118]. A recent review article outlines etiology, mechanisms, and possible new techniques for transcatheter ablation in CHD. Interestingly, the recurrence rate for ventricular arrhythmia is lower than atrial tachycardia [119].

Anesthetic considerations

As with other catheter procedures, it is possible to conduct EP studies in conscious patients or with minimal sedation. Both techniques are used for procedures in children and adolescents. Although only vascular access is likely to be painful, the procedures are often prolonged, multiple venous and arterial access points may be required, and periods of arrhythmia are inevitable that may be unpleasant for the patient. Deep sedation may offer no advantage to anesthesia and the additive effect of repeated doses of sedative drugs over a period of time must be considered. When vascular access sheaths are placed within the thorax in spontaneously breathing patients, there is more potential for air embolus.

Anesthetic considerations include the presence of CHD, and the consequences of repair, cardiomyopathy, or familial conditions associated with arrhythmia (long QT syndrome and arrhythmogenic right ventricular dysplasia). The patient should be questioned to the frequency of arrhythmia, factors that precipitate the arrhythmia, their symptoms during the arrhythmia, and whether treatment is required to terminate the arrhythmia. Arrhythmia associated with fainting or collapse of the patient is likely to be associated with greater hemodynamic compromise. If anxiety is a known precipitant of the arrhythmia, preoperative anxiolysis is relatively contraindicated due to the possibility of a false negative study. Antiarrhythmic drugs are usually stopped prior to the procedure unless the arrhythmia is frequent and poorly tolerated. The majority of patients will be adolescents and it is important to be aware of privacy issues, autonomy, and risk-taking behavior. Pregnancy testing preoperatively is routine in many institutions, and is particularly important in view of the radiation exposure. Drug and alcohol abuse can trigger arrhythmias, and smoking cessation should be counseled at any and every opportunity.

Often the electrophysiologist is aware of the likely mechanism of arrhythmia from surface EKG (e.g., delta waves indicate Wolf-Parkinson-White syndrome) or from Holter recording of the arrhythmia. This allows the anesthetic technique to be adapted to avoid suppression of the arrhythmia and to have minimal effects on the patient's EP. Specific agents may suppress abnormal pathways or foci to a point where their detection and induction of the arrhythmia is not possible. This leads to false-negative studies and failure of the procedure.

Other considerations are the length of the procedures, poor access to the patient, and the potential for hemodynamic compromise. EP studies are often scheduled for 4 hours and can take longer. X-ray tables are very firm and patient positioning can be awkward. Care needs to be taken to avoid injury to nerves and pressure areas. Large adolescent patients may be particularly difficult to position.

Access to the patient is reduced due to the use of the subclavian or internal jugular veins for vascular access. Upper body access is intimidating for awake patients, and may be more than some can tolerate. Intravenous lines, ventilator tubing, and anesthetic machines should be positioned accordingly.

Periods of tachycardia are to be expected during an EP study and healthy patients tolerate this well. Significant hemodynamic compromise occurs with very high ventricular rates or when the patient has a reduced cardiac reserve. Vasopressors may be used to improve perfusion pressure but α-adrenergic agonists have reflex effects on the EP of the heart. Discussion with the cardiologist prior to and during the procedure is vital in the management of more difficult patients. Rarely, temporary mechanical support may be required. Most arrhythmia can be terminated rapidly by overdrive pacing. Drugs (other than adenosine) or external cardioversion are rarely required and may force the cancellation of the procedure.

Anesthetic drugs and the cardiac conduction system

Anesthetic agents influence the EP of the heart. Effects are mediated via the sympathetic and parasympathetic systems or via the cardiac conduction systems and myocardium. The significance of these effects depends on the mechanism of the tachycardia. Anesthetic drugs also slow cardiac conduction and can be associated with significant bradycardia, which may due to vagal stimulation (fentanyl, remifentanil), or to α-adrenergic blockade (clonidine). It has been stated that dexmedetomidine is contraindicated in electrophysiological studies, or in situations where cardiac output is profoundly dependent on sympathetic tone [65,66].

Anesthetic drugs and preexcitation syndromes

SVT due to preexcitation syndromes requires conduction of impulses in a circuit involving functional atrioventricular node and accessory pathway. Effects upon the accessory pathway are most critical and can be characterized by two EP variables: the accessory pathway effective refractory period (APERP) and the coupling interval [120]. The APERP is the minimal time between two impulses that are still conducted by the accessory pathway. The coupling interval is the maximal time between two impulses that will precipitate an SVT. A false-negative EPS due to suppression of conduction via the accessory pathway is most critical following RF ablation, when it may lead to recurrence of SVT.

Isoflurane and halothane at one minimum alveolar concentration have been shown to cause prolongation of the APERP and it has been suggested that these agents be avoided during ablation of accessory pathways [120]. However, a further study of isoflurane and a study of sevoflurane failed to demonstrate significant EP effects at one minimum alveolar concentration [121,122]. Conversely, isoflurane and halothane prolong coupling interval potentially increasing susceptibility to SVT. From animal studies it is clear that inhalational agents do have a number of EP effects in sufficient dose; however, the clinical significance of this may be limited.

A number of clinical studies have demonstrated no direct effect of propofol on conduction at doses of 100–150 mcg/kg/min other than possibly slight prolongation of atrial refractory period [121,123,124]. In studies on isolated hearts, significant EP effects are apparent only at concentrations unlikely to be achieved clinically. Midazolam and alfentanil in combination has been shown not to have direct effects on cardiac conduction [125]. Droperidol produces a marked prolongation of APERP [126] and should be avoided. Vecuronium has no EP effects, but other neuromuscular blocking agents have not been studied.

Despite the EP effects of volatile agents, SVTs due to reentry will remain inducible in most patients. A technique utilizing opioids, nitrous oxide, and a low concentration of volatile agent is acceptable. Sevoflurane may be preferable to isoflurane in this circumstance. The successful use of TIVA with propofol for maintenance of anesthesia during EPS for reentry tachycardia has been described [127]. It remains uncertain whether the risk of false-negative studies is reduced in comparison to volatile anesthetics.

Anesthetic drugs and automatic tachycardia

Ectopic arrhythmia resulting from increased automaticity will behave differently under anesthesia. Many of the extrinsic factors, which promote automaticity, are minimized during steady state anesthesia. Typically, catecholamine levels are low and cardiac work is decreased.

The direct effects of inhalational anesthetics on automaticity are complex. As described above, the abnormal behavior of these foci is related to an acceleration of spontaneous depolarization of the cell membrane. Halothane will reduce the rate of depolarization in sinoatrial cells producing a predictable reduction in heart rate [128]. However, when uninjured Purkinje cells are exposed to halothane and epinephrine, the rate of spontaneous depolarization is increased [129]. The most likely substrate for tachycardia is injured Purkinje cells already demonstrating increased automaticity. It has been shown that these cells are not affected by volatile agents and their response to epinephrine is unaltered [129].

In a series of 150 patients with SVT, anesthetized with propofol infusions, seven patients had arrhythmia due to ectopic atrial tachycardia [130]. The arrhythmia could not be induced in four of these patients despite infusion of isoproterenol, though EP studies were successful in all of the 143 patients with reentry tachycardia. However, a 2006 study concluded that propofol was an appropriate choice for electrophysiological studies as it had no effect on AV nodal conduction [131].

Given this data, it is difficult to suggest a best anesthetic technique for EPS studies in patients with ectopic tachycardia. Limiting the dose of volatile anesthetics during attempts to induce the tachycardia and the replacement of endogenous sympathetic activity with sympathomimetic drugs such as isoproterenol is one approach. The avoidance of general anesthesia can be considered in older patients.

Implantation of pacemakers and defibrillators

Pacemaker implantation is less common in children than in adults [132] and is indicated for complete heart block or for sinus node dysfunction leading to symptomatic brady-cardia. Bradycardia may complicate CHD or surgery near the conduction pathways. Other indications include anti-tachycardia pacing for SVT, and placement of automatic defibrillator devices in long QT syndrome or late tetralogy of Fallot with ventricular tachycardia.

Placement of epicardial wires requires a sternotomy and general anesthesia. Anesthesia may be associated with worsening of bradycardia. Treatment with atropine and isoproterenol may be instituted followed by the rapid placement of a temporary pacemaker wire or transtho-racic or esophageal pacing. Transthoracic pacing is very disconcerting in the awake patient.

There are practical problems associated with placement of pacemakers in small children. The pacemaker systems are large, and thrombosis of central veins is a concern. It is difficult to accommodate for patient growth, and sub-cutaneous placement of the generator may be impossible (the abdomen is an alternative site). Therefore, epicardial wires are required in small infants and when access to heart via the venous system is not possible (e.g., follow-ing the Fontan procedure).

Implantation of defibrillators is indicated for life-threatening ventricular arrhythmia [133]. It is usual to test the defibrillator by induction of ventricular fibrillation. It is prudent to have mechanical support on standby in case the device fails and it is difficult to defibrillate the heart. Indications include isolated arrhythmia associated with long QT syndromes and patients with hypertrophic cardiomyopathy or arrhythmogenic right ventricular dys-plasia who may have more general myocardial disease [134–136]. Often patients present after near-miss sudden death or death of a close family member and they and their families are often extremely anxious. Preoperative anxiety can be sufficient to induce arrhythmia and premedication with an anxiolytic is advisable. There is a significant rate of inappropriate discharge of devices in young patients, as well as lead failure presumably due to growth. CHD ac-counted for the majority of young patients with automated internal cardiac defibrillator in a single center report in 2004 [137].

Conclusions

The trend toward more invasive therapeutic cardiac catheterization procedures in younger, smaller, and sicker patients increases the potential for hemodynamic and res-piratory instability. As such, preparation and vigilance for these procedures by the anesthesiologist is essential. Ap-proaching these procedures as if the patient were under-going surgery will help ensure the best outcome. Indeed, in the future an increasing number of combined surgical and catheter interventions may be performed at the same setting, in a modified catheterization laboratory that is fully equipped for surgery.

Acknowledgment

We acknowledge the help of Dr Joel Kirsh (Cardiology HSC), Dr Shi-Joon Yoo (Diagnostic Imaging HSC), and Dr Lee Benson (Cardiology HSC) for supplying figures for use in this chapter and Dr Joel Kirsh for help in preparation of the manuscript.

References

1. Rubio-Alvarez V, Limon R, Soni J (1953) Intracardiac valvu-lotomy by means of a catheter. Arch Inst Cardiol Mex 23: 183–192.
2. Rashkind WJ, Miller WW (1968) Transposition of the great arteries. Results of palliation by balloon atrioseptostomy in thirty-one infants. Circulation 38: 453–462.
3. Inglis JM (1954) Anaesthesia for cardiac catheterisation in children. Anaesthesia 9: 25–30.
4. Keown II, Fisher SM, Downing DF, Hitchcock P (1957) Anesthesia for cardiac catheterization in infants and chil-dren. Anesthesiology 18: 270–274.
5. Smith C (1958) Sedation of children for cardiac catheteriza-tion with an atretic mixture. Can Anaesth Soc J 5: 35–40.
6. Reddy K, Jaggar S, Gillbe C (2006) The anaesthetist and the cardiac catheterisation laboratory. Anaesthesia 61: 1175–1186.
7. Shook DC, Gross W (2007) Offsite anesthesiology in the cardiac catheterization lab. Curr Opin Anaesthesiol 20: 352–358.
8. Grifka RG (1997) Transcatheter intervention for the treat-ment of congenital cardiac defects. Tex Heart Inst J 24: 293–300.
9. Shim D, Lloyd TR, Crowley DC, Beekman RH (1999) Neona-tal cardiac catheterization: a 10-year transition from diag-nosis to therapy. Pediatr Cardiol 20: 131–133.
10. Allan CK, Thiagarajan RR, Armsby LR, et al. (2006) Emer-gent use of extracorporeal membrane oxygenation during pediatric cardiac catheterization. Pediatr Crit Care Med 7: 212–219.
11. Booth KL, Roth SJ, Perry SB, et al. (2002) Cardiac catheter-ization of patients supported by extracorporeal membrane oxygenation. J Am Coll Cardiol 40: 1681–1686.
12. Matern U, Koneczny S (2007) Safety, hazards and er-gonomics in the operating room. Surg Endosc 21: 1965–1969.
13. Wichert A, Marcos-Suarez P, Vereczkei A, et al. (2004) Im-provement of the ergonomic situation in the integrated op-erating room for laparoscopic operations. Int Cong Ser 1268: 842–846.
14. Wilson IH, Walker IA (2008) Theatre checklists and patient safety. Anaesthesia 63: 921–923.
15. Bashore TM, Bates ER, Berger PB, et al. (2001) American College of Cardiology/Society for Cardiac Angiography

and Interventions Clinical Expert Consensus Document on cardiac catheterization laboratory standards. A report of the American College of Cardiology Task Force on Clinical Expert Consensus Documents. J Am Coll Cardiol 37: 2170–2214.

16. Andreassi MG, Ait-Ali L, Botto N, et al. (2006) Cardiac catheterization and long-term chromosomal damage in children with congenital heart disease. Eur Heart J 27: 2703–2708.

17. Bacher K, Bogaert E, Lapere R, et al. (2005) Patient-specific dose and radiation risk estimation in pediatric cardiac catheterization. Circulation 111: 83–89.

18. Venneri L, Rossi F, Botto N, et al. (2009) Cancer risk from professional exposure in staff working in cardiac catheterization laboratory: insights from the National Research Council's Biological Effects of Ionizing Radiation VII Report. Am Heart J 157: 118–124.

19. Vano E, Gonzalez L, Fernández JM, Haskal ZJ (2008) Eye lens exposure to radiation in interventional suites: caution is warranted. Radiology 248: 945–953.

20. Andropoulos DB, Stayer S (2003) An anesthesiologist for all pediatric cardiac catheterizations: luxury or necessity? J Cardiothorac Vasc Anesth 17: 683–685.

21. Schneeweiss S, Saranapalan S (2007) Impact of a multifaceted pediatric sedation course: self directed learning versus a formal continuing medical education course to improve knowledge of sedation guidelines. Can J Emerg Med 9: 93–100.

22. American Academy of Pediatrics; American Academy of Pediatric Dentistry, Coté CJ, Wilson S; Work Group on Sedation (2006). Guidelines for monitoring and management of pediatric patients during and after sedation for diagnostic and therapeutic procedures: an update. Pediatrics 118: 2587–2602.

23. American Society of Anesthesiologists Task Force on Sedation and Analgesia by Non-Anesthesiologists (2002) Practice guidelines for sedation and analgesia by non-anesthesiologists. Anesthesiology 96: 1004–1017.

24. Scottish Intercollegiate Guidelines Network (2004) Safe sedation of children undergoing diagnostic and therapeutic procedures. Available at: http://www.sign.ac.uk/guidelines/fulltext/58/index.html. Accessed August 24, 2009.

25. Cote CJ, Notterman DA, Karl HW, et al. (2000) Adverse sedation events in pediatrics: a critical incident analysis of contributing factors. Pediatrics 105: 805–814.

26. Friesen RH, Alswang M (1996) End-tidal PCO_2 monitoring via nasal cannulae in pediatric patients: accuracy and sources of error. J Clin Monit 12: 155–159.

27. Simpson JM, Moore P, Teitel DF (2001) Cardiac catheterization of low birth weight infants. Am J Cardiol 87: 1372–1377.

28. Ryan CA, Robertson M, Coe JY (1993) Seizures due to lidocaine toxicity in a child during cardiac catheterization. Pediatr Cardiol 14: 116–118.

29. Deng M, Wang X, Wang L, et al. (2008) The hemodynamic effects of newborn caudal anesthesia assessed by transthoracic echocardiography: a randomized, double-blind, controlled study. Paediatr Anaesth 18: 1075–1081.

30. Pirat A, Karaaslan P, Candan S, et al. (2005) Topical EMLA cream versus prilocaine infiltration for pediatric cardiac catheterization. J Cardiothorac Vasc Anesth 19: 642–645.

31. Mehta R, Lee KJ, Chaturvedi R, Benson L (2008) Complications of pediatric cardiac catheterization: a review in the current era. Catheter Cardiovasc Interv 72: 278–285.

32. Hansen TG, Henneberg SW (1999) Brachial plexus injury during cardiac catheterisation in children. Acta Anaesthesiol Scand 43: 364–365.

33. Carmosino MJ, Friesen RH, Doran A, Ivy DD (2007) Perioperative complications in children with pulmonary hypertension undergoing noncardiac surgery or cardiac catheterization. Anesth Analg 104: 521–527.

34. Allen HD, Beekman RH III, Garson A Jr, et al. (1998) Pediatric therapeutic cardiac catheterization: a statement for healthcare professionals from the Council on Cardiovascular Disease in the Young, American Heart Association. Circulation 97: 609–625.

35. Section on Cardiology and Cardiac Surgery (2002) American Academy of Pediatrics. Guidelines for pediatric cardiovascular centers. Pediatrics 109: 544–549.

36. Vitiello R, McCrindle BW, Nykanen D, Freedom RM, Benson LN (1998) Complications associated with pediatric cardiac catheterization. J Am Coll Cardiol 32: 1433–1440.

37. Dubin AM, Van Hare GF (2000) Radiofrequency catheter ablation: indications and complications. Pediatr Cardiol 21: 551–556.

38. Van Hare GF, Colan SD, Javitz H, et al. (2007) Prospective assessment after pediatric cardiac ablation: fate of intracardiac structure and function, as assessed by serial echocardiography. Am Heart J 153: 815–820.

39. Kain ZN, Mayes LC, Wang SM, et al. (1998) Parental presence during induction of anesthesia versus sedative premedication: which intervention is more effective? Anesthesiology 89: 1147–1156; discussion 9A–10A.

40. Levine MF, Hartley EJ, Macpherson BA, et al. (1993) Oral midazolam premedication for children with congenital cyanotic heart disease undergoing cardiac surgery: a comparative study. Can J Anaesth 40: 934–938.

41. Cote CJ, Cohen IT, Suresh S, et al. (2002) A comparison of three doses of a commercially prepared oral midazolam syrup in children. Anesth Analg 94: 37–43.

42. Clark DJ (1999) Venous thromboembolism in paediatric practice. Paediatr Anaesth 9: 475–484.

43. Cote CJ, Karl HW, Notterman DA, et al. (2000) Adverse sedation events in pediatrics: analysis of medications used for sedation. Pediatrics 106: 633–644.

44. Coté CJ (1995) Monitoring guidelines: do they make a difference? AJR Am J Roentgenol 165: 910–912.

45. Auden SM, Sobczyk WL, Solinger RE, Goldsmith LJ (2000) Oral ketamine/midazolam is superior to intramuscular meperidine, promethazine, and chlorpromazine for pediatric cardiac catheterization. Anesth Analg 90: 299–305.

46. Wodey E, Pladys P, Copin C, et al. (1997) Comparative hemodynamic depression of sevoflurane versus halothane in infants: an echocardiographic study. Anesthesiology 87: 795–800.

47. Rivenes SM, Lewin MB, Stayer SA, et al. (2001) Cardiovascular effects of sevoflurane, isoflurane, halothane, and fentanyl-midazolam in children with congenital heart disease: an echocardiographic study of myocardial contractility and hemodynamics. Anesthesiology 94: 223–229.

48. Murray DJ, Forbes RB, Mahoney LT (1992) Comparative hemodynamic depression of halothane versus isoflurane in neonates and infants: an echocardiographic study. Anesth Analg 74: 329–337.

49. Laird TH, Stayer SA, Rivenes SM, et al. (2002) Pulmonary-to-systemic blood flow ratio effects of sevoflurane, isoflurane, halothane, and fentanyl/midazolam with 100% oxygen in children with congenital heart disease. Anesth Analg 95: 1200–1206.

50. Williams GD, Jones TK, Hanson KA, Morray JP (1999) The hemodynamic effects of propofol in children with congenital heart disease. Anesth Analg 89: 1411–1416.

51. Uezono S, Clarke WR (1995) The effect of propofol on normal and increased pulmonary vascular resistance in isolated perfused rabbit lung. Anesth Analg 80: 577–582.

52. Tramer MR, Moore RA, McQuay HJ (1997) Propofol and bradycardia: causation, frequency and severity. Br J Anaesth 78: 642–651.

53. Shekerdemian L, Bush A, Redington A (1997) Cardiovascular effects of intravenous midazolam after open heart surgery. Arch Dis Child 76: 57–61.

54. Li J, Zhang G, McCrindle BW, et al. (2007) Profiles of hemodynamics and oxygen transport derived by using continuous measured oxygen consumption after the Norwood procedure. J Thorac Cardiovasc Surg 133: 441–448.

55. Nguyen NK, Magnier S, Georget G, et al. (1991) Anesthesia for heart catheterization in children. Comparison of 3 techniques. Ann Fr Anesth Reanim 10: 522–528.

56. Sarkar M, Laussen PC, Zurakowski D, et al. (2005) Hemodynamic responses to etomidate on induction of anesthesia in pediatric patients. Anesth Analg 101: 645–650.

57. Mellon RD, Simone AF, Rappaport BA (2007) Use of anesthetic agents in neonates and young children. Anesth Analg 104: 509–520.

58. McGowan FX Jr, Davis PJ (2008) Anesthetic-related neurotoxicity in the developing infant: of mice, rats, monkeys and, possibly, humans. Anesth Analg 106: 1599–1602.

59. Jevtovic-Todorovic V, Olney JW (2008) PRO: anesthesia-induced developmental neuroapoptosis: status of the evidence. Anesth Analg 106: 1659–1663.

60. Loepke AW, McGowan FX Jr, Soriano SG (2008) CON: the toxic effects of anesthetics in the developing brain: the clinical perspective. Anesth Analg 106: 1664–1649.

61. Loepke AW, Soriano SG, Loepke AW, Soriano SG (2008) An assessment of the effects of general anesthetics on developing brain structure and neurocognitive function. Anesth Analg 106: 1681–1707.

62. Munro HM, Tirotta CF, Felix DE, et al. (2007) Initial experience with dexmedetomidine for diagnostic and interventional cardiac catheterization in children. Paediatr Anaesth 17: 109–112.

63. Easley RB, Tobias JD (2008) Pro: dexmedetomidine should be used for infants and children undergoing cardiac surgery. J Cardiothorac Vasc Anesth 22: 147–151.

64. Hammer GB (2008) Con: dexmedetomidine should not be used for infants and children during cardiac surgery. J Cardiothorac Vasc Anesth 22: 152–154.

65. Sichrovsky TC, Mittal S, Steinberg JS (2008) Dexmedetomidine sedation leading to refractory cardiogenic shock. Anesth Analg 106: 1784–1786.

66. Hammer GB, Drover DR, Cao H, et al. (2008) The effects of dexmedetomidine on cardiac electrophysiology in children. Anesth Analg 106: 79–83.

67. Donmez A, Kizilkan A, Berksun H, et al. (2001) One center's experience with remifentanil infusions for pediatric cardiac catheterization. J Cardiothorac Vasc Anesth 15: 736–739.

68. Rautiainen P (1991) Alfentanil infusion for sedation in infants and small children during cardiac catheterization. Can J Anaesth 38: 980–984.

69. Foubert L, Reyntjens K, De Wolf D, et al. (2002) Remifentanil infusion for cardiac catheterization in children with congenital heart disease. Acta Anaesthesiol Scand 46: 355–360.

70. Shekerdemian LS, Bush A, Lincoln C, et al. (1997) Cardiopulmonary interactions in healthy children and children after simple cardiac surgery: the effects of positive and negative pressure ventilation. Heart 78: 587–593.

71. Shekerdemian LS, Bush A, Shore DF, et al. (1997) Cardiopulmonary interactions after Fontan operations: augmentation of cardiac output using negative pressure ventilation. Circulation 96: 3934–3942.

72. Lofland GK (2001) The enhancement of hemodynamic performance in Fontan circulation using pain free spontaneous ventilation. Eur J Cardiothorac Surg 20: 114–118.

73. Friesen RH, Alswang M (1996) Changes in carbon dioxide tension and oxygen saturation during deep sedation for paediatric cardiac catheterization. Paediatr Anaesth 6: 15–20.

74. Javorski JJ, Hansen DD, Laussen PC, et al. (1995) Paediatric cardiac catheterization: innovations. Can J Anaesth 42: 310–329.

75. Pihkala J, Nykanen D, Freedom RM, Benson LN (1999) Interventional cardiac catheterization. Pediatr Clin North Am 46: 441–464.

76. O'laughlin MP (1995) Balloon-expandable stenting in pediatric cardiology. J Interv Cardiol 8: 463–475.

77. Tabatabaei H, Boutin C, Nykanen DG, et al. (1996) Morphologic and hemodynamic consequences after percutaneous balloon valvotomy for neonatal pulmonary stenosis: medium-term follow-up. J Am Coll Cardiol 27: 473–478.

78. Gournay V, Piechaud JF, Delogu A, et al. (1995) Balloon valvotomy for critical stenosis or atresia of pulmonary valve in newborns. J Am Coll Cardiol 26: 1725–1731.

79. Fedderly RT, Lloyd TR, Mendelsohn AM, Beekman RH (1995) Determinants of successful balloon valvotomy in infants with critical pulmonary stenosis or membranous pulmonary atresia with intact ventricular septum. J Am Coll Cardiol 25: 460–465.

80. Stanfill R, Nykanen DG, Osorio S, et al. (2008) Stent implantation is effective treatment of vascular stenosis in young

infants with congenital heart disease: acute implantation and long-term follow-up results. Catheter Cardiovasc Interv 71: 831–841.

81. O'Laughlin MP (1998) Catheterization treatment of stenosis and hypoplasia of pulmonary arteries. Pediatr Cardiol 19: 48–56.

82. Hosking MC, Thomaidis C, Hamilton R, et al. (1992) Clinical impact of balloon angioplasty for branch pulmonary arterial stenosis. Am J Cardiol 69: 1467–1470.

83. Butera G, Antonio LT, Massimo C, Mario C (2006) Expanding indications for the treatment of pulmonary artery stenosis in children by using cutting balloon angioplasty. Catheter Cardiovasc Interv 67: 460–465.

84. Sugiyama H, Veldtman GR, Norgard G, et al. (2004) Bladed balloon angioplasty for peripheral pulmonary artery stenosis. Catheter Cardiovasc Interv 62: 71–77.

85. Baerlocher L, Kretschmar O, Harpes P, et al. (2008) Stent implantation and balloon angioplasty for treatment of branch pulmonary artery stenosis in children. Clin Res Cardiol 97: 310–317.

86. Geggel RL, Gauvreau K, Lock JE (2001) Balloon dilation angioplasty of peripheral pulmonary stenosis associated with Williams syndrome. Circulation 103: 2165–2170.

87. Lurz P, Coats L, Khambadkone S, et al. (2008) Percutaneous pulmonary valve implantation: impact of evolving technology and learning curve on clinical outcome. Circulation 117: 1964–1972.

88. Ghanbari H, Kidane AG, Burriesci G, et al. (2008) Percutaneous heart valve replacement: an update. Trends Cardiovasc Med 18: 117–125.

89. Kostolny M, Tsang V, Nordmeyer J, et al. (2008) Rescue surgery following percutaneous pulmonary valve implantation. Eur J Cardiothorac Surg 33: 607–612.

90. Fedderly RT (1999) Left ventricular outflow obstruction. Pediatr Clin North Am 46: 369–384.

91. McCrindle BW (1996) Independent predictors of immediate results of percutaneous balloon aortic valvotomy in children. Valvuloplasty and Angioplasty of Congenital Anomalies (VACA) Registry Investigators. Am J Cardiol 77: 286–293.

92. Fratz S, Gildein HP, Balling G, et al. (2008) Aortic valvuloplasty in pediatric patients substantially postpones the need for aortic valve surgery: a single-center experience of 188 patients after up to 17.5 years of follow-up. Circulation 117: 1201–1206.

93. McCrindle BW, Blackstone EH, Williams WG, et al. (2001) Are outcomes of surgical versus transcatheter balloon valvotomy equivalent in neonatal critical aortic stenosis? Circulation 104: I152–I158.

94. Corno AF (2005) Borderline left ventricle. Eur J Cardiothorac Surg 27: 67–73.

95. Han RK, Gurofsky RC, Lee KJ, et al. (2007) Outcome and growth potential of left heart structures after neonatal intervention for aortic valve stenosis. J Am Coll Cardiol 50: 2406–2414.

96. Weber HS (2006) Catheter management of aortic valve stenosis in neonates and children. Catheter Cardiovasc Interv 67: 947–955.

97. Karagöz T, Aypar E, Erdoğan I, et al. (2008) Congenital aortic stenosis: a novel technique for ventricular pacing during valvuloplasty. Catheter Cardiovasc Interv 72: 527–530.

98. McCrindle BW, Jones TK, Morrow WR, et al. (1996) Acute results of balloon angioplasty of native coarctation versus recurrent aortic obstruction are equivalent. Valvuloplasty and Angioplasty of Congenital Anomalies (VACA) Registry Investigators. J Am Coll Cardiol 28: 1810–1817.

99. Tynan M, Finley JP, Fontes V, et al. (1990) Balloon angioplasty for the treatment of native coarctation: results of Valvuloplasty and Angioplasty of Congenital Anomalies Registry. Am J Cardiol 65: 790–792.

100. Rodés-Cabau J, Miró J, Dancea A, et al. (2007) Comparison of surgical and transcatheter treatment for native coarctation of the aorta in patients greater than or equal to 1 year old. The Quebec Native Coarctation of the Aorta study. Am Heart J 154: 186–192.

101. Hellenbrand WE, Allen HD, Golinko RJ, et al. (1990) Balloon angioplasty for aortic recoarctation: results of Valvuloplasty and Angioplasty of Congenital Anomalies Registry. Am J Cardiol 65: 793–797.

102. Auslender M, Beekman RH, Lloyd TR (1995) Transcatheter closure of atrial septal defects. J Interv Cardiol 8: 533–542.

103. Cowley CG, Lloyd TR, Bove EL, et al. (2001) Comparison of results of closure of secundum atrial septal defect by surgery versus Amplatzer septal occluder. Am J Cardiol 88: 589–591.

104. Hijazi ZM, Hakim F, Al-Fadley F, et al. (2000) Transcatheter closure of single muscular ventricular septal defects using the amplatzer muscular VSD occluder: initial results and technical considerations. Catheter Cardiovasc Interv 49: 167–172.

105. Laussen PC, Hansen DD, Perry SB, et al. (1995) Transcatheter closure of ventricular septal defects: hemodynamic instability and anesthetic management. Anesth Analg 80: 1076–1082.

106. Beekman RH, Shim D, Lloyd TR (1995) Embolization therapy in pediatric cardiology. J Interv Cardiol 8: 543–556.

107. Rashkind WJ, Miller WW (1966) Creation of an atrial septal defect without thoracotomy. A palliative approach to complete transposition of the great arteries. JAMA 196: 991–992.

108. Galantowicz M, Cheatham JP (2005) Lessons learned from the development of a new hybrid strategy for the management of hypoplastic left heart syndrome. Pediatr Cardiol 26: 190–199.

109. Galantowicz M, Cheatham JP, Phillips A, et al. (2008) Hybrid approach for hypoplastic left heart syndrome: intermediate results after the learning curve. Ann Thorac Surg 85: 2063–2070.

110. Caldarone CA, Benson L, Holtby H, et al. (2007) Initial experience with hybrid palliation for neonates with single-ventricle physiology. Ann Thorac Surg 84: 1294–1300.

111. Li J, Zhang G, Benson L, et al. (2007) Comparison of the profiles of postoperative systemic hemodynamics and oxygen transport in neonates after the hybrid or the Norwood procedure: a pilot study. Circulation 116 (Suppl 11): I179–I187.

112. De Oliveira NC, Ashburn DA, Khalid F, et al. (2004) Prevention of early sudden circulatory collapse after the Norwood operation. Circulation 110 (11 Suppl 1): II133–II138.

113. Sherlock RL, McQuillen PS, Miller SP (2009) Preventing brain injury in newborns with congenital heart disease: brain imaging and innovative trial designs. Stroke 40: 327–332.

114. Galli KK, Zimmerman RA, Jarvik GP, et al. (2004) Periventricular leukomalacia is common after neonatal cardiac surgery. J Thorac Cardiovasc Surg 127: 692–704.

115. Kugler JD, Danford DA, Houston K, Felix G (1997) Radiofrequency catheter ablation for paroxysmal supraventricular tachycardia in children and adolescents without structural heart disease. Pediatric EP Society, Radiofrequency Catheter Ablation Registry. Am J Cardiol 80: 1438–1443.

116. Renwick J, Kerr C, McTaggart R, Yeung J (1993) Cardiac electrophysiology and conduction pathway ablation. Can J Anaesth 40: 1053–1064.

117. Erickson CC, Walsh EP, Triedman JK, Saul JP (1994) Efficacy and safety of radiofrequency ablation in infants and young children <18 months of age. Am J Cardiol 74: 944–947.

118. Hebe J, Hansen P, Ouyang F, et al. (2000) Radiofrequency catheter ablation of tachycardia in patients with congenital heart disease. Pediatr Cardiol 21: 557–575.

119. Szili-Torok T, Kornyei L, Jordaens LJ (2008) Transcatheter ablation of arrhythmias associated with congenital heart disease. J Interv Card Electrophysiol 22: 161–166.

120. Sharpe MD, Dobkowski WB, Murkin JM, et al. (1994) The electrophysiologic effects of volatile anesthetics and sufentanil on the normal atrioventricular conduction system and accessory pathways in Wolff-Parkinson-White syndrome. Anesthesiology 80: 63–70.

121. Lavoie J, Walsh EP, Burrows FA, et al. (1995) Effects of propofol or isoflurane anesthesia on cardiac conduction in children undergoing radiofrequency catheter ablation for tachydysrhythmias. Anesthesiology 82: 884–887.

122. Sharpe MD, Cuillerier DJ, Lee JK, et al. (1999) Sevoflurane has no effect on sinoatrial node function or on normal atrioventricular and accessory pathway conduction in Wolff-Parkinson-White syndrome during alfentanil/midazolam anesthesia. Anesthesiology 90: 60–65.

123. Sharpe MD, Dobkowski WB, Murkin JM, et al. (1995) Propofol has no direct effect on sinoatrial node function or on normal atrioventricular and accessory pathway conduction in Wolff-Parkinson-White syndrome during alfentanil/midazolam anesthesia. Anesthesiology 82: 888–895.

124. Pires LA, Huang SK, Wagshal AB, Kulkarni RS (1996) Electrophysiological effects of propofol on the normal cardiac conduction system. Cardiology 87: 319–324.

125. Sharpe MD, Dobkowski WB, Murkin JM, et al. (1992) Alfentanil-midazolam anaesthesia has no electrophysiological effects upon the normal conduction system or accessory pathways in patients with Wolff-Parkinson-White syndrome. Can J Anaesth 39: 816–821.

126. Gomez-Arnau J, Marquez-Montes J, Avello F (1983) Fentanyl and droperidol effects on the refractoriness of the accessory pathway in the Wolff-Parkinson-White syndrome. Anesthesiology 58: 307–313.

127. Erb TO, Kanter RJ, Hall JM, et al. (2002) Comparison of electrophysiologic effects of propofol and isoflurane-based anesthetics in children undergoing radiofrequency catheter ablation for supraventricular tachycardia. Anesthesiology 96: 1386–1394.

128. Bosnjak ZJ, Kampine JP (1983) Effects of halothane, enflurane, and isoflurane on the SA node. Anesthesiology 58: 314–321.

129. Polic S, Atlee JL, Laszlo A, et al. (1991) Anesthetics and automaticity in latent pacemaker fibers. III. Effects of halothane and ouabain on automaticity of the sinoatrial node and subsidiary atrial pacemakers in the canine heart. Anesthesiology 75: 305–312.

130. Lai LP, Lin JL, Wu MH, et al. (1999) Usefulness of intravenous propofol anesthesia for radiofrequency catheter ablation in patients with tachyarrhythmias: infeasibility for pediatric patients with ectopic atrial tachycardia. Pacing Clin Electrophysiol 22: 1358–1364.

131. Warpechowski P, Lima GG, Medeiros CM, et al. (2006) Randomized study of propofol effect on electrophysiological properties of the atrioventricular node in patients with nodal reentrant tachycardia. Pacing Clin Electrophysiol 29: 1375–1382.

132. Bevilacqua L, Hordof A (1998) Cardiac pacing in children. Curr Opin Cardiol 13: 48–55.

133. Silka MJ, Kron J, Dunnigan A, Dick M (1993) Sudden cardiac death and the use of implantable cardioverter–defibrillators in pediatric patients. The Pediatric Electrophysiology Society. Circulation 87: 800–807.

134. Berger S, Dhala A, Friedberg DZ (1999) Sudden cardiac death in infants, children, and adolescents. Pediatr Clin North Am 46: 221–234.

135. McKenna WJ, Behr ER (2002) Hypertrophic cardiomyopathy: management, risk stratification, and prevention of sudden death. Heart 87: 169–176.

136. Harrison TC, Kessler D (2001) Arrhythmogenic right ventricular dysplasia/cardiomyopathy. Heart Lung 30: 360–369.

137. Alexander ME, Cecchin F, Walsh EP, et al. (2004) Implications of implantable cardioverter defibrillator therapy in congenital heart disease and pediatrics. J Cardiovasc Electrophysiol 15: 72–76.

28 Anesthesia for noncardiac surgery and magnetic resonance imaging

Laura K. Diaz, M.D.

Children's Hospital of Philadelphia, University of Pennsylvania School of Medicine, Philadelphia, Pennsylvania, USA

Introduction

In the USA each year nearly 32,000 children are born with congenital heart disease (CHD), with approximately 10,000 of these being critically ill infants [1]. Many of these children require the care of an anesthesiologist within the first year of life, as extracardiac anomalies are seen in up to 30% of infants with CHD [2,3] and may necessitate surgical intervention in the neonatal period prior to repair or palliation of their cardiac lesion. As a result of continuing advances in prenatal diagnosis, interventional cardiol-

ogy, pediatric cardiac surgery, anesthesia, and critical care, nearly all these children will survive to adulthood. These patients will subsequently return for additional palliative or reparative cardiac surgeries as well as more routine general surgeries.

Caring for young infants and children with underlying cardiac disease presents a unique set of challenges. Studies of morbidity and mortality in general pediatric anesthesia indicate that a greater risk of anesthesia exists for healthy infants and children, particularly those under 1 year of age, when compared with adults [4–6]. Flick et al. in a review of perioperative cardiac arrests (CA) occurring in pediatric patients at a tertiary care center also found the incidence of perioperative CA and the mortality after CA to be highest in neonates [7]. Studies of

Anesthesia for Congenital Heart Disease 2nd edition. Edited by Dean Andropoulos, Stephen Stayer, Isobel Russell and Emad Mossad.
© 2010 Blackwell Publishing.

closed malpractice claims in pediatric anesthesia also represent infants and young children as a particularly high-risk group, with claims involving children [8] and patients [9]. The Pediatric Perioperative Cardiac Arrest (POCA) Registry, formed in 1994, originally evaluated 289 cases of perioperative CA in children, which occurred between 1994 and 1997, with 150 of these arrests determined to be anesthetic related in origin. Patients [10]. Between 1998 and 2004, 397 reports of perioperative cardiac arrest in children were evaluated, with 49% of these judged to be anesthesia-related. Cardiovascular events replaced respiratory events as the primary etiology of cardiac arrest, with one-third of cardiovascular-related arrests classified as having an unclear etiology. Of these, 81% occurred in American Society of Anesthesiologists (ASA) physical status 3–5 children, one-third of who had CHD [11].

Studies have examined the incidence and spectrum of extracardiac malformations and chromosomal abnormalities associated with CHD. A necropsy study of 815 fetuses at a university hospital identified CHD in 16%, or 129 cases, with the most commonly observed defects being ventricular septal defect (VSD), atrial septal defect (ASD), hypoplastic left heart syndrome (HLHS), and double outlet right ventricle (DORV). In 66% of cases there were multiple associated cardiac malformations, and 66% had noncardiac malformations as well. The most common noncardiac malformations involved the central nervous (31%), genitourinary (GU) (26%), and gastrointestinal (GI) (24%) systems, with the respiratory (11%) and skeletal systems (8%) affected less frequently. Chromosomal anomalies were confirmed in 33% of cases, with all these cases complicated by additional cardiac (56%) or extracardiac (98%) malformations [12]. An analysis of pooled data from three large international birth defect databases found a similarly high incidence of associated noncardiac defects in infants with single ventricle, conotruncal anomalies, interrupted aortic arch (IAA), DORV, and endocardial cushion defects. Distribution of defects commonly involved the craniofacial, GI, GU, and musculoskeletal systems [13]. Noncardiac surgical interventions will be necessary in many of these children, often prior to repair or palliation of their CHD. Careful preoperative assessment and investigations are therefore required in order to plan a safe anesthetic, frequently involving multidisciplinary providers and recovery in a high acuity unit.

The influence of CHD on patient outcome after noncardiac surgery has also been described. A review of 191,261 inpatient anesthetics administered to children [14]. A 10-year study of patients with CHD undergoing inpatient and outpatient general surgery procedures in a university hospital showed the preoperative ASA classification to be the most accurate predictor of postoperative mortality, as no deaths were noted in ASA physical status 1 or 2 patients. Mortality was increased in patients with age [15]. Flick

et al. in evaluating the incidence of perioperative cardiac arrest in over 92,000 pediatric patients between 1988 and 2005 also found patients with CHD to be at significant risk as 87.5% of patients with perioperative CA had CHD [7]. In another retrospective study of children and adults with CHD undergoing noncardiac procedures, those patients with pulmonary hypertension, cyanosis, congestive heart failure (CHF), inpatient hospital status or age [16]. Patients with pulmonary hypertension and those with significant ventricular dysfunction are at particular risk for increased perioperative morbidity and postoperative monitoring in an intensive care setting is recommended [17,18].

Several common factors emerge from these studies. Although physiologically well-compensated patients may undergo non-cardiac surgery with minimal risk, certain patient groups have been identified as high risk: children less than 1 year or age, especially premature infants; patients with severe cyanosis, poorly compensated CHF or pulmonary hypertension; patients for emergency surgery and patients with multiple coexisting diseases.

A joint task force of the American College of Cardiology (ACC) and the American Heart Association (AHA) formulated practice guidelines for the perioperative care of adult patients with heart disease presenting for noncardiac surgery. [19] As increasing numbers of children and adults are surviving after palliative or reparative surgeries for CHD it will be important to develop similar strategies for their care.

Endocarditis prophylaxis

Infective endocarditis (IE) is the consequence of a set of complex preconditions whereby endothelial damage initially results in platelet deposition and subsequent formation of nonbacterial thrombotic endocarditis (NBTE). Bacteremia then allows adherence of bacteria to existent thrombi, with bacterial proliferation then occurring within the thrombi. Thus, in attempting to prevent IE two questions need to be addressed: does the patient manifest the requisite conditions for endothelial damage and formation of NBTE and is the proposed procedure generally associated with bacteremia of significant magnitude and composition to allow bacterial adherence and proliferation with the development of IE as the eventual outcome.

The goal of prophylaxis for IE is to provide appropriate antibiotic therapy to protect against organisms known to cause endocarditis during a period of time when the patient is at high risk for bacteremia with these organisms. The first recommendations for antibiotic prophylaxis against endocarditis were the result of the studies of Northrop and Crowley in 1943 [20], which showed a decrease in the incidence of bacteremia during dental extractions when the patients were given sulfathiazole prior to the procedure. Recommendations by the AHA for antibiotic prophylaxis prior to procedures likely to cause bacteremia followed several years later and have been regularly updated since. The AHA recommendations for the use of antibiotic prophylaxis were liberalized in 1997 due to an apparent increase in the incidence of bacterial endocarditis in the pediatric population over the preceding three decades [21]. However, the most recent AHA guidelines for antibiotic prophylaxis are more stringent [22], as the AHA committee is convinced that recommendations for the prophylaxis of IE should be evidence-based. Current opinion reflects the view that IE is more likely to result from frequent exposure to bacteremias that occur as a consequence of activities of daily living than those due to dental, GI, or GU tract procedures [23–26], as well as recognition of the development of virulent multidrug resistant bacteria in the community.

Current AHA recommendations address the question of whether IE prophylaxis should be recommended for patients at highest risk of acquiring IE or for patients at highest risk of adverse outcome from IE. Although its effectiveness has not been fully established, IE prophylaxis is recommended for cardiac conditions that are associated with the highest risk of adverse outcome for dental procedures (see Table 28.1). Dental procedures that mandate prophylaxis include those involving manipulation of gingival tissue, the periapical region of the teeth, and/or perforation of the oral mucosa. The recommendations also encourage choosing an antibiotic from a different class in patients who are receiving chronic antibiotic therapy. The current recommendations have also been approved by the American Dental Association [22]. A Cochrane review determined penicillin prophylaxis to be of no benefit with invasive dental procedures [27], and emphasis is now shifting toward appropriate oral hygiene rather than widespread antibiotic usage.

Except for the conditions listed in Table 28.1, the AHA no longer routinely recommends antibiotic prophylaxis for any other form of CHD. Institutional guidelines and practices often take precedence over the AHA guidelines

in determining individualized prophylaxis. Certain conditions are associated with the highest risk of acquisition of endocarditis over a lifetime. These include mitral valve prolapse (MVP), CHD, and rheumatic heart disease. The committee no longer recommends IE prophylaxis based solely on an increased lifetime risk of acquisition of IE. Other lesions associated with IE have historically included Marfan's syndrome with aortic valve disease, hypertrophic obstructive cardiomyopathy (HOCM), and any lesion producing high-velocity turbulent flow resulting in damage to the endocardial endothelium [28]. High-velocity flow lesions include VSDs, patent ductus arteriosus (PDA), aortic stenosis, and coarctation of the aorta. Interestingly, high-velocity regurgitant flow across a systemic atrioventricular (AV) or semilunar valve is considered a high-risk substrate, while high-velocity regurgitant flow across a tricuspid or pulmonary valve is of negligible risk [29].

Similar guidelines have been issued by the British Society for Antimicrobial Chemotherapy [30] and by the IE prophylaxis expert group in Australia [31]. The European Society of Cardiology has issued more liberal guidelines for IE prophylaxis. In addition to the list of conditions provided by the AHA, cardiac conditions for which the European Society advises IE prophylaxis include MVP with significant valvar regurgitation, valvar heart disease, noncyanotic CHD excluding ASD, and hypertrophic cardiomyopathy [32]. International recommendations have more liberal IE prophylaxis guidelines, and the suggested antibiotics are tailored to national usage. For a more comprehensive discussion, the reader is referred to the original publications [32, 33] (see Table 28.2).

Antibiotic regimens

The AHA recommends that a single dose of appropriate antibiotic be administered prior to the procedure. If inadvertently delayed, the dose should be administered up to 2 hours after the procedure. For dental procedures, prophylaxis is targeted toward streptococcus viridans and

Table 28.1 Cardiac conditions associated with the highest risk of adverse outcome from endocarditis for which prophylaxis with dental procedures is reasonable

Prosthetic cardiac valve
Previous infective endocarditis
Congenital heart disease
Unrepaired cyanotic CHD, including palliative shunts and conduits
Completely repaired congenital heart defect with prosthetic material or device, whether placed by surgery or catheter intervention during the first 6 mo after the procedure

Repaired CHD with residual defects at the site or adjacent to the site of a prosthetic patch or prosthetic device that inhibit endothelialization
Cardiac transplantation recipients who develop cardiac valvulopathy

CHD, congenital heart disease.
Source: Reproduced with permission from Reference [22]. See also the AHA Web site: www.americanheart.org.

Table 28.2 A comparison of recent guidelines reducing indications for infective endocarditis prophylaxis

Procedures listed	Predisposing conditions	
	High risk	Moderate risk
Dental procedures		
French (2002) [33]: Several procedures—extractions, scaling, etc.	Prophylaxis recommended	Prophylaxis optional
BSAC (2006) [30]: All dental procedures involving dento-gingival manipulations/endodontics	Prophylaxis recommended	Prophylaxis not recommended
AHA (2007) [21]: Any dental procedure that involves manipulation of oral mucosa	Prophylaxis recommended	Prophylaxis not recommended
ESC (2004) [32]: Dental procedures with risk of gingival/mucosal trauma	Prophylaxis recommended	Prophylaxis recommended
Australian (2008) [31]: Complex recommendations; extractions, periodontal procedures, reimplantation of avulsed teeth; surgical procedures involving periodontal/gingival tissue	Prophylaxis recommended	Prophylaxis not recommended/optional
Extradental procedures		
French (2002) [33]: Several procedures, e.g., colonoscopy	Prophylaxis recommended/optional	Prophylaxis optional/not recommended
BSAC (2006) [30]: Several procedures (esophageal laser therapy)	Prophylaxis recommended	Prophylaxis recommended
AHA (2007) [21]: Several procedures: diagnostic GI/GU procedure; any GI/GU procedures in the presence of intra-abdominal/GU infections; any procedure where antibiotic prophylaxis is indicated for surgical reasons	Prophylaxis not recommended Antibiotic regimen can be tailored to include an agent active against enterococci	Prophylaxis not recommended
ESC (2004) [32]: T&A, rigid bronchoscopy; surgery involving ENT/respiratory mucosa/urinary tract mucosa; any GI/GU procedures in the presence of intra abdominal/GU infections; instrumentation of GU/biliary tracts and esophageal dilation/sclerotherapy	Prophylaxis recommended	Prophylaxis optional/recommended
Australian (2008) [31]: T&A, rigid/flexible bronchoscopy with biopsy; surgery procedures in the presence of intra-abdominal/GU infections; any procedure where antibiotic prophylaxis is indicated for surgical reasons; localized abscesses; surgical procedures through infected skin	Prophylaxis recommended	Prophylaxis not recommended

GU, genitourinary; GI, gastrointestinal.
Source: Reproduced with permission and adapted from Reference [34].

typically use of a penicillin or cephalosporin would be recommended (see Table 28.3). However, high rates of resistance to penicillins, cephalosporins, and macrolides are being reported. For invasive procedures involving the respiratory tract, the antibiotic chosen (penicillins, cephalosporins, or vancomycin) should target *Staphylococcus aureus*. Vancomycin is appropriate for methicillin-resistant organisms. Although polymicrobial colonization or infection of the GI tract exists, enterococcus is the principal organism associated with GI or GU procedures that results in IE. In situations where an active GI or GU infection is present, it is recommended that a course of antibiotics to treat the infection should be completed prior to the procedure, and an infectious disease consultation obtained. Antibiotic therapy solely to prevent IE is not recommended for GI or GU procedures under the current guidelines. Only for infected lesions of the skin, subcutaneous tissues and/or musculoskeletal tissues is an antibiotic active against staphylococci and hemolytic streptococci recom-

mended. Patients receiving anticoagulant therapy should not receive intramuscular (IM) antibiotics. Perioperative antibiotic prophylaxis for cardiac surgery is targeted toward staphylococci, and should be initiated prior to surgical incision. Cephalosporins are most frequently utilized perioperatively for a period not exceeding 48 hours (see Table 28.4).

In summary, current AHA guidelines have been determined by two main factors:

1 IE is more often the consequence of bacteremias associated with activities of daily living, and even if prophylaxis was 100% effective, only an extremely small number of cases of IE might be prevented by antibiotic prophylaxis prior to dental or surgical procedures.

2 There has been an increase in the development of virulent multidrug resistant bacteria in the community.

Although the current guidelines were published in 2007, institutional practices vary and there is reluctance to avoid prophylaxis until further evidence is available. At the

Table 28.3 American Heart Association guidelines for dental procedure prophylaxis 2007

| Situation | Drug | Single dose 30–60 min before dental procedure | |
		Adults	Children
Oral	Amoxicillin	2 g	50 mg/kg
Unable to take oral medication	Ampicillin *OR*	2 g IM/IV	50 mg/kg IM/IV
	Cefazolin/ceftriaxone	1 g IM/IV	50 mg/kg IM/IV
Allergic to penicillins/oral	Cephalexin *OR*	2 g	50 mg/kg IM/IV
	Clindamycin *OR*	600 mg	20 mg/kg IM/IV
	Azithromycin/clarithromycin	500 mg	15 mg/kg
Allergic to penicillins/unable to take oral medication	Cefazolin/ceftriaxone *OR*	1 g IM/IV	50 mg/kg IM/IV
	Clindamycin	600 mg	20 mg/kg

Vancomycin is an alternative for patients who are unable to tolerate a β-lactam or where the infective agent is considered to be methicillin resistant *Staphylococcus aureus*.
Source: Reproduced with permission from Reference [22]. See also the AHA Web site: www.americanheart.org.

Table 28.4 Current American Heart Association guidelines for endocarditis prophylaxis 2007

Procedures	Organism targeted/antibiotics/considerations
Dental	

Dental procedures that involve
  Manipulation of gingival tissue
  Periapical region of the teeth
  Perforation of oral mucosa
	Viridans group streptococci

May be reasonable for
  Biopsies
  Orthodontic band
  Suture removal	

Respiratory tract	

Procedures involving incision of the respiratory mucosa
  Tonsillectomy
  Adenoidectomy
	Viridans group streptococci
	Viridans group streptococci
	Staphylococcus aureus (antibiotic regimen should include a antistaphylococcal penicillin/cephalosporin/vancomycin)

Bronchoscopy, when associated with incision of the mucosa Bronchoscopic biopsy	
Invasive respiratory tract procedure to treat established infection Empyema/pulmonary abscess	If MRSA is suspected vancomycin would be the antibiotic of choice
Gastrointestinal/genitourinary	Polymicrobial colonization; enterococcus is the organism most likely to cause IE.
General GI/GU procedures including diagnostic upper and lower GI endoscopy	Increasing incidence of drug resistance to penicillin/aminoglycosides and vancomycin.
Elective cystoscopy or GU procedures in the presence of urinary tract colonization with or active enterococcal UTI	Prophylaxis solely to prevent IE is not routinely recommended
Emergent procedures in the presence or enterococcal UTI	Prophylaxis to prevent surgical site/wound infections/sepsis should include antibiotic active against enterococcus, e.g., penicillin, ampicillin, piperacillin, and vancomycin Eradication of enterococcal infection prior to procedure Prophylaxis with agent active against enterococcus
Procedures on infected skin, skin structure, or musculoskeletal tissue	Polymicrobial infections. Possible IE pathogens include staphylococci and β-hemolytic streptococci; antistaphylococcal penicillin/cephalosporin/clindamycin/vancomycin

GU, genitourinary; GI, gastrointestinal, UTI, urinary tract infection.
Source: Reproduced with permission from Reference [22]. See also the AHA Web site: www.americanheart.org.

author's institution, cases are evaluated on an individual basis with the child's cardiologist, and administration of antibiotic prophylaxis is based on a consensus between the cardiologist and the anesthesiologist.

Preoperative preparation and evaluation

Preoperative assessment

The spectrum of congenital and acquired cardiac lesions is so varied and the type of noncardiac surgeries performed so diverse that formulating one set of rules for evaluation and perioperative care of these patients is extremely difficult. One may begin by asking: is the child's cardiac disease the primary consideration in his or her perioperative care, one of several considerations, or a relatively minor consideration? A premature newborn with single ventricle physiology presenting for repair of a tracheoesophageal fistula is representative of an unrepaired, critically ill patient whose cardiac disease will directly impact anesthetic and postoperative management. A 6-year-old child with Down syndrome, repaired AV canal defect, and obstructive sleep apnea requiring tonsillectomy and adenoidectomy presents both cardiac and airway management issues, while a child who has previously undergone successful close of an ASD does not even require endocarditis prophylaxis. Children with unrepaired or palliated heart disease, children requiring surgery as a result of their cardiac disease, and children undergoing emergent surgery tend to be more critically ill and require more intensive preoperative preparation and assessment. An understanding of the child's underlying lesion, the residua and sequelae of any reparative or palliative surgeries he or she has undergone, and his or her current functional status will aid in determining whether the patient requires a cardiology consultation before proceeding with surgery or whether information from the parents and records of previous hospitalizations and clinic visits will suffice.

A thorough history is essential, including both details of the present indication for surgery and the past history of cardiac disease (see Table 28.5) of previous surgeries or catheterizations may be obtained from old medical records, it is equally important to obtain information from the parents regarding the patient's current state of health, activity level, growth and development, exercise tolerance, and any recent changes from her or her baseline condition. In infants the ability to appropriately feed and gain weight usually indicates adequate cardiac reserve. Observation of the child during the preoperative interview often provides valuable information to supplement the verbal history: is the child active, playful, and age appropriate, or is he or she lethargic and failing to thrive compared to his or her peers? It is important to use

Table 28.5 Preoperative evaluation of the congenital heart disease patient

Review underlying anatomy and physiology of cardiac lesion
    Previous cardiac surgeries: palliative vs reparative
    Evaluate existing residua or sequelae

Assess other preexisting diseases or congenital anomalies
Review information from last cardiology examination
    Recent cardiac catheterization, echocardiography, or MRI

Functional status and reserve at time of last examination
Presence of high-risk factors
    Congestive heart failure
    Dysrhythmias
    Pulmonary hypertension
    Cyanosis

Review changes since last cardiology examination
    History and physical examination
    Laboratory data
    Current medications

Review proposed surgical procedure
    Elective vs emergent
    Expected length and invasiveness
    Need for endocarditis prophylaxis

Plan treatment of potential complications
    Dysrhythmias
    Pulmonary hypertension
    Ventricular dysfunction

Plan postoperative care
    Monitoring
    Pain management
    Cardiology follow-up as needed

Discuss anesthetic plan and risks with parents and/or guardians

as many sources of information as possible to assess the child, because the history obtained from a parent may not always be a reliable indicator of cardiac function. Parents may unwittingly minimize the child's symptoms or lack an adequate frame of reference for comparison with other children. In addition to the cardiac history, details of other medical problems must be solicited. Certain syndromes, such as Goldenhar's (hemifacial microsomia or facioauriculovertebral syndrome), may include both cardiac and airway malformations (see Table 28.6) and because airway management may be challenging in such patients, it is helpful to review any previous anesthetic records for problems with tracheal intubation. Details regarding feeding disorders, gastroesophageal reflux, frequent respiratory infections, reactive airway disease, seizure disorders, or developmental delay should also be sought. Obesity has also been found to be a common comorbidity in children with congenital or acquired heart disease, perhaps due in part to the real or perceived need for activity restriction. A cross-sectional review of children at two outpatient cardiology clinics found over 25% of patients to be overweight

Table 28.6 Common syndromes and chromosomal anomalies associated with congenital heart disease

Syndrome	Lesion	Cardiac lesion	Comments
Syndromes with airway issues and CHD			
CHARGE association		VSD, ASD, PDA, TOF	Micrognathia, possible difficult airway
Edwards syndrome	Trisomy 18	VSD, ASD, PDA	Micrognathia, small mouth, difficult intubation
DiGeorge sequence	Microdeletion 22q11.2	Aortic arch and conotruncal lesions	Short trachea—tendency to endobronchial intubation
Goldenhar syndrome		VSD, PDA, TOF, CoA	Maxillary and mandibular hypoplasia, C-spine anomalies—difficult intubation
Hurler syndrome	MPS 1, storage disorder	Multivalvular disease, CAD, cardiomyopathy	Macroglossia, short neck—extremely difficult intubation
Noonan syndrome		PS, ASD, cardiomyopathy	Short webbed neck, macrognathia—difficult intubation
Turner syndrome	Monosomy X	LVOTO, AS, HLHS, CoA	Micrognathia, webbed neck—difficult intubation
VATER association		VSD, TOF, ASD, PDA	Potential for difficult intubation
Chromosomal disorders associated with CHD			
Down syndrome	Trisomy 21	VSD, CAVC	Large tongue, atlanto occipital instability, duodenal atresia, hypothyroidism
Edwards syndrome	Trisomy 18	VSD, ASD, PDA	
Patau syndrome	Trisomy 13	VSD, PDA, ASD	
Turner syndrome	Monosomy X	LVOTO, AS, HLHS, CoA	
3p syndrome	Deletion 3p	CAVC	
Cri du Chat syndrome	Deletion 4p	Variable	
8p syndrome	Deletion 8p	CAVC	
9p syndrome	Deletion 9p	VSD, PDA, PS	
Williams syndrome	Microdeletion 7q11	SVAS, SVPS, branch PS	
Smith–Magenis syndrome	Microdeletion 17p11.2	ASD, VSD, PS, AV valve malformations	
Miller–Dieker syndrome	Microdeletion 17p13.3	TOF, VSD, PS	
CHARGE Association		VSD, ASD, PDA, TOF	cColoboma, heart, choanal atresia, retardation, genital and ear anomalies
DiGeorge sequence/catch 22	Microdeletion 22q11.2	Aortic arch and conotruncal lesions	Cardiac defects, abnormal facies, thymic aplasia, cleft palate, hypocalcemia
VATER association		VSD, TOF, ASD, PDA	Vertebral, anal, tracheo-esophageal, radial and renal anomalies
PHACE syndrome		VSD, PDA, CoA, arterial aneurysms	Posterior cranial fossa tumors, facial hemangiomas, arterial and cardiac and eye anomalies
Noonan syndrome		PS, ASD, cardiomyopathy	
Marfan syndrome		Aortic dissection, MVP, TVP	Joint laxity, pneumothorax, respiratory infections
Cornelia de Lange syndrome		VSD	
Ehler–Danlos syndrome		MVP, TVP, ASD, aortic root dilatation	Hyperextensible joints, hyperelastic skin
Ellis–Van Creveld syndrome		Single atrium, VSD	
Rubinstein–Taybi Syndrome		VSD	
Holt–Oram syndrome		ASD, VSD, CHB	
Scimitar syndrome		Anomalous PVR to IVC	Hypoplasia of right lung

VSD, ventricular septal defect; ASD, atrial septal defect; PDA, patent ductus arteriosus; TOF, tetralogy of Fallot; LVOTO, left ventricular outflow tract obstruction; HLHS, hypoplastic left heart syndrome; CHD, congenital heart disease; CAVC, complete atrioventricular canal; AV, atrioventricular; TVP, tricuspid valve prolapse; MVP, mitral valve prolapse; PVR, pulmonary venous return; IVC, inferior vena cava, CHB, complete heart block. PS, pulmonic stenosis; AS, aortic stenosis; SV, supravalvar

or obese [35], placing these children at additional risk for hypertension, type 2 diabetes, and asthma. A prospective study of 2025 children undergoing noncardiac surgery revealed that obese children demonstrated a higher incidence of difficult mask ventilation, airway obstruction, bronchospasm, major oxygen desaturation, and critical respiratory events during the perioperative period [36].

Recent illnesses should be noted, particularly respiratory tract infections. Upper and lower respiratory tract infections can cause changes in airway reactivity and pulmonary vascular resistance (PVR) which may be poorly tolerated in children with decreased pulmonary compliance or pulmonary hypertension. In particular, patients with bidirectional cavopulmonary shunt (Glenn) or total cavopulmonary anastomosis (Fontan) physiology may be compromised by changes in PVR. While studies suggest that active or recent upper respiratory infections (URIs) carry no increase in long-term morbidity or mortality [37], the increased likelihood of reversible morbidities such as laryngospasm, major desaturation events, or breath holding may pose an unacceptable risk in cardiac patients presenting for elective surgeries. Respiratory adverse events are common, and have been shown to occur in up to 53% of children undergoing noncardiac procedures under general anesthesia [38]. In a study of 713 children undergoing cardiac surgery, children with URIs had a significantly higher incidence of respiratory and postoperative complications when compared to children without URIs [39]. Similarly, in a case control study of 130 patients Flick et al. found the risk of laryngospasm to be increased in children with URIs or an airway anomaly, with the majority of events occurring either during induction or emergence from anesthesia [40]. Risk must be balanced against the possible benefit of surgery in patients who have frequent upper respiratory tract infections. This situation is most often observed in children presenting for ear, nose, and throat surgeries, because chronic otitis, sinusitis, or tonsillitis may be unresponsive to repeated courses of antibiotics and may require surgical intervention in order for improvement to occur.

Children with congenital cardiac lesions are often receiving numerous medications, including antiarrhythmics, angiotensin-converting enzyme (ACE) inhibitors, digitalis, and diuretics. Our practice is to continue cardiac medications throughout the perioperative period with as little interruption as possible with the possible exception of diuretics. Patients who have undergone cardiac transplantation should have arrangements made to assure continuance of their immunosuppressant medications throughout the perioperative period. Children on daily medications for reactive airway disease, severe gastroesophageal reflux and seizure disorders should also have these medications continued with as little interruption as possible.

Guidelines for the use of antithrombotic therapy for different clinical entities in children were recently published by the American College of Chest Physicians (ACCP) [41]. Patients with CHD may be receiving antithrombotic therapy for a variety of reasons, including the presence of systemic-to-PA (pulmonary artery) shunts, mechanical or biological prosthetic heart valves, a history of thrombosis involving a conduit or a shunt, recent transcatheter interventions or device placement, treatment of Kawasaki disease, and the presence of risk factors for thromboembolic events including Fontan physiology [42]. No specific pediatric guidelines exist for the discontinuation of antithrombotic medications prior to elective surgery, although the ACCP has recently formulated guidelines for perioperative management of antithrombotic therapy in adults [43].

Aspirin irreversibly inhibits cyclooxygenase (COX-1), and because platelets lack the synthetic machinery to regenerate significant amounts of COX, this inhibitory effect persists for the life of the platelet, approximately 10–14 days [44]. Clopidogrel, a thienopyridine derivative, is an irreversible inhibitor of platelet aggregation that is receiving increasing utilization in pediatric antithrombotic therapy. Recent studies have evaluated the safety and efficacy of clopidogrel in pediatric patients, as well as appropriate dosing regimens [42,45,46]. Clopidogrel's antiplatelet effects occur via modification of the platelet ADP receptor with subsequent activation of the glycoprotein IIb/IIIa complex, culminating in inhibition of platelet aggregation [47]. This pathway provides a level of platelet inhibition that is additive to the inhibition provided by aspirin. While surgeons frequently request that aspirin or clopidogrel therapy be stopped a week prior to elective surgery, this allows for only partial reversal of the antiplatelet effect. In patients who are dependent on a systemic-to-PA shunt for pulmonary blood flow (PBF), particularly patients who are exhibiting increasing levels of cyanosis, we do not routinely stop aspirin therapy preoperatively as the risk of increased bleeding is less severe than the risk of a thrombosed shunt [48]. We advocate awareness of the antiplatelet effects of aspirin or clopidogrel by avoidance of nasotracheal tubes and discussion regarding the need for possible platelet transfusion with the patient's family prior to surgery, particularly those surgeries where significant blood loss is anticipated. In order to optimize perioperative management of patients who are on combined antiplatelet (clopidogrel and aspirin) therapy, detailed discussions between the surgeon and anesthesiology team should be held regarding the appropriate timing for stopping these medications preoperatively, and platelets should be available for transfusion during surgery as profound bleeding may be seen.

The physical examination should include a detailed evaluation of the airway, chest, and heart, with any change from the child's baseline status carefully noted.

Wheezing, retractions, increased work of breathing, or a change in a cardiac murmur may require further investigation. If new onset arrhythmias are suspected, a 12-lead electrocardiogram (ECG) should be obtained along with a cardiology consultation prior to surgery. Examination of the extremities for cyanosis, edema, adequacy of perfusion, and possible vascular access sites is also important. Vital signs should include blood pressure measurements in all four extremities in patients with a history of coarctation of the aorta or aortic arch reconstruction. Height, weight, and baseline hemoglobin oxygen saturation should be recorded in all patients.

Recent chest radiographs should be reviewed for the presence of cardiomegaly, increased pulmonary vascular markings, and other abnormalities. A new chest radiograph should be obtained in any patient exhibiting new onset of cardiac or lower respiratory symptoms. Electrocardiogram may reveal ventricular hypertrophy or strain, residual bundle-branch block, and other rhythm disturbances.

While preoperative laboratory work is not universally required, a hematocrit is useful as an index for evaluating the degree of secondary erythrocytosis due to chronic hypoxemia among patients with cyanotic CHD. Severely cyanotic patients with hematocrits >60% may also demonstrate clotting factor abnormalities and/or thrombocytopenia [49]. Phlebotomy is not advocated for patients, however, unless they are experiencing severe symptoms of hyperviscosity syndrome (headache, dizziness, impaired mentation, visual disturbances, muscle weakness, or paresthesias) in the absence of dehydration or iron deficiency [50]. Repeated phlebotomies have been shown to increase the risk of cerebrovascular accident (CVA) by causing chronic iron deficiency, which in turn results in microcytosis and increased blood viscosity. While Ammash et al. found an increased incidence of CVAs in patients with cyanotic CHD, these events were not associated with increased hemoglobin or hematocrit but rather hypertension, atrial fibrillation, repeated phlebotomies, and iron deficiency [51]. Prior to elective phlebotomy volume replacement, low-dose iron therapy and consultation with the patient's cardiologist are recommended. Preoperative evaluation of serum electrolytes, particularly potassium, is recommended for patients receiving digoxin, ACE inhibitors, or diuretic therapy.

A review of all available information from previous surgeries, cardiac catheterizations, and cardiology clinic visits is imperative. Recent echocardiographic assessments of anatomy and ventricular function should be sought, and if the child's symptoms appear to be worsening, a cardiology consultation and follow-up echocardiogram may be advisable. Cardiac catheterization data are useful for reviewing intracardiac and PA pressures, saturations, and shunting. Whenever possible the patient's current physical status, anatomy, and physiology should be reviewed with his or her cardiologist in order to optimize anesthetic management and reassure parents who have frequently established a strong relationship with their child's cardiologist.

Emergency surgery presents additional management issues and often adds risk in several areas. Patients who have not been appropriately fasted or who present with bowel obstruction may be at increased risk for aspiration events. There may be little time preoperatively to optimize the patient's cardiac condition, along with difficulty obtaining complete cardiology and surgical records prior to the administration of an anesthetic. In these cases, the preoperative evaluation must be distilled into the most important factors: the nature and duration of the present illness, and the child's underlying cardiac disease, baseline status, and medications. Fasting status and the need for a rapid sequence induction must be considered in light of the child's cardiac lesion; pediatric patients who present for emergency surgery are at higher risk for pulmonary aspiration episodes regardless of fasting interval [52]. A patient who depends on a shunt for PBF, cyanotic patients, and patients who have undergone total cavopulmonary anastomosis (Fontan procedure) require intravenous (IV) hydration prior to induction of anesthesia if they are hypovolemic. Based on the child's condition and the nature of the emergency, a decision can be made as to whether to proceed with the case with no further workup and a review of available old records, or whether new consultations and studies should be obtained preoperatively. It should be recognized that in extreme cases the child's clinical status will make the decision for the anesthesiologist: the critically injured trauma patient cannot wait for a consultation with a cardiologist prior to entering the operating room. In many centers such patients are brought directly to the operating room for their initial resuscitation. In this situation maintaining preload, judiciously using inotropes to support ventricular function, and promptly treating acidosis are most important until more information can be obtained.

Fasting guidelines

Although a 6-hour or longer fast from solid foods is still recommended [53], NPO guidelines have been modified to allow ingestion of clear liquids until 2 hours prior to surgery. Studies in children undergoing cardiac surgery have shown no increase in gastric volume or acidity with this practice [54]. In addition to improved patient and parental satisfaction and avoidance of hypoglycemia, these guidelines offer clinical advantages to cyanotic and shunt-dependent patients who would be adversely affected by prolonged periods of fasting and possible dehydration. Children allowed clear liquids on the morning of surgery were found less likely to be dehydrated as measured by clinical findings of dry mucous membranes, delayed capillary refill, and unwell appearance [55]. It remains important to verify NPO times with parents prior to surgery as surgical delays can still occasionally result in patients who have been fasted for prolonged periods of time. These patients are best served by offering them clear liquids if time permits, or by starting an IV infusion prior to the induction of anesthesia if significant dehydration is suspected.

Premedication

Anesthetic care of the pediatric patient with heart disease begins with psychological preparation of the patient and his or her family for the proposed anesthetic and surgical procedure. Developing a rapport with the child and his or her family and identifying the child's specific needs can be as effective as a pharmacologic premedication in allaying anxiety prior to surgery; child life specialists and preoperative preparation programs can be helpful as well. Children who are at high risk for extreme preoperative anxiety include younger children, children with high baseline anxiety, and those who have had previous negative interactions with health care providers [56]. It is important to discuss the available alternatives for induction and maintenance of anesthesia and postoperative pain management so that both the child and the family feel comfortable with the proposed plans. Many of these patients have had previous heart surgeries or cardiac catheterizations, and their questions and concerns may be different from those of the family who has never visited the hospital before. Children who have had multiple surgical procedures have often developed strong personal preferences regarding the method of induction of anesthesia, and whenever possible these preferences should be respected.

There are multiple benefits to premedication for children with CHD. Certainly one of the major reasons for administering a pharmacologic premedication is to ease the child's separation from her or her parents. Even older children and teenagers often feel significant anxiety when the moment of separation arrives although they may maintain a calm facade until that time. Premedication may also facilitate the induction of anesthesia by decreasing the amount of inhalation or IV agents necessary for induction. In addition, it is safer and easier to induce a calm, cooperative child than an anxious, crying toddler or a combative older child. In cyanotic patients, the use of appropriate premedication may decrease their oxygen consumption, thereby increasing their oxygen saturation as they become calm and sedated. A study of children with CHD receiving IM scopolamine/morphine/secobarbital showed the effects of this premedication on SaO_2 in cyanotic children to be variable. Although the mean SaO_2 of the group increased, significant decreases in SaO_2 were noted in several individual patients [57]. Monitoring with continuous pulse oximetry and intermittent blood pressures is recommended after the administration of premedication. Personnel trained in airway management and necessary drugs and equipment for resuscitation should also be readily available.

In the pediatric cardiac population, the primary goals of premedication are to achieve sedation and anxiolysis with minimal hemodynamic or respiratory effects. A premedication that will not delay time to discharge is also desirable for patients undergoing outpatient surgery. The use of IM injections has been largely abandoned as oral premedications have been shown to be equally efficacious [58] and are better accepted by children. Intranasal midazolam provides effective anxiolysis and sedation with stable hemoglobin oxygen saturations and hemodynamic parameters but is poorly tolerated by children due to its bitter taste [59]. Intranasal administration of sufentanil, although better accepted than intranasal midazolam, was shown to have an unacceptably high incidence of desaturation and decreased chest wall compliance [60]. Oral transmucosal fentanyl citrate (Fentanyl Oralet) provides a pleasant vehicle for administration with a rapid onset of sedation but unfortunately is associated with a high incidence of undesirable side effects such as pruritus, vomiting, and occasional hypoxemia in children with CHD [61].

Midazolam has been used as an oral premedication by mixing the IV midazolam product with a variety of additives to enhance patient acceptance. Studies have shown a dose of 0.5 mg/kg will reliably produce sedation and anxiolysis at the time of separation from parents with no observed changes in heart rate (HR), systolic blood pressure, hemoglobin oxygen saturation, or respiratory rate. In addition, no increase in the incidence of postoperative vomiting or increase in time-to-discharge was noted. Although doses of 0.75 and 1 mg/kg were also efficacious in providing sedation and anxiolysis, an increase in loss of balance, blurred vision, and dysphoric reactions were observed at these higher doses [62]. Midazolam syrup (2 mg/mL, Roche Laboratories, Inc., Nutley, NJ) is available in a cherry flavored commercial preparation. In a comparison of ASA physical status 1–3 children receiving either 0.25, 0.5, or 1 mg/kg of the commercially prepared midazolam syrup, the smallest dose was found to be equally effective in providing sedation and anxiolysis, though a faster onset of sedation was noted with the larger doses. This is in contrast to previous studies utilizing nonstandard preparations, suggesting more consistent bioavailability of the commercial preparation [63]. For those children presenting with an IV line in place midazolam 0.05–0.2 mg/kg provides an effective premedication with minimal hemodynamic effects.

In patients who are unable or unwilling to accept an oral premedication and who have no IV access, IM ketamine provides a rapid and effective means of premedication. Ketamine 2–4 mg/kg IM will facilitate the acceptance of an inhalation induction of anesthesia within several minutes. With the lower dose of 2 mg/kg, excessive salivation has not been observed and the routine administration of an antisialogogue may not be necessary [64].

The risks of premedication include oversedation, which can result in airway obstruction, hypoxia, and hypercarbia. A statistically significant increase in PETCO$_2$ and decrease in SaO$_2$ was observed in children after they received either IM morphine and scopolamine or oral midazolam as premedication before cardiac surgery. Clinically significant changes in SaO$_2$ were seen both in children with and without preexisting pulmonary hypertension or cyanosis [65]. Care in avoiding hypercarbia is particularly important in patients with pulmonary hypertension because these patients have increased pulmonary vascular reactivity and are at risk for pulmonary hypertensive crises. These risks can be minimized by careful attention to patient selection and drug dosage along with appropriate monitoring after the premedication is administered. Often patients presenting for emergency surgery have received sedatives or narcotics in the emergency department, and this should be taken into account before additional medications are given.

Monitoring

Once the patient is in the operating room, standard noninvasive monitors are placed prior to induction of anesthesia. Occasionally, a crying patient will resist the placement of monitors, in which case a precordial stethoscope and pulse oximetry probe are applied and the remainder of the monitors are added as the child is going to sleep. Standard noninvasive monitors include pulse oximetry, oscillometric blood pressure measurement, precordial stethoscope, ECG, capnography, and temperature monitoring. An additional pulse oximetry probe should be placed to assure continuous monitoring of hemoglobin oxygen saturation particularly for infants, cyanotic children, or cases expected to be of long duration. In patients with vasoconstriction due to hypothermia or poor peripheral perfusion, a pulse oximetry probe may be placed on an ear lobe, the tongue, or the buccal mucosa [66]. Not only will a centrally located probe function more effectively during periods of hypothermia or vasoconstriction but it will also reflect periods of desaturation and recovery more quickly than peripheral sensors [67]. In the neonate, a pulse oximeter that "suddenly" stops working should warn of hypotension and/or poor peripheral perfusion. At these times, the presence of a second pulse oximetry probe is extremely useful to differentiate between failure of an individual probe versus a true inability of the oximetry probe to obtain a signal from the patient. Additional information to corroborate any acute changes in the patient's condition can be gained from examining trends in the patient's HR, blood pressure, and capnography tracing. Direct observation of the patient is also a critical source of monitoring information. Palpating arterial pulses, checking capillary refill, and feeling an infant's anterior fontanelle can yield important information regarding blood pressure, the quality of peripheral perfusion, as well as indirect assessment of fluid balance.

Depending on the duration and magnitude of the planned surgical procedure, as well as the child's cardiac lesion and preoperative condition, more invasive monitoring may be useful. Preoperative consultation with the surgeon can be helpful to discuss his or her expectations regarding the planned duration of surgery, potential blood loss, and the need for invasive monitoring intraoperatively and/or postoperatively. It is important to remember that many of these children have previously had arterial or central venous lines placed for cardiac procedures and that accessing these vessels again may be difficult. Cardiac catheterization diagrams often yield useful information regarding previously occluded vessels, and preoperative ultrasonography of central vessels can also provide valuable information regarding vessel patency. Should arterial or central venous line placement prove excessively difficult, the relative importance of such monitoring should be weighed against the risk and delays involved in multiple attempts. In cases where large fluid shifts or blood loss are expected, the placement of a urinary catheter aids in assessing ongoing urine output and fluid balance.

The presence of a classic or modified Blalock–Taussig (BT) shunt (systemic-to-PA shunt, often utilizing the subclavian artery), coarctation of the aorta, or previous radial artery cutdowns should be noted prior to attempting placement of a radial arterial line. Often this assessment may be more easily accomplished once anesthesia has been induced. The contralateral radial artery should be used for monitoring in the presence of a BT shunt or if a previous subclavian flap repair of coarctation of the aorta has been performed. The pulse oximetry probe should also be placed on the opposite side from the previous surgical intervention.

Central venous lines may be placed after reviewing the child's specific anatomy. In small infants with single ventricle physiology, it is usually advisable to avoid the right internal jugular vein if possible, because any stenosis of the superior vena cava would prove extremely detrimental to these children as they undergo their staged bidirectional cavopulmonary shunt (Glenn procedure) and total cavopulmonary anastomosis (Fontan procedure). Small (3 Fr) single lumen catheters may be placed if necessary.

In placing a central venous line in infants or children, audio Doppler or ultrasound guidance is very helpful both in facilitating cannulation of small vessels as well as in teaching successful cannulation techniques [68–70]. Such guidance may also decrease the incidence of arterial puncture [71] and the number of unsuccessful needle insertions [72]. Complications secondary to central venous catheter placement (pneumothorax, hemothorax, hypotension, and bradycardia) accounted for half of the equipment-related CA in the most recent POCA data [11]. Careful attention to positioning of internal jugular or subclavian venous lines is warranted as perforation of the heart with resultant pericardial tamponade is a devastating and potentially fatal complication [73, 74]. A simple formula utilizing the child's height as a guide for depth of insertion has been studied and validated in infants and children. Using this formula:

[Height in centimeters/10] − 1 for patients < 100 cm, and

[Height in centimeters/10] − 2 for children > 100 cm

yields placement of the central venous line above the right atrium in 97% of patients [75]. PA catheters are only rarely used in children and the utility of the information to be gained must be measured against the difficulty and risk of placing such a line.

Transesophageal echocardiography (TEE) can be used during major noncardiac surgeries and often proves helpful in evaluating ventricular filling and function. A prospective study of pediatric patients undergoing scoliosis surgery in the prone position found TEE to be more useful than central venous pressure monitoring in determining cardiac volume and function [76].

Monitoring considerations in cyanotic patients

Studies of children with cyanotic CHD have demonstrated that pulse oximetry is less accurate below an SpO_2 reading of 80% and may overestimate the actual hemoglobin oxygen saturation of the patient. Should extreme or prolonged desaturation occur, it is best to measure arterial blood gases to confirm the patient's actual PaO_2 [77]. Alternatively, the arterial hemoglobin oxygen saturation may be measured by analysis of an arterial blood sample in a laboratory CO-oximeter. It is also noteworthy that at lower saturations a higher degree of accuracy was noted when the sensor was placed on an ear rather than a finger [78].

Arterial desaturation due to intracardiac shunting is also associated with an increased arterial-to-end tidal ($PaCO_2$ to $PETCO_2$) difference, as a portion of mixed venous blood returning to the heart will bypass the lungs, adding blood that is low in oxygen and rich in carbon dioxide to the systemic circulation. Studies comparing acyanotic and cyanotic children with CHD have shown that $PETCO_2$ may significantly underestimate $PaCO_2$ in cyanotic children [79]. Individuals with unrepaired tetralogy of Fallot (TOF) (VSD, right ventricular outflow tract (RVOT) obstruction, overriding aorta, and right ventricular (RV) hypertrophy) may have varying degrees of right-to-left shunting depending on the degree of dynamic infundibular narrowing occurring and the resultant obstruction to PBF. In these patients, the relationship between $PETCO_2$ and $PaCO_2$ will also fluctuate, thus $PETCO_2$ will not reliably estimate $PaCO_2$ during surgery in this group of patients [80].

Special considerations for patients with pacemakers and implanted cardioverter-defibrillators

Indications for permanent pacemakers in patients with CHD include congenital complete heart block, surgically induced complete heart block, and sinus node or AV node dysfunction as a result of CHD. In recent years, increasing numbers of pediatric patients have had implantable cardioverter-defibrillators (ICDs) placed for prevention of sudden cardiac death (SCD) with indications of congenital or acquired long QT [81]. The risk of SCD in patients with CHD appears to be greatest in patients with repaired TOF, d-transposition of the great arteries (d-TGA), or aortic stenosis [82]. Epicardial pacing systems are employed in younger and smaller patients as well as those with residual intracardiac shunts.

Recently, published guidelines from the ACC/AHA advocate preoperative and postoperative interrogation of permanent pacemakers if at all possible [83]. Every patient with an ICD should undergo preoperative device interrogation. Previous recommendations to use a magnet to convert a pacemaker to asynchronous mode during surgery are no longer universally valid as most modern pacemakers are programmable and may be unpredictably affected by the placement of a magnet over the pacemaker, especially in the presence of electrocautery. Unipolar devices should be programmed to an asynchronous mode, and special algorithms such as rate-adaptive functions should be suspended prior to surgery [84]. Implanted cardioverter-defibrillators should have their antitachycardia and arrhythmia therapies disabled preoperatively by a cardiologist or other qualified individual and external methods of cardioversion or defibrillation should be available. Any necessary pacing function provided by the ICD should be reprogrammed for the duration of the procedure. Postoperatively, pacemakers and ICDs should be reinterrogated and reenabled [85] (see Table 28.7).

In patients with pacemakers or ICDs, it is important to monitor not only electrical but also mechanical evidence of cardiac activity. While the ECG gives indication of electrical activity, it does not guarantee that mechanical systoles are actually being generated with each QRS

Table 28.7 Evaluation and care of the patient with a pacemaker or implantable cardioverter-defibrillator

History
  Indication for placement of device
  Type of device
  Pacing mode
  Date device placed
  Date of last evaluation

Physical examination/laboratory
  Evaluate underlying rate, rhythm and hemodynamic stability: is
    patient device-dependent?
  Review recent ECG
  Determine anatomic position of generator
  Examination of leads on CXR

Interrogation of device by a trained individual
  Evaluate lead integrity
  Obtain current programming information
  Determine frequency of initiated therapies with ICDs
  Consult pacemaker representative if questions arise
  Reprogram device if necessary prior to surgery
  Disable antitachycardia therapies on ICDs preoperatively
  Disable rate-reponsive modes preoperatively

Intraoperative management
  Ensure electrical activity is converted to mechanical systole
  Have temporary pacing support available: transvenous vs transthoracic
  Ensure availability of trained personnel
  Electrocautery to be delivered in short bursts
    Consider use of bipolar electrocautery or ultrasonic scalpel
  Assure defibrillator capability
  Evaluate effects of anesthetic techniques on device function

Postoperative interrogation and reprogramming of device

CXR, chest X-ray; ICDs, implantable cardioverter-defibrillators.

complex. Manual palpation of the pulse, auscultation of heart sounds, pulse oximetry, plethysmography, and direct monitoring via arterial line are all useful methods to verify mechanical function of the heart. Continuous invasive arterial pressure monitoring is recommended for pacemaker-dependent patients with poorly tolerated escape rhythms. Backup methods to increase the HR or provide pacing should be available in the event of an emergency. External transcutaneous pacing systems should be in place for patients who have hemodynamic compromise without proper pacemaker function, but it is important to remember that only ventricular contractions will be generated. Patients who are dependent on atrial function, such as those who have undergone total cavopulmonary anastomosis (Fontan procedure), may remain hemodynamically compromised despite external pacing.

Electrocautery may inhibit or cause permanent changes in pacemaker function including asynchronous pacing, reprogramming, and/or damage to device circuitry [86]. Converting the pacemaker to the asynchronous mode will eliminate electrocautery-induced inhibition, but cir-

cuit damage may still occur [87]. Bipolar electrocautery should be utilized whenever possible in the patient with a pacemaker or ICD. If monopolar electrocautery is used, the electrocautery return pad should be placed as far away from the pacing generator as possible, and additionally the pacemaker generator/leads axis should not be located between the operative site and the grounding pad. If the pacemaker cannot be placed in an asynchronous mode and electrocautery adversely affects it, cautery current should be applied for not >1 second at a time with 10 seconds between burses of current to allow for maintenance of cardiac output (CO) [88]. Other potential sources of electromagnetic interference in addition to electrocautery include radiation therapy, magnetic resonance imaging (MRI), radio frequency (RF) ablation procedures, and lithotripsy. For further details, the reader is encouraged to refer to the ASA Practice Advisory for the Perioperative Management of Patients with Cardiac Rhythm Management Devices [89].

Intraoperative management

The anesthetic plan should be formulated prior to entering the operating room, taking into account the child's preoperative condition, the anticipated duration of surgery, the potential hemodynamic consequences of surgery, and the expected length of postoperative recovery.

Goals of anesthetic management include optimizing oxygen delivery and ventricular function within the range expected for an individual patient according to their preoperative assessment and underlying cardiac physiology. For most patients, a euvolemic state should be maintained. In general, efforts should be made to avoid increases in oxygen demand, HR, or contractility. Maintenance of normal sinus rhythm is especially important in patients with single ventricle physiology. Emergency cardiac resuscitation drugs should be immediately available for all patients; if complications arise due to hypotension or arrhythmias, immediate pharmacologic intervention is critical.

Induction

Induction of anesthesia may be accomplished in several ways. Many children will present without IV access prior to surgery and prefer not to have an IV started while awake. Hensley et al. [90] studied the effects of an inhalation induction with halothane and nitrous oxide in 25 children with cyanotic heart disease and found that oxygen saturation increased with induction, especially in those patients with dynamic RVOT obstruction. With the introduction of sevoflurane, an alternative to halothane finally existed for inhalation induction in children, with studies suggesting that sevoflurane provided improved hemodynamic stability in children with CHD. Russell et al. [91] compared the safety and efficacy of sevoflurane and halothane in 180 infants and children with CHD. Anesthesia was induced with either sevoflurane to a maximum of 8% or halothane to a maximum of 4%, with delivered concentrations decreased by half in children with CHF. Although episodes of hypotension were noted in both groups, patients receiving halothane experienced nearly twice as many episodes of severe hypotension. Moderate bradycardia and emergent drug use were also more prevalent in the group receiving halothane. Although appearing to offer hemodynamic advantages compared to halothane for inhalation induction of anesthesia in infants and children, sevoflurane has been associated with a 20% incidence of nodal rhythms in healthy infants [92]. Prolongation of the QTc interval in infants and children receiving sevoflurane has also been described [93] although the clinical significance of this is unclear, as sevoflurane does not appear to increase the propensity for torsadogenicity [94].

The presence of right-to-left shunting can slow the inhalation induction of anesthesia by decreasing the available flood flow to the lungs and therefore decreasing the rate of rise of inhaled anesthetic concentrations in the arterial blood [95]. Not only does the shunted blood not absorb any inhaled agent but it also dilutes the concentration of agent in systemic arterial blood as the two mix. This effect is more dramatic with poorly soluble agents such as sevoflurane and nitrous oxide in contrast to the more soluble agents, halothane and isoflurane [96]. A computer model demonstrated little effect on the speed of induction with left-to-right shunts or mixed right-to-left and left-to-right shunting [97].

For children presenting with existing IV access several alternatives exist. Propofol, a sedative-hypnotic, is a rapidly acting IV agent that can be utilized for both induction and maintenance of anesthesia. Its short half-life and antiemetic properties make it an ideal drug for day surgery patients. Doses ranging from 2.5 to 3.5 mg/kg are recommended for induction of anesthesia in pediatric patients [98]. Propofol can have significant hemodynamic effects, which must be considered carefully in more fragile patients. Williams et al. [99] compared the hemodynamic effects of propofol in 30 children with CHD. Sixteen patients had no intracardiac shunt, 6 had left-to-right shunts, and 8 had right-to-left shunts. Propofol was initially given as a 2 mg/kg bolus and then continued as an infusion. Both systemic mean arterial pressure (MAP) and systemic vascular resistance (SVR) decreased significantly, while systemic blood flow increased. In patients with cardiac shunts, this yielded an increase in right-to-left shunt flow, resulting in clinically important decreases in $PaCO_2$ and SpO_2 in cyanotic patients. Two patients with unrepaired TOF and left-to-right shunting exhibited reversal of shunt flow af-

ter administration of propofol. Propofol should be used with caution in patients whose PBF depends on balancing their systemic and PVRs and in patients who cannot tolerate systemic afterload reduction. Similarly, in comparing the hemodynamic effects of thiopental and propofol for IV induction in infants, Wodey et al. found that propofol decreased MAP to a greater degree than thiopental due to a more significant effect on afterload [100].

Etomidate, an imidazole derived sedative-hypnotic agent, is short-acting and has minimal cardiovascular effects, making it an extremely useful agent in critically ill patients undergoing short procedures. Due to its side effects of pain on injection, myoclonus, high incidence of postoperative nausea and vomiting, and possible adrenocorticoid suppression, its use has remained selective rather than widespread. Although prolonged use or multiple doses of etomidate may cause adrenal suppression, single doses of 0.3 mg/kg in children have not been shown to decrease cortisol levels below the lower limits of normal [101]. A prospective study of pediatric patients undergoing radio frequency ablation of SVT or device closure of ASD in the cardiac catheterization laboratory evaluated intracardiac pressures, oxygen saturations, and Qp:Qs pre- and postadministration of an induction dose of etomidate, finding no significant difference in any of the variables after drug administration [102]. In a study examining the effects of etomidate on failing and nonfailing human cardiac tissue, it was further shown that etomidate does not cause myocardial depression at clinically relevant concentrations [103], making etomidate an excellent alternative to propofol for the IV induction of anesthesia in children with marginal cardiac reserve.

Ketamine is a versatile drug that may be used for sedation, premedication, induction, or maintenance of anesthesia. It may be administered orally, intranasally, or rectally but is most commonly used via the IM or IV routes for induction of anesthesia. IM ketamine frequently proves useful for induction in severely developmentally delayed or autistic children who are unable to cooperate with an inhalation induction or placement of an IV preoperatively. When used intramuscularly for induction, doses of 4–10 mg/kg should be combined with an antisialogogue in order to avoid excess oral secretions. Although adult studies have shown conflicting results, ketamine has not been shown to increase PVR in children, even those with preexisting elevations in PVR, as long as the airway and ventilation are adequately maintained [104]. A recent study evaluated hemodynamic responses to ketamine in pediatric patients with documented pulmonary hypertension who were spontaneously breathing sevoflurane prior to placement of IV access and administration of ketamine. No change in mean PA pressure or PVR index was observed after administration of a 2 mg/kg ketamine bolus followed by a 10 μg/kg/min infusion. In addition, no changes were seen in arterial pH or PacO$_2$, demonstrating that ketamine does not augment respiratory depressant effects of sevoflurane [105]. While ketamine is a direct myocardial depressant, this effect is clinically manifest only in the catecholamine-depleted patient [106].

In critically ill patients, fentanyl and midazolam may be used for induction of anesthesia, particularly when tracheal extubation is not anticipated at the conclusion of surgery. Patients with poorly compensated CHF may not tolerate the myocardial depressant effects of inhaled agents, and an opioid–benzodiazepine anesthetic is more likely to provide hemodynamic stability during induction of anesthesia.

Maintenance of anesthesia

Shorter-acting muscle relaxants and narcotics have provided enhanced flexibility in planning an anesthetic without exclusive reliance on inhaled agents. In recent years, fentanyl has been the "gold standard" of narcotic anesthesia for pediatric cardiac patients. In a study of infants who had recently undergone congenital heart surgery, the administration of fentanyl 25 µg/kg over 1–2 minutes resulted in no significant changes in HR, mean PA pressure, PVR index, or cardiac index (CI) [107]. With the introduction of remifentanil, a nonspecific esterase-metabolized synthetic opioid, an anesthetic technique combining the hemodynamic stability of a high-dose opioid technique yet allowing tracheal extubation at the conclusion of surgery became possible. Pharmacokinetic studies of remifentanil in ASA physical status 1–4 pediatric patients ranging in age from 5 days to 17 years show a consistent half-life with means from 3.4 to 5.7 minutes [108]. Remifentanil's nonspecific esterase-based metabolism allows its elimination to be independent of CO, renal, or hepatic function [109]; in addition, it is not subject to the genetic variability and drug interactions seen with drugs that are dependent on plasma cholinesterase for clearance [110]. As with other potent opioids, however, remifentanil can be associated with bradycardia. Chavanaz et al., utilizing echocardiographic data in healthy pediatric patients, demonstrated that a remifentanil bolus (1 µg/kg) followed by an infusion (0.2–0.5 µg/kg/min) resulted in a significant decrease in HR and CI compared to baseline values. While atropine pretreatment prevented the decrease in HR, a dose-dependent decrease in MAP and CI was still observed, with spontaneous resolution as the infusion rate was decreased [111]. As remifentanil alone cannot reliability assure amnesia, the concomitant use of an inhaled agent, propofol infusion, or a benzodiazepine is important. Remifentanil is well suited for short procedure with intense stimulation followed by minimal postoperative pain such as bronchoscopy or foreign body removal. For procedure where

significant postoperative pain is anticipated plans should be made for the provision of postoperative analgesia prior to discontinuation of remifentanil in order to avoid the acute onset of pain in the postanesthesia care unit (PACU).

Many choices exist when considering the use of a neuromuscular blocking drug. For routine or rapid sequence induction of anesthesia, rocuronium 0.5–1.2 mg/kg may be used in place of succinylcholine [112]. Generally, the length of the surgical procedure and the cardiovascular profile of the individual drug will dictate the choice of blocking drug. For patients with compromised renal or hepatic function, cisatracurium is an excellent alternative, and in doses of 0.2 mg/kg has been shown to provide acceptable intubating conditions in 98% of pediatric patients in <2 minutes regardless of the anesthetic technique utilized, and without negatively impacting hemodynamic stability [113]. Although patients may breathe spontaneously for short procedures, controlled ventilation is optimal for most patients undergoing longer or more invasive procedures. Many patients with CHD cannot tolerate the high concentration of inhaled agent that is required during spontaneous ventilation. Appropriate mechanical ventilation can also help prevent the atelectasis and hypercarbia that often result from spontaneous ventilation while anesthetized. Postoperative ventilation should be considered for patients whose lungs were ventilated preoperatively, patients with poorly controlled CHF who have undergone major procedures, and patients who have had an unexpectedly complication intraoperative course.

Regional anesthesia is a useful adjunct to general anesthesia in children and may assist in providing both intraoperative and postoperative pain relief. Caudal blocks with bupivacaine or ropivacaine provide excellent postoperative pain relief for children undergoing lower extremity or urologic procedures [114]. Preservative free morphine (Duramorph™, Astromorph™) may be added for those children undergoing more extensive procedures who will have appropriate in-hospital monitoring postoperatively [115]. Preoperative coagulation studies should be obtained for severely cyanotic children who may be at risk for coagulation abnormalities if placement of an indwelling lumbar or thoracic epidural catheter is planned.

Emergence and postoperative management

Residual neuromuscular blockade should be reversed prior to tracheal extubation in patients who have received muscle relaxants. Adequate return of neuromuscular function should be assured prior to tracheal extubation by monitoring peripheral nerve stimulation, as well as by clinical observation of respiratory pattern, depth of respirations, and muscle tone.

Once tracheally extubated and transferred to the PACU, patients should be continuously monitored for adequacy of oxygenation and ventilation; it is important to remember that a pulse oximetry reading of 100% does not assure appropriate ventilation. Postoperative fluid management is especially important in patients with passive PBF (Glenn or Fontan physiology) and patients being treated for CHF. Control of postoperative nausea and vomiting allows patients to resume their oral medications as soon as possible. Postoperative pain may be controlled with incremental doses of fentanyl or morphine, and ketorolac 0.5 mg/kg may be utilized in patients without renal dysfunction or concerns regarding postoperative bleeding.

Considerations for outpatient surgery

Outpatient surgery provides many advantages to children and families, and the presence of CHD need not exclude children from consideration for day surgery. Even ASA physical status 3 patients may qualify for outpatient surgery if their cardiac disease is stable, their current condition optimized, and appropriate preoperative consultation with the child's cardiologist has occurred. In a series of 25 children with CHD undergoing outpatient surgery, including 4 with compensated CHF, only 2 adverse occurrences were noted in 27 anesthetics with neither occurrence related to the child's underlying heart disease [116]. It should be recognized, however, that children with chronic disease processes have limited physiologic reserve, and even when well controlled may be adversely affected by seemingly minor surgery. Prior to surgery, agreement should be reached between the family, surgeon, and anesthesiologist, ensuring that arrangements can be made for overnight observation should the surgery be protracted in length, blood loss more than minimal, or issues arise in postoperative management.

Children who have pacemakers or ICDs should not be cared for at freestanding surgery centers if personnel are not available to provide device interrogation and reprogramming, or if alternate methods of providing backup external pacing do not readily exist. Outpatient surgery should not include intrathoracic, intracranial, or major abdominal procedures, and the intraoperative blood loss and risk of postoperative hemorrhage should be minimal. No particular activity restriction or special care should be required postoperatively, and the child's parents should be able to follow care instructions and seek appropriate medical help if needed. Same-day discharge should be discouraged if the child cannot resume his or her home medications postoperatively or if the child will not have ready access to medical care once he or she has returned home. Families who live in remote areas several hours from the hospital are encouraged to stay overnight for observation or to stay close to the hospital for the first postoperative night before returning home. It is also preferable

for the outpatient surgery facility to be hospital-based or affiliated in the event that it is necessary to admit the child unexpectedly.

Upper respiratory tract infections occur frequently in children and can increase the risk of adverse respiratory events. Consequently, children with CHD should be evaluated with particular care prior to clearance for outpatient surgery. Factors to be considered include the child's overall appearance, activity level, and appetite; the onset and duration of symptoms; any fever or increase in white blood cell count; and the nature of the child's cough or nasal drainage. Children who snore, are exposed to passive smoke, have nasal congestion or a productive cough, or whose parents report they have a cold have been shown to have a higher probability of anesthetic complications than other children [117]. It is best in younger children or those requiring endotracheal intubation to reschedule surgery unless the symptoms are clearly noninfectious and related to seasonal or vasomotor rhinitis.

In order to be discharged home after same-day surgery specific criteria must be met. Vital signs including hemoglobin oxygen saturation must be stable and at baseline levels, and the child must be in no respiratory distress. An appropriate level of consciousness should be attained, pain well controlled, and age appropriate ambulation possible. Opinions vary on the advisability of forcing children to tolerate liquids prior to discharge from day surgery, as studies suggest that requiring children to drink in the PACU may increase the incidence of early vomiting and prolong their hospital stay [118]. If children are not willing to take oral liquids prior to discharge, they should receive appropriate IV fluid replacement to compensate for their hourly maintenance requirements during fasting, surgical, and PACU time. In addition, if nausea or vomiting has occurred it should be adequately treated and resolved prior to discharge. Children who are more compromised by their cardiac disease warrant more conservative treatment and should be able to tolerate oral fluids and take any necessary cardiac medications prior to discharge. The parents' comfort with the child's condition and readiness for discharge should be noted, and written instructions provided for the child's care after leaving the hospital.

Anesthetic management of specific lesions

A thorough understanding of the pathophysiology of each cardiac lesion is essential in order to provide optimal perioperative care for pediatric cardiac patients. Within each category of lesions, there exists a spectrum of severity and a variety of surgical treatments, resulting in varying pathophysiology even for children with the same anatomic diagnosis.

Paradoxical emboli are possible in any patient with a septal defect, and care should routinely be exercised to avoid air bubbles in IV tubing in any patient with CHD.

Tetralogy of Fallot

TOF with pulmonary atresia/TOF with absent pulmonary valve syndrome/TOF with complete AV canal defect

Anatomy/pathophysiology
TOF consists of an overriding aortic root, RVOT obstruction, a malalignment VSD or multiple VSDs, and RV hypertrophy. The RVOT obstruction may be valvar, subvalvar, supravalvar, or a combination. Both fixed and dynamic components of the RVOT obstruction may exist.

Variations/associated lesions
Absent pulmonary valve variant usually includes aneurysmal dilation of the PAs with resultant airway compression and tracheo/bronchomalacia. These patients may ultimately require tracheostomy and long-term ventilatory support. Patients who have TOF with pulmonary atresia require a systemic-to-pulmonary shunt in the newborn period to provide PBF. TOF may also be associated with complete AV canal, and may be seen in patients with CHARGE (coloboma, heart anomaly, choanal atresia, retardation, and genital and ear anomalies) association, velocardiofacial syndrome, DiGeorge syndrome, and Goldenhar's syndrome.

Issues in unrepaired patients
Symptomatology correlates with degree of RVOT obstruction. Dynamic obstruction results in hypercyanotic or "Tet" spells with right-to-left shunting of blood. Children commonly receive β-blockers, usually propranolol, to decrease infundibular spasm. Treatment of a hypercyanotic spell involves maneuvers to increase SVR or decrease infundibular spasm. These may include administration of oxygen, sedation, or deepening of the anesthetic level, augmentation of preload, and the use of phenylephrine to increase the SVR/PVR ratio. Abdominal compression may also result in increased venous return and an increase in SVR via compression of the aorta.

Issues in palliated patients
Modified BT (innominate or subclavian artery-to-PA) shunts are sometimes used to palliate children prior to definitive repair. Blood pressure monitoring may not be as accurate in the upper extremity ipsilateral to the shunt. The amount of PBF provided via a systemic-to-pulmonary shunt is directly related to the radius of the shunt and the pressure gradient between the systemic and PA pressures. If systemic blood pressure decreases, PBF will also decrease leading to hypoxemia. While a shunt that is too small will result in cyanosis, one that is too large can result in pulmonary edema and CHF.

Issues in repaired patients
Residual RVOT obstruction, residual VSD, and pulmonary insufficiency may exist postoperatively. Right bundle branch block is commonly seen on ECG. An increased prevalence of significant ventricular arrhythmias has been demonstrated in patients with severe pulmonary regurgitation and RV dysfunction [119]. Children who underwent repair later in life also have a higher risk of postoperative atrial and/or ventricular arrhythmias and SCD [120]. Patients with ventricular arrhythmias may require electrophysiologic studies and placement of an ICD.

Children with pulmonary atresia typically have right ventricle-to-pulmonary artery (RV-to-PA) conduits placed as part of their repair, and these may later become stenotic or regurgitant. Children with absent pulmonary valve syndrome often continue to have symptoms of tracheo/bronchomalacia and bronchospasm even after repair and plication of the PAs.

Special anesthetic concerns
Tachycardia, increased contractility, and dehydration can result in increased RVOT obstruction and should be avoided, especially in unrepaired patients. Care should be taken to avoid hypovolemia and hypotension in shunt-dependent children. Acute hypercyanotic events may be treated by increased SVR relative to PVR. A hypertrophied RV may have decreased compliance, and provision of adequate preload is necessary to maintain RV filling pressures. Eventual RV dysfunction secondary to free pulmonary insufficiency or continued hypertrophy due to RV-to-PA conduit stenosis may also be observed. Concerns after surgical repair of TOF include the presence of residual defects and the ability to detect and manage ventricular arrhythmias. New onset of arrhythmias noted prior to surgery requires a cardiology consult and evaluation. If the patient has an ICD, preoperative reprogramming is necessary and intraoperative placement of defibrillator and external pacing pads is recommended.

Atrial septal defects

Anatomy/pathophysiology

Left-to-right shunting results in atrial dilation, and RV volume overload along with increased PBF.

Variations/associated lesions

Sinus venosus defects are frequently associated with partial anomalous pulmonary venous connection, usually right sided. Primum ASDs are endocardial cushion defects and often associated with a cleft in the anterior leaflet of the mitral valve and resultant mitral regurgitation.

Issues in unrepaired patients

RV volume overload is commonly seen, but PA hypertension is rare. Atrial tachyarrhythmias are more common in older unrepaired patients.

Issues in repaired patients

Residual defects and atrial dysrhythmias may occur. Sinus node dysfunction is more likely after the repair of a sinus venosus defect, while residual mitral regurgitation is possible after repair of an ostium primum defect.

Ventricular septal defect

Anatomy/pathophysiology

Left-to-right shunting of blood results in ventricular volume overload, increased PBF, and possible CHF. The degree of shunting is determined by the size and location of the defect, along with the relative resistances of the pulmonary and systemic vascular beds.

Variations/associated lesions

Ventricular septal defects may occur as single or multiple defects; they are also associated with TOF, IAA, transposition of the great vessels, coarctation of the aorta, truncus arteriosus, and AV canal defects. Anterior malalignment defects as seen with TOF result in RVOT obstruction, while posterior malalignment defects can cause left ventricular outflow tract (LVOT) obstruction.

Issues in unrepaired patients

Ventricular septal defects result in increased PBF, potentially allowing the development of PA hypertension, pulmonary vascular occlusive disease (PVOD), and eventual Eisenmenger's syndrome. Increased respiratory infections, failure to thrive, and CHF may be seen. Aortic regurgitation is possible with subarterial defects.

Issues in palliated patients

Patients with multiple VSDs and severe CHF may have a PA band placed to limit PBF prior to definitive repair. Baseline preoperative hemoglobin oxygen saturations should be noted in these patients, as they may be relatively cyanotic due to limitation of their PBF.

Issues in repaired patients

Residual defects may exist. Right bundle branch block is frequently seen and may be secondary to right ventriculotomy or injury to the right bundle near the VSD [121]. Complete heart block may also occur after surgical repair. Postoperative ventricular arrhythmias are more likely in patients repaired later in life or in patients who have had ventriculotomies [122].

Special anesthetic concerns

Increased work of breathing, decreased pulmonary compliance, and frequent respiratory infections are commonly seen in unrepaired patients. Fluid overload should be avoided. Increasing the child's F_{IO_2} and lowering her or her P_{CO_2} will result in decreased PVR, and consequently increase PBF at the expense of systemic blood flow.

AV canal defect

Anatomy/pathophysiology

An ostium primum defect, common AV valve, and an interventricular communication result from failure of fusion of the endocardial cushions, with subsequent biatrial and biventricular hypertrophy.

Variations/associated lesions

This defect is often seen in children with trisomy 21 (Down syndrome). In the "unbalanced" form, hypoplasia of the right or left ventricle (LV) may make a two-ventricle repair difficult to achieve and single ventricle palliation may be required. A partial AV canal defect involves an ostium primum ASD and usually a cleft of the anterior leaflet of the mitral valve. Transitional AV canal defects include a partial AV canal defect as well as a smaller, restrictive VSD component.

Issues in unrepaired patients

Increased PBF, frequent respiratory infections, failure to thrive, and CHF are seen in these patients.

Issues in palliated patients

PA banding may be done on rare occasions prior to complete repair, and baseline oxygen saturations should be noted in these patients.

Issues in repaired patients

Residual atrial or ventricular defects, tricuspid, or mitral valve insufficiency, and ventricular dysfunction frequently exist. Heart block and residual PA hypertension may also be seen.

Special anesthetic considerations

Controlled ventilation is recommended due to decreased pulmonary compliance and possible PA hypertension. Patients with Down syndrome may also have an increased likelihood of upper airway obstruction.

Truncus arteriosus

Anatomy/pathophysiology

A single arterial trunk arises from both ventricles and supplies the coronary, pulmonary, and systemic circulations. A subarterial VSD is present. The truncal valve may have a varying number of leaflets (2–6) and may exhibit both stenosis and regurgitation.

Variations/associated lesions

IAA, coronary artery or PA anomalies, and a right aortic arch may be present. Truncus arteriosus is often associated with DiGeorge syndrome or microdeletion of the 22nd chromosome, which can also include hypocalcemia and T-cell deficiency.

Issues in unrepaired patients

As PVR falls, patients develop pulmonary overcirculation and manifest CHF with early development of PVOD. Truncal valve regurgitation may further worsen heart failure. Coronary ischemia may be seen due to low diastolic pressures. Alternatively, PA stenosis may be present, limiting PBF.

Issues in repaired patients

Residual ventricular dysfunction, VSDs, and pulmonary hypertension may exist postoperatively. An atrial defect may have been left as a "pop-off." Other possible postoperative sequelae include dysrhythmias and complete heart block. Right bundle branch block is nearly always seen on postoperative ECG due to the right ventriculotomy. The truncal valve may be stenotic or regurgitant, along with the RV-to-PA conduit.

Special anesthetic considerations

Neonatal patients with DiGeorge syndrome should have blood products irradiated and serum calcium levels checked. In addition, they may have associated findings of micrognathia, choanal atresia, esophageal atresia, imperforate anus, or diaphragmatic hernia.

Aortic stenosis

Anatomy/pathophysiology

The aortic valve may be unicommissural in neonates with critical aortic stenosis. Older children with aortic stenosis more frequently have a bicuspid aortic valve. Left ventricular pressure load and hypertrophy occur, and endocardial fibroelastosis may also be seen in neonates with aortic stenosis.

Variations/associated lesions

Other left-sided obstructive lesions such as mitral stenosis, hypoplastic ascending aorta, or hypoplastic LV may also be present. Aortic insufficiency may also be seen.

Issues in unrepaired patients

Pulmonary edema and pulmonary hypertension may be seen with severe aortic stenosis. Neonates may be ductal-dependent and can present in shock if ductal closure has occurred. Coronary ischemia may be seen. Older children may be asymptomatic despite moderate to severe aortic stenosis, or they may exhibit symptoms of angina, syncope, or easy fatiguability.

Issues in repaired patients

Patients who have undergone balloon valvuloplasty or surgical valvotomy may have resultant aortic insufficiency. Children may also undergo a Ross procedure, which involves replacement of the aortic valve with the native pulmonary valve, translocation of the coronaries to the new aortic valve, and placement of a valved homograft in the pulmonary position. Resultant complications can include coronary ischemia, RVOT conduit obstruction, aortic insufficiency, and ventricular dysfunction. A Ross–Konno procedure is performed when significant LVOT obstruction exists along with aortic stenosis, and involves patch enlargement of the LVOT along with the Ross procedure.

Special anesthetic considerations

Thickened myocardium will have an increased oxygen demand, and therefore, tachycardia, hypotension, dysrhythmias, and hypovolemia should be avoided along with decreases in SVR. Care should be exercised to maintain adequate coronary perfusion.

Subaortic stenosis, membrane-type subaortic stenosis, tunnel-type subaortic stenosis, dynamic/hypertrophic subaortic stenosis

Anatomy/pathophysiology

A discrete membrane or a long segment tunnel-type stenosis may exist beneath the aortic valve, resulting in left ventricular hypertrophy and aortic valve insufficiency.

Variations/associated lesions

Subaortic stenosis may be associated with coarctation of the aorta, aortic insufficiency, or VSD.

Issues in unrepaired patients

Patients with symptoms of chest pain, syncope, or new onset arrhythmias should be reevaluated by their cardiologist prior to elective surgery. A gradient >25 mm Hg is considered significant, and patients who are symptomatic or have a gradient >50 mm Hg are generally referred for surgical intervention. Patients with dynamic obstruction are often receiving β-blockers.

Issues in repaired patients

Patients with a discrete membrane may have resection of the membrane with possible injury to the mitral valve or creation of a VSD. A Konno procedure (aortoventriculoplasty) may be performed for tunnel-type stenosis, and postoperatively, these patients may demonstrate heart block, residual VSD, RVOT obstruction, and/or prosthetic valve complications. Recurrence of subaortic obstruction may also occur.

Special anesthetic considerations

It is important to maintain coronary perfusion pressure and normal SVR. Tachycardia, hypotension, and increased cardiac contractility should be avoided.

Supravalvar aortic stenosis

Anatomy/pathophysiology

Supravalvar aortic stenosis consists of a membranous or tubular supravalvar narrowing of the aorta with possible impairment of coronary filling and resultant left ventricular pressure overload and hypertrophy.

Variations/associated lesions

This lesion may be associated with Williams' syndrome, which also includes elfin facies, peripheral pulmonic stenosis, mental retardation, and neonatal hypercalcemia.

Issues in unrepaired patients

Patients may have chest pain, syncope, and ST-T wave segment changes on ECG. Sudden death with anesthesia has been reported in patients with Williams' syndrome due to myocardial ischemia, decreased CO, and/or ventricular arrhythmias [123–126].

Issues in repaired patients

Residual LVOT stenosis, aortic insufficiency, and coronary ischemia may occur.

Special anesthetic considerations

Avoid myocardial depressants and increases in PVR. Maintain preload, sinus rhythm, SVR, and coronary artery perfusion pressure.

Coarctation of the aorta

Anatomy/pathophysiology

Coarctation of the aorta is a constriction of the thoracic aorta, which may be either discrete or long segment, and usually occurs at the point of ductal insertion into the aorta. Left ventricular pressure overload and hypertrophy result with eventual development of upper extremity hypertension and aortic collaterals.

Variations/associated lesions

Coarctation of the aorta may be seen in Turner's syndrome along with webbed neck, short stature, and edematous hands and feet. It can also be associated with other left-sided obstructive lesions such as bicuspid aortic valve and aortic or subaortic stenosis. Coarctation of the aorta may also be associated with a VSD.

Issues in unrepaired patients

Patients with critical coarctation in the neonatal period are dependent on a PDA for distal aortic flow and frequently require a prostaglandin E_1 (PGE_1) infusion prior to repair in order to maintain ductal patency. Left ventricular overload and pulmonary edema may be evident. In older children, left ventricular hypertrophy, systemic hypertension, and development of collateral vessels are frequently seen. A blood pressure differential between the upper and lower extremities is usually evident.

Issues in repaired patients

Patients may have residual or recurrent coarctation and left ventricular hypertrophy. They may also continue to require antihypertensive therapy postrepair.

Special anesthetic considerations

Four extremity blood pressures should be noted in patients who have undergone coarctation repair to assess for potential restenosis. Left ventricular hypertrophy and systemic hypertension often persist after repair of coarctation. Blood pressures in the left arm may be inaccurate if subclavian flap angioplasty has been performed for repair of the coarctation.

Interrupted aortic arch

Anatomy/pathophysiology

IAA occurs when a complete interruption of the aortic arch exists, making distal perfusion dependent on the presence of a PDA. IAA is classified into three subtypes depending on the site of interruption.

Variations/associated lesions

A VSD is frequently present, especially in type B interruption (between the left subclavian and left carotid arteries). Other cardiac anomalies seen with IAA include bicuspid aortic valve, truncus arteriosus, TGA, and double inlet LV [127]. DiGeorge syndrome (22q11 microdeletion), which includes hypocalcemia, absent thymus, and abnormalities of the face, ears and palate, is commonly seen in patients with IAA, and appropriate diagnostic tests should be performed.

Issues in unrepaired patients

Unrepaired patients are dependent on a PDA for distal perfusion and require PGE_1 infusions until surgical repair is accomplished. Depending on the site of the interrup-

tion, hemoglobin oxygen saturations are generally noted to be higher in the right hand or upper extremity, as blood supply distal to the interruption will have mixed with PBF, yielding a lower SpO_2.

Issues in repaired patients

Residual VSD and heart block may be seen postoperatively, along with stenosis and a pressure gradient at the site of the arch repair. Late obstruction of the LVOT is possible.

Special anesthetic concerns

Velocardiofacial syndrome (Shprintzen syndrome) includes microcephaly, external ear anomalies, pharyngeal hypotonia, cleft palate, and micrognathia. It is due to the same chromosomal deletion as DiGeorge syndrome and has significant clinical overlap. Fluorescence in situ hybridization testing is usually but not always diagnostic. In addition to airway considerations, patients with DiGeorge or Shprintzen syndrome should have carefully monitored serum calcium levels. Blood products should be irradiated due to the likelihood of T-cell defects and the risk of graft versus host disease.

Single ventricle lesions and physiology

Anatomy/pathophysiology

The anatomy of patients classified as having single ventricle physiology may include any lesion or group of lesions in which a two-ventricle repair is not feasible. Generally, either both AV valves enter a single ventricular chamber, or there is atresia of an AV or semilunar valve. Intracardiac mixing of systemic and pulmonary venous blood flow occurs and ventricular output is shared between the pulmonary and systemic circulations. Patients with relative hypoplasia of one ventricle such as unbalanced AV canal defect or severe Ebstein's anomaly may also undergo single ventricle palliation.

The first stage in palliation involves establishing unobstructed blood flow from the systemic ventricle to both the systemic and pulmonary circuits with creation of a controlled source of PBF. This is usually accomplished by creating a modified BT shunt, but occasional patients may require PA banding to limit PBF. If the atrial septum is restrictive, an atrial septectomy is performed to assure adequate mixing. Certain patients may undergo a hybrid procedure instead of a traditional Stage I palliation. During a hybrid procedure the PDA is stented open during a cardiac catheterization procedure and, if restrictive, the atrial septum is ballooned and/or stented. The PAs are surgically banded and definitive aortic repair is deferred until the second stage palliative procedure is performed several months later. A bidirectional cavopulmonary shunt, generally performed as the second-stage palliative procedure, entails ligation of the systemic-to-pulmonary shunt and anastomosis of the superior vena cava to the PAs allowing bidirectional flow. The final palliative procedure for most single ventricle patients is a total cavopulmonary anastomosis, or Fontan procedure, which involves baffling the inferior vena cava flow to the PA-superior vena cava anastomosis, thus directing all venous return to the pulmonary circulation.

Issues in unoperated patients

Patients with single ventricle physiology have parallel circulations, and care requires appropriately managing systemic and PVRs in order to balance systemic and PBF. PGE_1 is generally used to maintain ductal patency prior to first-stage palliative surgery. Hemoglobin oxygen saturations should range between 75 and 85% when systemic and pulmonary circulations are appropriately balanced. In ventilated patients, the PCO_2 should be 40–45 mm Hg. Permissive hypercarbia with PCO_2 in the 50 seconds may occasionally be used for patients with pulmonary overcirculation in order to increase their PVR and decrease PBF. Generally, these patients are ventilated with an FIO_2 of 0.21 unless other pulmonary issues exist. Patients with persistently high oxygen saturations (>90%) typically have poor systemic perfusion and develop acidemia. The hematocrit should be kept at 40–45 in order to optimize oxygen carrying capacity.

Issues in patients after initial palliation

Patients may be dependent on a modified BT shunt for PBF, or alternately the "Sano modification" may have been utilized, providing PBF via an RV–PA connection. Saturations >85% indicate pulmonary overcirculation and patients may exhibit symptoms of CHF. Once the patient is anesthetized and mechanically ventilated their oxygen saturation often increases, requiring the adjustment of the FIO_2 and PCO_2 in order to maintain saturations between 75 and 85%. An acute drop in oxygen saturation along with the absence of a murmur indicates loss of shunt flow and is catastrophic.

Issues in patients after bidirectional cavopulmonary shunt (bidirectional Glenn procedure, or hemi-Fontan procedure)

Oxygen saturations will range from 75 to 85% as patients are still mixing oxygenated and deoxygenated blood for ejection from the systemic ventricle. Ventricular function is generally improved as the volume load has been removed from the heart. Systemic hypertension is frequently seen in these children.

Issues in patients after total cavopulmonary anastomosis (Fontan procedure)

Surgeons usually choose to place a fenestration in the atrial baffle allowing right-to-left shunting to occur, and these patients often have hemoglobin oxygen saturation of 80–90%. The presence of aortopulmonary collaterals or baffle leaks may also result in decreased systemic oxygen saturation. Atrial arrhythmias and ventricular dysfunction are frequently seen as late complications. Patients with Fontan physiology can also develop chronic complications of protein losing enteropathy and thrombus. The patient's volume status should be assessed preoperatively, and patients who are dehydrated should have an IV placed and adequate hydration assured prior to induction of anesthesia. Care should be taken to avoid hypovolemia, as PBF is dependent on preload. Normal sinus rhythm should be maintained if possible. A cardiologist or pacemaker representative should be available for patients with pacemakers, and external pacing or cardioversion should be available for patients who have a history of arrhythmias. Controlled ventilation is appropriate for most procedures as long as excessive airway pressures are avoided, and physiologic levels of positive end-expiratory pressure (PEEP) may be used to avoid atelectasis without impairing PBF.

Transposition of the great arteries: d-transposition of the great arteries with or without ventricular septal defect

Anatomy/pathophysiology

The PA arises from the morphologic LV, while the aorta is malpositioned anterior and rightward above the right ventricle. A PDA, ASD, and/or VSD must exist to allow mixing of pulmonary and systemic venous return prior to repair.

Variations/associated lesions

Ventricular septal defects, coarctation of the aorta, obstruction to PBF, and abnormal coronary artery anatomy may be seen with d-TGA.

Issues in unrepaired patients

Patients who do not have adequate mixing via an ASD or VSD are dependent on PGE_1 to maintain ductal patency prior to repair. If patients do not respond to PGE_1 a balloon atrial septostomy may be performed to improve mixing and reduce hypoxemia. Pulmonary vascular disease also develops quickly in unrepaired patients with TGA, especially in the presence of a VSD.

Issues in patients after atrial switch (Senning or Mustard)

Atrial arrhythmias, sinus node dysfunction, baffle leak or obstruction, and late right (systemic) ventricular dysfunction may be seen.

Issues in patients after arterial switch (Jatene procedure)

Arrhythmias may be a marker of coronary ischemia. Supravalvar aortic stenosis or pulmonic stenosis may be seen.

Issues in patients after Rastelli operation

The Rastelli operation is performed for children with d-TGA, VSD, and LVOT obstruction. Left ventricular outflow is baffled to the aorta, and a RV-to-PA conduit is placed. Late complications include residual VSD, subaortic stenosis, and conduit obstruction.

Special anesthetic considerations

Arrhythmias and late ventricular dysfunction are frequently seen in patients who have undergone an atrial switch. Ventricular function appears to be better preserved after an arterial switch operation.

Congenitally corrected TGA or l-TGA

Anatomy/pathophysiology

l-TGA or ventricular inversion implies that the morphologic LV is on the right side and the right ventricle is on the left side. TGA also exists such that the aorta arises from the left-sided, morphologic right ventricle, and the PA originates from the right-sided, morphologic LV. If no other defects exist the patient then has a series circulation, albeit with the right ventricle as the systemic ventricle. If no coexisting defects are present this lesion may go undetected for many years, although progressive RV dysfunction can occur.

Variations/associated lesions

Ventricular septal defect, LVOT (subpulmonic) obstruction, and tricuspid valve abnormalities may exist. Approximately 5–10% of children are born with complete heart block, and the incidence increases annually by about 2% [128].

Issues in unoperated patients

An increased incidence of complete heart block exists in patients with l-TGA. Depending on the presence or absence of pulmonary obstruction and a VSD, the patient may have cyanosis, pulmonary overcirculation, or be asymptomatic.

Issues in "repaired" patients

Heart block is common after repair of a VSD. Residual VSD and residual LVOT obstruction may be seen, along with late ventricular dysfunction.

Issues in anatomically repaired patients

A combined Senning (atrial switch)–arterial switch may be performed for patients without LVOT obstruction, and a combined Senning–Rastelli for patients with LVOT obstruction. These anatomic corrections result in the LV becoming the systemic ventricle. Residual VSD, systemic (tricuspid) valve regurgitation, baffle obstruction, and heart block may occur.

Special anesthetic considerations

Patients with pacemakers should be evaluated by the cardiologist or designated representative preoperatively and again postoperatively. The patient's underlying rate and rhythm should be known and pacing capability should be available intraoperatively. Late ventricular dysfunction is often seen in anatomically unrepaired patients.

Cardiac transplant patients

Initial etiology of heart failure/date of transplant

Patients are transplanted due to either cardiomyopathy, CHD, need for retransplantation, or acute myocarditis [129]. CHD is the most common indication for cardiac transplantation in patients <1 year of age, while cardiomyopathy is the most common in patients >1 year of age [130].

Special anesthetic considerations

Immunosuppressive regimens should be maintained during the perioperative period. Patients on cyclosporine, tacrolimus (FK506), or steroids frequently exhibit hypertension and may be taking ACE inhibitors or calcium channel antagonists. New onset arrhythmias are suggestive of acute rejection or coronary artery disease and should be investigated prior to surgery.

The denervated transplanted heart will not respond to atropine, thus isoproterenol should be available to increase the HR if necessary.

Long-term consequences of CHD

Pulmonary hypertension

Constant exposure of the pulmonary vascular bed to high flows due to left-to-right shunting lesions can lead to elevated PA pressures and the development of PVOD. Any prolonged obstruction to pulmonary venous drainage or exposure to high left atrial pressures can also result in increased pulmonary vascular pressures. The time to development of PVOD is variable according to the amount of flow and pressure the vessels are exposed to. Pulmonary veno-occlusive disease develops earlier in certain lesions, such as d-TGA with VSD, and in certain patient populations, such as children with Down syndrome [131]. Reversibility of these changes once a defect is repaired is variable as well.

While the structural changes affecting the pulmonary vascular bed may be fixed, a superimposed reactive component of vascular smooth muscle also exists that can be positively or negatively affected by a variety of factors. Increases in PVR are seen with acidosis, hypercarbia, hypoxia, hypothermia, increased sympathetic stimulation, and increased airway pressures, and these factors may act alone or in synergistic fashion [132]. PVR can be reduced, RV function improved, and the degree of intracardiac right-to-left shunting minimized by appropriate management of these variables. Conversely, acute increases in PVR can result in RV failure, hypoxemia, and death. Morray et al. [133] studied the effects of pH and PCO_2 on pulmonary hemodynamics in children with CHD, concluding that hypocarbic alkalosis decreases PA pressures and that higher PA pressures exhibit a more dramatic response to alkalosis. They also noted that hydrogen ion concentration, rather than carbon dioxide concentration, seems to be the most important factor mediating the decrease in PA pressures. Lung volumes and airway pressures also affect PVR. While lung volumes less than the patient's functional residual capacity can result in higher PVR due to hypoxic vasoconstriction, volumes above functional residual capacity can result in compression of intra-alveolar vessels.

Pulmonary arterial hypertension (PAH) has been shown to be a significant risk factor for postoperative in-hospital death in a study of >2000 infants and children undergoing cardiopulmonary bypass for the repair of CHD [134]. In two recent studies, the presence of PAH was shown to be a significant predictor of major perioperative car-

diovascular complications including pulmonary hypertensive crises, cardiac arrest, and death in pediatric patients undergoing cardiac catheterization or noncardiac surgery under anesthesia. Children with suprasystemic pulmonary arterial pressure were eight times more likely to experience adverse events than those with subsystemic pulmonary artery pressure (PAP) [135]. In adults with PAH undergoing noncardiac surgery, a history of pulmonary embolism, New York Heart Association (NYHA) functional class >II, intermediate to high-risk surgery (thoracic, abdominal, major orthopedic, vascular, and transplant), and duration of surgery >3 hours were independent predictors of increased short-term morbidity, including respiratory failure, arrhythmias, CHF, renal and hepatic insufficiency. RV hypertrophy, RV myocardial performance index >0.75, RV systolic pressure >2/3 systemic blood pressure, and the intraoperative use of vasopressors were predictive of increases in short-term mortality [136].

Current therapeutic strategies for the treatment of PAH are multiple and involve the use of pulmonary vasodilators such as calcium channel blockers, phosphodiesterase 5 (PDE5) inhibitors (sildenafil), prostacyclin and prostanoids, and endothelin receptor antagonists (bosentan), as well as heart failure therapy, oxygen, and anticoagulants. Severely affected patients require a constant central venous infusion of prostacyclin (epoprostenol or Flolan®) in order to lower PVR. Combination therapy is the norm, and patients are regularly reevaluated for disease progression or improvement. Patients with lung hypoplasia as part of their clinical spectrum are not infrequently ventilator dependent via a tracheostomy.

Patients with primary pulmonary hypertension may present for a variety of procedures while awaiting lung transplantation. Historically, this group of patients has been a very difficult population to safely sedate or anesthetize, and significant risk is associated with induction and emergence from general anesthesia. Preanesthetic assessment should include consultation with the patient's cardiologist and a review of the most recent cardiac catheterization or echocardiographic information in order to obtain a measure of PA pressures, PVR, and the degree of reactivity noted in the pulmonary vascular bed when exposed to 100% oxygen or other pulmonary vasodilators. RV performance, preservation of LV contractility, and position of the interventricular septum should also be assessed. The presence of preexisting cardiac disease and the direction of intracardiac shunting, if present, should be noted. It is important that a frank discussion of the high risk of anesthesia in these patients be held with the patient's family when anesthetic consent is obtained.

The pathophysiology and anesthetic implications of PAH have been well reviewed in the literature [137–139], and there is no "ideal" sedative/anesthetic agent for patients with PAH. Hypercarbia with exacerbation of pulmonary hypertension may be a risk in premedicated children during the preoperative period. Friesen et al. studied the effects of opiate versus benzodiazepine premedication on sedation and respiratory parameters. Forty-four children were randomly assigned to receive either IM morphine (0.2 mg/kg), scopolamine (0.01 mg/kg), or oral midazolam (0.75 mg/kg) 1 hour prior to anesthetic induction, with significant sedation noted after both regimens. $PtcCO_2$, $PETCO_2$, SpO_2, RR, and sedation score were monitored and clinically significant increases in $PtcCO_2$ (>45 mm Hg) and decreases in SpO_2 occurred in several patients, including those with pulmonary hypertension, suggesting that hypercarbia following premedication may pose a risk to children with CHD and pulmonary hypertension [140]. Another study of 50 infants undergoing cardiac catheterization compared three different sedation regimens used under conditions of spontaneous ventilation with a fourth regimen involving pancuronium, endotracheal intubation, and positive pressure ventilation. Regimens 1–3 were associated with clinically and statistically significant increases in $PETCO_2$ and decreases in SpO_2 [141]. Sedation regimens associated with respiratory depression in patients breathing spontaneously can exacerbate PAP and increase PVR in patients with pulmonary hypertension.

As noted by Burrows et al., anesthetic management should be guided by three considerations: (i) appropriate manipulation of those factors known to affect PVR; (ii) the effect of anesthetic agents on PVR; and (iii) maintenance of CO and coronary perfusion pressures [142]. Adequate depth of anesthesia should be assured prior to any airway manipulations such as tracheal intubation or suctioning in order to avoid acute increases in PVR that can lead to oxygen desaturation in patients who are able to shunt right-to-left or acute RV failure [143]. In patients without intracardiac shunting, increased PVR will cause hypotension secondary to decreased CO, frequently with resulting bradycardia. Treatment consists of hyperventilation with 100% oxygen, inotropic support of the right ventricle, administration of nitric oxide or other pulmonary vasodilators, and prompt treatment of any acidosis. Inhaled nitric oxide, an endothelium-derived vasodilator, may also be used to rapidly decrease PVR. Studies in infants and children have also demonstrated a blunting of the stress responses in the pulmonary circulation by the use of synthetic opioids such as fentanyl [144]. Ventilatory strategies, especially the use of PEEP, can profoundly alter cardiovascular pathophysiology by complex interactions that can influence cardiac function and output by altering RV preload and afterload. Resulting increases in PVR can potentially culminate in RV failure if excessive [145–147]. Given the propensity for desaturation and increases in PCO_2 with sedation and spontaneous ventilation, controlled ventilation is recommended in these patients, maintaining lung volumes at or around functional residual capacity with minimal PEEP and avoidance of high inspiratory pressures, hypercarbia, or hypoxemia. Preload should be maintained and hypotension avoided in these patients in order to provide normal CO along with adequate coronary artery flow and oxygen supply to the right ventricle. Dopamine, epinephrine, and milrinone should also be available to further improve cardiac function if necessary.

Postoperative pain management can be challenging in patients with significant PAH. Opioid mediated sedation and respiratory depression can have deleterious effects on PAP in the spontaneously breathing patient. Central neuraxial blockade carries significant risk in anticoagulated patients, and acute decreases in afterload can be deleterious, especially when the maintenance of SVR is critical for maintenance of RV perfusion. Local infiltration of the surgical site is often beneficial.

Our current approach to this patient population for sedation involves either the use of ketamine and/or midazolam. When possible, preservation of respiratory drive is a useful property as it allows avoidance of laryngoscopy and instrumentation of the airway, which are high-risk maneuvers in this patient population. If deeper levels of sedation are required however the risks of hypercarbia, hypoxemia, and/or potential airway obstruction may override the perceived advantages of avoiding general anesthesia. A laryngeal mask airway (LMA) may be useful for shorter procedures in order to minimize airway instrumentation, but in patients undergoing more extensive procedures, endotracheal intubation allows optimal control of oxygenation, ventilation, and the ability to aggressively manage a pulmonary hypertensive crisis. Carmosino et al. found the risk of complications in patients with PAH undergoing noncardiac surgery or cardiac catheterization to be independent of the method of airway management [17]. Induction of general anesthesia may be accomplished gently with small doses of ketamine, fentanyl, midazolam, and/or sevoflurane, followed by neuromuscular blockade and endotracheal intubation. Ketamine preserves SVR and left ventricular systolic pressure, thereby preserving coronary perfusion of the hypertrophied right ventricle and reducing the leftward septal shift, and preserving left ventricular filling and CO [137]. Postoperative management in an intensive care setting is recommended for all patients diagnosed with and undergoing treatment for PAH.

Congestive heart failure

CHF is the end product of continued increased pressure or volume load on the heart, resulting in signs and symptoms of jugular venous distention, hepatomegaly, poor peripheral perfusion, tachypnea, tachycardia, and failure to thrive. Chronic CHF also leads to increased work of breathing due to pulmonary congestion. Nonstructural causes of CHF in pediatric patients include idiopathic dilated cardiomyopathy, myocarditis, arrhythmias, muscular dystrophies, left ventricular noncompaction, metabolic disease, and drug toxicity [148]. An epidemiologic study of heart failure in pediatric patients found CHD to be the primary cause of heart failure during infancy, while arrhythmias, cardiomyopathies, and acquired heart disease were more likely etiologies in older children [149]. Patients are generally treated with digoxin, diuretics, and afterload reducing medications such as captopril or enalapril. Depending on the etiology of the heart failure, β-blockers and/or antiarrhythmic medications may also be utilized. Even after corrective cardiac surgery, many children remain on these medications in order to optimize cardiac function. Children with very poor cardiac function, particularly those awaiting cardiac transplantation, may be in the intensive care unit (ICU) preoperatively as they may require chronic milrinone infusions.

In children taking anticongestive medications, serum electrolytes should be checked prior to surgery. Loop diuretics such as furosemide can result in hypokalemia and hypochloremic alkalosis. Potassium sparing diuretics such as spironolactone and triamterene can result in hyperkalemia. Captopril, enalapril, and ACE inhibitors are also potassium sparing. Our practice is to give all cardiac medications on the morning of surgery and resume them as soon as possible after surgery in order to minimally disrupt the child's physiologic balance. Care should be taken to judiciously manage IV fluids in order to avoid electrolyte imbalance or fluid overload. When surgery is necessary for a patient with poorly controlled chronic CHF, consideration should be given to placing an arterial line for blood pressure and blood gas monitoring. For surgeries with significant anticipated blood loss or fluid shifts, central venous pressure monitoring is useful, along with placement of a urinary catheter for precise measurement of urine output. TEE may be considered for continuous monitoring of ventricular filling and function, and may provide better information for optimal intraoperative management of ventricular function than a PA catheter [150]. Dopamine may prove helpful intraoperatively to support CO and enhance renal blood flow. Mechanical ventilation should be utilized throughout surgery in patients with CHF and may also be necessary afterward in poorly compensated patients. Afterload reduction therapy should be reinstituted as soon as possible after surgery is completed.

Cyanosis and polycythemia

Cyanosis in patients with CHD can be the result of either right-to-left shunting with inadequate PBF or admixture of oxygenated and deoxygenated blood into the systemic circulation. Severe, long-standing cyanosis causes a variety of systemic derangements and hematologic, neurologic, vascular, respiratory, and coagulation abnormalities can all result.

One of the initial responses to cyanosis is an increase in erythropoietin levels with a subsequent increase in hemoglobin and hematocrit. Once the increase in red cell mass and hemoglobin in adequate to allay tissue hypoxemia the erythropoietin levels return to normal [151]. At hematocrit levels >65% increased blood viscosity can result in a decrease in the delivery of oxygen to tissues; this is especially true if iron deficiency is present, as it causes an increase in rigidity of the red cells which further increases the blood viscosity [152]. Hyperviscosity syndrome is characterized by symptoms of headache, dizziness, fatigue, visual disturbances, paresthesias, myalgias, and reduced mentation [153]. Increases in PVR, SVR, and a decrease in coronary blood flow can also be seen as blood viscosity increases. Preoperative phlebotomy is recommended only in patients who have hematocrits >65%, are experiencing symptoms of hyperviscosity, and are not dehydrated. Acute onset of symptomatic hyperviscosity syndrome can be seen in cyanotic patients whose hematocrit abruptly increases due to dehydration. In these patients, rehydration is recommended rather than phlebotomy. CVAs occur with greater frequency in cyanotic patients, particularly children under 4 years of age. Erythrocytosis alone is not felt to be a risk factor for cerebral arterial thrombosis, but dehydration in younger cyanotic patients can predispose to intracranial venous thrombosis with devastating consequences [154].

Increased bleeding tendencies and a wide variety of associated laboratory abnormalities have long been noted in cyanotic patients. When compared to acyanotic children a disproportionate number of cyanotic children are thrombocytopenic, with the degree of thrombocytopenia directly related to the severity of polycythemia. Abnormalities in prothrombin time, partial thromboplastin time, and individual factor deficiencies have also been described [155] and defy simple classification. Although these deficiencies may cause no symptoms other than easy bruising, severely cyanotic patients should have clotting studies prior to surgery. In surgeries expected to involve more than minimal blood loss fresh frozen plasma and platelets may be necessary to treat nonsurgical bleeding.

Cyanotic patients also exhibit respiratory abnormalities of importance to the anesthesiologist. The ventilatory response to hypoxia is significantly decreased in cyanotic children and directly proportional to the degree of cyanosis. This abnormality in ventilatory drive normalizes after surgical correction of cyanotic heart disease [156]. Patients with cyanotic heart disease also display chronic alveolar hyperventilation with abnormally high minute ventilation for a given amount of carbon dioxide production [157]; therefore, the metabolic and respiratory cost of eliminating carbon dioxide is very high in these children [158].

It is important that cyanotic children remain well hydrated throughout the perioperative period to avoid symptoms of hyperviscosity syndrome or thrombosis. This is particularly critical in those children who are dependent on a systemic-to-pulmonary shunt for their PBF. Children should be encouraged to take clear liquids until 2 hours prior to surgery, and an IV should be started on arrival to the hospital for provision of maintenance fluids until surgery. Due to their repeated need for IV access during hospitalizations and the tendency for neovascularization, these children often have small, tortuous veins. A 24 g IV may prove adequate for preoperative hydration, and induction of anesthesia and a larger IV may be placed after the child is anesthetized. During preoperative evaluation, the child's baseline range of hemoglobin oxygen saturation, HR, and blood pressure should be noted. Any history of stroke, seizure, or preexisting neurologic defects should also be documented. Care should be taken during the anesthetic to maintain normal fluid balance and cardiac function. The use of air filters in IV lines and meticulous attention to air in volume lines without filters is essential as paradoxical emboli may occur in children with right-to-left shunts. Controlled ventilation is recommended for all but the shortest procedures due to the ventilatory abnormalities in these patients. It is important to remember that end-tidal carbon dioxide monitoring underestimates $PaCO_2$ in cyanotic children and that this relationship may vary during surgery in those children whose cyanosis is due to mixing of oxygenated and deoxygenated blood [159].

Postoperative concerns include assurance of adequate respiratory drive, hemostasis, and control of nausea, and vomiting. IV fluids should be continued until the child's oral intake is adequate.

Arrhythmias

Many children who have undergone surgery for CHD are at increased risk for arrhythmias, particularly those who have had surgeries involving extensive atrial suture lines or ventriculotomies. Patients on medications for control of chronic arrhythmias should have these medications continued up to the time of surgery and restarted as soon postoperatively as feasible. Concerns have been raised regarding the safety of amiodarone in patients undergoing anesthesia [160], but given the extremely long elimination half-life of this drug it is not usually appropriate to discontinue it prior to surgery, as it would cause an unreasonable delay and possibly place the patient at risk for life-threatening arrhythmias. Preoperative consulta-

tion with the child's cardiologist is essential and a plan should be formulated for intraoperative monitoring and management of arrhythmias and potential hemodynamic complications.

Atrial arrhythmias are commonly seen in patients who have previously undergone surgery involving the atria or AV valves. Those who have had Mustard or Senning (atrial switch) procedures or a Fontan procedure (total cavopulmonary anastomosis) are at increasing risk for atrial dysrhythmias with each passing postoperative year. Ventricular dysrhythmias are more frequently seen in patients who have undergone ventriculotomies or had RV-to-PA conduits placed. Prior to the induction of anesthesia, the child's cardiologist should investigate any new onset of arrhythmias, particularly those causing dizziness, syncope, or chest pain.

In the rare patient with congenital complete heart block, the child's underlying rate, rhythm, and hemodynamic stability should be assessed with exercise studies or Holter monitoring prior to surgery [161]. The advisability of temporary transvenous pacing or the availability of intraoperative transcutaneous pacing should be discussed with the patient's surgeon and cardiologist preoperatively.

Anesthesia for MRI

MRI in pediatric patients is being used with increasing frequency as it provides excellent images of brain, spine, and soft tissue lesions without the use of ionizing radiation. Magnetic resonance (MR) is also an important modality for evaluation of patients with cardiac and vascular disease. Because all images are obtained in one time interval and because image quality depends on patient immobility to reduce motion artifact, pediatric anesthesiologists are frequently asked to provide sedation or general anesthesia for children undergoing MR scans.

MR scanners utilize high-strength magnetic fields and RF pulses to create tomographic images of the body. Patients are exposed to a static magnetic field, time-varying magnetic fields, and RF pulses. The patient is placed in a static magnetic field, typically at 1.5 T (approximately 30,000 times the intensity of the earth's magnetic field), and rapid minor variations of the magnetic field are then induced via transient application of magnetic field gradients during imaging. The static magnetic field causes a net orientation of protons along the long axis of the patient's body; when RF pulses are applied, the protons deviate away from the direction of the static magnetic field. When the transient RF pulse is removed the protons "relax" back to their original positions, resulting in the emission of an RF signal, which is then detected by a receiving coil. The necessary time for this realignment is known as the relaxation time and is specific for a given tissue. Evaluation of the varying rates of return of the different nuclei to their original alignment creates contrast between differential tissues in the image. Any movement of the patient during this process results in artifact and blurring of the desired images. Newer 3.0 T magnets with higher magnetic field strength can be used in children, allowing faster acquisition times and high spatial resolution but at the cost of substantially higher noise levels [162]. Gadolinium, a contrast agent, is a paramagnetic substance used to enhance proton relaxation, thus allowing improved image contrast between two adjacent tissues with differing amounts of perfusion. Although allergic reactions are rare, anaphylactoid reactions and death have been reported after use of gadolinium [163].

Due to the strength of the magnetic field and its ability to interfere with the function of implanted devices, certain contraindications exist for MR scanning. Absolute contraindications include electrically, magnetically, or mechanically activated implants such as pacemakers, implantable cardiac defibrillators, cochlear implants, neurostimulators, bone growth stimulators, and implantable drug infusion pumps. Although recent publications describe the use of MR in patients with pacemakers or ICDs, it is important to remember that changes in programming and lead thresholds have been described as a result of MR studies and no cardiac devices have been Food and Drug Administration (FDA) approved for use during MR scans [164]. Patients with external pacing wires, PA catheters, or other conductive wires should not undergo MRI due to the risk of the wire acting as an antenna and inducing burns or fibrillation [165]. Many aneurysm clips are ferromagnetic; if insufficient information regarding the nature of the clip is unavailable, the patient should not undergo an MR scan. Most prosthetic heart valves have been tested and found to safely tolerate MR scanning. Coils or stents placed in the catheterization laboratory should be attached sufficiently into the vessel wall after 6 weeks to make MR scanning possible without undue risk, although they can cause significant artifact on future scans. Nickel, stainless steel, titanium, and alloys are safe metals and may enter the scanner. Comprehensive lists of materials, devices, and implants that have been tested for ferromagnetic properties and deflection force may be found in various publications and Web sites that are regularly updated [166–168]. Appropriate screening forms for MR patients may also be accessed at www.MRIsafety.com [169].

Considerations for sedation and general anesthesia with MRI

The MR scanner is one of the most challenging environments anesthesiologists face, as it renders monitoring difficult and direct patient observation nearly impossible.

Multiple hazards exist in providing anesthesia for MR scanning, among them field avoidance, movement of the patient from the induction area to the scanner, hypothermia, possible injury from unsafe objects introduced into the scanner, and the administration of contrast material. Despite the complications of inducing anesthesia in a remote location and the difficulties in monitoring imposed by the magnetic field, the same standards of care apply as in the operating room. Patients requiring anesthesia for an MR scan should be given appropriate instructions for preanesthetic fasting and may be admitted through the ambulatory surgery area on the day of the procedure. Preoperative assessment should note the reasons for the scan, the information to be obtained, and any recent changes in the child's condition. After discussion of the anesthetic/sedation plan with the parents, an informed consent for sedation or general anesthesia should then be obtained and signed. In many institutions, consent is not obtained for the scan itself; it is incumbent on the anesthesiologist to be sure the appropriate documents have been signed and witnessed for provision of anesthesia. After completion of the scan, children return to the PACU for recovery and eventual discharge by the anesthesia staff.

Although MR scanning is not painful, it does require immobility for the duration of the scan and tolerance of a noisy, claustrophobic environment. For most infants and children, deep sedation or general anesthesia is necessary in order to obtain a successful scan. Teens and young adults with claustrophobia or anxiety disorders may also require sedation to tolerate a scan. The partial or complete loss of airway reflexes that accompanies deep sedation, coupled with the anesthesiologist's lack of immediate access to the patient, may make general anesthesia a safer alternative for patients with poorly controlled CHF, pulmonary hypertension, airway obstruction, or severe gastroesophageal reflux. Cardiac MR (CMR) places additional demands on the anesthesiologist as the scans tend to be longer in duration and can require periods of apnea during certain scan sequences. Depending on the number and length of breath-holding episodes necessary, general endotracheal anesthesia with controlled ventilation is often the only reasonable option [170]. CMR studies are also being requested with increasing frequency in infants and children from ICU settings, resulting in additional challenges for anesthesiologists in transporting and providing sedation or anesthesia for this patient population. Information gained from these studies is often critically important; however, as Sarikouch et al. found that 70% of ICU patients who underwent CMR studies had a subsequent catheter-based or surgical intervention based on the CMR findings [171].

Although rectally and orally administered drugs have been used for sedation, IV agents offer the advantage of increased flexibility should the scan take more time than originally anticipated or should the patient cough or move. Propofol is well suited for use in the MR scanner as it is easily titratable, does not require an MR compatible anesthetic machine or scavenging of gases, and allows the patient to maintain spontaneous ventilation and awaken promptly at the conclusion of the procedure. Frankville et al. [172] studied 30 ASA physical status 1 and 2 children undergoing MRI and found that after halothane induction and a propofol bolus of 2 mg/kg, a continuous infusion of propofol at 100 μg/kg/min provided good scanning conditions in all children with no episodes of desaturation noted during the scanning process. All children received supplemental oxygen by mask, remained breathing spontaneously throughout the study, and were able to maintain a patent airway with no intervention other than slight neck extension. It is important to note, however, that propofol may produce apnea after bolus doses and has a dose-dependent depressant effect on ventilation [173]; appropriate equipment to assist or control ventilation must always be readily available. In reviewing 258 infants who underwent MR studies utilizing either chloral hydrate, pentobarbital, or propofol for sedation, Dalal et al. found that infants who received propofol were ready to begin the scan sooner, had less movement inside the scanner, and were ready for discharge faster after conclusion of the scan when compared to the other two groups. A physician-supervised sedation nurse administered chloral hydrate and pentobarbital regimens, while propofol infusions were regulated by an anesthesiologist or a sedation-trained pediatrician. Even so, respiratory events were most common in the propofol group and on two occasions required the intervention of an anesthesiologist [174].

Barbiturates may also be successfully used for deep sedation and may be administered intravenously, orally, or rectally. IV pentobarbital was used by Galli et al. [175] for MR of the brain in infants [176]. Limitations to the use of IV pentobarbital also include the length of scan time required, as many CMR studies frequently take over an hour to complete, and the increased time to discharge in infants and children who have received pentobarbital [174].

Dexmedetomidine is a highly selective α2-adrenoreceptor agonist with sedative and analgesic properties. Although it does not have FDA approval for use in children, the use of dexmedetomidine for sedation of infants and children in multiple settings including the ICU and radiological imaging studies has been well described [177]. Dexmedetomidine is most commonly administered as a loading dose over 10 minutes followed by an infusion and has been successfully utilized for pediatric CT and MR sedation, although Mason and colleagues noted the need for higher infusion rates in children undergoing MR compared to CT [178–180]. The use of dexmedetomidine is considered to be contraindi-

cated in patients who are receiving digoxin, as it has been associated with bradycardia and cardiac arrest [181].

Many practitioners induce sedation or general anesthesia on the detachable scanner table outside the MR scanner room, which provides better proximity to an anesthesia car and drugs, and also allows the use of a metal laryngoscope and a conventional ferromagnetic stethoscope. Should resuscitation of the patient be necessary at any point, the child is brought out of the scanner so that standard equipment may be freely used without interference from the magnet. Once induction is complete and the patient is stable, the table is rolled into the scanner room and locked into place. Special attention is paid to positioning in order to optimally maintain the airway in patients whose tracheas have not been intubated. In smaller patients, a rolled sheet is often placed under the shoulders and rolled sheets on either side support the head. A variety of MR compatible anesthesia machines are now available with pneumatically or electronically driven ventilators capable of ventilating even premature infants. Alternatively, an MR compatible Siemens 900°C Servo ventilator (Siemens-Elema AB, Solna, Sweden) provides an effective means of ventilation for infants and children. Noninvasive (oscillometric) blood pressure monitoring, ECG, pulse oximetry, and capnography via endotracheal tube or nasal cannula are utilized. All MR scanners do not operate at the same frequency and therefore it is not only essential that monitoring equipment be MR compatible, but also that it has been tested to assure its proper functioning within each individual MR scanner [182]. The pulse oximeter probe should be placed as far from the scan site as possible, avoiding any loops in the cable which may act as an antenna and either absorb signal from the MR receiver or burn the patient due to induced current in the loop. Electrocardiogram wires should be braided to avoid looping of the cables and brought down the center of the table with a towel or blanket between the wires and the patient in order to protect against burns [183]. Remote visual monitoring via a television camera provides some opportunity to observe the patient should the anesthesiologist elect not to stay in the scanner with the patient. As noise levels in the scanner can reach 95–110 dB, earplugs should be placed in order to protect the patient's hearing during the scan, and should the anesthesiologist elect to stay in the scanner room during the study, he or she should wear protective earplugs as well. Temperature monitoring may be achieved by using liquid crystal temperature monitoring strips (CliniTemp, Hallcrest, Glenview, IL) or MR-compatible skin temperature monitors. Warm blankets and thermal packs are used to maintain body temperature, as the room must be kept cool to accommodate the magnet.

At the conclusion of the procedure, the patient is brought out of the scanning room on the scanner table and transferred to a PACU bed. Unless children are returning to an ICU, those who have received a general anesthesia may be extubated at this time. Depending on the proximity of the recovery area to the magnet, essential equipment for transport includes oxygen, a transport monitor capable of monitoring ECG, pulse oximetry and noninvasive (oscillometric) blood pressure, a "tackle box" with emergency drugs and airway equipment, and elevator override keys to ensure rapid, uninterrupted transport.

Cardiac MRI

MRI in the evaluation of CHD has evolved tremendously since its introduction in the 1980s. As technology continues to improve, CMR offers multiple advantages over cardiac catheterization, transthoracic echocardiography, and CT angiography for many patients. Although expensive, MR is less costly and invasive than cardiac catheterization and does not involve exposure to ionizing radiation or the risk of stroke, vascular compromise, or bleeding. In children who will require multiple surgeries, the ability to conserve vascular access is an important consideration. Compared to transthoracic echocardiography, MR does not rely on the need for certain acoustic windows and has superior ability to evaluate extracardiac thoracic and vascular anatomy, and is unparalleled in its ability to provide three-dimensional (3D) images of complex cardiac anatomy. While CT angiography can provide high-resolution 3D imaging and has the advantage of short acquisition times, it also requires exposure to significant amounts of ionizing radiation and is therefore not useful for children needing serial evaluations [184]. Disadvantages of CMR include difficulty in obtaining scanner time, the long examination times required (usually an hour or more), and the need for sedation or general anesthesia in most pediatric patients, especially those in whom breath-holding techniques will be used. The portability and rapid availability of echocardiography will continue to make it a valuable tool in assessing patients who are too critically ill to be transported to the MR scanner.

Combined cardiac catheterization/CMR procedures ("XMR") are becoming increasingly frequent. Due to the length of these procedures and the need for patient immobility, general anesthesia is required for all patients, including adults with CHD. An MR suite is connected to a cardiac catheterization laboratory via a sliding door, allowing each area to be independently utilized as well. Currently, the availability of MR-compatible catheters and wires are limited but MR-guided diagnostic catheterization is possible, allowing more detailed assessment of certain anatomical details. Postinterventional MR assessment is also possible [185].

Once the patient is sedated or anesthetized, ECG leads are placed in a cluster on the anterior chest to allow syn-

chronization of the acquisition of data with the R wave from the ECG signal. A coil is then positioned around the chest as snugly as possible in order to serve as the receiver. Examinations begin with localizing images in the axial, coronal, and sagittal planes. Depending on the information being sought, a variety of techniques may then be utilized, including cine-MR, phase-encoded velocity mapping, and gadolinium-enhanced angiography [186]. Electrocardiogram-gated spin echo yields basic anatomic and morphologic information and is well suited to analyze the segmental anatomy of the heart, including evaluation of atrial situs, AV, and ventriculoarterial connections. Gradient reversal or "cine" imaging looks at changes in the size and shape of the atria and ventricles, intracardiac and extracardiac shunts, and abnormal flow patterns in the cardiac chambers, valves, and great vessels. It is useful in assessing ventricular shortening, regional wall motion abnormalities, ejection fraction, and CI. Because CMR can measure indices of ventricular geometry in multiple planes, it is extremely useful in gathering data regarding end-diastolic volumes, regional wall motion abnormalities, ejection fraction, CI, and AV valve regurgitant fraction

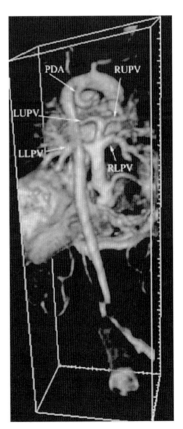

Figure 28.1 A neonate with infradiaphragmatic total anomalous pulmonary venous return. LLPV, left lower pulmonary vein; LUPV, left upper pulmonary vein; PDA, patent ductus arteriosus; RLPV, right lower pulmonary vein; RUPV, right upper pulmonary vein

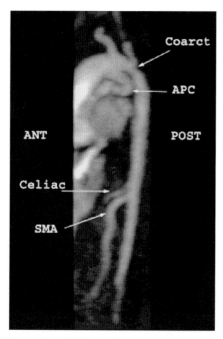

Figure 28.2 A 4-day-old infant with pulmonary atresia and ventricular septal defect. ANT, anterior; APC, aortopulmonary collateral vessel; Celiac, celiac axis; Coarct, coarctation of aorta; POST, posterior; SMA, superior mesenteric artery

in single ventricle patients [187]. Cine phase contrast can measure flow volumes and characteristics, estimating pressure gradients across valves and stenotic regions.

MRI is an excellent tool for evaluating the aorta and characterizing the precise anatomy of coarctation, arch anomalies, dilation of the aortic root, and vascular rings. In addition, the caliber of the trachea and bronchi in relation to a vascular ring can be clearly delineated, defining areas of vascular compression. Postoperative imaging of the reconstructed aorta can be useful in patients who have undergone a Norwood procedure (reconstruction/augmentation of a hypoplastic aorta, atrial septectomy, and systemic-to-pulmonary shunt) for HLHS [187]. Pulmonary arterial and venous anatomy is also well demonstrated with MR (see Figure 28.1). MR is superior to echocardiography in defining the subpulmonary region, delineating main, and branch PA anatomy, PA continuity, and assessing aortopulmonary shunts [188]. The presence of aneurysmal PAs and resultant bronchial compression may be seen in TOF with absent pulmonary valve syndrome. The patency of systemic-to-PA shunts, size and confluence of PAs, and anatomic variations of anomalous pulmonary venous return may all be well defined with MR [189]. Sources of collateral blood flow to the lungs can also be identified [190] (see Figure 28.2).

New generations of MR scanners with advanced technology allow faster image acquisition, development of new imaging strategies, and continue to move toward "real-time" evaluation of patients [191]. In utero evaluation of cardiac anomalies with CMR has also been described and aids in planning postnatal care for these infants [192,193]. CMR is the only imaging modality capable of yielding information on anatomy, function and tissue characterization, and as its utility in diagnosing cardiac disease continues to grow, pediatric anesthesiologists will be indispensable in providing or supervising sedation and general anesthetic services for children requiring these studies.

References

1. Moodie DS (1997) The future of pediatric cardiology: is there one? Clin Pediatr 36: 249–252.
2. Greenwood RD, Rosenthal A, Parisi L, et al. (1975) Extracardiac abnormalities in infants with congenital heart disease. Pediatrics 55: 485–492.
3. Hoffman JI, Christianson R (1978) Congenital heart disease in a cohort of 19 502 births with long-term follow-up. Am J Cardiol 42: 641–647.
4. Tiret L, Nivoche Y, Hatton F, et al. (1988) Complications related to anaesthesia in infants and children. A prospective survey of 40 240 anaesthetics. Br J Anaesth 61: 263–269.
5. Cohen MM, Cameron CB, Duncan PG (1990) Pediatric anesthesia morbidity and mortality in the perioperative period. Anesth Analg 70: 160–167.
6. Braz LG, Braz JR, Pinheiro NS, et al. (2006) Perioperative cardiac arrest and its mortality in children. A 9-year survey in a Brazilian tertiary teaching hospital. Ped Anesth 16: 860–866.
7. Flick RP, Sprung J, Harrison TE, et al. (2007) Perioperative cardiac arrests in children between 1988 and 2005 at a tertiary referral center: a study of 92 881 patients. Anesthesiology 106: 226–237.
8. Morray JP, Geiduschek JM, Caplan RA, et al. (1993) A comparison of pediatric and adult anesthesia closed malpractice claims. Anesthesiology 78: 461–467.
9. Jimenez N, Posner KL, Cheney, FW, et al. (2007) An update on pediatric anesthesia liability: a closed claims analysis. Anesth Analg 104: 147–153.
10. Morray JP, Geiduschek JM, Ramamoorthy C, et al. (2000) Anesthesia-related cardiac arrest in children: initial findings of the Pediatric Perioperative Cardiac Arrest (POCA) Registry. Anesthesiology 93: 6–14.
11. Bhananker SM, Ramamoorthy C, Geiduschek JM, et al. (2007) Anesthesia-related cardiac arrest in children: update from the pediatric perioperative cardiac arrest registry. Anesth Analg 105: 344–350.
12. Tennstedt C, Chaoui R, Korner H, et al. (1999) Spectrum of congenital heart defects and extracardiac malformations associated with chromosomal abnormalities: results of a seven year necropsy study. Heart 82: 34–39.
13. Pradat P, Francannet C, Harris JA (2003) The epidemiology of cardiovascular defects, part I: a study based on data from three large registries of congenital malformations. Pediatr Cardiol 24: 195–221.

14. Baum VC, Barton DM, Gutgesell HP (2000) Influence of congenital heart disease on mortality after noncardiac surgery in hospitalized children. Pediatrics 105: 332–335.

15. Hennein HA, Mendeloff EN, Cilley RE, et al. (1994) Predictors of postoperative outcome after general surgical procedures in patients with congenital heart disease. J Pediatr Surg 29: 866–870.

16. Warner MA, Lunn RJ, O'Leary PW, et al. (1998) Outcomes of noncardiac surgical procedures in children and adults with congenital heart disease. Mayo Clin Proc 73: 728–734.

17. Carmosino MJ, Friesen RH, Doran A, et al. (2007) Perioperative complications in children with pulmonary hypertension undergoing noncardiac surgery or cardiac catheterization. Anesth Analg 104: 521–527.

18. Kipps AK, Ramamoorthy C, Rosenthal DN, et al. (2007) Children with cardiomyopathy: complications after noncardiac procedures with anesthesia. Paediatr Anaesth 17: 775–781.

19. Eagle KA, Berger PB, Calkins H, et al. (2002) ACC/AHA Guidelines Update for Perioperative Cardiovascular Evaluation for Noncardiac Surgery—Executive Summary. A report of the American College of Cardiology/American Heart Association Task Force on Practice Guidelines (Committee to Update the 1996 Guidelines on Perioperative Cardiovascular Evaluation for Noncardiac Surgery). Anesth Analg 94: 1052–1064.

20. Northrop PM, Crowley MC (1943) The prophylactic use of sulfathiazole in transient bacteremia following the extraction of teeth. J Oral Surg 1: 19–29.

21. Dajani AS, Taubert KA, Wilson W, et al. (1997) Prevention of bacterial endocarditis. Recommendations by the American Heart Association. Circulation 96: 358–366.

22. Wilson W, Taubert KA, Gewitz M, et al. (2007) Prevention of infective endocarditis: recommendations by the American Heart Association Rheumatic Fever, Endocarditis and Kawasaki Disease Committee, Council on Cardiovascular Disease in the Young, and the Council on Clinical Cardiology, Council on Cardiovascular Surgery and Anesthesia, and the Quality of Care and Outcomes Research Interdisciplinary Working Group. Circulation 116: 1736–1754.

23. Strom BL, Abrutyn E, Berlin JA, et al. (1998) Dental and cardiac risk factors for infective endocarditis. A population based, case-control study. Ann Intern Med 129: 761–769.

24. Roberts GJ (1999) Dentists are innocent! Everyday bacteremia is the real culprit: a review and assessment of the evidence that dental surgical procedures are the principal cause of endocarditis in children. Paediatr Cardiol 20: 317–325.

25. Seymour RA, Lowry R, Whitworth JM, et al. (2000) Infective endocarditis, dentistry and antibiotic prophylaxis; time for a rethink? Br Dent J 189: 610–615.

26. Durack D (1998) Antibiotics for prevention of endocarditis during dentistry: time to scale back? Ann Intern Med 129: 829–831.

27. Oliver R, Roberts GJ, Hooper L, et al. (2004) Penicillins for the prophylaxis of bacterial endocarditis in dentistry. Cochrane Database Syst Rev (2): CD003813.

28. Steckleberg JM, Wilson WR (1993) Risk factors for infective endocarditis. Infect Dis Clin North Am 7: 9–19.

29. Child JS, Perloff JK, Kubak B (1998) Infective endocarditis: risks and prophylaxis. In: Perloff JK, Child JK (eds) Congenital Heart Disease in Adults, 2nd edn. Saunders, Philadelphia, pp. 129–143.

30. Gould FK, Elliott TSJ, Foweraker J, et al. (2006) Guidelines for the prevention of endocarditis: report of the working party of the British Society for Antimicrobial Chemotherapy. J Antimicrob Chemother 57: 1035–1042.

31. Infective Endocarditis Prophylaxis Expert Group (2008) Prevention of Endocarditis. 2008 Update from Therapeutic Guidelines; Antibiotic Version 13, and Therapeutic Guidelines: Oral and Dental Version 1. Melbourne: Therapeutic Guidelines Limited.

32. Horskotte D, Follath F, Gutschik E, et al. (2004) Guidelines on the prevention, diagnosis and treatment of infective endocarditis: executive summary. The task force on infective endocarditis of the European society of cardiology. Eur Heart J 25: 267–276.

33. Danchin N, Duval X, Leport C (2005) Prophylaxis of infective endocarditis: French recommendations 2002. Heart 91: 715–718.

34. Duval X, Leport C (2008) Prophylaxis of infective endocarditis: current tendencies, continuing controversies. Lancet Infect Dis 8: 225–232.

35. Pinto NM, Marino BS, Wernovsky G, et al. (2007) Obesity is a common comorbidity in children with congenital and acquired heart disease. Pediatrics 120: e1157–e1164.

36. Tait AR, Voepel-Lewis T, Burke C, et al. (2008) Incidence and risk factors for perioperative adverse respiratory events in children who are obese. Anesthesiology 108: 375–380.

37. Tait AR, Malviya S, Voepel-Lewis T, et al. (2001) Risk factors for perioperative adverse respiratory events in children with upper respiratory tract infections. Anesthesiology 95: 299–306.

38. Murat I, Constant I, Maud'huy H (2004) Perioperative anaesthetic morbidity in children: a database of 24 165 anaesthetics over a 30-month period. Paediatr Anaesth 14: 158–166.

39. Malviya S, Voepel-Lewis T, Siewert M, et al. (2003) Risk factors for adverse postoperative outcomes in children presenting for cardiac surgery with upper respiratory tract infections. Anesthesiology 98: 628–632.

40. Flick RP, Wilder RT, Pieper SF, et al. (2008) Risk factors for laryngospasm in children during general anesthesia. Paediatr Anaesth 18: 289–296.

41. Monagle P, Chalmers E, Chan A, et al. (2008) Antithrombotic therapy in neonates and children: American College of Chest Physicians evidence-based clinical practice guidelines (8th edn). Chest 133: 887S–968S.

42. Maltz LA, Gauvreau K, Connor JA, et al. (2009) Clopidogrel in a pediatric population: prescribing practice and outcomes from a single center. Pediatric Cardiol 30: 99–105.

43. Douketis JD, Berger PB, Dunn AS, et al. (2008) The Perioperative management of antithrombotic therapy: American College of Chest Physicians Evidence-Based Clinical Practice Guidelines (8th edn). Chest 133: 299S–339S.

44. Israels SJ, Michelson AD (2006) Antiplatelet therapy in children. Thromb Res 118: 75–83.

45. Li JS, Yow E, Berezny KY, et al. (2008) Dosing of clopidogrel for platelet inhibition in infants and young children: primary results of the Platelet Inhibition in Children On cLOpidogrel (PICOLO) trial. Circulation 117: 553–559.
46. Mertens L, Eyskens B, Boshoff D, et al. (2008) Safety and efficacy of clopidogrel in children with heart disease. J Pediatrics 153: 61–64.
47. Herbert JM, Tissinier A, Defreyn G, et al.(1993) Inhibitory effect of clopidogrel on platelet adhesion and intimal proliferation after arterial injury in rabbits. Arterioscler Thromb 13: 1171–1179.
48. Li JS, Yow E, Berezny KY, et al. (2007) Clinical outcomes of palliative surgery including a systemic-to-pulmonary artery shunt in infants with cyanotic congenital heart disease: does aspirin make a difference? Circulation 116: 293–297.
49. Colon-Otero G, Gilchrist GS, Holcomb GR, et al. (1987) Pre-operative evaluation of hemostasis in patients with congenital heart disease. Mayo Clin Proc 62: 379–385.
50. Perloff JK, Rosove MH, Sietsema KE, et al. (1998) Cyanotic congenital heart disease: a multisystem disorder. In: Perloff JK, Child JS (eds) Congenital Heart Disease in Adults, 2nd edn. Saunders, Philadelphia, pp. 199–226.
51. Ammash N, Warnes CA (1996) Cerebrovascular events in adult patients with cyanotic congenital heart disease. J Am Coll Cardiol 128: 768–772.
52. Warner MA, Warner ME, Warner DO, et al. (1999) Perioperative pulmonary aspiration in infants and children. Anesthesiology 90: 54–59.
53. (1999) Practice guidelines for preoperative fasting and the use of pharmacologic agents to reduce the risk of pulmonary aspiration: application to healthy patients undergoing elective procedures: a report by the American Society of Anesthesiologist Task Force on Preoperative Fasting. Anesthesiology 90: 896–905.
54. Nicolson SC, Betts EK, Jobes DR, et al. (1992) Shortened preanesthetic fasting interval in pediatric cardiac surgical patients. Anesth Analg 74: 694–697.
55. Castillo-Zamora C, Castillo-Peralta LA, Nava-Ocampo A (2005) Randomized trial comparing overnight preoperative fasting period vs. oral administration of apple juice at 06:00–06:30 AM in pediatric orthopedic surgical patients. Paediatr Anaesth 15: 638–642.
56. Kain Z, Mayes LC, O'Connor TZ, et al. (1996) Preoperative anxiety in children. Predictors and outcomes. Arch Pediatr Adolesc Med 150: 1238–1245.
57. DeBock TL, Davis PJ, Tome J, et al. (1990) Effect of premedication on arterial oxygen saturation in children with congenital heart disease. J Cardiothorac Anesth 4: 425–429.
58. Nicolson SC, Betts EK, Jobes DR, et al. (1989) Comparison of oral and intramuscular preanesthetic medication for pediatric inpatient surgery. Anesthesiology 71: 8–10.
59. Wilton NC, Leigh J, Rosen DR, et al. (1988) Preanesthetic sedation of preschool children using intranasal midazolam. Anesthesiology 69: 972–975.
60. Karl HW, Keifer AT, Rosenberger JL, et al. (1992) Comparison of the safety and efficacy of intranasal midazolam or sufentanil for preinduction of anesthesia in pediatric patients. Anesthesiology 76: 209–215.
61. Goldstein-Dresner MC, Davis PJ, Kretchman E, et al. (1991) Double-blind comparison of oral transmucosal fentanyl citrate with oral meperidine, diazepam, and atropine as pre-anesthetic medication in children with congenital heart disease. Anesthesiology 74: 28–33.
62. McMillan CO, Spahr-Schopfer IA, Sikich N, et al. (1992) Premedication of children with oral midazolam. Can J Anaesth 39: 545–550.
63. Cote CJ, Cohen IT, Suresh S, et al. (2002) A comparison of three doses of commercially prepared oral midazolam syrup in children. Anesth Analg 94: 37–43.
64. Hannallah RS, Patel RL (1989) Low-dose intramuscular ketamine for anesthesia pre-induction in young children undergoing brief outpatient procedures. Anesthesiology 70: 598–600.
65. Alswang M, Friesen RH, Bangert P (1990) Effect of premedication on arterial oxygen saturation in children with congenital heart disease. J Cardiothorac Anesth 4: 425–429.
66. Jobes DR, Nicolson SC (1988) Monitoring of arterial hemoglobin oxygen saturation using a tongue sensor. Anesth Analg 67: 186–188.
67. Reynolds LM, Nicolson SC, Steven JM, et al. (1993) Influence of sensor site location on pulse oximetry kinetics in children. Anesth Analg 76: 751–754.
68. Arai T, Yamashita M (2005) Central venous catheterization in infants and children—small caliber audio-Doppler probe versus ultrasound scanner. Paediatr Anaesth 15: 858–861.
69. Verghese ST, McGill WA, Patel RI, et al. (1999) Ultrasound-guided internal jugular venous cannulation in infants. Anesthesiology 91: 71–77.
70. Hosokawa K, Shime N, Kato Y, et al. (2007) A randomized trial of ultrasound image-based skin surface marking versus real-time ultrasound-guided internal jugular vein catheterization in infants. Anesthesiology 107: 720–724.
71. Iwashima S, Ishikawa T, Ohzeki T (2008) Ultrasound-guided versus landmark-guided femoral vein access in pediatric cardiac catheterization. Pediatric Cardiol 29: 339–342.
72. Domino KB, Bowdie TA, Posner KL, et al. (2004) Injuries and liability related to central vascular catheters. Anesthesiology 100: 1411–1418.
73. Bar-Joseph G, Galvis AG (1983) Perforation of the heart by central venous catheters in infants: guidelines to diagnosis and management. J Pediatr Surg 18: 284–287.
74. Bowdle TA (1996) Central line complications from the ASA closed claims project. ASA Newsl 60: 23–25.
75. Andropoulos DB, Bent ST, Skjonsby B, et al. (2001) The optimal length of insertion of central venous catheters for pediatric patients. Anesth Analg 93: 883–886.
76. Soliman DE, Maslow AD, Bokesch PM, et al. (1998) Transesophageal echocardiography during scoliosis repair: comparison with CVP monitoring. Can J Anaesth 45: 925–932.
77. Schmitt HJ, Schuetz WH, Proeschel PA, et al. (1993) Accuracy of pulse oximetry in children with cyanotic congenital heart disease. J Cardiothorac Vasc Anesth 7: 61–65.
78. Severinghaus JW, Naifeh KH (1987) Accuracy of response of six pulse oximeters to profound hypoxia. Anesthesiology 67: 551–558.

79. Burrows FA (1989) Physiologic dead space, venous admixture, and the arterial to end-tidal carbon dioxide difference in infants and children undergoing cardiac surgery. Anesthesiology 70: 219–225.

80. Lazzell VA, Burrows FA (1991) Stability of the intraoperative arterial to end-tidal carbon dioxide partial pressure difference in children with congenital heart disease. Can J Anaesth 38: 859–865.

81. Silka MJ, Bar-Cohen Y (2006) Pacemakers and implantable cardioverter-defibrillators in pediatric patients. Heart Rhythm 3: 1360–1366.

82. Pelech AN, Neish SR (2004) Sudden death in congenital heart disease. Ped Clin N Amer 51: 1257–1271.

83. Epstein AE, DiMarco JP, Ellenbogen KA, et al. (2008) ACC/AHA/HRS 2008 Guidelines for Device-Based Therapy of Cardiac Rhythm Abnormalities: a Report of the American College of Cardiology/American Heart Association Task Force on Practice Guidelines. Circulation 117: e350–e408.

84. Bourke ME (1996) The patient with a pacemaker or related device. Can J Anaesth 43: R24–R41.

85. Rozner M (2007) The patient with a cardiac pacemaker or implanted defibrillator and management during anaesthesia. Curr Opin Anesth 20: 261–268.

86. Salukhe TV, Dob D, Sutton R (2004) Pacemakers and defibrillators: anaesthetic implications. Br J Anaesth 93: 95–104.

87. Mangar D, Atlas GM, Kane PB (1991) Electrocautery-induced pacemaker malfunction during surgery. Can J Anaesth 38: 616–618.

88. Madigan JD, Choudhri AF, Chen J, et al. (1999) Surgical management of the patient with an implanted cardiac device: implications of electromagnetic interference. Ann Surg 230: 639–647.

89. American Society of Anesthesiologists Task Force (2005) Practice advisory for perioperative management of patients with cardiac rhythm management devices: pacemakers and implantable cardioverter-defibrillators: a report by the American Society of Anesthesiologists Task Force on Perioperative Management of Patients with Cardiac Rhythm Management Devices. Anesthesiology 103: 186–198.

90. Hensley FA, Larach DR, Martin DE, et al. (1987) The effect of halothane/nitrous oxide/oxygen mask induction on arterial hemoglobin saturation in cyanotic heart disease. J Cardiothorac Anesth 1: 289–296.

91. Russell IA, Miller-Hance WC, Gregory G, et al. (2001) The safety and efficacy of sevoflurane anesthesia in infants and children with congenital heart disease. Anesth Analg 92: 1152–1158.

92. Green DH, Townsend P, Bagshaw O, et al. (2000) Nodal rhythm and bradycardia during inhalation induction with sevoflurane in infants: a comparison of incremental and high-concentration techniques. Br J Anesth 85: 368–370.

93. Loeckinger A, Kleinsasser A, Maier S, et al. (2003) Sustained prolongation of the QTc interval after anesthesia with sevoflurane in infants during the first 6 months of life. Anesthesiology 98: 639–642.

94. Whyte S, Sanatani S, Lim J, et al. (2007) A Comparison of the effect on dispersion of repolarization of age-adjusted

95. Huntington J, Malviya S, Voepel-Lewis T, et al. (1999) The effect of a right-to-left intracardiac shunt on the rate of rise of arterial and end-tidal halothane in children. Anesth Analg 88: 759–762.

96. Zeyneloglu P, Donmez A (2008) Sevoflurane induction in cyanotic and acyanotic children with congenital heart disease. Adv Ther 25: 1–8.

97. Tanner GE, Angers DG, Barash PG, et al. (1985) Effect of left-to-right, mixed left-to-right, and right-to-left shunts on inhalational anesthetic induction in children: a computer model. Anesth Analg 64: 101–107.

98. Patel DK, Keeling PA, Newman GB, et al. (1988) Induction dose of propofol in children. Anaesthesia 43: 949–952.

99. Williams GD, Jones TK, Hanson KA, et al. (1999) The hemodynamic effects of propofol in children with congenital heart disease. Anesth Analg 89: 1411–1416.

100. Wodey E, Chonow L, Beneux X, et al. (1999) Haemodynamic effects of propofol vs thiopental in infants: an echocardiographic study. Br J Anaesth 82: 516–520.

101. Donmez A, Kaya H, Haberal A, et al. (1998) The effect of etomidate induction on plasma cortisol levels in children undergoing cardiac surgery. J Cardiothorac Vasc Anesth 12: 182–185.

102. Sarkar M, Laussen PC, Zurakowski D, et al. (2005) Hemodynamic responses to etomidate on induction of anesthesia in pediatric patients. Anesth Analg 101: 645–650.

103. Sprung J, Ogletree-Hughes ML, Moravec CS (2000) The effects of etomidate on the contractility of failing and nonfailing human heart muscle. Anesth Analg 91: 68–75.

104. Hickey PR, Hansen DD, Cramolini GM, et al. (1985) Pulmonary and systemic hemodynamic responses to ketamine in infants with normal and elevated pulmonary vascular resistance. Anesthesiology 62: 287–293.

105. Williams GD, Philip BM, Chu LF, et al. (2007) Ketamine does not increase pulmonary vascular resistance in children with pulmonary hypertension undergoing sevoflurane anesthesia and spontaneous ventilation. Anesth Analg 105: 1578–1584.

106. Christ G, Mundigler G, Merhaut C, et al. (1997) Adverse cardiovascular effects of ketamine infusion in patients with catecholamine-dependent heart failure. Anaesth Intensive Care 25: 255–259.

107. Hickey PR, Hansen DD, Wessel DL, et al. (1985) Pulmonary and systemic hemodynamic responses to fentanyl in infants. Anesth Analg 64: 483–486.

108. Ross AK, Davis PJ, Dear GDL, et al. (2001) Pharmacokinetics of remifentanil in anesthetized pediatric patients undergoing elective surgery or diagnostic procedures. Anesth Analg 93: 1393–1401.

109. Glass PS, Gan TJ, Howell S (1999) A review of the pharmacokinetics and pharmacodynamics of remifentanil. Anesth Analg 89: S7–S14.

110. Stiller RL (1985) In vitro metabolism of remifentanil: the effects of pseudocholinesterase deficiency. Anesthesiology 83: A381.

MAC values of sevoflurane in children. Anesth Analg 104: 277–282.

111. Chavanaz C, Tirel O, Wodey E, et al. (2005) Haemodynamic effects of remifentanil in children with and without intravenous atropine. Br J Anaesth 94: 74–79.

112. Fisher DM (1999) Neuromuscular blocking agents in paediatric anaesthesia. Br J Anaesth 83: 58–64.

113. Kenaan CA, Estacio RL, Bikhazi GB, (2000) Pharmacodynamics and intubating conditions of cisatracurium in children during halothane and opioid anesthesia. J Clin Anesth 12: 173–176.

114. DaConceicao MJ (1999) Ropivacaine 0.25% compared with bupivacaine 0.25% by the caudal route. Pediatr Anaesth 9: 229–233.

115. Valley RD, Bailey AG (1991) Caudal morphine for postoperative analgesia in infants and children: a report of 138 cases. Anesth Analg 72: 120–124.

116. Strafford MA, Henderson MH (1991) Anesthetic morbidity in congenital heart disease patients undergoing outpatient surgery. Anesthesiology 75: A866.

117. Parnis SJ, Barket DS, Van Der Walt JH (2001) Clinical predictors of anaesthetic complications in children with respiratory tract infections. Pediatr Anaesth 11: 29–40.

118. Schreiner MS, Nicolson SC, Martin T, et al. (1992) Should children drink before discharge from day surgery? Anesthesiology 76: 528–533.

119. Dietl CA, Cazzaniga ME, Dubner SJ, et al. (1994) Life-threatening arrhythmias and RV dysfunction after surgical repair of tetralogy of Fallot. Comparison between transventricular and transatrial approaches. Circulation 90: 117–122.

120. Gatzoulis MA, Balaji S, Weber SA, et al. (2000) Risk factors for arrhythmia and sudden cardiac death late after repair of tetralogy of Fallot: a multicentre study. Lancet 356: 975–981.

121. Okoroma EO, Guller B, Maloney JD, et al. (1975) Etiology of right bundle-branch pattern after surgical closure of ventricular-septal defects. Am Heart J 90: 14–18.

122. Houyel L, Vaksmann G, Fournier A, et al. (1990) Ventricular arrhythmias after correction of ventricular septal defects: importance of surgical approach. J Am Coll Cardiol 16: 1224–1228.

123. Burch TM, McGowan FX, Kussman B, et al. (2008) Congenital supravalvular aortic stenosis and sudden death associated with anesthesia: what's the mystery? Anesth Analg 107: 1848–1854.

124. Medley J, Russo P, Tobias JD (2005) Perioperative care of the patient with Williams syndrome. Paediatr Anaesth 15: 243–247.

125. Bird LM, Billman GF, Lacro RV, et al. (1996) Sudden death in Williams syndrome: report of ten cases. J Pediatr 129: 926–931.

126. Horowitz PE, Akhtar S, Wulff JA, et al. (2002) Coronary artery disease and anesthesia-related death in children with Williams syndrome. J Cardiothor Vasc Anesth 16: 739–741.

127. Van Mierop LH, Kutsche LM (1984) Interruption of the aortic arch and coarctation of the aorta: pathogenetic relations. Am J Cardiol 54: 829–834.

128. Huhta JC, Maloney JD, Ritter DG, et al. (1983) Complete atrioventricular block in patients with atrioventricular discordance. Circulation 67: 1374–1377.

129. Alkhaldi A, Chin C, Berstein D (2006) Pediatric cardiac transplantation. Semin Pediatr Surg 15: 188–198.

130. Boucek MM, Edwards LB, Keck BM, et al. (2005) Registry of the International Society for Heart and Lung Transplantation: eighth official pediatric report—2005. J Heart Lung Transplant 24: 968–982.

131. Clapp S, Perry BL, Farooki ZQ, et al. (1990) Down's syndrome, complete atrioventricular canal, and pulmonary vascular obstructive disease. J Thorac Cardiovasc Surg 100: 115–121.

132. Rudolph AM, Yuan S (1966) Response of the pulmonary vasculature to hypoxia and H^+ ion concentration changes. J Clin Invest 45: 399–411.

133. Morray JP, Lynn AM, Mansfield PB (1988) Effect of pH and PCO_2 on pulmonary and systemic hemodynamics after surgery in children with congenital heart disease and pulmonary hypertension. J Pediatr 113: 474–479.

134. Bando K, Turrentine MW, Sharp TG (1996) Pulmonary hypertension after operations for congenital heart disease: analysis of risk factors and management. J Thorac Cardiovasc Surg 112: 1600–1609.

135. Taylor CJ, Derrick G, McEwan A, et al. (2007) Risk of cardiac catheterization under anaesthesia in children with pulmonary hypertension. Br J Anaesth 98: 657–661.

136. Ramakrishna G, Sprung J, Ravi BS, et al. (2005) Impact of pulmonary hypertension on the outcomes of noncardiac surgery: predictors of perioperative morbidity and mortality. J Am Coll Cardiol 45: 1691–1699.

137. Blaise G, Langleben D, Hubert B (2003) Pulmonary arterial hypertension. Anesthesiology 99: 1415–1432.

138. Fischer LG, Van Aken H, Burkle H (2003) Management of pulmonary hypertension: physiological and pharmacological considerations for anesthesiologists. Anesth Analg 96: 1603–1616.

139. Friesen RH, Williams GD (2008) Anesthetic management of children with pulmonary arterial hypertension. Paediatr Anaesth 18: 208–216.

140. Alswang M, Friesen RH, Bangert P (1994) Effect of preanesthetic medication on carbon dioxide tension in children with congenital heart disease. J Cardiothorac Vasc Anesth 8: 415–419.

141. Friesen RH, Alswang M (1996) Changes in carbon dioxide tension and oxygen saturation during deep sedation for paediatric cardiac catheterization. Paediatr Anaesth 6: 15–20.

142. Burrows FA, Klinck JR, Rabinovitch M, et al. (1986) Pulmonary hypertension in children: perioperative management. Can J Anaesth J 33: 606–628.

143. Hickey PR, Retzack SM (1993) Acute right ventricular failure after pulmonary hypertensive responses to airway instrumentation: effect of fentanyl dose. Anesthesiology 78: 372–376.

144. Hickey PR, Hansen DD, Wessel DL (1985) Blunting of stress responses in the pulmonary circulation of infants by fentanyl. Anesth Analg 64: 1137–1142.

145. Hakim TS, Michel RP, Chang HK (1982) Effect of lung inflation on pulmonary vascular resistance by arterial and venous occlusion. J Appl Physiol 53: 1110–1115.

146. Luce JM (1984) The cardiovascular effects of mechanical ventilation and positive end expiratory pressure. JAMA 252: 807–811.

147. Jardin F, Vieillard-Baron A (2003) Right ventricular function and positive pressure ventilation in clinical practice: from hemodynamic subsets to respiratory settings. Intensive Care Med 29: 1426–1434.

148. Andrews RE, Fenton MJ, Ridout DA, et al. (2008) New-onset heart failure due to heart muscle disease in childhood: a prospective study in the United Kingdom and Ireland. Circulation 117: 79–84.

149. Massin MM, Astadicko I, Dessy H (2007) Noncardiac comorbidities of congenital heart disease in children. Acta Paediatr 96: 753–755.

150. Perloff JK, Sangwan S (1998) Noncardiac surgery. In: Perloff JK, Child JS (eds) Congenital Heart Disease in Adults, 2nd edn. Saunders, Philadelphia, pp. 291–299.

151. Gidding SS, Stockman JA III (1988) Erythropoietin in cyanotic heart disease. Am Heart J 116: 128–132.

152. Linderkamp O, Klose HJ, Betke K, et al. (1979) Increased blood viscosity in patients with cyanotic congenital heart disease and iron deficiency. J Pediatr 95: 567–569.

153. Territo MC, Rosove MH (1991) Cyanotic congenital heart disease: hematologic management. J Am Coll Cardiol 18: 320–322.

154. Wedemeyer AL, Edson JR, Krivit W (1972) Coagulation in cyanotic congenital heart disease. Am J Dis Child 124: 656–660.

155. Henriksson P, Varendh G, Lundstron MR (1979) Haemostatic defects in cyanotic congenital heart disease. Br Heart J 41: 23–27.

156. Edelman NH, Lahiri S, Braudo L, et al. (1970) The blunted ventilatory response to hypoxia in cyanotic congenital heart disease. N Engl J Med 282: 405–411.

157. Davies HHGN (1965) Dyspnoea in cyanotic congenital heart disease. Br Heart J 27: 28–41.

158. Strieder DJ, Mesko ZG, Zaver AG, et al. (1973) Exercise tolerance in chronic hypoxemia due to right-to-left shunt. J Appl Physiol 34: 853–858.

159. Fletcher R (1991) The relationship between the arterial to end-tidal PCO_2 difference and hemoglobin saturation in patients with congenital heart disease. Anesthesiology 75: 210–216.

160. Liberman BA, Teasdale SJ (1985) Anaesthesia and amiodarone. Can Anaesth Soc J 32: 629–638.

161. Teske DW, Caniano DA (2001) Noncardiac surgery in patients with heart disease. In: Allen HD, Clark EB, Cutgesell HP, et al. (eds) Moss and Adams' Heart Disease in Infants, Children, and Adolescents including the Fetus and Young Adult, 6th edn. Lippincott, Williams & Wilkins, Philadelphia, pp. 408–413.

162. Kuhl CK, Traber F, Gieseke J, et al. (2008) Whole-body high-field strength (3.0 T) MR imaging in clinical practice. Part II. Technical considerations and clinical applications. Radiology 247: 16–35.

163. Shellock FG, Kanal E (1996) Bioeffects and safety of MR procedures. In: Edelman R, Hesselink J, Zlatkin M (eds) Clinical Magnetic Resonance Imaging. Saunders, Philadelphia, pp. 391–433.

164. Nazarian S, Rogiun A, Zviman M, et al. (2006) Clinical utility and safety of a protocol for noncardiac and cardiac magnetic resonance imaging of patients with permanent pacemakers and implantable-cardioverter defibrillators at 1.5 Tesla. Circulation 114: 1277–1284.

165. Kanal E, Shellock FG, Talagala L (1990) Safety considerations in MR imaging. Radiology 176: 593–606.

166. Shellock FG, Spinazzi G (2008) MRI safety update 2008: part 2, screening patients for MRI. AJR Am J Roentgenol 191: 1140–1149.

167. Shellock FG (2008) Reference Manual for Magnetic Resonance Safety, Implants and Devices: 2008 Edition. Biomedical Research Publishing Group, Los Angeles.

168. Institute for Magnetic Resonance Safety, Education and Research (2008). www.IMRSER.org. Accessed January 29, 2009.

169. Shellock FG (2008) MRIsafety.com: MRI Safety, Bioeffects and Patient Management. www.mrisafety.com Accessed January 29, 2009.

170. Odegard KC, DiNardo JA, Tasi-Goodman B, et al. (2004) Anesthesia considerations for cardiac MRI in infants and small children. Paediatr Anaesth 14: 471–476.

171. Sarikouch S, Schaefler R, Korperich H, et al. (2009) Cardiovascular magnetic resonance imaging for intensive care infants: safe and effective? Pediatr Cardiol 30: 146–152.

172. Frankville DD, Spear RM, Dyck JB (1993) The dose of propofol required to prevent children from moving during magnetic resonance imaging. Anesthesiology 79: 953–958.

173. Hannallah RS, Baker SB, Casey W, et al. (1991) Propofol: effective dose and induction characteristics in unpremedicated children. Anesthesiology 74: 217–219.

174. Dalal PG, Murray D, Cox T, et al. (2006) Sedation and anesthesia protocols used for magnetic resonance imaging studies in infants: provider and pharmacologic considerations. Anesth Analg 103: 863–868.

175. Galli K, Gaynor W, Peterson K, et al. (2002) Safety and efficacy of intravenous pentobarbital for sedation in neonates and infants with natural airways for brain MRI in the early postoperative period following surgery for congenital heart disease involving cardiopulmonary bypass. Society for Pediatric Anesthesia Annual Scientific Program, 2002; unpublished abstract.

176. Pereira JK, Burrows PE, Richards HM, et al. (1993) Comparison of sedation regimens for pediatric outpatient CT. Pediatr Radiol 23: 341–344.

177. Phan H, Nahata MC (2008) Clinical uses of dexmedetomidine in pediatric patients. Pediatr Drugs 10: 49–69.

178. Mason KP (2008) The pediatric sedation service: who is appropriate to sedate, which medications should I use, who should prescribe the drugs, how do I bill? Pediatr Radiol 38: 5218–5224.

179. Mason KP, Zgleszewski SE, Prescilla R, et al. (2008) Hemodynamic effects of dexmedetomidine sedation for CT imaging studies. Paediatr Anaesth 18: 393–402.

180. Mason KP, Zurakowski D, Zgleszewski SE, et al. (2008) High dose dexmedetomidine as the sole sedative for pediatric MRI. Paediatr Anaesth 18: 403–411.

181. Berkenbosch JW, Tobias JD (2003) Development of bradycardia during sedation with Dexmedetomidine in an infant concurrently receiving digoxin. Ped Crit Care Med 4: 203–205.

182. Jorgensen NH, Messick JMJr, Gray J, et al. (1994) ASA monitoring standards and magnetic resonance imaging. Anesth Analg 79: 1141–1147.

183. Shellock FG, Slimp GL (1989) Severe burn of the finger caused by using a pulse oximeter during MR imaging. Am J Roentgenol 153: 1105.

184. Bailliard F, Hughes ML, Taylor AM (2008) Introduction to cardiac imaging in infants and children: techniques and role in the imaging work-up of various cardiac malformations and other pediatric heart conditions. Eur J Radiol 68: 191–198.

185. Moodie DS (2005) MRI and cardiac catheterization: seeing the heart in a new way. Catheter Cardiovasc Interv 66: 9.

186. Berlin SC (1997) Magnetic resonance imaging of the cardiovascular system and airway. Pediatr Clin North Am 44: 659–679.

187. Fogel MA (2006) Cardiac magnetic resonance of single ventricles. J Cardiovasc Magn Reson 8: 661–670.

188. Vick GWIII, Rokey R, Huhta JC, et al. (1990) Nuclear magnetic resonance imaging of the pulmonary arteries, subpulmonary region, and aorticopulmonary shunts: a comparative study with two-dimensional echocardiography and angiography. Am Heart J 119: 1103–1110.

189. Hubbard AM, Fellows KE, Weinberg PM, et al. (1998) Preoperative and postoperative MRI of congenital heart disease. Semin Roentgenol 33: 218–227.

190. Kellenberger CJ, Yoo S, Buchel ER (2007) Cardiovascular MR imaging in neonates and infants with congenital heart disease. Radiographics 27: 5–18.

191. Chung T (2000) Assessment of cardiovascular anatomy in patients with congenital heart disease by magnetic resonance imaging. Pediatr Cardiol 21: 18–26.

192. Whitham JKE, Hasan B, Schamberger M, et al. (2008) Use of cardiac magnetic resonance imaging to determine myocardial viability in an infant with in utero septal myocardial infarction and ventricular noncompaction. Pediatr Cardiol 29: 950–953.

193. McMahon CJ, Taylor MD, Cassady CI, et al. (2007) Diagnosis of pentalogy of Cantrell in the fetus using magnetic resonance imaging and ultrasound. Pediatr Cardiol 28: 172–175.

29 Cardiac intensive care

Peter C. Laussen, M.B.B.S.
Children's Hospital Boston, Harvard Medical School, Boston, Massachusetts, USA

Stephen J. Roth, M.D., M.P.H.
Lucile Packard Children's Hospital, Stanford University School of Medicine, Palo Alto, California, USA

Introduction

The primary aims of treatment strategies for managing children with congenital cardiac defects are to promote normal growth and development and to limit the pathophysiologic consequences of congenital cardiac defects such as volume overload, pressure overload, and chronic hypoxemia. As a result, there has been a distinct change in management philosophy over the past 10–20 years toward performing reparative operations on neonates and infants, rather than initial palliation and later repair [1]. However, because of a limited physiologic

reserve and the complications associated with cardiopulmonary bypass (CPB) and open-heart surgery, the risk for cardiorespiratory dysfunction in neonates and young infants in the immediate postoperative period may be increased.

The successful management of congenital heart defects requires detailed knowledge, experience, and technical expertise because of the significant heterogeneity in patient age, structural disease, and cardiorespiratory physiology. The range of operative procedures performed at Children's Hospital Boston during calendar year 2008 is shown in Chapter 1, Table 1.1. Many of the postoperative management problems are therefore quite different from those experienced in adults in the intensive care unit (ICU) following surgery for acquired heart disease. The wide age range of patients undergoing congenital cardiac surgery is another factor that has

Anesthesia for Congenital Heart Disease 2nd edition. Edited by Dean Andropoulos, Stephen Stayer, Isobel Russell and Emad Mossad.
© 2010 Blackwell Publishing.

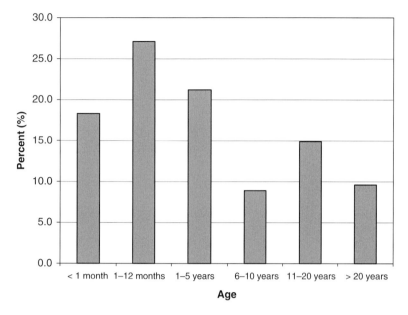

Figure 29.1 Age range of cardiac surgical and medical patients admitted to the Cardiac Intensive Care Unit at Children's Hospital Boston in 2008

had a substantial bearing on postoperative management. The age ranges for cardiac surgical or medical patients ($n = 1248$) admitted to the Cardiac Intensive Care Unit at Children's Hospital Boston in the calendar year 2008 are shown in Figure 29.1. Patients at the extremes of this age spectrum—low-birth-weight and premature newborns at one end, and adults with congenital cardiac disease at the other end—are providing new challenges for postoperative management and resource management in the ICU.

Virtually all congenital cardiac defects are now amenable to either an anatomic or functional correction, but while "corrected" may not be "cured." The optimal postoperative management of patients with congenital heart disease (CHD) requires a multidisciplinary approach, combining the disciplines of cardiology, cardiac surgery, anesthesia, critical care, and nursing. A thorough understanding of the precise anatomic diagnosis, pathophysiology, and details of the surgical technique, including the potential for residual defects, are necessary when managing pediatric cardiac patients in the ICU.

For most patients, postoperative recovery is uncomplicated, reflecting the improvements in preoperative diagnosis and stabilization, surgical techniques, and in particular, CPB management. In general, when the patient's clinical progress or postoperative cardiorespiratory function does not follow the expected course, the accuracy of the preoperative diagnosis should be questioned and the adequacy of the surgical repair or palliation investigated, either with echocardiography and/or cardiac catheterization.

Pathophysiology of congenital cardiac defects

A thorough understanding of the pathophysiology of congenital cardiac defects is essential when managing these patients in the ICU. Not only will this influence preoperative management strategies for stabilization and/or resuscitation prior to surgery, but the effects of preexisting cyanosis and pressure and volume overload may have a substantial impact on myocardial performance and recovery after surgery. Further, if there are hemodynamically significant residual intracardiac lesions or defects after surgery, the accompanying alterations in pulmonary blood flow, systemic perfusion, and ventricular compliance may significantly affect recovery in the ICU.

Mixing

Intra-atrial mixing of pulmonary and systemic venous return is essential for maintenance of cardiac output (CO) in defects with severe right or left atrioventricular valve stenosis or atresia, e.g., hypoplastic left heart syndrome (HLHS) or tricuspid atresia, those with an anatomically parallel pulmonary and systemic circulation, such as d-transposition of the great arteries (d-TGA), and postoperative patients who have undergone a Norwood-type procedure. If complete mixing occurs, the systemic arterial oxygen saturation (SaO_2) should be approximately 85% in room air, although this can be highly variable depending on the amount of pulmonary blood flow. Inadequate mixing across a restrictive atrial septal defect (ASD) can cause significant systemic desaturation secondary to reduced pulmonary blood flow or pulmonary edema from pulmonary venous hypertension. The septal defect can be enlarged either by catheter balloon septostomy or balloon dilation, or surgically by atrial septectomy.

Shunts

Shunting between the pulmonary and systemic circulations can be intracardiac occurring between the atria or ventricles (e.g., across an ASD or ventricular septal defect), or extracardiac occurring between the pulmonary arteries and aorta (e.g., across a patent ductus arteriosus (PDA), aortopulmonary window, or an aortopulmonary artery collateral vessel in patients with tetralogy of Fallot (TOF) and pulmonary atresia). Depending on the size of the communication and the pressure and resistance differences between the systemic and pulmonary circulations, patients may have an increased or decreased amount of pulmonary blood flow and be either acyanotic or cyanotic.

Increased pulmonary blood flow

Shunts that increase pulmonary blood flow may occur either between the ventricles, atria, or great arteries, and can be described as "simple" (either unrestricted or restricted) or "complex."

Simple shunt

The amount of flow across a "simple" left-to-right shunt depends on the size of the defect and balance between pulmonary and systemic vascular resistance (SVR). It is important to understand that this is a physiologic term and has no direct relationship to specific diagnoses (Table 29.1). Therefore, patients who have a simple shunt may have:

1 A normal SaO_2 with two ventricles, such as in a large ventricular septal defect (VSD), complete atrioventricular canal defect (CAVC), and large PDA.
2 A normal SaO_2 with single ventricular outflow trunk and two ventricles, such as in truncus arteriosus.
3 A low SaO_2 and two ventricles, such as in patients with d-TGA and VSD.
4 A low SaO_2 and a single ventricle, such as in atrioventricular valve atresia (tricuspid or mitral) and following placement of a systemic-to-pulmonary artery shunt as in the Norwood-type procedure.

If the simple shunt is "unrestrictive," the physiologic consequence for all the above diagnoses will be the same, i.e., excessive pulmonary blood flow and volume overload to the systemic ventricle. The clinical manifestation will also be the same, i.e., congestive cardiac failure and pulmonary hypertension, although some patients will be

Table 29.1 Simple shunts: defects or surgical procedures contributing to an increased Qp/Qs

	Acyanotic	Cyanotic
Two ventricles	ASD VSD CAVC DORV	d-TGA/VSD PA/VSD
Single ventricle		TA ± TGA HLHS DORV/MA Norwood procedure BT shunt
Aortopulmonary connection	PDA Truncus arteriosus A-P window	PA/MAPCA

Qp, pulmonary blood flow; Qs, systemic blood flow; ASD, atrial septal defect; VSD, ventricular septal defect; CAVC, complete atrioventricular canal; DORV, double outlet right ventricle; d-TGA, d-transposition of the great arteries; PA, pulmonary atresia; TA, tricuspid atresia; MA, mitral atresia; HLHS, hypoplastic left heart syndrome; BT, Blalock–Taussig; PDA, patent ductus arteriosus; MAPCA, major aortopulmonary collateral arteries; A-P, aortopulmonary.

cyanotic and others acyanotic depending on the amount of intracardiac mixing.

On the other hand, for a simple *"restrictive"* shunt, the orifice or size of the defect is small, and the pressure gradient across this now determines the magnitude of shunting rather than relative vascular resistances [2,3]. In this circumstance, there is less systemic ventricle volume overload and the pulmonary circulation is protected to some extent from excessive pressure and flow; as a result patients may be relatively asymptomatic and continue to thrive or present later for management.

Complex shunt

In the presence of additional pulmonary or systemic outflow obstruction, the ratio of pulmonary (Qp) to systemic (Qs) blood flow (Qp/Qs) is determined by the size of the orifice, the outflow gradient as well as the resistance across the pulmonary or systemic vascular bed. The obstruction may be fixed as with valvular stenosis, or dynamic as in subvalvar stenosis (some forms of TOF).

Clinical consequences of increased pulmonary to systemic blood flow ratio

If the increase in pulmonary blood flow and pressure persists over months to years, structural changes occur within the pulmonary vasculature until eventually pulmonary vascular resistance (PVR) becomes irreversibly elevated [2–4]. The time course for developing this pathology, termed pulmonary vascular obstructive disease, depends on the amount of shunting, but changes may be evident by 4–6 months of age in some lesions (e.g., truncus arteriosus). The progression is more rapid when both the volume and pressure load to the pulmonary circulation is increased, such as with a large VSD or CAVC defect. When pulmonary flow is increased in the absence of elevated pulmonary artery pressure, as with an ASD, persistently elevated PVR develops much more slowly, if at all.

As PVR decreases in the first few months after birth, and the hematocrit falls to its lowest physiologic value, the increased left-to-right shunt, and therefore volume load on the systemic ventricle, can lead to congestive cardiac failure and failure to thrive. A typical pressure–volume loop for a volume-loaded ventricle is shown in Figure 29.2 [5,6]. The end-diastolic volume is increased, and the end-systolic pressure–volume line displaced to the right indicating reduced contractility. The time course over which irreversible ventricular dysfunction develops is variable, but if surgical intervention to correct the volume overload is undertaken within the first 2 years of life, residual dysfunction is uncommon [6]. The volume load on the systemic ventricle and increased end-diastolic pressure contributes to increased lung water and pulmonary edema by increasing pulmonary venous and lymphatic pressures. Compliance of the lung is therefore decreased, and airway resistance increased secondary to small airway compression by distended vessels [7–9]. These infants typically have both tachypnea as well as increased work of breathing. If tracheally intubated for mechanical ventilation, the lungs may feel stiff on hand ventilation and deflate slowly.

Besides cardiomegaly on chest radiograph, the lung fields are usually congested as well as hyperinflated. Ventilation/perfusion mismatch contributes to an increased alveolar-to-systemic arterial O_2 (A–aO_2) gradient and dead space ventilation [10]. Minute ventilation is therefore increased, primarily by an increase in respiratory rate. Pulmonary artery and left atrial enlargement may compress mainstem bronchi causing lobar collapse.

It is important to appreciate that such clinical scenarios can be present after surgery in patients who have significant residual intracardiac shunts that cause an increase in Qp/Qs. It may be manifest during the early postoperative course as a low CO state (LCOS) (see below) or become apparent some days after surgery with an inability to wean from mechanical ventilation or persistent requirement for vasoactive support.

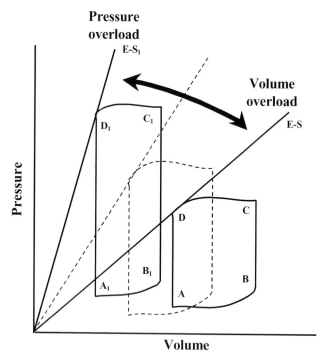

Figure 29.2 Comparison of pressure–volume loops between ventricles with a volume load (ABCD) or pressure load ($A_1B_1C_1D_1$). The end-systolic pressure–volume line is displaced to the right in a volume-loaded ventricle (E-S), reflecting decreased contractility. The end-systolic pressure–volume line is displaced to the left in a pressure-loaded ventricle (E-S_1), reflecting preserved systolic function. A, A_1, end isovolumetric relaxation (assuming no atrioventricular valve regurgitation); B, B_1, end diastole; C, C_1 onset ventricular ejection; D, D_1, end systole; E-S, E-S_1, end systolic pressure–volume lines

Decreased pulmonary blood flow

Pulmonary blood flow may be reduced either from pulmonary outflow obstruction or a right-to-left intracardiac shunt. While elevated PVR is the primary cause of an intracardiac right-to-left shunt at the atrial level via a patent foramen ovale (PFO) in neonates with noncardiac diseases, such as persistent pulmonary hypertension of the newborn or congenital diaphragmatic hernia, the shunt in newborns with congenital heart defects usually results from right ventricle (RV) outflow obstruction, such as in TOF and pulmonary atresia. Pulmonary blood flow is reduced, and PVR is usually normal in these patients. However, the decreased pulmonary flow during fetal development can lead to diminished arborization of the pulmonary vessels and a decrease in total cross-sectional area of the pulmonary vascular bed, resulting in a relatively increased and fixed PVR.

Pulmonary mechanics and lung volumes are generally normal in patients with reduced pulmonary blood flow. Dead space ventilation is increased, although minute ventilation is only slightly increased to maintain normocapnia. The lung fields appear oligemic on chest radiograph.

Target oxygen level

It is very important to know what the target SaO₂ should be in the immediate postoperative period. If the SaO₂ is lower than anticipated, there are a number of important causes that must be evaluated (Table 29.2). These include:

1 A reduction in pulmonary venous oxygen saturation indicating an intra-pulmonary shunt such as from pulmonary edema, lung collapse or pleural effusion.

2 A reduction in effective pulmonary blood flow, such as from pulmonary ventricle outflow tract obstruction or increased pulmonary artery resistance, an intra-cardiac right-to-left shunt across an ASD or VSD, or a decompressing vessel from the pulmonary artery to pulmonary vein.

Table 29.2 Factors to consider in a postcardiac surgery patient who has an arterial oxygen saturation lower than the anticipated range

Etiology	Considerations
Low Fio₂	Inappropriately low dialed oxygen concentration
	Failure of oxygen delivery device
Pulmonary vein desaturation	Impaired diffusion
	Alveolar process: edema
	Infectious
	Restrictive process: effusion
	Atelectasis
	Pneumothorax
	Intrapulmonary shunt
	RDS
	Pulmonary AVM
	PA-to-PV collateral vessel(s)
Reduced pulmonary blood flow	Anatomic RV outflow obstruction
	Anatomic pulmonary artery stenosis
	Increased PVR
	Atrial level right-to-left shunt
	RV hypertension
	Restrictive RV physiology (low compliance)
	Severe tricuspid regurgitation
	Large fenestration (modified Fontan operation)
	Intra-atrial baffle leak
	Ventricular level right-to-left shunt
	RV hypertension and residual VSD
Low dissolved oxygen content (mixing defects)	Low mixed venous oxygen level
	Increased O₂ extraction: hypermetabolic state
	Decreased O₂ delivery: low cardiac output state
	Anemia

Fio₂, fractional inspired concentration of oxygen; RDS, respiratory distress syndrome; PA, pulmonary artery; AVM, arteriovenous malformation; PV, pulmonary vein; RV, right ventricle; PVR, pulmonary vascular resistance; VSD, ventricular septal defect.

3 A reduction in oxygen content, principally in patients who have mixing of systemic and pulmonary venous blood at the atrial level. The reduction in O₂ content may be due to a low mixed venous oxygen level, such as reduced oxygen delivery secondary to an LCOS or increased oxygen extraction in a febrile or hypermetabolic state following surgery, or to a low hematocrit.

Outflow obstruction

Severe left or right ventricular outflow obstruction in the newborn may be associated with ventricular hypertrophy and vessel hypoplasia distal to the level of obstruction. The increased pressure load may cause ventricular failure, with mixing or shunting at the atrial and/or ventricular level necessary to maintain CO if there is complete outflow obstruction.

A typical pressure–volume loop from a chronic pressure load on the ventricle is shown in Figure 29.2 [6]. The end-diastolic pressure is elevated and the end-systolic pressure–volume line displaced to the left, reflecting increased contractility. Maintenance of preload, afterload, and normal sinus rhythm is important to prevent a fall in CO or coronary hypoperfusion. As the time course to develop significant ventricular dysfunction is longer in patients with a chronic pressure load compared to a chronic volume load, symptoms of congestive heart failure (CHF) are uncommon unless the obstruction is severe and prolonged.

In the immediate postoperative period, it is important to evaluate both systolic and diastolic ventricular function in a previously obstructed but still hypertrophied ventricle.

1 A hyperdynamic state may be present particularly following left ventricle (LV) outflow reconstruction. This will be manifest as systemic hypertension and should be treated promptly to reduce myocardial work and protect surgical suture lines, especially those in the aorta.

2 Systolic dysfunction of a hypertrophied ventricle may be apparent early after cardiac surgery secondary to myocardial ischemia and ventricular dysrhythmias. Ischemia may occur particularly if there has been a long aortic cross clamp time, or if there has been inadequate protection of the subendocardium with cardioplegia solution or by hypothermia. In the case of the RV, dysfunction may be also be present after surgery if an extended ventriculotomy has been performed (e.g., TOF or truncus repair) or there has been direct injury to a coronary artery across the right ventricular outflow tract.

3 Diastolic dysfunction is usually manifest as a poorly compliant or stiff ventricle that often contracts well but is unable to relax and fill effectively during diastole. On the left side of the heart, this is usually manifest as left atrial hypertension with either pulmonary edema, atrial dysrhythmias or pulmonary hypertension. On the right

side of the heart, an increase in RV end-diastolic pressure is demonstrated by right atrial hypertension along with clinical signs such as a lower SaO_2 from a right-to-left atrial shunt (in the presence of a PFO or residual ASD), hepatomegaly, pleural effusions (especially in neonates and young infants), and possibly ascites.

In all the above examples of mixing, shunting, and outflow obstruction, the mode and method of mechanical ventilation may have a substantial impact on hemodynamics and systemic perfusion. Particularly for neonates and infants, cardiorespiratory interactions are essential to recognize during postoperative management. In addition to evaluating the adequacy of mechanical ventilation settings by arterial blood gases and chest radiography, it is very important that ventilator settings be continually evaluated and adjusted according to hemodynamic response. This is completely different to the general concepts of mechanical ventilation used in general pediatric and neonatal ICUs. The application of standard or accepted practices for mechanical ventilation as applied to pediatric patients with respiratory disease, or as applied to the premature newborn or newborn with hyaline membrane disease, will often result in an ineffective matching of ventilation with perfusion in patients with congenital cardiac disease, and contribute to delayed postoperative recovery and possible adverse outcomes.

Airway and ventilation management

Altered respiratory mechanics and positive pressure ventilation may have a significant influence on hemodynamics following congenital heart surgery. While changes in alveolar O_2 (PaO_2), $PaCO_2$, and pH significantly affect PVR, the mean airway pressure and changes in lung volume during positive pressure ventilation will also affect PVR, preload, and ventricular afterload. Therefore, the approach to mechanical ventilation should not only be directed at achieving a desired gas exchange, but also influenced by the potential cardiorespiratory interactions of positive pressure ventilation and method of weaning.

Airway management

Intubation of the trachea in an awake neonate or young infant with CHD may illicit major undesirable hemodynamic and metabolic responses, and therefore, appropriate anesthetic techniques are necessary to secure the airway under most circumstances.

The narrowest part of the airway before puberty is below the vocal cords at the level of the cricoid cartilage, and the use of uncuffed endotracheal tubes has been generally recommended. While a leak around the endotracheal tube at an inflation pressure of approximately 20 cm

H_2O is desirable, a significant air leak may have a detrimental effect on mechanical ventilation and delivery of a consistent ventilation pattern. Examples include patients with extensive chest and abdominal wall edema following CPB and patients with labile PVR and increased Qp/Qs. If a significant air leak exists around the endotracheal tube, lung volume, and in particular functional residual capacity (FRC), will not be maintained and fluctuations in gas exchange can occur. During the weaning process, a significant leak will also increase the work of breathing for some neonates and infants. In these situations, it is therefore preferable to change the endotracheal tube to a larger size or to use a cuffed endotracheal tube.

In certain circumstances, a smaller than expected endotracheal tube may be necessary. This is particularly the case in patients with other congenital defects such as Down syndrome (Trisomy 21). Tracheal stenosis may also occur in association with some congenital cardiac defects such as a pulmonary artery sling. Extrinsic compression of the bronchi may occur secondary to pulmonary artery and left atrial dilation. This may be suspected by persistent hyperinflation or lobar atelectasis.

Mechanical ventilation

Altered lung mechanics and ventilation/perfusion abnormalities are common problems in the immediate postoperative period [11,12]. Patients who have an increased Qp/Qs > 2:1 may have cardiomegaly and congested lung fields on radiograph. Patients who have an elevated left atrial pressure from some form of outflow tract obstruction to the LV may demonstrate signs of pulmonary venous hypertension and pulmonary edema. Additional considerations include the surgical incision and lung retraction, increased lung water following CPB, possible pulmonary reperfusion injury, surfactant depletion in neonates and restrictive defects from atelectasis and pleural effusions.

In general, patients with known limited physiologic reserve should not be weaned from mechanical ventilation until hemodynamically stable, and problems contributing to an increase in intrapulmonary shunt and altered respiratory mechanics have improved.

Cardiorespiratory interactions

Cardiorespiratory interactions vary significantly between patients, and it is not possible to provide specific ventilation strategies or protocols that are appropriate for all patients. Rather, the mode of ventilation must be matched to the hemodynamic status of each patient to achieve the adequate CO and gas exchange. The influence of positive pressure ventilation on preload and afterload are shown in Table 29.3. Frequent modifications to the mode and pattern of ventilation may be necessary during recovery after

Table 29.3 The effect of a positive pressure mechanical breath on afterload and preload to the pulmonary and systemic ventricles

	Afterload	Preload
Pulmonary ventricle	Elevated Effect: ↑ RVEDp ↑ RVp ↓ Antegrade PBF ↑ PR and/or TR	Reduced Effect: ↓ RVEDV ↓ RAp
Systemic ventricle	Reduced Effect: ↓ LVEDp ↓ LAp ↓ Pulmonary edema	Reduced Effect: ↓ LVEDV ↓ LAp Hypotension

RVEDp, right ventricle end diastolic pressure; RVp, right ventricle pressure; RVEDV, right ventricle end diastolic volume; PBF, pulmonary blood flow; PR, pulmonary regurgitation; TR, tricuspid regurgitation; LVEDp, left ventricle end diastolic pressure; LVEDV, left ventricle end diastolic volume; LAp, left atrial pressure; RAp, right atrial pressure.

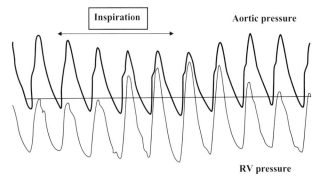

Figure 29.3 Simultaneous tracings of aortic and right ventricle (RV) pressure waveforms during positive pressure ventilation in a child with pulmonary artery stenosis. Note the increase in RV pressure to approximately systemic (aortic) level during inspiration when the afterload on the right ventricle is increased

surgery, with attention to changes in lung volume and airway pressure.

Influence of lung volume

Changes in lung volume have a major effect on PVR, which is lowest at FRC, while both hypo- or hyperinflation may result in a significant increase in PVR [13]. At low tidal volumes, alveolar collapse occurs because of reduced interstitial traction on alveolar septae. In addition, radial traction on extra-alveolar vessels such as the branch pulmonary arteries is reduced, therefore reducing the cross-sectional diameter. Conversely, hyperinflation of the lung may cause stretching of the alveolar septae and compression of extra-alveolar vessels.

An increase in PVR increases the afterload or wall stress on the RV, compromising RV function and contributing to decreased LV compliance secondary to interventricular septal shift (from right to left). In addition to low CO, signs of RV dysfunction including tricuspid regurgitation, hepatomegaly, ascites, and pleural effusions may be observed.

Influence of intrathoracic pressure

An increase in mean intrathoracic pressure during positive pressure ventilation decreases preload to both pulmonary and systemic ventricles, but has opposite effects on afterload to each ventricle [14,15].

Right ventricle

The increase in pressure in the right atrium (RA) and reduction in RV preload that occurs with positive pressure

ventilation may reduce CO. Normally, the RV diastolic compliance is extremely high, and the pulmonary circulation is able to accommodate changes in flow without a large change in pressure. An increase in mean intrathoracic pressure increases the afterload on the RV from direct compression of extra-alveolar and alveolar pulmonary vessels. This has a number of clinical consequences (Table 29.3). An increase in afterload causes an increase in RV end-diastolic pressure and myocardial work, which may lead to ischemia in a patient with limited coronary perfusion. An example of the increase in RV pressure during a positive pressure breath is demonstrated in Figure 29.3. The increase in afterload on the RV will also reduce antegrade pulmonary blood flow and therefore preload to the systemic ventricle. If there is pulmonary or tricuspid valve incompetence, the amount of regurgitant flow across these valves will also increase during positive pressure ventilation from the increase in RV afterload.

Patients with normal RV compliance and without residual volume load or pressure load on the ventricle following surgery usually show little change in RV function from the alteration in preload and afterload that occurs with positive pressure ventilation. However, these effects can be magnified in patients with RV hypertrophy and those with restrictive RV physiology following congenital heart surgery, in particular neonates who have required a right ventriculotomy for repair of TOF, pulmonary atresia, or truncus arteriosus, and patients with concentric RV hypertrophy. While systolic RV function may be preserved, the ventricles have diastolic dysfunction with increased RV end-diastolic pressure and impaired RV filling.

The potential deleterious effects of mechanical ventilation on RV function are important to emphasize. The aim should be to ventilate with a mode that enables the lowest possible mean airway pressure, yet maintaining a tidal volume of 10 cm^3/kg. While ventilating with a low peak inspiratory pressure, short inspiratory time, increased intermittent mandatory ventilation (IMV) rate, and low levels of positive end-expiratory pressure (PEEP) have been recommended as one ventilation strategy in patients with restrictive RV physiology, the smaller tidal volumes, e.g., 6–8 cm^3/kg, with this pattern of ventilation may reduce lung volume and FRC, thereby increasing PVR and afterload on the RV.

An alternative strategy in a pressure-limited mode of ventilation is to use larger tidal volumes of 12–15 cm^3/kg, with a longer inspiratory time of 0.9–1.0 seconds, increased peak inspiratory pressure of around 30 cm H_2O and low PEEP (i.e., wide ΔP), and slow IMV rate of 12–15 breaths/min. For the same mean airway pressure, RV filling is maintained and RV output augmented by maintaining lung volume and reduced RV afterload.

Left ventricle

Left ventricular preload is also affected by changes in lung volume. Pulmonary blood flow, and therefore preload to the systemic ventricle, may be reduced by an increase or decrease in lung volume secondary to alteration in radial traction on alveoli and extra-alveolar vessels.

The systemic arteries are under higher pressure and not exposed to radial traction effects during inflation or deflation of the lungs. Therefore, changes in lung volume will affect LV preload, but the effect on afterload is dependent on changes in intrathoracic pressure alone rather than changes in lung volume.

In contrast to the RV, a major effect of positive pressure ventilation on the LV is a reduction in afterload. Using La Place's law, wall stress is directly proportional to the transmural LV pressure and the radius of curvature of the LV. The transmural pressure across the LV is the difference between the intracavity LV pressure and surrounding intrathoracic pressure. Assuming a constant arterial pressure and ventricular dimension, an increase in intrathoracic pressure, as occurs during positive pressure ventilation, will reduce the transmural gradient and therefore wall stress on the LV. Therefore, positive pressure ventilation and PEEP can have significant beneficial effects in patients with left ventricular failure (Table 29.3).

Patients with LV dysfunction and increased end-diastolic volume and pressure can have impaired pulmonary mechanics secondary to increased lung water, decreased lung compliance, and increased airway resistance. The work of breathing is increased and neonates can fatigue early because of limited respiratory reserve. A significant proportion of total body oxygen consumption is directed at the increased work of breathing in neonates and infants with LV dysfunction, contributing to poor feeding and failure to thrive. Therefore, positive pressure ventilation has an additional benefit in patients with significant

volume overload and systemic ventricular dysfunction by reducing the work of breathing and oxygen demand.

Weaning from positive pressure ventilation may be difficult in patients with persistent systemic ventricular dysfunction. As spontaneous ventilation increases during the weaning process, swings in mean intrathoracic pressure may substantially alter afterload on the systemic ventricle. Once extubated, the subatmospheric intrapleural pressure means that the transmural pressure across the systemic ventricle is increased. This sudden increase in wall stress may contribute to an increase in end-diastolic pressure and volume, leading to pulmonary edema and a low output state. It may be difficult to determine which patients are likely to fail extubation because of ventricular failure; even a small amount of positive pressure as used during continuous positive airway pressure (CPAP) or pressure support modes of ventilation may be sufficient to reduce afterload and myocardial work. Inotropic agents, vasodilators, and diuretics should be continued throughout the weaning process and early after extubation to maintain stable ventricular function in these patients.

Positive end-expiratory pressure

The use of PEEP in patients with CHD has been controversial. It was initially perceived not to have a significant positive impact on gas exchange, and there was concern that the increased airway pressure could have a detrimental effect on hemodynamics and contribute to lung injury and air leak.

Nevertheless, PEEP increases FRC enabling lung recruitment and redistributes lung water from alveolar septal regions to the more compliant perihilar regions. Both of these actions will improve gas exchange and reduce PVR. PEEP should, therefore, be used in all mechanically ventilated patients following congenital heart surgery. However, excessive levels of PEEP can be detrimental by increasing afterload on the RV. Usually 3–5 cm H_2O of PEEP will help maintain FRC and redistribute lung water without causing hemodynamic compromise.

The use of PEEP in patients who have undergone a Fontan procedure or cavopulmonary anastomosis has also been debated. In this group of patients, pulmonary blood flow is nonpulsatile and depends on the pressure gradient between the superior vena cava (SVC) and the pulmonary venous atrium. During positive pressure ventilation, pulmonary blood flow can be diminished, and during a Valsava maneuver and at high levels of PEEP, retrograde pulmonary blood flow may be demonstrated by Doppler echocardiography. Nevertheless, the beneficial effects of PEEP to 5 cm H_2O as outlined above can be demonstrated following the Fontan procedure, and it rarely contributes to a significant clinical decrease in effective pulmonary blood flow.

Weaning from mechanical ventilation

Weaning from mechanical ventilation is a dynamic process that requires continued reevaluation. While most patients following congenital cardiac surgery who have had no complications with repair or CPB will wean without difficulty, some patients with borderline cardiac function and residual defects may require prolonged mechanical ventilation and a slow weaning process.

The method of weaning varies between patients. Most patients can be weaned using either a volume- or pressure-limited mode by simply decreasing the IMV rate. Guided by physical examination, hemodynamic criteria, respiratory pattern, and arterial blood gas measurements, the mechanical ventilator rate is gradually reduced. Patients with limited hemodynamic and respiratory reserve may demonstrate tachypnea, diaphoresis, and shallow tidal volumes as they struggle to breathe spontaneously against the resistance of the endotracheal tube. The addition of pressure- or flow-triggered pressure support above PEEP at a level related to the size of the endotracheal tube is often beneficial in reducing the work of breathing.

A flow-triggered mode of pressure- or volume-support, with a backup ventilator rate if the patient becomes apneic (assist-control mode), is particularly useful for neonates and infants who have either required prolonged ventilation following surgery or a residual volume or pressure load compromising ventricular function. Patients are often more comfortable weaning in this mode and have reduced work of breathing, and the level of pressure support is adjusted according to their gas exchange, respiratory rate, and tidal volume.

Numerous factors contribute to the inability to wean from mechanical ventilation following congenital heart surgery (Table 29.4). As a general rule, however, residual defects following surgery causing either a volume or pressure load must be excluded first by echocardiography or cardiac catheterization.

Restrictive defects

Pulmonary edema, pleural effusions, and persistent atelectasis may delay weaning from mechanical ventilation. Residual chest and abdominal wall edema, ascites, and hepatomegaly limit chest wall compliance and diaphragmatic excursion. Chest tubes and peritoneal catheters may be necessary to drain pleural effusions and ascites, respectively.

If atelectasis persists, bronchoscopy is often useful to remove secretions and to diagnose extrinsic compression from enlarged pulmonary arteries, a dilated left atrium, or conduits. Upper airway obstruction from vocal cord injury (e.g., recurrent laryngeal nerve damage during aortic

Table 29.4 Factors contributing to the inability to wean from mechanical ventilation after congenital heart surgery

Residual cardiac defects
   Volume and/or pressure overload
   Myocardial dysfunction
   Arrhythmias
Restrictive pulmonary defects
   Pulmonary edema
   Pleural effusion
   Atelectasis
   Pneumothorax
   Chest wall edema
   Phrenic nerve injury
   Ascites
   Hepatomegaly
Airway
   Subglottic edema and/or stenosis
   Retained secretions
   Vocal cord injury
   Extrinsic bronchial compression
   Tracheo-bronchomalacia
Metabolic
   Inadequate nutrition
   Diuretic therapy
   Sepsis
   Stress response

arch reconstruction), edema, or bronchomalacia can also be evaluated.

Phrenic nerve injury can occur during cardiac surgery, either secondary to traction, thermal injury from electrocautery, or direct transection as a complication of extensive aortic arch and pulmonary hilar dissection, particularly for repeat operations. Diaphragmatic paresis (no motion) or paralysis (paradoxical motion) should be investigated in any patient who fails to wean and extubate [16]. Increased work of breathing, increased $PaCO_2$, and/or an elevated hemidiaphragm on chest radiograph following extubation are all consistent with diaphragmatic dysfunction. Ultrasonography or fluoroscopy is useful for identifying abnormal diaphragmatic movement.

Fluid and nutrition

Fluid restriction and aggressive diuretic therapy can result in metabolic disturbances and limit nutritional intake. A hypochloremic, hypokalemic metabolic alkalosis with secondary respiratory acidosis is a common complication from high-dose diuretic use and can delay the ventilator weaning process. Diuretic therapy should be continually reevaluated based on fluid balance, daily weight (if possible), clinical examination, and measurement of electrolyte levels and blood urea nitrogen (BUN). Chloride and potassium supplementation are essential to correct the metabolic acidosis.

It is critical to maintain adequate nutrition, particularly as patients will be catabolic early following cardiac surgery and may have a limited reserve secondary to preoperative failure to thrive. Fluid restriction may limit parenteral nutrition, and enteral nutrition may be poorly tolerated from splanchnic hypoperfusion secondary to low CO or low diastolic pressure (e.g., with an aortopulmonary shunt).

Sedation

Sedation is often necessary to improve synchronization with the ventilator and maintain hemodynamic stability. However, excessive sedation and/or withdrawal symptoms from opioids and benzodiazepines will impair the weaning process.

Sepsis

Sepsis is a frequent cause of failure to wean from mechanical ventilation in the ICU. Invasive monitoring catheters are a common source for blood stream infections, and the increased utilization of invasive monitoring after cardiac surgery may increase the risk for catheter-associated blood stream infections (CA-BSI). In addition to sending surveillance blood cultures and initiation of antibiotic therapy, removal or replacement of central venous and arterial catheters should be considered as soon as possible during an episode of suspected or culture-proven sepsis. Following standardized protocols for catheter insertion, access, and maintenance can reduce the incidence of CA-BSI. More recently a subset of patients at increased risk following cardiac surgery have been identified who may benefit from additional strategies, such as the insertion of antibiotic-coated catheters (Table 29.5) [17,18].

Table 29.5 Factors associated with an increased risk for catheter-associated blood stream infection in patients with congenital cardiac defects before and after surgery

Risk factors at the time of admission
  Unscheduled admission
  Noncardiac comorbidities
  Weight ≤ 5 kg
  Greater surgical complexity (RACHS-1 category ≥3)
Risk factors developing after admission
  Greater initial severity of illness (PRISM-III score ≥ 15)
  Prolonged use of central venous catheters
  Hydrocortisone use for presumed adrenal insufficiency
  Greater blood product exposures
  Prolonged mechanical ventilation

The signs of sepsis may be subtle and nonspecific, and often broad-spectrum intravenous (IV) antibiotic coverage is started before culture results are known. Signs to note in neonates and infants include temperature instability (hyper- or hypothermia), hypoglycemia, unexplained metabolic acidosis, hypotension and tachycardia with poor extremity perfusion and oliguria, increased respiratory effort and ventilation requirements, altered consciousness, and leukocytosis with left shift on white blood cell count.

Colonization of the airway occurs frequently in patients mechanically ventilated for an extended period, but may not require IV antibiotic therapy unless there is evidence of either increased secretions with fever, leukocytosis, new chest radiograph abnormalities, or detection of an organism on Gram stain together with abundant neutrophils. Urinary tract infection and both superficial and deep surgical site infections must also be excluded in patients with clinical suspicion of sepsis (i.e., sternotomy or thoracotomy wounds), and in addition to careful insertion practices, early removal of the urinary catheter is recommended.

Tight glycemic control may help reduce the risk for infection after pediatric cardiac surgery, although definitive data for this subset of patients are not yet available. Further, a slightly higher range of glucose level may be acceptable without increasing the risk of infection, and thereby also helping to avoid the serious complication of hypoglycemia, which may occur in newborns and infants if an insulin infusion is used to achieve tight glycemic control [19].

Airway

Bronchospasm can complicate mechanical ventilation and the weaning process. While this may reflect intrinsic airway disease, bronchospasm can also result from increased airway secretions and extrinsic airway compression. Treatment with inhaled or systemic bronchodilators may be beneficial, although they should be used with caution because of their chronotropic and tachyarrhythmic potential.

The sudden onset of bronchospasm with increased peak inspiratory pressure and difficult hand ventilation should raise the immediate concern for acute endotracheal tube obstruction or pneumothorax. Bronchospasm in patients with labile PVR may reflect acute pulmonary hypertension, and treatment is directed at maneuvers to lower pulmonary artery pressure and improve CO.

Postextubation stridor may be due to mucosal swelling of the large airway, and treatment with dexamethasone before extubation can be beneficial to reduce edema in patients who have required prolonged ventilation. Stridor following extubation is initially treated with nebulized racemic epinephrine, which promotes vasoconstriction and decreases airway hyperemia and edema. If reintubation is necessary, a smaller endotracheal tube should be used. Vocal cord dysfunction should also be considered, particularly as surgery around the ductus arteriosus and left pulmonary artery may injure the recurrent laryngeal nerve.

The ability to clear secretions and potential for nosocomial infection are additional concerns in patients who have been ventilated for an extended period of time. Inability to clear secretions because of sedation, bulbar, and vocal cord dysfunction, ineffective cough following prolonged intubation and poor nutritional state with muscle fatigue will result in atelectasis and respiratory failure. Frequent chest physiotherapy, mask CPAP, and nasopharyngeal suction are beneficial, provided patients are hemodynamically stable with adequate gas exchange. In tachypneic patients, the use of nasopharyngeal CPAP can be beneficial by reducing the work of breathing; however, these patients have limited reserve and frequent reassessment is essential.

Myocardial dysfunction and monitoring

Assessment of cardiac output

The accurate assessment of the postoperative patient's CO should be a focus of management in the ICU. Establishing an adequate CO is important, because low CO is associated with longer duration of mechanical ventilatory support, ICU stay, and hospital stay, all of which can increase the risk of morbidity and/or mortality. Data from physical examination, routine laboratory testing, bedside hemodynamic monitoring, echocardiography, and occasionally bedside CO determination typically are sufficient to manage patients optimally. If patients are not progressing as expected and low CO persists, a cardiac catheterization should be performed to investigate and exclude the possibility of residual or undiagnosed structural defects.

The systemic CO is defined as the product of ventricular stroke volume (in liters/beat) multiplied by heart rate (in beats/min) [20]. The ventricular stroke volume is determined chiefly by three factors: afterload (the resistance to ventricular emptying), preload (the atrial filling pressure), and myocardial contractility. CO is usually indexed to body surface area (BSA, in m^2) because it is a function of body mass. Thus, CO/BSA is designated cardiac index (CI) (in L/min/m^2). The CI varies inversely with age so that normal values in children at rest are 4.0–5.0 L/min/m^2, whereas the normal resting CI at age 70 is 2.5 L/min/m^2 [21].

Postoperative patients with low CO can present with a variety of abnormalities on physical exam or of bedside monitoring and laboratory values. These manifesta-

Table 29.6 Manifestations of low cardiac output

Physical examination
Mental status: Lethargy or irritability

Vital signs: Core hyperthermia (often associated with peripheral vasoconstriction)
  Tachycardia or bradycardia
  Tachypnea
  Hypotension (for age and weight)
  Narrow pulse pressure

Peripheral perfusion: Pale or mottled skin color and cool skin temperature
  Prolonged (>3 s) distal extremity capillary refill
  Poorly palpable pulses

Signs of congestive heart failure: Failure to thrive, poor feeding and diaphoresis
  Increased respiratory work, chest wall retraction
  Tachypnea, grunting
  Gallop rhythm
  Hepatomegaly

Bedside monitoring data
ECG tracing: Rhythm other than normal sinus
Arterial waveform: Blunted upstroke and narrow pulse pressure
Atrial pressure change: See Table 29.7
Urine output: <1.0 mL/kg/h in neonates, infants, and children
  <25 mL/h in older patients

Laboratory and radiographic data
SvO_2: Decreased (<65–70%) with an increased (>25–30%)
  AV O_2 difference

Acid–base balance: Metabolic acidosis with increased anion gap
  Increased arterial lactate (>2.2 mM/L)

Electrolytes: Hyperkalemia
  Elevated BUN and Cr
  Increased liver transaminases

Chest radiography: Cardiac enlargement
  Abnormal (increased or decreased) pulmonary blood flow
  Pulmonary edema

AV, arteriovenous; BUN, blood urea nitrogen; Cr, creatinine; SvO_2, systemic venous oxygen saturation.

tions of low CO are listed in Table 29.6. Clinical signs on examination include cool extremities and diminished peripheral perfusion, tachycardia, hypotension, oliguria, and hepatomegaly. An increase in the arterial to mixed venous oxygen saturation difference (a–vO_2) of >30% and a metabolic acidosis provide biochemical evidence for an LCOS. The atrial pressure is a useful measure to follow, and both an increase and decrease could be observed in an LCOS. Factors that should be considered when evaluating the atrial pressure following surgery are shown in Table 29.7.

The mechanism(s) underlying low CO in a specific patient can be related to one or a combination of factors following surgery. Strategies for treating the patient with

Table 29.7 Factors that should be considered when there is a change in the measured atrial pressure outside of the anticipated range for a particular postoperative patient

Increased

Increased ventricular end-diastolic pressure
    Decreased ventricular systolic or diastolic function
    Myocardial ischemia
    Ventricular hypertrophy
    Ventricular outflow obstruction
    Semilunar valve disease

Mitral or tricuspid valve disease

Large left-to-right anatomic shunt
    Residual ventricular septal defect
    Systemic-to-pulmonary artery connection

Chamber hypoplasia
Intravascular or ventricular volume overload
Cardiac tamponade

Dysrhythmia
    Tachyarrhythmia
    Complete heart block

Artifactual
    Catheter tip not in the atrium (e.g., in a ventricle or wedged in a
        pulmonary vein)
    Pressure transducer below level of heart or improperly calibrated or
        zeroed
    Concomitant drug infusions through the atrial line

Decreased

Inadequate preload

Artifactual
    Catheter malfunction (e.g., cracked or clotted)
    Pressure transducer above level of heart, or improperly calibrated or
        zeroed

an LCOS should focus on optimizing the balance between oxygen delivery (DO_2) and consumption (VO_2). In an LCOS, oxygen and metabolic demand should be minimized by maintaining an adequate depth of analgesia and sedation, including chemical paralysis to avoid movement and reduce muscle tone and oxygen debt. Strict avoidance of hyperthermia from any cause is essential, and in some circumstances, mild hypothermia may be preferable, although the effect of peripheral vasoconstriction and increase in SVR could have an adverse effect on myocardial wall stress and oxygen requirement.

Surgical factors

Residual or unrecognized defects

A thorough understanding of the underlying cardiac anatomy, surgical findings, and surgical procedures is essential because this will direct the initial postoperative evaluation and examination. Residual lesions may be evident by auscultation, intracardiac pressures and waveforms, and oxygen saturation data. For example, a large V wave on the left atrial waveform may indicate significant residual mitral valve regurgitation. A step-up of the right atrial to pulmonary artery oxygen saturation of more than 10% may indicate a significant intracardiac shunt across a residual VSD.

However, if there are significant concerns for important residual lesions that are compromising CO and ventricular function, further evaluation with echocardiography and/or cardiac catheterization should be considered. Imaging of the heart may be difficult immediately after surgery because of limited transthoracic access and acoustic windows. During transthoracic echocardiography, it is important that hemodynamics be closely observed, because inadvertent pressure applied with the transducer may adversely affect filling pressures and mechanical ventilation. Similarly, vigorous antegrade flexion of a transesophageal echocardiography probe may alter left atrial filling or compromise ventilation by partial obstruction of a main stem bronchus.

Surgical procedure and technique

While surgery may be routine for many uncomplicated defects, such as ASD closure, the approach for more complex intracardiac repairs may cause specific postoperative problems. For example, if a ventriculotomy is performed to close the VSD in a patient with TOF, RV dyskinesia and poor contraction may be apparent. On the other hand, if a transatrial approach had been used to close the VSD in the same patient, the risk for atrioventricular valve injury or dysrhythmias such as junctional ectopic tachycardia and heart block is increased. Often unexpected findings or technical difficulties at the time of surgery mean that modifications to the approach or procedure are necessary. A difficult procedure may lead to a longer time on CPB or additional traction on cardiac structures.

Complications related to surgery

Failure to secure adequate hemostasis may expose the patient to significant volumes of tranfused blood products, and if there is inadequate drainage via chest drains placed at the time of surgery, the risk for cardiac tamponade is significant. This may be an acute event, but more commonly it is evident by progressive hypotension with a narrow pulse width, tachycardia, an increase in filling pressures and reduced peripheral perfusion with possible evolving metabolic acidosis. This is primarily a clinical diagnosis and treatment (i.e., opening of the sternum) should not be delayed while waiting for possible echocardiographic confirmation.

Myocardial ischemia from inadequate coronary perfusion is often an under-appreciated event in the postoperative pediatric patient. Nevertheless, there are a number of circumstances in which ischemia may occur, compromising ventricular function and CO. Myocardial ischemia may occur intraoperatively because of problems with cardioplegia delivery or insufficient hypothermic myocardial protection, and from intracoronary air embolism. In the ICU setting, mechanical obstruction of the coronary circulation is usually the cause of myocardial ischemia rather than coronary vasospasm. Examples include extrinsic compression of a coronary artery by an outflow tract conduit or annulus of a prosthetic valve, and kinking or distortion of a transferred coronary artery button. While electrocardiogram (ECG) changes may indicate ischemia (ST segment abnormalities), a sudden increase in left atrial pressure or sudden onset of a dysrhythmia such as ventricular fibrillation or complete heart block may be an earlier warning sign.

Cardiopulmonary bypass and the systemic inflammatory response

The effects of prolonged CPB relate in part to the interactions of blood components with the extracorporeal circuit. This is magnified in children due to the large bypass circuit surface area and priming volume relative to patient blood volume. Humoral responses include activation of complement, kallikrein, eicosinoid, and fibrinolytic cascades; cellular responses include platelet activation and an inflammatory response with an adhesion molecule cascade stimulating neutrophil activation and release of proteolytic and vasoactive substances [22,23].

The clinical consequences include increased interstitial fluid and generalized capillary leak, and potential multiorgan dysfunction. Total lung water is increased with an associated decrease in lung compliance and increase in A–aO$_2$ gradient. Myocardial edema results in impaired ventricular systolic and diastolic function. A secondary fall in CO by 20–30% is common in neonates in the first 6–12 hours following surgery, contributing to decreased renal function and oliguria [24]. Sternal closure may need to be delayed due to mediastinal edema and associated cardiorespiratory compromise when closure is attempted. Ascites, hepatic ingestion, and bowel edema may affect mechanical ventilation, causing a prolonged ileus and delay in enteral feeding. A coagulopathy post-CPB may contribute to delayed hemostasis. (See Chapter 8 for a detailed discussion of the inflammatory response to CPB.)

Dysrhythmias

The ECG is an essential component of the initial postoperative evaluation because the ICU team must identify whether the patient is in sinus rhythm early in the recovery period. If the rhythm cannot be determined with certainty from a surface 12- or 15-lead ECG, temporary epicardial atrial pacing wires, if present, can be used with the limb leads to generate an atrial ECG [25]. Also, right and left atrial waveforms are useful in diagnosing atrioventricular synchrony (see Chapter 17). Temporary epicardial atrial and/or ventricular pacing wires are routinely placed in most patients to allow mechanical pacing should sinus node dysfunction or heart block occur in the early postoperative period. Because atrial wires are applied directly to the atrial epicardium, the electrical signal generated by atrial depolarization is significantly larger and thus easy to distinguish compared to the P wave on a surface ECG. Sinus tachycardia, which is common and often secondary to medications (e.g., sympathomimetics), pain and anxiety, or diminished ventricular function, must be distinguished from a supraventricular, ventricular, or junctional tachycardia. Any of these tachyarrhythmias can lower CO by either compromising diastolic filling of the ventricles or depressing their systolic function [26,27]. High-grade second-degree heart block and third-degree (or complete) heart block can diminish CO by producing either bradycardia or loss of atrioventricular synchrony or both. Third-degree block is transient in approximately one-third of cases. If it persists beyond postoperative day 9–10, it is unlikely to resolve, and a permanent pacemaker is indicated [28] (see Chapter 17).

Low preload

The diagnosis of insufficient preload is usually made by monitoring the mean atrial pressure or central venous pressure. The most common cause in the ICU is hypovolemia secondary to blood loss from postoperative bleeding. Initially after surgery and CPB, the filling pressures may be in the normal range or slightly elevated, but this often reflects a centralized blood volume secondary to peripheral vaso- and venoconstriction following hypothermic CPB. As the patient continues to rewarm and vasodilate in the ICU, considerable IV volume may be necessary to maintain the circulating blood volume. There may also be significant third-space fluid loss in neonates and small infants who manifest the greatest systemic inflammatory response following CPB. The "leaking" of fluid into serous cavities (e.g., ascites) and the extracellular space (edema progressing to anasarca) requires that these patients receive close monitoring and volume replacement to maintain the circulating blood volume. Patients with a hypertrophied or poorly compliant ventricle, and those with lesions dependent on complete mixing at the atrial level, also often require additional preload in the early postoperative period.

High afterload

Elevated afterload in both the pulmonary and systemic circulations frequently follows surgery with CPB [29]. Excessive afterload in the systemic circulation is caused by elevated SVR and typically produces both diminished peripheral perfusion and low urine output. Treatment of elevated SVR includes recognizing and improving conditions that exacerbate vasoconstriction (e.g., pain and hypothermia) and administering a vasodilating agent. A vasodilator, which can be either a phosphodiesterase inhibitor (e.g., milrinone) or a nitric oxide donor (e.g., nitroprusside), is frequently added to an inotropic agent such as dopamine to augment CO [30–33]. Neonates, who tolerate increased afterload less well than older infants and children, appear to derive particular benefit from afterload reduction therapy.

Decreased myocardial contractility

Because decreased myocardial contractility occurs frequently after reparative or palliative surgery with CPB, pharmacologic enhancement of contractility is used routinely in the ICU. Before initiating treatment with an inotrope, however, the patient's intravascular volume status, serum ionized Ca^{++} level, and cardiac rhythm should be considered. Inotropic agents enhance CO more effectively if preload is adequate, so IV colloid or crystalloid administration should be given if preload is low. If hypocalcemia (normal serum ionized Ca^{++} levels are 1.14–1.30 mmol/L) [34] is detected, supplementation with IV calcium gluconate or calcium chloride is appropriate, because Ca^{++} is a potent positive inotrope itself, particularly in neonates and infants [35].

Dopamine is usually the first-line agent to treat of either mild (10–20% decrease in normal mean arterial blood pressure for age) or moderate (20–30% decrease in normal mean arterial blood pressure for age) hypotension. This sympathomimetic agent promotes myocardial contractility by elevating intracellular Ca^{++}, both via direct binding to myocyte β_1-adrenoceptors and by increasing norepinephrine levels. Dopamine is administered by a constant infusion because of its short half-life, and a usual starting dose for inotropy is 5 mcg/kg/min. At a dose >5 mcg/kg/min, dopamine should be infused through a central venous catheter to avoid superficial tissue damage should extravasation occur. The dose is titrated to achieve the desired systemic blood pressure, although some patients, especially older children and adults, may develop an undesirable dose-dependent tachycardia.

If a patient does not respond adequately to dopamine up to 10 mcg/kg/min or has severe hypotension (more than 30% decrease in mean arterial blood pressure for age), treatment with epinephrine should be considered.

Epinephrine should be given exclusively via a central venous catheter and can be added to dopamine at a starting dose of 0.03–0.0.05 mcg/kg/min, with subsequent titration of the infusion to achieve the target systemic blood pressure. At high doses (i.e., ≥ 0.3 mcg/kg/min), epinephrine can produce significant renal and peripheral vasoconstriction, tachycardia, and increased myocardial oxygen demand. Patients with severe ventricular dysfunction who require persistent or escalating doses of epinephrine >0.3–0.5 mcg/kg/min may benefit from opening of the sternum and/or should be evaluated for the possibility of mechanical circulatory support with a ventricular assist device (VAD) or extracorporeal membrane oxygenation (ECMO) (see below).

A combination of epinephrine at lower doses (e.g., <0.1 mcg/kg/min) or dopamine with an IV afterload reducing agent such as nitroprusside or milrinone is frequently beneficial to support patients with significant ventricular dysfunction accompanied by elevated afterload. Epinephrine is preferred to the equally potent inotrope norepinephrine because it generally is well tolerated in pediatric patients and causes less dramatic vasoconstriction. Norepinephrine is a direct-acting alpha agonist, primarily causing intense arteriolar vasoconstriction, but it also has positive inotropic actions. At doses of 0.01–0.2 mcg/kg/min, it can be considered in patients with severe hypotension and low SVR (e.g., "warm" or "distributive" shock), inadequate coronary artery perfusion or inadequate pulmonary blood flow with a systemic-to-pulmonary artery shunt. There can be a decrease in responsiveness to increasing doses of catecholamines over time, and vasopressin at a dose of 10–120 milliunits/kg/h is a potent vasopressor that may help improve the hemodynamics in advanced shock without compromising cardiac function [36].

Patients who have the clinical features of relative adrenal insufficiency may benefit from stress steroid therapy [37–39]. This is primarily a clinical finding of poor vascular tone with persistent hypotension and volume requirement that is refractory to increasing inotrope and/or vasopressor support. The serum cortisol level may be low or show a limited response to ACTH stimulation testing; however, the ranges of normal have not been established for pediatric patients, and in particular for newborns and infants after cardiac surgery, and there is no consistent correlation between serum cortisol level and LCOS. Nevertheless, stress doses of hydrocortisone (50 mg/m^2/day) have been demonstrated to increase systemic blood pressure and lower inotrope scores, although they have not been definitively demonstrated to improve eventual survival. The increased risk for infection and poor wound healing dictates that stress dosing of steroids should be for a brief period of time (e.g., over 3–5 days) rather than continuing with a longer taper.

Hypothyroidism is another cause for a persistent LCOS after cardiac surgery. Triiodothyronine (T_3) levels have been demonstrated to be low after CPB, and may remain low for up to 5 days after surgery, particularly if a sick euthyroid state develops and there is decreased conversion of thyroxine (T_4) to the biologically active T_3 in peripheral tissues [40, 41]. An infusion of T_3 at a dose of 0.05 mcg/kg/h has been shown to improve blood pressure and a composite score of recovery after cardiac surgery in newborns and infants [40].

Delayed sternal closure

Pericardial and sternal closure following cardiac surgery causes a restriction to cardiac function and can interfere with efficient mechanical ventilation. This is particularly important for neonates and infants in whom considerable capillary leak and edema can develop following CPB, and in whom cardiopulmonary interactions have a significant impact on immediate postoperative recovery. In the operating room, mediastinal edema, unstable hemodynamic conditions, and bleeding are indications for delayed sternal closure, although it may also be considered semi-electively for patients in whom hemodynamic or respiratory instability are anticipated in the immediate postoperative period (e.g., following a Norwood procedure for HLHS). Urgent reopening of the sternum in the ICU following surgery is associated with higher mortality compared to leaving the sternum open in the operating room, and successful sternal closure can be achieved for most patients by postoperative day 4 with a low risk for surgical site infection [42, 43].

Mechanical support of the circulation

Mechanical assist devices have an important role providing short-term circulatory support to enable myocardial recovery early after surgery and the potential for longer-term support while awaiting cardiac transplantation. Although a variety of assist devices are available for adult-sized patients, other than ECMO, the development of alternate pediatric VADs has lagged behind adult devices. A problem for pediatric patients is determining which method of support is optimal. While venoarterial ECMO provides biventricular support with oxygenation, a number of patients may benefit from univentricular support with a left or right VAD.

Extracorporeal membrane oxygenation

ECMO has become the most widely used mode of mechanical cardiopulmonary support for children with CHD. Venoarterial ECMO (venous cannula in the RA or SVC and

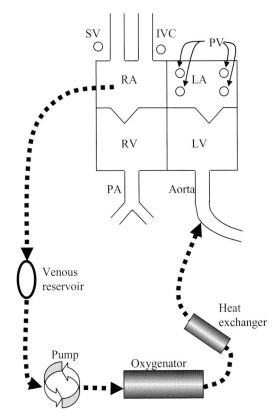

Figure 29.4 Extracorporeal membrane oxygenation (ECMO) circuit. The dashed lines represent flow through a venoarterial ECMO circuit. Blood is drained from the right atrium by direct atrial cannulation, or from an SVC catheter advanced into the right atrium. When using a roller pump, the blood is first drained to a small venous reservoir; with a centrifugal pump, a reservoir is not used. Blood then passes through a membrane oxygenator and heat exchanger before returning to the ascending aorta, which is cannulated directly or via the right carotid artery. SVC, superior vena cava; IVC, inferior vena cava; RA, right atrium; RV, right ventricle; PA, pulmonary artery; PV, pulmonary vein; LA, left atrium; LV, left ventricle

arterial cannula in the aorta or innominate artery) is the mode of support necessary for patients with cardiac failure. ECMO fully supports the heart and lungs, similar to conventional CPB, and requires significant systemic anticoagulation. Figure 29.4 depicts a standard ECMO circuit. Currently, there are over 300 children per year who receive ECMO for cardiac support reported to the Extracorporeal Life Support Registry, with the majority of patients placed on ECMO following cardiotomy [44–46]. However, the percentage of patients who are successfully decannulated from ECMO in the ICU (approximately 40–45% of all reported cases), and the percentage of patients subsequently discharged home after cardiac ECMO (approximately 37% of reported cases), has remained largely unchanged over the last 5 years [45,47]. Therefore, critical appraisal of indications and techniques is required if the success rate for cardiac ECMO is to increase to levels currently achieved in neonates with respiratory distress syndrome (approximately 90%).

Centers with an efficient and well-established ECMO service are more likely to utilize this form of support in patients with low CO. Furthermore, surgical technique and bypass management are additional, complicated factors which make comparisons of the use and indications for ECMO between institutions difficult to interpret. Nevertheless, this form of mechanical support clearly can be life-saving and must be available, if needed, for selected patients following congenital heart surgery.

ECMO may be useful for critically ill patients prior to cardiac surgery, thereby enabling preoperative stabilization and limiting end-organ dysfunction prior to repair. These patients form a small group, usually neonates, and indications include severe low output state, pulmonary hypertension, and severe hypoxemia.

The best outcomes from ECMO are in postoperative patients who have a period of relative stability after reparative surgery, but then develop progressive myocardial or respiratory failure, or have a sudden cardiac arrest. Hospital survival in this group of patients has been reported to be as high as 70% [45,48]. The outcome of patients who require ECMO because of inability to wean from CPB in the operating room is generally poor, with a reported survival between 10 and 33% [48–50]. Other than factors such as primary myocardial dysfunction, pulmonary hypertension, severe hypoxemia, and cardiac dysrhythmia after surgical repair, lack of a significant residual defect(s) is the major factor determining successful outcome.

Patients with a systemic-to-pulmonary artery shunt also have worse outcomes when ECMO is used [51]. Pulmonary runoff through the shunt will limit systemic flow and contribute to both pulmonary over circulation and ventricular volume overload. Therefore, partial occlusion of the shunt may be necessary while on ECMO. When attempting to discontinue ECMO, shunt flow is reestablished, potentially causing a reperfusion injury in the pulmonary vasculature and severe pulmonary hypertension. Reducing the shunt size to allow a limited amount of pulmonary flow while on ECMO will reduce the incidence of this complication.

The survival of pediatric patients who require in-hospital resuscitation following a cardiorespiratory arrest has been reported to be extremely poor [52,53]. Nevertheless, following pediatric cardiac surgery, ECMO has been used successfully to support children, even after prolonged cardiac arrest unresponsive to conventional closed or open chest cardiac massage [54–58]. Prolonged resuscitation, particularly when combined with the obligatory time taken to set up the ECMO circuit, obviously increases the likelihood of significant neurologic and other end-organ injury, and many centers have developed rapid deployment ECMO teams and circuits that are primed for immediate use in the ICU at all times. Patients without significant recovery of cardiac function within 10–15 minutes of the initiation of properly applied advanced life support measures following a witnessed cardiac arrest, and who have no contraindication to mechanical support, are cannulated either through the chest, neck, or groin and ECMO initiated.

ECMO may also be used as a bridge to cardiac transplantation. However, prolonged support from ECMO is associated with increasing complications such as bleeding, renal failure, and sepsis. In our experience, if there is no significant recovery of myocardial function after 48–72 hours on ECMO support, a cardiac transplant evaluation is performed [55].

A brief review of ECMO management principles follows. In emergency situations, an asanguinous prime is used, with blood added later after initiation of ECMO flow. Initially, the patient is supported with ECMO flows approaching full bypass flow, i.e., 100–150 mL/kg/min for patients less than 10 kg. This provides opportunity for a completely unloaded myocardium to recover from an ischemic insult and fully supports other organ systems. Inotropic agents are discontinued or minimized in order to prevent down regulation of adrenergic receptors in the myocardium and peripheral vasculature. Vasodilating agents such as milrinone, nitroprusside, or phentolamine are often required to maintain mean arterial pressure within desired limits. The left atrium may need to be decompressed with a small cannula in patients who have blood return to the left heart and an intact atrial septum (e.g., those with systemic to pulmonary collaterals). Left atrial pressure may also be elevated if ECMO flow is inadequate. The lungs are ventilated with "lung rest" settings to prevent atelectasis, but also to avoid oxygen toxicity and barotrauma (e.g., a rate of 10–20 breaths/min, FIO_2 less than 0.50, and PEEP of 5 cm H_2O or less with long inspiratory times and low peak inflating pressures). Anticoagulation is maintained with a heparin infusion, usually at 10–20 units/kg/h, and titrated to keep the activated clotting time (ACT) within 200–250 seconds. Ongoing bleeding and coagulopathy are common, and blood products must be readily available for infusion into the circuit. The need for surgical exploration is common in these patients due to accumulation of blood or clot in the mediastinum or under a patch covering an open sternum. The platelet count is maintained above 100,000, the hematocrit above 30, and the prothrombin time within the normal range. Aminocaproic acid has been shown to be effective at reducing blood loss and transfusion in cardiac ECMO [59]. Central nervous system (CNS) bleeding is a catastrophic complication and should be suspected when there is sudden volume loss without other explanation. Cranial ultrasonography in infants is adequate for screening or diagnostic purposes. Infectious complications are prevented by meticulous sterile technique, and in many cases, broad-spectrum antibiotics are administered. Inadequate ECMO circuit volume is indicated by excessive negative pressure readings on the venous side of the circuit, and an inability to maintain target flows and mean arterial pressures. Renal insufficiency can be managed by placing a hemofilter in the circuit for continuous hemofiltration. Sedation, analgesia, and paralysis are required for these patients, and tolerance develops rapidly. ECMO support is weaned when the compromised myocardium has recovered, which may vary from as little as 24–48 hours to 3–4 weeks. Transthoracic echocardiography may give an estimate of contractility if volume is added to the heart. Before weaning flow, inotropic agents must be restarted or increased, the hematocrit and electrolytes optimized, and ventilation increased. As ECMO flow is gradually reduced, additional cardiovascular support with intravascular volume and intropes may be required, and CO is assessed at lower levels of flow. If repeated attempts to wean are unsuccessful, the caregivers and parents/guardians must decide if support should be withdrawn or the patient listed for cardiac transplantation.

Ventricular assist devices

The experience with VADs in children remains relatively small primarily due to technical considerations and concerns regarding suitability of children with CHD for univentricular support [60]. A major limitation of the application of adult systems for pediatric patients is the risk of thromboembolism when lower flows are used.

The majority of pediatric patients reported have received left ventricular support, which has been particularly beneficial in patients with an ischemic myocardium secondary to an anomalous left coronary artery from the pulmonary artery, and in patients who require retraining of an "unprepared" LV in d-TGA and intact ventricular septum or a small VSD after an arterial switch procedure [48]. Survival results reported to date are similar to those achieved with cardiac ECMO.

A VAD has a number of advantages. The circuit is simple in design, takes less time to prime, and requires little technical manipulation once established. It may more effectively decompress the LV, and pulsatile flow is possible with some devices (e.g., Thoratec PVAD and Berlin Heart EXCOR). Bleeding complications and platelet consumption are often less problematic in patients on VADs compared to ECMO. Because of the lower complications associated with VADs, patients may be supported for a longer period (e.g., months) as a bridge to transplantation [61].

Management of the patient on VAD support is similar to ECMO in some respects, but the following important

differences exist. An oxygenator is not used with a VAD, requiring full ventilatory support. Decreased intravascular volume causes a reduction in flow; therefore, atrial filling pressures are monitored to establish a Starling curve for each patient. The circuit volume is smaller, and because there is no oxygenator in the circuit, a lower level of anticoagulation is required (ACT of 180–200 s). Consequently, bleeding complications are fewer with VADs. A patient receiving LVAD support must have a RV capable of pumping blood into the lungs. Inotropic support and RV afterload reduction to reduce PVR (e.g., milrinone or inhaled nitric oxide) may be necessary. If the RV fails, either a biventricular assist device or ECMO needs to be instituted. Since the patient's lungs provide oxygenation, ventilation and pulmonary toilet must be optimized. Patients with intracardiac shunts (e.g., a PFO) may not be suitable candidates for VAD because arterial desaturation may develop from R→L shunting, and there is increased risk of paradoxical emboli causing stroke. The principles for weaning attempts are similar to those discussed above for ECMO.

Application of adult VAD technology to larger pediatric patients and miniaturization of existing technology has increased the availability of VADs in children and the potential to provide longer periods of mechanical support of the circulation with fewer complications. Patients can potentially be extubated and ambulate. Two such devices are the Thoratec [62], available for patients down to approximately 17 kg, and the Berlin Heart [63], which has been miniaturized for patients to <5 kg. The survival rates for infants and children with application of these technologies is 50–70% [64,65]. (See Chapter 31 for a more detailed discussion of ECMO and VADs in children.)

Intra-aortic balloon pump

Intra-aortic balloon pumps have been used with success in infants and children, although experience is limited [66]. Problems in pediatric patients include size constraints of the device and balloon, difficulty synchronizing the balloon inflation–deflation cycle with faster heart rates, and the increased elasticity of the aorta, which makes effective counterpulsation difficult.

Fluid management and renal function

Because the inflammatory response to CPB often leads to an increase in total body water, fluid management in the immediate postoperative period is critical. Capillary leak and interstitial fluid accumulation continue for the first 24–48 hours following surgery, necessitating ongoing volume replacement with colloid or blood products. A fall in CO and increased antidiuretic hormone secretion contribute to delayed water clearance and potential prerenal dysfunction, which could progress to acute tubular necrosis and renal failure if an LCOS persists.

During bypass, optimizing the circuit prime hematocrit and oncotic pressure, possibly attenuating the inflammatory response with steroids, and the use of modified ultrafiltration techniques have all been recommended to limit interstitial fluid accumulation [67,68]. During the first 24 hours following surgery, maintenance fluids should be restricted to 50% of full maintenance, and volume replacement titrated to appropriate filling pressures and hemodynamic response.

Oliguria in the first 24 hours after complex surgery and CPB is common in neonates and infants, even when CO is adequate. While diuretics are commonly prescribed in the immediate postoperative period, CO must also be enhanced with volume replacement and vasoactive drug infusions for these to be most effective. In addition to supporting CO, low-dose dopamine (3 mcg/kg/min) may have the advantage of increasing renal blood flow and promoting diuresis. Fenoldopam mesylate, a selective dopamine receptor (DA_1) agonist, leads to both renal and splanchnic vasodilation, and at a dose of 0.1–0.5 mcg/kg/min, it may also have a role in postoperative ICU management to enhance renal perfusion by decreasing renal vascular resistance [69].

Furosemide (1 mg/kg IV every 8–12 h) is a commonly prescribed loop diuretic that must be excreted into the renal tubular system before producing diuresis. Low CO therefore reduces its efficacy. Bolus dosing may result in a significant diuresis over a short period, thereby causing changes in intravascular volume and possibly hypotension. Rapid boluses may also damage the hair cells of the inner ear in premature and full-term newborns, causing hearing loss. A continuous infusion of 0.2–0.3 mg/kg/h after an initial bolus of 1 mg/kg IV often provides a more consistent and sustained diuresis without sudden fluid shifts. Chlorothiazide (5–10 mg/kg IV or PO every 6–12 h) is also an effective diuretic, particularly when used in conjunction with loop diuretics.

Peritoneal dialysis, hemodialysis, and continuous venovenous hemofiltration provide alternate renal replacement therapy in patients with persistent oliguria and renal failure [70,71]. In addition to enabling water and solute clearance, fluids with increased nutritional content can be increased in volume to ensure adequate nutrition. The indications for renal support vary, but include BUN >100 mg/dL, life-threatening electrolyte imbalance such as severe hyperkalemia, ongoing metabolic acidosis, fluid restrictions limiting adequate nutrition, and increased mechanical ventilation requirements secondary to persistent pulmonary edema, reduced chest wall compliance, or ascites.

A peritoneal dialysis catheter can be placed into the peritoneal cavity at the completion of surgery or later in the ICU and used for simple drainage or dialysis. Indications in the ICU include the need for renal support or to reduce intra-abdominal pressure from ascites that may be compromising mechanical ventilation. Drainage may be significant in the immediate postoperative period as third space fluid losses continue, and replacement with albumin and/or fresh frozen plasma may be necessary to treat hypovolemia and hypoproteinemia.

To enhance fluid excretion if oliguria persists, "minivolume dialysis" may be effective using 10 cm^3/kg of 1.5 or 2.25% dialysate over a 30–40 minute cycle. A persistent communication between the peritoneum, mediastinum, and/or pleural cavities following surgery will limit the effectiveness of peritoneal dialysis and is a relative contraindication.

Arteriovenous hemofiltration or hemodialysis through double lumen femoral or subclavian vein catheters (typically 7 Fr in size) can be used effectively in neonates. Complications related to venous access, catheter-related thrombosis and hemodynamic instability are potential complications that require close monitoring.

Hemostasis

Hemostasis after surgery may be difficult to obtain, particularly if CPB has been prolonged, if there are extensive suture lines, and following repeat cardiac surgery. Prompt management and meticulous control of surgical bleeding is essential to prevent the complications associated with a massive transfusion. Generally, if postoperative bleeding >10 cm^3/kg/h persists in the immediate postoperative period with a normal coagulation profile and platelet count, surgical bleeding should be suspected and reexploration considered.

Factors contributing to a coagulopathy after CPB include hemodilution of coagulation factors and platelets from the bypass circuit prime, stimulation of the intrinsic coagulation pathway, and both platelet activation and aggregation. In addition, several preoperative factors may contribute to postoperative coagulopathy: chronic cyanosis, low CO with tissue hypoperfusion and disseminated intravascular coagulopathy, hepatic immaturity or dysfunction, and the use of platelet inhibitors such as prostaglandin E_1 (PGE_1) infusion and aspirin.

Transfusion of platelets and fresh frozen plasma or cryoprecipitate is often necessary. Priming the bypass circuit with reconstituted whole blood has been demonstrated to be beneficial in neonates and infants undergoing cardiac surgery to reduce postbypass bleeding [72,73]. Antifibrinolytic drugs such as E-aminocaproic acid and tranexamic acid are used intraoperatively to reduce postoperative bleeding, but may also be effective in the ICU if coagulopathy and fibrinolysis persists.

Hypothermia and hypocalcemia following bypass will also contribute to delayed hemostasis and should be corrected in conjunction with the above-mentioned maneuvers.

Neurologic injury

While patients with CHD may have coexisting abnormalities of the CNS, they are also at risk for acquired neurologic injury throughout the perioperative period. These injuries may occur from periods of hypoxia/ischemia, CNS hemorrhage, paradoxical air and thrombotic emboli, and cerebral abscess and venous or arterial thrombosis from erythrocytosis caused by chronic cyanosis [74,75]. Premature newborns are at risk for intraventricular hemorrhage (IVH); cerebral ultrasonography is recommended before and after CPB in these patients. Although there are no data to support an increased incidence of IVH related to CPB, this should be viewed with caution based on the ECMO experience with IVH.

Patients with CHD may develop circulatory collapse and/or severe hypoxemia, which may contribute to global hypoxic-ischemic neurologic damage. Encephalopathy and seizures are manifestations of neurologic injury; however, preoperative assessment is often difficult because of the need for mechanical ventilation, sedation, and paralysis. An electroencephalogram (EEG) and a computed tomography (CT) scan may help localize specific sites of neurologic injury, but there is poor correlation with longer-term neurologic outcome. The potential for neurologic recovery of the immature brain is greater compared to older children and adults [76]. Because of the risk (transport to radiology) and lack of proven benefit, these patients often proceed to surgery with an uncertain neurologic status.

The application of deep hypothermia provides protection of the CNS during periods of ischemia. However, prolonged periods (>45 min) of hypothermic arrest may cause an ischemic reperfusion injury to the brain. In addition, there are other variables that increase the risk for brain injury during CPB. These include problems related to aortic and venous cannula placement, the duration of bypass, the rate of cooling, perfusion pressure and flow rate, air embolism, pH and PCO_2 management during deep hypothermia, degree of hypothermia, type of oxygenator, circuit hematocrit, and duration of circulatory arrest. (For a more detailed discussion, see Chapters 7 and 10.)

Seizures are the most frequently observed neurologic complication following cardiac surgery using deep hypothermic circulatory arrest (DHCA) with a reported in-

cidence of 4–25% [77,78]. Both focal and generalized seizures have been described, usually occurring on the first or second postoperative day, and can usually be controlled with anticonvulsants; status epilepticus is uncommon. A brain CT scan is usually nondiagnostic, but it is indicated in patients with persistent focal seizures, because a larger area of damage, or a focal lesion such as an intracerebral hemorrhage, may be seen. Postoperative seizures do not increase the risk of seizures later in life, and in the past were thought to be benign. However, the randomized trial of DHCA versus low-flow bypass during the arterial switch operation for d-TGA demonstrated that seizures are a marker of neurologic damage and a prognostic indicator of worse neurodevelopmental outcome [79–81].

Detection of seizures in the postoperative period is a diagnostic challenge in the ICU. Clonic, tonic, or myoclonic manifestations of seizures may be difficult to detect because of sedation or paralysis. Autonomic manifestations such as the sudden onset of tachycardia, hypertension, and pupillary dilation are suggestive of seizure activity, although the cause of these signs is difficult to distinguish from other hemodynamic causes. Nevertheless, the early detection and management of seizures after DHCA and/or CPB is important, and they should not be considered a benign event, rather both a marker for and manifestation of ongoing neurologic injury. In the Boston Circulatory Arrest Study, clinical seizures were detected in 11% of infants, but continuous EEG monitoring detected seizure activity in 25% of these infants [78,82]. Over recent years, postoperative clinical seizures have become a rare event, with an incidence <4%, which is most likely secondary to improved techniques for neurological protection [83]. DHCA is now performed less frequently, and when used, the duration of cooling on CPB is longer, pH-stat blood gas management strategy is used, and circulatory arrest time kept <40 minutes, whenever possible [84,85].

Longitudinal follow-up of neonates and infants who have undergone cardiac surgery and hypothermic CPB demonstrate the risk for longer-term neurodevelopmental abnormalities [80,81,86,87]. At 1 year of age, scores on the Psychomotor Development Index of the Bayley Scales (a measure of fine and gross motor ability) were significantly lower in children randomized to circulatory arrest versus low-flow CPB and in those who developed seizures in the early postoperative period. At 4 years of age, lower verbal and performance intelligence quotient was also detected in this group of patients.

Postoperative factors contributing to neurologic injury include cerebral embolism, persistent low output state with low cerebral perfusion pressure, and hyperventilation with low $PaCO_2$ reducing cerebral blood flow. Postbypass hyperthermia may develop from low CO and peripheral vasoconstriction, or from aggressive rewarming practices, and may contribute to neurologic injury. Postischemia brain temperature has been shown to be important in influencing delayed neuronal death and subsequent neurologic recovery following traumatic brain injury. Recent data from a neonatal porcine model of circulatory arrest also demonstrated the detrimental effect of hyperthermia on neurologic outcome following DHCA [88]. Mild hypothermia may help attenuate neurologic injury following DHCA, and hyperthermia in the immediate postoperative period should be aggressively treated. A recent study of children after CPB documented cerebral hyperthermia (measured with jugular venous bulb thermistors) develops in a majority of patients. The mean cerebral temperature was 39.6°C (one patient with 41.4°C) and was underestimated by the use of rectal temperature monitoring (mean 37.7°C) [89].

Choreoathetosis is a rare, yet sometimes devastating complication following cardiac surgery in children with or without the use of DHCA. It has been reported in the neonate, but is more common in older infants. Factors that contribute to the development of choreoathetosis include inadequate brain cooling, particularly to deeper structures such as the basal ganglia and midbrain, a rapid rate of cooling, an alkaline (i.e., alpha-stat) blood gas strategy during cooling, and the presence of systemic-to-pulmonary artery collateral vessels that may result in a "cerebral steal [90, 91].

The importance of routine perioperative monitoring of the brain is increasingly recognized. Multimodality monitoring with continuous EEG monitoring, intermittent transcranial Doppler, and frontal lobe infrared spectroscopy [92–95] can be used to evaluate cerebral blood flow velocity and perfusion, and cerebral O_2 delivery and extraction in the immediate postoperative period.

Gastrointestinal problems

Splanchnic hypoperfusion may be secondary to low CO from ventricular dysfunction or from low diastolic pressure in patients with systemic-to-pulmonary artery runoff [96]. It often manifests as a persistent ileus or feeding intolerance; gut ischemia or necrotizing enterocolitis may also develop.

Besides splanchnic hypoperfusion, other causes of feeding intolerance include bowel edema following CPB, delayed gastric emptying secondary to opioids, gastroesophageal reflux, and small bowel obstruction secondary to malrotation, which occurs in some patients with heterotaxy syndrome. Patients with decreased ventricular function may be unable to increase their CO sufficiently to meet the metabolic demand associated with oral feeding and the absorption of food. Coexisting problems such as tachypnea also restrict oral intake. To ensure adequate

nutrition in these situations, placement of a transpyloric feeding tube should be considered [97].

As in adult ICUs, stress ulceration and gastritis occur in pediatric patients. Prophylaxis with H_2 receptor blocking drugs and/or antacids should be used in any patient requiring protracted hemodynamic and respiratory support. Early resumption of enteral nutrition is encouraged to reduce the risk of nosocomial pulmonary and blood infections by preventing bacterial overgrowth; feeding algorithms have been demonstrated to improve the introduction of enteral nutrition after cardiac surgery [98].

The onset of abdominal distension, ileus, blood within the stool, and pneumatosis intestinalis on abdominal radiograph suggests necrotizing enterocolitis. Severe cases manifest additional signs of abdominal wall cellulitis, sepsis, hemodynamic instability, and gut perforation. Initial treatment includes stopping enteral feeds and initiating IV maintenance fluids and broad-spectrum IV antibiotics. Hemodynamic support may be necessary, and occasionally laparotomy if perforation occurs or hemodynamic instability persists.

Factors contributing to postoperative liver dysfunction include complications during CPB secondary to low perfusion pressure or inadequate venous drainage, and persistent low CO causing ischemic hepatitis. Patients following a Fontan procedure may be at particular risk because of hepatic venous congestion from elevated central venous pressure. Marked elevations in liver transaminases may begin within hours of surgery and remain elevated for 2–3 days before gradually returning to normal. These patients also typically have significantly elevated prothrombin and partial thromboplastin times, and thus are at increased risk of bleeding complications. Fulminant hepatic failure is uncommon.

Chylothorax

Chylothorax may occur from injury to the thoracic duct anywhere along its course from the lower mediastinum to its drainage into the systemic venous system near the left innominate vein. Inadvertent surgical trauma is the most common cause of thoracic duct injury, particularly in repeat operations where identification of anatomic structures is difficult. Chylothorax is heralded by pleural effusions, often left sided, that do not clear with diuresis, and worsen with enteral feeding. First-line treatment involves eliminating or restricting enteral intake to non-fat-containing feedings, such as Portagen. Persistent chylothorax can be treated with octreotide, tube drainage, or in severe cases, pleurodesis or ligation of the thoracic duct. SVC thrombosis may also cause chylothorax. Most cases can be managed conservatively without surgery.

Sedation and analgesia

Maintenance of adequate analgesia and sedation is an essential component of patient management following congenital heart surgery. Besides relieving pain and anxiety after surgery and during procedures, attenuation of the stress response and promoting synchrony with mechanical ventilation are important considerations.

A number of patients, particularly newborns, require resuscitation and stabilization prior to surgery. Sedation and analgesia, with or without neuromuscular blockade, are often necessary to minimize cardiorespiratory work, assist with coordinated mechanical ventilation, and limit patient movement during painful procedures such as catheter placement and balloon septostomy. Drug doses should be titrated to the desired effect; however, children will develop tolerance after a few days of exposure to opioids and benzodiazepines and have increased dose requirements following surgery.

Early extubation

Recovery following cardiac surgery and the duration of mechanical ventilation depend on numerous factors, including the patient's preoperative clinical condition, type and duration of surgical procedure, hemodynamic stability, and complications such as postoperative bleeding and dysrhythmias [99]. For the majority of patients with stable preoperative hemodynamics undergoing uncomplicated surgical repair, postoperative ventilation is not necessary. Once hemodynamically stable, normothermic, and no longer bleeding, patients can be rapidly weaned and extubated. Examples include infants and older children undergoing uncomplicated ASD and VSD repair, RV outflow tract reconstruction and conduit replacement, and following LV outflow tract reconstruction such as aortic valve replacement. Low-dose opioid techniques are used to maintain anesthesia, and following repairs such as an ASD, extubation in the operating room or soon after transfer to the ICU is usually possible. A similar approach for early extubation is applicable to patients following a cavopulmonary anastomosis when early resumption of spontaneous ventilation is preferable because of the potential deleterious effects of positive pressure ventilation on preload and pulmonary blood flow.

Patients undergoing early extubation can be managed with intermittent doses of opioids to ensure adequate analgesia without respiratory depression, and may also benefit from sedation with benzodiazepines to treat restlessness or agitation to prevent dislodgment of transthoracic catheters, the arterial catheter, chest drains, and pacing wires.

Several problems should be anticipated following extubation in the operating room or soon after transfer to the ICU. A mild respiratory acidosis is common and usually resolves within the first 6 hours following surgery [100]. Hypertension and tachycardia may develop during emergence from anesthesia and sedation, increasing the risk for bleeding from operative suture lines; therefore, antihypertensive agents may be necessary. Warming blankets should be used to prevent hypothermia and shivering, and the patient closely observed for possible airway obstruction.

Stress response

Stress and adverse postoperative outcomes have been linked closely in critically ill newborns and infants [101]. This is not surprising given their precarious balance of limited metabolic reserve and increased resting metabolic rate. Metabolic derangements such as altered glucose homeostasis, metabolic acidosis, salt and water retention, and a catabolic state contributing to protein breakdown and lipolysis are commonly seen following major stress in sick neonates and infants. This complex of maladaptive processes may be associated with prolonged mechanical ventilation courses and ICU stay, as well as increased morbidity and mortality.

Newborns and infants can generate a significant stress response following cardiac surgery and CPB [102]. High-dose opioid anesthesia continuing into the initial postoperative recovery period has been demonstrated to significantly attenuate this stress response, leading to a reduction in morbidity and possibly mortality [103]. The patients who would most benefit from this approach include those with limited myocardial reserve, labile pulmonary hypertension, myocardial ischemia, and those undergoing complex repairs that have required prolonged CPB and aortic cross clamp times.

Improvements in preoperative assessment, earlier interventions, and modifications to surgical techniques and CPB have all contributed to improved patient outcome and reduced total ICU stay. Therefore, the notion of extending anesthesia into the ICU is not necessary for all patients, but rather should be considered on a case-by-case basis according to hemodynamic stability after surgery [104].

Prolonged ventilation may be necessary for some patients because of residual hemodynamic or respiratory complications. Examples include persistent cardiac failure, pulmonary disease, recurrent pleural effusions, sepsis, phrenic nerve injury with diaphragm paresis, and muscle weakness from inadequate nutrition and prolonged paralysis. A slow wean from mechanical ventilation is necessary, and appropriate analgesia and sedation are important. Commonly, a combination of benzodiazepines and opioids is effective, although this should be frequently reevaluated to avoid the complications of tolerance and dependence.

Assessment

The assessment of adequate analgesia in children can be difficult, particularly when paralyzed and ventilated. Primarily, autonomic signs such as hypertension, tachycardia, pupillary size, and diaphoresis are used. If unparalyzed, children will grimace and withdraw from a painful stimulus, and if breathing spontaneously, changes in respiratory pattern such as tachypnea, grunting, and splinting of the chest wall may be evident.

However, changes in autonomic signs do not only reflect pain. Other causes include awareness, fever, hypoxemia, hypercapnea, changes in vasoactive drug infusions, and seizures. If not diagnosed correctly, patients may receive additional opioid or benzodiazepine doses when hypertensive and tachycardic, which will only contribute to tolerance and possible withdrawal symptoms later.

Sedatives

Chloral hydrate is commonly used hypnotic agent to sedate children prior to medical procedures and imaging studies [105]. It can be administered orally or rectally in a dose ranging from 50 to 100 mg/kg (maximum dose 1 gm). Onset of action is within 15–30 minutes with a duration of action between 2 and 4 hours. Between 10 and 20% of children may have a dysphoric reaction following chloral hydrate, causing them to become excitable and uncooperative. On the other hand, some children may become excessively sedated with associated respiratory depression and inability to protect their airway.

The regular administration of chloral hydrate to provide sedation in the ICU is controversial. Administered intermittently, it can be used to supplement benzodiazepines and opioids, may assist sedation during drug withdrawal, and is useful as a nocturnal hypnotic when trying to establish normal sleep cycles. Repetitive dosing to maintain prolonged sedation is not recommended by the American Academy of Pediatrics and should be avoided in the ICU [106].

Benzodiazepines are the most commonly used sedatives in the ICU because of their anxiolytic, anticonvulsant, hypnotic, and amnestic properties. While providing excellent sedation, they may cause dose-dependent respiratory depression as well as myocardial depression, resulting in significant hypotension in patients with limited hemodynamic reserve. Following chronic administration, tolerance and withdrawal symptoms are common.

The benzodiazepine midazolam, when administered as a continuous infusion at 0.05–0.1 mg/kg/h, is useful in children following congenital heart surgery [107]. However, its use in neonates remains debated because of the concerns for neurological outcome and prolonged length of stay [108]. It is short-acting and water soluble, although if CO and splanchnic perfusion are diminished, hepatic metabolism is reduced and drug accumulation can occur. Tachyphylaxis can occur within days of commencing a continuous infusion, and withdrawal symptoms of restlessness, agitation, and visual hallucinations can occur following prolonged administration. A reversible encephalopathy has been reported following the abrupt discontinuation of midazolam and fentanyl infusions, characterized by movement disorders, dystonic posturing and poor social interaction [109].

Both diazepam and lorazepam can be effectively used within the ICU, and they possess the advantage of longer duration of action. Prescribed on a regular basis, lorazepam can provide useful longer-term sedation, supplementing an existing sedation regimen and assisting with withdrawal from opioids.

Opioid analgesics

Opioid analgesics are the mainstay of pain management in the ICU, and in high doses can provide anesthesia. They also provide sedation for patients while mechanically ventilated and blunt hemodynamic responses to procedures such as endotracheal tube suctioning. Hypercyanotic episodes associated with TOF and air hunger associated with CHF are also effectively treated with opioids.

Intermittent dosing of opioids can provide effective analgesia and sedation following surgery, although periods of over-sedation and under-medication can occur because of peaks and troughs in drug levels. A continuous infusion is therefore advantageous.

Intermittent morphine doses of 0.05–0.1 mg/kg IV or as a continuous infusion at 50–100 mcg/kg/h provides excellent postoperative analgesia for most patients. The sedative property of morphine is an advantage over the synthetic opioids; however, histamine release can cause systemic vasodilation and an increase in pulmonary artery pressure. It should therefore be used with caution in patients with limited myocardial reserve and labile pulmonary hypertension.

The synthetic opioids, fentanyl, sufentanil, and alfentanil have a shorter duration of action than morphine and do not cause histamine release, therefore producing less vasodilation and hypotension. Fentanyl is commonly prescribed following cardiac surgery. It blocks the stress response in a dose-related fashion while maintaining both systemic and pulmonary hemodynamic stability [110,111]. A bolus dose of 10–15 mcg/kg IV effectively ameliorates the hemodynamic response to intubation in neonates [112]. Patients with high endogenous cate-cholamine levels, e.g., severe cardiac failure or critical aortic stenosis in the neonate, can become hypotensive after a bolus induction dose, and fentanyl must be used with caution in these conditions. Chest wall rigidity is an idiosyncratic and dose-related reaction that can occur with a rapid bolus in newborns as well as older children.

A continuous infusion of fentanyl 1–3 mcg/kg/h pro-vides analgesia following surgery, although it often needs to be combined with a benzodiazepine to maintain seda-tion. Large variability between children in fentanyl clear-ance exists, making titration of an infusion difficult. The experience with ECMO indicates tolerance and depen-dence to a fentanyl infusion develops rapidly and signifi-cant increases in infusion rate may be required.

Sufentanil is more potent than fentanyl, although it has similar effects and offers no specific advantage. A con-tinuous infusion of the ultrashort-acting synthetic opioid, remifentanil, may be useful in the operating room or ICU for patients with limited hemodynamic reserve undergo-ing short procedures.

The development of tolerance is dose- and time-related, and is a particular problem following cardiac surgery in patients who received a high-dose opioid technique to maintain anesthesia. Physical dependence with with-drawal symptoms such as dysphoria, fussiness, crying, agitation, piloerection, tachypnea, tachycardia, and di-aphoresis may be seen in children and can be managed by gradually tapering the opioid dose or administering a longer-acting opioid such as methadone. Methadone has a similar potency to morphine with the advantage of a prolonged elimination half-life between 18 and 24 hours. It can be administered intravenously, but is also absorbed well orally. It is particularly useful, therefore, to treat pa-tients with opioid withdrawal.

Alternate methods of opioid delivery which are of-ten effective following cardiac surgery include patient-controlled analgesia and epidural opioids, either as a bolus or continuous infusion. Patients receiving epidural opi-oids must be closely monitored for potential respiratory depression, and side effects include pruritis, nausea, vom-iting, and urinary retention.

Nonsteroidal analgesics

Nonsteroidal anti-inflammatory drugs can provide effec-tive analgesia following cardiac surgery, either as a sole analgesic agent or in combination with opioids or local anesthetics. Ketorolac (0.5 mg/kg IV every 8 h) is partic-ularly useful as an adjunct to opioids for patients who are weaned and extubated in the early postoperative pe-riod. However, there are significant concerns regarding nephrotoxicity and inhibition of platelet aggregation. The incidence of acute renal failure is increased if ketorolac

administration is continued for more than 3 days postop-eratively, and in general, it should be avoided in patients potentially predisposed to renal failure, such as those with hypovolemia, preexisting renal disease, and low CO, and those receiving medications such as angiotensin-converting enzyme inhibitors. Acute renal failure is more commonly seen after initiation of treatment, or after an increase in dose, and is reversible in most cases [113].

Inhibition of platelet aggregation and increased bleed-ing time may occur following a single IV dose of ketorolac, although it has not been demonstrated to increase the risk of surgical site bleeding following cardiac surgery [114].

Acetaminophen can be given rectally, in an initial dose of 30–40 mg/kg, followed by 15–20 mg/kg every 6 hours for 24–48 hours following surgery. This regimen is de-sirable because of its adjunctive ability to treat pain and lower temperature without platelet inhibition effects or narcotic side effects.

Anesthetic agents

Barbiturates

Thiopental and methohexital are rarely used in the ICU because of direct myocardial depression and venodilation that may cause severe hypotension in patients with limited cardiac reserve.

Propofol

Propofol is an anesthesia induction agent and that can be suitable for use in the ICU for short procedures such as transesophageal echocardiography, pericardiocentesis, and cardioversion. Its use, however, is limited because of the potential for hypotension from a decrease in SVR and direct myocardial depression. Although it has short duration of action and rapid clearance, propofol is cur-rently not approved for longer-term continuous infusion for sedation in pediatric patients because of the potential risk for the propofol infusion syndrome. Nevertheless, it has a useful role in facilitating early extubation. Rather than relying on frequent intermittent doses of opioids and benzodiazepines in small children, a short-term (i.e., 4–6 h) continuous infusion of propofol up to 50 mcg/kg/min will keep the patient comfortable, allow for initial recovery after surgery (i.e., to achieve hemostasis and normother-mia), and permit rapid weaning and extubation after the infusion is discontinued.

Ketamine

Ketamine is a "dissociative" anesthetic agent with a rapid onset and short duration of action. It can be effectively ad-ministered intravenously or intramuscularly and provides adequate anesthesia for most ICU procedures including intubation, draining of pleural and pericardial effusions, and sternal wound exploration and closure. It produces a type of catalepsy whereby the eyes remain open, usually with nystagmus and intact corneal reflexes. Occasionally, nonpurposeful myoclonic movements occur. It causes cerebral vasodilation and should be avoided in patients with intracranial hypertension.

Because hemodynamic stability is generally maintained, it is commonly used in ICUs. Heart rate and blood pressure are usually increased through sympathomimetic actions secondary to central stimulation and reduced postganglionic catecholamine uptake. However, it is important to remember that this drug does have direct myocardial depressant effects and should be used with caution in patients with limited myocardial reserve, e.g., neonates with critical aortic stenosis and poor LV function.

Dose-related respiratory depression may occur, however, most patients continue to breathe spontaneously after an induction dose of 2–3 mg/kg IV. Airway secretions are increased, and even though airway reflexes seem intact, aspiration may occur. It is essential that patients be fasted prior to administration of ketamine and complete airway management equipment must be available. An increase in airway secretions may cause laryngospasm during airway manipulation, and an antisialagogue such as atropine or glycopyrrolate should be administered concurrently. Side effects of emergence delirium and hallucinations may be ameliorated with the concurrent use of benzodiazepines.

There are conflicting reports about the effect of ketamine on PVR. One small study in children undergoing cardiac catheterization concluded that PVR was increased following ketamine in patients predisposed to pulmonary hypertension [115]. However, another demonstrated minimal effects in young children either breathing spontaneously or during controlled ventilation [116]. On balance, ketamine has minimal effects on PVR and can be used safely in patients with pulmonary hypertension, provided secondary events such as airway obstruction and hypoventilation are avoided.

Etomidate

Etomidate is an anesthetic induction agent with the advantage of minimal cardiovascular and respiratory depression [117,118]. An IV dose of 0.3 mg/kg induces a rapid loss of consciousness with a duration of 3–5 minutes. It can cause pain on injection and is associated with spontaneous movements, hiccoughing and myoclonus. Etomidate may be used as an alternative to the synthetic opioids for induction of patients with limited myocardial reserve. It is not approved for continuous infusion because adrenal steroidogenesis can be inhibited [119].

Dexmedetomidine

The newer agent dexmedetomidine, an α_2-adrenergic agonist, is being used increasingly to provide sedation and analgesia in pediatric patients due to its favorable sedative and anxiolytic properties combined with its limited effect on respiratory function. In addition to sedation in the critical care unit and during noninvasive procedures, dexmedetomidine also has a potential role to prevent emergence delirium and help with opioid withdrawl [120]. Because of its adverse cardiovascular effects, including hypotension, bradycardia, and heart block, it should be used with caution in children with CHD [121].

Muscle relaxants

Muscle relaxants are more commonly used in pediatric ICUs compared to adult units. In addition to their ability to facilitate tracheal intubation and controlled mechanical ventilation, patients with limited cardiorespiratory reserve also benefit from paralysis because of reduced myocardial work and oxygen demand. However, prolonged paralysis carries the concomitant risks of prolonged ventilatory support and delayed establishment of enteral nutrition, and can result in tolerance and prolonged muscle weakness after discontinuance.

Succinylcholine is a depolarizing muscle relaxant with rapid onset and short duration of action. While frequently used in the pediatric ICU to facilitate tracheal intubation, the potential for bradycardia and hyperkalemia may be disastrous side effects following cardiac surgery. Its use should therefore be restricted to patients requiring a rapid sequence induction because of the risk for aspiration of gastric contents. The usual IV dose of 1 mg/kg should be increased in newborns and infants to 2 mg/kg because of the greater surface area-to-weight ratio in these patients. It can also be administered intramuscularly in an urgent situation where no vascular access is available at a dose usually double the IV dose (i.e., 3–4 mg/kg). The risk for bradycardia is exaggerated in children, especially after multiple doses, and atropine (20 mcg/kg IV) should be administered concurrently.

Rocuronium is an aminosteroid, nondepolarizing muscle relaxant with fast onset and intermediate duration of action. Time to complete neuromuscular blockade for an intubating dose of 0.6 mg/kg IV ranges from 30 to 180 seconds, although adequate intubating conditions are usually achieved within 60 seconds. It is therefore a suitable alternative to succinylcholine during rapid sequence induction. The duration of action averages 25 minutes, although recovery is slower in infants. It is a safe drug to administer to patients with limited hemodynamic reserve and does not cause histamine release.

Table 29.8 Criteria for ICU discharge

Cardiovascular

Stable and desired blood pressure without requiring intravenous vasoactive support

Invasive intravascular monitoring no longer required for monitoring or blood sampling

No requirement for mechanical pacing using temporary wires and an external pacemaker

Stable cardiac rhythm (preferably sinus) with a stable blood pressure and cardiac output

Respiratory

Not dependent on mechanical ventilatory support

Stable and adequate ventilation rate and pattern, and no signs of airway obstruction

Stable and adequate oxygenation (PaO_2 depends on lesion and physiology after repair or palliation) ± supplemental O_2 via nasal cannula, mask, or blow-by

Neurologic status adequate to protect airway from aspiration

Appropriate nursing intensity

Chest physical therapy or bronchodilator treatments at least 3 h apart in frequency

Established nutrition plan (enteral or parenteral)

Controlled analgesic or sedation requirements

Vecuronium and cis-atracurium are nondepolarizing muscle relaxants with intermediate durations of actions. They can be administered as an IV bolus or continuous infusion within the ICU. Both of these agents have minimal effect on the circulation and can be administered safely to patients with limited hemodynamic reserve.

Pancuronium is a commonly used, longer-acting, nondepolarizing relaxant that can be administered intermittently at a dose of 0.1 mg/kg IV. It can cause a mild tachycardia and increase in blood pressure, but is also safe to administer to patients with limited hemodynamic reserve.

Criteria for ICU discharge

As patients improve after surgery and require less intensive monitoring and therapy, the timing of discharge from the ICU becomes an important management decision. For the majority of patients who have stable hemodynamics without significant residual defects, and who have been weaned and extubated uneventfully after surgery, the decision to transfer out of the ICU is not difficult. The function of all organ systems should be assessed and considered in this decision, although the focus will be on cardiovascular and respiratory function. The cost of intensive care medicine is high, and early rather than delayed discharge is recommended. Indeed, as the mortality and

morbidity associated with congenital cardiac surgery have declined, length of ICU stay, total hospital stay, and cost-effectiveness have become important outcome variables.

In addition to poor CO and residual anatomic lesions, there are a variety of noncardiac problems that can complicate recovery and prolong ICU stay. Many of these problems affect respiratory function and cause inability to wean from mechanical ventilation (see mechanical ventilation). Table 29.8 provides a list of cardiovascular and respiratory criteria for consideration prior to patient discharge from the ICU. It is important to emphasize that this decision should be multidisciplinary, with particular attention paid to nursing availability and experience, and availability of adequate monitoring.

References

1. Castaneda AR, Mayer JE, Jonas RA, et al. (1989) The neonate with critical congenital heart disease: repair—a surgical challenge. J Thorac Cardiovasc Surg 98:869–875.
2. Rabinovitch M, Haworth SG, Castaneda AR, et al. (1978) Lung biopsy in congenital heart disease: a morphometric approach to pulmonary vascular disease. Circulation 58:1107–1122.
3. Hoffman JIE, Rudolph AM, Heymann MA (1981) Pulmonary vascular disease with congenital heart lesions: pathologic features and causes. Circulation 64:873–877.
4. Heath D, Edwards JE (1958) The pathology of hypersensitive pulmonary vascular disease: a description of six grades of structural changes in the pulmonary arteries with special reference to congenital cardiac septal defects. Circulation 18:533–547.
5. Sagawa K (1981) The end-systolic pressure-volume relation of the ventricle: definition, modifications and clinical use. Circulation 63:1223–1227.
6. Graham TP (1991) Ventricular performance in congenital heart disease. Circulation 84:2259–2274.
7. Howlett G (1972) Lung mechanics in normal infants and infants with congenital heart disease. Arch Dis Child 47:707–715.
8. Bancalari E, Jesse MJ, Gelband H, Garcia O (1977) Lung mechanics in congenital heart disease with increased and decreased pulmonary blood flow. J Pediatr 90:192–195.
9. Lees MH, Way RC, Ross BB (1967) Ventilation and respiratory gas transfer of infants with increased pulmonary blood flow. Pediatrics 40:259–271.
10. Levin AR, Ho E, Auld PA (1973) Alveolar-arterial oxygen gradients in infants and children with left-to-right shunts. J Pediatr 83:979–987.
11. Lister G, Talner N (1981) Management of respiratory failure of cardiac origin. In: Gregory GA (ed.) Respiratory Failure in the Child. Churchill Livingstone, New York, pp. 67–87.
12. Jenkins J, Lynn A, Edmonds J, Barker GA (1985) Effects of mechanical ventilation on cardiopulmonary function in children after open-heart surgery. Crit Care Med 13:77–80.

13. West JB (1995) Respiratory Physiology: The Essentials. Williams & Wilkins, Baltimore.
14. Robotham JL, Lixfeld W, Holland L, et al. (1980) The effects of positive end-expiratory pressure on right and left ventricular performance. Am Rev Resp Dis 121:677–683.
15. Pinsky MR, Summer WR, Wise RA, et al. (1983) Augmentation of cardiac function by elevation of intrathoracic pressure. J Appl Physiol 54:950–955.
16. Watanabe T, Trusler GA, Williams WG, et al. (1987) Phrenic nerve paralysis after pediatric cardiac surgery. Retrospective study of 125 cases. J Thorac Cardiovasc Surg 94:383–388.
17. Costello JM, Morrow DF, Graham DA, et al. (2008) A systematic intervention to reduce blood stream infections in a cardiac intensive care unit. Pediatrics 121:915–923.
18. Costello JM, Graham DA, Morrow DF, et al. (2009) Risk factors for central line-associated bloodstream infection in a pediatric cardiac intensive care unit. Ped Crit Care Med 10:453–459.
19. Polito A, Thiagarajan RR, Laussen PC, et al. (2008) Association between intra-operative and early postoperative glucose levels and adverse outcomes following complex congenital heart surgery. Circulation 118:2235–2242.
20. Grossman W (1996) Blood flow measurement: the cardiac output. In: Grossman W, Baim D (eds) Cardiac Catheterization, Angiography, and Intervention. Williams & Wilkins, Baltimore, pp. 109–124.
21. Guyton A, Jones C, Coleman TG (eds) (1973) Circulatory Physiology: Cardiac Output and its Regulation. WB Saunders, Philadelphia, pp. 4–80.
22. Verrier ED, Boyle EM (1997) Endothelial cell injury in cardiovascular surgery: an overview. Ann Thorac Surg 64:S2–S8.
23. Hall RI, Smith MS, Rocker G (1997) Systemic inflammatory response to cardiopulmonary bypass: pathophysiological, therapeutic and pharmacological considerations. Anesth Analg 85:766–782.
24. Wernovsky G, Wypij D, Jonas RA, et al. (1995) Postoperative course and hemodynamic profile after the arterial switch operation in neonates and infants. A comparison of low-flow cardiopulmonary bypass and circulatory arrest. Circulation 92:2226–2235.
25. Perry JC, Walsh EP (1998) Diagnosis and management of cardiac arrhythmias. In: Chang AC, Hanley FL, Wernovsky G, Wessel DL (eds) Pediatric Cardiac Intensive Care. Williams & Wilkins, Baltimore, p. 469.
26. Mukharji J, Rehr RB, Hastillo A, et al. (1990) Comparison of atrial contribution to cardiac hemodynamics in patients with normal and severely compromised cardiac function. Clin Cardiol 13:639–643.
27. Leinbach RC, Chamberlain DA, Kastor JA, et al. (1969) A comparison of the hemodynamic effects of ventricular and sequential A-V pacing in patients with heart block. Am Heart J 78:502–508.
28. Weindling SN, Saul JP, Gamble WJ, et al. (1998) Duration of complete atrioventricular block after congenital heart disease surgery. Am J Cardiol 82:525–527.
29. Wessel DL (1993) Hemodynamic responses to perioperative pain and stress in infants. Crit Care Med 21:S361–S362.
30. Lawless ST, Zaritsky A, Miles M (1991) The acute pharmacokinetics and pharmacodynamics of amrinone in pediatric patients. J Clin Pharmacol 31:800–803.
31. Benzing G, Helmsworth JA, Schreiber JT, et al. (1979) Nitroprusside and epinephrine for treatment of low output in children after open heart surgery. Ann Thorac Surg 27:523–528.
32. Chang AC, Atz AM, Wernovsky G, et al. (1995) Milrinone: systematic and pulmonary hemodynamic effects in neonates after cardiac surgery. Crit Care Med 23:1907–1914.
33. Hoffman TN, Wernovsky G, Atz AM, et al. (2002) Prophylactic intravenous use of milrinone after cardiac operation in pediatrics (PRIMACORP) study. Prophylactic intravenous use of milrinone after cardiac operation in pediatrics. Am Heart J 143:15–21.
34. Loughead JL, Mimouni F, Tsang RC (1988) Serum ionized calcium concentrations in normal neonates. Am J Dis Child 142:516–518.
35. Opie LH (1995) Regulation of myocardial contractility. J Cardiovasc Pharmacol 26:S1–S9.
36. Jerath N, Frndova H, McCrindle BW, et al. (2008) Clinical impact of vasopressin infusion on hemodynamics, liver and renal function in pediatric patients. Intensive Care Med 34:1274–1280.
37. Millar KJ, Thiagarajan RR, Laussen PC (2007) Glucocorticoid therapy for hypotension in the cardiac intensive care unit. Pediatr Cardiol 28:176–182.
38. Suominen PK, Dickerson HA, Moffet BS, et al. (2005) Hemodynamic effects of rescue protocol hydrocortisone in neonates with low cardiac output syndrome after cardiac surgery. Pediatr Crit Care Med 6:655–659.
39. Shore S, Nelson DP, Pearl JM, et al. (2001) Usefulness of corticosteroid therapy in decreasing epinephrine requirements in critically infants with congenital heart disease. Am J Cardiol 88:591–594.
40. Mackie AS, Booth KL, Newburger JW, et al. (2005) A randomized, double-blind, placebo-controlled pilot trial of triiodothyronine in neonatal heart surgery. J Thorac Cardiovasc Surg 130:810–816.
41. Bettendorf M, Schmidt KG, Grulich-Henn J, et al. (2000) Triiodothyronine treatment in children after cardiac surgery: a double-blind, randomized, placebo-controlled study. Lancet 356(9229):529–534.
42. Tabbutt S, Duncan BW, McLaughlin D, et al. (1997) Delayed sternal closure after cardiac operations in the pediatric population. J Thorac Cardiovasc Surg 113:886–893.
43. Alexi-Meskishvili V, Weng Y, Uhlemann F, et al. (1995) Prolonged open sternotomy after pediatric open heart operation: experience with 113 patients. Ann Thorac Surg 59:379–383.
44. Zwischenberger JB, Bartlett RH (eds) (1995) ECMO in Critical Care. Extracorporeal Life Support Registry: Ann Arbor MI, pp. 445–468.
45. Salvin JW, Laussen PC, Thiagarajan RR (2008) Extracorporeal membrane oxygenation for postcardiotomy mechanical cardiovascular support in children with congenital heart disease. Paediatr Anaesth 18:1157–1162.

46. Cooper DS, Jacobs JP, Moore L, et al. (2007) Cardiac extra-corporeal life support: state of the art in 2007. Cardiol Young 17(Suppl 2):104–115.

47. Chan T, Thiagarajan RR, Frank D, Bratton SL (2008) Survival after extracorporeal cardiopulmonary resuscitation in infants and children with heart disease. J Thorac Cardiovasc Surg 136:984–992.

48. Duncan BW (2002) Mechanical circulatory support for infants and children with cardiac disease. Ann Thorac Surg 73:1670–1677.

49. Thiagarajan RR, Nelson DP (2005) Should we be satisfied with current outcomes for cardiac extracorporeal life support? Pediatr Crit Care Med 6:89–90.

50. Pennington DG, Swartz MT (1993) Circulatory support in infants and children. Ann Thorac Surg 55:233–237.

51. Allan CK, Thiagarajan RR, del Nido PJ, et al. (2007) Indication for initiation of mechanical circulatory support impacts survival of infants with shunted single-ventricle circulation supported with extracorporeal membrane oxygenation. J Thorac Cardiovasc Surg 133:660–667.

52. Slonim AD, Patel KM, Ruttimann UE, Pollack MM (1997) Cardiopulmonary resuscitation in pediatric intensive care units. Crit Care Med 25:1951–1955.

53. Schindler MB, Bohn D, Cox PN, et al. (1996) Outcome of out-of-hospital cardiac or respiratory arrest in children. N Engl J Med 335:1473–1479.

54. Parra DA, Totapally BR, Zahn E, et al. (2000) Outcome of cardiopulmonary resuscitation in a pediatric cardiac intensive care unit. Crit Care Med 28:3296–3300.

55. Duncan BW, Ibrahim AE, Hraska V, et al. (1998) Use of rapid deployment extracorporeal membrane oxygenation for the resuscitation of pediatric patients with heart disease after cardiac arrest. J Thorac Cardiovasc Surg 116:305–311.

56. Duncan BW, Hraska V, Jonas RA, et al. (1996) Mechanical circulatory support for pediatric cardiac patients. Circulation 94:173.

57. Fiser RT, Morris MC (2008) Extracorporeal cardiopulmonary resuscitation in refractory pediatric cardiac arrest. Pediatr Clin North Am 55:929–941.

58. Thiagarajan RR, Laussen PC, Rycus PT, et al. (2007) Extracorporeal membrane oxygenation to aid cardiopulmonary resuscitation in infants and children. Circulation 116:1693–1700.

59. Downard CD, Betit P, Chang RW, et al. (2003) Impact of AMICAR of hemorrhagic complications of ECMO: a ten-year review. J Pediatr Surg 38:1212–1216.

60. Karl TR (1994) Extracorporeal circulatory support in infants and children. Semin Thorac Cardiovasc Surg 6:154–160.

61. Warnecke H, Berdjis F, Hennig E, et al. (1991) Mechanical left ventricular support as a bridge to cardiac transplantation in childhood. Eur J Cardiothorac Surg 5:330–333.

62. Reinhartz O, Keith FM, El Banayosy A, et al. (2001) Multicenter experience with the thoratec ventricular assist device in children and adolescents. J Heart Lung Transplant 20:439–448.

63. Reinhartz O, Stiller B, Eilers R, Farrar DJ (2002) Current clinical status of pulsatile pediatric circulatory support. ASAIO J 48:455–459.

64. Malaisrie SC, Pelletier MP, Yun JJ, et al. (2008) Pneumatic paracorporeal ventricular assist device in infants and children: initial Stanford experience. J Heart Lung Transplant 27:173–177.

65. Blume ED, Naftel DC, Bastardi HJ, et al. (2006) Pediatric Heart Transplant Study Investigators. Outcomes of children bridged to heart transplantation with ventricular assist devices: a multi-institutional study. Circulation 113:2313–2319.

66. Booker PD (1997) Intra-aortic balloon pumping in young children. Paediatr Anaesth 7:501–507.

67. Davies MJ, Nguyen K, Gaynor JW, Elliott MJ (1998) Modified ultrafiltration improves left ventricular systolic function in infants after cardiopulmonary bypass. J Thorac Cardiovasc Surg 115:361–370.

68. Elliot MJ (1993) Ultrafiltration and modified ultrafiltration in pediatric open heart operations. Ann Thorac Surg 56:1518–1522.

69. Costello JM, Thiagarajan RR, Dionne RE, et al. (2006) Initial experience with fenoldopam after cardiac surgery in neonates with an insufficient response to conventional diuretics. Pediatr Crit Care Med 7:28–33.

70. Giuffre RM, Tam KH, Williams WW, et al. (1992) Acute renal failure complicating pediatric cardiac surgery: a comparison of survivors and non-survivors following acute peritoneal dialysis. Pediatr Cardiol 13:208–213.

71. Paret G, Cohen AJ, Bohn DJ, et al. (1992) Continuous arteriovenous hemofiltration after cardiac operations in infants and children. J Thorac Cardiovasc Surg 104:1225–1230.

72. Mou SS, Giroir BP, Molitor-Kirsch EA, et al. (2004) Fresh whole blood versus reconstituted blood for pump priming in heart surgery in infants. N Engl J Med 351:1635–1644.

73. Gruenwald CE, McCrindle BW, Crawford-Lean L, et al. (2008) Reconstituted fresh whole blood improves clinical outcomes compared with stored component blood therapy for neonates undergoing cardiopulmonary bypass for cardiac surgery: a randomized controlled trial. J Thorac Cardiovasc Surg 136:1442–1449.

74. Jonas RA (1998) Neurological protection during cardiopulmonary bypass/deep hypothermia. Pediatr Cardiol 19:321–330.

75. Dominguez TE, Wernovsky G, Gaynor JW (2007) Cause and prevention of central nervous system injury in neonates undergoing cardiac surgery. Semin Thorac Cardiovasc Surg 19:269–277.

76. Johnston MV (1996) Brain development and its relationship to pattern of injury. In: Jonas RA, Newburger JW, Volpe JJ (eds) Cardiopulmonary Bypass in Neonates, Infants and Young Children. Butterworth-Heineman, Oxford, pp. 237–300.

77. Jonas RA, Wernovsky G, Ware JH, et al. (1992) The Boston circulatory arrest study: perioperative neurologic outcome after the arterial switch operation. Circulation 86:360A.

78. Newburger JW, Jonas RA, Wernovsky G, et al. (1993) A comparison of the perioperative neurologic effects of hypothermic circulatory arrest versus low-flow cardiopulmonary bypass in infant heart surgery. The Boston Circulatory Arrest Study. N Engl J Med 329:1057–1064.

79. Bellinger DC, Jonas RA, Rappaport LA, et al. (1995) Developmental and neurologic status of children after heart surgery with hypothermic circulatory arrest or low flow cardiopulmonary bypass. N Engl J Med 332:549–555.

80. Bellinger DC, Wypij D, Kuban KC, et al. (1999) Developmental and neurological status of children at 4 years of age after heart surgery with hypothermic circulatory arrest or low-flow cardiopulmonary bypass. Circulation 100:526–532.

81. Bellinger DC, Rappaport LA, Wypij D, et al. (1997) Patterns of developmental dysfunction after surgery during infancy to correct transposition of the great arteries. J Dev Behav Pediatr 18:75–83.

82. Rappaport LA, Wypij D, Bellinger DC, et al. (1998) Relation of seizures after cardiac surgery in early infancy to neurodevelopmental outcome. Boston circulatory arrest study group. Circulation 97:773–779.

83. Menache CC, du Plessis AJ, Wessel DL, et al. (2002) Current incidence of acute neurologic complications after open-heart operations in children. Ann Thorac Surg 73:1752–1758.

84. du Plessis AJ, Jonas RA, Wypij D, et al. (1997) Perioperative effects of alpha-stat versus pH-stat strategies for deep hypothermic cardiopulmonary bypass in infants. J Thorac Cardiovasc Surg 114:991–1001.

85. Newburger JW, Jonas RA, Soul J, et al. (2008) Randomized trial of hematocrit 25% versus 35% during hypothermic cardiopulmonary bypass in infant heart surgery. J Thorac Cardiovasc Surg 135:347–354.

86. Ballweg JA, Wernovsky G, Gaynor JW (2007) Neurodevelopmental outcomes following congenital heart surgery. Pediatr Cardiol 28:126–133.

87. Bellinger DC, Newburger JW, Wypij D, et al. (2008) Behaviour at eight years in children with surgically corrected transposition: The Boston Circulatory Arrest Trial. Cardiol Young 11:1–12.

88. Shum-Tim D, Nagashima M, Shinoka T, et al. (1998) Postischemic hyperthermia exacerbates neurologic injury after deep hypothermic circulatory arrest. J Thorac Cardiovasc Surg 116:780–792.

89. Bissonnette B, Holtby HM, Davis AJ, et al. (2000) Cerebral hyperthermia in children after cardiopulmonary bypass. Anesthesiology 93:611–618.

90. DeLeon S, Ilbawi M, Arcilla R, et al. (1990) Choreoathetosis after deep hypothermia without circulatory arrest. Ann Thorac Surg 50:714–719.

91. Wong PC, Barlow CF, Hickey PR, et al. (1992) Factors associated with choreoathetosis after cardiopulmonary bypass in children with congenital heart disease. Circulation 86:III118–III126.

92. Andropoulos DB, Stayer SA, Diaz LK, Ramamoorthy C (2004) Neurological monitoring for congenital heart surgery. Anesth Analg 99:1365–1375.

93. Hoffman GM, Stuth EA, Jaquiss RD, et al. (2004) Changes in cerebral and somatic oxygenation during stage 1 palliation of hypoplastic left heart syndrome using continuous regional cerebral perfusion. J Thorac Cardiovasc Surg 127:223–233.

94. Kussman BD, Wypij D, DiNardo JA, et al. (2009) Cerebral oximetry during infant cardiac surgery: evaluation and relationship to early postoperative outcomes. Anesth Analg 108:1122–1131.

95. Kussman BD, Gauvreau K, DiNardo JA, et al. (2007) Cerebral perfusion and oxygenation after the Norwood procedure: comparison of right ventricle to pulmonary artery conduit with modified Blalock–Taussig shunt. J Thoracic Cardiovasc Surg 133:648–655.

96. Kelleher DK, Laussen PC, Teixeira-Pinto A, Duggan C (2006) Growth and correlates of nutritional status among infants with hypoplastic left heart syndrome (HLHS) following the Stage One Norwood Procedure. Nutrition 22:23–44.

97. Sánchez C, López-Herce J, Carrillo A, et al. (2006) Transpyloric enteral feeding in the postoperative of cardiac surgery in children. J Pediatr Surg 41:1096–1102.

98. Braudis NJ, Curley MA, Beaupre K, et al. (2009) Enteral feeding algorithm for infants with hypoplastic left heart syndome poststage 1 palliation. Ped Crit Care Med 10:460–466.

99. Shi S, Zhao Z, Liu X, et al. (2008) Perioperative risk factors for prolonged mechanical ventilation following cardiac surgery in neonates and young infants. Chest 134:768–774.

100. Laussen PC, Reid RW, Stene RA, et al. (1996) Tracheal extubation of children in the operating room after atrial septal defect repair as part of a clinical practice guideline. Anesth Analg 82:988–993.

101. Shew SB, Jaksic T (1999) The metabolic needs of critically ill children and neonates. Semin Pediatr Surg 8:131–139.

102. Anand KJ, Hansen DD, Hickey PR (1990) Hormonal-metabolic stress responses in neonates undergoing cardiac surgery. Anesthesiology 73:661–670.

103. Anand KJ, Hickey PR (1992) Halothane-morphine compared with high-dose sufentanil for anesthesia and postoperative analgesia in neonatal cardiac surgery. N Engl J Med 326:1–9.

104. Gruber EM, Laussen PC, Casta A, et al. (2001) Stress response in infants undergoing cardiac surgery: a randomized study of fentanyl bolus, fentanyl infusion and fentanyl-midazolam infusion. Anesth Analg 92:882–890.

105. Cote CJ (1994) Sedation for the pediatric patient. A review. Pediatr Clin N Am 41:31–58.

106. American Academy of Pediatrics, Committee on Drugs (1992) Guidelines for monitoring and management of pediatric patients during and after sedation for diagnostic and therapeutic procedures. Pediatrics 89:1110–1115.

107. Lloyd-Thomas AR, Booker PD (1986) Infusion of midazolam in paediatric patients after cardiac surgery. Br J Anaesth 58:1109–1115.

108. Ng E, Taddio A, Ohlsson A (2003) Intravenous midazolam infusion for sedation of infants in the neonatal intensive care unit. Cochrane Database Syst Rev (1): CD002052.

109. Bergman I, Steeves M, Burckart G, et al. (1991) Reversible neurologic abnormalities associated with prolonged intravenous midazolam and fentanyl administration. J Pediatr 119:644–649.

110. Hickey PR, Hansen DD, Wessel DL, et al. (1985) Blunting of stress responses in the pulmonary circulation of infants by fentanyl. Anesth Analg 64:1137–1142.

111. Hickey PR, Hansen DD, Wessel DL, et al. (1985) Pulmonary and systemic hemodynamic responses to fentanyl in infants. Anesth Analg 64:483–486.

112. Yaster M (1987) The dose response of fentanyl in neonatal anesthesia. Anesth 66:433–435.

113. Tarkkila P, Rosenberg PH (1998) Perioperative analgesis with non-steroidal analgesics. Curr Opin Anaesthesiol 11:407–410.

114. Gupta A, Daggett C, Drant S, et al. (2004) Prospective randomized trial of ketorolac after congenital heart surgery. J Cardiothorac Vasc Anesth 18:454–457.

115. Morray JP, Lynn AM, Stamm SJ, et al. (1984) Hemodynamic effects of ketamine in children with congenital heart disease. Anesth Analg 63:895–899.

116. Hickey PR, Hansen DD, Cramolini GM, et al. (1985) Pulmonary and systemic hemodynamic responses to ketamine in infants with normal and elevated pulmonary vascular resistance. Anesthesiology 62:287–293.

117. Ostwald P, Doenicke AW (1998) Etomidate revisited. Curr Opin Anaesthesiol 11:391–398.

118. Sarker M, Odegard KC, Laussen PC (2002) Cardiac surgery in a child with sacral and intrasacral hemangioma. Paediatr Anaesth 12:552–555.

119. Dönmez A, Kaya H, Haberal A, et al. (1998) The effect of etomidate induction on plasma cortisol levels in children undergoing cardiac surgery. J Cardiothorac Vasc Anesth 12:182–185.

120. Tobias JD (2007) Dexmedetomidine: applications in pediatric critical care and pediatric anesthesiology. Pediatr Crit Care Med 8:115–131.

121. Hammer GB, Drover DR, Cao H et al. (2008) The effects of dexmedetomidine on cardiac electrophysiology in children. Anesth Analg 106:79–83.

30 Mechanical support of the circulation

Pablo Motta, M.D.
Texas Children's Hospital, Baylor College of Medicine, Houston, Texas, USA

Brain W. Duncan, M.D.
Cleveland Clinic, Cleveland, Ohio, USA

Stephen Stayer, M.D.
Texas Children's Hospital, Baylor College of Medicine, Houston, Texas, USA

Background/introduction/history

The successful use of extracorporeal membrane oxygenation (ECMO) in children began in the late 1970s when Bartlett et al. applied this technology to term newborn infants with respiratory failure. Sixteen patients were treated with ECMO for up to 8 days and their survival rate was higher than infants treated with conventional ventilator therapy (37.5% vs 10%, respectively). Intracranial bleeding was the most common complication in both groups: 43 and 57%, respectively. These authors concluded that in high mortality risk infants, the rate of survival is higher and intracranial bleeding lower with ECMO compared to optimal ventilator management [1].

Soeter was the first to describe the use of ECMO for cardiorespiratory failure after tetralogy of Fallot correction [2], and Kanter reported the first series of 13 patients with postoperative cardiac failure treated with ECMO. Seven patients (53%) were weaned from ECMO and 5 (38%) survived long term [3]. The complication rate was high, and included bleeding (69%), renal insufficiency (38%), and neurologic injury (23%).

The utilization of ECMO for cardiac support has increased steadily since the 1980s [4–6]. Improved perfusion and anticoagulation techniques make the support safer so that it may be initiated earlier and not as a last resort. Data from the Extracorporeal Life Support Organization (ELSO) reveal an increase in ECMO support for cardiac failure across all age groups with higher survival rates for neonatal and pediatric patients than adults: 38, 43, and 33%, respectively [6].

The first successful use of a ventricular assist device (VAD) as a bridge to heart transplant in an adult was reported by Cooley in 1969 [7]. The first description of VAD

Anesthesia for Congenital Heart Disease 2nd edition. Edited by
Dean Andropoulos, Stephen Stayer, Isobel Russell and Emad Mossad.
© 2010 Blackwell Publishing.

use in children was 20 years later [8], and the authors concluded that, like adults, VAD could be used as a bridge to cardiac transplantation in children. In the 1990s VAD use in children was sporadic. However, due to improvements and miniaturization of equipment, VAD implantation in children has grown exponentially in recent years [9].

Classification/types of devices

Mechanical support of the circulation can be provided by ECMO, VAD, or aortic balloon pump; however, balloon pumps are rarely used in children because the small size and increased elasticity of a child's aorta makes this device less effective and more difficult to effectively time balloon inflations at high heart rates. ECMO is capable of supporting both circulatory and respiratory failure, whereas VAD only provides support of the circulation. In children, unlike adults, isolated left ventricular dysfunction is rare. The need for circulatory support in children is often due to a combination of right ventricular failure, hypoxemia, and pulmonary hypertension [10, 11]. For this reason, ECMO is more commonly used in the pediatric population. Left VAD (LVAD) is used in patients with predominantly left ventricular failure and normal lung function. Biventricular support is more commonly required in children with heart failure secondary to congenital heart disease. The main differences between these devices are presented in Table 30.1.

Indications for circulatory support

The indications for ECMO include cardiac failure, respiratory failure unresponsive to optimal ventilator and medical management, pulmonary hypertensive crisis, and resuscitation, whereas VAD is only indicated for circulatory support. When used for cardiac failure, one goal of initiating circulatory support is to rest and unload the heart, allowing the myocardium to recover from injury, referred to as "bridge to recovery." If the myocardium does not recover, the patient may be transitioned to a long-term means of circulatory support until heart transplant, referred to as "bridge to transplant" [12, 13]. In pediatrics, currently there is no "destination therapy" device as there is in adults, referring to permanent long-term circulatory support for the remainder of the patient's life.

Clinical criteria are used to determine the need for ECMO or VAD and include progressive increase in inotropic and/or vasopressor support (e.g., epinephrine $>1\,\mu g/kg/min$) with poor end-organ perfusion evidenced by acidosis, oliguria ($<1\,mL/kg/h$), decreased mixed venous ($<40\%$), or near-infrared cerebral saturation ($>20\%$ below baseline). The ideal timing for initiating circula-

tory support is before circulatory collapse, avoiding long-term end-organ injury, in particular irreversible neurologic damage. Early initiation of mechanical support has yielded better outcomes [12].

The two populations in which circulatory support is indicated are postcardiotomy (postsurgical) cardiac dysfunction and medical cardiac failure (Table 30.2).

The most common cardiac indication for circulatory support is failure to wean from cardiopulmonary bypass (CPB) after repair or palliation of congenital heart disease [6]. Patients may fail to wean from CPB due to ventricular dysfunction, respiratory failure, and/or pulmonary hypertension. Ventricular dysfunction after CPB in children is associated with complex surgical repairs that require long CPB times and/or inadequate myocardial protection [14]. There is no one single diagnosis associated with the need of postoperative ECMO; however, in some published series, single ventricle physiology and cyanotic heart lesions more commonly require support [11–16]. The reported frequency of ECMO use after CPB in children is 3–5% [17–19]. The location for initiation of ECMO varies between the intensive care unit (ICU) and the operating room (OR), depending on the urgency. Chaturvedi has

Table 30.1 Types of mechanical support devices

	ECMO	VAD
Circuit complexity	High	Low
Trauma to red blood cells	High	Low
Flow type	Nonpulsatile	Pulsatile or nonpulsatile
Ventricular decompression	Not always achieved*	Usually achieved
Cannulation	Peripheral or central†	Central‡
Need for anticoagulation	Full heparinization (ACT >180 s)	Heparinization/ antiaggregation
Respiratory support	Yes	No
Biventricular support	Always	Possible§
Maximum support duration (days)	15—21	>400
Complications	High	Low
Neurologic injury**	60%	20%

*May require left atrial venting to achieve ventricular decompression.
†Peripheral cannulation includes neck cannulation in infants or femoral in older children (>30 kg), central cannulation is achieved through sternotomy.
‡New VAD system Tandem Heart allows peripheral cannulation.
§Requires two devices and four cannulae.
**ECMO-supported patient includes higher proportion of critically ill neonates undergoing complex congenital heart disease repair or palliation.
ACT, activated clotting time; ECMO, extracorporeal membrane oxygenation; VAD, ventricular assist device.

PART 6 Anesthesia outside the cardiac operating room

Table 30.2 Mechanical circulatory support indications

	Device of choice
Surgical (postcardiotomy)	
Inability to wean from CPB	
• Ventricular dysfunction	VAD or ECMO
• Respiratory failure	ECMO
○ Oxygenation	
○ Ventilation	
○ Both	
• Increased pulmonary vascular resistance	ECMO
Hemodynamic instability in PICU	
• Low cardiac output syndrome	VAD or ECMO
• Pulmonary hypertensive crisis	ECMO
• Postoperative cardiopulmonary arrest	ECMO
Medical (nonsurgical)	
• Acute myocarditis/cardiomyopathy	VAD or ECMO
• Arrhythmias	ECMO
• Catheterization laboratory instability	ECMO
• Preoperative stabilization	VAD or ECMO
• Intoxications	ECMO
• Hypothermic arrest	ECMO

CPB, cardiopulmonary bypass; ECMO, extracorporeal membrane oxygenation; VAD, ventricular assist device.

shown better survival in patients placed on ECMO in the OR versus the ICU, with a survival rate 64% versus 29%, respectively [11]. This author supports the concept of early initiation of ECMO and attributes the better outcome to the more controlled environment of the OR setting and the lack of end-organ damage with early initiation of support. LVAD may also be used for circulatory support after failure to wean from CPB. However, survival data show that postcardiotomy patients requiring LVAD have worse outcomes than patients requiring LVAD for myocarditis or cardiomyopathy [19,20]. This difference in recovery reflects the difference in recovery of these patient populations, not a difference between ECMO and VAD. LVAD is preferable over ECMO for patients suspected to need circulatory support longer (>2 wk), those who do not have pulmonary hypertension or respiratory dysfunction, and among those where recovery is not expected (heart transplant candidates). Patients with anomalous origin of the left coronary artery from the pulmonary artery (ALCAPA) have good outcomes from VAD support since their primary problem is left ventricular dysfunction. del Nido reported the successful use of LVAD in 7 infants with ALCAPA and associated severe left ventricular failure and severe mitral regurgitation; 5 patients survived and regained left ventricular function [21]. Among patients whose right ventricular function is also affected, biventricular support may be needed.

ECMO, either venovenous or venoarterial, is the only lifesaving treatment option for patients with primary graft dysfunction after lung transplant, which occurs in 5–25% of patients. ECMO provides respiratory and circulatory support while the lungs recover from an acute injury. Data from the ELSO registry reveal outcomes similar to other groups receiving ECMO support, with 62% successfully weaning and 42% survival [22].

Viral myocarditis is the leading cause of acute heart failure in children without congenital heart disease and is the most common indication of nonsurgical ECMO. Chen et al. were the first to report successful use of ECMO for patients with acute myocarditis presenting with shock, with an 80% survival rate [23]. Duncan found the same survival rate (12/15, 80%) in 15 pediatric patients with acute fulminant myocarditis. Twelve patients received ECMO and 3 VAD support, with 7 survivors recovering function (bridged to recovery) and 5 requiring a heart transplant (bridged to transplant) [24]. In children bridged to transplant, VAD support appears to result in improved outcomes over ECMO, with a lesser incidence of neurologic complications [19,20].

ECMO is used for cardiopulmonary resuscitation during cardiac arrest. The 2005 American Heart Association (AHA) recommendations suggest that ECMO be considered for patients during CPR in situations of in-hospital cardiac arrest refractory to initial resuscitation attempts if the condition leading to cardiac arrest is reversible or amenable to heart transplantation, if excellent conventional CPR has been performed after no more than several minutes of no-flow cardiac arrest (arrest time without CPR), and if the institution is able to rapidly perform ECMO. The level of evidence supporting this recommendation is based on case series without a control group, and is considered to be Class IIb where the benefits seem to outweigh the risk and its use should be considered [25]. The evidence for this guideline is based on an initial work by del Nido, which reports that ECMO use in witnessed sudden cardiac arrest had a better outcome than ECMO for cardiac failure [26]. This observation was confirmed by Duncan who successfully used a rapid-deployment ECMO system for the resuscitation of pediatric patients with heart disease after cardiac arrest. The rapid-deployment ECMO system consisted of a simplified preprimed circuit with in-house personnel available for placement, and initiated after 10 minutes of lack of response to standard resuscitative measures. This approach shortened the resuscitation times and improved survival [27]. The AHA guidelines do not discourage the use of ECMO in longer CPR periods since long-term survival is possible even after >50 minutes of CPR in selected patients [28]. The advantage of ECMO over conventional CPR is that it provides a steady blood flow supplying adequate tissue perfusion and allowing myocardial and pulmonary function to recover [29]. The effectiveness of ECMO to resuscitate patients following critical cardiac events in the catheterization laboratory has also been described [30,31]. In this population the incidence of reported neurologic injury was high (47%), and patients in which the device was placed semielectively had significant lower neurologic injury. See Chapter 29 for further discussion of ECMO-CPR (E-CPR).

Life-threatening arrhythmias are another indication for ECMO use. Walker reported the use of ECMO in two pediatric patients with cardiogenic shock due to intractable supraventricular tachycardia. While on ECMO one patient's medical management was optimized and the other underwent a successful radioablative procedure [32], and both were weaned from ECMO and discharged from the hospital. Darst successfully treated an infant with congenital junctional ectopic tachycardia. ECMO allowed arrhythmia control and myocardial rest, leading to functional recovery [33].

ECMO is used in other situations of circulatory collapse. It has been used to support the circulation after severe intoxications with cardiovascular collapse, and should be considered early in cases of near-fatal intoxications with cardiodepressive drugs [34–36]. Active rewarming with ECMO can also be lifesaving after hypothermic cardiac arrest from exposure with core temperatures <28°C, usually due to cold water drowning. Hypothermic arrest offers the possibility of survival without major neurologic damage due to the neuroprotective effect of rapid cooling on the brain [37], and has resulted in 50% survival in this population. Hyperkalemia is a potential prognostic indicator that can be used to avoid ECMO when there is a very poor chance of recovery since potassium is released when there is irreversible cell damage [38].

Contraindications to mechanical circulatory support

The absolute contraindications for initiation of circulatory support are related to severe central nervous system injuries [11], and patients with suspected injuries should be evaluated by a neurologist and have appropriate imaging studies. Because of the need for anticoagulation, active central nervous system bleeding must be ruled out. Other absolute contraindications are extreme prematurity and very low weight because of the risk of intracranial hemorrhage.

Relative contraindications to the institution of mechanical circulatory support are palliative congenital cardiac operations in single ventricle patients and in patients with coexisting congenital diaphragmatic hernia. Decisions about the use of ECMO in such patients are made on a case-by-case basis since some of these pa-

tients have been successfully resuscitated with ECMO [11]. There is limited experience in circulatory support in single ventricle physiology, and the outcomes are worse than biventricular patients. Early application of the circulatory support is advised since the use of ECMO for resuscitation in this population carries a high risk of mortality [39].

Devices

Extracorporeal membrane oxygenation

ECMO circuits are composed of a centrifugal or roller pump with a hollow-fiber or a membrane oxygenator, oxygen blender, pump console, heat exchanger, and pump cart (Color Plate 30.1). At Texas Children's Hospital, our circuit is composed of a Rotaflow centrifugal pump (Maquet, Inc., Wayne, NJ, USA; www.maquet.com, accessed September 26, 2009) with membrane oxygenator (Avecor ECMO Membrane Oxygenator, Avecor Cardiovascular, Inc., Plymouth, MN, USA). This pump drives the blood by force vortex pumping, is preload and afterload dependent, and drainage is independent of gravity. Roller pump flow systems are also dependent on gravity drainage. Both pump systems require continuous circuit pressure monitoring to avoid excessive negative pressure in the circuit which could produce blood microcavitation and hemolysis. Centrifugal pumps cause less cellular damage and activation of the immune system than roller head pumps [40,41]. There are two types of oxygenators: membrane and hollow fiber. In membrane oxygenators gas exchange is produced across a diffusion membrane, and in hollow-fiber oxygenators, across microporous fibers. Membrane oxygenators have higher resistance to blood flow than hollow-fiber oxygenators. Heat exchangers are placed distally in the circuit to warm the blood just before returning it to the patient. The cannulae used depend on the cannulation site, patient weight, vessel size, and desired flow rate (Tables 30.3 and 30.4). Wire-reinforced cannulae are preferred since they are incompressible and resist kinking. Heparin-bonded circuits and cannulae (Carmeda® BioActive Surface Medtronic, Minneapolis, MN, USA) are used to reduce but not eliminate the need for systemic anticoagulation. Additional information about the ECMO equipment components is available at the ELSO Web site: www.elso.med.umich.edu/ [42].

The site of cannulation varies with the indication for ECMO. Patients requiring support in the immediate postoperative period are cannulated through a sternotomy, via aortic, right atrial, and often left atrial cannulae, the latter for decompression of the left ventricle. This approach is especially useful to expedite the institution of support

Table 30.3 ECMO cannula sizing

Flow (mL/min)	Sizes (Fr)					
	Arterial		Venous			
	Aortic	Femoral	Single polystan®	Single DLP®	Single atrial	
0–500	8		18	14/16	12/14	
500–1000	10	10	21	18/20	16/18	
1000–1800	12	14	24/28	20/24	18/20	
1800–2500	14	14	32/36	24/28	20/22	
2500–4000	16	18	36	28	24	
4000–5000	18	24	36	28	24	
4500–↑	20/21	24	36	28	24	

ECMO, extracorporeal membrane oxygenation.

in postcardiac surgical patients after cardiac arrest. Peripheral cannulation via the neck (right carotid artery, right internal jugular vein) or femoral (artery and vein) vessels is preferred in nonsurgical patients or in patients who required ECMO later in the postoperative period. Neck cannulation is the peripheral site of choice in infants and young children due to the larger caliber vessel, whereas older children and young adults are cannulated via the femoral vessels [11]. A left atrial vent is used in patients with biventricular anatomy when there is echocardiographic evidence of poor left ventricular decompression [17]. Insertion of the left atrial vent can be performed surgically in patients who fail to wean from CPB or percutaneously in the catheterization laboratory or under echocardiography guidance.

The prime volume and components for ECMO are individualized based on patient size. The prime volume is kept to an absolute minimum to decrease the effect of hemodilution. Use of a low prime (99 mL) ECMO circuit has been reported in sudden cardiopulmonary collapse in pediatric patients, including postcardiotomy patients

Table 30.4 Flow rate calculator

Patients weighing <10 kg
  Flow = Weight (kg) × 150 mL/min

Patients weighing >10 kg
  Flow = BSA × cardiac index (age specific)

0–2 yr 3.0–3.2 × BSA
2–4 yr 2.8 × BSA
4–6 yr 2.6 × BSA
6–10 yr 2.5 × BSA
>10 yr 2.4 × BSA

BSA, body surface area.

[43]. Since hyperkalemia and lactic acidosis are common as stored red blood cells age, we most commonly use blood collected within 48 hours to prime the circuit of neonatal patients.

Mechanical ventilatory support should be continued while on ECMO to avoid atelectasis, improve pulmonary venous saturation, and improve the delivered PaO$_2$ to the coronaries [17,18]. Low settings should be used to avoid lung injury, with peak airway pressures less than 30 cm H$_2$O, end expiratory pressure under 10 cm H$_2$O, FiO$_2$ of less than 40%, and a respiratory rate of 10–15 breaths/min.

Ventricular assist devices

VAD circuits are composed of inflow and outflow cannulae, pump system (axial or pulsatile), power source, and a system controller (Color Plate 30.2) [9,10,44–47]. The inflow cannula is attached to the left atrium or to the apex of the left ventricle, and blood is pumped by the device into the outflow cannula, which is sutured to the ascending aorta. Ventricular inflow cannulae achieve better unloading of the heart reducing wall stress and allowing better recovery, and they have a decreased incidence of thrombosis. When a right VAD (RVAD) is indicated, the inflow cannula is attached to the right atrium and the outflow cannula into the main pulmonary artery. Right atrial inflow cannula insertion is used for RVAD implantation if right ventricular function recovery is expected.

The VAD devices can be classified as short or long term, with 2 weeks being the usual limit for short-term VADs (Table 30.5). Another classification is based on the pumping mode. The ejection can be achieved with centrifugal pump (e.g., Biomedicus), pneumatic pusher plate (e.g., Berlin Heart), or axial flow (e.g., MicroMed DeBakey). The available VAD systems for pediatric use in the USA are described in Table 30.5.

Centrifugal pumps

There are several devices available: Biomedicus Biopump® (Medtronic Corp., Minneapolis, MN, USA), CentriMag® (Levitronix, Zürich, Switzerland), RotaFlow® (Jostra, Hirrigen, Germany), and Capiox® (Terumo, Ann Arbor, MI, USA) (Figure 30.1). The centrifugal pumps provide nonpulsatile flow by a constrained vortex design that is both preload and afterload sensitive. The Biopumps® are available in two different volumes (50 and 80 mL), with the 80 mL capable of flowing up to 10 L/min. Centrifugal pumps require a flow probe for monitoring since the pump is preload dependent, and revolutions per minute do not correlate exactly with the flow. Compared to an ECMO circuit, this VAD circuit has the advantage of a lower priming volume

Table 30.5 Ventricular assist device systems available in the USA

	Flow type	Stroke volume (mL) or pump speed (rpm)	Flow range (L/min)	BSA range (m²)	Device type
Short term (<14 days)					
Centrifugal pumps	Nonpulsatile	0–4500 rpm	0 to 5–6	No minimum*	Rotational
TandemHeart	Nonpulsatile	3000–7500 rpm	Up to 5	>1.3	Rotational
Abiomed	Pulsatile	80 mL	>2	>0.7	Pusher plate
Long term (> 14 days)					
Pneumatic pulsatile ventricular assist devices					
Berlin Heart	Pulsatile	12, 15, 25, 30, 50, 60, and 80 mL	Variable†	0.2	Pusher plate
Adult-size pulsatile devices impanted in children					
Thoratec	Pulsatile	65 mL	5–6	> 0.7	Pusher plate
Continous-flow ventricular assist device					
Heart Mate II	Axial	6,000–15,000 rpm	>2.5	>1.4	Axial
DeBakey	Axial	7,500–12,500 rpm	1–10	>07–<1.5	Axial

*Smaller patient reported 1.9 kg neonate.
†Depends on pump size and set rate.
BSA, body surface area.

and applicability to patients of all ages. In addition, due to the lack of an oxygenator or venous reservoirs, heparin requirements and trauma to red cells are reduced in comparison to ECMO. Limitations of the centrifugal pumps are that only short-term support is provided and there is continued need for sedation and mechanical ventilation [9,10,45–47]. The Biopump® system has been the most frequently used VAD for pediatric support in the USA, and is successfully used after congenital heart surgery in children less than 6 kg [48].

The TandemHeart

The TandemHeart (Cardiac Assist Inc, Pittsburgh, PA, USA; http://www.cardiacassist.com/TandemHeart/, accessed February 1 2009) (Color Plate 30.3) is a centrifugal pump that has been used for LVAD and RVAD support for short periods of time. The advantages of this system are its simplicity and that it can be inserted percutaneously without the need for CPB. The venous cannula is placed transseptally in the left atrium and the arterial cannula is placed in the femoral artery percutaneously or by surgical

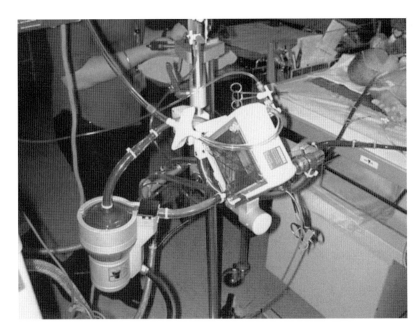

Figure 30.1 Centrifugal ECMO pump showing (a) Rotaflow® centrifugal pump (Maquet, Harlingen, Germany) with (b) hollow-fiber polymethylpentene oxygenator (QuadroxD, Jostra Medizintechnik AG, Hirrlingen, Germany)

cutdown. Its use in pediatric is limited to older, larger children due to the size of the cannulae: 21 Fr (French) venous and a 15–17-Fr arterial cannulae [49], but it has been used to support the failing right ventricle in single ventricle patients and posttransplant patients with right ventricular dysfunction [50].

Abiomed BVS 5000

Abiomed BVS 5000 (Abiomed Cardiovascular, Inc., Danvers, MA, USA; http://www.abiomed.com/products/index.cfm, accessed February 1, 2009) (Figure 30.2) is another paracorporeal pneumatic VAD. It is capable of providing univentricular or biventricular short-term support. It has two sets of polyurethane chambers, both atrial and ventricular. The atrial chambers fill passively and the ventricular chambers are emptied by air drive power. Ashton et al. published the successful use of this device for pediatric patients with a body surface area (BSA) >1.2 m² bridged to transplant or to recovery [51]. Similar to the Thoratec VAD, this device is associated with an increased thromboembolic risk.

The Berlin Heart VAD or EXCOR

The Berlin Heart VAD or EXCOR (Berlin Heart AG, Berlin, Germany; http://www.berlinheart.de/englisch/medpro/excor-pediatric, accessed February 1, 2009) (Color Plates 30.4 and 30.5) is a pulsatile, paracorporeal

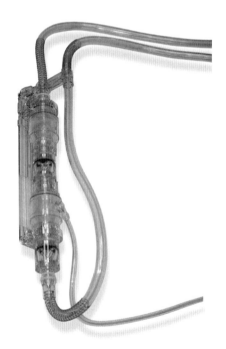

Figure 30.2 Abiomed BVS 5000 two-chambered pneumatically driven device

VAD that is suitable for all pediatric patients including neonates. It is available with several pumping chamber sizes (10–80 mL) and provides pulsatile flow delivered through pneumatically driven thin membrane pump. In systole the pump moves compressed air into the diaphragm, causing the ejection. In diastole, negative pressure is generated to aid in the filling of the chamber. The maximum systolic positive pressure generated is 350 mm Hg and the maximum negative driving pressure is −100 mm Hg. High pressure is sometimes needed to overcome the resistance of small pediatric cannulae. The pump rate can be adjusted between 30 and 150 beats/min, and the systolic time can be adjusted between 20 and 70% of the cycle. The blood pump is transparent, allowing visual control of filling, emptying, and thrombus formation. If there is any thrombus formation in the pump or cannulae, the pump must be exchanged to avoid systemic embolization. The blood-contacting surfaces of the pump including the polyurethane valves are heparin coated through the Carmeda® process (Carmeda, Upplands Väsby, Sweden), reducing anticoagulation requirements. It also has silicon cannulae with a Dacron covering that works as a biologic barrier against ascending infections. When using this, VAD patients are not dependent on mechanical ventilation, can resume enteral feeding, are ambulatory, and can be discharged from the ICU [52]. The rate of neurologic complications of 5% is much lower than ECMO and other adult-sized VADs [53,54]. At the time this chapter was written, the use of this device in the USA was limited to an investigational Food and Drug Adminstration (FDA) protocol and was available only in 10 centers.

MEDOS HIA-VAD system

The MEDOS HIA-VAD System (Medizintechnik AG, Stolberg Germany; available at www.medos-ag.com, accessed August 24, 2009) is a paracorporeal pneumatically driven device similar to the Berlin Heart VAD. The ventricles are made of polyurethane with a double-layer inner displacement membrane. It generates up to 300 mm Hg of positive pressure, −80 mm Hg negative pressure, and rates up to 180 beats/min. It is available in 10, 25, 60, and 80 mL size chambers for LVAD support and 9, 22.5, 54, and 72 mL size chambers for RVAD support. Like the Berlin Heart, it is also transparent, allowing visual control of filling, emptying and thrombus formation. Konertz published the first pediatric series describing a 66% survival rate [55]. It has been extensively used in Europe but is only approved in the USA for compassionate use.

Thoratec VAD

Thoratec VAD (Thoratec Corporation, Pleasanton, CA, USA; http://www.thoratec.com/medical-professionals/

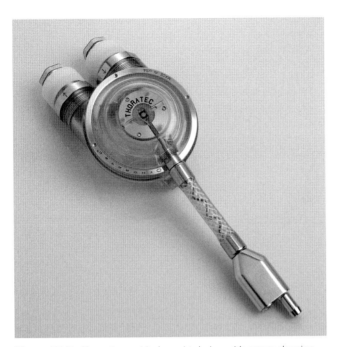

Figure 30.3 Thoractec ventricular assist device, with arrows showing the direction of the blood flow and the pneumatic line

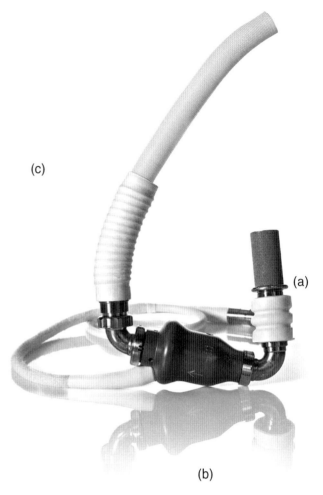

Figure 30.4 Heart Mate II showing (a) inflow cannula, (b) axial pump, and (c) outflow cannula

vad-product-information/index.aspx, accessed February 1, 2009) (Figure 30.3) is another paracorporeal pneumatic VAD. The prosthetic ventricle has a 65-mL stroke volume chamber with a maximum output flow of 7 L/min. It works on three different modes: fixed rate, synchronous (for weaning), or fill to empty mode. Like other paracorporeal pneumatic devices, it can be used as a LVAD or biventricular VAD. The lower limits for implantation are a BSA of 0.7 m^2 and an age of 7 years or older. Reinhartz reported a 68% survival to transplant or recovery in 209 pediatric patients (range 5–18 yr, BSA 0.7–2.3 m^2) [56]. Patients with cardiomyopathies or myocarditis had better outcome than patients with congenital heart disease, with a survival rate of 74, 86, and 27% respectively [56,57]. The risk of thromboembolism in children is higher than in adults (27% vs 5–12%, respectively) [58]. This increased risk is due to reduced flow velocities, blood stasis in the device, and systolic hypertension due to mismatch of the pump size and the patient aorta.

Heart Mate II

Heart Mate II (Thoratec Corp., Pleasanton, CA, USA) (Figure 30.4 and Color Plate 30.6) is an axial-flow LVAD. Axial-flow devices are smaller and simpler than pulsatile pumps. They have only one moving component, with no valves, vent, or compliance chamber, reducing the complexity. Because of their small size, axial-flow LVADs can be used in smaller patients (BSA $\geq$ 1.4 m^2). Frazier published the first series using Heart Mate II in adult and

teenage patients with an 81% survival rate [59]. Three patients in this series were under 18 years of age.

MicroMed DeBakey VAD Child

The MicroMed DeBakey VAD Child (MicroMed Technology, Inc., Houston, TX, USA; http://www.micromedcv.com/united_states/index.html, accessed February 1, 2009) (Figure 30.5 and Color Plate 30.7) employs the same axial-flow pump used in the adult version but has reduced lateral space requirement, making its implantation in children easier. Under the current Humanitarian Device Exemption status by the US FDA, the VAD Child is indicated as a bridge to cardiac transplantation for children in heart failure New York Class IV from 5 to 16 years of age with a BSA of >0.7 and <1.5 m^2. It is designed to be fully implantable in this age range. This device allows ambulation and rehabilitation during support. Fraser recently summarized the experience with the VAD Child in 6 patients. The average patient age was

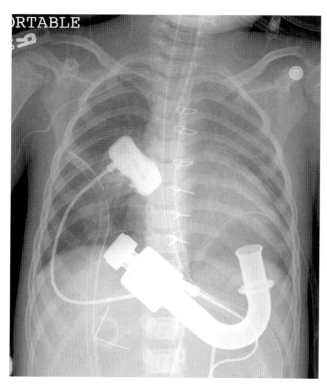

Figure 30.5 MicroMed DeBakey VAD Child radiographic view

11 years (range 6–15 yr), with a BSA of 0.8–1.7 m² [60]. The average duration of support was 39 days, with 84 days being the longest duration of support. Half of these patients were successfully transplanted, while half died during support awaiting transplantation.

Role of transesophageal echocardiography in VAD insertion

Transesophageal echocardiography (TEE) provides a useful guide during cannula insertion and the initiation of VAD, and is a Class I indication according to the ACC/AHA/ASE 2003 guidelines (Table 30.6) [61–64]. Before CPB, TEE is a valuable tool in detecting valvular disease that will affect the device function. Mitral stenosis and aortic insufficiency, if severe, are two conditions that must be addressed before initiating VAD. The former will limit the device filling and the latter will cause blood to flow back to the heart, decreasing forward output and impeding left ventricular unloading (Color Plate 30.8). Mitral regurgitation and aortic stenosis do not affect device function with pulsatile devices. Axial-flow devices provide partial support requiring the aortic valve to open and contribute to cardiac output, and are therefore less effective in patients with severe aortic stenosis. Mitral insufficiency typically improves after left ventricular unloading, with an associated decrease in left ventricular chamber size.

Table 30.6 Role of transesophageal echocardiography in ventricular assist device insertion

Prebypass
Monitor
- Optimize left ventricular filling
- Right ventricular function

Diagnose
- Right–left shunting (PFO, ASD, VSD)
- Aortic insufficiency
- Mitral stenosis
- Characterize baseline tricuspid regurgitation
- Thrombi
- Pulmonary insufficiency (RVAD)

On bypass
Monitor
- Inlet–outlet cannula alignment
- Deairing
- Aorta (ascending and descending)
- Degree of decompression of LV and LA

Diagnose
- Residual right-to-left atrial shunting
- Exclude aortic regurgitation

Postbypass
Monitor
- Right ventricular function
- Tricuspid regurgitation
- Pericardial effusion/cardiac tamponade
- Aortic dissection
- Decompression of LV and LA
- Air entrainment

PFO, patent foramen ovale; ASD, atrial septal defect; VSD, ventricular septal defect; LV, left ventricle; LA, left atrium; RVAD, right ventricular assist device.

The inflow cannula is easily identified by transesophageal echocardiography (Figure 30.6), and should be aligned with in the mitral inflow to produce laminar flow entering the cannula. A peak flow velocity > 2.3 m/s and evidence of turbulent flow are indicative of inflow cannula obstruction (Color Plate 30.9). Echocardiography is also used to assess left-to-right shunting lesions that must be closed before VAD insertion because after VAD initiation an unloaded (low-pressure) left chambers with continued high right-sided pressures will produce right-to-left shunting with desaturation. Right ventricular function and the severity of tricuspid regurgitation should be assessed before LVAD placement to assist in determining the need for biventricular support. Thorough surveillance for intracardiac thrombi should also be completed before VAD placement since thromboembolic events are potentially devastating complication of these procedures [20,21].

During the procedure, TEE is useful for monitoring right ventricular function, detecting air, and monitoring

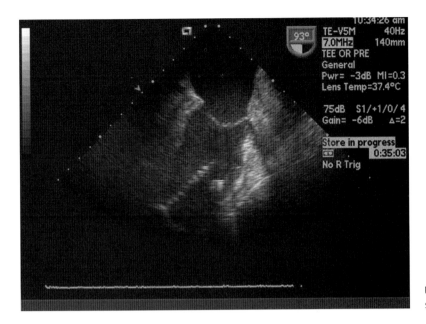

Figure 30.6 Mid-esophageal two-chamber view showing the inflow cannula and the mitral valve

left ventricular decompression. Air entering through suture lines is possible if the left ventricle completely collapses and a subatmospheric intradevice pressure develops. While weaning from CPB, the early detection of right ventricular failure will determine the need for biventricular support. Severe septal shifting of the intraventricular septum to the left is an indicator of right-sided heart failure. On the other hand, an intraventricular septum that is shifted to the right is suspicious of device malfunction or cannula obstruction. Hypovolemia is a common cause for flow reduction since these devices are preload dependent and TEE will clearly show ventricular filling. The aorta should be carefully scanned after device implantation to rule out the possibility of dissection distal to the outlet cannula insertion site. After chest closure a final scan should be performed to exclude any kinking of the cannulae and right ventricular compression.

Weaning from circulatory support

ECMO

Patients are weaned from mechanical support when their cardiac function has recovered (bridge to recovery). In situations where there is no long-term damage to the heart-like acute myocarditis or a stunned myocardium from a long CPB period or aortic cross-clamp, patients can usually weaned 48–72 hours after the initiation of support. Besides regaining cardiac function, respiratory function should be adequate to ventilate and oxygenate with conventional mechanical ventilation. Typically, weaning would be delayed until renal and liver function has re-

covered. Before attempting to wean from mechanical support, inotropic support and ventilatory support are optimized. Similar to weaning from CPB, flow is gradually reduced while following TEE, hemodynamics, and cerebral oximetry. Once flow is stopped the bridge between the arterial and venous systems is unclamped and the circuit allowed to recirculate. The cannulae remain in place for about 1 hour after weaning from circulatory support until there is evidence that the patient has stable hemodynamics [18].

VADs: weaning from cardiopulmonary bypass to VAD

Almost all VAD cannulations in children are performed when the child is on full CPB. The two main problems during weaning from CPB are air embolism and right ventricular failure. Intracardiac air commonly occurs during assist device insertion since air can be hidden in the cannulae or the device itself. The right coronary sinus is anterior–superior when the patient is supine and is a common site for air emboli, which will produce right ventricular dysfunction. While on CPB, air that was trapped in the pulmonary veins may become dislodged when pulmonary blood flow and ventilation are resumed and therefore continuous ST-segment monitoring and TEE should be used to detect this. Deairing the heart can be achieved by placing the patient in steep Trendelenburg position and by using an aortic vent until the air disappears [63].

In many patients the right ventricular function improves after the left ventricle is supported and the pulmonary capillary pressure decreases. However, right ventricular function should be carefully monitored with TEE, right and left atrial pressures, and systemic pressure monitored as the patient is converted from CPB support to VAD. Patients may benefit from prophylactic inodilator pharmacologic support of the right ventricle with milrinone, nitroglycerin, prostaglandin E_1, and nitrous oxide [64].

Hypertension is also frequently seen after VAD implantation, especially if there is a mismatch between the pump size and the patient vasculature, and should be aggressively treated with short-acting vasodilators, such as sodium nitroprusside, phentolamine, or nicardipine.

VADs: weaning from VAD to recovery

Assist device weaning to recovery is possible in self-limited injuries as stated above. The same principles mentioned for ECMO apply to VAD. In the OR, once inotropic and ventilatory support are started the mechanical circulatory support is decreased while monitoring TEE and systemic perfusion. If the patient tolerates the weaning process, the cannulae are removed after about an hour of stable hemodynamics.

Anesthesia, sedation, and analgesia for ECMO/LVAD insertion

Most patients requiring ECMO are intubated, have invasive hemodynamic monitors, and are deeply sedated. In cases in which airway needs to be controlled before instituting ECMO or VAD, the hemodynamic consequences of the administration of anesthetics and the conversion from spontaneous ventilation to positive pressure ventilation can result in circulatory collapse. In a recent study from the Children's Hospital in Boston, the frequency of cardiac arrests in patients with congenital heart disease undergoing cardiac surgery was 0.79%. Eleven cardiac arrests were related to the anesthesia for an incidence of 21.1 per 10,000 anesthetics (0.21%). None of the arrests were during ECMO or VAD insertion [65]. Before the induction of anesthesia, the anesthesia care team should be prepared for immediate resuscitation and the surgical team should be at the bedside.

ECMO produces several pharmacokinetic changes (Table 30.7) [66,67]. The circuit expands the circulating volume, increases intracellular water, and reduces plasma protein concentrations. Sequestration of drugs has also been described by the polymeric components of the circuit. Hemofiltration is required in 25% of patients on ECMO, which also affects drug pharmacokinetics.

All patients supported with ECMO and many patients supported by VAD require sedation with or without muscle relaxation, and benzodiazepines with opioids are used most commonly [68,69]. Patients develop tolerance and dependence to both these groups of medications and their pharmacokinetics are affected mostly by ECMO [70,71]. In addition, neonatal patients have a reduction in hepatic CYP3A activity, resulting in reduced midazolam clearance. The short half-life and variable pharmacokinetics make midazolam a poor choice as a first-line sedative for children requiring mechanical circulatory support [70]. Similarly, neonates rapidly develop tolerance from a continuous infusion of fentanyl while on ECMO, and exhibit neonatal abstinence syndrome when total fentanyl doses exceed 1.6 mg/kg and/or ECMO duration is of more that 5 days [71].

Table 30.7 ECMO physiology, pharmacokinetic changes, and therapeutic implications

ECMO physiology	Pharmacokinetic change	Therapeutic implication	Drugs affected
Priming solution/transfusion			
• Volume expansion	Increased volume of distribution	Higher loading doses	Hydrophilic drugs
○ Effect inversely related to BSA	Decreased serum protein	Increased dosing interval	Gentamycin
• Changes in serum protein concentration	binding—increasing free drug		Vancomycin
	Prolonged elimination half-life		Nondepolarizing muscle relaxants
Biomaterials			
• Cannulae	Adhesion to circuit component	Decreased bioavailability	Propofol
• Oxygenator	Drug loss during circuit changes	Redosing needed after circuit changes	Benzodiazepines
			Heparin
			Morphine
			Fentanyl
			Furosemide
			Phenytoin
			Phenobarbital

BSA, body surface area; ECMO, extracorporeal membrane oxygenation.

Morphine has an increased clearance and distribution volume in patients on ECMO. Even though tolerance can develop after prolonged morphine exposure, the long duration of action make this analgesic preferable over fentanyl. The initial morphine dosing should be guided by age and weight, but due to both pharmacokinetic changes and the development of tolerance, further morphine therapy should be guided by clinical monitoring [72].

Dexmedetomidine, an α_2-agonist, has sedative properties with minimal respiratory depression. It is not currently approved for use in pediatric patients. There are several reports of safe and effective use of dexedetomidine in children, including patients with congenital heart disease. However, the only reported use related to ECMO is to facilitate the weaning of opioids after ECMO and subsequent heart transplantation [73–75].

Neuromuscular relaxants may be used to avoid movement and potential injury, especially for ECMO patients. In our practice we avoid continuous use of muscle relaxants in order to facilitate neurologic evaluation and reduce the risk of myopathy.

Due to all pharmacokinetic changes on ECMO and the interpatient variability, there is a need to frequently reassess the depth of sedation and analgesia. The Bispectral Index monitor (BIS monitor, Aspect Medical, Newton, MA, USA) may be a useful adjunct to this assessment [76–78].

Anticoagulation, antifibrinolytics, and platelet antiaggregation therapies

ECMO

Anticoagulation is required during ECMO support, and the challenge is to achieve adequate anticoagulation without developing hemorrhagic complications. We utilize a heparin bolus dose of 100 U/kg to achieve an activated clotting time (ACT) of 180–200 seconds at the initiation of ECMO, followed by an infusion of 8 U/kg/h (range 6–60 U/kg/h), and heparin is added to the ECMO prime depending on the total volume. Even though ACT is an easy measurement with point of care testing, the activated partial thromboplastin timeprovides a more accurate assessment of anticoagulation and heparin levels are also useful. If the patient is actively bleeding, platelets are transfused to keep platelet count >100,000 mm^3 and cryoprecipitate administered to maintain the fibrinogen >150 mg/dL. Platelets are administered into the circuit after blood has passed through the oxygenator to avoid platelet damage and to preserve the life of the oxygenator. Thromboelastography is a useful tool to aid in decision making, especially when the patient is bleeding [79–81] (Table 30.8).

Table 30.8 Treatment protocol for citrated thromboelastography

TEG value	Clinical cause	Suggested treatment
R > 14 min	↓clotting factors	FFP 4 mL/kg
R > 18 min	↓↓clotting factors	FFP 8 mL/kg
MA < 46	↓platelet function	Platelets 1 U/5 kg
Angle < 55°	↓↓fibrinogen level	Cryoprecipitate 0.6 U/kg

R, the time from when the sample is put on the TEG until the first significant levels of detectable clot formation; MA, maximum amplitude; FFP, fresh frozen plasma; TEG, thromboelastography.

VAD

Most commonly, VADs are initiated when the patient is on full CPB and therefore fully anticoagulated with heparin. After transitioning the patient from CPB to VAD, the heparin may be partially reversed with protamine using an ACT of approximately 180 seconds as a guide. Once the patient is stable in the ICU and surgical bleeding is under control, the patient can be transitioned to Coumadin. Platelet aggregation studies are useful in guiding the administration of antiplatelet agents such as aspirin, dipyridamole, or clopidogrel. The Berlin group has shown a reduction in the incidence of bleeding complications with this approach to anticoagulation–antiaggregation [81]. Another important factor to consider is infection, which may significantly alter clotting, and patient coagulation status monitoring should be increased when infection is suspected [52].

Anti-infective therapy

ECMO patients are a high-risk group for nosocomial infection, in particular patients with an open sternum for whom antibiotic prophylaxis is recommended [82]. As noted above, antibiotics adhere to ECMO circuit biomaterials (cannulae, oxygenator), decreased bioavailability, and require redosing after circuit changes. First- or second-generation cephalosporins provide reasonable prophylaxis in populations that do not have a high incidence of methicillin-resistant *Staphylococcus aureus* [83]; otherwise vancomycin is indicated.

VAD infections have been classified in four groups: Class I, patient-related nonblood infections; Class II, blood-borne infections; Class III, percutaneous site infections; and Class IV, intracorporeal VAD component infections [84]. Bloodstream infections can usually be controlled with adequate intravenous therapy, but intracorporeal infections usually require surgical debridement, drainage of infected fluids, and device replacement.

Outcome and complications

Compared to many surgical therapies, mechanical support of the circulation is associated with a high incidence of morbidity and mortality, most commonly related to tissue ischemia from inadequate perfusion, trauma to blood elements, and activation of systemic inflammatory and coagulation cascades. The presence of and oxygenator in the ECMO circuit increases the risk for red blood cell damage. Multiple connector sites increase the risk of air and particulate embolism. Complications associated with these devices include stroke, intracerebral hemorrhage, bleeding, infection, and multisystem organ failure. Diaphragmatic paralysis has also been reported and related to multiple thoracic explorations to investigate bleeding [11]. Failure to regain ventricular function within 72 hours of the initiation of support is an ominous sign that the heart will not recover in patients supported with either ECMO or VAD [10].

The long-term outcome of pediatric patients requiring mechanical circulatory support who survive to hospital discharge is good [84,85]. Ibrahim reported over a 90% survival in discharged patients who received ECMO or VAD for cardiac failure of different etiologies [87]. More than 80% of the patients were in New York Heart Association Class I or II. Unfortunately, the incidence of neurologic sequela is high and is significantly higher in ECMO compared to VAD patients (59% vs 25%).

ECMO

Kovolos reported a 50% survival to discharge from ECMO after pediatric cardiac surgery. Risk factors for mortality were single ventricle physiology and the need for dialysis [85]. Aharon reported similar survival of 50% [17], finding that renal failure, extended periods of circulatory support (>72 h), and prolonged CPR time (>45 min) were risk factors for early mortality. Shunt-dependent flow lesion did not affect survival in a report from Balsiam, in which patients with single ventricle physiology and repaired truncus arteriosus had an increased risk of death [86].

VAD

Arabia reported a 70% survival in a small series of pediatric patients bridged to transplant with a variety of VADs (Berlin Heart, Medos and Thoratec); however, the rate of complications was high: thromboembolic event, 40%; bleeding, 40%; and infection rate, 30% [88]. Hetzer reported a 76.7% survival rate with the Berlin Heart VAD in 205 pediatric patients during a 3-year follow-up. From these survivors, 9.8% were successfully bridged to recovery, 53.2% underwent heart transplantation, and 13.7%

Table 30.9 Mechanical support complications

Incidence	ECMO (%)	VAD (%)
CNS		
Stroke	7.8	8.5*
Coagulopathy		
Reexploration	15.4	12.7[‡]
Infections		
Drug-treated infection	48.2	32.1[‡]
Renal failure		
Dialysis	17.2	9.1[‡]

* Not significant difference.
[‡] $p \leq 0.005$ between the groups.
ECMO, extracorporeal membrane oxygenation; VAD, ventricular assist device.
Source: Adapted from United Network for Organ Sharing database Report (21).

were awaiting transplant at the time of publication [9]. The same authors reported a survival rate of 70% in infants less than 1 year of age supported with the Berlin Heart [54]. A multi-institutional prospective study also showed a high survival rate of 83%, 77% survived to transplantation, and 6% were weaned to recovery [18]. Patients with congenital heart disease, female gender, and earlier year of implantation had a worse prognosis. There was also a high incidence of stroke (20%) and it was higher with the use of short-term devices compared to long-term ones (35% vs 13%, respectively). The United Network for Organ Sharing database also reported a 10-year survival of 50–60% for pediatric patients bridged to transplant. The greatest risk for mortality is in the immediate postoperative period [19]. Patients bridged on ECMO had higher incidence of complications and worse overall outcome than patients who did not need mechanical support or those bridged with VAD (Table 30.9).

The future

Due to limitations in the current technology of mechanical support devices available for children, the National Heart, Lung and Blood Institute launched a "Pediatric Circulatory Support Program," with the aim of developing novel circulatory support device for children ranging from 2 to 25 kg. The technical requirements for these devices were:

(a) Rapid deployment (<1 h after decision to initiate support)
(b) Minimal priming volume and blood product exposure
(c) Flexible cannulation to accommodate anatomic variants
(d) Minimize risk of complications, including infection, bleeding, hemolysis, and thrombosis
(e) Long-term support up to 6 months after insertion

Five contracts were awarded to develop five new families of devices, which include mixed-flow, axial-flow, and pulsatile VAD [89].

References

1. Bartlett RH, Gazzaniga AB, Huxtable RF, et al. (1977) Extracorporeal circulation (ECMO) in neonatal respiratory failure. J Thorac Cardiovasc Surg 74:826–833.
2. Soeter JR, Mamiya RT, Sprague AY, et al. (1973) Prolonged extracorporeal oxygenation for cardiorespiratory failure after tetralogy correction. J Thorac Cardiovasc Surg 66:214–218.
3. Kanter KR, Pennington DG, Weber TR, et al. (1987) Extracorporeal membrane oxygenation for postoperative cardiac support in children. J Thorac Cardiovasc Surg 93:27–35.
4. Bartlett RH, Roloff DW, Custer JR, et al. (2000) Extracorporeal life support: the University of Michigan experience. JAMA 283:904–908.
5. Hintz SR, Benitz WE, Colby CE, et al. (2005) Utilization and outcomes of neonatal cardiac extracorporeal life support: 1996–2000. Pediatr Crit Care 6:33–38.
6. Conrad SA, Rycus PT, Dalton H (2005) Extracorporeal Life Support Registry Report 2004. ASAIO J 5:4–10.
7. Cooley DA, Hallman GL, Bloodwell RD, et al. (1969) First human implantation of a cardiac prosthesis for staged total replacement of the heart. Trans Am Soc Artif Intern Organs 15:252–266.
8. Frazier OH, Bricker JT, Macris MP, et al. (1989) Use of a left ventricular assist device as a bridge to transplantation in a pediatric patient. Tex Heart Inst J 16:46–50.
9. Hetzer R, Stiller B, Potapov E, et al. (2007) Ventricular assist device and mechanical circulatory support for children. Curr Opin Organ Transplant 12:522–528.
10. Duncan BW (2002) Mechanical circulatory support for infants and children with cardiac disease. Ann Thorac Surg 73:1670–1677.
11. Chaturvedi RR, Macrae D, Brown KL, et al. (2004) Cardiac ECMO for biventricular hearts after paediatric open heart surgery. Heart 90:545–551.
12. del Nido P, Armitage JM, Fricker FJ, et al. (1994) Extracorporeal membrane oxygenation support as a bridge to pediatric heart transplantation. Circulation 90 (Part 2):II-66–II-69.
13. Davies LK (2005) Management of postbypass myocardial dysfunction. In: Lake CL, Booker PD (eds), Pediatric Cardiac Anesthesia, 4th edn. Lippincott, Williams & Wilkins, Philadelphia, pp. 291–303.
14. del Nido PJ (1996) Extracorporeal membrane oxygenation for cardiac support in children. Ann Thorac Surg 61:336–339.
15. Duncan BW, Hraska V, Jonas RA, et al. (1999) Mechanical circulatory support in children with cardiac disease. J Thorac Cardiovasc Surg 117:529–542.
16. Jaggers JJ, Forbess JM, Shah AS, et al. (2000) Extracorporeal membrane oxygenation for infant postcardiotomy support: significance of shunt management. Ann Thorac Surg 69:1476–1483.
17. Aharon AS, Drinkwater DC, Churchwell KB, et al. (2001) Extracorporeal membrane oxygenation in children after repair of congenital cardiac lesions. Ann Thorac Surg 72:2095–2102.
18. Thourani VH, Krishbom PM, Kanter KR, et al. (2006) Venoarterial extracorporeal membrane oxygenation (VA-ECMO) in pediatric cardiac support. Ann Thorac Surg 82:138–145.
19. Blume ED, Naftel DC, Bastardi HJ, et al. (2006) Outcomes of children bridged to heart transplantation with ventricular assist devices: a multi-institutional study. Circulation 113:2313–2319.
20. Davies RR, Russo MJ, Hong KN, et al. (2008) The use of mechanical circulatory support as a bridge to transplantation in pediatric patients: an analysis of the United Network for Organ Sharing database. J Thorac Cardiovasc Surg 135:421–427.
21. del Nido PJ, Duncan BW, Mayer JE, et al. (1999) Left ventricular assist device improves survival in children with left ventricular dsyfunction after repair of anomalous origin of left coronary artery form the pulmonary artery. Ann Thorac Surg 67:169–172.
22. Fischer S, Bohn D, Rycus P, et al. (2007) Extracorporeal membrane oxygenation for primary graft dysfunction after lung transplantation: analysis of the Extracorporeal Life Support Organization (ELSO) Registry. J Heart Lung Transplant 26:472–477.
23. Chen YS, Wang MJ, Chou NK, et al. (1999) Rescue for acute myocarditis with shock by extracorporeal membrane oxygenation. Ann Thorac Surg 68:220–224.
24. Duncan BW, Bohn DJ, Atz AM (2001) Mechanical circulatory support for the treatment of children with acute fulminant myocarditis. J Thorac Cardiovasc Surg 122:440–448.
25. American Heart Association (2005) American Heart Association guidelines for cardiopulmonary resuscitation and emergency cardiovascular care. Circulation 112:IV-167–IV-187.
26. del Nido PJ, Dalton HJ, Thompson AE, et al. (1992) Extracorporeal membrane oxygenator rescue in children during cardiac arrest after cardiac surgery. Circulation 86 (Suppl II): II-300–II-304.
27. Duncan BW, Ibrahim AE, Hraska V, et al. (1998) Use of rapid-deployment extracorporeal membrane oxygenation for the resuscitation of pediatric patients with heart disease after cardiac arrest. J Thorac Cardiovasc Surg 116:305–311.
28. Morris MC, Wernovsky G, BNadkarni VM (2004) Survival outcomes after extracorporeal cardiopulmonary resuscitation instituted during active chest compressions following refractory in-hospital pediatric cardiac arrest. Pediatr Crit Care Med 5:440–446.
29. Morris MC, Fiser RT (2008) Extracorporeal cardiopulmonary resuscitation in refractory pediatric cardiac arrest. Pediatr Clin North Am 55:929–941.
30. Allan CK, Thiagarajan RR, Armsby LR, et al. (2006) Emergent use of extracorporeal membrane oxygenation during pediatric cardiac catheterization. Pediatr Crit Care Med 7:212–219.
31. Vitiello R, McCrindle BW, Nykanen D, et al. (1998) Complications associated with pediatric cardiac catheterization. J Am Coll Cardiol 32:1433–1440.
32. Walker GM, McLeod K, Brown KL, et al. (2003) Extracorporeal life support as a treatment of supraventricular tachycardia in infants. Pediatric Crit Care Med 4:52–54.

33. Darst JR, Kaufman J (2007) Case report: an infant with congenital junctional ectopic tachycardia requiring extracorporeal mechanical oxygenation. Curr Opin Pediatr 19:597–600.

34. Durward A, Guerguerian AM, Lefebvre M, et al. (2003) Massive diltiazem overdose treated with extracorporeal membrane oxygenation. Pediatr Crit Care Med 4:372–376.

35. Marciniak KE, Thomas IH, Brogan TV, et al. (2007) Massive ibuprofen overdose requiring extracorporeal membrane oxygenation for cardiovascular support. Pediatr Crit Care Med 8:180–182.

36. Kolcz J, Pietrzyk J, Januszewska K, et al. (2007) Extracorporeal life support in severe propranolol and verapamil intoxication. J Intensive Care Med 22:381–385.

37. Walpoth BH, Walpoth-Aslan BN, Mattle HP, et al. (1997) Outcome of survivors of accidental deep hypothermia and circulatory arrest treated with extracorporeal blood warming. N Engl J Med 337:1500–1505.

38. Scaife ER, Connors RC, Morris SE, et al. (2007) An established extracorporeal membrane oxygenation protocol promotes survival in extreme hypothermia. J Pediatr Surg 42:2012–2016.

39. Ravishankar C, Gaynor JW (2006) Mechanical support of the functionally single ventricle. Cardiol Young 16 (Suppl 1): 55–60.

40. Morgan IS, Codispoti M, Sanger K, et al. (1998) Superiority of centrifugal pump over roller pump in paediatric cardiac surgery: prospective randomised trial. Eur J Cardiothorac Surg 13:526–532.

41. Mc Mullan DM, Elliot MJ, Cohen GA (2007) ECMO for infants and children. In: Gravlee GP, Davis RF, Stammers AH, Ungerleider RM (eds) Cardiopulmonary Bypass Principles and Practice, 3rd edn. Lippincott Williams & Wilkins, Philadelphia, pp. 735–755.

42. ELSO Database. Available at: http://www.elso.med. umich.edu/support.htm. Accessed February 1, 2009.

43. Yamasaki Y, Hayashi T, Nakatani T, et al. (2006) Early experience with low-prime (99 mL) extracorporeal membrane oxygenation support in children. ASAIO J 52:110–114.

44. Goldstein DJ, Oz MC, Rose EA (1998) Implantable left ventricular assist devices. N Eng J Med 339:1522–1533.

45. Fuchs A, Netz H (2002) Ventricular assist devices in pediatrics. Images Paediatr Cardiol 9:924–954.

46. Baldwin JT, Duncan BW (2006) Ventricular assist device for children. Prog Pediatr Cardiol 21:173–184.

47. Pauliks LB, Ündar A (2008) New devices for pediatric mechanical circulatory support. Curr Opin Cardiol 23:91–96.

48. Thuys CA, Mullaly RJ, Horton SB, et al. (1998) Centrifugal ventricular assist device in children under 6 kg. Eur J Cardiothorac Surg 13:130–134.

49. Windecker S (2007) Percutaneous left ventricular assist devices for treatment of patients with cardiogenic shock. Curr Opin Crit Care 13:521–527.

50. Ricci M, Gaughan CB, Rossi M, et al. (2008) Initial experience with the Tandem Heart circulatory support system in children. ASAIO J 54:542–545.

51. Ashton RC, Oz MC, Michler RE, et al. (1995) Left ventricular assist device options in pediatric patients. ASAIO J 41:277–280.

52. Potapov EV, Stiller B, Hertzer R (2007) Ventricular assist devices in children: current achievements and future perspectives. Pediatr Transplant 11:241–235.

53. Stiller B, Hertzer R, Weng Y, et al. (2003) Heart transplantation in children after mechanical circulatory support with pulsatile pneumatic assist device. J Heart Lung Transplant 22:1201–1208.

54. Stiller B, Weng Y, Hübler M, et al. (2005) Pneumatic pulsatile ventricular assist devices in children under 1 year of age. Eur J Cardiothorac Surg 28:234–239.

55. Konertz W, Hotz H, Schneider M, et al. (1997) Clinical experience with the MEDOS HIA-VAD System in infants and children: a preliminary report. Ann Thorac Surg 63:1138–1144.

56. Reinhartz O, Hill JD, Al-Khaldi A, et al. (2005) Thoratec ventricular assist devices in pediatric patients: update on clinical results. ASAIO J 51:501–503.

57. Reinhartz O, Keith FM, El-Banayosy A, et al. (2001) Multicenter experience with the Thoratec ventricular assist device in children and adolescents. J Heart Lung Transplant 20:439–448.

58. Sharma MS, Webber SA, Gandhi SK, et al. (2005) Pulsatile paracorporeal assist devices in children and adolescents with biventricular failure. ASAIO J 51:490–494.

59. Frazier OH, Gemmato C, Myers TJ, et al. (2007) Initial clinical experience with the Heartmate® II axial-flow left ventricular assist device. Tex Heart Inst J 34:275–281.

60. Fraser CD Jr, Carberry KE, Owens WR, et al. (2006) Preliminary experience with the MicroMed DeBakey pediatric ventricular assist device. Semin Thorac Cardiovasc Surg Pediatr Card Surg Annu 109–114.

61. Cheitlin MD, Armstrong WF, Aurigemma GP, et al. (2003) ACC/AHA/ASE 2003 guideline update for the clinical application of echocardiography: summary article. Circulation 108:1146–1162.

62. Augostides J, Mancini J, Horak J, et al. (2000) The use of intraoperative echocardiography during insertion of ventricular assist devices. J Cardiothorac Vasc Anesth 14:316–326.

63. Mets B (2000) Anesthesia for left ventricular assist device placement. J Cardiothorac Vasc Anesth 14:316–326.

64. Chumnanvej S, Wood MJ, Mac Gillivray TE, et al. (2007) Perioperative echocardiographic examination for ventricular assist device implantation. Anesth Analg 105:583–601.

65. Odegard KC, DiNardo JA, Kussman BD, et al. (2007) The frequency of anesthesia-related cardiac arrests in patients with congenital heart disease undergoing cardiac surgery. Anesth Analg 105:335–343.

66. Burda G, Trittenwein G (1999) Issues of pharmacology in pediatric extracorporeal membrane oxygenation with special reference to analgesia and sedation. Artif Organs 23:1015–1019.

67. Buck ML (2003) Pharmacokinetic changes during extracorporeal membrane oxygenation. Clin Pharmacokinet 42:403–417.

68. Tobias JD (2005) Sedation and analgesia in the pediatric intensive care unit. Pediatr Ann 34:636–645.

69. De Berry BB, Lych JE, Chernin J, et al. (2005) A survey for pain and sedation medications in pediatric patients during extracorporeal membrane oxygenation. Perfusion 20:139–143.

70. Mulla H, Mc Cormack P, Lawson G, et al. (2003) Pharmacokinetics of midazolam in neonates undergoing extracorporeal membrane oxygenation. Anesthesiology 99:275–282.

71. Arnold JH, Truog RD, Orav EJ, et al. (1990) Tolerance and dependence in neonates sedated with fentanyl during extracorporeal memembrane oxygenation. Anesthesiology 73:1136–1140.

72. Peters JW, Anderson BJ, Simons SH, et al. (2005) Morphine pharmacokinetics during venoarterial extracorporeal membrane oxygenation in neonates. Intensive Care Med 31:257–263.

73. Tobias JD, Berkenbosch JW (2004) Sedation during mechanical ventilation in infants and children: dexmedetomidine versus midazolam. South Med J 97:451–455.

74. Chrysostomou C, Di Filippo S, Manrique AM, et al. (2006) Use of dexmedetomidine in children after cardiac and thoracic surgery. Pediatr Crit Care Med 7:126–131.

75. Finkel JC, Johnson Y J, Quezado ZMN (2005) The use of dexmedetomidine to facilitate acute discontinuation of opioids after cardiac transplantation in children. Crit Care Med 33:2110–2112.

76. Tobias JD (2005) Monitoring the depth of sedation in the pediatric ICU patient: where are we, or more importantly, where are our patients? Pediatr Crit Care Med 6:715–718.

77. Crean P (2004) Sedation and neuromuscular blockade in paeditaric intensive care; practice in the United Kingdom and North America. Pediatr Anesth 14:439–442.

78. Playfor S, Jenkins I, Boyles C, et al. (2006) Consensus guidelines on sedation and analgesia in critically ill children. Intensive Care Med 32:1125–1136.

79. Miller BE, Guzzetta NA, Tosone SR, et al. (2000) Rapid evaluation of coagulopathies after cardiopulmonary bypass in children using modified thromboelastography. Anesth Analg 90:1324–1330.

80. Ganter MT, Hofer CK (2008) Coagulation monitoring: current techniques and clinical use of viscoelastic point-of-care coagulation devices. Anesth Analg 106:1366–1375.

81. Drews T, Stiller B, Hübler M, et al. (2007) Coagulation management in pediatric mechanical circulatory support. ASAIO J 53:640–645.

82. Brown KL, Ridout DA, Shaw M, et al. (2006) Healthcare-associated infection in pediatric patients on extracorporeal life support: the role of multidisciplinary surveillance. Pediatr Crit Care Med 7:546–550.

83. Engelman R, Shahian D, Shermin R, et al. (2007) The Society of Thoracic Surgeons practice guidelines in cardiac surgery. Part II: Antibiotic choice. Ann Thorac Surg 83:1569–1576.

84. Holam WL, Skinner JL, Waites KB, et al. (1999) Infection during circulatory support with ventricular assist devices. Ann Thorac Surg 68:711–716.

85. Kovolos NK, Bratton SL, Moler FW, et al. (2003) Outcome of pediatric patients treated with extracorporeal life support after cardiac surgery. Ann Thorac Surg 76:1453–1460.

86. Balsiam G, Bshore J Al-Malki F, et al. (2006) Can the outcome of pediatric extracorporeal membrane oxygenation after cardiac surgery be predicted? Ann Thorac Surg 12:21–27.

87. Ibrahim AE, Duncan BW, Blume ED, et al. (2000) Long term follow up of pediatric cardiac patients requiring mechanical circulatory support. Ann Thorac Surg 69:186–192.

88. Arabia FA, Tsau PH, Smith RG, et al. (2006) Pediatric bridge to heart transplantation: application of the Berlin Heart, Medos and Thoratec ventricular assist devices. J Heart Lung Transplant 25:16–21.

89. Baldwin JT, Borovetz HS, Duncan BW, et al. (2006) The National Heart, Lung, and Blood Institute Pediatric Circulatory Support Program. Circulation 113:147–155.

Appendix: Texas Children's Hospital Pediatric Cardiovascular Anesthesia Drug Sheet (March 2009)

Vasoactive infusions

Dopamine	3–20 mcg/kg/min	
Dobutamine	3–20 mcg/kg/min	
Milrinone	0.375–0.75 mcg/kg/min	Loading: 50–75 mcg/kg over 15 min
Epinephrine	0.03–1 mcg/kg/min	
Norepinephrine	0.05–1 mcg/kg/min	
Isoproterenol	0.03–1 mcg/kg/min	
Phenylephrine	0.05–0.5 mcg/kg/min	
Sodium nitroprusside	0.5–5 mcg/kg/min	
Nitroglycerine	0.5–5 mcg/kg/min	
Prostaglandin E1	0.03–0.1 mcg/kg/min	
Lidocaine	20–50 mcg/kg/min	Loading: 1–2 mg/kg
Procainamide	20–80 mcg/kg/min	Loading: 10–15 mg/kg over 60 min
Esmolol	50–100 mcg/kg/min	Loading: 250–500 mcg/kg over 1 min
Vasopressin	0.02–0.05 units/kg/h	
Fenoldopam	0.025–0.3 mcg/kg/min initially, titrate to max 1.6 mcg/kg/min	
Nesiritide	0.01–0.03 mcg/kg/min	Loading: 2 mcg/kg
Nicardipine	0.1–0.3 mg/kg/h; max 15 mg/h	

Vasoactive bolus drugs

Epinephrine	0.5–10 mcg/kg
Atropine	10–20 mcg/kg IV; 20–40 mcg/kg IM
Phenylephrine	0.5–3 mcg/kg
$CaCl_2$	10 mg/kg
Ca gluconate	30 mg/kg
Adenosine	25–50 mcg/kg—double if ineffective
Labetalol	0.25–0.5 mg/kg
Amiodarone	5 mg/kg over 10–15 min, may repeat 2 times to max 15 mg/kg
Verapamil	0.1–0.3 mg/kg
Propranolol	0.01–0.1 mg/kg
Bretylium	5 mg/kg; increase to 10 mg/kg if ineffective

Phenoxybenzamine	0.25 -1 mg/kg
Hydralazine	0.1–0.2 mg/kg
Phentolamine	0.1–0.2 mg/kg on CPB
Ephedrine	0.1 mg/kg, max 5 mg

Miscellaneous drugs for cardiac anesthesia

Heparin (100 units = 1 mg)	300–400 U/kg for CPB; 100 U/kg for heparinization for closed cases
Protamine	1–1.3 times the heparin dose in mg
Furosemide	0.5–1 mg/kg, max 20 mg
Sodium Bicarbonate	1–3 mEq/kg; dilute 1:1 sterile H_2O for newborns
THAM	3–6 mL/kg
Cefazolin	25–30 mg/kg
Naficillin	50 mg/kg, max 2 g
Gentamicin	1.5–2.5 mg/kg, max 120 mg
Ampicillin	50 mg/kg, max 2 g
Clindamycin	20 mg/kg, max 600 mg
Cefuroxime	25–30 mg/kg
Methylprednisolone	30 mg/kg in CPB circuit
Dexamethasone	0.25 mg/kg for airway edema
Hydrocortisone	1–2 mg/kg for adrenal suppression
Digoxin	8–10 mcg/kg first loading dose
Vancomycin	10–15 mg/kg, max 1 g
Naloxone	1–10 mcg/kg, repeat as necessary
Flumazenil	1–5 mcg/kg, repeat as necessary
Dextrose 50%	0.5–1 mL/kg; dilute 1:1 sterile H_2O
Mannitol	0.25–0.5 g/kg
Amicar	75 mg/kg load over 5–10 min, then 75/mg/kg/h infusion; and 75 mg/kg into CPB circuit; 75 mg/kg/h after CPB
Tranexamic acid	50–100 mg/kg load over 5–10 min, then 10/mg/kg/h infusion; and 50–100 mg/kg into CPB circuit; 10 mg/kg/h after CPB
Aprotinin*	28,000–60,000 KIU/kg load, then 3500–7000 KIU/kg/h infusion
Recombinant factor VIIa	90 mcg/kg; repeat Q1–2h, max 3 doses
KCL	0.5–1 meq/kg over 1 h
MgSO4	25–50 mg/kg/over 1 h
Bumetanide	0.1 mg/kg/dose
Ranitindine	1 mg/kg
Diphenhydramine	1–2 mg/kg
Levoalbuterol	8–16 puffs MDI per ETT
Metaclopromide	0.15–0.3 mg/kg; max 10 mg
Ondansetron	0.1–0.15 mg/kg; max 4 mg

Anesthetic agents and muscle relaxants

Fentanyl	1–10 mcg/kg bonus; 50–200 mcg/kg total dose; 5–20 mcg/kg/h infusion
Remifentanil	0.05–2 mcg/kg/min IV infusion
Midazolam	0.03–0.1 mg/kg per dose; 0.5–1 mg/kg total dose
Pancuronium	0.1–0.2 mg/kg intubation
Vecuronium	0.1–0.4 mg/kg intubation
Rocuronium	0.6–1.2 mg/kg IV; 2 mg/kg IM intubation
Atracurium	0.4–0.5 mg/kg intubation
Cisatracurium	0.15–0.2 mg/kg intubation
Succinylcholine	1–2 mg/kg IV; 4 mg/kg IM
Neostigmine	70 mcg/kg
Glycopyrrolate	14 mcg/kg
Thiopental	1–4 mg/kg
Ketamine	1–2 mg/kg IV; 5–10 mg/kg IM
Etomidate	0.1–0.3 mg/kg
Propofol	1–3 mg/kg induction; 50–200 mcg/kg/min maintenance
Dexmedetomidine	0.3–1 mcg/kg load; 0.2–0.7 mcg/kg/h infusion

Blood products and volume expanders

5% albumin	10–20 mL/kg
25% albumin	2–4 mL/kg; 0.5–1 g/kg
Platelets	1 unit per 5 kg will increase platelet count by approximately 50,000
FFP	10–20 mL/kg
PRBCs	10–15 mL/kg
Cryoprecipitate	1 unit per 5 kg; max 4 units
Whole blood	10–15 mL/kg
Hetastarch	5–10 mL/kg; max 15 mL/kg per 24 h

DC defibrillation/synchronized cardioversion

Internal defibrillation: 5 J; increase to 10
External defibrillation: 2–5 J/kg; increase if ineffective
External synchronized cardioversion: 0.5 J/kg

*Aprotinin was not available in the USA in March 2009.

Index

Index

Index